The Maudsley
Prescribing Guidelines
in Psychiatry

LRM

The Maudsley Prescribing Guidelines in Psychiatry

13th Edition

David M. Taylor, BSc, MSc, PhD, FFRPS, FRPharmS

Director of Pharmacy and Pathology at the Maudsley Hospital and
Professor of Psychopharmacology at King's College, London, UK

Thomas R. E. Barnes, MBBS, MD, FRCPsych, DSc

Emeritus Professor of Clinical Psychiatry at Imperial College London and
joint-head of the Prescribing Observatory for Mental Health at the
Royal College of Psychiatrists' Centre for Quality Improvement, London, UK

Allan H. Young, MB, ChB, MPhil, PhD, FRCPC, FRCPsych

Chair of Mood Disorders and Director of the Centre for Affective Disorders in the
Department of Psychological Medicine in the Institute of Psychiatry at
King's College London, UK

WILEY Blackwell

This thirteenth edition first published 2018
© 2018 David M. Taylor

The right of David M. Taylor, Thomas R. E. Barnes and Allan H. Young to be identified as the author(s) of this work has been asserted in accordance with law.

Registered Office(s)
John Wiley & Sons, Inc., 111 River Street, Hoboken, NJ 07030, USA
John Wiley & Sons Ltd, The Atrium, Southern Gate, Chichester, West Sussex, PO19 8SQ, UK

Editorial Office
The Atrium, Southern Gate, Chichester, West Sussex, PO19 8SQ, UK

For details of our global editorial offices, customer services, and more information about Wiley products visit us at www.wiley.com.

Wiley also publishes its books in a variety of electronic formats and by print-on-demand. Some content that appears in standard print versions of this book may not be available in other formats.

Library of Congress Cataloging-in-Publication Data

Names: Taylor, David M., 1963– author. | Barnes, Thomas R. E., author. | Young, Allan H., 1938– author.
Title: The Maudsley prescribing guidelines in psychiatry / David M. Taylor, Thomas R. E. Barnes, Allan H. Young.
Other titles: Prescribing guidelines in psychiatry
Description: 13th edition. | Hoboken, NJ : Wiley, 2019. | Includes bibliographical references and index. |
Identifiers: LCCN 2018013198 (print) | LCCN 2018013542 (ebook) | ISBN 9781119442561 (pdf) |
    ISBN 9781119442585 (epub) | ISBN 9781119442608 (pbk.) | ISBN 9781119442561 (ePDF)
Subjects: | MESH: Mental Disorders–drug therapy | Psychotropic Drugs–therapeutic use |
    Psychotropic Drugs–administration & dosage | Psychopharmacology–methods
Classification: LCC RC483 (ebook) | LCC RC483 (print) | NLM WM 402 | DDC 616.89/18–dc23
LC record available at https://lccn.loc.gov/2018013198

Cover design by Wiley

Set in 10/12pt Sabon by SPi Global, Pondicherry, India

Printed and bound in Spain by Graphycems

4   2019

Contents

For this 13th edition of *The Maudsley Prescribing Guidelines in Psychiatry* I am honoured to welcome Thomas Barnes and Allan Young as co-authors. Thomas and Allan are of course internationally renowned for their expertise in the treatment of psychosis and mood disorders, respectively. They take over from Carol Paton, who has edged perceptibly towards retirement, and Shitij Kapur, who has moved on to become the Dean of the faculty of Medicine, Dentistry and Health Sciences at the University of Melbourne. My sincere and substantial gratitude is due to Carol and Shitij for their considerable contributions to several previous editions of *The Guidelines*. Carol in particular has written a great many sections (reflecting her very wide knowledge) and has been an honest and candid critic of submissions from me and other contributors.

The Guidelines have grown somewhat organically since they were first produced as a 16-page pamphlet in 1994. For this edition we have reorganised sections into 14 chapters, each consisting of a more or less consistent theme of subject areas. Tables listing licensed uses and doses of antidepressants (a relic from the very first edition) have been removed – this information is readily available elsewhere – and new sections have been added. These include antipsychotics and thromboembolism, ECT augmentation of antipsychotics, psychotropics after bariatric surgery and re-starting psychotropics after a period of non-compliance. Although we have tried to a great extent to limit the length of each section and the number of references cited, this edition is inevitably bigger than the last. In order to maintain some semblance of portability, we have reduced by one notch the weight of paper used. The increase in size and weight will be of no significance to the increasing numbers who use *The Guidelines* as an app or (more rarely these days) as a pdf.

The Guidelines originated as a local document and gradually grew in size and scope into a reference used throughout the UK. More recent editions have been translated into several languages, including Japanese and Chinese, and *The Guidelines* have seen increased use in other English-speaking countries, particularly the USA. Because of this we have tried more than ever in this edition to make *The Guidelines* of worldwide relevance by including advice on the use of a range of psychotropics commonly prescribed in countries outside the UK.

The clinical validity of *The Guidelines* depends to a great extent on expert contributions from a broad array of specialist psychiatrists and pharmacists. I extend my heartfelt thanks to these colleagues, listed in the Acknowledgements section that follows. I would like to express particular gratitude to Shubhra Mace, Ian Osborne and Siobhan Gee who have made numerous and excellent contributions to this edition. Special thanks are also rightly due to Maria O'Hagan and Sandy Chang, Managing Editors of this 13th edition of *The Guidelines*.

David M. Taylor
London
March 2018

Acknowledgements

The following have contributed to the 13th edition of *The Maudsley Prescribing Guidelines in Psychiatry.*

Andrea Danese
Anne Connolly
Anthony Cleare
Argyris Stringaris
Bruce Clark
Cristal Oxley
Daniel Harwood
Daniel Hayes
Darren Schwartz
David Game
David McLaughlan
David Veale
Deborah Robson
Delia Bishara
Emily Finch
Emmert Roberts
Eromona Whiskey
Farinaz Keshavarzi
Flora Coker
Georgina Boon
Gordana Milavic
Hind Kalifeh
Hubertus Himmerich
Ian Osborne

Iris Rathwell
Jane Marshall
Jonathan Rogers
Justin Sauer
Kwame Peprah
Loren Bailey
Louise Howard
Marinos Kyriakopoulos
Mike Kelleher
Nada Zahreddine
Nicola Kalk
Nilou Nourishad
Olubanke Dzahini
Oluwakemi Oduniyi
Paramala Santosh
Paul Gringras
Paul Moran
Petrina Douglas-Hall
Philip Asherson
Philip Collins
Seema Varma
Shubhra Mace
Siobhan Gee
Ulrike Schmidt

Notes on using *The Maudsley Prescribing Guidelines in Psychiatry*

The main aim of *The Guidelines* is to provide clinicians with practically useful advice on the prescribing of psychotropic agents in both commonly and less commonly encountered clinical situations. The advice contained in this handbook is based on a combination of literature review, clinical experience and expert contribution. We do not claim that this advice is necessarily 'correct' or that it deserves greater prominence than guidance provided by other professional bodies or special interest groups. We hope, however, to have provided guidance that helps to assure the safe, effective and economic use of medicines in psychiatry. We hope also to have made clear precisely the sources of information used to inform the guidance given.

Please note that many of the recommendations provided here go beyond the licensed or labelled indications of many drugs, both in the UK and elsewhere. Note also that, while we have endeavoured to make sure all quoted doses are correct, clinicians should always consult statutory texts before prescribing. Users of *The Guidelines* should also bear in mind that the contents of this handbook are based on information available to us in March 2018. Much of the advice contained here will become out-dated as more research is conducted and published.

No liability is accepted for any injury, loss or damage, however caused.

Notes on inclusion of drugs

The Guidelines are used in many other countries outside the UK. With this in mind, we have included in this edition those drugs in widespread use throughout the Western world in March 2018. These include drugs not marketed in the UK such as brexipiprazole, cariprazine, desvenlafaxine and vilazodone, amongst several others. Many older drugs or those not widely available (for example levomepromazine, pericyazine, maprotiline, zotepine, oral loxapine, etc.) are either only briefly mentioned or not included on the basis that these drugs are not in widespread use at the time of writing.

Contributors' conflict of interest

Most of the contributors to *The Guidelines* have received funding from pharmaceutical manufacturers for research, consultancy or lectures. Readers should be aware that these relationships inevitably colour opinions on such matters as drug selection or preference. We cannot therefore guarantee that guidance provided here is free of indirect influence of the pharmaceutical industry but hope to have mitigated this risk by providing copious literature support for statements made. As regards direct influence, no pharmaceutical company has been allowed to view or comment on any drafts or proofs of *The Guidelines* and none has made any request for the inclusion or omission of any topic, advice or guidance. To this extent, *The Guidelines* have been written independent of the pharmaceutical industry.

List of abbreviations

AACAP	American Academy of Child and Adolescent Psychiatry	BAC	blood alcohol concentration
ACE	angiotensin-converting enzyme	BAP	British Association for Psychopharmacology
ACh	acetylcholine	BBB	blood–brain barrier
AChE	acetylcholinesterase	bd	*bis die* (twice a day)
AChE-I	acetylcholinesterase inhibitor	BDD	body dysmorphic disorder
ACR	albumin:creatinine ratio	BDI	Beck Depression Inventory
AD	Alzheimer's disease	BDNF	brain-derived neurotrophic factor
ADAS-cog	Alzheimer's Disease Assessment Scale – cognitive subscale	BED	binge eating disorder
		BEN	benign ethnic neutropenia
ADH	alcohol dehydrogenase	BMI	body mass index
ADHD	attention deficit hyperactivity disorder	BN	bulimia nervosa
		BP	blood pressure
ADIS	Anxiety Disorders Interview Schedule	BPD	borderline personality disorder
		BPSD	behavioural and psychological symptoms of dementia
ADL	activities of daily living		
ADR	adverse drug reaction	BuChE	butyrylcholinesterase
AF	atrial fibrillation	CAM	Confusion Assessment Method
AIDS	acquired immune deficiency syndrome	CAMS	Childhood Anxiety Multimodal Study
AIMS	Abnormal Involuntary Movement Scale	CATIE	Clinical Antipsychotic Trials of Intervention Effectiveness
ALP	alkaline phosphatase	CBT	cognitive behavioural therapy
ALT	alanine transaminase/aminotransferase	CBZ	carbamazepine
		CDRS	Children's Depression Rating Scale
ANC	absolute neutrophil count	CDT	carbohydrate-deficient transferrin
ANNSERS	Antipsychotic Non-Neurological Side-Effects Rating Scale	CES-D	Centre for Epidemiological Studies Depression scale
APA	American Psychological Association	CGAS	Children's Global Assessment Scale
ARB	angiotensin II receptor blocker	CGI	Clinical Global Impression scales
ASD	autism spectrum disorders	CI	confidence interval
ASEX	Arizona Sexual Experience Scale	CIBIC-Plus	Clinician's Interview-Based Impression of Change
AST	aspartate aminotransferase		
AUDIT	Alcohol Use Disorders Identification Test	CIGH	clozapine-induced gastrointestinal hypomotility

CIWA-Ar	Clinical Institute Withdrawal Assessment of Alcohol scale revised
CK	creatine kinase
CKD	chronic kidney disease
CKD-EPI	Chronic Kidney Disease Epidemiology Collaboration
CNS	central nervous system
COMT	catechol-O-methyltransferase
COPD	chronic obstructive pulmonary disease
COX	cyclo-oxygenase
CPK	creatinine phosphokinase
CPP	child–parent psychotherapy
CPSS	Child PTSD Symptom Scale
CrCl	creatinine clearance
CREB	cAMP response element-binding protein
CRP	C-reactive protein
CUtLASS	Cost Utility of the Latest Antipsychotic Drugs in Schizophrenia Study
CVA	cerebrovascular accident
CY-BOCS	Children's Yale-Brown Obsessive Compulsive Scale
CYP	cytochrome P
DAI	drug attitude inventory
DESS	Discontinuation–Emergent Signs and Symptoms scale
DEXA	dual-energy X-ray absorptiometry
DHEA	dehydroepiandrosterone
DIVA	Diagnostic Interview for DSM-IV ADHD
DLB	dementia with Lewy bodies
DMDD	disruptive mood dysregulation disorder
DOAC	direct-acting oral anticoagulant
DoLS	Deprivation of Liberty Safeguards
DSM	*Diagnostic and Statistical Manual of Mental Disorders*
DVLA	Driver and Vehicle Licensing Agency
EAD	early after depolarisation
ECG	electrocardiogram
ECT	electroconvulsive therapy
EDTA	ethylenediaminetetra-acetic acid
EEG	electroencephalogram
eGFR	estimated glomerular filtration rate
EMDR	eye movement desensitisation and reprocessing
EOSS	early-onset schizophrenia-spectrum
EPA	eicosapentanoic acid
EPS	extrapyramidal symptoms
ER	extended release
ERK	extracellular signal-regulated kinase
ERP	exposure and response prevention
ES	effect size
ESR	erythrocyte sedimentation rate
FAST	functional assessment staging
FBC	full blood count
FDA	Food and Drug Administration (USA)
FGA	first-generation antipsychotic
FPG	fasting plasma glucose
FTI	Fatal Toxicity Index
GABA	γ-aminobutyric acid
GAD	generalised anxiety disorder
GASS	Glasgow Antipsychotic Side-effect Scale
GBL	γ-butaryl-lactone
G-CSF	granulocyte colony-stimulating factor
GFR	glomerular filtration rate
GGT	γ-glutamyl transferase
GHB	γ-hydroxybutyrate
GI	gastrointestinal
GM-CSF	granulocyte-macrophage colony-stimulating factor
GSK3	glycogen synthase kinase 3
HADS	Hospital Anxiety and Depression Scale
HAMA	Hamilton Anxiety Rating Scale
HAND	HIV-associated neurocognitive disorders
HD	Huntington's disease
HDL	high-density lipoprotein
HDRS	Hamilton Depression Rating Scale
HIV	human immunodeficiency virus
5-HMT	5-hydroxy-methyl-tolterodine
HPA	hypothalamic-pituitary-adrenal
HR	hazard ratio
IADL	instrumental activities of daily living
ICD	International Classification of Diseases
ICH	intracerebral haemorrhage
IFG	impaired fasting glucose
IG	intra-gastric
IJ	intra-jejunal
IM	intramuscular
IMCA	independent mental capacity advocate
IMHP	intramuscular high potency
INR	international normalised ratio
IR	immediate release
IV	intravenous

IVHP	intravenous high potency	PANS	Paediatric Acute-onset
Kiddie-SADS	Kiddie-Schedule for Affective		Neuropsychiatric Syndrome
	Disorders and Schizophrenia	PANSS	Positive and Negative Syndrome Scale
LAI	long-acting injection	PBA	pseudobulbar affect
LD	learning disability	PCP	phencyclidine
LDL	low-density lipoprotein	PD	Parkinson's disease
LFTs	liver function tests	PDD	pervasive developmental disorders
LGIB	lower gastrointestinal bleeding	PDD-NOS	pervasive developmental disorders
LSD	lysergic acid diethylamide		not otherwise specified
MADRS	Montgomery-Asberg Depression	P-gp	P-glycoprotein
	Rating Scale	PHQ-9	Patient Health Questionnaire-9
mane	morning	PICU	psychiatric intensive care unit
MAOI	monoamine oxidase inhibitor	PLC	pathological laughter and crying
MARS	Medication Adherence Rating Scale	PLWH	people living with HIV
MASC	Multidimensional Anxiety Scale	PMR	post-mortem redistribution
	for Children	po	*per os* (by mouth)
MCA	Mental Capacity Act	POMH-UK	Prescribing Observatory for Mental
MCI	mild cognitive impairment		Health
MDA	3,4-methylenedioxyamphetamine	PPH	post-partum haemorrhage
MDMA	3,4-methylenedioxymeth-	PPI	proton pump inhibitor
	amphetamine	prn	*pro re nata* (as required)
MDRD	Modification of Diet in Renal	PT	prothrombin time
	Disease	PTSD	post-traumatic stress disorder
MHRA	Medicines and Healthcare	PWE	people with epilepsy
	Products Regulatory Agency	qds	*quarter die sumendum* (four times
MI	myocardial infarction		a day)
MMSE	Mini Mental State Examination	QTc	QT interval adjusted for heart rate
MR	modified release	RC	responsible clinician
MS	mood stabilisers/multiple sclerosis	RCADS	Revised Children's Anxiety and
NAS	neonatal abstinence syndrome		Depression Scale
NICE	National Institute for Health and	RCT	randomised controlled trial
	Care Excellence	RID	relative infant dose
NMDA	N-methyl-D-aspartate	RIMA	reversible inhibitor of monoamine
NMS	neuroleptic malignant syndrome		oxidase A
NNH	number needed to harm	RLAI	risperidone long-acting injection
NNT	number needed to treat	ROMI	Rating of Medication Influences
nocte	at night		scale
NPI	neuropsychiatric inventory	RPG	random plasma glucose
NRT	nicotine replacement therapy	RR	relative risk
NSAID	non-steroidal anti-inflammatory drug	RRBI	restricted repetitive behaviours and
NVC	neurovascular coupling		interests
OCD	obsessive compulsive disorder	RT	rapid tranquillisation
od	*omni die* (once a day)	RTA	road traffic accident
OD	overdose	rTMS	repetitive transcranial magnetic
OGTT	oral glucose tolerance test		stimulation
OOWS	Objective Opiate Withdrawal Scale	RUPP	Research Units on Paediatric
OST	opioid substitution treatment		Psychopharmacology
PANDAS	Paediatric Autoimmune	RYGB	Roux-en-Y gastric bypass
	Neuropsychiatric Disorder	SADQ	Severity of Alcohol Dependence
	Associated with Streptococcus		Questionnaire

SAWS	Short Alcohol Withdrawal Scale
SCARED	Screen for Child Anxiety and Related Emotional Disorders
SCIRS	Severe Cognitive Impairment Rating Scale
SCRA	synthetic cannabinoid receptor agonist
SGA	second-generation antipsychotics
SIADH	syndrome of inappropriate antidiuretic hormone
SIB	severe impairment battery
SJW	St John's wort
SLE	systemic lupus erythematosus
SNRI	serotonin–noradrenaline reuptake inhibitor
SOAD	second opinion appointed doctor
SPC	summary of product characteristics
SPECT	single photon emission computed tomography
SROM	slow release oral morphine
SS	steady state
SSRI	selective serotonin reuptake inhibitor
STAR*D	Sequenced Treatment Alternatives to Relieve Depression programme
STS	selegiline transdermal system
TADS	Treatment of Adolescents with Depression Study
TCA	tricyclic antidepressant
TD	tardive dyskinesia
tDCS	transcranial direct current stimulation
TDP	torsades de pointes
tds	*ter die sumendum* (three times a day)
TEAM	Treatment of Early Age Mania
TF-CBT	trauma-focused cognitive behavioural therapy
TFT	thyroid function test
THC/CBD	tetrahydrocannabinol/cannabidiol
TIA	transient ischaemic attack
TMS	transcranial magnetic stimulation
TORDIA	Treatment of Resistant Depression in Adolescence
TPR	temperature, pulse, respiration
TRS	treatment-resistant schizophrenia
TS	Tourette syndrome
U&Es	urea and electrolytes
UGIB	upper gastrointestinal bleeding
UGT	UDP-glucuronosyl transferase
VaD	vascular dementia
VNS	vagal nerve stimulation
VTE	venous thromboembolism
WBC	white blood cell
WCC	white cell count
WHO	World Health Organization
XL	extended release
YMRS	Young Mania Rating Scale
ZA	zuclopenthixol acetate

Part 1

Drug treatment of major psychiatric conditions

Chapter 1

Schizophrenia and related psychoses

ANTIPSYCHOTIC DRUGS

General introduction

Classification of antipsychotics

Before the 1990s, antipsychotics (or major tranquillisers as they were then known) were classified according to their chemistry. The first antipsychotic, chlorpromazine, was a phenothiazine compound – a tricyclic structure incorporating a nitrogen and a sulphur atom. Further phenothiazines were generated and marketed, as were chemically similar thioxanthenes such as flupentixol. Later, entirely different chemical structures were developed according to pharmacological paradigms. These included butyrophenones (haloperidol), diphenylbutylpiperidines (pimozide) and substituted benzamides (sulpiride, amisulpride).

Chemical classification remains useful but is rendered somewhat redundant by the broad range of chemical entities now available and by the absence of any clear structure–activity relationships for newer drugs. The chemistry of some older drugs does relate to their propensity to cause movement disorders. Piperazine phenothiazines (e.g. fluphenazine, trifluoperazine), butyrophenones and thioxanthenes are most likely to cause extrapyramidal symptoms (EPS) while piperidine phenothiazines (e.g. pipotiazine) and benzamides are the least likely. Aliphatic phenothiazines (e.g. chlorpromazine) and diphenylbutylpiperidines (pimozide) are perhaps somewhere in between.

Relative liability for inducing EPS was originally the primary factor behind the typical/atypical classification. Clozapine had long been known as an atypical antipsychotic on the basis of its low liability to cause EPS and its failure in animal-based antipsychotic screening tests. Its re-marketing in 1990 signalled the beginning of a series of new

The Maudsley Prescribing Guidelines in Psychiatry, Thirteenth Edition. David M. Taylor,
Thomas R. E. Barnes and Allan H. Young.
© 2018 David M. Taylor. Published 2018 by John Wiley & Sons Ltd.

medications, all of which were introduced with claims (of varying degrees of accuracy) of 'atypicality'. Of these medications, perhaps only clozapine and quetiapine are 'fully' atypical, seemingly having a very low liability for EPS. Others show dose-related effects, although, unlike with typical drugs, therapeutic activity can usually be achieved without EPS. This is possibly the real distinction between typical and atypical drugs: the ease with which a dose can be chosen (within the licensed dosage range) which is effective but which does not cause EPS (for example, compare haloperidol with olanzapine).

The typical/atypical dichotomy does not lend itself well to classification of antipsychotics in the middle ground of EPS liability. Thioridazine was widely described as atypical in the 1980s but is a 'conventional' phenothiazine. Sulpiride was marketed as an atypical but is often classified as typical. Risperidone, at its maximum dose of 16 mg/day (10 mg in the USA), is just about as 'typical' as a drug can be. Alongside these difficulties is the fact that there is nothing, either pharmacologically or chemically, which clearly binds these so-called 'atypicals' together as a group, save perhaps a general but not universal finding of preference for D_2 receptors outside the striatum. Nor are atypicals characterised by improved efficacy over older drugs (clozapine and one or two others excepted) or the absence of hyperprolactinaemia (which is worse with risperidone, paliperidone and amisulpride than with typical drugs).

In an attempt to get round some of these problems, typicals and atypicals were re-classified as first- or second-generation antipsychotics (FGA/SGA). All drugs introduced since 1990 are classified as SGAs (i.e. all atypicals) but the new nomenclature dispenses with any connotations regarding atypicality, whatever that may mean. However the FGA/SGA classification remains problematic because neither group is defined by anything other than time of introduction – hardly the most sophisticated pharmacological classification system. Perhaps more importantly, date of introduction is often wildly distant from date of first synthesis. Clozapine is one of the oldest antipsychotics (synthesised in 1959) while olanzapine is hardly in its first flush of youth, having first been patented in 1971. These two drugs are of course SGAs, apparently the most modern of antipsychotics.

In this edition of *The Guidelines* we conserve the FGA/SGA distinction more because of convention than some scientific basis. Also we feel that most people know which drugs belong to each group – it thus serves as a useful shorthand. However, it is clearly more sensible to consider the properties of *individual* antipsychotics when choosing drugs to prescribe or in discussions with patients and carers. With this in mind, the use of neuroscience-based nomenclature (NbN)[1] – a naming system that reflects pharmacological activity – is strongly recommended.

Choosing an antipsychotic

The NICE guideline for medicines adherence[2] recommends that patients should be as involved as possible in decisions about the choice of medicines that are prescribed for them, and that clinicians should be aware that illness beliefs and beliefs about medicines influence adherence. Consistent with this general advice that covers all of healthcare, the NICE guideline for schizophrenia emphasises the importance of patient choice rather than specifically recommending a class or individual antipsychotic as first-line treatment.[3]

Antipsychotics are effective in both the acute and maintenance treatment of schizophrenia and other psychotic disorders. They differ in their pharmacology, pharmacokinetics, overall efficacy/effectiveness and tolerability, but perhaps more importantly, response and tolerability differ between patients. This variability of individual response means that there is no clear first-line antipsychotic medication that is preferable for all.

Relative efficacy

Further to the publication of CATIE[4] and CUtLASS,[5] the World Psychiatric Association reviewed the evidence relating to the relative efficacy of 51 first-generation antipsychotics (FGAs) and 11 second-generation antipsychotics (SGAs) and concluded that, if differences in EPS could be minimised (by careful dosing) and anticholinergic use avoided, there was no convincing evidence to support any advantage for SGAs over FGAs.[6] As a class, SGAs may have a lower propensity to cause EPS and tardive dyskinesia[7] but this is somewhat offset by a higher propensity to cause metabolic adverse effects. A meta-analysis of antipsychotic medications for first-episode psychosis[8] found few differences between FGAs and SGAs as groups of drugs but minor advantages for olanzapine and amisulpride individually. A more recent network meta-analysis of first-episode studies found small efficacy advantages for olanzapine and amisulpride and overall poor performance for haloperidol.[9]

When individual non-clozapine SGAs are compared with each other, it would appear that olanzapine is more effective than aripiprazole, risperidone, quetiapine and ziprasidone, and that risperidone has the edge over quetiapine and ziprasidone.[10] Differences were small. FGA-controlled trials also suggest an advantage for olanzapine, risperidone and amisulpride over older drugs.[11,12] A network meta-analysis[13] broadly confirmed these findings, ranking amisulpride second behind clozapine and olanzapine third. These three drugs were the only ones to show clear efficacy advantages over haloperidol. The magnitude of differences was again small (but potentially substantial enough to be clinically important)[13] and must be weighed against the very different adverse-effect profiles associated with individual antipsychotics.

Clozapine is clearly the drug of choice in refractory schizophrenia[14] although, bizarrely, this is not a universal finding,[15] probably because of the nature and quality of many active-comparator trials.[16,17]

Both FGAs and SGAs are associated with a number of adverse effects. These include weight gain, dyslipidaemia, increases in plasma glucose/diabetes,[18,19] hyperprolactinaemia, hip fracture,[20] sexual dysfunction, EPS including neuroleptic malignant syndrome,[21] anticholinergic effects, venous thromboembolism (VTE),[22] sedation and postural hypotension. The exact profile is drug-specific (see individual sections on specific adverse effects), although comparative data are not robust[23] (see the meta-analysis by Leucht et al.[13] for rankings of some adverse-effect risks). Adverse effects are a common reason for treatment discontinuation,[24] particularly when efficacy is poor.[13] Patients do not always spontaneously report adverse effects, however,[25] and psychiatrists' views of the prevalence and importance of adverse effects differ markedly from patient experience.[26] Systematic enquiry along with a physical examination and appropriate biochemical tests is the only way accurately to assess their presence and severity or perceived severity. Patient-completed checklists such as the Glasgow Antipsychotic

Side-effect Scale (GASS)[27] can be a useful first step in this process. The clinician-completed Antipsychotic Non-Neurological Side-Effects Rating Scale (ANNSERS) facilitates more detailed and comprehensive assessment.[28]

Non-adherence to antipsychotic treatment is common and here the guaranteed medication delivery associated with depot/long-acting injectable (LAI) antipsychotic preparations is potentially advantageous. In comparison with oral antipsychotics, there is strong evidence that depots are associated with a reduced risk of relapse and rehospitalisation.[29–31] The introduction of SGA long-acting injections has to some extent changed the image of depots, which were sometimes perceived as punishments for miscreant patients. Their tolerability advantage probably relates partly to the better definition of their therapeutic dose range, meaning that the optimal dose is more likely to be prescribed (compare aripiprazole, with a licensed dose of 300 mg or 400 mg a month, with flupentixol, which has a licensed dose in the UK of 50 mg every 4 weeks to 400 mg a week).

As already mentioned, for patients whose symptoms have not responded sufficiently to adequate, sequential trials of two or more antipsychotic drugs, clozapine is the most effective treatment[32–34] and its use in these circumstances is recommended by NICE.[3] The biological basis for the superior efficacy of clozapine is uncertain.[35] Olanzapine should probably be one of the two drugs used before clozapine.[10,36]

This chapter covers the treatment of schizophrenia with antipsychotic drugs, the relative adverse-effect profile of these drugs and how adverse effects can be managed.

References

1. Zohar J et al. A review of the current nomenclature for psychotropic agents and an introduction to the neuroscience-based nomenclature. Eur Neuropsychopharmacol 2015; 25:2318–325.
2. National Institute for Health and Care Excellence. Medicines adherence: involving patients in decisions about prescribed medicines and supporting adherence. Clinical Guideline CG76, 2009. https://www.nice.org.uk/guidance/cg76
3. National Institute for Health and Care Excellence. Schizophrenia: core interventions in the treatment and management of schizophrenia in adults in primary and secondary care (update). Clinical Guideline 82, 2009. https://www.nice.org.uk/guidance/cg82.
4. Lieberman JA et al. Effectiveness of antipsychotic drugs in patients with chronic schizophrenia. N Engl J Med 2005; 353:1209–1223.
5. Jones PB et al. Randomized controlled trial of the effect on Quality of Life of second- vs first-generation antipsychotic drugs in schizophrenia: Cost Utility of the Latest Antipsychotic Drugs in Schizophrenia Study (CUtLASS 1). Arch Gen Psychiatry 2006; 63:1079–1087.
6. Tandon R et al. World Psychiatric Association Pharmacopsychiatry Section statement on comparative effectiveness of antipsychotics in the treatment of schizophrenia. Schizophr Res 2008; 100:20–38.
7. Tarsy D et al. Epidemiology of tardive dyskinesia before and during the era of modern antipsychotic drugs. Handb Clin Neurol 2011; 100:601–616.
8. Zhang JP et al. Efficacy and safety of individual second-generation vs. first-generation antipsychotics in first-episode psychosis: a systematic review and meta-analysis. Int J Neuropsychopharmacol 2013; 16:1205–1218.
9. Zhu Y et al. Antipsychotic drugs for the acute treatment of patients with a first episode of schizophrenia: a systematic review with pairwise and network meta-analyses. Lancet Psychiatry 2017; 4:694–705.
10. Leucht S et al. A meta-analysis of head-to-head comparisons of second-generation antipsychotics in the treatment of schizophrenia. Am J Psychiatry 2009; 166:152–163.
11. Davis JM et al. A meta-analysis of the efficacy of second-generation antipsychotics. Arch Gen Psychiatry 2003; 60:553–564.
12. Leucht S et al. Second-generation versus first-generation antipsychotic drugs for schizophrenia: a meta-analysis. Lancet 2009; 373:31–41.
13. Leucht S et al. Comparative efficacy and tolerability of 15 antipsychotic drugs in schizophrenia: a multiple-treatments meta-analysis. Lancet 2013; 382:951–962.
14. Siskind D et al. Clozapine v. first- and second-generation antipsychotics in treatment-refractory schizophrenia: systematic review and meta-analysis. Br J Psychiatry 2016; 209:385–392.
15. Samara MT et al. Efficacy, acceptability, and tolerability of antipsychotics in treatment-resistant schizophrenia: a network meta-analysis. JAMA Psychiatry 2016; 73:199–210.
16. Taylor DM. Clozapine for treatment-resistant schizophrenia: still the gold standard? CNS Drugs 2017; 31:177–180.
17. Kane JM et al. The role of clozapine in treatment-resistant schizophrenia. JAMA Psychiatry 2016; 73:187–188.

18. Manu P et al. Prediabetes in patients treated with antipsychotic drugs. J Clin Psychiatry 2012; 73:460–466.

19. Rummel-Kluge C et al. Head-to-head comparisons of metabolic side effects of second generation antipsychotics in the treatment of schizophrenia: a systematic review and meta-analysis. Schizophr Res 2010; 123:225–233.

20. Sorensen HJ et al. Schizophrenia, antipsychotics and risk of hip fracture: a population-based analysis. Eur Neuropsychopharmacol 2013; 23:872–878.

21. Trollor JN et al. Comparison of neuroleptic malignant syndrome induced by first- and second-generation antipsychotics. Br J Psychiatry 2012; 201:52–56.

22. Masopust J et al. Risk of venous thromboembolism during treatment with antipsychotic agents. Psychiatry Clin Neurosci 2012; 66:541–552.

23. Pope A et al. Assessment of adverse effects in clinical studies of antipsychotic medication: survey of methods used. Br J Psychiatry 2010; 197:67–72.

24. Falkai P. Limitations of current therapies: why do patients switch therapies? Eur Neuropsychopharmacol 2008; 18 Suppl 3:S135–S139.

25. Yusufi B et al. Prevalence and nature of side effects during clozapine maintenance treatment and the relationship with clozapine dose and plasma concentration. Int Clin Psychopharmacol 2007; 22:238–243.

26. Day JC et al. A comparison of patients' and prescribers' beliefs about neuroleptic side-effects: prevalence, distress and causation. Acta Psychiatr Scand 1998; 97:93–97.

27. Waddell L et al. A new self-rating scale for detecting atypical or second-generation antipsychotic side effects. J Psychopharmacol 2008; 22:238–243.

28. Ohlsen RI et al. Interrater reliability of the Antipsychotic Non-Neurological Side-Effects Rating Scale measured in patients treated with clozapine. J Psychopharmacol 2008; 22:323–329.

29. Tiihonen J et al. Effectiveness of antipsychotic treatments in a nationwide cohort of patients in community care after first hospitalisation due to schizophrenia and schizoaffective disorder: observational follow-up study. BMJ 2006; 333:224.

30. Leucht C et al. Oral versus depot antipsychotic drugs for schizophrenia – a critical systematic review and meta-analysis of randomised long-term trials. Schizophr Res 2011; 127:83–92.

31. Leucht S et al. Antipsychotic drugs versus placebo for relapse prevention in schizophrenia: a systematic review and meta-analysis. Lancet 2012; 379:2063–2071.

32. Kane J et al. Clozapine for the treatment-resistant schizophrenic. A double-blind comparison with chlorpromazine. Arch Gen Psychiatry 1988; 45:789–796.

33. McEvoy JP et al. Effectiveness of clozapine versus olanzapine, quetiapine, and risperidone in patients with chronic schizophrenia who did not respond to prior atypical antipsychotic treatment. Am J Psychiatry 2006; 163:600–610.

34. Lewis SW et al. Randomized controlled trial of effect of prescription of clozapine versus other second-generation antipsychotic drugs in resistant schizophrenia. Schizophr Bull 2006; 32:715–723.

35. Stone JM et al. Review: the biological basis of antipsychotic response in schizophrenia. J Psychopharmacol 2010; 24:953–964.

36. Agid O et al. An algorithm-based approach to first-episode schizophrenia: response rates over 3 prospective antipsychotic trials with a retrospective data analysis. J Clin Psychiatry 2011; 72:1439–1444.

General principles of prescribing*

- The **lowest possible** dose should be used. For each patient, the dose should be titrated to the lowest known to be effective (see section on 'Minimum effective doses' in this chapter); dose increases should then take place only after 2 weeks of assessment during which the patient is clearly showing poor or no response. (There is gathering evidence that lack of response at 2 weeks is a potent predictor of later poor outcome, unless dose or drug is changed.)
- With regular dosing of **depot medication,** plasma levels rise for at least 6–12 weeks after initiation, even without a change in dose (see section on 'Depot antipsychotics – pharmacokinetics' in this chapter). Dose increases during this time are therefore difficult to evaluate. The preferred method is to establish efficacy and tolerability of oral medication at a particular dose and then give the equivalent dose of that drug in LAI form. Where this is not possible, the target dose of LAI for an individual should be that established to be optimal in clinical trials (although such data are not always available for older LAIs).
- For the large majority of patients, the use of a **single antipsychotic** (with or without additional mood stabiliser or sedatives) is recommended. Apart from exceptional circumstances (e.g. clozapine augmentation) antipsychotic polypharmacy should generally be avoided because of the risks associated with QT prolongation and sudden cardiac death (see section on 'Combined antipsychotics' in this chapter).
- **Combinations** of antipsychotics should only be used where response to a single antipsychotic (including clozapine) has been clearly demonstrated to be inadequate. In such cases, the effect of the combination against target symptoms and adverse effects should be carefully evaluated and documented. Where there is no clear benefit, treatment should revert to single antipsychotic therapy.
- In general, **antipsychotics should not be used as** *pro re nata* **('PRN', as required) sedatives.** Short courses of benzodiazepines or general sedatives (e.g. promethazine) are recommended (see section on 'Acutely disturbed or violent behaviour').
- Responses to antipsychotic drug treatment should be **assessed by recognised rating scales** and be documented in patients' records.
- Those receiving antipsychotics should undergo close monitoring of physical health (including blood pressure, pulse, electrocardiogram [ECG], plasma glucose and plasma lipids) (see appropriate sections in this chapter).

---

* This section is not referenced. Please see relevant individual sections in this chapter for detailed and referenced guidance.

Minimum effective doses

Table 1.1 suggests the minimum dose of antipsychotic likely to be effective in first- or multi-episode schizophrenia. Most patients will respond to the dose suggested, although others may require higher doses. Given the variation in individual response, all doses should be considered approximate. Primary references are provided where available, but consensus opinion has also been used. Only oral treatment with commonly used drugs is covered.

Table 1.1 Antipsychotics: minimum effective dose/day

Drug	First episode	Multi-episode
FGAs		
Chlorpromazine[1]	200 mg*	300 mg
Haloperidol[2–6]	2 mg	4 mg
Sulpiride[7]	400 mg*	800 mg
Trifluoperazine[8,9]	10 mg*	15 mg
SGAs		
Amisulpride[10–15]	300 mg*	400 mg*
Aripiprazole[16–20]	10 mg	10 mg
Asenapine[21]	10 mg*	10 mg
Brexpiprazole[22]	2 mg*	2 mg
Cariprazine[23]	1.5 mg*	1.5 mg
Iloperidone[20,24]	4 mg*	8 mg
Lurasidone[25,26]	40 mg HCl/37 mg base*	40 mg HCl/37 mg base
Olanzapine[4,27–29]	5 mg	7.5 mg
Quetiapine[30–35]	150 mg* (but higher doses often used[36])	300 mg
Risperidone[3,37–40]	2 mg	4 mg
Sertindole[41,42]	Not appropriate	12 mg
Ziprasidone[20,43–45]	40 mg*	80 mg

*Estimate – too few data available.
FGA, first-generation antipsychotic; HCl, hydrochloride; SGA, second-generation antipsychotic.

References

1. Dudley K et al. Chlorpromazine dose for people with schizophrenia. Cochrane Database Syst Rev 2017; 4:CD007778.
2. McGorry PD. Recommended haloperidol and risperidone doses in first-episode psychosis. J Clin Psychiatry 1999; 60:794–795.
3. Schooler N et al. Risperidone and haloperidol in first-episode psychosis: a long-term randomized trial. Am J Psychiatry 2005; 162:947–953.
4. Keefe RS et al. Long-term neurocognitive effects of olanzapine or low-dose haloperidol in first-episode psychosis. Biol Psychiatry 2006; 59:97–105.
5. Donnelly L et al. Haloperidol dose for the acute phase of schizophrenia. Cochrane Database Syst Rev 2013; CD001951.
6. Oosthuizen P et al. A randomized, controlled comparison of the efficacy and tolerability of low and high doses of haloperidol in the treatment of first-episode psychosis. Int J Neuropsychopharmacol 2004; 7:125–131.
7. Soares BG et al. Sulpiride for schizophrenia. Cochrane Database Syst Rev 2000; CD001162.
8. Armenteros JL et al. Antipsychotics in early onset schizophrenia: systematic review and meta-analysis. Eur Child Adolesc Psychiatry 2006; 15:141–148.
9. Koch KE et al. Trifluoperazine versus placebo for schizophrenia. Cochrane Database Syst Rev 2014; CD010226.
10. Mota NE et al. Amisulpride for schizophrenia. Cochrane Database Syst Rev 2002; CD001357.
11. Puech A et al. Amisulpride, an atypical antipsychotic, in the treatment of acute episodes of schizophrenia: a dose-ranging study vs. haloperidol. The Amisulpride Study Group. Acta Psychiatr Scand 1998; 98:65–72.
12. Moller HJ et al. Improvement of acute exacerbations of schizophrenia with amisulpride: a comparison with haloperidol. PROD-ASLP Study Group. Psychopharmacology (Berl) 1997; 132:396–401.
13. Sparshatt A et al. Amisulpride – dose, plasma concentration, occupancy and response: implications for therapeutic drug monitoring. Acta Psychiatr Scand 2009; 120:416–428.
14. Buchanan RW et al. The 2009 schizophrenia PORT psychopharmacological treatment recommendations and summary statements. Schizophr Bull 2010; 36:71–93.
15. Galletly C et al. Royal Australian and New Zealand College of Psychiatrists clinical practice guidelines for the management of schizophrenia and related disorders. Aust N Z J Psychiatry 2016; 50:410–472.
16. Taylor D. Aripiprazole: a review of its pharmacology and clinical utility. Int J Clin Pract 2003; 57:49–54.
17. Cutler AJ et al. The efficacy and safety of lower doses of aripiprazole for the treatment of patients with acute exacerbation of schizophrenia. CNS Spectr 2006; 11:691–702.
18. Mace S et al. Aripiprazole: dose-response relationship in schizophrenia and schizoaffective disorder. CNS Drugs 2008; 23:773–780.
19. Sparshatt A et al. A systematic review of aripiprazole – dose, plasma concentration, receptor occupancy and response: implications for therapeutic drug monitoring. J Clin Psychiatry 2010; 71:1447–1456.
20. Liu CC et al. Aripiprazole for drug-naive or antipsychotic-short-exposure subjects with ultra-high risk state and first-episode psychosis: an open-label study. J Clin Psychopharmacol 2013; 33:18–23.
21. Citrome L. Role of sublingual asenapine in treatment of schizophrenia. Neuropsychiatr Dis Treat 2011; 7:325–339.
22. Correll CU et al. Efficacy of brexpiprazole in patients with acute schizophrenia: review of three randomized, double-blind, placebo-controlled studies. Schizophr Res 2016; 174:82–92.
23. Garnock-Jones KP. Cariprazine: a review in schizophrenia. CNS Drugs 2017; 31:513–525.
24. Crabtree BL et al. Iloperidone for the management of adults with schizophrenia. Clin Ther 2011; 33:330–345.
25. Leucht S et al. Dose equivalents for second-generation antipsychotics: the minimum effective dose method. Schizophr Bull 2014; 40:314–326.
26. Meltzer HY et al. Lurasidone in the treatment of schizophrenia: a randomized, double-blind, placebo- and olanzapine-controlled study. Am J Psychiatry 2011; 168:957–967.
27. Sanger TM et al. Olanzapine versus haloperidol treatment in first-episode psychosis. Am J Psychiatry 1999; 156:79–87.
28. Kasper S. Risperidone and olanzapine: optimal dosing for efficacy and tolerability in patients with schizophrenia. Int Clin Psychopharmacol 1998; 13:253–262.
29. Bishara D et al. Olanzapine: a systematic review and meta-regression of the relationships between dose, plasma concentration, receptor occupancy, and response. J Clin Psychopharmacol 2013; 33:329–335.
30. Small JG et al. Quetiapine in patients with schizophrenia. A high- and low-dose double-blind comparison with placebo. Seroquel Study Group. Arch Gen Psychiatry 1997; 54:549–557.
31. Peuskens J et al. A comparison of quetiapine and chlorpromazine in the treatment of schizophrenia. Acta Psychiatr Scand 1997; 96:265–273.
32. Arvanitis LA et al. Multiple fixed doses of "Seroquel" (quetiapine) in patients with acute exacerbation of schizophrenia: a comparison with haloperidol and placebo. Biol Psychiatry 1997; 42:233–246.
33. Kopala LC et al. Treatment of a first episode of psychotic illness with quetiapine: an analysis of 2 year outcomes. Schizophr Res 2006; 81:29–39.
34. Sparshatt A et al. Quetiapine: dose-response relationship in schizophrenia. CNS Drugs 2008; 22:49–68.
35. Sparshatt A et al. Relationship between daily dose, plasma concentrations, dopamine receptor occupancy, and clinical response to quetiapine: a review. J Clin Psychiatry 2011; 72:1108–1123.
36. Pagsberg AK et al. Quetiapine extended release versus aripiprazole in children and adolescents with first-episode psychosis: the multicentre, double-blind, randomised tolerability and efficacy of antipsychotics (TEA) trial. Lancet Psychiatry 2017; 4:605–618.

37. Lane HY et al. Risperidone in acutely exacerbated schizophrenia: dosing strategies and plasma levels. J Clin Psychiatry 2000; **61**:209–214.
38. Williams R. Optimal dosing with risperidone: updated recommendations. J Clin Psychiatry 2001; **62**:282–289.
39. Ezewuzie N et al. Establishing a dose-response relationship for oral risperidone in relapsed schizophrenia. J Psychopharm 2006; **20**:86–90.
40. Li C et al. Risperidone dose for schizophrenia. Cochrane Database Syst Rev 2009; CD007474.
41. Lindstrom E et al. Sertindole: efficacy and safety in schizophrenia. Expert Opin Pharmacother 2006; **7**:1825–1834.
42. Lewis R et al. Sertindole for schizophrenia. Cochrane Database Syst Rev 2005; CD001715.
43. Bagnall A et al. Ziprasidone for schizophrenia and severe mental illness. Cochrane Database Syst Rev 2000; CD001945.
44. Taylor D. Ziprasidone – an atypical antipsychotic. Pharm J 2001; **266**:396401.
45. Joyce AT et al. Effect of initial ziprasidone dose on length of therapy in schizophrenia. Schizophr Res 2006; **83**:285–292.

Further reading

Davis JM et al. Dose response and dose equivalence of antipsychotics. J Clin Psychopharmacol 2004; **24**:192–208.

Licensed maximum doses

Table 1.2 lists the EU licensed maximum doses of antipsychotics, according to the EMA labelling (as of March 2018).

Table 1.2 EU-licensed maximum doses of antipsychotics, according to the EMA labelling (March 2018)

Drug	Maximum dose
FGAs – oral	
Chlorpromazine	1000 mg/day
Flupentixol	18 mg/day
Haloperidol	20 mg/day
Levomepromazine	1000 mg/day
Pericyazine	300 mg/day
Perphenazine	24 mg/day
Pimozide	20 mg/day
Sulpiride	2400 mg/day
Trifluoperazine	None (suggest 30 mg/day)
Zuclopenthixol	150 mg/day
SGAs – oral	
Amisulpride	1200 mg/day
Aripiprazole	30 mg/day
Asenapine	20 mg (sublingual)
Clozapine	900 mg/day
Lurasidone	160 mg (HCl)/148 mg (base)/day
Olanzapine	20 mg/day
Paliperidone	12 mg/day
Quetiapine	750 mg/day schizophrenia (800 mg/day for MR preparation) 800 mg/day bipolar disorder
Risperidone	16 mg/day
Sertindole	24 mg/day
Depots	
Aripiprazole depot	400 mg/month
Flupentixol depot	400 mg/week
Fluphenazine depot	100 mg every 2 weeks
Haloperidol depot	300 mg every 4 weeks
Paliperidone depot – 1 monthly	150 mg/month
Paliperidone depot – 3 monthly	525 mg every 3 months
Pipotiazine depot	200 mg every 4 weeks
Risperidone	50 mg every 2 weeks
Zuclopenthixol depot	600 mg/week

FGA, first-generation antipsychotic; HCl, hydrochloride; MR, modified-release; SGA, second-generation antipsychotic.

Table 1.3 Licensed maximum doses of antipsychotics available outside the EU, according to FDA labelling (March 2018)

Drug	Maximum dose
SGAs – oral	
Brexpiprazole	4 mg/day
Cariprazine	6 mg/day
Iloperidone	24 mg/day
Molindone	225 mg/day
Ziprasidone	160 mg/day

FDA, US Food and Drug Administration; SGA, second-generation antipsychotic.

Table 1.3 lists the licensed maximum doses of antipsychotics available outside the EU, according to FDA labelling (as of March 2018).

Equivalent doses

Knowledge of equivalent dosages is useful when switching between FGAs. Estimates of 'neuroleptic' or 'chlorpromazine' equivalence, in mg/day, between these medications are based on clinical experience, expert panel opinion and/or early dopamine binding studies.

Table 1.4 provides approximate equivalent doses for FGAs.[1-4] The values given should be seen as a rough guide when switching from one FGA to another and are no substitute for clinical titration of the new medication dose against adverse effects and response.

Equivalent doses of SGAs may be less clinically relevant as these medications tend to have tighter, evidence-based licensed dose ranges. Nevertheless, a rough guide to equivalent SGA daily dosages is given in Table 1.5.[3-7] Clozapine is not included as this has a distinct initial titration schedule, partly for safety and tolerability reasons, and because it probably has a different mechanism of action.

Comparing potencies of FGAs with SGAs introduces yet more uncertainty with respect to dose equivalence. Very approximately, 100 mg chlorpromazine is equivalent to 1.5 mg risperidone.[3]

Table 1.4 First-generation antipsychotics: equivalent doses[1-4]

Drug	Equivalent dose (consensus)		Range of values in literature	
Chlorpromazine	100	mg/day	Reference	
Flupentixol	3	mg/day	2–3	mg/day
Flupentixol depot	10	mg/week	10–20	mg/week
Fluphenazine	2	mg/day	1–5	mg/day
Fluphenazine depot	5	mg/week	1–12.5	mg/week
Haloperidol	2	mg/day	1.5–5	mg/day
Haloperidol depot	15	mg/week	5–25	mg/week
Pericyazine	10	mg/day	10	mg/day
Perphenazine	10	mg/day	5–10	mg/day
Pimozide	2	mg/day	1.33–2	mg/day
Pipotiazine depot	10	mg/week	10–12.5	mg/week
Sulpiride	200	mg/day	133–300	mg/day
Trifluoperazine	5	mg/day	2.5–5	mg/day
Zuclopenthixol	25	mg/day	25–60	mg/day
Zuclopenthixol depot	100	mg/week	40–100	mg/week

Drug	Approximate equivalent dose
Amisulpride	400 mg
Aripiprazole	15 mg
Asenapine	10 mg
Brexpiprazole*	2 mg
Cariprazine*	3 mg
Clotiapine†	100 mg
Iloperidone*	12 mg
Lurasidone	80 mg (74 mg)
Molindone*	100 mg
Olanzapine	10 mg
Paliperidone LAI	75 mg/month
Quetiapine	300 mg
Risperidone oral	3 mg
Risperidone LAI	37.5 mg/2 weeks
Ziprasidone	80 mg

Table 1.5 Second-generation antipsychotics: approximate equivalent doses[3-7]

* Not available in EU at time of writing.
† Limited availability (not UK/USA).
LAI, long-acting injection.

References

1. Foster P. Neuroleptic equivalence. Pharm J 1989; **243**:431–432.
2. Atkins M et al. Chlorpromazine equivalents: a consensus of opinion for both clinical and research implications. Psychiatr Bull 1997; **21**:224–226.
3. Patel MX et al. How to compare doses of different antipsychotics: a systematic review of methods. Schizophr Res 2013; **149**:141–148.
4. Gardner DM et al. International consensus study of antipsychotic dosing. Am J Psychiatry 2010; **167**:686–693.
5. Woods SW. Chlorpromazine equivalent doses for the newer atypical antipsychotics. J Clin Psychiatry 2003; **64**:663–667.
6. Leucht S et al. Dose equivalents for second-generation antipsychotics: the minimum effective dose method. Schizophr Bull 2014; **40**:314–326.
7. Leucht S et al. Dose equivalents for second-generation antipsychotic drugs: the classical mean dose method. Schizophr Bull 2015; **41**:1397–1402.

CHAPTER 1

High-dose antipsychotics: prescribing and monitoring

'High-dose' antipsychotic medication can result from the prescription of either a single antipsychotic medication at a dose above the recommended maximum, or two or more antipsychotic medications concurrently that, when expressed as a percentage of their respective maximum recommended doses and added together, result in a cumulative dose of more than 100%.[1] In clinical practice, antipsychotic polypharmacy and PRN antipsychotic medication are strongly associated with high-dose prescribing.[2,3]

Efficacy

There is no firm evidence that high doses of antipsychotic medication are any more effective than standard doses for schizophrenia. This holds true for the use of antipsychotic medication for rapid tranquillisation, relapse prevention, persistent aggression and management of acute psychotic episodes.[1] Despite this, in the UK, approximately a quarter to a third of hospitalised patients on antipsychotic medication have been observed to be on a high dose,[2] while the national audit of schizophrenia in 2013, reporting on prescribing practice for over 5000 predominantly community-based patients, found that, overall, 10% were prescribed a high dose of antipsychotics.[4]

Review of the dose–response effects of a variety of antipsychotic medications has not found any evidence of greater efficacy for doses above accepted licensed ranges.[5,6] Efficacy appears to be optimal at relatively low doses: 4 mg/day risperidone;[7] 300 mg/day quetiapine;[8] olanzapine 10 mg[9,10] etc. Similarly, 100 mg 2-weekly risperidone depot offers no benefits over 50 mg 2-weekly,[11] and 320 mg/day ziprasidone[12] is no better than 160 mg/day. All currently available antipsychotics (with the possible exception of clozapine) exert their antipsychotic effect primarily through antagonism (or partial agonism) at post-synaptic dopamine receptors. There is increasing evidence that in some patients with schizophrenia, refractory symptoms do not seem to be driven through dysfunction of dopamine pathways,[13–15] and so increasing dopamine blockade in such patients is of uncertain value.

Dold et al.[16] conducted a meta-analysis of randomised controlled trials (RCTs) that compared continuation of standard-dose antipsychotic medication with dose escalation in patients whose schizophrenia had proved to be unresponsive to a prospective trial of standard-dose pharmacotherapy with the same antipsychotic medication. In this context, there was no evidence of any benefit associated with the increased dosage. There are a small number of RCTs that have examined the efficacy of high versus standard dosage in patients with a diagnosis of treatment-resistant schizophrenia (TRS).[1] Some demonstrated benefit[17] but the majority of these studies are old, the number of patients randomised is small and study design is poor by current standards. Some studies used daily doses equivalent to more than 10 g of chlorpromazine. In a study of patients with first-episode schizophrenia, increasing the dose of olanzapine up to 30 mg/day and the dose of risperidone up to 10 mg/day in non-responders to standard doses yielded only a 4% absolute increase in overall response rate; switching to an alternative antipsychotic, including clozapine, was considerably more successful.[18] One small (n = 12) open study of high-dose quetiapine (up to 1400 mg/day) found modest benefits in a third of subjects[19] but other, larger studies of quetiapine have shown no benefit for higher doses.[8,20,21] A further RCT of high-dose olanzapine (up to 45 mg/day) versus clozapine for TRS found similar efficacy for the two treatments but concluded that, given the small sample size, it would be premature to conclude that they were equivalent.[22] A systematic review of relevant studies comparing olanzapine at above standard dosage with clozapine for TRS concluded that while olanzapine, particularly in higher dosage, might be considered as an alternative to clozapine in TRS, clozapine still had the most robust evidence for efficacy.[23]

Adverse effects

The majority of adverse effects associated with antipsychotic treatment are dose-related. These include EPS, sedation, postural hypotension, anticholinergic effects, QTc prolongation and coronary heart disease mortality.[24–27] High-dose antipsychotic treatment is clearly associated with a greater adverse-effect burden.[12,21,27–29] There is some evidence that antipsychotic dose reduction from very high (mean 2253 mg chlorpromazine equivalents per day) to high (mean 1315 mg chlorpromazine equivalents per day) leads to improvements in cognition and negative symptoms.[30]

Recommendations

- The use of high-dose antipsychotic medication should be an exceptional clinical practice and only ever employed when adequate trials of standard treatments, including clozapine, have failed.
- Documentation of target symptoms, response and adverse effects, ideally using validated rating scales, should be standard practice so that there is ongoing consideration of the risk–benefit ratio for the patient. Close physical monitoring (including ECG) is essential.

Prescribing high-dose antipsychotic medication

Before using high doses, ensure that:

- Sufficient time has been allowed for response (see section on 'Antipsychotic response – to increase the dose, to switch, to add or wait?' in this chapter).
- At least two different antipsychotic medications have been tried sequentially (including, if possible, olanzapine).
- Clozapine has failed or not been tolerated due to agranulocytosis or other serious adverse effect. Most other adverse effects can be managed. A very small proportion of patients may also refuse clozapine.
- Medication adherence is not in doubt (use of blood tests, liquids/dispersible tablets, depot preparations, etc).
- Adjunctive medications such as antidepressants or mood stabilisers are not indicated.
- Psychological approaches have failed or are not appropriate.

The decision to use high doses should:

- Be made by a senior psychiatrist.
- Involve the multidisciplinary team.
- Be done, if possible, with a patient's informed consent.

Practice points

- Rule out contraindications (ECG abnormalities, hepatic impairment).
- Consider and minimise any risks posed by concomitant medication (e.g. potential to cause QTc prolongation, electrolyte disturbance or pharmacokinetic interactions via CYP inhibition).
- Document the decision to prescribe high dosage in the clinical notes along with a description of target symptoms. The use of an appropriate rating scale is advised.
- Adequate time for response should be allowed after each dosage increment before a further increase is made.

Monitoring

- Physical monitoring should be carried out as outlined in the section on 'Monitoring' in this chapter.
- All patients on high doses should have regular ECGs (baseline, when steady-state serum levels have been reached after each dosage increment, and then every 6–12 months). Additional biochemical/ECG monitoring is advised if drugs that are known to cause electrolyte disturbances or QTc prolongation are subsequently co-prescribed.
- Target symptoms should be assessed after 6 weeks and 3 months. If insufficient improvement in these symptoms has occurred, the dose should be decreased to the normal range.

References

1. Royal College of Psychiatrists. Consensus statement on high-dose antipsychotic medication. College Report CR190. RCP, London; 2014.
2. Paton C et al. High-dose and combination antipsychotic prescribing in acute adult wards in the UK: the challenges posed by p.r.n. prescribing. Br J Psychiatry 2008; 192:435–439.
3. Roh D et al. Antipsychotic polypharmacy and high dose prescription in schizophrenia: a 5-year comparison. Aust N Z J Psychiatry 2014; 48:52–60.
4. Patel MX et al. Quality of prescribing for schizophrenia: evidence from a national audit in England and Wales. Eur Neuropsychopharmacol 2014; 24:499–509.
5. Davis JM et al. Dose response and dose equivalence of antipsychotics. J Clin Psychopharmacol 2004; 24:192–208.
6. Gardner DM et al. International consensus study of antipsychotic dosing. Am J Psychiatry 2010; 167:686–693.
7. Ezewuzie N et al. Establishing a dose-response relationship for oral risperidone in relapsed schizophrenia. J Psychopharmacol 2006; 20:86–90.
8. Sparshatt A et al. Quetiapine: dose-response relationship in schizophrenia. CNS Drugs 2008; 22:49–68.
9. Kinon BJ et al. Standard and higher dose of olanzapine in patients with schizophrenia or schizoaffective disorder: a randomized, double-blind, fixed-dose study. J Clin Psychopharmacol 2008; 28:392–400.
10. Bishara D et al. Olanzapine: a systematic review and meta-regression of the relationships between dose, plasma concentration, receptor occupancy, and response. J Clin Psychopharmacol 2013; 33:329–335.
11. Meltzer HY et al. A six month randomized controlled trial of long acting injectable risperidone 50 and 100 mg in treatment resistant schizophrenia. Schizophr Res 2014; 154:14–22.
12. Goff DC et al. High-dose oral ziprasidone versus conventional dosing in schizophrenia patients with residual symptoms: the ZEBRAS study. J Clin Psychopharmacol 2013; 33:485–490.

13. Kapur S et al. Relationship between dopamine D2 occupancy, clinical response, and side effects: a double-blind PET study of first-episode schizophrenia. Am J Psychiatry 2000; **157**:514–520.

14. Demjaha A et al. Dopamine synthesis capacity in patients with treatment-resistant schizophrenia. Am J Psychiatry 2012; **169**:1203–1210.

15. Gillespie AL et al. Is treatment-resistant schizophrenia categorically distinct from treatment-responsive schizophrenia? A systematic review. BMC Psychiatry 2017; **17**:12.

16. Dold M et al. Dose escalation of antipsychotic drugs in schizophrenia: a meta-analysis of randomized controlled trials. Schizophr Res 2015; **166**:187–193.

17. Aubree JC et al. High and very high dosage antipsychotics: a critical review. J Clin Psychiatry 1980; **41**:341–350.

18. Agid O et al. An algorithm-based approach to first-episode schizophrenia: response rates over 3 prospective antipsychotic trials with a retrospective data analysis. J Clin Psychiatry 2011; **72**:1439–1444.

19. Boggs DL et al. Quetiapine at high doses for the treatment of refractory schizophrenia. Schizophr Res 2008; **101**:347–348.

20. Lindenmayer JP et al. A randomized, double-blind, parallel-group, fixed-dose, clinical trial of quetiapine at 600 versus 1200 mg/d for patients with treatment-resistant schizophrenia or schizoaffective disorder. J Clin Psychopharmacol 2011; **31**:160–168.

21. Honer WG et al. A randomized, double-blind, placebo-controlled study of the safety and tolerability of high-dose quetiapine in patients with persistent symptoms of schizophrenia or schizoaffective disorder. J Clin Psychiatry 2012; **73**:13–20.

22. Meltzer HY et al. A randomized, double-blind comparison of clozapine and high-dose olanzapine in treatment-resistant patients with schizophrenia. J Clin Psychiatry 2008; **69**:274–285.

23. Souza JS et al. Efficacy of olanzapine in comparison with clozapine for treatment-resistant schizophrenia: evidence from a systematic review and meta-analyses. CNS Spectr 2013;**18**:82–89.

24. Ray WA et al. Atypical antipsychotic drugs and the risk of sudden cardiac death. N Engl J Med 2009; **360**:225–235.

25. Barbui C et al. Antipsychotic dose mediates the association between polypharmacy and corrected QT interval. PLoS One 2016;**1**:e0148212.

26. Weinmann S et al. Influence of antipsychotics on mortality in schizophrenia: systematic review. Schizophr Res 2009; **113**:1–11.

27. Osborn DP et al. Relative risk of cardiovascular and cancer mortality in people with severe mental illness from the United Kingdom's General Practice Research Database. Arch Gen Psychiatry 2007; **64**:242–249.

28. Bollini P et al. Antipsychotic drugs: is more worse? A meta-analysis of the published randomized control trials. Psychol Med 1994; **24**:307–316.

29. Baldessarini RJ et al. Significance of neuroleptic dose and plasma level in the pharmacological treatment of psychoses. Arch Gen Psychiatry 1988; **45**:79–90.

30. Kawai N et al. High-dose of multiple antipsychotics and cognitive function in schizophrenia: the effect of dose-reduction. Prog Neuropsychopharmacol Biol Psychiatry 2006; **30**:1009–1014.

Combined antipsychotics

A systematic review of the efficacy of monotherapy with an antipsychotic medication concluded that the magnitude of the clinical improvement achieved is generally modest.[1] It is therefore unsurprising that the main clinical rationale for prescribing combined antipsychotics is to improve residual psychotic symptoms.[2,3] Nonetheless, there is no robust objective evidence that treatment with combined antipsychotics is superior to a single antipsychotic. A meta-analysis of 16 randomised trials in schizophrenia, comparing augmentation with a second antipsychotic with continued antipsychotic monotherapy, found that combining antipsychotic medication lacked double-blind/high-quality evidence for overall efficacy.[4] However, in patients with schizophrenia, the effects of a change from antipsychotic polypharmacy to monotherapy, even when carefully conducted, are uncertain. While the findings of two randomised studies suggested that the majority of patients may be successfully switched from antipsychotic polypharmacy to monotherapy without loss of symptom control,[5,6] another reported greater increases in symptoms after 6 months in those participants who had switched to antipsychotic monotherapy.[7]

Much of the evidence supporting antipsychotic combination therapy consists of small open studies and case series.[8,9] Placebo response and reporting bias (nobody reports the failure of polypharmacy) are clearly important factors in this flimsy evidence base. However, some antipsychotic polypharmacy has a valid rationale. It has been shown that co-prescribed aripiprazole reduces weight in patients receiving clozapine[10,11] and normalises prolactin in those on haloperidol[12] and risperidone LAI[13] (although not amisulpride[14]). Polypharmacy with aripiprazole in such circumstances may thus represent worthwhile, evidence-based practice, albeit in the absence of regulatory trials demonstrating safety. In many cases, however, using aripiprazole alone might be a more logical choice.

Evidence for harm is perhaps more compelling. There are a number of published reports of clinically significant adverse effects associated with combined antipsychotics, such as an increased prevalence of EPS,[15] severe EPS,[16] increased metabolic adverse effects and diabetes,[17,18] sexual dysfunction,[19] increased risk of hip fracture,[20] paralytic ileus,[21] grand mal seizures,[22] prolonged QTc[23] and arrhythmias.[3] Switching from antipsychotic polypharmacy to monotherapy has been shown to lead to worthwhile improvements in cognitive functioning.[6] With respect to systematic studies, one that followed a cohort of patients with schizophrenia prospectively over a 10-year period found that receiving more than one antipsychotic concurrently was associated with substantially increased mortality.[24] But there was no association between mortality and any measure of illness severity, suggesting that the increased mortality was related to the co-prescription of antipsychotic medication rather than the more severe or refractory illness for which the combined antipsychotics may have been prescribed. Another study, which involved the follow-up of 99 patients with schizophrenia over a 25-year period, found that those prescribed three antipsychotics simultaneously were twice as likely to die as those who had been prescribed only one.[25] Overall, however, the evidence regarding increased mortality is inconclusive: a negative case-control study and a negative database study have also been published.[26,27] Further, combined antipsychotics have been associated with longer admissions to hospital alongside more frequent adverse effects[28].

It follows that it should be standard practice to document the rationale for combined antipsychotics in individual cases in the clinical records, along with a clear account of any benefits and adverse effects. Medico-legally, this would seem to be prudent although in practice it is rarely done.[29]

Despite the adverse risk–benefit balance, prescriptions for combined antipsychotics are common[30–32] and often long term.[33] Combined antipsychotics are likely to involve depots/LAIs,[34,35] quetiapine[36] and FGAs,[37] the last of these perhaps reflecting their frequent use as PRN medications. Focused, assertive interventions can reduce the prevalence of prescribing of antipsychotic polypharmacy[38] but persistence with such programmes over several years may be required to achieve a significant change in practice.[39,40] In the UK there may have been some gradual reduction in the use of antipsychotic polypharmacy over recent years. National clinical audits conducted as part of a Prescribing Observatory for Mental Health (POMH-UK) quality improvement programme[40] found that combined antipsychotics were prescribed for 43% of patients on acute adult wards in the UK in 2006 while the respective figure in 2017 was 32%. It should be noted that only half of the in-patients receiving combined antipsychotics in the 2017 sample were prescribed more than one regular antipsychotic medication; the other half were prescribed a single regular antipsychotic plus PRN antipsychotic medication. The most common clinical reasons for prescribing regular, combined antipsychotics were a poor response to antipsychotic monotherapy and a period of crossover while switching from one antipsychotic to another. The use of combined antipsychotics has been found to be associated with younger patient age, male gender, and increased illness severity, acuity, complexity and chronicity, as well as poorer functioning, in-patient status and a diagnosis of schizophrenia.[2,31,36,41,42] These associations largely reinforce the notion that polypharmacy is used where monotherapy proves inadequate.[43]

The situation in the community appears to be different. A systematic audit conducted in the UK in 2011 involved 5000 adult patients with a diagnosis of schizophrenia or schizoaffective disorder who were living in the community, from nearly 60 different NHS Trusts. It found that just over 60% of these patients were receiving a single antipsychotic (FGA or SGA; oral or injectable) and a further 18% were receiving clozapine, while 5% were not prescribed any antipsychotic medication.[44] Thus, in this large sample of community patients, around one in six (16%) received combined antipsychotic medication. These data suggest some disparity between in-patient and out-patient practice, which probably reflects factors such as patient selection, disease severity and prescribing culture.

On the basis of the lack of evidence for efficacy and the potential for serious adverse effects, the routine use of combined antipsychotics should be avoided. But antipsychotic polypharmacy is clearly an established custom and practice. A questionnaire survey of US psychiatrists[45] found that for illnesses that had failed to respond to a single antipsychotic, two-thirds of psychiatrists switched to another single antipsychotic, while a third added a second antipsychotic. Those who switched were more positive about clinical outcomes than those who had augmented. Another questionnaire study, conducted in Denmark, revealed that almost two-thirds of psychiatrists would rather combine antipsychotics than prescribe clozapine.[46] An observational study found that patients whose illnesses had derived no benefit from antipsychotic monotherapy were likely to be switched to an alternative antipsychotic while those with a partial response were more likely to have a second antipsychotic added.[47] Such findings may partly explain why some patients are prescribed combined antipsychotics early in a treatment episode[3,48] and the use of combined antipsychotics in up to a third of patients prior to the initiation of clozapine.[49,50] They also indicate that the general consensus across treatment guidelines that the use of combined antipsychotic medication for the treatment of refractory psychotic illness should be considered only after other, evidence-based, pharmacological treatments such as clozapine have been exhausted is not consistently followed in clinical practice.[9] A UK study of patients newly prescribed continuing, combined, antipsychotic medication found that only a third had previously been trialled on clozapine.[42] However, it should be noted that clozapine augmentation strategies often involve combining antipsychotics and this is perhaps the sole therapeutic area where such practice is supportable[51-55] (see section on 'Optimising clozapine treatment' in this chapter). While there is little evidence to support starting polypharmacy, stopping may not always be easy. Switching to monotherapy, even when done in a graded fashion, may involve some increase in the risk of exacerbation of psychiatric symptoms, though it is usually rewarded with fewer/less severe adverse effects and the expectation is that such exacerbations can be successfully managed.[5]

Summary

- There is very little evidence supporting the efficacy of combined, non-clozapine, antipsychotic medications.
- There is substantial evidence supporting the potential for harm and so the use of combined antipsychotics should generally be avoided.
- Combined antipsychotics are commonly prescribed and this practice seems to be relatively resistant to change.
- As a minimum requirement, all patients who are prescribed combined antipsychotics should be systematically monitored for adverse effects (including an ECG) and any beneficial effect on symptoms should be carefully documented.
- Some antipsychotic polypharmacy (e.g. combinations with aripiprazole) shows clear benefits for tolerability but not efficacy.

References

1. Lepping P et al. Clinical relevance of findings in trials of antipsychotics: systematic review. Br J Psychiatry 2011; **198**:341–345.
2. Correll CU et al. Antipsychotic polypharmacy: a comprehensive evaluation of relevant correlates of a long-standing clinical practice. Psychiatr Clin North Am 2012; **35**:661–681.
3. Grech P et al. Long-term antipsychotic polypharmacy: how does it start, why does it continue? Ther Adv Psychopharmacol 2012; **2**:5–11.
4. Galling B et al. Antipsychotic augmentation vs. monotherapy in schizophrenia: systematic review, meta-analysis and meta-regression analysis. World Psychiatry 2017; **16**:77–89.
5. Essock SM et al. Effectiveness of switching from antipsychotic polypharmacy to monotherapy. Am J Psychiatry 2011; **168**:702–708.
6. Hori H et al. Switching to antipsychotic monotherapy can improve attention and processing speed, and social activity in chronic schizophrenia patients. J Psychiatr Res 2013; **47**:1843–1848.
7. Constantine RJ et al. The risks and benefits of switching patients with schizophrenia or schizoaffective disorder from two to one antipsychotic medication: a randomized controlled trial. Schizophr Res 2015; **166**:194–200.
8. Tracy DK et al. Antipsychotic polypharmacy: still dirty, but hardly a secret. A systematic review and clinical guide. Curr Psychopharmacol 2013; **2**:143–171.
9. Barnes TR et al. Antipsychotic polypharmacy in schizophrenia: benefits and risks. CNS Drugs 2011; **25**:383–399.
10. Fleischhacker WW et al. Effects of adjunctive treatment with aripiprazole on body weight and clinical efficacy in schizophrenia patients treated with clozapine: a randomized, double-blind, placebo-controlled trial. Int J Neuropsychopharmacol 2010; **13**:1115–1125.

11. Cooper SJ et al. BAP guidelines on the management of weight gain, metabolic disturbances and cardiovascular risk associated with psychosis and antipsychotic drug treatment. J Psychopharmacol 2016; 30:717–748.

12. Shim JC et al. Adjunctive treatment with a dopamine partial agonist, aripiprazole, for antipsychotic-induced hyperprolactinemia: a placebo-controlled trial. Am J Psychiatry 2007; 164:1404–1410.

13. Trives MZ et al. Effect of the addition of aripiprazole on hyperprolactinemia associated with risperidone long-acting injection. J Clin Psychopharmacol 2013; 33:538–541.

14. Chen CK et al. Differential add-on effects of aripiprazole in resolving hyperprolactinemia induced by risperidone in comparison to benzamide antipsychotics. Prog Neuropsychopharmacol Biol Psychiatry 2010; 34:1495–1499.

15. Carnahan RM et al. Increased risk of extrapyramidal side-effect treatment associated with atypical antipsychotic polytherapy. Acta Psychiatr Scand 2006; 113:135–141.

16. Gomberg RF. Interaction between olanzapine and haloperidol. J Clin Psychopharmacol 1999; 19:272–273.

17. Suzuki T et al. Effectiveness of antipsychotic polypharmacy for patients with treatment refractory schizophrenia: an open-label trial of olanzapine plus risperidone for those who failed to respond to a sequential treatment with olanzapine, quetiapine and risperidone. Hum Psychopharmacol 2008; 23:455–463.

18. Gallego JA et al. Safety and tolerability of antipsychotic polypharmacy. Expert Opin Drug Saf 2012; 11:527–542.

19. Hashimoto Y et al. Effects of antipsychotic polypharmacy on side-effects and concurrent use of medications in schizophrenic outpatients. Psychiatry Clin Neurosci 2012; 66:405–410.

20. Sorensen HJ et al. Schizophrenia, antipsychotics and risk of hip fracture: a population-based analysis. Eur Neuropsychopharmacol 2013; 23:872–878.

21. Dome P et al. Paralytic ileus associated with combined atypical antipsychotic therapy. Prog Neuropsychopharmacol Biol Psychiatry 2007; 31:557–560.

22. Hedges DW et al. New-onset seizure associated with quetiapine and olanzapine. Ann Pharmacother 2002; 36:437–439.

23. Beelen AP et al. Asymptomatic QTc prolongation associated with quetiapine fumarate overdose in a patient being treated with risperidone. Hum Exp Toxicol 2001; 20:215–219.

24. Waddington JL et al. Mortality in schizophrenia. Antipsychotic polypharmacy and absence of adjunctive anticholinergics over the course of a 10-year prospective study. Br J Psychiatry 1998; 173:325–329.

25. Joukamaa M et al. Schizophrenia, neuroleptic medication and mortality. Br J Psychiatry 2006; 188:122–127.

26. Baandrup L et al. Antipsychotic polypharmacy and risk of death from natural causes in patients with schizophrenia: a population-based nested case-control study. J Clin Psychiatry 2010; 71:103–108.

27. Tiihonen J et al. Polypharmacy with antipsychotics, antidepressants, or benzodiazepines and mortality in schizophrenia. Arch Gen Psychiatry 2012; 69:476–483.

28. Centorrino F et al. Multiple versus single antipsychotic agents for hospitalized psychiatric patients: case-control study of risks versus benefits. Am J Psychiatry 2004; 161:700–706.

29. Taylor D et al. Co-prescribing of atypical and typical antipsychotics – prescribing sequence and documented outcome. Psychiatr Bull 2002; 26:170–172.

30. Harrington M et al. The results of a multi-centre audit of the prescribing of antipsychotic drugs for in-patients in the UK. Psychiatr Bull 2002; 26:414–418.

31. Gallego JA et al. Prevalence and correlates of antipsychotic polypharmacy: a systematic review and meta-regression of global and regional trends from the 1970s to 2009. Schizophr Res 2012; 138:18–28.

32. Sneider B. Frequency and correlates of antipsychotic polypharmacy among patients with schizophrenia in Denmark: a nation-wide pharmacoepidemiological study. Eur Neuropsychopharmacol 2015; 25:1669–1676.

33. Procyshyn RM et al. Persistent antipsychotic polypharmacy and excessive dosing in the community psychiatric treatment setting: a review of medication profiles in 435 Canadian outpatients. J Clin Psychiatry 2010; 71:566–573.

34. Aggarwal NK et al. Prevalence of concomitant oral antipsychotic drug use among patients treated with long-acting, intramuscular, antipsychotic medications. J Clin Psychopharmacol 2012; 32:323–328.

35. Barnes TRE et al. Treatment of schizophrenia by long-acting depot injections in the UK. Br J Psychiatry 2009; 195:s37–s42.

36. Novick D et al. Antipsychotic monotherapy and polypharmacy in the treatment of outpatients with schizophrenia in the European Schizophrenia Outpatient Health Outcomes Study. J Nerv Ment Dis 2012; 200:637–643.

37. Paton C et al. High-dose and combination antipsychotic prescribing in acute adult wards in the UK: the challenges posed by p.r.n. prescribing. Br J Psychiatry 2008; 192:435–439.

38. Tani H et al. Interventions to reduce antipsychotic polypharmacy: a systematic review. Schizophr Res 2013; 143:215–220.

39. Mace S et al. Reducing the rates of prescribing high dose antipsychotics and polypharmacy on psychiatric inpatient and intensive care units: results of a 6-year quality improvement programme. Ther Adv Psychopharmacol 2015; 5:4–12.

40. Prescribing Observatory for Mental Health. Topic 1g & 3d. Prescribing high dose and combined antipsychotics on adult psychiatric wards. Prescribing Observatory for Mental Health, CCQI1272, 2017 (data on file).

41. Baandrup L et al. Association of antipsychotic polypharmacy with health service cost: a register-based cost analysis. Eur J Health Econ 2012; 13:355–363.

42. Kadra G et al. Predictors of long-term (≥6 months) antipsychotic polypharmacy prescribing in secondary mental healthcare. Schizophr Res 2016; 174:106–112.

43. Malandain L et al. Correlates and predictors of antipsychotic drug polypharmacy in real-life settings: results from a nationwide cohort study. Schizophr Res 2018; 192:213–218.

44. Patel MX et al. Quality of prescribing for schizophrenia: evidence from a national audit in England and Wales. Eur Neuropsychopharmacol 2014; 24:499–509.
45. Kreyenbuhl J et al. Adding or switching antipsychotic medications in treatment-refractory schizophrenia. Psychiatr Serv 2007; 58:983–990.
46. Nielsen J et al. Psychiatrists' attitude towards and knowledge of clozapine treatment. J Psychopharmacol 2010; 24:965–971.
47. Ascher-Svanum H et al. Comparison of patients undergoing switching versus augmentation of antipsychotic medications during treatment for schizophrenia. Neuropsychiatr Dis Treat 2012; 8:113–118.
48. Goren JL et al. Antipsychotic prescribing pathways, polypharmacy, and clozapine use in treatment of schizophrenia. Psychiatr Serv 2013; 64:527–533.
49. Howes OD et al. Adherence to treatment guidelines in clinical practice: study of antipsychotic treatment prior to clozapine initiation. Br J Psychiatry 2012; 201:481–485.
50. Thompson JV et al. Antipsychotic polypharmacy and augmentation strategies prior to clozapine initiation: a historical cohort study of 310 adults with treatment-resistant schizophrenic disorders. J Psychopharmacol 2016; 30:436–443.
51. Shiloh R et al. Sulpiride augmentation in people with schizophrenia partially responsive to clozapine. A double-blind, placebo-controlled study. Br J Psychiatry 1997; 171:569–573.
52. Josiassen RC et al. Clozapine augmented with risperidone in the treatment of schizophrenia: a randomized, double-blind, placebo-controlled trial. Am J Psychiatry 2005; 162:130–136.
53. Paton C et al. Augmentation with a second antipsychotic in patients with schizophrenia who partially respond to clozapine: a meta-analysis. J Clin Psychopharmacol 2007; 27:198–204.
54. Barbui C et al. Does the addition of a second antipsychotic drug improve clozapine treatment? Schizophr Bull 2009; 35:458–468.
55. Taylor DM et al. Augmentation of clozapine with a second antipsychotic – a meta-analysis of randomized, placebo-controlled studies. Acta Psychiatr Scand 2009; 119:419–425.

Antipsychotic prophylaxis

First episode of psychosis

Antipsychotics provide effective protection against relapse, at least in the short to medium term.[1] A meta-analysis of placebo-controlled trials found that 26% of first-episode patients randomised to receive maintenance antipsychotics relapsed after 6–12 months compared with 61% randomised to receive placebo.[2] Although the current consensus is that antipsychotics should be prescribed for 1–2 years after a first episode of schizophrenia,[3,4] Gitlin et al.[5] found that withdrawing antipsychotic treatment in line with this consensus led to a relapse rate of almost 80% after 1 year medication-free and 98% after 2 years. Other studies in first-episode patients have found that discontinuing antipsychotics increases the risk of relapse five-fold[6] and confirmed that only a small minority of patients who discontinue remain well 1–2 years later.[7–10] However, a 5-year follow-up of a 2-year RCT, during which patients received either maintenance antipsychotic treatment or had their antipsychotic dose reduced or discontinued completely, found that while there was a clear advantage for maintenance treatment with respect to reducing short-term relapse this advantage was lost in the medium term. Further, the dose-reduction/discontinuation group were receiving lower doses of antipsychotic drugs at follow-up and had better functional outcomes.[11] There are numerous interpretations of these outcomes but the most that can be concluded at this stage is that dose reduction is a possible option in first-episode psychosis. There are certainly other studies showing disastrous outcomes from antipsychotic discontinuation,[12] albeit over shorter periods with fewer subjects.

Clearly some patients with first-episode psychosis will not need long-term antipsychotics to stay well – figures of 18–30% have been quoted.[13] However, there are no reliable patient factors linked to good outcome following discontinuation of antipsychotics and there remains more evidence in favour of continuing antipsychotics than for stopping them.[14]

It should be noted that definitions of relapse usually focus on the severity of positive symptoms, and largely ignore cognitive and negative symptoms: positive symptoms are more likely to lead to hospitalisation while cognitive and negative symptoms (which respond less well, and in some circumstances may even be exacerbated by antipsychotic treatment) have a greater overall impact on quality of life.

With respect to antipsychotic choice, in the context of an RCT, clozapine did not offer any advantage over chlorpromazine in the medium term in first-episode patients with non-refractory illness.[15] However, in a large naturalistic study of patients with a first admission for schizophrenia, clozapine and olanzapine fared better with respect to preventing re-admission than other oral antipsychotics.[16] In this same study, the use of a long-acting antipsychotic injection seemed to offer advantages over oral antipsychotics despite confounding by indication (depots will have been prescribed to those considered to be poor adherers, oral to those perceived to have good adherence[16]). Later studies show a huge advantage for long-acting risperidone over oral risperidone in first-episode patients[17] and a smaller but substantial benefit for paliperidone LAI over oral antipsychotics in 'recently diagnosed schizophrenia'.[18]

In practice, a firm diagnosis of schizophrenia is rarely made after a first episode and the majority of prescribers and/or patients will have at least attempted to stop antipsychotic treatment within 1 year.[19] Ideally, patients should have their dose reduced gradually and all relevant family members and health-care staff should be aware of the discontinuation (such a situation is most likely to be achieved by using LAI). It is vital that patients, carers and key-workers are aware of the early signs of relapse and how to access help. Antipsychotics should not be considered the only intervention. Evidence-based psychosocial and psychological interventions are clearly also important.[20]

Multi-episode schizophrenia

The majority of those who have one episode of schizophrenia will go on to have further episodes. Patients with residual symptoms, a greater adverse-effect burden and a less positive attitude to treatment are at greater risk of relapse.[21] With each subsequent episode, the baseline level of functioning can deteriorate[22] and the majority of this decline is seen in the first decade of illness. Suicide risk (10%) is also concentrated in the first decade of illness. Antipsychotic drugs, when taken regularly, protect against relapse in the short, medium and (with less certainty) long term.[2,23] Those who receive targeted antipsychotics (i.e. only when symptoms re-emerge) seem to have a worse outcome than those who receive prophylactic antipsychotics[24,25] and the risk of tardive dyskinesia (TD) may also be higher. Similarly, low-dose antipsychotics are less effective than standard doses.[26]

Table 1.6 summarises the known benefits and harms associated with maintenance antipsychotic treatment as reported in a meta-analysis by Leucht et al. (2012).[2]

Depot preparations may have an advantage over oral in maintenance treatment, most likely because of guaranteed medication delivery (or at least guaranteed awareness of medication delivery). Meta-analyses of clinical trials have shown that the relative and absolute risks of relapse with depot maintenance treatment were 30% and

Table 1.6 Known benefits and harms associated with maintenance antipsychotic treatment

Benefits				Harms			
Outcome	Antipsychotic	Placebo	NNT	Adverse effect	Antipsychotic	Placebo	NNH*
Relapse at 7–12 months	27%	64%	3	Movement disorder	16%	9%	17
Re-admission	10%	26%	5	Anticholinergic effects	24%	16%	11
Improvement in mental state	30%	12%	4	Sedation	13%	9%	20
Violent/ aggressive behaviour	2%	12%	11	Weight gain	10%	6%	20

NNT, number needed to treat for one patient to benefit; NNH, number treated for one patient to be harmed.
* Likely to be a considerable underestimate as adverse effects are rarely systematically assessed in clinical trials.[27]

10% lower, respectively, than with oral treatment.[2,28] Long-acting preparations of antipsychotics may thus be preferred by both prescribers and patients.

A large meta-analysis concluded that the risk of relapse with newer antipsychotics is similar to that associated with older drugs.[2] (Note that lack of relapse is not the same as good functioning.[29]) The proportion of multi-episode patients who achieve remission is small and may differ between antipsychotic drugs. The CATIE study reported that only 12% of patients treated with olanzapine achieved remission for at least 6 months, compared with 8% treated with quetiapine and 6% with risperidone.[30] The advantage seen here for olanzapine is consistent with that seen in an acute efficacy network meta-analysis.[31]

Patients with schizophrenia often receive a number of sequential antipsychotic drugs during the maintenance phase.[32] Such switching is a result of a combination of suboptimal efficacy and poor tolerability. In both CATIE[33] and SOHO,[34,35] the attrition rate from olanzapine was lower than the attrition rate from other antipsychotic drugs, suggesting that olanzapine may be more effective than other antipsychotic drugs (except clozapine). However, prescribing choice should be based on potential risk–benefit and it should be noted that olanzapine is associated with a high propensity for metabolic adverse effects. In the SOHO study, the relapse rate over a 3-year period was relatively constant, supporting the benefit for maintenance treatment.[36,37]

Summary

- Relapse rates in patients discontinuing antipsychotics are extremely high.
- Antipsychotics significantly reduce relapse, re-admission and violence/aggression.
- Long-acting depot formulations provide the best protection against relapse.

Adherence to antipsychotic treatment

Amongst people with schizophrenia, non-adherence with antipsychotic treatment is high. Only 10 days after discharge from hospital up to 25% are partially or non-adherent, rising to 50% at 1 year and 75% at 2 years.[38] Not only does non-adherence increase the risk of relapse, it may also increase the severity of relapse and the duration of hospitalisation.[38] The risk of suicide attempts also increases four-fold[38] (see Chapter 14 'Enhancing medication adherence').

Dose for prophylaxis

Many patients probably receive higher doses than necessary (particularly of the older drugs) when acutely psychotic.[39,40] In the longer term, a balance needs to be struck between effectiveness and adverse effects. Lower doses of the older drugs (8 mg haloperidol/day or equivalent) are, when compared with higher doses, associated with less severe adverse effects,[41] better subjective state and better community adjustment.[42] Very low doses increase the risk of psychotic relapse.[39,43,44] There are no data to support the use of lower than standard doses of the newer drugs as prophylaxis. Doses that are acutely effective should generally be continued as prophylaxis[45,46] although an exception to this is prophylaxis after a first episode where very careful dose reduction is supportable.

How and when to stop antipsychotic treatment[47]

The decision to stop antipsychotic drugs requires a thorough risk–benefit analysis for each patient. Withdrawal of antipsychotic drugs after long-term treatment should be gradual and closely monitored. The relapse rate in the first 6 months after abrupt withdrawal is double that seen after gradual withdrawal (defined as slow taper down over at least 3 weeks for oral antipsychotics or abrupt withdrawal of depot preparations).[48] One analysis of incidence of relapse after switch to placebo found time to relapse to be very much longer for 3-monthly paliperidone than for 1-monthly and oral.[49] Overall percentage relapse was also reduced. Abrupt withdrawal of oral treatment may also lead to discontinuation symptoms (e.g. headache, nausea, insomnia) in some patients.[50]

The following factors should be considered:[47]

- Is the patient symptom-free, and, if so, for how long? Long-standing, non-distressing symptoms which have not previously been responsive to medication may be excluded.
- What is the severity of adverse effects (EPS, TD, sedation, obesity, etc.)?
- What was the previous pattern of illness? Consider the speed of onset, duration and severity of episodes and any danger posed to self and others.
- Has dosage reduction been attempted before, and, if so, what was the outcome?
- What are the patient's current social circumstances? Is it a period of relative stability, or are stressful life events anticipated?
- What is the social cost of relapse (e.g. is the patient the sole breadwinner for a family)?
- Is the patient/carer able to monitor symptoms, and, if so, will they seek help?

As with first-episode patients, patients, carers and key-workers should be aware of the early signs of relapse and how to access help. Be aware that targeted relapse treatment is much less effective than continuous prophylaxis.[9] Those with a history of aggressive behaviour or serious suicide attempts and those with residual psychotic symptoms should be considered for life-long treatment.

Key points that patients should know

- Antipsychotics do not 'cure' schizophrenia. They treat symptoms in the same way that insulin treats diabetes.
- Some antipsychotic drugs may be more effective than others.
- Many antipsychotic drugs are available. Different drugs suit different patients. Perceived adverse effects should always be discussed, so that the best tolerated drug can be found.
- Long-term treatment is generally required to prevent relapses.
- Antipsychotics should never be stopped suddenly.
- Psychological and psychosocial interventions increase the chance of staying well.[20]

Alternative views

While it is clear that antipsychotics effectively reduce symptom severity and rates of relapse, a minority view is that antipsychotics might also sensitise patients to psychosis. The hypothesis is that relapse on withdrawal can be seen as a type of discontinuation reaction resulting from super-sensitivity of dopamine receptors, although the evidence for this remains uncertain.[51] This phenomenon might explain better outcomes seen in first-episode patients who receive lower doses of antipsychotics but it also suggests the possibility that the use of antipsychotics might ultimately worsen outcomes.

The concept of 'super-sensitivity psychosis' was much discussed decades ago[52,53] and has recently seen a resurgence.[51] It is also striking that dopamine antagonists used for non-psychiatric conditions can induce withdrawal psychosis[54–56] (although, to our knowledge, these three references are the only ones in the medical literature). Whilst these theories and observations do not alter recommendations made in this section, they do emphasise the need for using the lowest possible dose of antipsychotic in all patients and the balancing of observed benefit with adverse outcomes, including those that might be less clinically obvious (e.g. the possibility of structural brain changes[57]).

References

1. Karson C et al. Long-term outcomes of antipsychotic treatment in patients with first-episode schizophrenia: a systematic review. Neuropsychiatr Dis Treat 2016; **12**:57–67.
2. Leucht S et al. Antipsychotic drugs versus placebo for relapse prevention in schizophrenia: a systematic review and meta-analysis. Lancet 2012; **379**:2063–2071.
3. American Psychiatric Association. Guideline Watch (September 2009): Practice Guideline for the Treatment of Patients With Schizophrenia. 2009. http://www.psychiatryonline.com/content.aspx?aid=501001
4. Sheitman BB et al. The evaluation and treatment of first-episode psychosis. Schizophr Bull 1997; **23**:653–661.
5. Gitlin M et al. Clinical outcome following neuroleptic discontinuation in patients with remitted recent-onset schizophrenia. Am J Psychiatry 2001; **158**:1835–1842.
6. Robinson D et al. Predictors of relapse following response from a first episode of schizophrenia or schizoaffective disorder. Arch Gen Psychiatry 1999; **56**:241–247.
7. Wunderink L et al. Guided discontinuation versus maintenance treatment in remitted first-episode psychosis: relapse rates and functional outcome. J Clin Psychiatry 2007; **68**:654–661.
8. Chen EY et al. Maintenance treatment with quetiapine versus discontinuation after one year of treatment in patients with remitted first episode psychosis: randomised controlled trial. BMJ 2010; **341**:c4024.
9. Gaebel W et al. Relapse prevention in first-episode schizophrenia – maintenance vs intermittent drug treatment with prodrome-based early intervention: results of a randomized controlled trial within the German Research Network on Schizophrenia. J Clin Psychiatry 2011; **72**:205–218.
10. Caseiro O et al. Predicting relapse after a first episode of non-affective psychosis: a three-year follow-up study. J Psychiatr Res 2012; **46**:1099–1105.
11. Wunderink L et al. Recovery in remitted first-episode psychosis at 7 years of follow-up of an early dose reduction/discontinuation or maintenance treatment strategy: long-term follow-up of a 2-year randomized clinical trial. JAMA Psychiatry 2013; **70**:913–920.
12. Boonstra G et al. Antipsychotic prophylaxis is needed after remission from a first psychotic episode in schizophrenia patients: results from an aborted randomised trial. Int J Psychiatry Clin Pract 2011; **15**:128–134.
13. Murray RM et al. Should psychiatrists be more cautious about the long-term prophylactic use of antipsychotics? Br J Psychiatry 2016; **209**:361–365.
14. Emsley R et al. How long should antipsychotic treatment be continued after a single episode of schizophrenia? Curr Opin Psychiatry 2016; **29**:224–229.
15. Girgis RR et al. Clozapine v. chlorpromazine in treatment-naive, first-episode schizophrenia: 9-year outcomes of a randomised clinical trial. Br J Psychiatry 2011; **199**:281–288.
16. Tiihonen J et al. A nationwide cohort study of oral and depot antipsychotics after first hospitalization for schizophrenia. Am J Psychiatry 2011; **168**:603–609.
17. Subotnik KL et al. Long-acting injectable risperidone for relapse prevention and control of breakthrough symptoms after a recent first episode of schizophrenia. a randomized clinical trial. JAMA Psychiatry 2015; **72**:822–829.
18. Schreiner A et al. Paliperidone palmitate versus oral antipsychotics in recently diagnosed schizophrenia. Schizophr Res 2015; **169**:393–399.
19. Johnson DAW et al. Professional attitudes in the UK towards neuroleptic maintenance therapy in schizophrenia. Psychiatr Bull 1997; **21**:394–397.
20. National Institute for Health and Care Excellence. Psychosis and schizophrenia in adults: prevention and management. Clinical Guideline 178, 2014. https://www.nice.org.uk/guidance/cg178
21. Schennach R et al. Predictors of relapse in the year after hospital discharge among patients with schizophrenia. Psychiatr Serv 2012; **63**:87–90.
22. Wyatt RJ. Neuroleptics and the natural course of schizophrenia. Schizophr Bull 1991; **17**:325–351.
23. Almerie MQ et al. Cessation of medication for people with schizophrenia already stable on chlorpromazine. Schizophr Bull 2008; **34**:13–14.

24. Jolley AG et al. Trial of brief intermittent neuroleptic prophylaxis for selected schizophrenic outpatients: clinical and social outcome at two years. Br Med J 1990; 301:837–842.

25. Herz MI et al. Intermittent vs maintenance medication in schizophrenia. Two-year results. Arch Gen Psychiatry 1991; 48:333–339.

26. Schooler NR et al. Relapse and rehospitalization during maintenance treatment of schizophrenia. The effects of dose reduction and family treatment. Arch Gen Psychiatry 1997; 54:453–463.

27. Pope A et al. Assessment of adverse effects in clinical studies of antipsychotic medication: survey of methods used. Br J Psychiatry 2010; 197:67–72.

28. Leucht C et al. Oral versus depot antipsychotic drugs for schizophrenia – a critical systematic review and meta-analysis of randomised long-term trials. Schizophr Res 2011; 127:83–92.

29. Schooler NR. Relapse prevention and recovery in the treatment of schizophrenia. J Clin Psychiatry 2006; 67 Suppl 5:19–23.

30. Levine SZ et al. Extent of attaining and maintaining symptom remission by antipsychotic medication in the treatment of chronic schizophrenia: evidence from the CATIE study. Schizophr Res 2011; 133:42–46.

31. Leucht S et al. Comparative efficacy and tolerability of 15 antipsychotic drugs in schizophrenia: a multiple-treatments meta-analysis. Lancet 2013; 382:951–962.

32. Burns T et al. Maintenance antipsychotic medication patterns in outpatient schizophrenia patients: a naturalistic cohort study. Acta Psychiatr Scand 2006; 113:126–134.

33. Lieberman JA et al. Effectiveness of antipsychotic drugs in patients with chronic schizophrenia. N Engl J Med 2005; 353:1209–1223.

34. Haro JM et al. Three-year antipsychotic effectiveness in the outpatient care of schizophrenia: observational versus randomized studies results. Eur Neuropsychopharmacol 2007; 17:235–244.

35. Haro JM et al. Antipsychotic type and correlates of antipsychotic treatment discontinuation in the outpatient treatment of schizophrenia. Eur Psychiatry 2006; 21:41–47.

36. Ciudad A et al. The Schizophrenia Outpatient Health Outcomes (SOHO) study: 3-year results of antipsychotic treatment discontinuation and related clinical factors in Spain. Eur Psychiatry 2008; 23:1–7.

37. Suarez D et al. Overview of the findings from the European SOHO study. Expert Rev Neurother 2008; 8:873–880.

38. Leucht S et al. Epidemiology, clinical consequences, and psychosocial treatment of nonadherence in schizophrenia. J Clin Psychiatry 2006; 67 Suppl 5:3–8.

39. Baldessarini RJ et al. Significance of neuroleptic dose and plasma level in the pharmacological treatment of psychoses. Arch Gen Psychiatry 1988; 45:79–90.

40. Harrington M et al. The results of a multi-centre audit of the prescribing of antipsychotic drugs for in-patients in the UK. Psychiatr Bull 2002; 26:414–418.

41. Geddes J et al. Atypical antipsychotics in the treatment of schizophrenia: systematic overview and meta-regression analysis. Br Med J 2000; 321:1371–1376.

42. Hogarty GE et al. Dose of fluphenazine, familial expressed emotion, and outcome in schizophrenia. Results of a two-year controlled study. Arch Gen Psychiatry 1988; 45:797–805.

43. Marder SR et al. Low- and conventional-dose maintenance therapy with fluphenazine decanoate. Two-year outcome. Arch Gen Psychiatry 1987; 44:518–521.

44. Uchida H et al. Low dose vs standard dose of antipsychotics for relapse prevention in schizophrenia: meta-analysis. Schizophr Bull 2011; 37:788–799.

45. Rouillon F et al. Strategies of treatment with olanzapine in schizophrenic patients during stable phase: results of a pilot study. Eur Neuropsychopharmacol 2008; 18:646–652.

46. Wang CY et al. Risperidone maintenance treatment in schizophrenia: a randomized, controlled trial. Am J Psychiatry 2010; 167:676–685.

47. Wyatt RJ. Risks of withdrawing antipsychotic medications. Arch Gen Psychiatry 1995; 52:205–208.

48. Viguera AC et al. Clinical risk following abrupt and gradual withdrawal of maintenance neuroleptic treatment. Arch Gen Psychiatry 1997; 54:49–55.

49. Weiden PJ et al. Does half-life matter after antipsychotic discontinuation? A relapse comparison in schizophrenia with 3 different formulations of paliperidone. J Clin Psychiatry 2017; 78:e813–e820.

50. Chouinard G et al. Withdrawal symptoms after long-term treatment with low-potency neuroleptics. J Clin Psychiatry 1984; 45:500–502.

51. Yin J et al. Antipsychotic induced dopamine supersensitivity psychosis: a comprehensive review. Curr Neuropharmacol 2017; 15:174–183.

52. Chouinard G et al. Neuroleptic-induced supersensitivity psychosis: clinical and pharmacologic characteristics. Am J Psychiatry 1980; 137:16–21.

53. Kirkpatrick B et al. The concept of supersensitivity psychosis. J Nerv Ment Dis 1992; 180:265–270.

54. Chaffin DS. Phenothiazine-induced acute psychotic reaction: the "psychotoxicity" of a drug. Am J Psychiatry 1964; 121:26–32.

55. Lu ML et al. Metoclopramide-induced supersensitivity psychosis. Ann Pharmacother 2002; 36:1387–1390.

56. Roy-Desruisseaux J et al. Domperidone-induced tardive dyskinesia and withdrawal psychosis in an elderly woman with dementia. Ann Pharmacother 2011; 45:e51.

57. Huhtaniska S et al. Long-term antipsychotic use and brain changes in schizophrenia – a systematic review and meta-analysis. Hum Psychopharmacol 2017; 32.

Negative symptoms

Negative symptoms in schizophrenia represent the absence or diminution of normal behaviours and functions and constitute an important dimension of psychopathology. A subdomain of 'expressive deficits' manifests as a decrease in verbal output or verbal expressiveness and flattened or blunted affect, assessed by diminished facial emotional expression, poor eye contact, decreased spontaneous movement and lack of spontaneity. A second 'avolition/amotivation' subdomain is characterised by a subjective reduction in interests, desires and goals, and a behavioural reduction in purposeful acts, including a lack of self-initiated social interactions.[1,2]

Persistent negative symptoms are held to account for much of the long-term morbidity and poor functional outcome of patients with schizophrenia.[3–6] However, the aetiology of negative symptoms is complex and it is important to determine the most likely cause in any individual case before embarking on a treatment regimen. An important clinical distinction is between primary negative symptoms, which comprise an enduring deficit state, predict a poor prognosis and are stable over time, and secondary negative symptoms, which are consequent upon positive psychotic symptoms, depression or demoralisation, or medication adverse effects such as bradykinesia as part of drug-induced parkinsonism.[5,7] Other sources of secondary negative symptoms may include chronic substance/alcohol use, high-dose antipsychotic medication, social deprivation, lack of stimulation and hospitalisation.[8] Secondary negative symptoms may be best tackled by treating the relevant underlying cause. In people with established schizophrenia, negative symptoms are seen to a varying degree in up to three-quarters, with up to 20% having persistent primary negative symptoms.[9,10]

The literature pertaining to the pharmacological treatment of negative symptoms largely consists of sub-analyses of acute efficacy studies, correlational analysis and path analyses.[11] There is often no reliable distinction between primary and secondary negative symptoms or between the two subdomains of expressive deficits and avolition/amotivation, and few studies specifically recruit patients with persistent negative symptoms. While the evidence suggests short-term efficacy for a few interventions, there is no robust evidence for an effective treatment for persistent primary negative symptoms.

In general:

- In first-episode psychosis, the presence of negative symptoms has been related to poor outcome in terms of recovery and level of social functioning.[4,9] There is evidence to suggest that the earlier a psychotic illness is effectively treated, the less likely is the development of negative symptoms over time.[12–14] However, when interpreting such data it should be borne in mind that an early clinical picture characterised by negative symptoms, being less socially disruptive and more subtle as signs of psychotic illness than positive symptoms, may contribute to delay in presentation to clinical services and thus be associated with a longer duration of untreated psychosis. In other words, patients with an inherently poorer prognosis in terms of persistent negative symptoms may be diagnosed and treated later.
- While antipsychotic medication has been shown to improve negative symptoms, this benefit seems to be limited to secondary negative symptoms in acute psychotic

episodes.[15] There is no consistent evidence for any superiority of SGAs over FGAs in the treatment of negative symptoms.[16–20] Similarly, there is no consistent evidence for the superiority of any individual SGA.[21] While a meta-analysis of 38 RCTs found a statistically significant reduction in negative symptoms with SGAs, the effect size did not reach a threshold for 'minimally detectable clinical improvement over time'.[22]

- Nevertheless, there are some data suggesting efficacy for negative symptoms with certain antipsychotic treatment strategies, such as amisulpride,[23–26] cariprazine,[27,28] and augmentation with aripiprazole.[29,30]

- While clozapine remains the only medication with convincing superiority for TRS, whether it has superior efficacy for negative symptoms, at least in the short term, in such cases remains uncertain.[31–33] One potential confounder in studies of clozapine for negative symptoms is that the medication has a low liability for parkinsonian adverse effects, including bradykinesia, which have a phenomenological overlap with negative symptoms, particularly the subdomain of expressive deficits.

- With respect to non-antipsychotic pharmacological interventions, several drugs that modulate glutamate pathways have been directly tested as adjuncts, but this approach has proved disappointing. Metabotropic glutamate 2/3 (mGlu2/3) receptor agonists have not been found to have any clear effect on negative symptoms over placebo.[34,35] Drugs modulating N-methyl-D-aspartate (NMDA) receptors in other ways have been tested: for example, there are negative RCTs of glycine,[36] D-serine,[37] modafinil,[38] armodafinil,[39] and bitopertin[40,41] augmentation of antipsychotic medication. There is a small preliminary positive RCT of pregnenolone.[42] With respect to decreasing glutamate transmission, there are inconsistent meta-analysis findings for lamotrigine augmentation of clozapine[43,44] and one positive[45] and one negative[46] RCT of memantine (the negative study being much larger). The antibiotic minocycline may have neuroprotective effects and modulate glutamate neurotransmission. There is some suggestion from meta-analyses of relevant studies that adding minocycline may improve negative symptoms, but the total sample size remains small.[47,48]

- With respect to antidepressant augmentation of an antipsychotic for negative symptoms, a Cochrane review concluded that this may be an effective strategy for reducing affective flattening, alogia and avolition,[49] although RCT findings for antidepressant augmentation of antipsychotic medication have found only inconsistent evidence of modest efficacy.[50–53] One review of meta-analyses of relevant studies concluded that the evidence supported the efficacy of mirtazapine and mianserin (postulated to be related to their α_2-adrenergic antagonist effects).[15] Another review concluded from the results of meta-analyses that adjunctive topiramate (a noradrenaline reuptake inhibitor) was effective for negative symptoms in schizophrenia spectrum disorders, being perhaps more efficacious when used to augment clozapine than non-clozapine antipsychotic medication.[54,55]

- Meta-analyses support the efficacy of augmentation of an antipsychotic with *Ginkgo biloba*[56] and a COX-2 inhibitor (albeit with a small effect size)[57] while small RCTs have demonstrated some benefit for selegiline,[58,59] pramiprexole,[60] testosterone (applied topically),[61] ondansetron[62] and granisetron.[63] The findings from studies of repetitive transcranial magnetic stimulation (rTMS) are mixed but promising.[64–66] The evidence for transcranial direct current stimulation (tDCS) as a treatment for negative symptoms is limited and inconclusive.[15,67] A large (n = 250) RCT in adults[68] and a smaller RCT in elderly patients[69] each found no benefit for donepezil and there is a further negative RCT of galantamine.[70]

Patients who misuse psychoactive substances experience fewer negative symptoms than patients who do not.[54] But rather than any pharmacological effect, it may be that this association at least partly reflects that those people who develop psychosis in the context of substance use, specifically cannabis, have fewer neurodevelopmental risk factors and thus better cognitive and social function.[71,72]

Summary and recommendations

The following recommendations are derived from the BAP schizophrenia guideline,[73] Veerman et al. 2017,[8] Aleman et al. 2017[15] and Remington et al.[74]

- There are no well-replicated, large trials, or meta-analyses of trials, with negative symptoms as the primary outcome measure that have yielded convincing evidence for enduring and clinically significant benefit.
- Where some improvement has been demonstrated in clinical trials, this may be limited to secondary negative symptoms.
- Psychotic illness should be identified and treated as early as possible as this may offer some protection against the development of negative symptoms.
- For any given patient, the antipsychotic medication that provides the best balance between overall efficacy and adverse effects should be used, at the lowest dose that maintains control of positive symptoms.
- Where negative symptoms persist beyond an acute episode of psychosis:
  - Ensure EPS (specifically bradykinesia) and depression are detected and treated if present, and consider the contribution of the environment to negative symptoms (e.g. institutionalisation, lack of stimulation).
  - There is insufficient evidence at present to support a recommendation for any specific pharmacological treatment for negative symptoms. Nevertheless, a trial of add-on medication for which there is some RCT evidence for efficacy, such as an antidepressant, may be worth considering in some cases, ensuring that the choice of the augmenting agent is based on minimising the potential for compounding adverse effects through pharmacokinetic or pharmacodynamic drug interactions.

References

1. Messinger JW et al. Avolition and expressive deficits capture negative symptom phenomenology: implications for DSM-5 and schizophrenia research. Clin Psychol Rev 2011; 31:161–168.
2. Foussias G et al. Dissecting negative symptoms in schizophrenia: opportunities for translation into new treatments. J Psychopharmacol 2015; 29:116–126.
3. Carpenter WT. The treatment of negative symptoms: pharmacological and methodological issues. Br J Psychiatry 1996; 168:17–22.
4. Galderisi S et al. Persistent negative symptoms in first episode patients with schizophrenia: results from the European First Episode Schizophrenia Trial. Eur Neuropsychopharmacol 2013; 23:196–204.
5. Buchanan RW. Persistent negative symptoms in schizophrenia: an overview. Schizophr Bull 2007; 33:1013–1022.
6. Rabinowitz J et al. Negative symptoms have greater impact on functioning than positive symptoms in schizophrenia: analysis of CATIE data. Schizophr Res 2012; 137:147–150.
7. Barnes TRE et al. How to distinguish between the neuroleptic-induced deficit syndrome, depression and disease-related negative symptoms in schizophrenia. Int Clin Psychopharmacol 1995; 10 (Suppl. 3):115–121.
8. Veerman RT et al. Treatment for negative symptoms in schizophrenia: a comprehensive review. Drugs 2017; 77:1423–1459.

9. Rammou A et al. Negative symptoms in first-episode psychosis: clinical correlates and 1-year follow-up outcomes in London Early Intervention Services. Early Interv Psychiatry 2017, Nov 16. doi: 10.1111/eip.12502. [Epub ahead of print]

10. Bobes J et al. Prevalence of negative symptoms in outpatients with schizophrenia spectrum disorders treated with antipsychotics in routine clinical practice: findings from the CLAMORS study. J Clin Psychiatry 2010; 71:280–286.

11. Buckley PF et al. Pharmacological treatment of negative symptoms of schizophrenia: therapeutic opportunity or cul-de-sac? Acta Psychiatr Scand 2007; 115:93–100.

12. Waddington JL et al. Sequential cross-sectional and 10-year prospective study of severe negative symptoms in relation to duration of initially untreated psychosis in chronic schizophrenia. Psychol Med 1995; 25:849–857.

13. Melle I et al. Prevention of negative symptom psychopathologies in first-episode schizophrenia: two-year effects of reducing the duration of untreated psychosis. Arch Gen Psychiatry 2008; 65:634–640.

14. Perkins DO et al. Relationship between duration of untreated psychosis and outcome in first-episode schizophrenia: a critical review and meta-analysis. Am J Psychiatry 2005; 162:1785–1804.

15. Aleman A et al. Treatment of negative symptoms: where do we stand and where do we go? Schizophr Res 2017; 186:55–62.

16. Darba J et al. Efficacy of second-generation-antipsychotics in the treatment of negative symptoms of schizophrenia: a meta-analysis of randomized clinical trials. Rev Psiquiatr Salud Ment 2011; 4:126–143.

17. Leucht S et al. Second-generation versus first-generation antipsychotic drugs for schizophrenia: a meta-analysis. Lancet 2009; 373:31–41.

18. Erhart SM et al. Treatment of schizophrenia negative symptoms: future prospects. Schizophr Bull 2006; 32:234–237.

19. Harvey RC et al. A systematic review and network meta-analysis to assess the relative efficacy of antipsychotics for the treatment of positive and negative symptoms in early-onset schizophrenia. CNS Drugs 2016; 30:27–39.

20. Zhang JP et al. Efficacy and safety of individual second-generation vs first-generation antipsychotics in first episode psychosis: a systematic review and meta-analysis. Int J Neuropsychopharmacol 2013; 16:1205–1218.

21. Leucht S et al. A meta-analysis of head-to-head comparisons of second-generation antipsychotics in the treatment of schizophrenia. Am J Psychiatry 2009; 166:152–163.

22. Fusar-Poli P et al. Treatments of negative symptoms in schizophrenia: meta-analysis of 168 randomized placebo-controlled trials. Schizophr Bull 2015; 41:892–899.

23. Danion JM et al. Improvement of schizophrenic patients with primary negative symptoms treated with amisulpride. Amisulpride Study Group. Am J Psychiatry 1999; 156:610–616.

24. Speller JC et al. One-year, low-dose neuroleptic study of in-patients with chronic schizophrenia characterised by persistent negative symptoms. Amisulpride v. haloperidol. Br J Psychiatry 1997; 171:564–568.

25. Leucht et al. Amisulpride, an unusual "atypical" antipsychotic: a meta-analysis of randomized controlled trials. Am J Psychiatry 2002; 159:180–190.

26. Liang Y et al. Effectiveness of amisulpride in Chinese patients with predominantly negative symptoms of schizophrenia: a subanalysis of the ESCAPE study. Neuropsychiatr Dis Treat 2017; 13:1703–1712.

27. Nemeth B et al. Quality-adjusted life year difference in patients with predominant negative symptoms of schizophrenia treated with cariprazine and risperidone. J Comp Eff Res 2017; 6:639–648.

28. Németh G et al. Cariprazine versus risperidone monotherapy for treatment of predominant negative symptoms in patients with schizophrenia: a randomised, double-blind, controlled trial. Lancet 2017; 389:1103–1113.

29. Zheng W et al. Efficacy and safety of adjunctive aripiprazole in schizophrenia: meta-analysis of randomized controlled trials. J Clin Psychopharmacol 2016; 36:628–636.

30. Galling B et al. Antipsychotic augmentation vs. monotherapy in schizophrenia: systematic review, meta-analysis and meta-regression analysis. World Psychiatry 2017; 16:77–89.

31. Siskind D et al. Clozapine v. first- and second-generation antipsychotics in treatment-refractory schizophrenia: systematic review and meta-analysis. Br J Psychiatry 2016; 209:385–392.

32. Souza JS et al. Efficacy of olanzapine in comparison with clozapine for treatment-resistant schizophrenia: evidence from a systematic review and meta-analyses. CNS Spectr 2013; 18:82–89.

33. Asenjo Lobos C et al. Clozapine versus other atypical antipsychotics for schizophrenia. Cochrane Database Syst Rev 2010; 11:CD006633.

34. Adams DH et al. Pomaglumetad methionil (LY2140023 monohydrate) and aripiprazole in patients with schizophrenia: a phase 3, multi-center, double-blind comparison. Schizophr Res Treat 2014; 2014:758212.

35. Stauffer VL et al. Pomaglumetad methionil: no significant difference as an adjunctive treatment for patients with prominent negative symptoms of schizophrenia compared to placebo. Schizophr Res 2013; 150:434–441.

36. Buchanan RW et al. The Cognitive and Negative Symptoms in Schizophrenia Trial (CONSIST): the efficacy of glutamatergic agents for negative symptoms and cognitive impairments. Am J Psychiatry 2007; 164:1593–1602.

37. Weiser M et al. A multicenter, add-on randomized controlled trial of low-dose d-serine for negative and cognitive symptoms of schizophrenia. J Clin Psychiatry 2012; 73:e728–e734.

38. Pierre JM et al. A randomized, double-blind, placebo-controlled trial of modafinil for negative symptoms in schizophrenia. J Clin Psychiatry 2007; 68:705–710.

39. Kane JM et al. Adjunctive armodafinil for negative symptoms in adults with schizophrenia: a double-blind, placebo-controlled study. Schizophr Res 2012; 135:116–122.

40. Bugarski-Kirola D et al. A phase II/III trial of bitopertin monotherapy compared with placebo in patients with an acute exacerbation of schizophrenia – results from the CandleLyte study. Eur Neuropsychopharmacol 2014; 24:1024–1036.

41. Goff DC. Bitopertin: the good news and bad news. JAMA Psychiatry 2014; 71:621–622.

42. Marx CE et al. Proof-of-concept trial with the neurosteroid pregnenolone targeting cognitive and negative symptoms in schizophrenia. Neuropsychopharmacology 2009; 34:1885–1903.

43. Tiihonen J et al. The efficacy of lamotrigine in clozapine-resistant schizophrenia: a systematic review and meta-analysis. Schizophr Res 2009; 109:10–14.

44. Veerman SR et al. Clozapine augmented with glutamate modulators in refractory schizophrenia: a review and metaanalysis. Pharmacopsychiatry 2014; 47:185–194.

45. Rezaei F et al. Memantine add-on to risperidone for treatment of negative symptoms in patients with stable schizophrenia: randomized, double-blind, placebo-controlled study. J Clin Psychopharmacol 2013; 33:336–342.

46. Lieberman JA et al. A randomized, placebo-controlled study of memantine as adjunctive treatment in patients with schizophrenia. Neuropsychopharmacology 2009; 34:1322–1329.

47. Oya K et al. Efficacy and tolerability of minocycline augmentation therapy in schizophrenia: a systematic review and meta-analysis of randomized controlled trials. Hum Psychopharmacol 2014; 29:483–491.

48. Xiang YQ et al. Adjunctive minocycline for schizophrenia: a meta-analysis of randomized controlled trials. Eur Neuropsychopharmacol 2017; 27:8–18.

49. Rummel C et al. Antidepressants for the negative symptoms of schizophrenia. Cochrane Database Syst Rev 2006; 3:CD005581.

50. Kishi T et al. Meta-analysis of noradrenergic and specific serotonergic antidepressant use in schizophrenia. Int J Neuropsychopharmacol 2014; 17:343–354.

51. Sepehry AA et al. Selective serotonin reuptake inhibitor (SSRI) add-on therapy for the negative symptoms of schizophrenia: a meta-analysis. J Clin Psychiatry 2007; 68:604–610.

52. Singh SP et al. Efficacy of antidepressants in treating the negative symptoms of chronic schizophrenia: meta-analysis. Br J Psychiatry 2010; 197:174–179.

53. Barnes TRE et al. Antidepressant Controlled Trial For Negative Symptoms In Schizophrenia (ACTIONS): a double-blind, placebo-controlled, randomised clinical trial. Health Technol Assess 2016; 20:1–46.

54. Veerman SRT et al. Treatment for negative symptoms in schizophrenia: a comprehensive review. Drugs 2017; 77:1423–1459.

55. Zheng W et al. Efficacy and safety of adjunctive topiramate for schizophrenia: a meta-analysis of randomized controlled trials. Acta Psychiatr Scand 2016; 134:385–398.

56. Singh V et al. Review and meta-analysis of usage of ginkgo as an adjunct therapy in chronic schizophrenia. Int J Neuropsychopharmacol 2010; 13:257–271.

57. Sommer IE et al. Nonsteroidal anti-inflammatory drugs in schizophrenia: ready for practice or a good start? A meta-analysis. J Clin Psychiatry 2012; 73:414–419.

58. Amiri A et al. Efficacy of selegiline add on therapy to risperidone in the treatment of the negative symptoms of schizophrenia: a double-blind randomized placebo-controlled study. Hum Psychopharmacol 2008; 23:79–86.

59. Bodkin JA et al. Double-blind, placebo-controlled, multicenter trial of selegiline augmentation of antipsychotic medication to treat negative symptoms in outpatients with schizophrenia. Am J Psychiatry 2005; 162:388–390.

60. Kelleher JP et al. Pilot randomized, controlled trial of pramipexole to augment antipsychotic treatment. Eur Neuropsychopharmacol 2012; 22:415–418.

61. Ko YH et al. Short-term testosterone augmentation in male schizophrenics: a randomized, double-blind, placebo-controlled trial. J Clin Psychopharmacol 2008; 28:375–383.

62. Zhang ZJ et al. Beneficial effects of ondansetron as an adjunct to haloperidol for chronic, treatment-resistant schizophrenia: a double-blind, randomized, placebo-controlled study. Schizophr Res 2006; 88:102–110.

63. Khodaie-Ardakani MR et al. Granisetron as an add-on to risperidone for treatment of negative symptoms in patients with stable schizophrenia: randomized double-blind placebo-controlled study. J Psychiatr Res 2013; 47:472–478.

64. Shi C et al. Revisiting the therapeutic effect of rTMS on negative symptoms in schizophrenia: a meta-analysis. Psychiatry Res 2014; 215:505–513.

65. Wobrock T et al. Left prefrontal high-frequency repetitive transcranial magnetic stimulation for the treatment of schizophrenia with predominant negative symptoms: a sham controlled, randomized multicenter trial. Biol Psychiatry 2015; 77:979–988.

66. Wang J et al. Efficacy towards negative symptoms and safety of repetitive transcranial magnetic stimulation treatment for patients with schizophrenia: a systematic review. Shanghai Arch Psychiatry 2017; 29:61–76.

67. Mondino M et al. Transcranial direct current stimulation for the treatment of refractory symptoms of schizophrenia. Current evidence and future directions. Curr Pharm Des 2015; 21:3373–3383.

68. Keefe RSE et al. Efficacy and safety of donepezil in patients with schizophrenia or schizoaffective disorder: significant placebo/practice effects in a 12-week, randomized, double-blind, placebo-controlled trial. Neuropsychopharmacology 2007; 33:1217–1228.

69. Mazeh D et al. Donepezil for negative signs in elderly patients with schizophrenia: an add-on, double-blind, crossover, placebo-controlled study. Int Psychogeriatr 2006; 18:429–436.

70. Conley RR et al. The effects of galantamine on psychopathology in chronic stable schizophrenia. Clin Neuropharmacol 2009; 32:69–74.

71. Arndt S et al. Comorbidity of substance abuse and schizophrenia: the role of pre-morbid adjustment. Psychol Med 1992; 22:388.

72. Leeson V et al. The effect of cannabis use and cognitive reserve on age at onset and psychosis outcomes in first-episode schizophrenia. Schizophr Bull 2012; 38:873–880.

73. Barnes TR. Evidence-based guidelines for the pharmacological treatment of schizophrenia: recommendations from the British Association for Psychopharmacology. J Psychopharmacol 2011; 25:567–620.

74. Remington G et al. Treating negative symptoms in schizophrenia: an update. Curr Treat Options Psychiatry 2016; 3:133–150.

CHAPTER 1

Monitoring

Table 1.7 summarises suggested monitoring for those receiving antipsychotic drugs. More detail and background are provided in specific sections in this chapter.

References

1. Burckart GJ et al. Neutropenia following acute chlorpromazine ingestion. Clin Toxicol 1981; **18**:797–801.
2. Grohmann R et al. Agranulocytosis and significant leucopenia with neuroleptic drugs: results from the AMUP program. Psychopharmacology (Berl) 1989; **99 Suppl**:S109–S112.
3. Esposito D et al. Risperidone-induced morning pseudoneutropenia. Am J Psychiatry 2005; **162**:397.
4. Montgomery J. Ziprasidone-related agranulocytosis following olanzapine-induced neutropenia. Gen Hosp Psychiatry 2006; **28**:83–85.
5. Cowan C et al. Leukopenia and neutropenia induced by quetiapine. Prog Neuropsychopharmacol Biol Psychiatry 2007; **31**:292–294.
6. Buchman N et al. Olanzapine-induced leukopenia with human leukocyte antigen profiling. Int Clin Psychopharmacol 2001; **16**:55–57.
7. Marder SR et al. Physical health monitoring of patients with schizophrenia. Am J Psychiatry 2004; **161**:1334–1349.
8. Fenton WS et al. Medication-induced weight gain and dyslipidemia in patients with schizophrenia. Am J Psychiatry 2006; **163**:1697–1704.
9. Weissman EM et al. Lipid monitoring in patients with schizophrenia prescribed second-generation antipsychotics. J Clin Psychiatry 2006; **67**:1323–1326.
10. Cohn TA et al. Metabolic monitoring for patients treated with antipsychotic medications. Can J Psychiatry 2006; **51**:492–501.
11. Paton C et al. Obesity, dyslipidaemias and smoking in an inpatient population treated with antipsychotic drugs. Acta Psychiatr Scand 2004; **110**:299–305.
12. Taylor D et al. Undiagnosed impaired fasting glucose and diabetes mellitus amongst inpatients receiving antipsychotic drugs. J Psychopharmacol 2005; **19**:182–186.
13. Citrome L et al. Incidence, prevalence, and surveillance for diabetes in New York State psychiatric hospitals, 1997-2004. Psychiatr Serv 2006; **57**:1132–1139.
14. Novotny T et al. Monitoring of QT interval in patients treated with psychotropic drugs. Int J Cardiol 2007; **117**:329–332.
15. Ray WA et al. Atypical antipsychotic drugs and the risk of sudden cardiac death. N Engl J Med 2009; **360**:225–235.
16. Hummer M et al. Hepatotoxicity of clozapine. J Clin Psychopharmacol 1997; **17**:314–317.
17. Erdogan A et al. Management of marked liver enzyme increase during clozapine treatment: a case report and review of the literature. Int J Psychiatry Med 2004; **34**:83–89.
18. Regal RE et al. Phenothiazine-induced cholestatic jaundice. Clin Pharm 1987; **6**:787–794.
19. Centorrino F et al. EEG abnormalities during treatment with typical and atypical antipsychotics. Am J Psychiatry 2002; **159**:109–115.
20. Gross A et al. Clozapine-induced QEEG changes correlate with clinical response in schizophrenic patients: a prospective, longitudinal study. Pharmacopsychiatry 2004; **37**:119–122.
21. Twaites BR et al. The safety of quetiapine: results of a post-marketing surveillance study on 1728 patients in England. J Psychopharmacol 2007; **21**:392–399.
22. Kelly DL et al. Thyroid function in treatment-resistant schizophrenia patients treated with quetiapine, risperidone, or fluphenazine. J Clin Psychiatry 2005; **66**:80–84.

Table 1.7 Monitoring of physical parameters for patients receiving antipsychotic medications

Parameter/test	Suggested frequency	Action to be taken if results outside reference range	Drugs with special precautions	Drugs for which monitoring is not required
Urea and electrolytes (including creatinine or estimated GFR)	Baseline and yearly as part of a routine physical health check	Investigate all abnormalities detected	Amisulpride and sulpiride renally excreted – consider reducing dose if GFR reduced	None
Full blood count (FBC)[1-6]	Baseline and yearly as part of a routine physical health check and to detect chronic bone marrow suppression (small risk associated with some antipsychotics)	Stop suspect drug if neutrophils fall below 1.5 × 10⁹/L Refer to specialist medical care if neutrophils below 0.5 × 10⁹/L. Note high frequency of benign ethnic neutropenia in certain ethnic groups	Clozapine – FBC weekly for 18 weeks, then fortnightly up to 1 year, then monthly (schedule varies from country to country)	None
Blood lipids[7,8] (cholesterol; triglycerides) Fasting sample, if possible	Baseline, at 3 months then yearly to cetect antipsychotic-induced changes, and generally monitor physical health	Offer lifestyle advice. Consider changing antipsychotic and/or initiating statin therapy	Clozapine, olanzapine – 3-monthly for first year, then yearly	Some antipsychotics (e.g. aripiprazole, lurasidone) not clearly associated with dyslipidaemia but prevalence is high in this patient group[9-11] so all patients should be monitored
Weight[7,8,11] (include waist size and BMI, if possible)	Baseline, frequently for 3 months then yearly to detect antipsychotic-induced changes, and generally monitor physical health	Offer lifestyle advice. Consider changing antipsychotic and/or dietary/pharmacological intervention	Clozapine, olanzapine – frequently for 3 months then 3-monthly for first year, then yearly	Aripiprazole, ziprasidone, brexpiprazole, cariprazine and lurasidone not clearly associated with weight gain but monitoring recommended nonetheless – obesity prevalence high in this patient group
Plasma glucose (fasting sample, if possible)	Baseline, at 4–6 months, then yearly to detect antipsychotic-induced changes and generally monitor physical health	Offer lifestyle advice. Obtain fasting sample or non-fasting and HbA₁c Refer to GP or specialist	Clozapine, olanzapine, chlorpromazine – test at baseline, 1 month, then 4–6-monthly	Some antipsychotics not clearly associated with IFG but prevalence is high in this patient group[12,13] so all patients should be monitored
ECG	Baseline and when target dose is reached (ECG changes rare in practice[14]) on admission to hospital and before discharge if drug regimen changed	Discuss with/refer to cardio ogist if abnormality detected	Haloperidol, pimozide, sertindole – ECG mandatory Ziprasidone – ECG mandatory in some situations	Risk of sudden cardiac death increased with most antipsychotics.[15] Ideally, all patients should be offered an ECG at least yearly

(Continued)

Table 1.7 *(Continued)*

Parameter/test	Suggested frequency	Action to be taken if results outside reference range	Drugs with special precautions	Drugs for which monitoring is not required
Blood pressure	Baseline; frequently during dose titration to detect antipsychotic-induced changes, and generally monitor physical health	If severe hypotension or hypertension (clozapine) observed, slow rate of titration. Consider switching to another antipsychotic if symptomatic postural hypotension. Treat hypertension in line with NICE guidelines	Clozapine, chlorpromazine and quetiapine most likely to be associated with postural hypotension	Amisulpride, aripiprazole, brexpiprazole, cariprazine, lurasidone, trifluoperazine, sulpiride
Prolactin	Baseline, then at 6 months, then yearly to detect antipsychotic-induced changes	Switch drugs if hyperprolactinaemia confirmed and symptomatic. Consider tests of bone mineral density (e.g. DEXA scanning) for those with chronically raised prolactin	Amisulpride, sulpiride, risperidone and paliperidone particularly associated with hyperprolactinaemia	Asenapine, aripiprazole, brexpiprazole, cariprazine, clozapine, lurasidone, quetiapine, olanzapine (<20 mg), ziprasidone usually do not elevate prolactin, but worth measuring if symptoms arise
Liver function tests (LFTs)[16–18]	Baseline, then yearly as part of a routine physical health check and to detect chronic antipsychotic-induced changes (rare)	Stop suspect drug if LFTs indicate hepatitis (transaminases × 3 normal) or functional damage (PT/albumin change)	Clozapine and chlorpromazine associated with hepatic failure	Amisulpride, sulpiride
Creatinine phosphokinase (CPK)	Baseline, then if NMS suspected	See section on 'Neuroleptic malignant syndrome' in this chapter	NMS more likely with first-generation antipsychotics	None

Other tests:

Patients on clozapine may benefit from an EEG[19,20] as this may help determine the need for anticonvulsant treatment (although interpretation is obviously complex). Those on quetiapine should have thyroid function tests yearly although the risk of abnormality is very small.[21,22]

Note: this table is a summary – see individual sections for detail and discussion.

BMI, body mass index; DEXA, dual-energy X-ray absorptiometry; ECG, electrocardiograph; EEG, electroencephalogram; GFR, glomerular filtration rate; IFG, impaired fasting glucose; NMS, neuroleptic malignant syndrome; PT, prothrombin time.

Relative adverse effects – a rough guide

Table 1.8 is made up of approximate estimates of relative incidence and/or severity, based on clinical experience, manufacturers' literature and published research. This is a very rough guide – see individual sections for more precise information.

Other adverse effects not mentioned in Table 1.8 do occur. Please see dedicated sections on other adverse effects included in this book for more information.

Table 1.8 Relative adverse effects of antipsychotic drugs

Drug	Sedation	Weight gain	Akathisia	Parkinsonism	Anti cholinergic	Hypotension	Prolactin elevation
Amisulpride*	–	+	+	+	–	–	+++
Aripiprazole	–	–	+	–	–	–	–
Asenapine*	+	+	+	–	–	–	+
Benperidol*	+	+	+	+++	+	+	+++
Brexpiprazole*	–	+	+	–	–	–	–
Cariprazine*	–	+	+	–	–	–	–
Chlorpromazine	+++	++	+	++	++	+++	+++
Clozapine	+++	+++	–	–	+++	+++	–
Flupentixol	+	++	++	++	++	+	+++
Fluphenazine*	+	+	++	+++	+	+	+++
Haloperidol	+	+	+++	+++	+	+	++
Iloperidone*	–	++	+	+	–	+	–
Loxapine*	++	+	+	+++	+	++	+++
Lurasidone	+	–	+	+	–	–	–
Olanzapine	++	+++	–	–	+	+	+
Paliperidone	+	++	+	+	+	++	+++
Perphenazine	+	+	++	+++	+	+	+++
Pimozide*	+	+	+	+	+	+	+++
Pipotiazine*	++	++	+	++	++	++	+++
Promazine*	+++	++	+	+	++	++	++
Quetiapine	++	++	–	–	+	++	–
Risperidone	+	++	+	+	+	++	+++
Sertindole*	–	+	+	–	–	+++	–
Sulpiride*	–	+	+	+	–	–	+++
Trifluoperazine	+	+	+	+++	+	+	+++
Ziprasidone*	+	–	+	–	–	+	+
Zuclopenthixol*	++	++	++	++	++	+	+++

*Availability varies from country to country.

+++ high incidence/severity; ++ moderate; + low; – very low.

Treatment algorithms for schizophrenia

First-episode schizophrenia

See Figure 1.1.

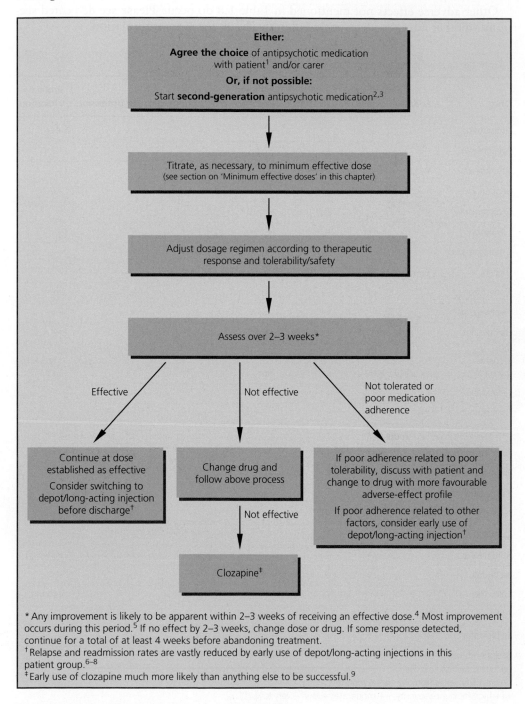

Either:
Agree the choice of antipsychotic medication with patient[1] and/or carer
Or, if not possible:
Start **second-generation** antipsychotic medication[2,3]

Titrate, as necessary, to minimum effective dose
(see section on 'Minimum effective doses' in this chapter)

Adjust dosage regimen according to therapeutic response and tolerability/safety

Assess over 2–3 weeks*

Effective

Not effective

Not tolerated or poor medication adherence

Continue at dose established as effective
Consider switching to depot/long-acting injection before discharge[†]

Change drug and follow above process

Not effective

If poor adherence related to poor tolerability, discuss with patient and change to drug with more favourable adverse-effect profile
If poor adherence related to other factors, consider early use of depot/long-acting injection[†]

Clozapine[‡]

*Any improvement is likely to be apparent within 2–3 weeks of receiving an effective dose.[4] Most improvement occurs during this period.[5] If no effect by 2–3 weeks, change dose or drug. If some response detected, continue for a total of at least 4 weeks before abandoning treatment.
[†] Relapse and readmission rates are vastly reduced by early use of depot/long-acting injections in this patient group.[6–8]
[‡] Early use of clozapine much more likely than anything else to be successful.[9]

Figure 1.1 Treatment algorithm for first-episode schizophrenia.

Relapse or acute exacerbation of schizophrenia (full adherence confirmed)

See Figure 1.2.

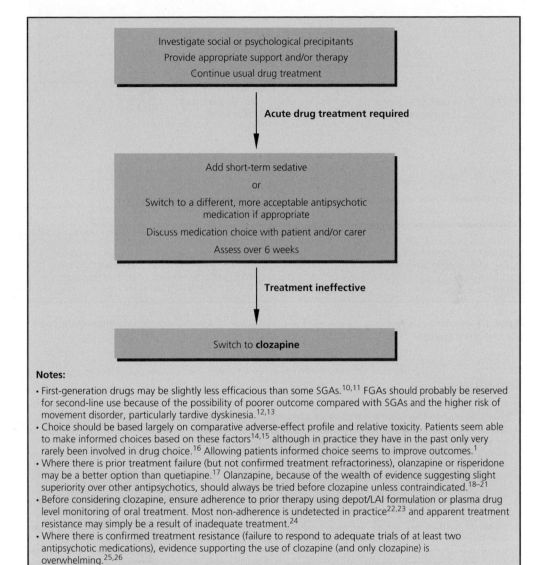

Notes:
- First-generation drugs may be slightly less efficacious than some SGAs.[10,11] FGAs should probably be reserved for second-line use because of the possibility of poorer outcome compared with SGAs and the higher risk of movement disorder, particularly tardive dyskinesia.[12,13]
- Choice should be based largely on comparative adverse-effect profile and relative toxicity. Patients seem able to make informed choices based on these factors[14,15] although in practice they have in the past only very rarely been involved in drug choice.[16] Allowing patients informed choice seems to improve outcomes.[1]
- Where there is prior treatment failure (but not confirmed treatment refractoriness), olanzapine or risperidone may be a better option than quetiapine.[17] Olanzapine, because of the wealth of evidence suggesting slight superiority over other antipsychotics, should always be tried before clozapine unless contraindicated.[18-21]
- Before considering clozapine, ensure adherence to prior therapy using depot/LAI formulation or plasma drug level monitoring of oral treatment. Most non-adherence is undetected in practice[22,23] and apparent treatment resistance may simply be a result of inadequate treatment.[24]
- Where there is confirmed treatment resistance (failure to respond to adequate trials of at least two antipsychotic medications), evidence supporting the use of clozapine (and only clozapine) is overwhelming.[25,26]

Figure 1.2 Treatment algorithm for relapse or acute exacerbation of schizophrenia (full adherence to medication confirmed). FGA, first-generation antipsychotic; LAI, long-acting injection; SGA, second-generation antipsychotic.

Relapse or acute exacerbation of schizophrenia (adherence in doubt)

See Figure 1.3.

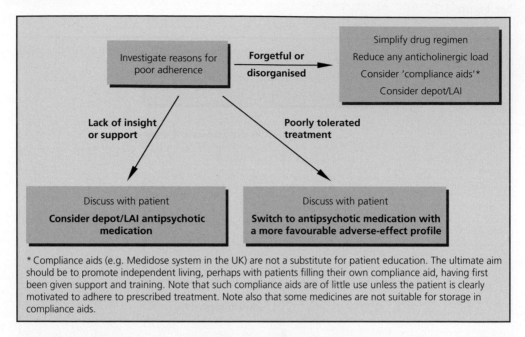

* Compliance aids (e.g. Medidose system in the UK) are not a substitute for patient education. The ultimate aim should be to promote independent living, perhaps with patients filling their own compliance aid, having first been given support and training. Note that such compliance aids are of little use unless the patient is clearly motivated to adhere to prescribed treatment. Note also that some medicines are not suitable for storage in compliance aids.

Figure 1.3 Treatment of relapse or acute exacerbation of schizophrenia (adherence doubtful or known to be poor). LAI, long-acting injection.

References

1. Robinson DG et al. Psychopharmacological treatment in the RAISE-ETP Study: outcomes of a manual and computer decision support system based intervention. Am J Psychiatry 2018; **175**:169–179.

2. Zhu Y et al. Antipsychotic drugs for the acute treatment of patients with a first episode of schizophrenia: a systematic review with pairwise and network meta-analyses. Lancet Psychiatry 2017; **4**:694–705.

3. Zhang JP et al. Efficacy and safety of individual second-generation vs. first-generation antipsychotics in first-episode psychosis: a systematic review and meta-analysis. Int J Neuropsychopharmacol 2013; **16**:1205–1218.

4. Leucht S et al. Early-onset hypothesis of antipsychotic drug action: a hypothesis tested, confirmed and extended. Biol Psychiatry 2005; **57**:1543–1549.

5. Agid O et al. The "delayed onset" of antipsychotic action – an idea whose time has come and gone. J Psychiatry Neurosci 2006; **31**:93–100.

6. Subotnik KL et al. Long-acting injectable risperidone for relapse prevention and control of breakthrough symptoms after a recent first episode of schizophrenia. A randomized clinical trial. JAMA Psychiatry 2015; **72**:822–829.

7. Schreiner A et al. Paliperidone palmitate versus oral antipsychotics in recently diagnosed schizophrenia. Schizophr Res 2015; **169**:393–399.

8. Alphs L et al. Treatment effect with paliperidone palmitate compared with oral antipsychotics in patients with recent-onset versus more chronic schizophrenia and a history of criminal justice system involvement. Early Interv Psychiatry 2018; **12**:55–65.

9. Agid O et al. An algorithm-based approach to first-episode schizophrenia: response rates over 3 prospective antipsychotic trials with a retrospective data analysis. J Clin Psychiatry 2011; **72**:1439–1444.

10. Davis JM et al. A meta-analysis of the efficacy of second-generation antipsychotics. Arch Gen Psychiatry 2003; **60**:553–564.

11. Leucht S et al. Second-generation versus first-generation antipsychotic drugs for schizophrenia: a meta-analysis. Lancet 2009; **373**:31–41.

12. Schooler N et al. Risperidone and haloperidol in first-episode psychosis: a long-term randomized trial. Am J Psychiatry 2005; **162**:947–953.

13. Oosthuizen PP et al. Incidence of tardive dyskinesia in first-episode psychosis patients treated with low-dose haloperidol. J Clin Psychiatry 2003; **64**:1075–1080.

14. Whiskey E et al. Evaluation of an antipsychotic information sheet for patients. Int J Psychiatry Clin Pract 2005; **9**:264–270.

15. Stroup TS et al. Results of phase 3 of the CATIE schizophrenia trial. Schizophr Res 2009; **107**:1–12.

16. Olofinjana B et al. Antipsychotic drugs – information and choice: a patient survey. Psychiatr Bull 2005; **29**:369–371.

17. Stroup TS et al. Effectiveness of olanzapine, quetiapine, risperidone, and ziprasidone in patients with chronic schizophrenia following discontinuation of a previous atypical antipsychotic. Am J Psychiatry 2006; **163**:611–622.

18. Haro JM et al. Remission and relapse in the outpatient care of schizophrenia: three-year results from the Schizophrenia Outpatient Health Outcomes study. J Clin Psychopharmacol 2006; **26**:571–578.

19. Novick D et al. Recovery in the outpatient setting: 36-month results from the Schizophrenia Outpatients Health Outcomes (SOHO) study. Schizophr Res 2009; **108**:223–230.

20. Tiihonen J et al. Effectiveness of antipsychotic treatments in a nationwide cohort of patients in community care after first hospitalisation due to schizophrenia and schizoaffective disorder: observational follow-up study. BMJ 2006; **333**:224.

21. Leucht S et al. A meta-analysis of head-to-head comparisons of second-generation antipsychotics in the treatment of schizophrenia. Am J Psychiatry 2009; **166**:152–163.

22. Remington G et al. The use of electronic monitoring (MEMS) to evaluate antipsychotic compliance in outpatients with schizophrenia. Schizophr Res 2007; **90**:229–237.

23. Stephenson JJ et al. Adherence to oral second-generation antipsychotic medications in patients with schizophrenia and bipolar disorder: physicians' perceptions of adherence vs. pharmacy claims. Int J Clin Pract 2012; **66**:565–573.

24. McCutcheon R et al. Antipsychotic plasma levels in the assessment of poor treatment response in schizophrenia. Acta Psychiatr Scand 2018; **137**:39–46.

25. McEvoy JP et al. Effectiveness of clozapine versus olanzapine, quetiapine, and risperidone in patients with chronic schizophrenia who did not respond to prior atypical antipsychotic treatment. Am J Psychiatry 2006; **163**:600–610.

26. Lewis SW et al. Randomized controlled trial of effect of prescription of clozapine versus other second-generation antipsychotic drugs in resistant schizophrenia. Schizophr Bull 2006; **32**:715–723.

First-generation antipsychotics – place in therapy

Nomenclature

First-generation ('typical') and second-generation ('atypical') antipsychotic medications are not categorically differentiated, the medications in both groups being heterogeneous in terms of pharmacological and adverse-effect profiles. First-generation medications tend to be associated with acute EPS, hyperprolactinaemia and, in the longer term, TD. There are expectations that such adverse effects are less likely with SGAs although in practice most show dose-related EPS, some induce hyperprolactinaemia (often to a greater extent than with FGAs) and all may eventually give rise to TD. Second-generation medications tend to be associated with metabolic and cardiac complications.[1-3] To complicate matters further, it has been suggested that the therapeutic and adverse effects of FGAs can be separated by careful dosing[4] – essentially turning them into SGAs if used in small doses (although there is much evidence to the contrary[5-7]).

Given these observations, it seems unwise and unhelpful to consider so-called 'FGAs' and 'SGAs' as distinct groups of drugs. Perhaps the essential difference between the two groups is the size of the therapeutic index in relation to acute EPS: for instance haloperidol has an extremely narrow index (probably less than 0.5 mg/day); olanzapine a wide index (20–40 mg/day).

The use of neuroscience-based nomenclature (NbN)[8,9] (for which there is a free app for iPhone and other devices) obviates the need for classification as FGA or SGA and describes an individual drug by its pharmacological activity. The wider use of NbN will undoubtedly improve understanding of individual drug effects and perhaps forestall future redundant categorisation.

Role of older antipsychotics

FGAs still play an important role in schizophrenia: for example, chlorpromazine and haloperidol are frequent choices for PRN medication, and depot preparations of fluphenazine, zuclopenthixol and flupentixol are commonly prescribed. FGAs can offer a valid alternative to SGAs where these are poorly tolerated (usually because of metabolic changes) or where FGAs are preferred by patients themselves. Some FGAs may be less effective than some non-clozapine SGAs (amisulpride, olanzapine and risperidone may be more efficacious[10,11]) but any differences in therapeutic efficacy seem to be modest. Two large pragmatic studies, CATIE[12] and CUtLASS,[13] found few important differences between SGAs and FGAs (mainly perphenazine and sulpiride, respectively).

The main drawbacks of FGAs are, inevitably, acute EPS, hyperprolactinaemia and TD. Hyperprolactinaemia is probably unavoidable in practice (the dose that achieves efficacy is too close to the dose that causes hyperprolactinaemia) and, even when not symptomatic, may grossly affect hypothalamic function.[14] It is also associated with sexual dysfunction,[15] but be aware that the autonomic effects of some SGAs may also cause sexual dysfunction.[16] Also, some SGAs (risperidone, paliperidone, amisulpride) increase prolactin to a greater extent than FGAs.[17]

Some FGAs, like haloperidol, are potent dopamine antagonists and are liable to induce dysphoria.[18] Perhaps as a consequence, some FGAs may produce smaller benefits in quality of life than some SGAs.[19]

TD probably occurs more frequently with FGAs than with SGAs[20–23] (notwithstanding difficulties in defining what is 'atypical'), although there remains some uncertainty[23–25] and the dose of FGA used is a crucial factor. Careful observation of patients and the prescribing of the lowest effective dose are essential to help reduce the risk of this serious adverse event.[26,27] Even with these precautions, the risk of TD with some FGAs may be unacceptably high.[28]

A good example of the relative merits of SGAs and a carefully dosed FGA comes from a trial comparing paliperidone palmitate with low-dose haloperidol decanoate.[29] Paliperidone produced more weight gain and prolactin change but haloperidol was associated with significantly more akathisia and parkinsonism, and numerically more TD. Efficacy was identical.

References

1. Musil R et al. Weight gain and antipsychotics: a drug safety review. Expert Opin Drug Saf 2015; 14:73–96.

2. Vancampfort D et al. Risk of metabolic syndrome and its components in people with schizophrenia and related psychotic disorders, bipolar disorder and major depressive disorder: a systematic review and meta-analysis. World Psychiatry 2015; 14:339–347.

3. Khasawneh FT et al. Minimizing cardiovascular adverse effects of atypical antipsychotic drugs in patients with schizophrenia. Cardiol Res Pract 2014; 2014:273060.

4. Oosthuizen P et al. Determining the optimal dose of haloperidol in first-episode psychosis. J Psychopharm 2001; 15:251–255.

5. Zimbroff DL et al. Controlled, dose-response study of sertindole and haloperidol in the treatment of schizophrenia. Sertindole Study Group. Am J Psychiatry 1997; 154:782–791.

6. Jeste DV et al. Incidence of tardive dyskinesia in early stages of low-dose treatment with typical neuroleptics in older patients. Am J Psychiatry 1999; 156:309–311.

7. Meltzer HY et al. The effect of neuroleptics on serum prolactin in schizophrenic patients. Arch Gen Psychiatry 1976; 33:279–286.

8. Blier P et al. Progress on the neuroscience-based nomenclature (NbN) for psychotropic medications. Neuropsychopharmacology 2017; 42:1927–1928.

9. Caraci F et al. A new nomenclature for classifying psychotropic drugs. Br J Clin Pharmacol 2017; 83:1614–1616.

10. Davis JM et al. A meta-analysis of the efficacy of second-generation antipsychotics. Arch Gen Psychiatry 2003; 60:553–564.

11. Leucht S et al. Second-generation versus first-generation antipsychotic drugs for schizophrenia: a meta-analysis. Lancet 2009; 373:31–41.

12. Lieberman JA et al. Effectiveness of antipsychotic drugs in patients with chronic schizophrenia. N Engl J Med 2005; 353:1209–1223.

13. Jones PB et al. Randomized controlled trial of the effect on Quality of Life of second- vs first-generation antipsychotic drugs in schizophrenia: Cost Utility of the Latest Antipsychotic Drugs in Schizophrenia Study (CUtLASS 1). Arch Gen Psychiatry 2006; 63:1079–1087.

14. Smith S et al. The effects of antipsychotic-induced hyperprolactinaemia on the hypothalamic-pituitary-gonadal axis. J Clin Psychopharmacol 2002; 22:109–114.

15. Smith SM et al. Sexual dysfunction in patients taking conventional antipsychotic medication. Br J Psychiatry 2002; 181:49–55.

16. Aizenberg D et al. Comparison of sexual dysfunction in male schizophrenic patients maintained on treatment with classical antipsychotics versus clozapine. J Clin Psychiatry 2001; 62:541–544.

17. Leucht S et al. Comparative efficacy and tolerability of 15 antipsychotic drugs in schizophrenia: a multiple-treatments meta-analysis. Lancet 2013; 382:951–962.

18. King DJ et al. Antipsychotic drug-induced dysphoria. Br J Psychiatry 1995; 167:480–482.

19. Grunder G et al. Effects of first-generation antipsychotics versus second-generation antipsychotics on quality of life in schizophrenia: a double-blind, randomised study. Lancet Psychiatry 2016; 3:717–729.

20. Tollefson GD et al. Blind, controlled, long-term study of the comparative incidence of treatment-emergent tardive dyskinesia with olanzapine or haloperidol. Am J Psychiatry 1997; 154:1248–1254.

21. Beasley C et al. Randomised double-blind comparison of the incidence of tardive dyskinesia in patients with schizophrenia during long-term treatment with olanzapine or haloperidol. Br J Psychiatry 1999; 174:23–30.

22. Correll CU et al. Lower risk for tardive dyskinesia associated with second-generation antipsychotics: a systematic review of 1-year studies. Am J Psychiatry 2004; 161:414–425.

23. Novick D et al. Tolerability of outpatient antipsychotic treatment: 36-month results from the European Schizophrenia Outpatient Health Outcomes (SOHO) study. Eur Neuropsychopharmacol 2009; 19:542–550.

24. Halliday J et al. Nithsdale Schizophrenia Surveys 23: movement disorders. 20-year review. Br J Psychiatry 2002; 181:422–427.

25. Miller DD et al. Extrapyramidal side-effects of antipsychotics in a randomised trial. Br J Psychiatry 2008; 193:279–288.

26. Jeste DV et al. Tardive dyskinesia. Schizophr Bull 1993; 19:303–315.

27. Cavallaro R et al. Recognition, avoidance, and management of antipsychotic-induced tardive dyskinesia. CNS Drugs 1995; 4:278–293.

28. Oosthuizen P et al. A randomized, controlled comparison of the efficacy and tolerability of low and high doses of haloperidol in the treatment of first-episode psychosis. Int J Neuropsychopharmacol 2004; 7:125–131.

29. McEvoy JP et al. Effectiveness of paliperidone palmitate vs haloperidol decanoate for maintenance treatment of schizophrenia: a randomized clinical trial. JAMA 2014; 311:1978–1987.

NICE guidelines for the treatment of schizophrenia[1]

The 2009 NICE guidelines[1] differed importantly from previous guidelines. There was no longer an imperative to prescribe an 'atypical' as first-line treatment and it was recommended only that clozapine be 'offered' (rather than prescribed) after the prior failure of two antipsychotics. These differences pointed respectively towards disillusionment with SGAs and recognition of the delay in prescribing clozapine in practice. Much emphasis was placed on involving patients and their carers in prescribing decisions. There is some evidence that this is rarely done[2] but that it can be done.[3] New NICE guidelines appeared in February 2014 and were reviewed in November 2017. Few changes were made to recommendations regarding drug treatment but psychological treatments are now more strongly promoted (perhaps reflecting the make-up of the NICE review panel).

NICE guidelines – a summary

- For people with newly diagnosed schizophrenia, offer oral antipsychotic medication. Provide information and discuss the benefits and adverse-effect profile of each drug with the service user. The choice of drug should be made by the service user and health-care professional together, considering:
    - the relative potential of individual antipsychotic drugs to cause EPS (including akathisia), cardiovascular adverse effects, metabolic adverse effects (including weight gain), hormonal adverse effects and other adverse effects (including unpleasant subjective experiences)
    - the views of the carer where the service user agrees.
- Before starting antipsychotic medication, undertake and record the following baseline investigations:
    - weight
    - waist circumference
    - pulse and blood pressure
    - fasting blood glucose, HbA_{1c}, blood lipid profile, prolactin
    - assessment of movement disorders
    - assessment of nutritional status, diet and level of physical activity.
- Before starting antipsychotic medication, offer the person with schizophrenia an electrocardiogram (ECG) if:
    - specified in the summary of product characteristics (SPC)
    - a physical examination has identified specific cardiovascular risk (such as diagnosis of high blood pressure)
    - there is personal history of cardiovascular disease, or
    - the service user is being admitted as an in-patient.
- Treatment with antipsychotic medication should be considered an explicit individual therapeutic trial. Include the following:
    - Record the indications and expected benefits and risks of oral antipsychotic medication, and the expected time for a change in symptoms and appearance of adverse effects.

- At the start of treatment give a dose at the lower end of the licensed range and slowly titrate upwards within the dose range given in the British National Formulary (BNF) or SPC.
- Justify and record reasons for dosages outside the range given in the BNF or SPC.
- Record the rationale for continuing, changing or stopping medication and the effects of such changes.
- Carry out a trial of medication at optimum dosage for 4–6 weeks (although half of this period is probably sufficient if no effect at all is seen).
- Monitor and record the following regularly and systematically throughout treatment, but especially during titration:
  - efficacy, including changes in symptoms and behaviour
  - adverse effects of treatment, taking into account overlap between certain adverse effects and clinical features of schizophrenia, for example the overlap between akathisia and agitation or anxiety
  - adherence
  - weight, weekly for the first 6 weeks, then at 12 weeks, 1 year and annually
  - waist circumference annually
  - pulse and blood pressure at 12 weeks, 1 year and annually
  - fasting blood glucose, HbA_{1c} and blood lipids at 12 weeks, 1 year and annually
  - nutritional status, diet and physical activity.
- Physical monitoring is to be the responsibility of the secondary care team for 1 year or until the patient is stable.
- Do not use a loading dose of antipsychotic medication (often referred to as 'rapid neuroleptisation'). (Note that this does not apply to loading doses of depot forms of olanzapine and paliperidone.)
- Do not routinely initiate regular combined antipsychotic medication, except for short periods (for example, when changing medication).
- If prescribing chlorpromazine, warn of its potential to cause skin photosensitivity. Advise using sunscreen if necessary.
- Consider offering depot/LAI antipsychotic medication to people with schizophrenia:
  - who would prefer such treatment after an acute episode
  - where avoiding covert non-adherence (either intentional or unintentional) to antipsychotic medication is a clinical priority within the treatment plan.
- Offer clozapine to people with schizophrenia whose illness has not responded adequately to treatment despite the sequential use of adequate doses of at least two different antipsychotic drugs alongside psychological therapies. At least one of the drugs should be a non-clozapine SGA. (See Figure 1.1 – we recommend that one of the drugs should be olanzapine).
- For people with schizophrenia whose illness has not responded adequately to clozapine at an optimised dose, health-care professionals should establish prior compliance with optimised antipsychotic treatment (including measuring drug levels) and engagement with psychological treatment before adding a second antipsychotic to augment treatment with clozapine. An adequate trial of such an augmentation may need to be up to 8–10 weeks (some data suggest 6 weeks may be enough[4]). Choose a drug that does not compound the common adverse effects of clozapine.

References

1. National Institute for Health and Care Excellence. Psychosis and schizophrenia in adults: prevention and management. Clinical Guideline 178, 2014. https://www.nice.org.uk/guidance/cg178
2. Olofinjana B et al. Antipsychotic drugs – information and choice: a patient survey. Psychiatr Bull 2005; 29:369–371.
3. Whiskey E et al. Evaluation of an antipsychotic information sheet for patients. Int J Psychiatry Clin Pract 2005; 9:264–270.
4. Taylor D et al. Augmentation of clozapine with a second antipsychotic. A meta analysis. Acta Psychiatr Scand 2012; 125:15–24.

Antipsychotic response – to increase the dose, to switch, to add or just wait – what is the right move?

For any clinician taking active care of patients with schizophrenia, the single most common clinical dilemma is what to do when the current antipsychotic medication is not optimal for the patient. This may be for two broad reasons: first, while the symptoms are well controlled, the adverse effects are problematic and, second, there is an inadequate therapeutic response. Fortunately, with regard to the first reason, the diversity of the available antipsychotic medications means that it is usually possible to find one that has an adverse-effect profile that is appropriate and acceptable to the patient. What to do next is a more difficult question with regard to the second reason – an insufficient symptom response. If the patient has already had adequate trials, in terms of dosage, duration and adherence, of two antipsychotic medications then clozapine should clearly be considered. However, the majority of the patients in the clinic are those who are either not yet ready for clozapine or unwilling to choose that option. In those instances, the clinician has four main choices: to increase the dose of the current medication; to switch to another antipsychotic; to add an adjunct medication; or just to wait.

When to increase the dose?

While optimal doses of FGAs were always a matter of debate, the recommended doses of the SGAs were generally based on careful and extensive clinical trials, but even then the consensus on optimal doses has changed with time. For example, when risperidone was first launched it was suggested that optimal titration was from 2 mg to 4 mg to 6 mg or more for all patients; however, the field has tended towards lower doses.[1] On the other hand, when quetiapine was introduced, 300 mg was considered the optimal dose and the overall consensus now is towards higher doses,[2] although RCT and other evidence does not support this shift.[2,3] Nonetheless, most clinicians feel comfortable in navigating within the recommended clinical dose range. The more critical question is what should be done if one has hit the upper limit of these dose ranges and the patient is tolerating the medication well but with limited benefit.

Dose–response observations

Davis and Chen performed a systematic meta-analysis of relevant dose–response data available up to 2004 and concluded that the average dose that produces maximal benefit was 4 mg for risperidone, 16 mg of olanzapine, 120 mg of ziprasidone and 10–15 mg of aripiprazole (they could not determine such a dose for quetiapine using their method).[4] More recent trials have tried to compare 'high-dose' with standard dosage. For example, one group[5] studied the dose–response relationship of standard and higher doses of olanzapine in a randomised, double-blind, 8-week, fixed-dose study comparing olanzapine 10 mg, 20 mg and 40 mg and found no additional benefit with the higher doses (i.e. 40 mg was no better than 10 mg) but clear evidence for an increasing adverse-effect burden (weight gain and prolactin) with dose. Similarly, the initial licensing studies of risperidone compared the usual doses of 2–6 mg with higher doses of 8–16 mg/day. While they found no additional benefit with the higher doses, there was a clear signal for a greater risk of adverse effects (EPS and increased prolactin). The findings of these studies are in accord with older studies involving fixed doses of haloperidol.[6] However, it is important to keep in mind that these doses are extracted from group evidence where patients are assigned to different doses, which is a different situation from the clinical one where the prescriber considers increasing the dose only in those patients whose illnesses have failed to respond to the initial dosage regimen. The potential benefits and risks of such a strategy remain uncertain and warrant further investigation.[7] Kinon et al.[8] examined patients who failed to respond to the (then) standard dose of fluphenazine (20 mg) and tested three strategies: increasing the dose to 80 mg, switching to haloperidol or watchful waiting (on the original dose). All three strategies proved to be equivalent in terms of efficacy. These findings provide little supportive evidence at a group level (as opposed to an individual level) for treatment beyond the recommended dose range. Such RCT evidence is corroborated by the clinical practice norms – Hermes and colleagues examined the CATIE data to identify clinical factors that predicted a prescriber's decision to increase the dose and found that decisions for dose change (within the therapeutic ranges) were only weakly associated with clinical measures.[9] More recently a trial of lurasidone[10] showed that patients failing to respond at 2 weeks did somewhat better if their dose was doubled than if the dose was kept the same. It is not clear if these results are generalisable to other antipsychotics.

Plasma level variations

Group level evidence cannot completely determine individual decisions. There are significant inter-individual variations in plasma drug levels in patients treated with antipsychotic medication. One can often encounter a patient who, when receiving medication at the higher end of the dose range (say 6 mg of risperidone or 20 mg of olanzapine), would have plasma drug levels that are well below the range expected for 2 mg risperidone or 10 mg of olanzapine, respectively. In such patients, a rational case could be made for increasing the dose, provided the patient is informed and the adverse effects are tolerable, to bring the plasma levels to the median optimal range for the particular medication. (More details on plasma levels and their interpretation are provided in Chapter 11.) However, one often encounters an unresponsive patient, adherent to their medication, whose dose has reached the ceiling and plasma levels are also sufficient – what next?

Treatment choices

There are essentially three options here: clozapine, switch to another drug or add another (non-clozapine) drug. If the patient meets the criteria for clozapine it is undoubtedly the preferred option. Yet, in a clinical audit of community (not in-patient) practice in the UK, covering some 5000 patients in 60 different NHS Trusts, it was found that nearly 40% of the patients who met criteria for treatment resistance did not receive clozapine; of those who did, the vast majority (85%) received their clozapine after a much longer wait after the failure of two serial trials of antipsychotic medication than is advised in most guidelines.[11]

Nonetheless, there is a group of patients who do not like the idea of regular blood testing, the adverse-effect profile and the regular appointments required to receive clozapine. In such patients, the choice is to switch to another medication or to add another antipsychotic. The data on switching are sparse. While almost every clinical trial in patients with established schizophrenia has entailed the patient switching from one antipsychotic medication to another, there are no rigorous studies of preferred switch combinations (e.g. if risperidone fails – what next: olanzapine, quetiapine, aripiprazole or ziprasidone?). If one looks at only the switching trials that have been sponsored by the drug companies it leads to a rather confusing picture, with the trial results being very closely linked to the sponsor's interest (see Heres et al. 'Why olanzapine beats risperidone, risperidone beats quetiapine, and quetiapine beats olanzapine: an exploratory analysis of head-to-head comparison studies of second-generation antipsychotics'[12]).

CATIE, the major US-based publicly-funded comparative trial, examined patients who had failed their first SGA and were then randomly assigned to a different second one.[13] Patients switched to olanzapine and risperidone did better than those switched to quetiapine and ziprasidone. This greater effectiveness is supported by a meta-analysis that compared a number of SGAs with FGAs and concluded that, other than clozapine, only amisulpride, risperidone and olanzapine were superior to FGAs in efficacy,[14] and a meta-analysis comparing SGAs amongst themselves which suggests that olanzapine and risperidone (in that order) may be more effective than the others,[15] although these differences in efficacy between medications may be judged as modest. Nevertheless, if a patient has not tried olanzapine or risperidone as yet, it would be a reasonable decision to switch to these drugs provided the adverse-effect balance is favourable. Comparing these two drugs the data are somewhat limited. However, a number of controlled but open-label studies do show an asymmetrical advantage (i.e. switching to olanzapine being more effective than risperidone), providing some direction, albeit incomplete.[16,17]

The best medication regimen (aside from clozapine) to choose for a patient who fails on olanzapine and risperidone remains unclear. Should one switch (to, say, aripiprazole or ziprasidone or even an older FGA) or should one add another antipsychotic medication? It should be borne in mind that after 'switching', adding another antipsychotic is probably the second most common clinical move as around 40% of patients in routine care are on more than one antipsychotic.[18] Often a second antipsychotic is added to get an additional profile (e.g. sedation with quetiapine, or decrease in prolactin with the addition of aripiprazole) – these matters are discussed elsewhere. Here we are concerned solely with the addition of an antipsychotic to another antipsychotic to increase efficacy. From a theoretical point of view, because all antipsychotics block D_2 receptors (unlike, say, antihypertensives which use different mechanisms), there is limited rationale for addition. Studies of add-ons have often chosen combinations of convenience or those based on clinical lore. Perhaps the most systematic evidence is available for the addition of a second antipsychotic to clozapine,[19] possibly supported by the rationale that because clozapine has low D_2 occupancy, increasing its D_2 occupancy may yield additional benefits.[20] However, a meta-analysis of RCTs comparing augmentation with a second antipsychotic with continuing antipsychotic monotherapy in schizophrenia[21] found a lack of double-blind/high-quality evidence for efficacy for the combination in terms of treatment response and symptom improvement. Further, compared with antipsychotic monotherapy, combined antipsychotics seem to be associated with an increased adverse-effect burden and a greater risk of high-dose prescribing.[22,23]

Although augmentation with another antipsychotic as a treatment strategy should probably be avoided, under some conditions of acute exacerbation or agitation the prescriber may see this as the only practicable solution. Or quite often the prescriber may inherit the care of a patient on antipsychotic polypharmacy. Most RCT evidence suggests that such a regimen can be safely switched back to antipsychotic monotherapy without symptom exacerbation, at least in the majority of patients,[24-26] although this is not a universal finding.[27] Essock et al.[26] conducted a relatively large trial involving 127 patients with schizophrenia who were stable on antipsychotic polypharmacy. Over a 12-month period, a switch to monotherapy was successful in about two-thirds of the patients in whom it was tested. In those cases where the move to monotherapy resulted in a return of symptoms, the most common recourse was a return to the original polypharmacy; this was achieved without any significant worsening in this group. The advantages for the monotherapy group were exposure to less medication, equivalent symptom severity and some loss of weight.

So, when should the prescriber just continue with the current regimen? The evidence reviewed above suggests that no one strategy, such as increasing the dose or switching or augmenting, is the clear winner in all situations. Increase the dose if plasma drug levels are low; switch if the patient has not tried olanzapine or risperidone; and if treatment with clozapine is failing, augmentation may help. Given the limited efficacy of these manoeuvres, perhaps an equally important call by the treating doctor is to just stay with the current pharmacotherapy and focus on non-pharmacological means: engagement in case management, targeted psychological treatments and vocational rehabilitation as means of enhancing patient well-being. While it may seem a passive option, staying may often do less harm than aimless switching.

Summary – when treatment fails

- If the dose has been optimised, consider watchful waiting.
- Consider increasing the antipsychotic dose according to tolerability and plasma levels (little supporting evidence).
- If this fails, consider switching to olanzapine or risperidone (if not already used).
- If this fails, use clozapine (supporting evidence very strong).
- If clozapine fails, use time-limited augmentation strategies (supporting evidence variable).

References

1. Ezewuzie N et al. Establishing a dose-response relationship for oral risperidone in relapsed schizophrenia. J Psychopharmacol 2006; 20:86–90.
2. Sparshatt A et al. Quetiapine: dose-response relationship in schizophrenia. CNS Drugs 2008; 22:49–68.
3. Honer WG et al. A randomized, double-blind, placebo-controlled study of the safety and tolerability of high-dose quetiapine in patients with persistent symptoms of schizophrenia or schizoaffective disorder. J Clin Psychiatry 2012; 73:13–20.
4. Davis JM et al. Dose response and dose equivalence of antipsychotics. J Clin Psychopharmacol 2004; 24:192–208.
5. Kinon BJ et al. Standard and higher dose of olanzapine in patients with schizophrenia or schizoaffective disorder: a randomized, double-blind, fixed-dose study. J Clin Psychopharmacol 2008; 28:392–400.
6. Van PT et al. A controlled dose comparison of haloperidol in newly admitted schizophrenic patients. Arch Gen Psychiatry 1990; 47:754–758.

7. Helfer B et al. Increasing antipsychotic dose for non response in schizophrenia (Protocol). Cochrane Database Syst Rev 2015; 10:CD011883.

8. Kinon BJ et al. Treatment of neuroleptic-resistant schizophrenic relapse. Psychopharmacol Bull 1993; 29:309–314

9. Hermes E et al. Predictors of antipsychotic dose changes in the CATIE schizophrenia trial. Psychiatry Res 2012; 199:1–7

10. Loebel A et al. Treatment of early non-response in patients with schizophrenia: assessing the efficacy of antipsychotic dose escalation. BMC Psychiatry 2015; 15:271.

11. Patel MX et al. Quality of prescribing for schizophrenia: evidence from a national audit in England and Wales. Eur Neuropsychopharmacol 2014; 24:499–509.

12. Heres S et al. Why olanzapine beats risperidone, risperidone beats quetiapine, and quetiapine beats olanzapine: an exploratory analysis of head-to-head comparison studies of second-generation antipsychotics. Am J Psychiatry 2006; 163:185–194.

13. Stroup TS et al. Effectiveness of olanzapine, quetiapine, risperidone, and ziprasidone in patients with chronic schizophrenia following discontinuation of a previous atypical antipsychotic. Am J Psychiatry 2006; 163:611–622.

14. Leucht S et al. Second-generation versus first-generation antipsychotic drugs for schizophrenia: a meta-analysis. Lancet 2009; 373:31–41.

15. Leucht S et al. A meta-analysis of head-to-head comparisons of second-generation antipsychotics in the treatment of schizophrenia. Am J Psychiatry 2009; 166:152–163.

16. Hong J et al. Clinical consequences of switching from olanzapine to risperidone and vice versa in outpatients with schizophrenia: 36-month results from the Worldwide Schizophrenia Outpatients Health Outcomes (W-SOHO) study. BMC Psychiatry 2012; 12:218.

17. Agid O et al. Antipsychotic response in first-episode schizophrenia: efficacy of high doses and switching. Eur Neuropsychopharmacol 2013; 23:1017–1022.

18. Paton C et al. High-dose and combination antipsychotic prescribing in acute adult wards in the UK: the challenges posed by p.r.n. prescribing. Br J Psychiatry 2008; 192:435–439.

19. Taylor DM et al. Augmentation of clozapine with a second antipsychotic – a meta-analysis of randomized, placebo-controlled studies. Acta Psychiatr Scand 2009; 119:419–425.

20. Kapur S et al. Increased dopamine D2 receptor occupancy and elevated prolactin level associated with addition of haloperidol to clozapine. Am J Psychiatry 2001; 158:311–314.

21. Galling B et al. Antipsychotic augmentation vs. monotherapy in schizophrenia: systematic review, meta-analysis and meta-regression analysis. World Psychiatry 2017; 16:77–89.

22. Gallego JA et al. Safety and tolerability of antipsychotic polypharmacy. Expert Opin Drug Saf 2012; 11:527–542.

23. Barnes TR et al. Antipsychotic polypharmacy in schizophrenia: benefits and risks. CNS Drugs 2011; 25:383–399.

24. Borlido C et al. Switching from 2 antipsychotics to 1 antipsychotic in schizophrenia: a randomized, double-blind, placebo-controlled study. J Clin Psychiatry 2016; 77:e14–20.

25. Hori H et al. Switching to antipsychotic monotherapy can improve attention and processing speed, and social activity in chronic schizophrenia patients. J Psychiatr Res 2013; 47:1843–1848.

26. Essock SM et al. Effectiveness of switching from antipsychotic polypharmacy to monotherapy. Am J Psychiatry 2011; 168:702–708.

27. Constantine RJ et al. The risks and benefits of switching patients with schizophrenia or schizoaffective disorder from two to one antipsychotic medication: a randomized controlled trial. Schizophr Res 2015; 166:194–200.

Acutely disturbed or violent behaviour

Acute behavioural disturbance can occur in the context of psychiatric illness, physical illness, substance abuse or personality disorder. Psychotic symptoms are common and the patient may be aggressive towards others secondary to persecutory delusions or auditory, visual or tactile hallucinations.

The clinical practice of rapid tranquillisation (RT) is used when appropriate psychological and behavioural approaches have failed to de-escalate acutely disturbed behaviour. It is, essentially, a treatment of last resort. Patients who require RT are often too disturbed to give informed consent and therefore participate in randomised controlled trials (RCTs), but with the use of a number of creative methodologies, the evidence base with respect to the efficacy and tolerability of pharmacological strategies has grown substantially in recent years. However, recommendations remain based partly on research data, partly on theoretical considerations and partly on clinical experience.

Several studies supporting the efficacy of oral SGAs have been published.[1-4] The level of behavioural disturbance exhibited by the patients in these studies was moderate at best, and all subjects accepted oral treatment (this degree of compliance would be unusual in clinical practice). Note too that patients recruited to these studies received the SGA as antipsychotic monotherapy. The efficacy and safety of adding a second antipsychotic as 'PRN' has not been explicitly tested in formal RCTs.

A single-dose RCT showed sublingual asenapine to be more effective than placebo for acute agitation.[5] The efficacy of inhaled loxapine (in behavioural disturbance that is moderate in severity) is also supported by RCTs[6-8] and case series.[9,10] Note that use of this preparation requires the co-operation of the patient, and that bronchospasm is an established but rare adverse effect.

Large, placebo-controlled RCTs support the efficacy of intramuscular (IM) preparations of olanzapine, ziprasidone and aripiprazole. When considered together, these trials suggested that IM olanzapine is more effective than IM haloperidol, which in turn is more effective than IM aripiprazole.[11] Again, the level of behavioural disturbance in these studies was moderate at most.

A large observational study supported the efficacy and tolerability of IM olanzapine in clinical emergencies (where disturbance was severe).[12] A study comparing IM haloperidol with a combination of IM midazolam and IM haloperidol found the combination more effective than haloperidol alone for controlling agitation in palliative care patients.[13]

Several RCTs have now investigated the effectiveness of parenteral medication in 'real-life' acutely disturbed patients. Overall:

- Compared with intravenous (IV) midazolam alone, a combination of IV olanzapine or IV droperidol with IV midazolam was more rapidly effective and resulted in fewer subsequent doses of medication being required.[14]
- IM midazolam 7.5–15 mg was more rapidly sedating than a combination of haloperidol 5–10 mg and promethazine 50 mg (TREC 1).[15]
- Olanzapine 10 mg was as effective as a combination of haloperidol 10 mg and promethazine 25–50 mg in the short term, but the effect did not last as long (TREC 4).[16]
- A combination of haloperidol 5–10 mg and promethazine 50 mg was more effective and better tolerated than haloperidol 5–10 mg alone (TREC 3).[17]

- A combination of haloperidol 10 mg and promethazine 25–50 mg was more effective than lorazepam 4 mg (TREC 2).[18]
- A combination of IV midazolam and IV droperidol was more rapidly sedating than either IV droperidol or IV olanzapine alone. Fewer patients in the midazolam–droperidol group required additional medication doses to achieve sedation.[19]
- IM olanzapine was more effective than IM aripiprazole in the treatment of agitation in schizophrenia in the short term (at 2 hours) but there was no significant difference between treatments at 24 hours.[20]
- In an open-label study the combination of IM haloperidol and IM lorazepam was found to be similar in efficacy to IM olanzapine.[21]
- IM droperidol and IM haloperidol were equally effective.[22]

Note that TREC 3[17] found IM haloperidol alone to be poorly tolerated; 6% of patients had an acute dystonic reaction. A Cochrane review concluded that haloperidol alone is effective in the management of acute behavioural disturbance but poorly tolerated, and that co-administration of promethazine but not lorazepam improves tolerability.[23,24] However, NICE considers the evidence relating to the use of promethazine for this purpose to be inconclusive.[25] When assessing haloperidol plus promethazine, Cochrane concluded that the combination is effective for use in patients who are aggressive due to psychosis and its use is based on good evidence. The resumption of aggression and need for further injections was more likely with olanzapine than with the haloperidol–promethazine combination. The authors also state that 'haloperidol used on its own without something to offset its frequent and serious adverse effects does seem difficult to justify'.[26] Cochrane recently concluded that available data for aripiprazole are rather poor. Available evidence suggests that aripiprazole is more effective than placebo and haloperidol, but not olanzapine. However, the authors advise caution when generalising these results to real-world practice.[27] A systematic review and meta-analysis of IM olanzapine for agitation found IM olanzapine and IM haloperidol to be equally effective, but IM olanzapine was associated with a lower incidence of EPS.[28] Cochrane suggests that droperidol is effective and may be used to control people with very disturbed and aggressive behaviours caused by psychosis.[29] Having become available again, droperidol is seeing a resurgence in use in some countries (its initial withdrawal was voluntary, so reintroduction is not prohibited).

In a meta-analysis that examined the tolerability of IM antipsychotics when used for the treatment of agitation, the incidence of acute dystonia with haloperidol was reported to be 5%, with SGAs faring considerably better.[30] Acute EPS may adversely affect longer-term compliance.[31] In addition, the SPC for haloperidol requires a pre-treatment ECG[32,33] and recommends that concomitant antipsychotics are not prescribed. The mean increase in QTc after 10 mg IM haloperidol has been administered has been reported to be 15 ms but the range is wide.[34] Note that promethazine may inhibit the metabolism of haloperidol,[35] a pharmacokinetic interaction that is potentially clinically significant given the potential of haloperidol to prolong QTc. While this is unlikely to be problematic if a single dose is administered, repeat dosing may confer risk.

Droperidol is also associated with QT changes (the reason for its withdrawal). In an observational study set in hospital emergency departments, of the 1009 patients administered parenteral droperidol only 13 patients (1.28%) had an abnormal QT recorded after dose administration. However, in seven of these cases another contributory factor was identified. There were no cases of torsades de pointes.[22]

Intravenous treatment is now rarely used in RT but where benefits are thought to outweigh risks it may be considered as a last resort. A small study comparing high-dose IV haloperidol with IV diazepam found both drugs to be effective at 24 hours.[36] Two large observational studies have examined the safety of IV olanzapine when used in the emergency department. The indications for its use varied, agitation being the most common. In one study,[37] in the group treated for agitation (n = 265), over a third of patients required an additional sedative dose after the initial IV olanzapine dose. Hypoxia was reported in 17.7% of cases and supplemental oxygen was used in 20.4% of cases. Six patients required intubation: in two this was likely to have been due to olanzapine treatment. In the other study,[38] IV olanzapine (n = 295) was compared with IM olanzapine (n = 489). Additional doses were not required for 81% of patients in the IV group and 84% of patients in the IM group. Respiratory depression was more commonly observed in the group receiving IV olanzapine. Five patients in the IM group and two in the IV group required intubation.

In an acute psychiatric setting, high-dose sedation (defined as a dose of more than 10 mg of haloperidol, droperidol or midazolam) was not more effective than lower doses but was associated with more adverse effects (hypotension and oxygen desaturation).[39] Consistent with this, a small RCT supports the efficacy of low-dose haloperidol, although both efficacy and tolerability were superior when midazolam was co-prescribed.[40] These data support the use of standard doses in clinical emergencies.

A small observational study supports the effectiveness of buccal midazolam in a psychiatric intensive care unit (PICU) setting.[41] Parenteral administration of midazolam, particularly in higher doses, may cause over-sedation accompanied by respiratory depression.[42] Lorazepam IM is an established treatment and TREC 2[18] supports its efficacy, although combining all results from the TREC studies suggests midazolam 7.5–15 mg is probably more effective. A Cochrane review of benzodiazepines for psychosis-induced aggression and agitation concluded that most trials were too small to highlight differences in either positive or negative effects and that although adding a benzodiazepine to another drug may not be clearly advantageous it may lead to unnecessary adverse effects.[43]

With respect to those who are behaviourally disturbed secondary to acute intoxication with alcohol or illicit drugs, there are fewer data to guide practice. A large observational study of IV sedation in patients intoxicated with alcohol found that combination treatment (most commonly haloperidol 5 mg and lorazepam 2 mg) was more effective and reduced the need for subsequent sedation than either drug given alone.[44] A case series (n = 59) of patients who received modest doses of oral, IM or IV haloperidol to manage behavioural disturbance in the context of phencyclidine (PCP) consumption reported that haloperidol was effective and well tolerated (one case each of mild hypotension and mild hypoxia).[45]

Data are emerging from hospital emergency departments on the use of ketamine for agitation. IM ketamine was shown to be effective, with minimal adverse effects, in a small group of patients who failed to respond to IM droperidol.[46] A small retrospective study found ketamine to be associated with few major adverse effects. However, many patients in the study (62%) required additional sedation.[47] An observational study comparing ketamine (IM or IV) first line with midazolam, lorazepam, haloperidol or a combination of haloperidol and benzodiazepine found that significantly more patients in the ketamine group were no longer agitated at 5, 10 and 15 minutes. Two patients receiving ketamine were intubated compared with one patient in the other group.[48] In a prospective study comparing IM ketamine with IM haloperidol, mean time to adequate sedation was significantly shorter with IM ketamine. Complications, including intubation, vomiting, hypersalivation and laryngospasm, were higher in the ketamine group.[49]

Practical measures

Plans for the management of individual patients should ideally be made in advance. The aim is to prevent disturbed behaviour and reduce risk of violence. Nursing interventions (de-escalation, time out, seclusion[50]), increased nursing levels, transfer of the patient to a PICU and pharmacological management are options that may be employed. Care should be taken to avoid combinations and high cumulative doses of antipsychotic drugs. The monitoring of routine physical observations after RT is essential. Note that RT is often viewed as punitive by patients. There is little research into the patient experience of RT.

The aims of RT are three-fold:

- to reduce suffering for the patient – psychological or physical (through self-harm or accidents)
- to reduce risk of harm to others by maintaining a safe environment
- to do no harm (by prescribing safe regimes and monitoring physical health).

Note: Despite the need for rapid and effective treatment, concomitant use of two or more antipsychotics (antipsychotic polypharmacy) should be avoided on the basis of risk associated with QT prolongation (common to almost all antipsychotics). This is a particularly important consideration in RT where the patient's physical state predisposes to cardiac arrhythmia.

Zuclopenthixol acetate

Zuclopenthixol acetate (ZA) is widely used in the UK and elsewhere and is best known by its trade name Acuphase. Zuclopenthixol itself is a thioxanthine dopamine antagonist and was first introduced in the early 1960s. Its elimination half-life is around 20 hours. IM injection of zuclopenthixol base results in rapid absorption and a duration of action of 12–24 hours. By slowing absorption after IM injection, the biological half-life (and so duration of action) becomes dependent on the rate of release from the IM reservoir. This can be achieved by esterification of the zuclopenthixol molecule, the rate of release being broadly in proportion to the length of the ester carbon chain. Thus, zuclopenthixol decanoate is slow to act but very long-acting as a result of retarded release after IM injection. ZA (with eight fewer carbon atoms) would be expected to provide relatively prompt release but with an intermediate duration of action. The intention of the manufacturers was that the use of ZA would obviate the need for repeated IM injections in disturbed patients.

An initial pharmacokinetic study of ZA included 19 patients 'in whom calming effect by parenteral neuroleptic was considered necessary'.[51] Zuclopenthixol was detectable in the plasma after 1–2 hours but did not reach peak concentrations until around 36 hours after dosing. At 72 hours, plasma levels were around a third of those at 36 hours. The clinical effect of ZA was not rapid – 10 of 17 patients exhibited minimal or no change in psychotic symptoms at 4 hours. Sedation was evident at 4 hours but it had effectively abated by 72 hours.

A follow-up study by the same research group[52] examined more closely the clinical effects of ZA in 83 patients. The authors concluded that ZA produced 'pronounced and rapid reduction in psychotic symptoms'. In fact, psychotic symptoms were first assessed only after 24 hours and so a claim of rapid effect is not reasonably supported. Sedative effects were measured after 2 hours, when a statistically significant effect was observed – at baseline mean sedation score was 0.0 (0 = no sign of sedation) and at 2 hours 0.6 (1 = slightly sedated). Maximum sedation was observed at 8 hours (mean score 2.2; 2 = moderately sedated). At 72 hours mean score was 1.1. Dystonia and rigidity were the most commonly reported adverse effects.

Two independently conducted open studies produced similar results – a slow onset of effect peaking at 24 hours and still being evident at 72 hours.[53,54] The first UK study was reported in 1990.[55] In the trial, a significant reduction in psychosis score was first evident at 8 hours and scores continued to fall until the last measurement at 72 hours. Of 25 patients assessed, only 4 showed signs of tranquillisation at 1 hour (19 at 2 hours and 22 at 24 hours).

A comparative trial of ZA[56] examined its effects and those of IM/oral haloperidol and IM/oral zuclopenthixol base (in multiple doses over 6 days). The two non-ester, IM/oral preparations produced a greater degree of sedation at 2 hours than did ZA but the effect of ZA and zuclopenthixol was more sustained than with haloperidol over 144 hours (although patients received more zuclopenthixol doses). No clear differences between treatments were detected with the exception of the slow onset of effect of ZA. The number of doses given varied substantially: ZA 1–4, haloperidol 1–26 and zuclopenthixol 1–22. This is the key (and perhaps unique) advantage of ZA – it reduces the need for repeat doses in acute psychosis. Indeed, this was the principal finding of the first double-blind study of ZA.[57] Participants were given either ZA or haloperidol IM and assessed over 3 days. Changes in Brief Psychiatric Rating Scale (BPRS) and Clinical Global Impression (CGI) scores were near identical on each daily assessment. However, only 1 of 23 ZA patients required a second injection whereas 7 of 21 haloperidol patients required a repeat dose. Speed of onset was not examined. Similar findings were reported by Thai researchers comparing the same treatments[58] and in three other studies of moderate size (n = 44,[59] n = 40,[60] n = 50[61]). In each study, the timing of assessments was such that time to onset of effect could not be determined.

A Cochrane review[62] included all of the above comparative studies as well as three further studies[63–65] for which the authors were unable to obtain full details. The Cochrane authors concluded that all studies were methodologically flawed and poorly reported and that ZA did not appear to have a 'rapid onset of action'. They noted that

---

Box 1.1 Guidelines for the use of zuclopenthixol acetate (Acuphase)

Zuclopenthixol acetate (ZA) is not a rapidly tranquillising agent. It should be used only after an acutely psychotic patient has required **repeated** injections of short-acting antipsychotic drugs such as haloperidol or olanzapine, or sedative drugs such as lorazepam. It is perhaps best reserved for those few patients who have a prior history of good response to Acuphase.

ZA should be given only when enough time has elapsed to assess the full response to previously injected drugs: allow 15 minutes after IV injections, 60 minutes after IM.

ZA should **never** be administered:

- in an attempt to 'hasten' the antipsychotic effect of other antipsychotic therapy
- for rapid tranquillisation (onset of effect is too slow)
- at the same time as other parenteral antipsychotics or benzodiazepines (may lead to over-sedation which is difficult to reverse)
- as a 'test dose' for zuclopenthixol decanoate depot
- to a patient who is physically resistant (risk of intravasation and oil embolus).

ZA should **never** be used for, or in, the following:

- patients who accept oral medication
- patients who are neuroleptic-naïve
- patients who are sensitive to EPS
- patients who are unconscious
- patients who are pregnant
- those with hepatic or renal impairment
- those with cardiac disease.

ZA was probably no less effective than other treatments and that its use might 'result in less numerous coercive injections'.

Overall, the utility of ZA in RT is limited by a somewhat delayed onset of both sedative and antipsychotic actions. Sedation may be apparent in a minority of patients after 2–4 hours, but antipsychotic action is evident only after 8 hours. If ZA is given to a restrained patient, their behaviour on release from restraint is likely to be unchanged and will remain as such for several hours. ZA has a role in reducing the number of restraints for IM injection but it has no role in RT.

Guidelines for the use of ZA are summarised in Box 1.1.

Summary – rapid tranquillisation

A summary of rapid tranquillisation is provided in Box 1.2.

Rapid tranquillisation – physical monitoring

A summary of physical monitoring in RT is provided in Box 1.3.

Remedial measures in rapid tranquillisation

Remedial measures in RT are summarised in Table 1.9 and the use of flumazenil in Box 1.4.

Box 1.2 Rapid tranquillisation – summary

In an emergency situation

Assess to see if there may be a medical cause.[66] Optimise regular prescription. The aim of pharmacological treatment is to calm the patient but not to oversedate. Note: lower doses should be used for children, adolescents and older adults. Patients' levels of consciousness and physical health should be monitored after administration of parenteral medication (see Box 1.3).

Step intervention

1. **De-escalation**, time out, placement, etc., as appropriate.

2. **Offer oral treatment**

If patient is prescribed a regular antipsychotic: **Lorazepam** 1–2 mg **Promethazine** 25–50 mg. Monotherapy with **buccal midazolam** may avoid the need for IM treatment. Dose: 10 mg. *Note that this preparation is unlicensed.*	If patient is not already taking a regular oral or depot antipsychotic: ■ **Olanzapine** 10 mg, or ■ **Risperidone** 1–2 mg, or ■ **Quetiapine** 50–100 mg, or ■ **Haloperidol** 5 mg (best with promethazine 25 mg). Note that the SPC for haloperidol recommends a pre-treatment ECG and to avoid concomitant antipsychotics. ■ **Inhaled loxapine** 10 mg. Note that use of this preparation requires the co-operation of the patient, and that bronchospasm is a rare adverse effect (have a salbutamol inhaler to hand).

Repeat after 45–60 minutes, if necessary. Consider combining sedative and antipsychotic treatment. Go to step 3 if two doses fail or sooner if the patient is placing themselves or others at significant risk.

3. **Consider IM treatment**

Lorazepam 2 mg[a,b]	Have flumazenil to hand in case of benzodiazepine-induced respiratory depression.
Promethazine 50 mg[c]	IM promethazine is a useful option in a benzodiazepine-tolerant patient.
Olanzapine 10 mg[d]	IM olanzapine should **not** be combined with an IM benzodiazepine, particularly if alcohol has been consumed.[67]
Aripiprazole 9.75 mg	Less hypotension than olanzapine, but possibly less effective.[3,11,68]
Haloperidol 5 mg	**Haloperidol should be the last drug considered** ■ The incidence of acute dystonia is high; combine with IM promethazine and ensure IM procyclidine is available. ■ The SPC recommends a pre-treatment ECG. ■ Recommended by NICE.

Repeat after 30–60 minutes if insufficient effect. Combinations of haloperidol and lorazepam or haloperidol and promethazine may be considered if single-drug treatment fails. Drugs must not be mixed in the same syringe. IM olanzapine must never be combined with IM benzodiazepine.

4. **Consider IV treatment**

■ Diazepam 10 mg over at least 2 minutes.[b,e]
■ Repeat after 5–10 minutes if insufficient effect (up to 3 times).
■ Have flumazenil to hand.

5. **Seek expert advice** from the consultant or senior clinical pharmacist on call.[f]

---

[a] Carefully check administration instructions, which differ between manufacturers. With respect to Ativan (the most commonly used preparation), mix lorazepam 1:1 with water for injections before injecting. Some centres use 2–4 mg. An alternative is midazolam 7.5–15 mg. The risk of respiratory depression is dose-related with both but generally greater with midazolam.

Box 1.2 (*Continued*)

[b] Caution in the very young and elderly and those with pre-existing brain damage or impulse control problems, as disinhibition reactions are more likely.[69]

[c] Promethazine has a slow onset of action but is often an effective sedative. Dilution is not required before IM injection. May be repeated up to a maximum of 100 mg/day. Wait 1–2 hours after injection to assess response. Note that promethazine alone has been reported, albeit very rarely, to cause neuroleptic malignant syndrome[70] although it is an extremely weak dopamine antagonist. Note the potential pharmacokinetic interaction between promethazine and haloperidol (reduced metabolism of haloperidol) which may confer risk if repeated doses of both are administered.

[d] Recommended by NICE only for moderate behavioural disturbance, but data from a large observational study also support efficacy in clinical emergencies.

[e] Use Diazemuls to avoid injection site reactions. IV therapy may be used instead of IM when a very rapid effect is required. IV therapy also ensures near immediate delivery of the drug to its site of action and effectively avoids the danger of inadvertent accumulation of slowly absorbed IM doses. Note also that IV doses can be repeated after only 5–10 minutes if no effect is observed.

[f] Options at this point are limited. IM amylobarbitone and paraldehyde have been used in the past but are used now only extremely rarely and are generally not readily available. IV olanzapine, IV/IM droperidol and IV haloperidol are possible but serious adverse effects are fairly common. Ketamine is an option in medical units. Electroconvulsive therapy (ECT) is probably a better option. Behavioural disturbance secondary to the use of illicit drugs can be very difficult to manage. Time and supportive care may be safer than administering more sedative medication.

Box 1.3 Physical monitoring in rapid tranquillisation – summary

After any parenteral drug administration, monitor as follows:

- **Temperature**
- **Pulse**
- **Blood pressure**
- **Respiratory rate.**

Every 15 minutes for 1 hour, and then hourly until the patient is ambulatory. Patients who refuse to have their vital signs monitored or who remain too behaviourally disturbed to be approached should be observed for signs/symptoms of pyrexia, hypoxia, hypotension, oversedation and general physical well-being.

If the patient is asleep or **unconscious**, the continuous use of pulse oximetry to measure oxygen saturation is desirable. A nurse should remain with the patient until ambulatory.

ECG and haematological monitoring are also strongly recommended when parenteral antipsychotics are given, especially when higher doses are used.[71,72] Hypokalaemia, stress and agitation place the patient at risk of cardiac arrhythmia[73] (see section on 'QT prolongation' in this chapter). ECG monitoring is formally recommended for all patients who receive haloperidol.

Table 1.9 Remedial measures in rapid tranquillisation – summary

Problem	Remedial measures
Acute dystonia (including oculogyric crises)	Give **procyclidine** 5–10 mg IM or IV
Reduced respiratory rate (<10/minutes) or oxygen saturation (<90%)	Give oxygen, raise legs, ensure patient is not lying face down
	Give **flumazenil** if benzodiazepine-induced respiratory depression suspected (see Box 1.4)
	If induced by any other sedative agent: **transfer to a medical bed and ventilate mechanically**
Irregular or slow (<50/minutes) **pulse**	**Refer** to specialist medical care immediately
Fall in blood pressure (>30 mmHg orthostatic drop or <50 mmHg diastolic)	**Have patient lie flat**, tilt bed towards head
	Monitor closely
Increased temperature	**Withold antipsychotics** (risk of NMS and perhaps arrhythmia). Check creatine kinase urgently

IM, intramuscular; IV, intravenous; NMS, neuroleptic malignant syndrome.

Box 1.4 Guidelines for the use of flumazenil

- **Indication for use.** If, after the administration of lorazepam, midazolam or diazepam, respiratory rate falls below 10/minute.
- **Contraindications.** Patients with epilepsy who have been receiving long-term benzodiazepines.
- **Caution.** Dose should be carefully titrated in hepatic impairment.
- **Dose and route of administration:**
  - *Initial:* 200 µg *intravenously* over 15 seconds
  - If required level of consciousness not achieved after 60 seconds, then *subsequent dose:* 100 µg over 15 seconds
- **Time before dose can be repeated.** 60 seconds.
- **Maximum dose.** 1 mg in 24 hours (one initial dose and eight subsequent doses).
- **Adverse effects.** Patients may become agitated, anxious or fearful on awakening. Seizures may occur in regular benzodiazepine users.
- **Management.** Adverse effects usually subside.

Monitoring

- **What to monitor?** Respiratory rate.
- **How often?** Continuously until respiratory rate returns to baseline level.
  Flumazenil has a short half-life (much shorter than diazepam) and respiratory function may recover and then deteriorate again.

Note: If respiratory rate does not return to normal or patient is not alert after initial doses given, assume that sedation is due to some other cause.

References

1. Currier GW et al. Acute treatment of psychotic agitation: a randomized comparison of oral treatment with risperidone and lorazepam versus intramuscular treatment with haloperidol and lorazepam. J Clin Psychiatry 2004; 65:386–394.
2. Ganesan S et al. Effectiveness of quetiapine for the management of aggressive psychosis in the emergency psychiatric setting: a naturalistic uncontrolled trial. Int J Psychiatry Clin Pract 2005; 9:199–203.

3. Simpson JR, Jr. et al. Impact of orally disintegrating olanzapine on use of intramuscular antipsychotics, seclusion, and restraint in an acute inpatient psychiatric setting. J Clin Psychopharmacol 2006; 26:333–335.

4. Hsu WY et al. Comparison of intramuscular olanzapine, orally disintegrating olanzapine tablets, oral risperidone solution, and intramuscular haloperidol in the management of acute agitation in an acute care psychiatric ward in Taiwan. J Clin Psychopharmacol 2010; 30:230–234.

5. Pratts M et al. A single-dose, randomized, double-blind, placebo-controlled trial of sublingual asenapine for acute agitation. Acta Psychiatr Scand 2014; 130:61–68.

6. Lesem MD et al. Rapid acute treatment of agitation in individuals with schizophrenia: multicentre, randomised, placebo-controlled study of inhaled loxapine. Br J Psychiatry 2011; 198:51–58.

7. Kwentus J et al. Rapid acute treatment of agitation in patients with bipolar I disorder: a multicenter, randomized, placebo-controlled clinical trial with inhaled loxapine. Bipolar Disord 2012; 14:31–40.

8. Allen MH et al. Efficacy and safety of loxapine for inhalation in the treatment of agitation in patients with schizophrenia: a randomized, double-blind, placebo-controlled trial. J Clin Psychiatry 2011; 72:1313–1321.

9. Kahl KG et al. Inhaled loxapine for acute treatment of agitation in patients with borderline personality disorder: a case series. J Clin Psychopharmacol 2015; 35:741–743.

10. Roncero C et al. Effectiveness of inhaled loxapine in dual-diagnosis patients: a case series. Clin Neuropharmacol 2016; 39:206–209.

11. Citrome L. Comparison of intramuscular ziprasidone, olanzapine, or aripiprazole for agitation: a quantitative review of efficacy and safety. J Clin Psychiatry 2007; 68:1876–1885.

12. Perrin E et al. A prospective, observational study of the safety and effectiveness of intramuscular psychotropic treatment in acutely agitated patients with schizophrenia and bipolar mania. Eur Psychiatry 2012; 27:234–239.

13. Ferraz Goncalves JA et al. comparison of haloperidol alone and in combination with midazolam for the treatment of acute agitation in an inpatient palliative care service. J Pain Palliat Care Pharmacother 2016; 30:284–288.

14. Chan EW et al. Intravenous droperidol or olanzapine as an adjunct to midazolam for the acutely agitated patient: a multicenter, randomized, double-blind, placebo-controlled clinical trial. Ann Emerg Med 2013; 61:72–81.

15. TREC Collaborative Group. Rapid tranquillisation for agitated patients in emergency psychiatric rooms: a randomised trial of midazolam versus haloperidol plus promethazine. BMJ 2003; 327:708–713.

16. Raveendran NS et al. Rapid tranquillisation in psychiatric emergency settings in India: pragmatic randomised controlled trial of intramuscular olanzapine versus intramuscular haloperidol plus promethazine. BMJ 2007; 335:865.

17. Huf G et al. Rapid tranquillisation in psychiatric emergency settings in Brazil: pragmatic randomised controlled trial of intramuscular haloperidol versus intramuscular haloperidol plus promethazine. BMJ 2007; 335:869.

18. Alexander J et al. Rapid tranquillisation of violent or agitated patients in a psychiatric emergency setting. Pragmatic randomised trial of intramuscular lorazepam v. haloperidol plus promethazine. Br J Psychiatry 2004; 185:63–69.

19. Taylor DM et al. Midazolam-droperidol, droperidol, or olanzapine for acute agitation: a randomized clinical trial. Ann Emerg Med 2017; 69:318–326.e311.

20. Kittipeerachon M et al. Intramuscular olanzapine versus intramuscular aripiprazole for the treatment of agitation in patients with schizophrenia: a pragmatic double-blind randomized trial. Schizophr Res 2016; 176:231–238.

21. Huang CL et al. Intramuscular olanzapine versus intramuscular haloperidol plus lorazepam for the treatment of acute schizophrenia with agitation: an open-label, randomized controlled trial. J Formos Med Assoc 2015; 114:438–445.

22. Calver L et al. The safety and effectiveness of droperidol for sedation of acute behavioral disturbance in the emergency department. Ann Emerg Med 2015; 66:230–238.e231.

23. Powney MJ et al. Haloperidol for psychosis-induced aggression or agitation (rapid tranquillisation). Cochrane Database Syst Rev 2012; 11:CD009377.

24. Ostinelli EG et al. Haloperidol for psychosis-induced aggression or agitation (rapid tranquillisation). Cochrane Database Syst Rev 2017; 7:CD009377.

25. National Institute for Health and Care Excellence. Evidence Summary of Unlicensed/Off-Label Medicines: Rapid tranquillisation in mental health settings: promethazine hydrochloride. ESUOM 28, 2014. http://www.nice.org.uk/

26. Huf G et al. Haloperidol plus promethazine for psychosis-induced aggression. Cochrane Database Syst Rev 2016; 11:CD005146.

27. Ostinelli EG et al. Aripiprazole (intramuscular) for psychosis-induced aggression or agitation (rapid tranquillisation). Cochrane Database Syst Rev 2018; 1:CD008074.

28. Kishi T et al. Intramuscular olanzapine for agitated patients: a systematic review and meta-analysis of randomized controlled trials. J Psychiatr Res 2015; 68:198–209.

29. Khokhar MA et al. Droperidol for psychosis-induced aggression or agitation. Cochrane Database Syst Rev 2016; 12:CD002830.

30. Satterthwaite TD et al. A meta-analysis of the risk of acute extrapyramidal symptoms with intramuscular antipsychotics for the treatment of agitation. J Clin Psychiatry 2008; 69:1869–1879.

31. van Harten PN et al. Acute dystonia induced by drug treatment. Br Med J 1999; 319:623–626.

32. Pharmacovigilance Working Party. Public Assessment Report on Neuroleptics and Cardiac safety, in particular QT prolongation, cardiac arrhythmias, ventricular tachycardia and torsades de pointes. 2006. http://www.mhra.gov.uk/home/groups/s-par/documents/websiteresources/con079326.pdf

33. Janssen-Cilag Ltd. Summary of Product Characteristics. Haldol Injection. 2014. https://www.medicines.org.uk/

34. Miceli JJ et al. Effects of high-dose ziprasidone and haloperidol on the QTc interval after intramuscular administration: a randomized, single-blind, parallel-group study in patients with schizophrenia or schizoaffective disorder. Clin Ther 2010; 32:472–491.

35. Suzuki A et al. Histamine H1-receptor antagonists, promethazine and homochlorcyclizine, increase the steady-state plasma concentrations of haloperidol and reduced haloperidol. Ther Drug Monit 2003; 25:192–196.

36. Lerner Y et al. Acute high-dose parenteral haloperidol treatment of psychosis. Am J Psychiatry 1979; **136**:1061–1064.

37. Martel ML et al. A large retrospective cohort of patients receiving intravenous olanzapine in the emergency department. Acad Emerg Med 2016; **23**:29–35.

38. Cole JB et al. A prospective observational study of patients receiving intravenous and intramuscular olanzapine in the emergency department. Ann Emerg Med 2017; **69**:327–336.e322.

39. Calver L et al. A prospective study of high dose sedation for rapid tranquilisation of acute behavioural disturbance in an acute mental health unit. BMC Psychiatry 2013; **13**:225.

40. Mantovani C et al. Are low doses of antipsychotics effective in the management of psychomotor agitation? A randomized, rated-blind trial of 4 intramuscular interventions. J Clin Psychopharmacol 2013; **33**:306–312.

41. Taylor D et al. Buccal midazolam for rapid tranquillisation. Int J Psychiatry Clin Pract 2008; **12**:309–311.

42. Spain D et al. Safety and effectiveness of high-dose midazolam for severe behavioural disturbance in an emergency department with suspected psychostimulant-affected patients. Emerg Med Australas 2008; **20**:112–120.

43. Zaman H et al. Benzodiazepines for psychosis-induced aggression or agitation. Cochrane Database Syst Rev 2017; **12**:CD003079.

44. Li SF et al. Safety and efficacy of intravenous combination sedatives in the ED. Am J Emerg Med 2013; **31**:1402–1404.

45. MacNeal JJ et al. Use of haloperidol in PCP-intoxicated individuals. Clin Toxicol (Phila) 2012; **50**:851–853.

46. Isbister GK et al. Ketamine as rescue treatment for difficult-to-sedate severe acute behavioral disturbance in the emergency department. Ann Emerg Med 2016; **67**:581–587.e581.

47. Hopper AB et al. Ketamine use for acute agitation in the emergency department. J Emerg Med 2015; **48**:712–719.

48. Riddell J et al. Ketamine as a first-line treatment for severely agitated emergency department patients. Am J Emerg Med 2017; **35**:1000–1004.

49. Cole JB et al. A prospective study of ketamine versus haloperidol for severe prehospital agitation. Clin Toxicol (Phila) 2016; **54**:556–562.

50. Huf G et al. Physical restraints versus seclusion room for management of people with acute aggression or agitation due to psychotic illness (TREC-SAVE): a randomized trial. Psychol Med 2012; **42**:2265–2273.

51. Amdisen A et al. Serum concentrations and clinical effect of zuclopenthixol in acutely disturbed, psychotic patients treated with zuclopenthixol acetate in Viscoleo. Psychopharmacology (Berl) 1986; **90**:412–416.

52. Amdisen A et al. Zuclopenthixol acetate in Viscoleo – a new drug formulation. An open Nordic multicentre study of zuclopenthixol acetate in Viscoleo in patients with acute psychoses including mania and exacerbation of chronic psychoses. Acta Psychiatr Scand 1987; **75**:99–107.

53. Lowert AC et al. Acute psychotic disorders treated with 5% zuclopenthixol acetate in 'Viscoleo' ('Cisordinol-Acutard'), a global assessment of the clinical effect: an open multi-centre study. Pharmatherapeutica 1989; **5**:380–386.

54. Balant LP et al. Clinical and pharmacokinetic evaluation of zuclopenthixol acetate in Viscoleo. Pharmacopsychiatry 1989; **22**:250–254.

55. Chakravarti SK et al. Zuclopenthixol acetate (5% in 'Viscoleo'): single-dose treatment for acutely disturbed psychotic patients. Curr Med Res Opin 1990; **12**:58–65.

56. Baastrup PC et al. A controlled Nordic multicentre study of zuclopenthixol acetate in oil solution, haloperidol and zuclopenthixol in the treatment of acute psychosis. Acta Psychiatr Scand 1993; **87**:48–58.

57. Chin CN et al. A double blind comparison of zuclopenthixol acetate with haloperidol in the management of acutely disturbed schizophrenics. Med J Malaysia 1998; **53**:365–371.

58. Taymeeyapradit U et al. Comparative study of the effectiveness of zuclopenthixol acetate and haloperidol in acutely disturbed psychotic patients. J Med Assoc Thai 2002; **85**:1301–1308.

59. Brook S et al. A randomized controlled double blind study of zuclopenthixol acetate compared to haloperidol in acute psychosis. Hum Psychopharmacol Clin Exp 1998; **13**:17–20.

60. Chouinard G et al. A double-blind controlled study of intramuscular zuclopenthixol acetate and liquid oral haloperidol in the treatment of schizophrenic patients with acute exacerbation. J Clin Psychopharmacol 1994; **14**:377–384.

61. Al-Haddad MK et al. Zuclopenthixol versus haloperidol in the initial treatment of schizophrenic psychoses, affective psychoses and paranoid states: a controlled clinical trial. Arab J Psychiatry 1996; **7**:44–54.

62. Jayakody K et al. Zuclopenthixol acetate for acute schizophrenia and similar serious mental illnesses. Cochrane Database Syst Rev 2012; **4**:CD000525.

63. Liu P et al. Observation of clinical effect of clopixol acuphase injection for acute psychosis. Chinese J Pharmacoepidemiol 1997; **6**:202–204.

64. Ropert R et al. Where zuclopenthixol acetate stands amid the "modified release" neuroleptics. Congres de Psychiatrie et de Neurologie de Langue Francaise, LXXXVIth Session, Jun 13–17 Chambery, France; 1988.

65. Berk M. A controlled double blind study of zuclopenthixol acetate compared with clothiapine in acute psychosis including mania and exacerbation of chronic psychosis. Proceedings of XXth Collegium Internationale Neuro-psychopharmacologicum. Jun 23–27 Melbourne, Australia; 1996.

66. Garriga M et al. Assessment and management of agitation in psychiatry: expert consensus. World J Biol Psychiatry 2016; **17**:86–128.

67. Wilson MP et al. Potential complications of combining intramuscular olanzapine with benzodiazepines in emergency department patients. J Emerg Med 2012; **43**:889–896.

68. Villari V et al. Oral risperidone, olanzapine and quetiapine versus haloperidol in psychotic agitation. Prog Neuropsychopharmacol Biol Psychiatry 2008; **32**:405–413.

69. Paton C. Benzodiazepines and disinhibition: a review. Psychiatr Bull 2002; **26**:460–462.

70. Chan-Tack KM. Neuroleptic malignant syndrome due to promethazine. South Med J 1999; **92**:1017–1018.

71. Appleby L et al. Sudden unexplained death in psychiatric in-patients. Br J Psychiatry 2000; **176**:405–406.

72. Yap YG et al. Risk of torsades de pointes with non-cardiac drugs. Doctors need to be aware that many drugs can cause QT prolongation. BMJ 2000; **320**:1158–1159.

73. Taylor DM. Antipsychotics and QT prolongation. Acta Psychiatr Scand 2003; **107**:85–95.

Further reading

National Institute for Clinical Excellence. Violence and aggression: short-term management in mental health, health and community settings. Guideline No 10, 2015. https://www.nice.org.uk/guidance/ng10

Antipsychotic depots/long-acting injections (LAIs)

Antipsychotic depots/long-acting injections (LAIs) are recommended where a patient has expressed a preference for such a formulation because of its convenience or where avoidance of covert non-adherence is a clinical priority.[1,2] LAIs do not assure compliance but they do assure awareness of compliance. With the advent of better tolerated SGA LAIs, these formulations are increasingly seen as treatments of choice by both patients and health professionals. Another advantage for LAIs over oral medication is that they provide the opportunity for regular scrutiny of a patient's mental state and adverse effects by the health-care professional administering the injection. It has been estimated that, in the UK, between a quarter and a third of people with schizophrenia are prescribed an LAI, depending on the clinical setting.[3] This prevalence varies from country to country. Some years ago, approximately half were also prescribed an oral antipsychotic drug, one possible reason being to allow for more rapid dose titration, but the combination of an oral and LAI antipsychotic preparation often resulted in high-dose prescribing[3] which is associated with an increased adverse-effect burden and has implications for physical health monitoring. It goes without saying that monotherapy with an LAI is likely to be optimal.

Advice on prescribing depots/LAIs

- **For FGAs, give a test dose.** Because of its long half-life, any adverse effects that result from the administration of an LAI are likely to be long-lived. Therefore, LAIs should be avoided in patients with a history of serious adverse effects that would warrant immediate discontinuation of the medication, such as neuroleptic malignant syndrome (NMS). For FGAs, a test dose consisting of a small dose of active drug in a small volume of oil serves a dual purpose: it is a test both of the patient's sensitivity to EPS and of any sensitivity to the base oil. For SGAs, test doses may not be required (less propensity to cause EPS and aqueous base not known to be allergenic) although they could be considered appropriate where a patient is suspected of being non-adherent to oral antipsychotic medication and the LAI will be the first exposure to guaranteed antipsychotic medication delivery. For both types of LAI prior treatment with the equivalent oral formulation is preferred, to assess efficacy and tolerability.
- **Begin with the lowest therapeutic dose.** There are few data showing clear dose–response effects for LAIs. There is some information indicating that low doses (within the licensed range) are at least as effective as higher ones.[4–6] Low doses are likely to be better. Perhaps the key problem with FGA LAIs is that, unlike with SGAs, the optimal dose range is not known.
- **Administer at the longest possible licensed interval.** All LAIs can be safely administered at their licensed dosing intervals, bearing in mind the maximum recommended single dose. There is no evidence to suggest that shortening the dose interval improves efficacy. Moreover, the injection site can be a cause of discomfort and pain, so less frequent administration is desirable. Although some patients are reported to deteriorate in the days before their next LAI is due, plasma levels may continue to fall, albeit slowly, for some hours (or even days with some preparations) after each injection (see Figure 1.11). Thus, patients may conceivably be most at risk of deterioration

immediately after an LAI. Moreover, in trials, relapse seems only to occur 3–6 months after withdrawing LAI therapy, roughly the time required to clear steady-state drug levels from the blood.

- **Adjust doses only after an adequate period of assessment.** Attainment of peak plasma levels, therapeutic effect and steady-state plasma levels are all delayed with LAIs. Doses may be **reduced** if adverse effects occur, but should only be increased after careful assessment over at least 1 month, and preferably longer. The use of adjunctive oral medication to assess dosage requirements of LAIs may be helpful, but is complicated by the slow emergence of antipsychotic effects. Note that at the start of therapy, plasma levels of antipsychotic released from a LAI increase over several weeks to months without increasing the given dose. (This is due to accumulation: steady state is only achieved after at least 6–8 weeks.) Dose increases during this time to steady-state plasma levels are thus illogical and impossible to evaluate properly. The monitoring and recording of therapeutic efficacy, adverse effects and any impact on physical health during therapy are recommended.
- **LAIs are not recommended for those who are antipsychotic-naïve.** Tolerance to some LAIs can be established by using the oral form of the same drug for 2 weeks before starting the LAI. Good examples here are haloperidol, aripiprazole and paliperidone (using oral risperidone).

Differences between LAIs

There are few differences between individual FGA LAIs. Pipotiazine (now withdrawn in most countries) may be associated with relatively less frequent EPS, and fluphenazine (which also has limited availability) with relatively more EPS but perhaps less weight gain.[7] Cochrane reviews have been completed for pipotiazine,[8] flupentixol,[9] zuclopenthixol,[10] haloperidol[11] and fluphenazine.[12] With the exception of zuclopenthixol,[10] these preparations are equally effective with respect to each other. Standard doses are said to be as effective as high doses for flupentixol.[9]

Two differences that possibly do exist between FGA LAIs are:

- Zuclopenthixol may be more effective in preventing relapses than others, although this may be at the expense of an increased burden of adverse effects.[13,14]
- Flupentixol decanoate can be given in very much higher 'neuroleptic equivalent' doses than the other LAI preparations and still remain 'within licensed dosing limits'. It is doubtful that this confers any real therapeutic advantage.

Aripiprazole, paliperidone, risperidone and olanzapine LAIs have a relatively lower propensity for EPS compared with FGA LAIs. At least some of this difference is a result of higher equivalent doses being used with FGAs but even when low doses are used there is still an advantage for SGAs.[6] Risperidone, however, increases prolactin, and dosage adjustment can be complex because of its pharmacokinetic profile. Olanzapine can cause significant weight gain and is associated with inadvertent intravascular injection or post-injection syndrome.[15] Unlike risperidone LAI, it is effective within a few days. Paliperidone 1-monthly is also rapidly released and effective within a few days, as is aripiprazole LAI.

Table 1.10 Antipsychotic LAIs: suggested doses and frequencies[2]

Drug	UK trade name	Licensed injection site	Test dose (mg)	Dose range (mg/week)	Dosing interval (weeks)	Comments
Aripiprazole	Abilify Maintena	Buttock	Not required[†]	300–400 mg monthly	Monthly	Does not increase prolactin Oral loading required
Flupentixol decanoate	Depixol	Buttock or thigh	20	50 mg every 4 weeks to 400 mg a week	2–4	Maximum licensed dose is high relative to other LAIs
Fluphenazine decanoate	Modecate	Gluteal region	12.5	12.5 mg every 2 weeks to 100 mg every 2 weeks	2–5	High EPS
Haloperidol decanoate	Haldol	Gluteal region	25*	50–300 mg every 4 weeks	4	High EPS
Olanzapine pamoate	ZypAdhera	Gluteal	Not required[†]	150 mg every 4 weeks to 300 mg every 2 weeks	2–4	Risk of post-injection syndrome
Paliperidone palmitate (monthly)	Xeplion	Deltoid or gluteal	Not required[†]	50–150 mg monthly	Monthly	Loading dose required at treatment initiation
Paliperidone palmitate (3-monthly)	Trevicta	Deltoid or gluteal	Not required[‡]	175–525 mg every 3 months	3 months	
Pipotiazine palmitate	Piportil	Gluteal region	25	50–200 mg every 4 weeks	4	? Lower incidence of EPS (relative to other FGAs)
Risperidone microspheres	Risperdal Consta	Deltoid or gluteal	Not required[†]	25–50 mg every 2 weeks	2	Drug release delayed for 2–3 weeks – oral therapy required
Zuclopenthixol decanoate	Clopixol	Buttock or thigh	100	200 mg every 3 weeks to 600 mg a week	2–4	? Slightly better efficacy than FGA LAIs

Notes:

- The doses in the table are for adults. Check formal labelling for appropriate doses in the elderly.
- After a test dose, wait 4–10 days then titrate to maintenance dose according to response (see product information for individual drugs).
- Avoid using shorter dose intervals than those recommended except in exceptional circumstances (e.g. long interval necessitates high-volume [>3–4 mL] injection). Maximum licensed single dose overrides longer intervals and lower volumes. For example, zuclopenthixol 500 mg every week is licensed whereas 1000 mg every 2 weeks is not (more than the licensed maximum of 600 mg is administered). Always check official manufacturer's information.

* Test dose not stated by manufacturer.

[†] Tolerability and response to the oral preparation should be established before administering the LAI. With respect to paliperidone LAI, oral risperidone can be used for this purpose.

[‡] May not be started until the completion of 4 months' treatment with monthly LAI.

EPS, extrapyramidal symptoms; FGA, first-generation antipsychotic; LAI, long-acting injection.

The use of LAIs does not guarantee good treatment adherence, and there is a lack of robust and consistent RCT evidence that LAIs offer better efficacy or tolerability than oral preparations.[16–18] Nevertheless, non-randomised, observational, 'real-world' data have suggested an overall better global outcome with LAIs compared with oral anti-psychotics, with a reduced risk of relapse and rehospitalisation.[19,20] It has been argued that adherence to oral antipsychotic medication decreases over time and that relapse rates in patients prescribed LAIs decrease in comparison with oral antipsychotics only in the longer term.[21] That is, LAIs reveal advantages over oral treatment only after several years. It is also probably true that patients volunteering for RCTs do not properly represent those treated in everyday practice.

Table 1.10 summarises suggested doses and frequencies for administration of anti-psychotic LAIs.

Intramuscular anticholinergic medication and depots/LAIs

Antipsychotic LAIs do not produce acute movement disorders at the time of administration:[22] this may take hours to days. The administration of IM procyclidine routinely with each dose is illogical as the effects of the anticholinergic drug will have worn off before plasma antipsychotic levels rise or peak.

References

1. National Institute for Health and Care Excellence. Psychosis and schizophrenia in adults: prevention and management. Clinical Guideline 178, 2014. https://www.nice.org.uk/guidance/cg178
2. Barnes TR. Evidence-based guidelines for the pharmacological treatment of schizophrenia: recommendations from the British Association for Psychopharmacology. J Psychopharmacol 2011; 25:567–620.
3. Barnes T et al. Antipsychotic long acting injections: prescribing practice in the UK. Br J Psychiatry Suppl 2009; 52:S37–S42.
4. Kane JM et al. A multidose study of haloperidol decanoate in the maintenance treatment of schizophrenia. Am J Psychiatry 2002; 159:554–560.
5. Taylor D. Establishing a dose-response relationship for haloperidol decanoate. Psychiatr Bull 2005; 29:104–107.
6. McEvoy JP et al. Effectiveness of paliperidone palmitate vs haloperidol decanoate for maintenance treatment of schizophrenia: a randomized clinical trial. JAMA 2014; 311:1978–1987.
7. Taylor D. Psychopharmacology and adverse effects of antipsychotic long acting injections. Br J Psychiatry 2009; 195:S13–S19.
8. Dinesh M et al. Depot pipotiazine palmitate and undecylenate for schizophrenia. The Cochrane Database Syst Rev 2004; CD001720.
9. Mahapatra J et al. Flupenthixol decanoate (depot) for schizophrenia or other similar psychotic disorders. Cochrane Database Syst Rev 2014; 6:CD001470.
10. Coutinho E et al. Zuclopenthixol decanoate for schizophrenia and other serious mental illnesses. Cochrane Database Syst Rev 2000; CD001164.
11. Quraishi S et al. Depot haloperidol decanoate for schizophrenia. Cochrane Database Syst Rev 2000; CD001361.
12. Maayan N et al. Fluphenazine decanoate (depot) and enanthate for schizophrenia. Cochrane Database Syst Rev 2015 CD000307.
13. da Silva Freire Coutinho E et al. Zuclopenthixol decanoate for schizophrenia and other serious mental illnesses. Cochrane Database Syst Rev 2006; CD001164.
14. Shajahan P et al. Comparison of the effectiveness of depot antipsychotics in routine clinical practice. Psychiatrist 2010; 34:273–279.
15. Citrome L. Olanzapine pamoate: a stick in time? Int J Clin Pract 2009; 63:140–150.
16. Ostuzzi G et al. Does formulation matter? A systematic review and meta-analysis of oral versus long-acting antipsychotic studies. Schizophr Res 2017; 183:10–21.
17. Kishimoto T et al. Long-acting injectable vs oral antipsychotics for relapse prevention in schizophrenia: a meta-analysis of randomized trials. Schizophr Bull 2014; 40:192–213.
18. Leucht C et al. Oral versus depot antipsychotic drugs for schizophrenia – a critical systematic review and meta-analysis of randomised long-term trials. Schizophr Res 2011; 127:83–92.
19. Tiihonen J et al. Real-world effectiveness of antipsychotic treatments in a nationwide cohort of 29823 patients with schizophrenia. JAMA Psychiatry 2017; 74:686–693.

20. Kirson NY et al. Efficacy and effectiveness of depot versus oral antipsychotics in schizophrenia: synthesizing results across different research designs. J Clin Psychiatry 2013; **74**:568–575.
21. Schooler NR. Relapse and rehospitalization: comparing oral and depot antipsychotics. J Clin Psychiatry 2003; **64 Suppl 16**:14–17.
22. Kane JM et al. Guidelines for depot antipsychotic treatment in schizophrenia. European Neuropsychopharmacology Consensus Conference in Siena, Italy. Eur Neuropsychopharmacol 1998; **8**:55–66.

Further reading

Patel MX et al. Antipsychotic long-acting (depot) injections for the treatment of schizophrenia. Br J Psychiatry 2009; **195 Suppl 52**:S1–S67.

Depot/LAI antipsychotics – pharmacokinetics

Table 1.11 summarises the pharmacokinetics of depot antipsychotics.

Table 1.11 Pharmacokinetics of depot/LAI antipsychotics

Drug	UK trade name	Time to peak (days)*	Plasma half-life (days)	Time to steady state (weeks)[†]
Aripiprazole[1]	Abilify Maintena	7	30–46	~20
Aripiprazole lauroxil[2,3]	Aristada (in US)	44–50	~30	~16
Flupentixol decanoate[4]	Depixol	7	8–17	~9
Fluphenazine decanoate[5–7]	Modecate	8–12[‡]	10	~8
Haloperidol decanoate[8,9]	Haldol	7	21	~14
Olanzapine pamoate[10,11]	ZypAdhera	2–3	30	~12
Paliperidone palmitate[12] (monthly)	Xeplion	13	29–45	~20
Paliperidone palmitate[13] (3-monthly)	Trevicta	25	~75	~52
Pipotiazine palmitate[14,15]	Piportil	7–14	15	~9
Risperidone microspheres[16,17]	Risperidal Consta	~30	4	~8
Zuclopenthixol decanoate[4,14,18]	Clopixol	4–7	19	~12

*Time to peak is not the same as time to reach therapeutic plasma concentration but both are dependent on dose. For large (loading) doses, therapeutic activity is often seen before peak levels are attained. For low (test) doses, the initial peak level may be subtherapeutic.

[†] Attainment of steady state (SS) follows logarithmic, not linear characteristics: around 90% of SS levels are achieved in three half-lives. Time to attain steady state is independent of dose and dosing frequency (i.e. you cannot hurry it up by giving more, more often). Loading doses can be used to produce prompt therapeutic plasma levels but time to SS remains the same.

[‡] Some estimates suggest peak concentrations after only a few hours.[18,19] It is likely that fluphenazine decanoate produces two peaks – one on the day of injection and a second slightly higher peak a week or so later.[8]

References

1. Mallikaarjun S et al. Pharmacokinetics, tolerability and safety of aripiprazole once-monthly in adult schizophrenia: an open-label, parallel-arm, multiple-dose study. Schizophr Res 2013; 150:281–288.
2. Hard ML et al. Aripiprazole lauroxil: pharmacokinetic profile of this long-acting injectable antipsychotic in persons with schizophrenia. J Clin Psychopharmacol 2017; 37:289–295.
3. Turncliff R et al. Relative bioavailability and safety of aripiprazole lauroxil, a novel once-monthly, long-acting injectable atypical antipsychotic, following deltoid and gluteal administration in adult subjects with schizophrenia. Schizophr Res 2014; 159:404–410.
4. Jann MW et al. Clinical pharmacokinetics of the depot antipsychotics. Clin Pharmacokinet 1985; 10:315–333.
5. Simpson GM et al. Single-dose pharmacokinetics of fluphenazine after fluphenazine decanoate administration. J Clin Psychopharmacol 1990; 10:417–421.
6. Balant-Gorgia AE et al. Antipsychotic drugs. Clinical pharmacokinetics of potential candidates for plasma concentration monitoring. Clin Pharmacokinet 1987; 13:65–90.
7. Gitlin MJ et al. Persistence of fluphenazine in plasma after decanoate withdrawal. J Clin Psychopharmacol 1988; 8:53–56.
8. Wiles DH et al. Pharmacokinetics of haloperidol and fluphenazine decanoates in chronic schizophrenia. Psychopharmacology (Berl) 1990; 101:274–281.
9. Nayak RK et al. The bioavailability and pharmacokinetics of oral and depot intramuscular haloperidol in schizophrenic patients. J Clin Pharmacol 1987; 27:144–150.

10. Heres S et al. Pharmacokinetics of olanzapine long-acting injection: the clinical perspective. Int Clin Psychopharmacol 2014; 29:299–312.

11. Mitchell M et al. Single- and multiple-dose pharmacokinetic, safety, and tolerability profiles of olanzapine long-acting injection: an open-label, multicenter, nonrandomized study in patients with schizophrenia. Clin Ther 2013; 35:1890–1908.

12. Hoy SM et al. Intramuscular paliperidone palmitate. CNS Drugs 2010; 24:227–244.

13. Ravenstijn P et al. Pharmacokinetics, safety, and tolerability of paliperidone palmitate 3-month formulation in patients with schizophrenia: a phase-1, single-dose, randomized, open-label study. J Clin Pharmacol 2016; 56:330–339.

14. Barnes TR et al. Long-term depot antipsychotics. A risk-benefit assessment. Drug Saf 1994; 10:464–479.

15. Ogden DA et al. Determination of pipothiazine in human plasma by reversed-phase high-performance liquid chromatography. J Pharm Biomed Anal 1989; 7:1273–1280.

16. Ereshefsky L et al. Pharmacokinetic profile and clinical efficacy of long-acting risperidone: potential benefits of combining an atypical antipsychotic and a new delivery system. Drugs RD 2005; 6:129–137.

17. Meyer JM. Understanding depot antipsychotics: an illustrated guide to kinetics. CNS Spectr 2013; 18 Suppl 1:58–67.

18. Viala A et al. Comparative study of the pharmacokinetics of zuclopenthixol decanoate and fluphenazine decanoate. Psychopharmacology (Berl) 1988; 94:293–297.

19. Soni SD et al. Plasma levels of fluphenazine decanoate. Effects of site of injection, massage and muscle activity. Br J Psychiatry 1988; 153:382–384.

Management of patients on long-term depots/LAIs

All patients receiving long-term treatment with antipsychotic medication should be seen by the psychiatrist responsible for them at least once a year (ideally more frequently) in order to review their progress and treatment. A systematic assessment of tolerability and safety should constitute part of this review. The assessment of adverse effects should include EPS (principally parkinsonism, akathisia and TD). TD can be assessed by recording the score on the Abnormal Involuntary Movement Scale (AIMS).[1] Some study findings have suggested that depot/LAI antipsychotic medication is more likely to cause TD but this remains uncertain[2] and not all studies confirm these observations.[3]

For most people with multi-episode schizophrenia, continuing antipsychotic treatment, even lifelong, may be necessary. However, with long-term LAI treatment, dose reduction may be considered in stable patients. There is some evidence to suggest that FGA depots are sometimes prescribed in excessive doses: haloperidol decanoate is optimally effective at 75 mg every 4 weeks,[4,5] paliperidone palmitate at 50 mg a month.[6] Further to this, dopamine occupancy required for relapse prevention may be lower than that for acute treatment – continuous occupancy above 65% may not be necessary.[7]

Long-term follow-up is required when antipsychotic dosage is decreased as such reduction, at least to very low doses, is associated with a greater risk of treatment failure, hospitalisation and relapse,[8] which may only become evident over the longer term. One study[9] comparing fluphenazine decanoate at 5 mg or 25 mg every 2 weeks found no difference in outcome at 1 year but a substantial disadvantage for the lower dose at 2 years (69% vs 36% relapse). In the same study, the facility to increase dose when symptoms emerged removed the advantage for the higher dose. Interestingly, in another trial which used low-dose (5 mg every 2 weeks) fluphenazine decanoate, this dose was substantially inferior to standard doses (56% vs 7% relapse at 1 year, respectively).[10] The lowest dose at which fluphenazine decanoate can be shown to be effective is 25 mg every 6 weeks.[11]

There is no simple formula for deciding when or whether to reduce the dose of maintenance antipsychotic treatment; therefore, a risk–benefit analysis must be done for every patient. Many patients, it should be noted, prefer to receive depots/LAIs.[12] When considering dose reduction, the following prompts may be helpful:

- Is the patient symptom-free and, if so, for how long? Long-standing, non-distressing symptoms which have not previously been responsive to medication may be excluded.
- What is the severity of the adverse effects (EPS including TD, metabolic adverse effects including obesity, etc.)? When patients report no or minimal adverse effects it is usually sensible to continue treatment and monitor closely for signs of TD.
- What is the previous pattern of illness? Consider the speed of onset, duration and severity of past relapses and any dangers or risks posed to self or others.
- Has dosage reduction been attempted before? If so, what was the outcome?
- What are the patient's current social circumstances? Is it a period of relative stability, or are stressful life events anticipated?
- What is the potential social cost of relapse (e.g. is the patient the sole breadwinner for a family)?
- Is the patient able to monitor his/her own symptoms? If so, will he/she seek help?

If, after consideration of the above, the decision is taken to reduce medication dose, the patient's family should be involved and a clear explanation given of what should be done if symptoms return or worsen. It would then be reasonable to proceed in the following manner:

- If it has not already been done, any co-prescribed oral antipsychotic medication should be discontinued.
- Where the product labelling allows, the interval between injections should be increased to up to 4 weeks before decreasing the dose given each time.
- The dose should be reduced by no more than a third at any one time. Note: special considerations apply to risperidone.
- Decrements should, if possible, be made no more frequently than every 3 months, preferably every 6 months. The slower the rate of withdrawal, the longer the time to relapse.[13]
- Discontinuation should not be seen as the ultimate aim of the above process although it sometimes results. NICE[14] (2014) now suggests that intermittent treatment (symptom-triggered) is preferable to no treatment.

If the patient becomes symptomatic, this should be seen not as a failure, but rather as an important step in determining the minimum effective dose that the patient requires.

For more discussion see section on 'Antipsychotic long-acting injections' in this chapter.

References

1. National Institute of Mental Health. Abnormal Involuntary Movement Scale (AIMS). (U.S. Public Health Service Publication No. MH-9-17). Washington, DC: US Government Printing Office; 1974.
2. Novick D et al. Incidence of extrapyramidal symptoms and tardive dyskinesia in schizophrenia: thirty-six-month results from the European schizophrenia outpatient health outcomes study. J Clin Psychopharmacol 2010; 30:531–540.
3. Barnes TR et al. Long-term depot antipsychotics. A risk-benefit assessment. Drug Saf 1994; 10:464–479.
4. Taylor D. Establishing a dose-response relationship for haloperidol decanoate. Psychiatr Bull 2005; 29:104–107.
5. McEvoy JP et al. Effectiveness of paliperidone palmitate vs haloperidol decanoate for maintenance treatment of schizophrenia: a randomized clinical trial. JAMA 2014; 311:1978–1987.
6. Rothe PH et al. Dose equivalents for second generation long-acting injectable antipsychotics: the minimum effective dose method. Schizophr Res 2017. doi: 10.1016/j.schres.2017.07.033. [Epub ahead of print]
7. Uchida H et al. Dose and dosing frequency of long-acting injectable antipsychotics: a systematic review of PET and SPECT data and clinical implications. J Clin Psychopharmacol 2014; 34:728–735.
8. Uchida H et al. Low dose vs standard dose of antipsychotics for relapse prevention in schizophrenia: meta-analysis. Schizophr Bull 2011; 37:788–799.
9. Marder SR et al. Low- and conventional-dose maintenance therapy with fluphenazine decanoate. Two-year outcome. Arch Gen Psychiatry 1987; 44:518–521.
10. Kane JM et al. Low-dose neuroleptic treatment of outpatient schizophrenics: I. preliminary results for relapse rates. Arch Gen Psychiatry 1983; 40:893–896.
11. Carpenter WT, Jr. et al. Comparative effectiveness of fluphenazine decanoate injections every 2 weeks versus every 6 weeks. Am J Psychiatry 1999; 156:412–418.
12. Heres S et al. The attitude of patients towards antipsychotic depot treatment. Int Clin Psychopharmacol 2007; 22:275–282.
13. Weiden PJ et al. Does half-life matter after antipsychotic discontinuation? a relapse comparison in schizophrenia with 3 different formulations of paliperidone. J Clin Psychiatry 2017; 78:e813–e820.
14. National Institute for Health and Care Excellence. Psychosis and schizophrenia in adults: prevention and management. Clinical Guideline 178, 2014. https://www.nice.org.uk/guidance/cg178

Aripiprazole long-acting injection

Aripiprazole lacks the prolactin-related and metabolic adverse effects of other SGA LAIs and so is a useful alternative to them. Placebo-controlled studies show a good acute and longer-term effect[1] but aripiprazole LAI has not been compared with other depots. For most patients, a suitable dosing regimen is oral aripiprazole 10 mg/day for 14 days (to establish tolerability and response) then 400 mg aripiprazole LAI once monthly. Oral aripiprazole should be continued for 14 days after the first injection. In such a regimen, peak plasma levels are seen 7 days after injection and the lowest trough at 4 weeks.[2] At steady state, peak plasma levels are up to 50% higher than the first dose peak and trough plasma levels only slightly below the first dose peak.[2] Dose adjustments should take this into account. A lower dose of 300 mg a month can be used in those not tolerating 400 mg. A dose of 200 mg a month may only be used for those patients receiving particular enzyme-inhibiting drugs. The incidence of akathisia, insomnia, nausea and restlessness is similar to that seen with oral aripiprazole.[3,4]

There are no formal recommendations for switching to aripiprazole but Table 1.12 presents recommendations based on our interpretation of available pharmacokinetic data.

A new long-acting formulation of aripiprazole has been approved by the FDA for the treatment of schizophrenia. Aripiprazole lauroxil is a pro-drug formulated to be administered at monthly, 6-weekly or 2-monthly intervals by IM injection into the deltoid or gluteal muscle depending on the dose.[5,6] It is available as four strengths: 441 mg, 662 mg, 882 mg and 1064 mg doses to deliver 300 mg, 450 mg, 600 mg and 724 mg of aripiprazole respectively (see section on 'Depot antipsychotics – pharmacokinetics' in this chapter).

Table 1.12 Switching to aripiprazole LAI

Switching from	Aripiprazole LAI regimen
Oral antipsychotics	Cross taper antipsychotic with oral aripiprazole* over 2 weeks. Start LAI, continue aripiprazole oral for 2 weeks then stop
Depot antipsychotics (not risperidone LAI)	Start oral aripiprazole* on day last depot injection was due. Start aripiprazole LAI after 2 weeks then stop oral aripiprazole 2 weeks later
Risperidone LAI	Start oral aripiprazole* 4–6 weeks after the last risperidone injection. Start aripiprazole LAI 2 weeks later; discontinue oral aripiprazole 2 weeks after that

*If prior response and tolerability to aripiprazole is known, oral aripiprazole may not be strictly required but attainment of effective aripiprazole plasma levels is dependent upon 4 weeks of oral supplementation so this is recommended in every situation.
LAI, long-acting injection.

References

1. Shirley M et al. Aripiprazole (ABILIFY MAINTENA®): a review of its use as maintenance treatment for adult patients with schizophrenia. Drugs 2014; 74:1097–1110.
2. Mallikaarjun S et al. Pharmacokinetics, tolerability and safety of aripiprazole once-monthly in adult schizophrenia: an open-label, parallel-arm, multiple-dose study. Schizophr Res 2013; 150:281–288.

3. Kane JM et al. Aripiprazole intramuscular depot as maintenance treatment in patients with schizophrenia: a 52-week, multicenter, randomized, double-blind, placebo-controlled study. J Clin Psychiatry 2012; 73:617–624.
4. Potkin SG et al. Safety and tolerability of once monthly aripiprazole treatment initiation in adults with schizophrenia stabilized on selected atypical oral antipsychotics other than aripiprazole. Curr Med Res Opin 2013; 29:1241–1251.
5. Hard ML et al. Aripiprazole lauroxil: pharmacokinetic profile of this long-acting injectable antipsychotic in persons with schizophrenia. J Clin Psychopharmacol 2017; 37:289–295.
6. Turncliff R et al. Relative bioavailability and safety of aripiprazole lauroxil, a novel once-monthly, long-acting injectable atypical antipsychotic, following deltoid and gluteal administration in adult subjects with schizophrenia. Schizophr Res 2014; 159:404–410.

Olanzapine long-acting injection

Like all esters, olanzapine pamoate (embonate, in some countries) is very poorly water soluble. An aqueous suspension of olanzapine pamoate, when injected intramuscularly, affords both prompt and sustained release of olanzapine. Peak plasma levels are seen within a week of injection (in most people within 2–4 days[1]) and efficacy can be demonstrated after only 3 days.[2] Only gluteal injection is licensed; deltoid injection is less effective.[3] Olanzapine LAI is effective when given every 4 weeks, with 2-weekly administration only required when the highest dose is prescribed. Half-life is around 30 days.[1] It has not been compared with other LAIs in RCTs but naturalistic data suggest similar effectiveness to paliperidone LAI.[4,5] Loading doses are recommended in some dose regimens (see Table 1.13). Formal labelling/SPC suggests that patients be given oral olanzapine to assess response and tolerability. This rarely happens in practice but is strongly recommended. Oral supplementation after the first depot injection is not necessary.

Switching

Direct switching to olanzapine LAI, ideally following an oral trial, is usually possible. So, when switching from another LAI (but not risperidone), olanzapine oral or LAI can be started on the day the last LAI was due. Likewise for switching from oral treatment – a direct switch is possible but prior antipsychotics are probably best reduced slowly after starting olanzapine (either oral or LAI). When switching from risperidone LAI, olanzapine should be started, we suggest, 2 weeks after the last injection was due (peak risperidone plasma levels can be expected 4–6 weeks after the last injection).

Post-injection syndrome

Post-injection syndrome occurs when olanzapine pamoate is inadvertently exposed to high blood volumes (probably via accidental intravasation[6]). Olanzapine plasma levels may reach 600 µg/L and delirium and somnolence result.[7] The incidence of post-injection syndrome is less than 0.1% of injections; almost all reactions (86%) occur within 1 hour of injection.[8] A more recent study suggested an incidence of 0.044% of injections (less than 1 in 2000) with 91% of reactions being apparent within 1 hour.[9] In most countries, olanzapine LAI may only be given in health-care facilities under

Table 1.13 Olanzapine LAI: dosing schedules

Oral olanzapine equivalent	Loading dose	Maintenance dose (given 8 weeks after the first dose)
10 mg/day	210 mg every 2 weeks	300 mg/4 weeks
	405 mg every 4 weeks	(or 150 mg every 2 weeks)
15 mg/day	300 mg every 2 weeks	405 mg/4 weeks
		(or 210 mg every 2 weeks)
20 mg/day	None – give 300 mg every 2 weeks	300 mg every 2 weeks

supervision and patients need to be kept under observation for 3 hours after the injection is given. Given the tiny number of cases appearing only after 2 hours, a good case can be made for shortening the observation period to 2 hours (as is the situation in New Zealand[10] and some other countries).

In the EU, the exact wording of the SPC[11] is as follows:

After each injection, patients should be observed in a healthcare facility by appropriately qualified personnel for at least 3 hours for signs and symptoms consistent with olanzapine overdose.

Immediately prior to leaving the healthcare facility, it should be confirmed that the patient is alert, oriented, and absent of any signs and symptoms of overdose. If an overdose is suspected, close medical supervision and monitoring should continue until examination indicates that signs and symptoms have resolved. The 3-hour observation period should be extended as clinically appropriate for patients who exhibit any signs or symptoms consistent with olanzapine overdose.

For the remainder of the day after injection, patients should be advised to be vigilant for signs and symptoms of overdose secondary to post-injection adverse reactions, be able to obtain assistance if needed, and should not drive or operate machinery.

This monitoring requirement undoubtedly has adversely affected the popularity of olanzapine LAI. No patient or medical factor has been identified that might predict post-injection syndrome[7] except that those experiencing the syndrome are more likely to have previously had an injection-site-related adverse effect.[12] Male gender and higher doses have more recently been suggested to be risk factors for post-injection syndrome (the study examined 46 events occurring in 103,505 injections).[9]

References

1. Heres S et al. Pharmacokinetics of olanzapine long-acting injection: the clinical perspective. Int Clin Psychopharmacol 2014; 29:299–312.

2. Lauriello J et al. An 8-week, double-blind, randomized, placebo-controlled study of olanzapine long-acting injection in acutely ill patients with schizophrenia. J Clin Psychiatry 2008; 69:790–799.

3. Mitchell M et al. Single- and multiple-dose pharmacokinetic, safety, and tolerability profiles of olanzapine long-acting injection: an open-label, multicenter, nonrandomized study in patients with schizophrenia. Clin Ther 2013; 35:1890–1908.

4. Denee TR et al. Treatment continuation and treatment characteristics of four long acting antipsychotic medications (paliperidone palmitate, risperidone microspheres, olanzapine pamoate and haloperidol decanoate) in the Netherlands. Value Health 2015; 18:A407.

5. Taipale H et al. Comparative effectiveness of antipsychotic drugs for rehospitalization in schizophrenia – a nationwide study with 20-year follow-up. Schizophr Bull 2017; doi: 10.1093/schbul/sbx176. [Epub ahead of print]

6. Luedecke D et al. Post-injection delirium/sedation syndrome in patients treated with olanzapine pamoate: mechanism, incidence, and management. CNS Drugs 2015; 29:41–46.

7. McDonnell DP et al. Post-injection delirium/sedation syndrome in patients with schizophrenia treated with olanzapine long-acting injection, II: investigations of mechanism. BMC Psychiatry 2010; 10:45.

8. Bushes CJ et al. Olanzapine long-acting injection: review of first experiences of post-injection delirium/sedation syndrome in routine clinical practice. Eli Lilly personal communication. 2013.

9. Meyers KJ et al. Postinjection delirium/sedation syndrome in patients with schizophrenia receiving olanzapine long-acting injection: results from a large observational study. BJPsych Open 2017; 3:186–192.

10. Eli Lilly and Company (NZ) Limited. ZYPREXA RELPREVV® (olanzapine pamoate monohydrate). 2016. http://www.medsafe.govt.nz/profs/Datasheet/z/zyprexarelprevvinj.pdf

11. Eli Lilly and Company Limited. Summary of Product Characteristics. ZYPADHERA 210 mg powder and solvent for prolonged release suspension for injection. 2017. https://www.medicines.org.uk/emc/product/6429

12. Atkins S et al. A pooled analysis of injection site-related adverse events in patients with schizophrenia treated with olanzapine long-acting injection. BMC Psychiatry 2014; 14:7.

Paliperidone palmitate long-acting injection

Paliperidone is the major active metabolite of risperidone: 9-hydroxyrisperidone.

Paliperidone LAI 1-monthly

Following an IM injection, active paliperidone plasma levels are seen within a few days, therefore co-administration of oral paliperidone or risperidone during initiation is not required.[1] Dosing consists of two initiation doses (deltoid) followed by monthly maintenance doses (deltoid or gluteal) (Table 1.14). Following administration of a single IM dose to the deltoid muscle, on average 28% higher peak concentration is observed compared with IM injection to the gluteal muscle.[1] Thus the two deltoid muscle injections on days 1 and 8 help to quickly attain therapeutic drug concentrations.

Paliperidone LAI has been compared with haloperidol depot given in a loading dose schedule matching that of paliperidone.[2] The two formulations were equally effective in preventing relapse but paliperidone increased prolactin to a greater extent and caused more weight gain. Haloperidol caused more akathisia and more acute movement disorder, and there was a trend for a higher incidence of TD. The average dose of haloperidol was around 75 mg a month, a dose rarely used in practice.

The second initiation dose may be given 4 days before or after day 8 (after the first initiation dose on day 1).[3] Similarly, the manufacturer recommends that patients may be given maintenance doses up to 7 days before or after the monthly time point.[3] This flexibility should help minimise the number of missed doses. See manufacturer's information for full recommendations around missed doses.[3]

Points to note:

- No test dose is required for paliperidone palmitate (but patients should ideally be currently stabilised on or have previously responded to oral paliperidone or risperidone).
- The median time to maximum plasma concentrations is 13 days.[3]

The approximate dose equivalents of different formulations of risperidone and paliperidone are shown in Table 1.15. Switching to paliperidone palmitate is shown in Table 1.16.

Table 1.14 Paliperidone dose and administration information[1]

	Dose	Route
Initiation		
Day 1	150 mg IM	Deltoid only
Day 8 (±4 days)	100 mg IM	Deltoid only
Maintenance		
Every month (±7 days) thereafter	50–150 mg IM*	Deltoid or gluteal

*The maintenance dose is perhaps best judged by consideration of what might be a suitable dose of oral risperidone and then giving paliperidone palmitate in an equivalent dose (see Table 1.15).
IM, intramuscularly.

Table 1.15 Approximate dose equivalence[1,3]

Risperidone oral (mg/day) (bioavailability = 70%)[4]	Paliperidone oral (mg/day) (bioavailability = 28%)[5]	Risperidone LAI (Consta) (mg/2 weeks)	Paliperidone palmitate (mg/monthly)
2	4	25	50
3	6	37.5	75
4	9	50	100
6	12	–	150

Table 1.16 Switching to paliperidone palmitate 1-monthly LAI

Switching from	Recommended method of switching	Comments
No treatment	Give the two initiation doses: 150 mg IM deltoid on day 1 and 100 mg IM deltoid on day 8 Maintenance dose starts 1 month later	In general the lowest most effective maintenance dose should be used The manufacturer recommends a dose of 75 mg monthly for the general adult population.[1] This is approximately equivalent to 3 mg/day oral risperidone (see Table 1.15). In practice the modal dose is 100 mg/month[6] Maintenance dose adjustments should be made monthly. However, the full effect of the dose adjustment may not be apparent for several months[3]
Oral paliperidone/ risperidone	Give the two initiation doses followed by the maintenance dose (see Table 1.15 and prescribe equivalent dose)	Oral paliperidone/risperidone supplementation during initiation is not necessary
Oral antipsychotics	Reduce the dose of the oral antipsychotic over 1–2 weeks following the first injection of paliperidone. Give the two initiation doses followed by the maintenance dose	
Depot antipsychotic	Start paliperidone (at the maintenance dose) when the next injection is due N.B. No initiation doses are required	Doses of paliperidone palmitate IM may be difficult to predict. The manufacturer recommends a dose of 75 mg monthly for the general adult population. If switching from risperidone LAI see Table 1.15 and prescribe equivalent dose Maintenance dose adjustments should be made monthly. However, the full effect of the dose adjustment may not be apparent for several months[3]
Antipsychotic polypharmacy with depot	Start paliperidone (at the maintenance dose) when the next injection is due N.B. No initiation doses are required Reduce the dose of the oral antipsychotic over 1–2 weeks following the first injection of paliperidone	Aim to treat the patient with paliperidone palmitate IM as the sole antipsychotic The maintenance dose should be governed as far as possible by the total dose of oral and injectable antipsychotic (see Table 1.15)

Paliperidone LAI 3-monthly

Paliperidone LAI 3-monthly is indicated for patients who are clinically stable on paliperidone LAI 1-monthly (preferably for 4 months or more) and do not require dose adjustment.[7]

Paliperidone LAI 3-monthly is generally well tolerated, with a tolerability profile similar to the 1-monthly preparation,[8,9] and is non-inferior to paliperidone 1-monthly in terms of relapse rate.[8]

When initiating paliperidone LAI 3-monthly, give the first dose in place of the next scheduled dose of paliperidone LAI 1-monthly. The dose of paliperidone LAI 3-monthly should be based on the previous paliperidone LAI 1-monthly dose, see Table 1.17.

Table 1.17 Dosing of paliperidone LAI 3-monthly[7]

Dose of paliperidone LAI 1-monthly	Dose of paliperidone LAI 3-monthly
50 mg	175 mg
75 mg	263 mg
100 mg	350 mg
150 mg	525 mg

References

1. Janssen Pharmaceutical Companies. Highlights of Prescribing Information. INVEGA SUSTENNA (paliperidone palmitate) extended-release injectable suspension, for intramuscular use. 2017. http://www.janssenlabels.com/package-insert/product-monograph/prescribing-information/INVEGA+SUSTENNA-pi.pdf

2. McEvoy JP et al. Effectiveness of paliperidone palmitate vs haloperidol decanoate for maintenance treatment of schizophrenia: a randomized clinical trial. JAMA 2014; 311:1978–1987.

3. Janssen-Cilag Ltd. Summary of Product Characteristics. Xeplion 25 mg, 50 mg, 75 mg, 100 mg, and 150 mg prolonged-release suspension for injection. 2016. https://www.medicines.org.uk/emc/medicine/31329

4. Janssen-Cilag Ltd. Summary of Product Characteristics. Risperdal Tablets, Liquid & Quicklet. 2018. https://www.medicines.org.uk/emc/product/6857

5. Janssen-Cilag Ltd. Summary of Product Characteristics. INVEGA 1.5 mg, 3 mg, 6 mg, 9 mg, 12 mg prolonged-release tablets. 2018. https://www.medicines.org.uk/emc/product/6816

6. Attard A et al. Paliperidone palmitate long-acting injection – prospective year-long follow-up of use in clinical practice. Acta Psychiatr Scand 2014; 130:46–51.

7. Janssen-Cilag Ltd. Summary of Product Characteristics. TREVICTA 175 mg, 263 mg, 350 mg, 525 mg prolonged release suspension for injection. 2017. https://www.medicines.org.uk/emc/medicine/32050

8. Lamb YN et al. Paliperidone palmitate intramuscular 3-monthly formulation: a review in schizophrenia. Drugs 2016; 76:1559–1566.

9. Ravenstijn P et al. Pharmacokinetics, safety, and tolerability of paliperidone palmitate 3-month formulation in patients with schizophrenia: a phase-1, single-dose, randomized, open-label study. J Clin Pharmacol 2016; 56:330–339.

Risperidone long-acting injection

Risperidone was the first 'atypical' drug to be made available as a depot, or LAI, formulation. Doses of 25–50 mg every 2 weeks appear to be as effective as oral doses of 2–6 mg/day.[1] The long-acting injection (RLAI) also seems to be well tolerated – fewer than 10% of patients experienced EPS and fewer than 6% withdrew from a long-term trial because of adverse effects.[2] Oral risperidone increases prolactin,[3] as does RLAI,[4] but levels appear to reduce somewhat following a switch from oral to injectable risperidone.[5-7] Rates of TD are said to be low.[8] There are no direct comparisons with standard depots using randomised controlled designs but comparisons from observational studies are available and results have been mixed. Switching from FGA depots in stable patients to RLAI has been shown to be less successful than remaining on the FGA depot;[9] in contrast, discontinuation rates were lower with RLAI when compared with FGAs.[10]

Uncertainty remains over the dose–response relationship for RLAI. Studies randomising subjects to different fixed doses of RLAI show no differences in response according to dose.[11] One randomised, fixed-dose, year-long study suggested better outcome for 50 mg every 2 weeks than with 25 mg, although no observed difference reached statistical significance.[12] Naturalistic studies indicate doses higher than 25 mg/2 weeks are frequently used.[13,14] One study suggested higher doses were associated with better outcome.[15,16]

Plasma levels afforded by 25 mg/2 weeks seem to be similar to, or even lower than, levels provided by 2 mg/day oral risperidone.[17,18] (One study found that 9.5% of plasma samples from people apparently receiving risperidone LAI contained no risperidone or 9-hydroxyrisperidone[19].) Striatal dopamine D_2 occupancies are similarly low in people receiving 25 mg/2 weeks.[20,21] So, although fixed-dose studies have not revealed clear advantages for doses above 25 mg/2 weeks, other indicators cast doubt on the assumption that 25 mg/2 weeks will be adequate for all or even most patients. While this conundrum remains unresolved the need for careful dose titration becomes of great importance. Titration is perhaps most efficiently achieved by establishing the required dose of oral risperidone and converting this dose into the equivalent injection dose. Trials have clearly established that switching from 2 mg oral to 25 mg injection and 4 mg oral to 50 mg injection is usually successful[2,22,23] (switching from 4 mg/day to 25 mg/2 weeks increases the risk of relapse[24]). There remains a question over the equivalent dose for 6 mg oral: in theory, patients should be switched to 75 mg injection but this showed no advantage over lower doses in clinical trials and is in any case above the licensed maximum dose. Nevertheless, an observational study reported successful outcomes in patients treated with doses in excess of 75 mg/2 weeks (range 75–200 mg) with continuation rates of 95% after 3 years.[25] Paliperidone palmitate 150 mg a month is equivalent to oral risperidone 6 mg/day. In fact, for many reasons, paliperidone palmitate (9-hydroxyrisperidone) may be preferred to risperidone injection: it acts acutely, can be given monthly, does not require cold storage and has a wider, more useful dose range (see section on 'Paliperidone palmitate long-acting injection' in this chapter).

RLAI differs importantly from other depots and the following should be noted:

- Risperidone depot is not an esterified form of the parent drug. It contains risperidone coated in polymer to form microspheres. These microspheres have to be suspended in an aqueous base immediately before use.

Table 1.18 Switching to risperidone long-acting injection (RLAI)

Switching from	Recommended method of switching	Comments
No treatment (new patient or recently non-compliant)	Start risperidone oral at 2 mg/day and titrate to effective dose. If tolerated, prescribe equivalent dose of RLAI Continue with oral risperidone for at least 3 weeks then taper over 1–2 weeks. Be prepared to continue oral risperidone for longer	Use oral risperidone before giving injection to assure good tolerability Those stabilised on 2 mg/day, start on 25 mg/2 weeks Those on higher doses, start on 37.5 mg/2 weeks and be prepared to use 50 mg/2 weeks (Manufacturer advice may differ from this – our guidance is based on numerous studies of dose-related outcome and on comparative plasma levels)
Oral risperidone	Prescribe equivalent dose of RLAI	See above
Oral antipsychotics (not risperidone)	*Either:* a. Switch to oral risperidone and titrate to effective dose. If tolerated, prescribe equivalent dose of RLAI Continue with oral risperidone for at least 3 weeks then taper over 1–2 weeks. Be prepared to continue oral risperidone for longer *Or:* b. Give RLAI and then slowly discontinue oral antipsychotics after 3–4 weeks. Be prepared to continue oral antipsychotics for longer	Dose assessment is difficult in those switching from another antipsychotic. Broadly speaking, those on low oral doses should be switched to 25 mg/2 weeks 'Low' in this context means towards the lower end of the licensed dose range or around the minimum dose known to be effective Those on higher oral doses should receive 37.5 mg or 50 mg every 2 weeks. The continued need for oral antipsychotics after 3–4 weeks may indicate that higher doses of RLAI are required
Depot antipsychotic	Give RLAI 1 week *before* the last depot injection is given	Dose of RLAI difficult to predict. For those on low doses (see above) start at 25 mg/2 weeks and then adjust as necessary Start RLAI at 37.5 mg/2 weeks in those previously maintained on doses in the middle or upper range of licensed doses. Be prepared to increase to 50 mg/2 weeks
Antipsychotic polypharmacy with depot	Give RLAI 1 week before the last depot injection is given Slowly taper oral antipsychotics 3–4 weeks later. Be prepared to continue oral antipsychotics for longer	Aim to treat patient with RLAI as the sole antipsychotic. As before, RLAI dose should be dictated, as far as is possible, by the total dose of oral and injectable antipsychotic

RLAI, risperidone long-acting injection.

- The injection must be stored in a fridge (consider the practicalities for community staff).
- It is available as doses of 25, 37.5 and 50 mg. The whole vial must be used (because of the nature of the suspension). This means that there is limited flexibility in dosing.

- A test dose is not required or sensible. (Testing tolerability with oral risperidone is desirable but not always practical.)
- It takes 3–4 weeks for the first injection to produce therapeutic plasma levels. Patients must be maintained on a full dose of their previous antipsychotic for at least 3 weeks after the administration of the first risperidone injection. Oral antipsychotic cover is sometimes required for longer (6–8 weeks). If the patient is not already receiving an oral antipsychotic, oral risperidone should be prescribed. (See Table 1.18 for advice on switching from depots.) **Patients who refuse oral treatment and are acutely ill should not be given RLAI because of the long delay in drug release.**
- Risperidone depot must be administered every 2 weeks. The product licence does not allow longer intervals between doses. There is little flexibility to negotiate with patients about the frequency of administration, although monthly injections may be effective.[26]
- The most effective way of predicting response to RLAI is to establish dose and response with oral risperidone.
- Risperidone injection is not considered suitable for patients with treatment-refractory schizophrenia, although there are studies showing positive effects.[27,28]

For guidance on switching to RLAI see Table 1.18.

Two new RLAIs are in development at the time of writing and are designed to deliver risperidone through monthly injections. RBP-7000 is a subcutaneous injection that has been approved by the FDA for the treatment of schizophrenia. Risperidone-ISM, which is undergoing Phase 3 trials, is designed to be given via the IM route. Both preparations form a biodegradable implant after injection to deliver risperidone in a sustained-release fashion.[29,30]

References

1. Chue P et al. Comparative efficacy and safety of long-acting risperidone and risperidone oral tablets. Eur Neuropsychopharmacol 2005; 15:111–117.
2. Fleischhacker WW et al. Treatment of schizophrenia with long-acting injectable risperidone: a 12-month open-label trial of the first long-acting second-generation antipsychotic. J Clin Psychiatry 2003; 64:1250–1257.
3. Kleinberg DL et al. Prolactin levels and adverse events in patients treated with risperidone. J Clin Psychopharmacol 1999; 19:57–61.
4. Fu DJ et al. Paliperidone palmitate versus oral risperidone and risperidone long-acting injection in patients with recently diagnosed schizophrenia: a tolerability and efficacy comparison. Int Clin Psychopharmacol 2014; 29:45–55.
5. Bai YM et al. A comparative efficacy and safety study of long-acting risperidone injection and risperidone oral tablets among hospitalized patients: 12-week randomized, single-blind study. Pharmacopsychiatry 2006; 39:135–141.
6. Bai YM et al. Pharmacokinetics study for hyperprolactinemia among schizophrenics switched from risperidone to risperidone long-acting injection. J Clin Psychopharmacol 2007; 27:306–308.
7. Peng PW et al. The disparity of pharmacokinetics and prolactin study for risperidone long-acting injection. J Clin Psychopharmacol 2008; 28:726–727.
8. Gharabawi GM et al. An assessment of emergent tardive dyskinesia and existing dyskinesia in patients receiving long-acting, injectable risperidone: results from a long-term study. Schizophr Res 2005; 77:129–139.
9. Covell NH et al. Effectiveness of switching from long-acting injectable fluphenazine or haloperidol decanoate to long-acting injectable risperidone microspheres: an open-label, randomized controlled trial. J Clin Psychiatry 2012; 73:669–675.
10. Suzuki H et al. Comparison of treatment retention between risperidone long-acting injection and first-generation long-acting injections in patients with schizophrenia for 5 years. J Clin Psychopharmacol 2016; 36:405–406.
11. Kane JM et al. Long-acting injectable risperidone: efficacy and safety of the first long-acting atypical antipsychotic. Am J Psychiatry 2003; 160:1125–1132.
12. Simpson GM et al. A 1-year double-blind study of 2 doses of long-acting risperidone in stable patients with schizophrenia or schizoaffective disorder. J Clin Psychiatry 2006; 67:1194–1203.
13. Turner M et al. Long-acting injectable risperidone: safety and efficacy in stable patients switched from conventional depot antipsychotics. Int Clin Psychopharmacol 2004; 19:241–249.

14. Taylor DM et al. Early clinical experience with risperidone long-acting injection: a prospective, 6-month follow-up of 100 patients. J Clin Psychiatry 2004; 65:1076–1083.

15. Taylor DM et al. Prospective 6-month follow-up of patients prescribed risperidone long-acting injection: factors predicting favourable outcome. Int J Neuropsychopharmacol 2006; 9:685–694.

16. Taylor DM et al. Risperidone long-acting injection: a prospective 3-year analysis of its use in clinical practice. J Clin Psychiatry 2009; 70:196–200.

17. Nesvag R et al. Serum concentrations of risperidone and 9-OH risperidone following intramuscular injection of long-acting risperidone compared with oral risperidone medication. Acta Psychiatr Scand 2006; 114:21–26.

18. Castberg I et al. Serum concentrations of risperidone and 9-hydroxyrisperidone after administration of the long-acting injectable form of risperidone: evidence from a routine therapeutic drug monitoring service. Ther Drug Monit 2005; 27:103–106.

19. Bowskill SV et al. Risperidone and total 9-hydroxyrisperidone in relation to prescribed dose and other factors: data from a therapeutic drug monitoring service, 2002-2010. Ther Drug Monit 2012; 34:349–355.

20. Gefvert O et al. Pharmacokinetics and D2 receptor occupancy of long-acting injectable risperidone (Risperdal Consta™) in patients with schizophrenia. Int J Neuropsychopharmacol 2005; 8:27–36.

21. Remington G et al. A PET study evaluating dopamine D2 receptor occupancy for long-acting injectable risperidone. Am J Psychiatry 2006; 163:396–401.

22. Lasser RA et al. Clinical improvement in 336 stable chronically psychotic patients changed from oral to long-acting risperidone: a 12-month open trial. Int J Neuropsychopharmacol 2005; 8:427–438.

23. Lauriello J et al. Long-acting risperidone vs. placebo in the treatment of hospital inpatients with schizophrenia. Schizophr Res 2005; 72:249–258.

24. Bai YM et al. Equivalent switching dose from oral risperidone to risperidone long-acting injection: a 48-week randomized, prospective, single-blind pharmacokinetic study. J Clin Psychiatry 2007; 68:1218–1225.

25. Fernandez-Miranda JJ et al. Effectiveness, good tolerability, and high compliance of doses of risperidone long-acting injectable higher than 75 mg in people with severe schizophrenia: a 3-year follow-up. J Clin Psychopharmacol 2015; 35:630–634.

26. Uchida H et al. Monthly administration of long-acting injectable risperidone and striatal dopamine D2 receptor occupancy for the management of schizophrenia. J Clin Psychiatry 2008; 69:1281–1286.

27. Meltzer HY et al. A six month randomized controlled trial of long acting injectable risperidone 50 and 100 mg in treatment resistant schizophrenia. Schizophr Res 2014; 154:14–22.

28. Kimura H et al. Risperidone long-acting injectable in the treatment of treatment-resistant schizophrenia with dopamine supersensitivity psychosis: results of a 2-year prospective study, including an additional 1-year follow-up. J Psychopharmacol 2016; 30:795–802.

29. Llaudo J et al. Phase I, open-label, randomized, parallel study to evaluate the pharmacokinetics, safety, and tolerability of one intramuscular injection of risperidone ISM at different dose strengths in patients with schizophrenia or schizoaffective disorder (PRISMA-1). Int Clin Psychopharmacol 2016; 31:323–331.

30. Laffont CM et al. Population pharmacokinetics and prediction of dopamine D2 receptor occupancy after multiple doses of RBP-7000, a new sustained-release formulation of risperidone, in schizophrenia patients on stable oral risperidone treatment. Clin Pharmacokinet 2014; 53:533–543.

Electroconvulsive therapy and psychosis

A Cochrane systematic review[1] reviewed randomised controlled clinical trials that compared ECT with placebo (sham ECT), non-pharmacological interventions and antipsychotic medication for patients with schizophrenia, schizoaffective disorder or chronic mental disorder. Where ECT was compared with placebo or sham ECT, more people improved in the real ECT group and there was a suggestion that real ECT resulted in fewer relapses in the short term and a greater likelihood of being discharged from hospital. The review concluded that ECT combined with continuing antipsychotic medication is a valid treatment option for schizophrenia, particularly when rapid global improvement and reduction of symptoms were desired, and where the illness had shown only a limited response to medication alone. Treatment guidelines for schizophrenia suggest the use of ECT for catatonia[2,3] and treatment-resistant illness.[1,4]

Recent studies have focussed on ECT augmentation of antipsychotic medication for treatment-resistant schizophrenia (TRS).[5-9] For example, in a relatively small sample of patients with TRS characterised by 'dominant negative symptoms', ECT augmentation of a variety of antipsychotic medications produced a significant decrease in symptom severity.[10] A meta-analysis of RCTs[8] examined the efficacy of the combination of ECT and (non-clozapine) antipsychotic medication versus the same antipsychotic medication as monotherapy, in TRS. The combination proved to be superior in terms of symptom improvement, study-defined response and remission rate.

Augmentation of clozapine may be at least as effective as ECT augmentation of other antipsychotic medications, if not more so.[9,11,12] In a retrospective study[6] assessing the effectiveness and safety of the combination of clozapine and ECT in a sample of patients with TRS, almost two-thirds were responders (defined as a 30% or greater reduction in PANSS total score). Follow-up data on a sub-sample of these patients, over a mean of 30 months, revealed that the majority had maintained their symptomatic improvement or improved further. In a randomised, single-blind study,[7] patients with clozapine-refractory schizophrenia either continued solely on their clozapine treatment or had it augmented with a course of bilateral ECT. After 8 weeks, a predefined response criterion (including a 40% or greater reduction in symptoms) was met by half the patients receiving clozapine plus ECT but none of the group on clozapine alone. When the non-responders from the clozapine-alone group crossed over to an 8-week, open trial of ECT, nearly half met the response criterion. A systematic review and meta-analysis[13] looking specifically at ECT augmentation of clozapine found a paucity of controlled studies, although the authors acknowledged the methodological challenges of such investigations. Analysis of the data from the controlled and open trials and case reports identified suggested that ECT augmentation of clozapine may be an efficacious and safe strategy in TRS, but the authors considered that double-blind studies of ECT augmentation were required, particularly given the potentially strong placebo effect.

Although ECT augmentation of continuing antipsychotic medication appears to be generally well tolerated, adverse effects such as transient memory impairment and headache have been reported for a minority of cases[8-10,14] and there are reports of an increase in blood pressure after ECT and prolonged seizures.[6]

In summary, the evidence supports ECT augmentation of pharmacotherapy, particularly clozapine, as an effective combination to improve mental state in TRS,[15] although further, well-controlled trials are required to establish the benefit–risk balance of the combination in both the short and long term.

References

1. Tharyan P et al. Electroconvulsive therapy for schizophrenia. Cochrane Database Syst Rev 2005; **2**:CD000076.
2. Pompili M et al. Indications for electroconvulsive treatment in schizophrenia: a systematic review. Schizophr Res 2013; **146**:1–9.
3. The National Institute for Health and Care Excellence. Guidance on the use of electroconvulsive therapy. Technology appraisal guidance (TA)59, 2003. https://www.nice.org.uk/guidance/ta59/documents
4. Weiner RD et al. *The Practice of Electroconvulsive Therapy: Recommendations for Treatment, Training, and Privileging: a Task Force Report of the American Psychiatric Association*, 2nd edn. Washington, DC: American Psychiatric Association; 2001.
5. Masoudzadeh A et al. Comparative study of clozapine, electroshock and the combination of ECT with clozapine in treatment-resistant schizophrenic patients. Pak J Biol Sci 2007; **10**:4287–4290.
6. Grover S et al. Effectiveness of electroconvulsive therapy in patients with treatment resistant schizophrenia: a retrospective study. Psychiatry Res 2017; **249**:349–353.
7. Petrides G et al. Electroconvulsive therapy augmentation in clozapine-resistant schizophrenia: a prospective, randomized study. Am J Psychiatry 2015; **172**:52–58.
8. Zheng W et al. Electroconvulsive therapy added to non-clozapine antipsychotic medication for treatment resistant schizophrenia: meta-analysis of randomized controlled trials. PLoS One 2016; **11**:e0156510.
9. Kaster TS et al. Clinical effectiveness and cognitive impact of electroconvulsive therapy for schizophrenia: a large retrospective study. J Clin Psychiatry 2017; **78**:e383–e389.
10. Pawełczyk T et al. Augmentation of antipsychotics with electroconvulsive therapy in treatment-resistant schizophrenia patients with dominant negative symptoms: a pilot study of effectiveness. Neuropsychobiology 2014; **70**:158–164.
11. Amed S et al. Combined use of electroconvulsive therapy and antipsychotics (both clozapine and non-clozapine) in treatment resistant schizophrenia: a comparative meta-analysis. Heliyon 2017; **3**:e00429.
12. Kim HS et al. Effectiveness of electroconvulsive therapy augmentation on clozapine-resistant schizophrenia. Psychiatry Investig 2017; **14**:58–62.
13. Lally J et al. Augmentation of clozapine with electroconvulsive therapy in treatment resistant schizophrenia: a systematic review and meta-analysis. Schizophr Res 2016; **171**:215–224.
14. Zheng W et al. Memory impairment following electroconvulsive therapy in Chinese patients with schizophrenia: meta-analysis of randomized controlled trials. Perspect Psychiatr Care 2017. doi: 10.1111/ppc.12206. [Epub ahead of print]
15. Zervas IM et al. Using ECT in schizophrenia: a review from a clinical perspective. World J Biol Psychiatry 2012; **13**:96–105.

Omega-3 fatty acid (fish oils) in schizophrenia

Fish oils contain the omega-3 fatty acids, eicosapentaenoic acid (EPA) and docosahexaenoic acid (DHA), also known as polyunsaturated fatty acids or PUFAs. These compounds are thought to be involved in maintaining neuronal membrane structure, in the modulation of membrane proteins and in the production of prostaglandins and leukotrienes.[1] High dietary intake of PUFAs may protect against psychosis[2] and antipsychotic treatment seems to normalise PUFA deficits.[3] Animal models suggest a protective effect for PUFAs.[4] PUFAs have been suggested as treatments for a variety of psychiatric illnesses;[5,6] in schizophrenia, case reports,[7–9] case series[10] and prospective trials originally suggested useful efficacy.[11–15]

A meta-analysis of these RCTs[16] concluded that EPA has 'no beneficial effect in established schizophrenia', although the estimate of effect size (0.242) approached statistical significance. Since then, an RCT comprising 71 patients with first-episode schizophrenia given 2.2 g EPA + DHA daily for 6 months showed a reduction in symptom severity for patients in the active arm, finding an NNT (number needed to treat for one patient to benefit) of 4 to produce a 50% reduction in symptoms measured by Positive and Negative Syndrome Scale (PANSS).[17] However, a further RCT of 97 subjects with acute psychosis showed no advantage for EPA 2 g daily[18] and a relapse prevention study of EPA 2 g + DHA 1 g a day failed to demonstrate any value for PUFAs over placebo (relapse rate was 90% with PUFAs, 75% with placebo).[19]

On balance, evidence now suggests that EPA (2–3 g daily) is unlikely to be a worthwhile option in schizophrenia when added to standard treatment. Set against doubts over efficacy are the observations that fish oils are relatively cheap, well tolerated (mild gastrointestinal symptoms may occur) and benefit physical health.[1,20–23] In addition, a study of 700 mg EPA + 480 mg DHA in adolescents and young adults at high risk of psychosis showed that such treatment greatly reduced emergence of psychotic symptoms compared with placebo[24] (although a review described this study as 'very low quality evidence'[25]). Since this single-site study, the large, multisite NEURAPRO trial[26] gave adult patients at high risk of psychosis 840 mg EPA + 560 mg DHA for 6 months, and failed to find any evidence of efficacy either for reduction in transition to psychosis or improvement in symptoms. Two further multisite trials are currently ongoing.

PUFAs are no longer recommended for the treatment of residual symptoms of schizophrenia or for the prevention of transition to psychosis in young people at high risk. If used, careful assessment of response is important and fish oils should be withdrawn if no effect is observed after 3 months' treatment unless they are required for their beneficial metabolic effects.

Recommendations

- **Patients at high risk of first-episode psychosis.** Not recommended. If used, suggest EPA 700 mg/day (2 × Omacor or 6 × Maxepa capsules).
- **Residual symptoms of multi-episode schizophrenia (added to antipsychotic).** Not recommended. If used, suggest dose of **EPA 2 g/day** (5 × Omacor or 10 × Maxepa capsules).

References

1. Fenton WS et al. Essential fatty acids, lipid membrane abnormalities, and the diagnosis and treatment of schizophrenia. Biol Psychiatry 2000; 47:8–21.
2. Hedelin M et al. Dietary intake of fish, omega-3, omega-6 polyunsaturated fatty acids and vitamin D and the prevalence of psychotic-like symptoms in a cohort of 33,000 women from the general population. BMC Psychiatry 2010; 10:38.
3. Sethom MM et al. Polyunsaturated fatty acids deficits are associated with psychotic state and negative symptoms in patients with schizophrenia. Prostaglandins Leukot Essent Fatty Acids 2010; 83:131–136.
4. Zugno AI et al. Omega-3 prevents behavior response and brain oxidative damage in the ketamine model of schizophrenia. Neuroscience 2014; 259:223–231.
5. Freeman MP. Omega-3 fatty acids in psychiatry: a review. Ann Clin Psychiatry 2000; 12:159–165.
6. Ross BM et al. Omega-3 fatty acids as treatments for mental illness: which disorder and which fatty acid? Lipids Health Dis 2007; 6:21.
7. Richardson AJ et al. Red cell and plasma fatty acid changes accompanying symptom remission in a patient with schizophrenia treated with eicosapentaenoic acid. Eur Neuropsychopharmacol 2000; 10:189–193.
8. Puri BK et al. Eicosapentaenoic acid treatment in schizophrenia associated with symptom remission, normalisation of blood fatty acids, reduced neuronal membrane phospholipid turnover and structural brain changes. Int J Clin Pract 2000; 54:57–63.
9. Su KP et al. Omega-3 fatty acids as a psychotherapeutic agent for a pregnant schizophrenic patient. Eur Neuropsychopharmacol 2001; 11:295–299.
10. Sivrioglu EY et al. The impact of omega-3 fatty acids, vitamins E and C supplementation on treatment outcome and side effects in schizophrenia patients treated with haloperidol: an open-label pilot study. Prog Neuropsychopharmacol Biol Psychiatry 2007; 31:1493–1499.
11. Mellor JE et al. Schizophrenic symptoms and dietary intake of n-3 fatty acids. Schizophr Res 1995; 18:85–86.
12. Peet M et al. Two double-blind placebo-controlled pilot studies of eicosapentaenoic acid in the treatment of schizophrenia. Schizophr Res 2001; 49:243–251.
13. Fenton WS et al. A placebo-controlled trial of omega-3 fatty acid (ethyl eicosapentaenoic acid) supplementation for residual symptoms and cognitive impairment in schizophrenia. Am J Psychiatry 2001; 158:2071–2074.
14. Emsley R et al. Randomized, placebo-controlled study of ethyl-eicosapentaenoic acid as supplemental treatment in schizophrenia. Am J Psychiatry 2002; 159:1596–1598.
15. Berger GE et al. Ethyl-eicosapentaenoic acid in first-episode psychosis: a randomized, placebo-controlled trial. J Clin Psychiatry 2007; 68:1867–1875.
16. Fusar-Poli P et al. Eicosapentaenoic acid interventions in schizophrenia: meta-analysis of randomized, placebo-controlled studies. J Clin Psychopharmacol 2012; 32:179–185.
17. Pawelczyk T et al. A randomized controlled study of the efficacy of six-month supplementation with concentrated fish oil rich in omega-3 polyunsaturated fatty acids in first episode schizophrenia. J Psychiatr Res 2016; 73:34–44.
18. Bentsen H et al. A randomized placebo-controlled trial of an omega-3 fatty acid and vitamins E + C in schizophrenia. Transl Psychiatry 2013; 3:e335.
19. Emsley R et al. A randomized, controlled trial of omega-3 fatty acids plus an antioxidant for relapse prevention after antipsychotic discontinuation in first-episode schizophrenia. Schizophr Res 2014; 158:230–235.
20. Scorza FA et al. Omega-3 fatty acids and sudden cardiac death in schizophrenia: if not a friend, at least a great colleague. Schizophr Res 2007; 94:375–376.
21. Caniato RN et al. Effect of omega-3 fatty acids on the lipid profile of patients taking clozapine. Aust N Z J Psychiatry 2006; 40:691–697.
22. Emsley R et al. Safety of the omega-3 fatty acid, eicosapentaenoic acid (EPA) in psychiatric patients: results from a randomized, placebo-controlled trial. Psychiatry Res 2008; 161:284–291.
23. Das UN. Essential fatty acids and their metabolites could function as endogenous HMG-CoA reductase and ACE enzyme inhibitors, anti-arrhythmic, anti-hypertensive, anti-atherosclerotic, anti-inflammatory, cytoprotective, and cardioprotective molecules. Lipids Health Dis 2008; 7:37.
24. Amminger GP et al. Long-chain omega-3 fatty acids for indicated prevention of psychotic disorders: a randomized, placebo-controlled trial. Arch Gen Psychiatry 2010; 67:146–154.
25. Stafford MR et al. Early interventions to prevent psychosis: systematic review and meta-analysis. BMJ 2013; 346:f185.
26. McGorry PD et al. Effect of omega-3 polyunsaturated fatty acids in young people at ultrahigh risk for psychotic disorders: The NEURAPRO Randomized Clinical Trial. JAMA Psychiatry 2017; 74:19–27.

CHAPTER 1

ANTIPSYCHOTIC ADVERSE EFFECTS

Extrapyramidal symptoms

Details of the extrapyramidal symptoms (EPS) caused by antipsychotic drug treatment are shown in Table 1.19.

EPS are:

- dose-related
- most likely with high doses of high-potency FGAs
- less common with other antipsychotics, particularly clozapine, olanzapine, quetiapine and aripiprazole,[38] but once present may be persistent.[39] Note that CUtLASS reported no difference in EPS between FGAs and SGAs[40] (although sulpiride was widely used in the FGA group). Vulnerability to EPS may be genetically determined.[41]

Note that in never-medicated patients with first-episode schizophrenia, 1% have dystonia, 8% parkinsonian symptoms and 11% akathisia.[42] Parkinsonian symptoms in such patients are associated with cognitive impairment.[43] In never-treated patients with established illness, 9% exhibit spontaneous dyskinesias and 17% parkinsonian symptoms.[44] Patients who experience one type of EPS may be more vulnerable to developing others.[45] Substance misuse increases the risk of dystonia, akathisia and TD.[46] There is some evidence for an association between alcohol use and akathisia.[47,48]

References

1. Barnes TR et al. Akathisia variants and tardive dyskinesia. Arch Gen Psychiatry 1985; 42:874–878.
2. Gervin M et al. Assessment of drug-related movement disorders in schizophrenia. Adv Psychiatr Treat 2000; 6:332–341.
3. Seemuller F et al. Akathisia and suicidal ideation in first-episode schizophrenia. J Clin Psychopharmacol 2012; 32:694–698.
4. Leong GB et al. Neuroleptic-induced akathisia and violence: a review. J Forensic Sci 2003; 48:187–189.
5. Simpson GM et al. A rating scale for extrapyramidal side effects. Acta Psychiatr Scand 1970; 212:11–19.
6. Barnes TRE. A rating scale for drug-induced akathisia. Br J Psychiatry 1989; 154:672–676.
7. Guy W. ECDEU Assessment Manual for Psychopharmacology. Washington, DC: US Department of Health, Education, and Welfare; 1976, pp. 534–537.
8. American Psychiatric Association. Practice guideline for the treatment of patients with schizophrenia. Am J Psychiatry 1997; 154 Suppl 4:1–63.
9. van Harten PN et al. Acute dystonia induced by drug treatment. Br Med J 1999; 319:623–626.
10. Bollini P et al. Antipsychotic drugs: is more worse? A meta-analysis of the published randomized control trials. Psychol Med 1994; 24:307–316.
11. Halstead SM et al. Akathisia: prevalence and associated dysphoria in an in-patient population with chronic schizophrenia. Br J Psychiatry 1994; 164:177–183.
12. Hirose S. The causes of underdiagnosing akathisia. Schizophr Bull 2003; 29:547–558.
13. Caligiuri M. Tardive dyskinesia: a task force report of the American Psychiatric Association. Hosp Community Psychiatry 1993; 44:190.
14. Caroff SN et al. Treatment outcomes of patients with tardive dyskinesia and chronic schizophrenia. J Clin Psychiatry 2011; 72:295–303.
15. Miller CH et al. Managing antipsychotic-induced acute and chronic akathisia. Drug Saf 2000; 22:73–81.
16. Hennings JM et al. Successful treatment of tardive lingual dystonia with botulinum toxin: case report and review of the literature. Prog Neuropsychopharmacol Biol Psychiatry 2008; 32:1167–1171.
17. Jankovic J. Treatment of hyperkinetic movement disorders. Lancet Neurol 2009; 8:844–856.
18. Poyurovsky M et al. Efficacy of low-dose mirtazapine in neuroleptic-induced akathisia: a double-blind randomized placebo-controlled pilot study. J Clin Psychopharmacol 2003; 23:305–308.
19. Stryjer R et al. Treatment of neuroleptic-induced akathisia with the 5-HT2A antagonist trazodone. Clin Neuropharmacol 2003; 26:137–141.
20. Stryjer R et al. Trazodone for the treatment of neuroleptic-induced acute akathisia: a placebo-controlled, double-blind, crossover study. Clin Neuropharmacol 2010; 33:219–222.
21. Stryjer R et al. Mianserin for the rapid improvement of chronic akathisia in a schizophrenia patient. Eur Psychiatry 2004; 19:237–238.

Table 1.19 Most common extrapyramidal symptoms

	Dystonia (uncontrolled muscular spasm)	Pseudoparkinsonism (bradykinesia, tremor, etc.)	Akathisia (restlessness)[1]	Tardive dyskinesia (abnormal involuntary movements)
Signs and symptoms[2]	Muscle spasm in any part of the body, e.g.: ■ eyes rolling upwards (oculogyric crisis) ■ head and neck twisted to the side (torticollis) The patient may be unable to swallow or speak clearly. In extreme cases, the back may arch or the jaw dislocate Acute dystonia can be both painful and very frightening	■ Tremor and/or rigidity ■ Bradykinesia (decreased facial expression, flat monotone voice, slow body movements, inability to initiate movement) ■ Bradyphrenia (slowed thinking) ■ Salivation Pseudoparkinsonism can be mistaken for depression or the negative symptoms of schizophrenia	A subjectively unpleasant state of inner restlessness where there is a strong desire or compulsion to move, e.g.: ■ foot stamping when seated ■ constantly crossing/uncrossing legs ■ rocking from foot to foot ■ constantly pacing up and down Akathisia can be mistaken for psychotic agitation and has been linked with suicidal ideation[3] and aggression towards others[4]	A wide variety of movements can occur such as: ■ lip smacking or chewing ■ tongue protrusion (fly catching) ■ choreiform hand movements (pill rolling or piano playing) ■ pelvic thrusting Severe orofacial movements can lead to difficulty speaking, eating or breathing. Movements are worse when under stress
Rating scales	No specific scale Small component of general EPS scales	Simpson–Angus EPS Rating Scale[5]	Barnes Akathisia Scale[6]	Abnormal Involuntary Movement Scale[7] (AIMS)
Prevalence (with older drugs)	Approximately 10%,[8] but more common:[9] ■ in young males ■ in the neuroleptic-naïve ■ with high-potency drugs (e.g. haloperidol) Dystonic reactions are rare in the elderly	Approximately 20%,[10] but more common in: ■ elderly females ■ those with pre-existing neurological damage (head injury, stroke, etc.)	Wide variation but approximately 25%[11] for acute akathisia with FGAs; lower with SGAs In decreasing order: aripiprazole, risperidone, olanzapine, quetiapine and clozapine[12]	5% of patients per year of antipsychotic exposure.[13] More common in: ■ elderly females ■ those with affective illness ■ those who have had acute EPS early in treatment TD may be associated with neurocognitive deficits[14]

(Continued)

Table 1.19 (*Continued*)

	Dystonia (uncontrolled muscular spasm)	Pseudoparkinsonism (bradykinesia, tremor, etc.)	Akathisia (restlessness)[1]	Tardive dyskinesia (abnormal involuntary movements)
Time taken to develop	Acute dystonia can occur within hours of starting antipsychotics (minutes if the IM or IV route is used) TD occurs after months to years of antipsychotic treatment	Days to weeks after antipsychotic drugs are started or the dose is increased	Acute akathisia occurs within hours to weeks of starting antipsychotics or increasing the dose Akathisia that has persisted for several months or so is called 'chronic akathisia'. Tardive akathisia tends to occur later in treatment and may be exacerbated or provoked by antipsychotic dose reduction or withdrawal[1]	Months to years Approximately 50% of cases are reversible[13,14]
Treatment	■ Anticholinergic drugs given orally, IM or IV depending on the severity of symptoms[9] ■ Remember the patient may be unable to swallow ■ Response to IV administration will be seen within 5 minutes ■ Response to IM administration takes around 20 minutes ■ TD may respond to ECT[15] ■ Where symptoms do not respond to simpler measures, including switching to an antipsychotic with a low propensity for EPS, botulinum toxin may be effective[16] ■ rTMS may be helpful[17]	Several options are available depending on the clinical circumstances: ■ Reduce the antipsychotic dose ■ Change to an antipsychotic with lower propensity for pseudoparkinsonism (see section on 'Relative adverse effects – a rough guide') ■ Prescribe an anticholinergic. The majority of patients do not require long-term anticholinergic agents. Use should be reviewed at least every 3 months. Do not prescribe at night (symptoms usually absent during sleep)	■ Reduce the antipsychotic dose ■ Change to an antipsychotic drug with lower propensity for akathisia (see sections on 'Akathisia' and 'Relative adverse effects – a rough guide') ■ A reduction in symptoms may be seen with:[18] propranolol 30–80mg/day (evidence poor); clonazepam (low dose) ■ 5-HT$_2$ antagonists such as cyproheptadine,[15] mirtazapine,[18] trazodone,[19,20] mianserin[21] and cyproheptadine[15] may help, as may diphenhydramine[22] All are unlicensed for this indication Anticholinergics are generally unhelpful[23]	■ Stop anticholinergic if prescribed ■ Reduce dose of antipsychotic medication ■ Change to an antipsychotic with lower propensity for TD[24-27] (note that data are conflicting[28,29]) ■ Clozapine is the antipsychotic most likely to be associated with resolution of symptoms.[30] Quetiapine may also be useful in this regard[31] ■ Both valbenazine and deutetrabenazine have a positive risk–benefit balance as add-on treatments[32-35] ■ There is also some evidence for tetrabenazine and *Ginkgo biloba*[36] as add-on treatments. For other treatment options see the review by the American Academy of Neurology[37] and the section on 'Tardive dyskinesia'

ECT, electroconvulsive therapy; EPS, extrapyramidal symptoms; IM, intramuscularly; IV, intravenously; rTMS, repetitive transcranial magnetic stimulation; TD, tardive dyskinesia.

22. Vinson DR. Diphenhydramine in the treatment of akathisia induced by prochlorperazine. J Emerg Med 2004; **26**:265–270.

23. Rathbone J et al. Anticholinergics for neuroleptic-induced acute akathisia. Cochrane Database Syst Rev 2006; CD003727.

24. Glazer WM. Expected incidence of tardive dyskinesia associated with atypical antipsychotics. J Clin Psychiatry 2000; **61 Suppl 4**:21–26.

25. Kinon BJ et al. Olanzapine treatment for tardive dyskinesia in schizophrenia patients: a prospective clinical trial with patients randomized to blinded dose reduction periods. Prog Neuropsychopharmacol Biol Psychiatry 2004; **28**:985–996.

26. Bai YM et al. Risperidone for severe tardive dyskinesia: a 12-week randomized, double-blind, placebo-controlled study. J Clin Psychiatry 2003; **64**:1342–1348.

27. Tenback DE et al. Effects of antipsychotic treatment on tardive dyskinesia: a 6-month evaluation of patients from the European Schizophrenia Outpatient Health Outcomes (SOHO) Study. J Clin Psychiatry 2005; **66**:1130–1133.

28. Woods SW et al. Incidence of tardive dyskinesia with atypical versus conventional antipsychotic medications: a prospective cohort study. J Clin Psychiatry 2010; **71**:463–474.

29. Pena MS et al. Tardive dyskinesia and other movement disorders secondary to aripiprazole. Mov Disord 2011; **26**:147–152.

30. Simpson GM. The treatment of tardive dyskinesia and tardive dystonia. J Clin Psychiatry 2000; **61 Suppl 4**:39–44.

31. Peritogiannis V et al. Can atypical antipsychotics improve tardive dyskinesia associated with other atypical antipsychotics? Case report and brief review of the literature. J Psychopharmacol 2010; **24**:1121–1125.

32. Hauser RA et al. KINECT 3: a phase 3 randomized, double-blind, placebo-controlled trial of valbenazine for tardive dyskinesia. Am J Psychiatry 2017; **174**:476–484.

33. Josiassen RC et al. Long-term safety and tolerability of valbenazine (NBI-98854) in subjects with tardive dyskinesia and a diagnosis of schizophrenia or mood disorder. Psychopharmacol Bull 2017; **47**:61–68.

34. Fernandez HH et al. Randomized controlled trial of deutetrabenazine for tardive dyskinesia: the ARM-TD study. Neurology 2017; **88**:2003–2010.

35. Citrome L. Deutetrabenazine for tardive dyskinesia: a systematic review of the efficacy and safety profile for this newly approved novel medication What is the number needed to treat, number needed to harm and likelihood to be helped or harmed? Int J Clin Pract 2017; **71**.

36. Zhang WF et al. Extract of ginkgo biloba treatment for tardive dyskinesia in schizophrenia: a randomized, double-blind, placebo-controlled trial. J Clin Psychiatry 2010; **72**:615–621.

37. Bhidayasiri R et al. Evidence-based guideline: treatment of tardive syndromes: report of the Guideline Development Subcommittee of the American Academy of Neurology. Neurology 2013; **81**:463–469.

38. Leucht S et al. Comparative efficacy and tolerability of 15 antipsychotic drugs in schizophrenia: a multiple-treatments meta-analysis. Lancet 2013; **382**:951–962.

39. Tenback DE et al. Incidence and persistence of tardive dyskinesia and extrapyramidal symptoms in schizophrenia. J Psychopharmacol 2010; **24**:1031–1035.

40. Peluso MJ et al. Extrapyramidal motor side-effects of first- and second-generation antipsychotic drugs. Br J Psychiatry 2012; **200**:387–392.

41. Zivkovic M et al. The association study of polymorphisms in DAT, DRD2, and COMT genes and acute extrapyramidal adverse effects in male schizophrenic patients treated with haloperidol. J Clin Psychopharmacol 2013; **33**:593–599.

42. Rybakowski JK et al. Extrapyramidal symptoms during treatment of first schizophrenia episode: results from EUFEST. Eur Neuropsychopharmacol 2014; **24**:1500–1505.

43. Cuesta MJ et al. Spontaneous Parkinsonism is associated with cognitive impairment in antipsychotic-naive patients with first-episode psychosis: a 6-month follow-up study. Schizophr Bull 2014; **40**:1164–1173.

44. Pappa S et al. Spontaneous movement disorders in antipsychotic-naive patients with first-episode psychoses: a systematic review. Psychol Med 2009; **39**:1065–1076.

45. Kim JH et al. Prevalence and characteristics of subjective akathisia, objective akathisia, and mixed akathisia in chronic schizophrenic subjects. Clin Neuropharmacol 2003; **26**:312–316.

46. Potvin S et al. Substance abuse is associated with increased extrapyramidal symptoms in schizophrenia: a meta-analysis. Schizophr Res 2009; **113**:181–188.

47. Hansen LK et al. Movement disorders in patients with schizophrenia and a history of substance abuse. Hum Psychopharmacol 2013; **28**:192–197.

48. Duke PJ et al. South Westminster schizophrenia survey. Alcohol use and its relationship to symptoms, tardive dyskinesia and illness onset. Br J Psychiatry 1994; **164**:630–636.

Further reading

Dayalu P et al. Antipsychotic-induced extrapyramidal symptoms and their management. Expert Opin Pharmacother 2008; **9**:1451–1462.

El Sayeh HG et al. Non-neuroleptic catecholaminergic drugs for neuroleptic induced tardive dyskinesia. Cochrane Database Syst Rev 2006; CD000458.

CHAPTER 1

Akathisia

Akathisia is a relatively common adverse effect of most antipsychotic medications although some SGAs have a lower liability for the condition. The core feature of akathisia is mental unease and dysphoria characterised by a sense of restlessness.[1,2] This is usually accompanied by observable motor restlessness, which, when severe, can cause patients to pace up and down and be unable to stay seated for more than a short time.[1,2] An association between the discomfiting subjective experience of akathisia and suicidal ideation has been postulated[3,4] but remains uncertain.

There is some evidence to suggest that akathisia may be prevented by avoiding high-dose antipsychotic medication, antipsychotic polypharmacy and rapid increase in dosage.[1,5,6] There is limited evidence for efficacy for any pharmacological treatment for akathisia, even those most commonly used, such as switching to an antipsychotic medication with a lower liability for the condition, or adding a beta-adrenergic blocker, a 5-HT$_{2A}$ antagonist or an anticholinergic agent. Figure 1.4 suggests a programme of treatment options for persistent, drug-induced akathisia.

References

1. Braude WM et al. Clinical characteristics of akathisia. A systematic investigation of acute psychiatric inpatient admissions. Br J Psychiatry 1983; **143**:139–150.
2. Barnes TRE. A rating scale for drug-induced akathisia. Br J Psychiatry 1989; **154**:672–676.
3. Seemuller F et al. Akathisia and suicidal ideation in first-episode schizophrenia. J Clin Psychopharmacol 2012; **32**:694–698.
4. Seemuller F et al. The relationship of akathisia with treatment emergent suicidality among patients with first-episode schizophrenia treated with haloperidol or risperidone. Pharmacopsychiatry 2012; **45**:292–296.
5. Miller CH et al. Managing antipsychotic-induced acute and chronic akathisia. Drug Saf 2000; **22**:73–81.
6. Berardi D et al. Clinical correlates of akathisia in acute psychiatric inpatients. Int Clin Psychopharmacol 2000; **15**:215–219.
7. Fleischhacker WW et al. The pharmacologic treatment of neuroleptic-induced akathisia. J Clin Psychopharmacol 1990; **10**:12–21.
8. Sachdev P. The identification and management of drug-induced akathisia. CNS Drugs 1995; **4**:28–46.
9. Kumar R et al. Akathisia and second-generation antipsychotic drugs. Curr Opin Psychiatry 2009; **22**:293–299.
10. Miller DD et al. Extrapyramidal side-effects of antipsychotics in a randomised trial. Br J Psychiatry 2008; **193**:279–288.
11. Rummel-Kluge C et al. Second-generation antipsychotic drugs and extrapyramidal side effects: a systematic review and meta-analysis of head-to-head comparisons. Schizophr Bull 2012; **38**:167–177.
12. Kane JM et al. Akathisia: an updated review focusing on second-generation antipsychotics. J Clin Psychiatry 2009; **70**:627–643.
13. Adler L et al. A controlled assessment of propranolol in the treatment of neuroleptic-induced akathisia. Br J Psychiatry 1986; **149**:42–45.
14. Fischel T et al. Cyproheptadine versus propranolol for the treatment of acute neuroleptic-induced akathisia: a comparative double-blind study. J Clin Psychopharmacol 2001; **21**:612–615.
15. Laoutidis ZG et al. 5-HT2A receptor antagonists for the treatment of neuroleptic-induced akathisia: a systematic review and meta-analysis. Int J Neuropsychopharmacol 2014; **17**:823–832.
16. Poyurovsky M et al. Mirtazapine – a multifunctional drug: low dose for akathisia. CNS Spectr 2011; **16**:63.
17. Poyurovsky M. Acute antipsychotic-induced akathisia revisited. Br J Psychiatry 2010; **196**:89–91.
18. Rathbone J et al. Anticholinergics for neuroleptic-induced acute akathisia. Cochrane Database Syst Rev 2006; CD003727.
19. Baskak B et al. The effectiveness of intramuscular biperiden in acute akathisia: a double-blind, randomized, placebo-controlled study. J Clin Psychopharmacol 2007; **27**:289–294.
20. Weiss D et al. Cyproheptadine treatment in neuroleptic-induced akathisia. Br J Psychiatry 1995; **167**:483–486.
21. Zubenko GS et al. Use of clonidine in treating neuroleptic-induced akathisia. Psychiatry Res 1984; **13**:253–259.
22. Gervin M et al. Assessment of drug-related movement disorders in schizophrenia. Adv Psychiatr Treat 2000; **6**:332–341.
23. Cunningham Owens D. *A Guide to the Extrapyramidal Side Effects of Antipsychotic Drugs*. Cambridge: Cambridge University Press; 1999.
24. Miodownik C et al. Vitamin B6 versus mianserin and placebo in acute neuroleptic-induced akathisia: a randomized, double-blind, controlled study. Clin Neuropharmacol 2006; **29**:68–72.
25. Lerner V et al. Vitamin B6 treatment in acute neuroleptic-induced akathisia: a randomized, double-blind, placebo-controlled study. J Clin Psychiatry 2004; **65**:1550–1554.
26. De Berardis D et al. Reversal of aripiprazole-induced tardive akathisia by addition of pregabalin. J Neuropsychiatry Clin Neurosci 2013; **25**:E9–10.

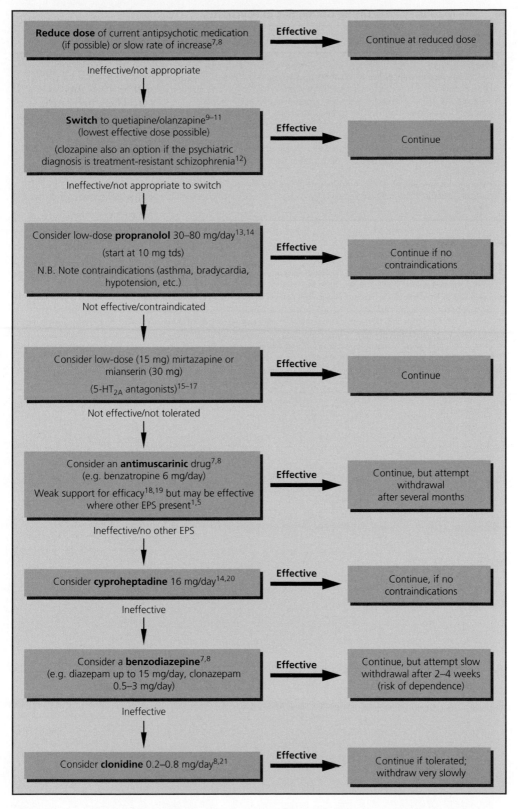

Figure 1.4 Suggested treatment options for persistent, drug-induced akathisia. EPS, extrapyramidal symptoms; tds, *ter die sumendum* (three times a day).

Notes:
- Akathisia is sometimes difficult to diagnose with certainty. Clinical physical examination schedules for EPS have been proposed.[22,23] A careful history of symptoms, medication and co-morbid substance use is essential.
- Evaluate the efficacy of each treatment option over at least 1 month. Some effect may be seen after a few days but it may take much longer to become apparent in those with chronic akathisia.
- Withdraw previously ineffective akathisia treatments before starting the next option in the algorithm.
- Combinations of treatment may be considered for refractory cases if carefully monitored.
- Other possible treatments for acute akathisia that have been investigated include vitamin B_6,[24,25] pregabalin,[26] diphenhydramine,[27] trazodone[15,28] and zolmitriptan.[29,30] Always read the primary literature before considering any of the treatment options.
- Parenteral midazolam (1.5 mg) has been successfully used to prevent akathisia associated with IV metoclopramide,[31] suggesting a specific therapeutic effect for midazolam and perhaps benzodiazepines more generally.

Figure 1.4 (*Continued*)

27. Friedman BW et al. A randomized trial of diphenhydramine as prophylaxis against metoclopramide-induced akathisia in nauseated emergency department patients. Ann Emerg Med 2009; 53:379–385.

28. Stryjer R et al. Trazodone for the treatment of neuroleptic-induced acute akathisia: a placebo-controlled, double-blind, crossover study. Clin Neuropharmacol 2010; 33:219–222.

29. Gross-Isseroff R et al. The 5-HT1D receptor agonist zolmitriptan for neuroleptic-induced akathisia: an open label preliminary study. Int Clin Psychopharmacol 2005; 20:23–25.

30. Avital A et al. Zolmitriptan compared to propranolol in the treatment of acute neuroleptic-induced akathisia: a comparative double-blind study. Eur Neuropsychopharmacol 2009; 19:476–482.

31. Erdur B et al. A trial of midazolam vs diphenhydramine in prophylaxis of metoclopramide-induced akathisia. Am J Emerg Med 2012; 30:84–91.

Weight gain

Antipsychotics have long been recognised as weight-inducing agents. Suggested mechanisms include 5-HT_{2C} antagonism, H_1 antagonism, D_2 antagonism, and increased serum leptin (leading to leptin desensitisation).[1-3] There is no evidence that drugs exert any direct metabolic effect: weight gain seems to result from increased food intake and, in some cases, reduced energy expenditure.[4] Risk of weight gain appears to be related to clinical response[5] (although the association is too small to be clinically important[6]) and may also have a genetic basis.[7] Weight gain may also be more pronounced in antipsychotic-naïve patients.[8]

All available antipsychotics have been associated with weight gain, although mean weight gained varies substantially between drugs. With all drugs, some patients lose weight, some gain no weight and some gain a great deal of weight. Knowledge of the mean weight gained is often not useful in predicting how much weight an individual might gain. Assessment of relative risk for different drugs is based largely on short-term studies. Notwithstanding these limitations, the results of indirect and direct meta-analyses suggest that antipsychotics can be clustered into three groups based on their weight gain liability.[9] Table 1.20 suggests approximate relative risk of weight gain and the extent of mean weight gain.

Table 1.20 Antipsychotic-induced weight gain[10-16]

Drug	Risk/extent of weight gain
Clozapine	**High**
Olanzapine	
Chlorpromazine	**Moderate**
Iloperidone	
Sertindole	
Quetiapine	
Risperidone	
Paliperidone	
Amisulpride	**Low**
Asenapine	
Brexpiprazole	
Aripiprazole	
Cariprazine	
Haloperidol	
Lurasidone	
Sulpiride	
Trifluoperazine	
Ziprasidone	

See section on 'Treatment of antipsychotic-induced weight gain' in this chapter for advice on treating drug-induced weight gain.

References

1. Nielsen MO et al. Striatal reward activity and antipsychotic-associated weight change in patients with schizophrenia undergoing initial treatment. JAMA Psychiatry 2016; 73:121–128.

2. Ragguett RM et al. Association between antipsychotic treatment and leptin levels across multiple psychiatric populations: an updated meta-analysis. Hum Psychopharmacol 2017; 32.

3. Reynolds GP et al. Mechanisms underlying metabolic disturbances associated with psychosis and antipsychotic drug treatment. J Psychopharmacol 2017; 31:1430–1436.

4. Benarroch L et al. Atypical antipsychotics and effects on feeding: from mice to men. Psychopharmacology (Berl) 2016; 233:2629–2653.

5. Sharma E et al. Association between antipsychotic-induced metabolic side-effects and clinical improvement: a review on the evidence for "metabolic threshold". Asian J Psychiatr 2014; 8:12–21.

6. Hermes E et al. The association between weight change and symptom reduction in the CATIE schizophrenia trial. Schizophr Res 2011; 128:166–170.

7. Zhang JP et al. Pharmacogenetic associations of antipsychotic drug-related weight gain: a systematic review and meta-analysis. Schizophr Bull 2016; 42:1418–1437.

8. Bak M et al. Almost all antipsychotics result in weight gain: a meta-analysis. PLoS One 2014; 9:e94112.

9. Cooper SJ et al. BAP guidelines on the management of weight gain, metabolic disturbances and cardiovascular risk associated with psychosis and antipsychotic drug treatment. J Psychopharmacol 2016; 30:717–748.

10. Rummel-Kluge C et al. Head-to-head comparisons of metabolic side effects of second generation antipsychotics in the treatment of schizophrenia: a systematic review and meta-analysis. Schizophr Res 2010; 123:225–233.

11. Leucht S et al. Comparative efficacy and tolerability of 15 antipsychotic drugs in schizophrenia: a multiple-treatments meta-analysis. Lancet 2013; 382:951–962.

12. Cutler AJ et al. Long-term safety and tolerability of iloperidone: results from a 25-week, open-label extension trial. CNS Spectr 2013; 18:43–54.

13. McEvoy JP et al. Effectiveness of paliperidone palmitate vs haloperidol decanoate for maintenance treatment of schizophrenia: a randomized clinical trial. JAMA 2014; 311:1978–1987.

14. Lao KS et al. Tolerability and safety profile of cariprazine in treating psychotic disorders, bipolar disorder and major depressive disorder: a systematic review with meta-analysis of randomized controlled trials. CNS Drugs 2016; 30:1043–1054.

15. Leucht S et al. Sixty years of placebo-controlled antipsychotic drug trials in acute schizophrenia: systematic review, bayesian meta-analysis, and meta-regression of efficacy predictors. Am J Psychiatry 2017; 174:927–942.

16. Garay RP et al. Therapeutic improvements expected in the near future for schizophrenia and schizoaffective disorder: an appraisal of phase III clinical trials of schizophrenia-targeted therapies as found in US and EU clinical trial registries. Expert Opin Pharmacother 2016; 17:921–936.

Treatment of antipsychotic-induced weight gain

Weight gain is an important adverse effect of nearly all antipsychotics with obvious consequences for self-image, morbidity and mortality. Prevention and treatment are therefore matters of clinical urgency.

Monitoring

Patients starting antipsychotic treatment or changing drugs should, as an absolute minimum, be weighed and their weight clearly recorded. Estimates of body mass index (BMI) and waist circumference should, ideally, also be made at baseline and at least every 6 months.[1] Weekly monitoring of weight is recommended early in treatment, for the first 3 months at least. Rapid weight gain in early treatment ($\geq 5\%$ above baseline after 1 month of treatment) strongly predicts long-term weight gain and should prompt consideration of preventative or remedial measures.[2,3]

There is somewhat dated evidence that only a minority of patients have anywhere near adequate monitoring of weight.[4] Clearly, monitoring of weight parameters is essential to assess the value of preventative and remedial measures.

Treatment and prevention

Most of the relevant literature in this area relates to attempts at reversing antipsychotic-related weight gain, although there are now useful data suggesting that early interventions can prevent or mitigate weight gain.[5,6]

When weight gain occurs, initial options involve switching drugs or instituting behavioural programmes (or both). Switching always presents a risk of relapse and treatment discontinuation[7] but there is fairly strong support for switching to aripiprazole,[8,9] ziprasidone[10–12] or lurasidone[13,14] as a method for reversing weight gain. It is possible that switching to other drugs with a low propensity for weight gain is also beneficial.[15,16]

Another option is to add aripiprazole to existing treatment: weight loss has been observed when aripiprazole was added to clozapine and to olanzapine.[6] Stopping antipsychotic treatment altogether will reverse weight gain[17,18] but this course of action would not be sensible for the large majority of people with multi-episode schizophrenia. Note that, while some switching and augmentation strategies may minimise further weight gain or facilitate weight loss, the overall effect is generally modest and many patients continue to be overweight. Additional lifestyle interventions are often required if BMI is to remain in/move towards the normal range.

A variety of lifestyle interventions have been proposed and evaluated with good results.[5,19,20] Interventions vary, but they are mainly 'behavioural lifestyle programmes' aimed at improving diet and increasing physical activity. Meta-analyses of RCTs have shown a robust effect for both prevention and intervention with these non-pharmacological interventions.[5,20] Pharmacological methods should be considered only where behavioural methods or switching have failed or where obesity presents clear, immediate physical risk to the patient. Some options are described in Table 1.21. Metformin is now probably considered to be the drug of choice for the prevention and treatment of

Table 1.21 Drug treatment of antipsychotic-induced weight gain

Drug	Comments
Amantadine[23,24] (100–300 mg/day)	May attenuate olanzapine-related weight gain. Seems to be well tolerated apart from insomnia and abdominal discomfort. May (theoretically, at least) exacerbate psychosis. Evidence base too limited to recommend[22]
Alpha-lipoic acid[25–27] (1200 mg/day)	Supplementation may lead to a small short-term weight loss. Limited data for antipsychotic-induced weight gain. Not recommended
Aripiprazole[6,28] (5–15 mg/day)	Three RCTs show beneficial effects on weight loss and possibly other metabolic parameters when used as an adjunct to clozapine or olanzapine. Adjunctive use appears to be safe and unlikely to worsen psychosis. Recommended as a possible option for weight gain associated with clozapine or olanzapine. Not recommended with other antipsychotics
Betahistine[29,30] (48 mg/day)	May attenuate olanzapine-induced weight gain. Limited data. Not recommended
Bupropion[31,32] (amfebutamone)	Seems to be effective in obesity when combined with calorie-restricted diets. Appears not to exacerbate psychosis symptoms, at least when used for smoking cessation.[33] Few data on its effects on drug-induced weight gain. Not recommended
Bupropion + naltrexone (Contrave/Mysimba)[34]	Combination approved for weight management as an adjunct to diet and exercise. No data in drug-induced weight gain. Not recommended, but should not be ruled out
Fluoxetine[6] (20–60 mg/day)	Two negative RCTs. Not recommended
Fluvoxamine[35–37] (50 mg/day)	Earlier conflicting data but one short-term RCT shows attenuated clozapine-induced weight gain (possibly related to a higher clozapine to norclozapine ratio). Co-administration markedly increases clozapine levels, requiring extreme caution. Evidence base is too limited to recommend
H_2 antagonists[38] (e.g. nizatidine 300 mg bd, ranitidine 300 mg bd or famotidine 40 mg/day)	Meta-analysis of RCTs suggests no effect on weight gain
Liraglutide[39,40] (3 mg/day via subcutaneous injection)	GLP-1 agonist that was previously approved for type 2 diabetes and more recently approved as an anti-obesity agent in non-diabetic patients. Dose for weight loss (3 mg/day) is higher than the dose used for diabetes (≤1.8 mg). Limited data in drug-induced weight gain. One RCT shows significant weight loss in overweight pre-diabetic patients stable on olanzapine or clozapine.[39] Beneficial effects on other metabolic parameters. Well tolerated but can cause gastrointestinal disturbances. Recommended option in pre-diabetic/diabetic patients and clozapine-induced weight gain

Other GLP-1 agonists are currently only approved for diabetes and have a more limited dose range. Exenatide LA (a once-weekly GLP-1 agonist) may be effective for weight loss in clozapine-treated patients[41] but not with other antipsychotics[42] |
| Metformin[43] (500–2000 mg/day) | Now a substantial database (in non-diabetic patients) supporting the use of metformin in both reducing and reversing weight gain caused by antipsychotics (mainly olanzapine). Beneficial effects on other metabolic parameters. Some negative studies, but clear and significant effect in meta-analyses. One positive RCT[44] and extension study[45] in children and adolescents with ASD published since then. Ideal for those with weight gain and diabetes or polycystic ovary syndrome. Note that metformin treatment increases the risk of vitamin B_{12} deficiency[46] |

Table 1.21 (*Continued*)

Drug	Comments
Melatonin[47–49] (up to 5 mg at night)	One small RCT showing attenuation of olanzapine-induced weight gain. Other studies show negative results. Effect, if any, is small
Methylcellulose (1500 mg ac)	Old-fashioned and rather unpalatable preparation. No data in drug-induced weight gain but once fairly widely used. Also acts as a laxative so may be suitable for clozapine-related weight gain
Modafinil[50,51] (up to 300 mg/day)	Limited positive data and one negative RCT for clozapine-induced weight gain. Not recommended
Naltrexone[52,53] (25–50 mg/day)	Some positive results but evidence is limited to two small pilot RCTs. Not recommended
Orlistat[54–59] (120 mg tds ac/pc)	Reliable effect in obesity, especially when combined with calorie restriction. Few published data in drug-induced weight gain but widely used in practice with some success. In trials for clozapine or olanzapine-induced weight gain, effect was only seen for men.[58,59] When used without calorie restriction in psychiatric patients effects are very limited. Failure to adhere to a low-fat diet will result in fatty diarrhoea and possible malabsorption of orally administered medication. Overall, a good choice for clozapine-induced weight gain where it reduces both weight and the incidence of constipation[60]
Reboxetine[6] (4–8 mg daily)	Attenuates olanzapine-induced weight gain. Reverses some metabolic changes.[61] Effective when combined with betahistine
Topiramate[62,63] (up to 300 mg daily)	Reliably reduces weight even when drug-induced. Meta-analyses of RCTs suggest a greater effect for prevention rather than treatment. Problems may arise because of topiramate's propensity for causing sedation, confusion and cognitive impairment. May have antipsychotic properties
Zonisamide[64] (100–600 mg/day)	Anticonvulsant drug with weight-reducing properties. An RCT of 150 mg a day showed significant weight reduction in people receiving SGAs. Another RCT (up to 600 mg/day) showed attenuated olanzapine-induced weight gain. Sedation, diarrhoea and cognitive impairment are the most common problems. Not recommended

ac, *ante cibum* (before meals); ASD, autism spectrum disorders; bd, *bis in die* (twice a day); pc, *post cibum* (after meals); RCT, randomised controlled trial; SGA, second-generation antipsychotic; tds, *ter die sumendum* (three times a day).

antipsychotic-induced weight gain although GLP-1 agonists may ultimately prove more effective and better tolerated. Bariatric surgery may rarely have a role in severe cases when all else fails.[21] However, the efficacy of bariatric surgery for drug-induced weight gain is not known.[22] Table 1.21 lists drug treatment options for antipsychotic-induced weight gain (in alphabetical order).

References

1. Marder SR et al. Physical health monitoring of patients with schizophrenia. Am J Psychiatry 2004; **161**:1334–1349.
2. American Diabetes Association et al. Consensus Development Conference on antipsychotic drugs and obesity and diabetes. Diabetes Care 2004; **27**:596–601.
3. Vandenberghe F et al. Importance of early weight changes to predict long-term weight gain during psychotropic drug treatment. J Clin Psychiatry 2015; **76**:e1417–1423.

4. Mitchell AJ et al. Guideline concordant monitoring of metabolic risk in people treated with antipsychotic medication: systematic review and meta-analysis of screening practices. Psychol Med 2012; 42:125–147.

5. Bruins J et al. The effects of lifestyle interventions on (long-term) weight management, cardiometabolic risk and depressive symptoms in people with psychotic disorders: a meta-analysis. PLoS One 2014; 9:e112276.

6. Mizuno Y et al. Pharmacological strategies to counteract antipsychotic-induced weight gain and metabolic adverse effects in schizophrenia: a systematic review and meta-analysis. Schizophr Bull 2014; 40:1385–1403.

7. Stroup TS et al. A randomized trial examining the effectiveness of switching from olanzapine, quetiapine, or risperidone to aripiprazole to reduce metabolic risk: comparison of antipsychotics for metabolic problems (CAMP). Am J Psychiatry 2011; 168:947–956.

8. Mukundan A et al. Antipsychotic switching for people with schizophrenia who have neuroleptic-induced weight or metabolic problems. Cochrane Database Syst Rev 2010; CD006629.

9. Barak Y et al. Switching to aripiprazole as a strategy for weight reduction: a meta-analysis in patients suffering from schizophrenia. J Obes 2011;2011.

10. Weiden PJ et al. Improvement in indices of health status in outpatients with schizophrenia switched to ziprasidone. J Clin Psychopharmacol 2003; 23:595–600.

11. Montes JM et al. Improvement in antipsychotic-related metabolic disturbances in patients with schizophrenia switched to ziprasidone. Prog Neuropsychopharmacol Biol Psychiatry 2007; 31:383–388.

12. Karayal ON et al. Switching from quetiapine to ziprasidone: a sixteen-week, open-label, multicenter study evaluating the effectiveness and safety of ziprasidone in outpatient subjects with schizophrenia or schizoaffective disorder. J Psychiatr Pract 2011; 17:100–109.

13. McEvoy JP et al. Effectiveness of lurasidone in patients with schizophrenia or schizoaffective disorder switched from other antipsychotics: a randomized, 6-week, open-label study. J Clin Psychiatry 2013; 74:170–179.

14. Stahl SM et al. Effectiveness of lurasidone for patients with schizophrenia following 6 weeks of acute treatment with lurasidone, olanzapine, or placebo: a 6-month, open-label, extension study. J Clin Psychiatry 2013; 74:507–515.

15. Gupta S et al. Weight decline in patients switching from olanzapine to quetiapine. Schizophr Res 2004; 70:57–62.

16. Ried LD et al. Weight change after an atypical antipsychotic switch. Ann Pharmacother 2003; 37:1381–1386.

17. de Kuijper G et al. Effects of controlled discontinuation of long-term used antipsychotics on weight and metabolic parameters in individuals with intellectual disability. J Clin Psychopharmacol 2013; 33:520–524.

18. Chen EY et al. Maintenance treatment with quetiapine versus discontinuation after one year of treatment in patients with remitted first episode psychosis: randomised controlled trial. BMJ 2010; 341:c4024.

19. Werneke U et al. Behavioural management of antipsychotic-induced weight gain: a review. Acta Psychiatr Scand 2003; 108:252–259.

20. Caemmerer J et al. Acute and maintenance effects of non-pharmacologic interventions for antipsychotic associated weight gain and metabolic abnormalities: a meta-analytic comparison of randomized controlled trials. Schizophr Res 2012; 140:159–168.

21. Manu P et al. Weight gain and obesity in schizophrenia: epidemiology, pathobiology, and management. Acta Psychiatr Scand 2015; 132:97–108.

22. Cooper SJ et al. BAP guidelines on the management of weight gain, metabolic disturbances and cardiovascular risk associated with psychosis and antipsychotic drug treatment. J Psychopharmacol 2016; 30:717–748.

23. Praharaj SK et al. Amantadine for olanzapine-induced weight gain: a systematic review and meta-analysis of randomized placebo-controlled trials. Ther Adv Psychopharmacol 2012; 2:151–156.

24. Zheng W et al. Amantadine for antipsychotic-related weight gain: meta-analysis of randomized placebo-controlled trials. J Clin Psychopharmacol 2017; 37:341–346.

25. Kucukgoncu S et al. Alpha-lipoic acid (ALA) as a supplementation for weight loss: results from a meta-analysis of randomized controlled trials. Obes Rev 2017; 18:594–601.

26. Kim E et al. A preliminary investigation of alpha-lipoic acid treatment of antipsychotic drug-induced weight gain in patients with schizophrenia. J Clin Psychopharmacol 2008; 28:138–146.

27. Ratliff JC et al. An open-label pilot trial of alpha-lipoic acid for weight loss in patients with schizophrenia without diabetes. Clin Schizophr Relat Psychoses 2015; 8:196–200.

28. Zheng W et al. Efficacy and safety of adjunctive aripiprazole in schizophrenia: meta-analysis of randomized controlled trials. J Clin Psychopharmacol 2016; 36:628–636.

29. Barak N et al. A randomized, double-blind, placebo-controlled pilot study of betahistine to counteract olanzapine-associated weight gain. J Clin Psychopharmacol 2016; 36:253–256.

30. Lian J et al. Ameliorating antipsychotic-induced weight gain by betahistine: mechanisms and clinical implications. Pharmacol Res 2016; 106:51–63.

31. Gadde KM et al. Bupropion for weight loss: an investigation of efficacy and tolerability in overweight and obese women. Obes Res 2001; 9:544–551.

32. Jain AK et al. Bupropion SR vs. placebo for weight loss in obese patients with depressive symptoms. Obes Res 2002; 10:1049–1056.

33. Tsoi DT et al. Interventions for smoking cessation and reduction in individuals with schizophrenia. Cochrane Database Syst Rev 2013; 2:CD007253.

34. Greig SL et al. Naltrexone ER/Bupropion ER: a review in obesity management. Drugs 2015; 75:1269–1280.

35. Hinze-Selch D et al. Effect of coadministration of clozapine and fluvoxamine versus clozapine monotherapy on blood cell counts, plasma levels of cytokines and body weight. Psychopharmacology (Berl) 2000; 149:163–169.

36. Lu ML et al. Effects of adjunctive fluvoxamine on metabolic parameters and psychopathology in clozapine-treated patients with schizophrenia: a 12-week, randomized, double-blind, placebo-controlled study. Schizophr Res 2017; doi: 10.1016/j.schres.2017.06.030. [Epub ahead of print].

37. Lu ML et al. Adjunctive fluvoxamine inhibits clozapine-related weight gain and metabolic disturbances. J Clin Psychiatry 2004; 65:766–771.

38. Kishi T et al. Efficacy and tolerability of histamine-2 receptor antagonist adjunction of antipsychotic treatment in schizophrenia: a meta-analysis of randomized placebo-controlled trials. Pharmacopsychiatry 2015; 48:30–36.

39. Larsen JR et al. Effect of liraglutide treatment on prediabetes and overweight or obesity in clozapine- or olanzapine-treated patients with schizophrenia spectrum disorder: a randomized clinical trial. JAMA Psychiatry 2017; 74:719–728.

40. Mayfield K et al. Glucagon-like peptide-1 agonists combating clozapine-associated obesity and diabetes. J Psychopharmacol 2016; 30:227–236.

41. Siskind D et al. Treatment of clozapine-associated obesity and diabetes with exenatide (CODEX) in adults with schizophrenia: a randomised controlled trial. Diabetes Obes Metab 2017: doi: 10.1111/dom.13167. [Epub ahead of print].

42. Ishoy PL et al. Effect of GLP-1 receptor agonist treatment on body weight in obese antipsychotic-treated patients with schizophrenia: a randomized, placebo-controlled trial. Diabetes Obes Metab 2017; 19:162–171.

43. Zheng W et al. Metformin for weight gain and metabolic abnormalities associated with antipsychotic treatment: meta-analysis of randomized placebo-controlled trials. J Clin Psychopharmacol 2015; 35:499–509.

44. Anagnostou E et al. Metformin for treatment of overweight induced by atypical antipsychotic medication in young people with autism spectrum disorder: a randomized clinical trial. JAMA Psychiatry 2016; 73:928–937.

45. Handen BL et al. A randomized, placebo-controlled trial of metformin for the treatment of overweight induced by antipsychotic medication in young people with autism spectrum disorder: open-label extension. J Am Acad Child Adolesc Psychiatry 2017; 56:849–856.e6.

46. Chapman LE et al. Association between metformin and vitamin B12 deficiency in patients with type 2 diabetes: a systematic review and meta-analysis. Diabetes Metab 2016; 42:316–327.

47. Agahi M et al. Effect of melatonin in reducing second-generation antipsychotic metabolic effects: a double blind controlled clinical trial. Diabetes Metab Syndr 2017; 12:9–15.

48. Wang HR et al. The role of melatonin and melatonin agonists in counteracting antipsychotic-induced metabolic side effects: a systematic review. Int Clin Psychopharmacol 2016; 31:301–306.

49. Porfirio MC et al. Can melatonin prevent or improve metabolic side effects during antipsychotic treatments? Neuropsychiatr Dis Treat 2017; 13:2167–2174.

50. Henderson DC et al. Effects of modafinil on weight, glucose and lipid metabolism in clozapine-treated patients with schizophrenia. Schizophr Res 2011; 130:53–56.

51. Roerig JL et al. An exploration of the effect of modafinil on olanzapine associated weight gain in normal human subjects. Biol Psychiatry 2009; 65:607–613.

52. Taveira TH et al. The effect of naltrexone on body fat mass in olanzapine-treated schizophrenic or schizoaffective patients: a randomized double-blind placebo-controlled pilot study. J Psychopharmacol 2014; 28:395–400.

53. Tek C et al. A randomized, double-blind, placebo-controlled pilot study of naltrexone to counteract antipsychotic-associated weight gain: proof of concept. J Clin Psychopharmacol 2014; 34:608–612.

54. Sjostrom L et al. Randomised placebo-controlled trial of orlistat for weight loss and prevention of weight regain in obese patients. European Multicentre Orlistat Study Group. Lancet 1998; 352:167–172.

55. Hilger E et al. The effect of orlistat on plasma levels of psychotropic drugs in patients with long-term psychopharmacotherapy. J Clin Psychopharmacol 2002; 22:68–70.

56. Pavlovic ZM. Orlistat in the treatment of clozapine-induced hyperglycemia and weight gain. Eur Psychiatry 2005; 20:520.

57. Carpenter LL et al. A case series describing orlistat use in patients on psychotropic medications. Med Health R I 2004; 87:375–377.

58. Joffe G et al. Orlistat in clozapine- or olanzapine-treated patients with overweight or obesity: a 16-week randomized, double-blind, placebo-controlled trial. J Clin Psychiatry 2008; 69:706–711.

59. Tchoukhine E et al. Orlistat in clozapine- or olanzapine-treated patients with overweight or obesity: a 16-week open-label extension phase and both phases of a randomized controlled trial. J Clin Psychiatry 2011; 72:326–330.

60. Chukhin E et al. In a randomized placebo-controlled add-on study orlistat significantly reduced clozapine-induced constipation. Int Clin Psychopharmacol 2013; 28:67–70.

61. Amrami-Weizman A et al. The effect of reboxetine co-administration with olanzapine on metabolic and endocrine profile in schizophrenia patients. Psychopharmacology (Berl) 2013; 230:23–27.

62. Correll CU et al. Efficacy for psychopathology and body weight and safety of topiramate-antipsychotic cotreatment in patients with schizophrenia spectrum disorders: results from a meta-analysis of randomized controlled trials. J Clin Psychiatry 2016; 77:e746–756.

63. Zheng W et al. Efficacy and safety of adjunctive topiramate for schizophrenia: a meta-analysis of randomized controlled trials. Acta Psychiatr Scand 2016; 134:385–398.

64. Buoli M et al. The use of zonisamide for the treatment of psychiatric disorders: a systematic review. Clin Neuropharmacol 2017; 40:85–92.

Neuroleptic malignant syndrome

Neuroleptic malignant syndrome (NMS) is an acute disorder of thermoregulation and neuromotor control. It is characterised by muscular rigidity, hyperthermia, altered consciousness and autonomic dysfunction following exposure to antipsychotic medication, although there is considerable heterogeneity in the clinical presentation.[1–4] Although widely seen as an acute, severe syndrome, NMS may, in many cases, have few signs and symptoms and 'full-blown' NMS may thus represent the extreme of a range of non-malignant-related symptoms.[5] Certainly, asymptomatic rises in plasma creatine kinase (CK) are fairly common.[6]

Table 1.22 Diagnosis and management of neuroleptic malignant syndrome

Signs and symptoms[9,47–49] (presentation varies considerably)[50]	Fever, diaphoresis, rigidity, confusion, fluctuating level of consciousness
	Fluctuating blood pressure, tachycardia
	Elevated CK, leukocytosis, altered liver function tests
Risk factors[8,10,45,48,49,51–53]	High potency FGAs, recent or rapid dose increase, rapid dose reduction, abrupt withdrawal of anticholinergic agents, antipsychotic polypharmacy
	Psychosis, organic brain disease, alcoholism, Parkinson's disease, hyperthyroidism, psychomotor agitation, mental retardation
	Male gender, younger age
	Agitation, dehydration
Treatments[9,48,54–57]	**In the psychiatric unit:**
	Withdraw antipsychotic medication, monitor temperature, pulse, blood pressure. Consider benzodiazepines if not already prescribed – IM lorazepam has been used[58]
	In the medical/A&E unit:
	Rehydration, bromocriptine + dantrolene, sedation with benzodiazepines, artificial ventilation if required
	L-dopa, apomorphine and carbamazepine have also been used, among many other drugs. Consider ECT for treatment of psychosis
Re-starting antipsychotics[39,48,54,59]	Antipsychotic treatment will be required in most instances and re-challenge is associated with acceptable risk
	Stop antipsychotics for at least 5 days, preferably longer. Allow time for symptoms and signs of NMS to resolve completely
	Begin with very small dose and increase very slowly with close monitoring of temperature, pulse and blood pressure. CK monitoring may be used, but is controversial.[49,60] Close monitoring of physical and biochemical parameters is effective in reducing progression to 'full-blown' NMS[61,62]
	Consider using an antipsychotic medication structurally unrelated to that previously associated with NMS or a drug with low dopamine affinity (quetiapine or clozapine). Aripiprazole may also be considered[63] but it has a long plasma half-life and has been linked to an increased risk of NMS[10]
	Avoid depot/LAI antipsychotic preparations (of any kind) and high potency FGAs

A&E, accident and emergency; CK, creatine kinase; ECT, electroconvulsive therapy; FGA, first-generation antipsychotic; IM, intramuscular; LAI, long-acting injection; NMS, neuroleptic malignant syndrome.

NMS occurs as a rare but potentially serious or even fatal adverse effect of antipsychotics, as medications with dopamine receptor-antagonist properties.[1] Risk factors include being male, dehydration, exhaustion and confusion/agitation.[4,7] Young adult males seem to be particularly at risk, while the condition is most likely to be lethal in older people.[4,8]

The incidence and mortality rates of NMS are difficult to establish and probably vary as drug use changes and recognition of NMS increases. It has been estimated that fewer than 1% of all patients treated with FGAs will experience NMS.[9] NMS is probably less common with SGAs[3,10] but most have been reported to be associated with the syndrome,[11–18] including later SGAs such as ziprasidone,[19,20] iloperidone,[21] aripiprazole,[22–25] paliperidone[26] (including paliperidone palmitate[27]), asenapine[28] and risperidone injection.[29] Mortality is probably lower with SGAs than with FGAs,[3,30–32] although the clinical picture is essentially similar[31] except that rigidity and fever may be less common.[3,31]

NMS is also sometimes seen with other medications, such as antidepressants,[33–36] valproate,[37,38] phenytoin[39] and lithium.[40] Combinations of antipsychotics with SSRIs[41] or cholinesterase inhibitors[42,43] may increase the risk of NMS. NMS-type syndromes induced by SGA/SSRI combinations may share their symptoms and pathogenesis with serotonin syndrome.[44] The use of benzodiazepines has been linked to an important increase in the risk of NMS.[10,45] NMS is also occasionally seen in people given non-psychotropic dopamine antagonists such as metoclopramide.[46]

The characteristics of NMS and its management are summarised in Table 1.22.

References

1. Caroff SN et al. Neuroleptic malignant syndrome. Med Clin North Am 1993; 77:185–202.
2. Gurrera RJ et al. Thermoregulatory dysfunction malignant syndrome. Biol Psychiatry 1996; 39:207–212.
3. Murri MB et al. Second-generation antipsychotics and neuroleptic malignant syndrome: systematic review and case report analysis. Drugs R D 2015; 15:45–62.
4. Ware MR et al. Neuroleptic malignant syndrome: diagnosis and management. Prim Care Companion CNS Disord 2018; 20:17r02185.
5. Bristow MF et al. How "malignant" is the neuroleptic malignant syndrome? BMJ 1993; 307:1223–1224.
6. Meltzer HY et al. Marked elevations of serum creatine kinase activity associated with antipsychotic drug treatment. Neuropsychopharmacology 1996; 15:395–405.
7. Keck PE et al. Risk-factors for neuroleptic malignant syndrome—a case-control study. Arch Gen Psychiatry 1989; 46:914–918.
8. Gurrera RJ. A systematic review of sex and age factors in neuroleptic malignant syndrome diagnosis frequency. Acta Psychiatr Scand 2017; 135:398–408.
9. Guze BH et al. Current concepts. Neuroleptic malignant syndrome. N Engl J Med 1985; 313:163–166.
10. Su YP et al. Retrospective chart review on exposure to psychotropic medications associated with neuroleptic malignant syndrome. Acta Psychiatr Scand 2014; 130:52–60.
11. Sing KJ et al. Neuroleptic malignant syndrome and quetiapine (Letter). Am J Psychiatry 2002; 159:149–150.
12. Suh H et al. Neuroleptic malignant syndrome and low-dose olanzapine (Letter). Am J Psychiatry 2003; 160:796.
13. Gallarda T et al. Neuroleptic malignant syndrome in an 72-year-old-man with Alzheimer's disease: a case report and review of the literature. Eur Neuropsychopharmacol 2000; 10 Suppl 3:357.
14. Stanley AK et al. Possible neuroleptic malignant syndrome with quetiapine. Br J Psychiatry 2000; 176:497.
15. Sierra-Biddle D et al. Neuroleptic malignant syndrome and olanzapine. J Clin Psychopharmacol 2000; 20:704–705.
16. Hasan S et al. Novel antipsychotics and the neuroleptic malignant syndrome: a review and critique. Am J Psychiatry 1998; 155:1113–1116.
17. Tsai JH et al. Zotepine-induced catatonia as a precursor in the progression to neuroleptic malignant syndrome. Pharmacotherapy 2005; 25:1156–1159.
18. Gortney JS et al. Neuroleptic malignant syndrome secondary to quetiapine. Ann Pharmacother 2009; 43:785–791.
19. Leibold J et al. Neuroleptic malignant syndrome associated with ziprasidone in an adolescent. Clin Ther 2004; 26:1105–1108.
20. Borovicka MC et al. Ziprasidone- and lithium-induced neuroleptic malignant syndrome. Ann Pharmacother 2006; 40:139–142.
21. Guanci N et al. Atypical neuroleptic malignant syndrome associated with iloperidone administration. Psychosomatics 2012; 53:603–605.
22. Spalding S et al. Aripiprazole and atypical neuroleptic malignant syndrome. J Am Acad Child Adolesc Psychiatry 2004; 43:1457–1458.
23. Chakraborty N et al. Aripiprazole and neuroleptic malignant syndrome. Int Clin Psychopharmacol 2004; 19:351–353.

24. Rodriguez OP et al. A case report of neuroleptic malignant syndrome without fever in a patient given aripiprazole. J Okla State Med Assoc 2006; 99:435–438.

25. Srephichit S et al. Neuroleptic malignant syndrome and aripiprazole in an antipsychotic-naive patient. J Clin Psychopharmacol 2006; 26:94–95.

26. Duggal HS. Possible neuroleptic malignant syndrome associated with paliperidone. J Neuropsychiatry Clin Neurosci 2007; 19:477–478.

27. Langley-DeGroot M et al. Atypical neuroleptic malignant syndrome associated with paliperidone long-acting injection: a case report. J Clin Psychopharmacol 2016; 36:277–279.

28. Singh N et al. Neuroleptic malignant syndrome after exposure to asenapine: a case report. Prim Care Companion J Clin Psychiatry 2010; 12:e1.

29. Mall GD et al. Catatonia and mild neuroleptic malignant syndrome after initiation of long-acting injectable risperidone: case report. J Clin Psychopharmacol 2008; 28:572–573.

30. Ananth J et al. Neuroleptic malignant syndrome and atypical antipsychotic drugs. J Clin Psychiatry 2004; 65:464–470.

31. Trollor JN et al. Comparison of neuroleptic malignant syndrome induced by first- and second-generation antipsychotics. Br J Psychiatry 2012; 201:52–56.

32. Nakamura M et al. Mortality of neuroleptic malignant syndrome induced by typical and atypical antipsychotic drugs: a propensity-matched analysis from the Japanese Diagnosis Procedure Combination database. J Clin Psychiatry 2012; 73:427–430.

33. Kontaxakis VP et al. Neuroleptic malignant syndrome after addition of paroxetine to olanzapine. J Clin Psychopharmacol 2003; 23:671–672.

34. Young C. A case of neuroleptic malignant syndrome and serotonin disturbance. J Clin Psychopharmacol 1997; 17:65–66.

35. June R et al. Neuroleptic malignant syndrome associated with nortriptyline. Am J Emerg Med 1999; 17:736–737.

36. Lu TC et al. Neuroleptic malignant syndrome after the use of venlafaxine in a patient with generalized anxiety disorder. J Formos Med Assoc 2006; 105:90–93.

37. Verma R et al. An atypical case of neuroleptic malignant syndrome precipitated by valproate. BMJ Case Rep 2014; 2014: doi:10.1136/bcr-2013-202578.

38. Menon V et al. Atypical neuroleptic malignant syndrome in a young male precipitated by oral sodium valproate. Aust N Z J Psychiatry 2016; 50:1208–1209.

39. Shin HW et al. Neuroleptic malignant syndrome induced by phenytoin in a patient with drug-induced Parkinsonism. Neurol Sci 2014; 35:1641–1643.

40. Gill J et al. Acute lithium intoxication and neuroleptic malignant syndrome. Pharmacotherapy 2003; 23:811–815.

41. Stevens DL. Association between selective serotonin-reuptake inhibitors, second-generation antipsychotics, and neuroleptic malignant syndrome. Ann Pharmacother 2008; 42:1290–1297.

42. Stevens DL et al. Olanzapine-associated neuroleptic malignant syndrome in a patient receiving concomitant rivastigmine therapy. Pharmacotherapy 2008; 28:403–405.

43. Warwick TC et al. Neuroleptic malignant syndrome variant in a patient receiving donepezil and olanzapine. Nat Clin Pract Neurol 2008; 4:170–174.

44. Odagaki Y. Atypical neuroleptic malignant syndrome or serotonin toxicity associated with atypical antipsychotics? Curr Drug Saf 2009; 4:84–93.

45. Nielsen RE et al. Neuroleptic malignant syndrome – an 11-year longitudinal case-control study. Can J Psychiatry 2012; 57:512–518.

46. Wittmann O et al. Neuroleptic malignant syndrome associated with metoclopramide use in a boy: case report and review of the literature. Am J Ther 2016; 23:e1246–1249.

47. Gurrera RJ. Sympathoadrenal hyperactivity and the etiology of neuroleptic malignant syndrome. Am J Psychiatry 1999; 156:169–180.

48. Levenson JL. Neuroleptic malignant syndrome. Am J Psychiatry 1985; 142:1137–1145.

49. Hermesh H et al. High serum creatinine kinase level: possible risk factor for neuroleptic malignant syndrome. J Clin Psychopharmacol 2002; 22:252–256.

50. Picard LS et al. Atypical neuroleptic malignant syndrome: diagnostic controversies and considerations. Pharmacotherapy 2008; 28:530–535.

51. Viejo LF et al. Risk factors in neuroleptic malignant syndrome. A case-control study. Acta Psychiatr Scand 2003; 107:45–49.

52. Spivak B et al. Neuroleptic malignant syndrome during abrupt reduction of neuroleptic treatment. Acta Psychiatr Scand 1990; 81:168–169.

53. Spivak B et al. Neuroleptic malignant syndrome associated with abrupt withdrawal of anticholinergic agents. Int Clin Psychopharmacol 1996; 11:207–209.

54. Olmsted TR. Neuroleptic malignant syndrome: guidelines for treatment and reinstitution of neuroleptics. South Med J 1988; 81:888–891.

55. Shoop SA et al. Carbidopa/levodopa in the treatment of neuroleptic malignant syndrome (Letter). Ann Pharmacother 1997; 31:119.

56. Terao T. Carbamazepine in the treatment of neuroleptic malignant syndrome (Letter). Biol Psychiatry 1999; 45:381–382.

57. Lattanzi L et al. Subcutaneous apomorphine for neuroleptic malignant syndrome. Am J Psychiatry 2006; 163:1450–1451.

58. Francis A et al. Is lorazepam a treatment for neuroleptic malignant syndrome? CNS Spectr 2000; 5:54–57.

59. Wells AJ et al. Neuroleptic rechallenge after neuroleptic malignant syndrome: case report and literature review. Drug Intell Clin Pharm 1988; 22:475–480.

60. Klein JP et al. Massive creatine kinase elevations with quetiapine: report of two cases. Pharmacopsychiatry 2006; 39:39–40.

61. Shiloh R et al. Precautionary measures reduce risk of definite neuroleptic malignant syndrome in newly typical neuroleptic-treated schizophrenia inpatients. Int Clin Psychopharmacol 2003; 18:147–149.

62. Hatch CD et al. Failed challenge with quetiapine after neuroleptic malignant syndrome with conventional antipsychotics. Pharmacotherapy 2001; 21:1003–1006.

63. Trutia A et al. Neuroleptic rechallenge with aripiprazole in a patient with previously documented neuroleptic malignant syndrome. J Psychiatr Pract 2008; 14:398–402.

Catatonia

The term 'catatonia' usually refers to a state of stupor (akinetic mutism) occurring in the context of a psychotic illness. There are two problems with this. First, catatonic schizophrenia may manifest as immobile stupor or a state of chaotic physical and psychological agitation.[1] Second, stupor is seen in many other non-organic conditions such as depression, mania and conversion disorder.[2–6]

Catatonia is thus one type of stupor, characterised by at least two of the following symptoms:

- marked psychomotor retardation, sometimes with complete immobility
- mutism
- waxy flexibility (no resistance from a patient to an attempt to move a limb into the most awkward position and maintenance of its position)
- negativism (strong opposite direction movement responses to an attempt to move a patient's limb) or automatic obedience
- peculiar voluntary movements, e.g. posturing, mannerisms, stereotyped movements and grimacing
- echolalia, echopraxia
- refusal to eat and/or drink.

If psychiatric stupor is left untreated, physical health complications are unavoidable and develop rapidly. Prompt treatment is crucial as it may prevent complications, which include dehydration, venous thrombosis, pulmonary embolism, pneumonia, and ultimately death.[7]

There are three major psychiatric illnesses that can present with stupor. Amongst them, stupor is mostly seen in psychotic illness. As outlined earlier, catatonic schizophrenia presents not only with an immobile mute picture of stupor, but also with a catatonic excitement, when a patient experiences the opposite of stupor – a chaotic psychomotor agitation and pronouncedly increased volume of speech, most of which is incoherent. The second psychiatric cause of stupor is affective illness, where an immobile mute clinical picture can occur in both depressive and, less commonly, manic states.[2,4,8–11] The third cause is one of the most intriguing and rare psychiatric conditions – conversion disorder stupor, which sometimes is referred to as psychosomatic or hysterical catatonia.[12–15]

There are also developmental disorders such as autism, as well as neurodegenerative[16,17] and organic disorders, which can present with a catatonia-like picture of a mute and immobile patient. These include a number of medical disorders such as:

- subarachnoid haemorrhages
- basal ganglia disorders
- non-convulsive status epilepticus
- locked-in and akinetic mutism states
- endocrine and metabolic disorders, e.g. Wilson's disease[18]
- Prader–Willi syndrome
- antiphospholipid syndrome[19]
- systemic lupus erythematosus (SLE)[20]

- infections
- dementia
- drug withdrawal and toxic drug states – can precipitate catatonic symptoms, e.g. after abrupt withdrawal of clozapine and withdrawal of zolpidem, temazepam and many non-psychotropics including the medicines used in oncology.

The treatment of stupor is dependent on its cause. Benzodiazepines are the drugs of choice for stupor occurring in the context of affective and conversion disorders.[8,9,21] It is postulated that benzodiazepines may act by increasing GABAergic transmission or reducing levels of brain-derived neurotropic factor.[22] There is most clinical experience with lorazepam. Many patients will respond to standard doses (up to 4 mg per day), but repeated and higher doses (between 8 and 24 mg per day) may be needed.[23] One observational study lasting 9 years in patients with stupor of a mood disorder causality,[8] either major depressive episodes or bipolar I, reported an 83.3% response to IM lorazepam 2 mg administered within the first 2 hours of presentation and a 100% response if 10 mg diazepam IV in 500 mL normal saline was added in cases of IM treatment failure. A very similar protocol achieved an 85.7% success rate in catatonia caused by general medical conditions or substance misuse.[24]

Where benzodiazepines are effective, their benefit is seen very quickly. A test dose of zolpidem (10 mg) is said to predict response to benzodiazepines[25] and frequent dosing of zolpidem may provide effective treatment.[26,27]

Catatonia in schizophrenia is somewhat less likely to respond to benzodiazepines, with a response in the range of 40–50%.[28] A double-blind, placebo-controlled, crossover trial with lorazepam up to 6 mg per day demonstrated no effect on catatonic symptoms in patients with chronic schizophrenia,[29] similar to the poor effect of lorazepam in a non-randomised trial.[30] A further complication in schizophrenia is that of differential diagnosis. Debate continues on the similarities and differences between catatonic stupor in psychosis and NMS.[31,32] Two terms, lethal catatonia and malignant catatonia,[33] have been coined to describe stupor that is accompanied by autonomic instability or hyperthermia. This potentially fatal condition cannot be distinguished either clinically or by laboratory testing from NMS, leading to a suggestion that NMS is a variant form of malignant catatonia.[34] However, the absence of any prior or recent administration of a dopamine antagonist can help rule out NMS.

In stupor associated with schizophrenia, ECT and benzodiazepines remain the treatments of first choice (Figure 1.5). The vast majority of evidence published recently as well as over previous decades suggests that prompt ECT remains the most successful treatment.[30,35–49] As with benzodiazepines, response to ECT may be lower in patients with schizophrenia (or in those who have been treated with antipsychotics) than in patients with mood disorders.[50] In malignant catatonia, every effort should be made to maximise the effect of ECT by using liberal stimulus dosing to induce well-generalised seizures.[51] Physical health needs should also be a priority and in-patient medical care obtained when necessary, especially for those showing autonomic imbalance and those whose dietary intake cannot be managed in psychiatric care.

The use of antipsychotic medication should be carefully considered (Table 1.23). Some authors recommend that antipsychotics should be avoided altogether in catatonic patients, although there are case reports of successful treatment with aripiprazole,

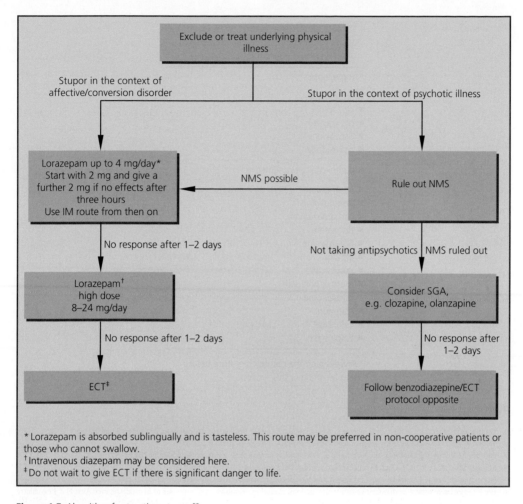

Figure 1.5 Algorithm for treating stupor.[58]

risperidone, olanzapine, ziprasidone and clozapine.[52–57] There is probably most evidence supporting clozapine and olanzapine.

Simple guidance on the usage of antipsychotic medication is to consider the history of a patient, their previous diagnosis and previous response to antipsychotic treatment, and the likelihood that non-adherence precipitated stupor. It needs to be noted that physical health problems, as in the examples listed in the beginning of this section, can present as a catatonia-like clinical picture, warranting treatment of the underlying medical condition. Antipsychotic medication should be avoided where there are clear signs of NMS: where stupor develops during treatment with antipsychotics and muscle rigidity is accompanied by autonomic instability. Where NMS can be ruled out and stupor occurs in the context of non-adherence to antipsychotic treatment, early re-establishment of antipsychotic medication is recommended. This is particularly important where stupor represents a withdrawal syndrome (as sometimes seen with clozapine).

Table 1.23 Alternatives to benzodiazepines in catatonia/stupor (listed in alphabetical order – no preference implied by order)

Antipsychotics[52–57,59–62]

- aripiprazole
- clozapine
- olanzapine
- risperidone
- ziprasidone

Experimental treatments* [9,10,26,27,45,63–68]

- amantadine
- amitriptyline
- carbamazepine
- fluoxetine
- fluvoxamine
- lithium
- memantine
- methylphenidate
- mirtazapine
- tramadol
- valproate
- zolpidem

* Always read the primary literature before using anything in this section.

References

1. Walther S. Dysfunctions of the motor system in schizophrenia. Eur Arch Psychiatry Clin Neurosci 2013; **263 Suppl 1**:S16.
2. Takacs R et al. Catatonia in affective disorders. Current Psychiatry Reviews 2013; **9**:101–105.
3. Fink M. Rediscovering catatonia: the biography of a treatable syndrome. Acta Psychiatr Scand Suppl 2013:1–47.
4. Mangas MCC et al. P-167 – Catatonia in bipolar disorder. Eur Psychiatry 2012; **27 Suppl 1**:1.
5. Bartolommei N et al. Catatonia: a critical review and therapeutic recommendation. J Psychopathol 2012; **18**:234–246.
6. Lee J. Dissociative catatonia: dissociative-catatonic reactions, clinical presentations and responses to benzodiazepines. Aust N Z J Psychiatry 2011; **45**:A42.
7. Petrides G et al. Synergism of lorazepam and electroconvulsive therapy in the treatment of catatonia. Biol Psychiatry 1997; **42**:375–381.
8. Huang YC et al. Rapid relief of catatonia in mood disorder by lorazepam and diazepam. Biomed J 2013; **36**:35–39.
9. Vasudev K et al. What works for delirious catatonic mania? BMJ Case Rep 2010; **2010**:1–5.
10. Neuhut R et al. Resolution of catatonia after treatment with stimulant medication in a patient with bipolar disorder. Psychosomatics 2012; **53**:482–484.
11. Ghaffarinejad AR et al. Periodic catatonia. Challenging diagnosis for psychiatrists. Neurosciences (Riyadh) 2012; **17**:156–158.
12. Suzuki K et al. Hysteria presenting as a prodrome to catatonic stupor in a depressive patient resolved with electroconvulsive therapy. J ECT 2006; **22**:276.
13. Alwaki A et al. Catatonia: an elusive diagnosis. Neurology 2013; **80 Suppl 1**:P05.127.
14. Dhadphale M. Eye gaze diagnostic sign in hysterical stupor. Lancet 1980; **2**:374–375.
15. Gomez J. Hysterical stupor and death. Br J Psychiatry 1980; **136**:105–106.
16. Mazzone L et al. Catatonia in patients with autism: prevalence and management. CNS Drugs 2014; **28**:205–215.
17. Dhossche DM et al. Catatonia in psychiatric illnesses. In: Fatemi SH, Clayton PJ, eds. *The Medical Basis of Psychiatry*. Totowa, NJ: Humana Press; 2008, pp. 471–486.
18. Shetageri VN et al. Case report: catatonia as a presenting symptom of Wilsons disease. Indian J Psychiatry 2011; **53 Suppl 5**:S93–S94.
19. Cardinal RN et al. Psychosis and catatonia as a first presentation of antiphospholipid syndrome. Br J Psychiatry 2009; **195**:272.
20. Pustilnik S et al. Catatonia as the presenting symptom in systemic lupus erythematosus. J Psychiatr Pract 2011; **17**:217–221.
21. Sienaert P et al. Adult catatonia: etiopathogenesis, diagnosis and treatment. Neuropsychiatry 2013; **3**:391–399.
22. Huang TL et al. Lorazepam reduces the serum brain-derived neurotrophic factor level in schizophrenia patients with catatonia. Prog Neuropsychopharmacol Biol Psychiatry 2009; **33**:158–159.

23. Fink M et al. Neuroleptic malignant syndrome is malignant catatonia, warranting treatments efficacious for catatonia. Prog Neuropsychopharmacol Biol Psychiatry 2006; 30:1182–1183.

24. Lin CC et al. The lorazepam and diazepam protocol for catatonia due to general medical condition and substance in liaison psychiatry. PLoS One 2017; 12:e0170452.

25. Javelot H et al. Zolpidem test and catatonia. J Clin Pharm Ther 2015; 40:699–701.

26. Bastiampillai T et al. Treatment refractory chronic catatonia responsive to zolpidem challenge. Aust N Z J Psychiatry 2016; 50:98.

27. Peglow S et al. Treatment of catatonia with zolpidem. J Neuropsychiatry Clin Neurosci 2013; 25:E13.

28. Rosebush PI et al. Catatonia: re-awakening to a forgotten disorder. Mov Disord 1999; 14:395–397.

29. Ungvari GS et al. Lorazepam for chronic catatonia: a randomized, double-blind, placebo-controlled cross-over study. Psychopharmacology (Berl) 1999; 142:393–398.

30. Dutt A et al. Phenomenology and treatment of catatonia: a descriptive study from north India. Indian J Psychiatry 2011; 53:36–40.

31. Luchini F et al. Catatonia and neuroleptic malignant syndrome: two disorders on a same spectrum? Four case reports. J Nerv Ment Dis 2013; 201:36–42.

32. Mishima T et al. [Diazepam-responsive malignant catatonia in a patient with an initial clinical diagnosis of neuroleptic malignant syndrome: a case report]. Brain Nerve 2011; 63:503–507.

33. Mann SC et al. Catatonia, malignant catatonia, and neuroleptic malignant syndrome. Current Psychiatry Reviews 2013; 9:111–119.

34. Taylor MA et al. Catatonia in psychiatric classification: a home of its own. Am J Psychiatry 2003; 160:1233–1241.

35. Bush G et al. Catatonia. II. Treatment with lorazepam and electroconvulsive therapy. Acta Psychiatr Scand 1996; 93:137–143.

36. Cristancho P et al. Successful use of right unilateral ECT for catatonia: a case series. J ECT 2014; 30:69–72.

37. Philbin D et al. Catatonic schizophrenia: therapeutic challenges and potentially a new role for electroconvulsive therapy? BMJ Case Rep 2013; 2013.

38. Takebayashi M. [Electroconvulsive therapy in schizophrenia]. Nihon Rinsho 2013; 71:694–700.

39. Oviedo G et al. Trends in the administration of electroconvulsive therapy for schizophrenia in Colombia. Descriptive study and literature review. Eur Arch Psychiatry Clin Neurosci 2013; 263 Suppl 1:S98.

40. Pompili M et al. Indications for electroconvulsive treatment in schizophrenia: a systematic review. Schizophr Res 2013; 146:1–9.

41. Ogando Portilla N et al. Electroconvulsive therapy as an effective treatment in neuroleptic malignant syndrome: purposely a case. Eur Psychiatry 2013; 28 Suppl 1:1.

42. Unal A et al. Effective treatment of catatonia by combination of benzodiazepine and electroconvulsive therapy. J ECT 2013; 29:206–209.

43. Kaliora SC et al. The practice of electroconvulsive therapy in Greece. J ECT 2013; 29:219–224.

44. Girardi P et al. Life-saving electroconvulsive therapy in a patient with near-lethal catatonia. Riv Psichiatr 2012; 47:535–537.

45. Kumar V et al. Electroconvulsive therapy in pregnancy. Indian J Psychiatry 2011; 53 Suppl 5:S100–S101.

46. Weiss M et al. Treatment of catatonia with electroconvulsive therapy in adolescents. J Child Adolesc Psychopharmacol 2012; 22:96–100.

47. Bauer J et al. Should the term catatonia be explicitly included in the ICD-10 description of acute transient psychotic disorder F23.0? Nord J Psychiatry 2012; 66:68–69.

48. Mohammadbeigi H et al. Electroconvulsive therapy in single manic episodes: a case series. Afr J Psychiatry 2011; 14:56–59.

49. Dragasek J. [Utilisation of electroconvulsive therapy in treatment of depression disorders]. Psychiatrie 2011; 15:1211–1219.

50. van Waarde JA et al. Electroconvulsive therapy for catatonia: treatment characteristics and outcomes in 27 patients. J ECT 2010; 26:248–252.

51. Kellner CH et al. Electroconvulsive therapy for catatonia. Am J Psychiatry 2010; 167:1127–1128.

52. Van Den EF et al. The use of atypical antipsychotics in the treatment of catatonia. Eur Psychiatry 2005; 20:422–429.

53. Caroff SN et al. Movement disorders associated with atypical antipsychotic drugs. J Clin Psychiatry 2002; 63 Suppl 4:12–19.

54. Guzman CS et al. Treatment of periodic catatonia with atypical antipsychotic, olanzapine. Psychiatry Clin Neurosci 2008; 62:482.

55. Babington PW et al. Treatment of catatonia with olanzapine and amantadine. Psychosomatics 2007; 48:534–536.

56. Bastiampillai T et al. Catatonia resolution and aripiprazole. Aust N Z J Psychiatry 2008; 42:907.

57. Strawn JR et al. Successful treatment of catatonia with aripiprazole in an adolescent with psychosis. J Child Adolesc Psychopharmacol 2007; 17:733–735.

58. Rosebush PI et al. Catatonia and its treatment. Schizophr Bull 2010; 36:239–242.

59. Voros V et al. [Use of aripiprazole in the treatment of catatonia]. Neuropsychopharmacol Hung 2010; 12:373–376.

60. Yoshimura B et al. Is quetiapine suitable for treatment of acute schizophrenia with catatonic stupor? A case series of 39 patients. Neuropsychiatr Dis Treat 2013; 9:1565–1571.

61. Todorova K. Olanzapine in the treatment of catatonic stupor – two case reports and discussion. Eur Neuropsychopharmacol 2012; 22 Suppl 2:S326.

62. Prakash O et al. Catatonia and mania in patient with AIDS: treatment with lorazepam and risperidone. Gen Hosp Psychiatry 2012; 34:321–326.

63. Daniels J. Catatonia: clinical aspects and neurobiological correlates. J Neuropsychiatry Clin Neurosci 2009; 21:371–380.

64. Obregon DF et al. Memantine and catatonia: a case report and literature review. J Psychiatr Pract 2011; 17:292–299.

65. Hervey WM et al. Treatment of catatonia with amantadine. Clin Neuropharmacol 2012; 35:86–87.

66. Consoli A et al. Lorazepam, fluoxetine and packing therapy in an adolescent with pervasive developmental disorder and catatonia. J Physiol Paris 2010; 104:309–314.

67. Lewis AL et al. Malignant catatonia in a patient with bipolar disorder, B12 deficiency, and neuroleptic malignant syndrome: one cause or three? J Psychiatr Pract 2009; 15:415–422.

68. Padhy SK et al. The catatonia conundrum: controversies and contradictions. Asian J Psychiatry 2014; 7:6–9.

ECG changes – QT prolongation

Introduction

Many psychotropic drugs are associated with ECG changes and some are causally linked to serious ventricular arrhythmia and sudden cardiac death. Specifically, some antipsychotics block cardiac potassium channels and are linked to prolongation of the cardiac QT interval, a risk factor for the ventricular arrhythmia torsades de pointes, which is often fatal. Case-control studies have suggested that the use of most antipsychotics is associated with an increase in the rate of sudden cardiac death.[1-7] This risk is probably a result of the arrhythmogenic potential of antipsychotics[8,9] although schizophrenia itself may be associated with QT prolongation.[10] Nonetheless, a study in first-episode patients showed that the use of antipsychotics produced clear prolongation of the QT interval after 2–4 weeks.[11] Overall risk is probably dose-related and, although the absolute risk is low, it is substantially higher than, say, the risk of fatal agranulocytosis with clozapine.[8] The effect of antipsychotic polypharmacy on QT is somewhat uncertain,[12] but the extent of QT prolongation is probably a function of overall dose.[13]

ECG monitoring of drug-induced changes in mental health settings is complicated by a number of factors. Psychiatrists may have limited expertise in ECG interpretation, for example, and still less expertise in manually measuring QT intervals. Even cardiologists show an inter-rater reliability in QT measurement of up to 20 ms.[14] Self-reading, computerised ECG devices are available and to some extent compensate for some lack of expertise, but different models use different algorithms and different correction formulae.[15] In addition, ECG machines may not be as readily available in all clinical areas as they are in general medicine. Also, time for ECG determination may not be available in many areas (e.g. out-patients). Lastly, ECG determination may be difficult to perform in acutely disturbed, physically uncooperative patients.

ECG monitoring is essential for all patients prescribed antipsychotics. An estimate of QT_C interval should be made on admission to in-patient units (in the UK this is recommended in the NICE schizophrenia guideline[16]) and yearly thereafter.

QT prolongation

- The cardiac QT interval (usually cited as QTc – QT corrected for heart rate) is a useful, but imprecise indicator of risk of torsades de pointes and of increased cardiac mortality.[17] Different correction factors and methods may give markedly different values.[18]
- The QT interval broadly reflects the duration of cardiac repolarisation. Lengthening of repolarisation duration induces heterogeneity of electrical phasing in different ventricular structures (a phenomenon known as dispersion) which in turn allows the emergence of early afterdepolarisations (EADs) which may provoke ventricular extrasystole and torsades de pointes.
- There is some controversy over the exact association between QTc and risk of arrhythmia. Very limited evidence suggests that risk is exponentially related to the extent of prolongation beyond normal limits (440 ms for men, 470 ms for women), although there are well-known exceptions that appear to disprove this theory[19] (some

drugs prolong QT without increasing dispersion). Rather stronger evidence links QTc values over 500 ms to a clearly increased risk of arrhythmia.[20] QT intervals of >650 ms may be more likely than not to induce torsades.[21] Despite some uncertainties, QTc determination remains an important measure in estimating risk of arrhythmia and sudden death.

- Individual components of the QT interval may have particular importance. The time from the start of the T wave to T-wave peak has been shown to be the only aspect of QT prolongation associated with sudden cardiac deaths.[22]
- QTc measurements and evaluation are complicated by:
  - difficulty in determining the end of the T wave, particularly where U waves are present (this applies both to manual and self-reading ECG machines)[20]
  - normal physiological variation in QTc interval: QT varies with gender, time of day, food intake, alcohol intake, menstrual cycle, ECG lead, etc.[18,19]
  - variation in the extent of drug-induced prolongation of QTc because of changes in plasma levels. QTc prolongation is most prominent at peak drug plasma levels and least obvious at trough levels.[18,19]

Other ECG changes

Other reported antipsychotic-induced changes include atrial fibrillation, giant P waves, T-wave changes and heart block.[19]

Quantifying risk

Drugs are categorised in Table 1.24 according to data available on their effects on the cardiac QTc interval (as reported; mostly using Bazett's correction formula). 'No-effect' drugs are those with which QTc prolongation has not been reported either at therapeutic doses or in overdose. 'Low-effect' drugs are those for which severe QTc prolongation has been reported only following overdose or where only small average increases (<10 ms) have been observed at clinical doses. 'Moderate-effect' drugs are those which have been observed to prolong QTc by >10 ms on average when given at normal clinical doses or where ECG monitoring is officially recommended in some circumstances. 'High-effect' drugs are those for which extensive average QTc prolongation (usually >20 ms at normal clinical doses).

Note that, as outlined previously, effect on QTc may not necessarily equate directly to risk of torsades de pointes or sudden death,[68] although this is often assumed. (A good example here is ziprasidone – a drug with a moderate effect on QTc but with no evidence of cardiac toxicity.[69]) Note also that categorisation is inevitably approximate given the problems associated with QTc measurements. Lastly, keep in mind that differences in the effects of different antipsychotics on the QT interval rarely reach statistical significance even in meta-analyses.[70]

Outside these guidelines, readers are directed to the RISQ-PATH study[71] which provides a scoring system for the prediction of QT prolongation (to above normal ranges) in any patient. RISQ-PATH has a 98% negative predictive value, so allowing a reduction in monitoring in low-risk patients. The RISQ-PATH method uses CredibleMeds categorisation for drug effects on QT – this, too, is recommended.[72]

Table 1.24 Effects of antipsychotics on QTc[18,19,23–51]

No effect	Low effect	Moderate effect	High effect	Unknown effect
Brexpiprazole*	Aripiprazole[†]	Amisulpride[§]	Any intravenous antipsychotic	Pipotiazine
Cariprazine*	Asenapine	Chlorpromazine	Pimozide	Trifluoperazine
Lurasidone	Clozapine	Haloperidol	Sertindole	Zuclopenthixol
	Flupentixol	Iloperidone	Any drug or combination of	
	Fluphenazine	Levomepromazine	drugs used in doses exceeding	
	Loxapine	Melperone	recommended maximum	
	Perphenazine	Quetiapine		
	Prochlorperazine	Ziprasidone		
	Olanzapine[‡]			
	Paliperidone			
	Risperidone			
	Sulpiride			

* Limited clinical experience (association with QT prolongation may emerge).

[†] One case of torsades de pointes (TDP) reported,[52] two cases of QT prolongation[53,54] and an association with TDP found in database study.[55] Recent data suggest aripiprazole causes QTc prolongation of around 8 ms.[56] Aripiprazole may increase QT dispersion.[57]

[‡] Isolated cases of QTc prolongation[27,58] and has effects on cardiac ion channel, I_{Kr},[59] other data suggest no effect on QT_c.[19,25,26,60]

[§] TDP common in overdose;[21,61] strong association with TDP in clinical doses.[55]

Note: Since the last edition aripiprazole has moved from 'no effect' to 'low effect'. Data are rather contradictory, with most studies showing a decrease in QTc associated with aripiprazole use[52] even in children and adolescents.[62] However more recent data[52,53,55,56,63] cast doubt on assumptions of cardiac safety. Lurasidone remains in the 'no effect' group[42] although one study mentioned in the US labelling[64] reports a QT lengthening of 7.5 mg in people receiving 120 mg (111 mg) a day. Those receiving 600 mg (555 mg) daily showed a lower change (+4.6 ms). These findings are in some contrast with those from studies in patients which uniformly suggest no or minimal effect.[65–67] This disparity is probably explained by the use of different correction factors and by random change, as often seen in placebo-treated patients[67] and as suggested by the apparent lack of dose-related effect. No cases of QTc > 500 ms or TDP have been reported with lurasidone to our knowledge.

Other risk factors

A number of physiological/pathological factors are associated with an increased risk of QT changes and of arrhythmia (Table 1.25) and many non-psychotropic drugs are linked to QT prolongation (Table 1.26).[20] These additional risk factors seem almost always to be present in cases of antipsychotic-induced TDP.[73]

ECG monitoring

Measure QTc in all patients prescribed antipsychotics:

- on admission
- if previous abnormality or known additional risk factor, at annual physical health check.

Consider measuring QTc within a week of achieving a therapeutic dose of a newly pre-scribed antipsychotic that is associated with a moderate or high risk of QTc prolongation or of newly prescribed combined antipsychotics. See Table 1.27 for the management of QT prolongation in patients receiving antipsychotic drugs.

Table 1.25 Physiological risk factors for QTc prolongation and arrhythmia

Factor	Symptom
Cardiac	Long QT syndrome Bradycardia Ischaemic heart disease Myocarditis Myocardial infarction Left ventricular hypertrophy
Metabolic	Hypokalaemia Hypomagnesaemia Hypocalcaemia
Others	Extreme physical exertion Stress or shock Anorexia nervosa Extremes of age – children and elderly people may be more susceptible to QT changes Female gender

Hypokalaemia-related QTc prolongation is more commonly observed in acute psychotic admissions.[74] Also, be aware that there are a number of physical and genetic factors which may not be discovered on routine examination but which probably predispose patients to arrhythmia.[75,76]

Table 1.26 Non-psychotropics associated with QT prolongation (see Crediblemeds.org for latest information)

Drug class	Drug
Antibiotics	Erythromycin Clarithromycin Ampicillin Co-trimoxazole Pentamidine (Some 4 quinolones affect QTc – see manufacturers' literature)
Antimalarials	Chloroquine Mefloquine Quinine
Antiarrhythmics	Quinidine Disopyramide Procainamide Sotalol Amiodarone Bretylium
Others	Amantadine Cyclosporin Diphenhydramine Hydroxyzine Methadone Nicardipine Tamoxifen

Beta-2 agonists and sympathomimetics may provoke torsades de pointes in patients with prolonged QTc.

Table 1.27 Management of QT prolongation in patients receiving antipsychotic drugs

QTc	Action	Refer to cardiologist
<440 ms (men) or <470 ms (women)	None unless abnormal T-wave morphology	Consider if in doubt
>440 ms (men) or >470 ms (women) but <500 ms	Consider reducing dose or switching to drug of lower effect; repeat ECG	Consider
>500 ms	Repeat ECG. Stop suspected causative drug(s) and switch to drug of lower effect	Immediately
Abnormal T-wave morphology	Review treatment. Consider reducing dose or switching to drug of lower effect	Immediately

Metabolic inhibition

The effect of drugs on the QTc interval is usually plasma level-dependent. Drug interactions are therefore important, especially when metabolic inhibition results in increased plasma levels of the drug affecting QTc. Commonly used metabolic inhibitors include fluvoxamine, fluoxetine, paroxetine and valproate.

Other cardiovascular risk factors

The risk of drug-induced arrhythmia and sudden cardiac death with psychotropics is an important consideration. With respect to cardiovascular disease, note that other risk factors such as smoking, obesity and impaired glucose tolerance present a much greater risk to patient morbidity and mortality than the uncertain outcome of QT changes. See relevant sections for discussion of these problems.

Summary

- In the absence of conclusive data, assume all antipsychotics are linked to sudden cardiac death.
- Prescribe the lowest dose possible and avoid polypharmacy/metabolic interactions.
- Perform ECG on admission, and, if previous abnormality or additional risk factor, at yearly check-up.
- Consider measuring QTc within a week of achieving a therapeutic dose of a moderate-/high-risk antipsychotic.

References

1. Reilly JG et al. Thioridazine and sudden unexplained death in psychiatric in-patients. Br J Psychiatry 2002; 180:515–522.
2. Murray-Thomas T et al. Risk of mortality (including sudden cardiac death) and major cardiovascular events in atypical and typical antipsychotic users: a study with the general practice research database. Cardiovasc Psychiatry Neurol 2013; 2013:247486.
3. Ray WA et al. Antipsychotics and the risk of sudden cardiac death. Arch Gen Psychiatry 2001; 58:1161–1167.
4. Hennessy S et al. Cardiac arrest and ventricular arrhythmia in patients taking antipsychotic drugs: cohort study using administrative data. BMJ 2002; 325:1070.
5. Straus SM et al. Antipsychotics and the risk of sudden cardiac death. Arch Intern Med 2004; 164:1293–1297.
6. Liperoti R et al. Conventional and atypical antipsychotics and the risk of hospitalization for ventricular arrhythmias or cardiac arrest. Arch Intern Med 2005; 165:696–701.

7. Ray WA et al. Atypical antipsychotic drugs and the risk of sudden cardiac death. N Engl J Med 2009; **360**:225–235.

8. Schneeweiss S et al. Antipsychotic agents and sudden cardiac death – how should we manage the risk? N Engl J Med 2009; **360**:294–296.

9. Nakagawa S et al. Antipsychotics and risk of first-time hospitalization for myocardial infarction: a population-based case-control study. J Intern Med 2006; **260**:451–458.

10. Fujii K et al. QT is longer in drug-free patients with schizophrenia compared with age-matched healthy subjects. PLoS One 2014; **9**: e98555.

11. Zhai D et al. QTc interval lengthening in first-episode schizophrenia (FES) patients in the earliest stages of antipsychotic treatment. Schizophr Res 2017; **179**:70–74.

12. Takeuchi H et al. Antipsychotic polypharmacy and corrected QT interval: a systematic review. Can J Psychiatry 2015; **60**:215–222.

13. Barbui C et al. Antipsychotic dose mediates the association between polypharmacy and corrected QT interval. PLoS One 2016; **11**:e0148212.

14. Goldenberg I et al. QT interval: how to measure it and what is "normal". J Cardiovasc Electrophysiol 2006; **17**:333–336.

15. Nielsen J et al. Assessing QT interval prolongation and its associated risks with antipsychotics. CNS Drugs 2011; **25**:473–490.

16. National Institute for Health and Care Excellence. Psychosis and schizophrenia in adults: prevention and management. Clinical Guideline 178, 2014. https://www.nice.org.uk/guidance/cg178.

17. Malik M et al. Evaluation of drug-induced QT interval prolongation: implications for drug approval and labelling. Drug Saf 2001; **24**:323–351.

18. Haddad PM et al. Antipsychotic-related QTc prolongation, torsade de pointes and sudden death. Drugs 2002; **62**:1649–1671.

19. Taylor DM. Antipsychotics and QT prolongation. Acta Psychiatr Scand 2003; **107**:85–95.

20. Botstein P. Is QT interval prolongation harmful? A regulatory perspective. Am J Cardiol 1993; **72**:50B–52B.

21. Joy JP et al. Prediction of torsade de pointes from the QT interval: analysis of a case series of amisulpride overdoses. Clin Pharmacol Ther 2011; **90**:243–245.

22. O'Neal WT et al. Association between QT-interval components and sudden cardiac death: The ARIC Study (atherosclerosis risk in communities). Circ Arrhythm Electrophysiol 2017; **10**.

23. Glassman AH et al. Antipsychotic drugs: prolonged QTc interval, torsade de pointes, and sudden death. Am J Psychiatry 2001; **158**:1774–1782.

24. Warner B et al. Investigation of the potential of clozapine to cause torsade de pointes. Adverse Drug React Toxicol Rev 2002; **21**:189–203.

25. Harrigan EP et al. A randomized evaluation of the effects of six antipsychotic agents on QTc, in the absence and presence of metabolic inhibition. J Clin Psychopharmacol 2004; **24**:62–69.

26. Lindborg SR et al. Effects of intramuscular olanzapine vs. haloperidol and placebo on QTc intervals in acutely agitated patients. Psychiatry Res 2003; **119**:113–123.

27. Dineen S et al. QTc prolongation and high-dose olanzapine (Letter). Psychosomatics 2003; **44**:174–175.

28. Gupta S et al. Quetiapine and QTc issues: a case report (Letter). J Clin Psychiatry 2003; **64**:612–613.

29. Su KP et al. A pilot cross-over design study on QTc interval prolongation associated with sulpiride and haloperidol. Schizophr Res 2003; **59**:93–94.

30. Chong SA et al. Prolonged QTc intervals in medicated patients with schizophrenia. Hum Psychopharmacol 2003; **18**:647–649.

31. Stollberger C et al. Antipsychotic drugs and QT prolongation. Int Clin Psychopharmacol 2005; **20**:243–251.

32. Isbister GK et al. Amisulpride deliberate self-poisoning causing severe cardiac toxicity including QT prolongation and torsades de pointes. Med J Aust 2006; **184**:354–356.

33. Ward DI. Two cases of amisulpride overdose: a cause for prolonged QT syndrome. Emerg Med Australas 2005; **17**:274–276.

34. Vieweg WV et al. Torsade de pointes in a patient with complex medical and psychiatric conditions receiving low-dose quetiapine. Acta Psychiatr Scand 2005; **112**:318–322.

35. Huang BH et al. Sulpiride induced torsade de pointes. Int J Cardiol 2007; **118**:e100–e102.

36. Kane JM et al. Long-term efficacy and safety of iloperidone: results from 3 clinical trials for the treatment of schizophrenia. J Clin Psychopharmacol 2008; **28**:S29–S35.

37. Kim MD et al. Blockade of HERG human K+ channel and IKr of guinea pig cardiomyocytes by prochlorperazine. Eur J Pharmacol 2006; **544**:82–90.

38. Meltzer H et al. Efficacy and tolerability of oral paliperidone extended-release tablets in the treatment of acute schizophrenia: pooled data from three 6-week placebo-controlled studies. J Clin Psychiatry 2006; **69**:817–829.

39. Chapel S et al. Exposure-response analysis in patients with schizophrenia to assess the effect of asenapine on QTc prolongation. J Clin Pharmacol 2009; **49**:1297–1308.

40. Ozeki Y et al. QTc prolongation and antipsychotic medications in a sample of 1017 patients with schizophrenia. Prog Neuropsychopharmacol Biol Psychiatry 2010; **34**:401–405.

41. Girardin FR et al. Drug-induced long QT in adult psychiatric inpatients: the 5-year cross-sectional ECG Screening Outcome in Psychiatry study. Am J Psychiatry 2013; **170**:1468–1476.

42. Leucht S et al. Comparative efficacy and tolerability of 15 antipsychotic drugs in schizophrenia: a multiple-treatments meta-analysis. Lancet 2013; **382**:951–962.

43. Grande I et al. QTc prolongation: is clozapine safe? Study of 82 cases before and after clozapine treatment. Hum Psychopharmacol 2011; **26**:397–403.

44. Hong HK et al. Block of hERG K+ channel and prolongation of action potential duration by fluphenazine at submicromolar concentration. Eur J Pharmacol 2013; **702**:165–173.

45. Vieweg WV et al. Risperidone, QTc interval prolongation, and torsade de pointes: a systematic review of case reports. Psychopharmacology (Berl) 2013; **228**:515–524.

CHAPTER 1

46. Suzuki Y et al. QT prolongation of the antipsychotic risperidone is predominantly related to its 9-hydroxy metabolite paliperidone. Hum Psychopharmacol 2012; 27:39–42.

47. Polcwiartek C et al. The cardiac safety of aripiprazole treatment in patients at high risk for torsade: a systematic review with a meta-analytic approach. Psychopharmacology (Berl) 2015; 232:3297–3308.

48. Danielsson B et al. Antidepressants and antipsychotics classified with torsades de pointes arrhythmia risk and mortality in older adults – a Swedish nationwide study. Br J Clin Pharmacol 2016; 81:773–783.

49. Citrome L. Cariprazine in schizophrenia: clinical efficacy, tolerability, and place in therapy. Adv Ther 2013; 30:114–126.

50. Das S et al. Brexpiprazole: so far so good. Ther Adv Psychopharmacol 2016; 6:39–54.

51. Meyer JM et al. Lurasidone: a new drug in development for schizophrenia. Expert Opin Investig Drugs 2009; 18:1715–1726.

52. Nelson S et al. Torsades de pointes after administration of low-dose aripiprazole. Ann Pharmacother 2013; 47:e11.

53. Hategan A et al. Aripiprazole-associated QTc prolongation in a geriatric patient. J Clin Psychopharmacol 2014; 34:766–768.

54. Suzuki Y et al. Dose-dependent increase in the QTc interval in aripiprazole treatment after risperidone. Prog Neuropsychopharmacol Biol Psychiatry 2011; 35:643–644.

55. Raschi E et al. The contribution of national spontaneous reporting systems to detect signals of torsadogenicity: issues emerging from the ARITMO project. Drug Saf 2016; 39:59–68.

56. Belmonte C et al. Evaluation of the relationship between pharmacokinetics and the safety of aripiprazole and its cardiovascular effects in healthy volunteers. J Clin Psychopharmacol 2016; 36:608–614.

57. Germano E et al. ECG parameters in children and adolescents treated with aripiprazole and risperidone. Prog Neuropsychopharmacol Biol Psychiatry 2014; 51:23–27.

58. Su KP et al. Olanzapine-induced QTc prolongation in a patient with Wolff-Parkinson-White syndrome. Schizophr Res 2004; 66:191–192.

59. Morissette P et al. Olanzapine prolongs cardiac repolarization by blocking the rapid component of the delayed rectifier potassium current. J Psychopharmacol 2007; 21:735–741.

60. Bar KJ et al. Influence of olanzapine on QT variability and complexity measures of heart rate in patients with schizophrenia. J Clin Psychopharmacol 2008; 28:694–698.

61. Berling I et al. Prolonged QT risk assessment in antipsychotic overdose using the QT nomogram. Ann Emerg Med 2015; 66:154–164.

62. Jensen KG et al. Corrected QT changes during antipsychotic treatment of children and adolescents: a systematic review and meta-analysis of clinical trials. J Am Acad Child Adolesc Psychiatry 2015; 54:25–36.

63. Karz AJ et al. Effects of aripiprazole on the QTc: a case report. J Clin Psychiatry 2015; 76:1648–1649.

64. Sunovion Pharmaceuticals Inc. Highlights of Prescribing Information: LATUDA (lurasidone hydrochloride) tablets. 2017. http://www.latuda.com/LatudaPrescribingInformation.pdf

65. Potkin SG et al. Double-blind comparison of the safety and efficacy of lurasidone and ziprasidone in clinically stable outpatients with schizophrenia or schizoaffective disorder. Schizophr Res 2011; 132:101–107.

66. Nakamura M et al. Lurasidone in the treatment of acute schizophrenia: a double-blind, placebo-controlled trial. J Clin Psychiatry 2009; 70:829–836.

67. Meltzer HY et al. Lurasidone in the treatment of schizophrenia: a randomized, double-blind, placebo- and olanzapine-controlled study. Am J Psychiatry 2011; 168:957–967.

68. Witchel HJ et al. Psychotropic drugs, cardiac arrhythmia, and sudden death. J Clin Psychopharmacol 2003; 23:58–77.

69. Strom BL et al. Comparative mortality associated with ziprasidone and olanzapine in real-world use among 18,154 patients with schizophrenia: The Ziprasidone Observational Study of Cardiac Outcomes (ZODIAC). Am J Psychiatry 2011; 168:193–201.

70. Chung AK et al. Effects on prolongation of Bazett's corrected QT interval of seven second-generation antipsychotics in the treatment of schizophrenia: a meta-analysis. J Psychopharmacol 2011; 25:646–666.

71. Vandael E et al. Development of a risk score for QTc-prolongation: the RISQ-PATH study. Int J Clin Pharm 2017; 39:424–432.

72. CredibleMeds®. CredibleMeds. 2018. https://www.crediblemeds.org/

73. Hasnain M et al. Quetiapine, QTc interval prolongation, and torsade de pointes: a review of case reports. Ther Adv Psychopharmacol 2014; 4:130–138.

74. Hatta K et al. Prolonged QT interval in acute psychotic patients. Psychiatry Res 2000; 94:279–285.

75. Priori SG et al. Low penetrance in the long-QT syndrome: clinical impact. Circulation 1999; 99:529–533.

76. Frassati D et al. Hidden cardiac lesions and psychotropic drugs as a possible cause of sudden death in psychiatric patients: a report of 14 cases and review of the literature. Can J Psychiatry 2004; 49:100–105.

Effect of antipsychotic medications on plasma lipids

Morbidity and mortality from cardiovascular disease are higher in people with schizophrenia than in the general population.[1] Dyslipidaemia is an established risk factor for cardiovascular disease along with obesity, hypertension, smoking, diabetes and sedentary lifestyle. The majority of patients with schizophrenia have several of these risk factors and can be considered at 'high risk' of developing cardiovascular disease. Dyslipidaemia is treatable and intervention is known to reduce morbidity and mortality.[2] Aggressive treatment is particularly important in people with diabetes, the prevalence of which is increased two- to three-fold over population norms in people with schizophrenia (see section on 'Diabetes and impaired glucose tolerance' in this chapter).

Effect of antipsychotic drugs on lipids

First-generation antipsychotics

Phenothiazines are known to be associated with increases in triglycerides and low-density lipoprotein (LDL) cholesterol and decreases in high-density lipoprotein (HDL)[3] cholesterol, but the magnitude of these effects is poorly quantified.[4] Haloperidol seems to have minimal effect on lipid profiles.[3]

Second-generation antipsychotics

Although there are relatively more data pertaining to some SGAs, they are derived from a variety of sources and are reported in different ways, making it difficult to compare drugs directly. While cholesterol levels can rise, the most profound effect of these drugs seems to be on triglycerides. Raised triglycerides are, in general, associated with obesity and diabetes. From the available data, olanzapine[5] would seem to have the greatest propensity to increase lipids, and quetiapine and risperidone moderate propensity.[6,7] Aripiprazole, lurasidone and ziprasidone have minimal adverse effect on blood lipids[5,8–13] and may even modestly reverse dyslipidaemias associated with previous antipsychotics.[12,14,15] For cariprazine and brexpiprazole, the effects on plasma lipids would also appear to be limited.[16–19] Iloperidone causes some weight gain but may not adversely affect cholesterol or triglycerides.[20,21]

Olanzapine has been shown to increase triglyceride levels by 40% over the short (12 weeks) and medium (16 months) term.[22,23] Levels may continue to rise for up to a year.[24] Up to two-thirds of olanzapine-treated patients have raised triglycerides[25] and just under 10% may develop severe hypertriglyceridaemia.[26] While weight gain with olanzapine is generally associated with both increases in cholesterol[23,27] and triglycerides,[26] severe hypertriglyceridaemia can occur independently of weight gain.[26] In one study, patients treated with olanzapine and risperidone gained a similar amount of weight, but in olanzapine patients serum triglyceride levels increased by four times as much (80 mg/dL) as in risperidone patients (20 mg/dL).[26] Quetiapine[28] seems to have more modest effects than olanzapine, although data are conflicting.[29]

A case-control study conducted in the UK found that patients with schizophrenia who were treated with olanzapine were five times more likely to develop hyperlipidaemia than controls and three times more likely to develop hyperlipidaemia than patients receiving typical antipsychotics.[30] Risperidone-treated patients could not be distinguished from controls.

Clozapine

Mean triglyceride levels have been shown to double and cholesterol levels to increase by at least 10% after 5 years' treatment with clozapine.[31] Patients treated with clozapine have triglyceride levels that are almost double those of patients who are treated with FGA drugs.[32,33] Cholesterol levels are also increased.[5]

Particular care should be taken before prescribing clozapine or olanzapine for patients who are obese, diabetic or known to have pre-existing hyperlipidaemia.[34]

Screening and monitoring

All patients should have their lipids measured at baseline, 3 months after starting treatment with a new antipsychotic, and then annually. Those prescribed clozapine and olanzapine should ideally have their serum lipids measured every 3 months for the first year of treatment, and then annually. Clinically significant changes in cholesterol are unlikely over the short term but triglycerides can increase dramatically.[35] In practice, dyslipidaemia is widespread in patients taking long-term antipsychotics irrespective of drug prescribed or of diagnosis.[36-38] Screening for this potentially serious adverse effect of antipsychotics is not yet routine in clinical practice,[39] but is strongly recommended by NICE.[40]

Severe hypertriglyceridaemia (fasting level of >5 mmol/L) is a risk factor for pancreatitis. Note that antipsychotic-induced dyslipidaemia can occur independent of weight gain.[41]

Treatment of dyslipidaemia

If moderate to severe hyperlipidaemia develops during antipsychotic treatment, a switch to another antipsychotic less likely to cause this problem should be considered in the first instance. Although not recommended as a strategy in patients with treatment-resistant illness, clozapine-induced hypertriglyceridaemia has been shown to reverse after a switch to risperidone.[42] This may hold true with other switching regimens but data are scarce.[43] Aripiprazole (or ziprasidone outside the UK) seems at present to be the treatment of choice in those with prior antipsychotic-induced dyslipidaemia.[15,44]

Patients with raised cholesterol may benefit from dietary advice, lifestyle changes and/or treatment with statins.[45,46] Statins seem to be effective in this patient group but interactions are possible.[47] Risk tables and treatment guidelines can be found in the *British National Formulary* (BNF). Evidence supports the treatment of cholesterol concentrations as low as 4 mmol/L in high-risk patients[48] and this is the highest level recommended by NICE for secondary prevention of cardiovascular events.[49] NICE makes no recommendations on target levels for primary prevention but recent advice

Table 1.28 Monitoring lipid concentrations in patients on antipsychotic drugs

Drug	Suggested monitoring
Clozapine Olanzapine	Fasting lipids at baseline, then every 3 months for a year, then annually
Other antipsychotics	Fasting lipids at baseline and at 3 months, and then annually

promotes the use of statins for anyone with a >10% 10-year risk of cardiovascular disease.[49] Coronary heart disease and stroke risk can be reduced by a third by reducing cholesterol to as low as 3.5 mmol/L.[2] When triglycerides alone are raised, diets low in saturated fats and the taking of fish oil and fibrates are effective treatments[24,50,51] although there is no proof that mortality is reduced. Such patients should be screened for impaired glucose tolerance and diabetes.

The recommended procedure for monitoring lipid levels in patients on antipsychotics is summarised in Table 1.28.

References

1. Brown S et al. Causes of the excess mortality of schizophrenia. Br J Psychiatry 2000; **177**:212–217.

2. Durrington P. Dyslipidaemia. Lancet 2003; **362**:717–731.

3. Sasaki J et al. Lipids and apolipoproteins in patients treated with major tranquilizers. Clin Pharmacol Ther 1985; **37**:684–687.

4. Henkin Y et al. Secondary dyslipidemia. Inadvertent effects of drugs in clinical practice. JAMA 1992; **267**:961–968.

5. Chaggar PS et al. Effect of antipsychotic medications on glucose and lipid levels. J Clin Pharmacol 2011; **51**:631–638.

6. Smith RC et al. Effects of olanzapine and risperidone on lipid metabolism in chronic schizophrenic patients with long-term antipsychotic treatment: a randomized five month study. Schizophr Res 2010; **120**:204–209.

7. Perez-Iglesias R et al. Glucose and lipid disturbances after 1 year of antipsychotic treatment in a drug-naive population. Schizophr Res 2009; **107**:115–121.

8. Olfson M et al. Hyperlipidemia following treatment with antipsychotic medications. Am J Psychiatry 2006; **163**:1821–1825.

9. L'Italien GJ et al. Comparison of metabolic syndrome incidence among schizophrenia patients treated with aripiprazole versus olanzapine or placebo. J Clin Psychiatry 2007; **68**:1510–1516.

10. Fenton WS et al. Medication-induced weight gain and dyslipidemia in patients with schizophrenia. Am J Psychiatry 2006; **163**:1697–1704.

11. Meyer JM et al. Change in metabolic syndrome parameters with antipsychotic treatment in the CATIE Schizophrenia Trial: prospective data from phase 1. Schizophr Res 2008; **101**:273–286.

12. Potkin SG et al. Double-blind comparison of the safety and efficacy of lurasidone and ziprasidone in clinically stable outpatients with schizophrenia or schizoaffective disorder. Schizophr Res 2011; **132**:101–107.

13. Correll CU et al. Long-term safety and effectiveness of lurasidone in schizophrenia: a 22-month, open-label extension study. CNS Spectr 2016; **21**:393–402.

14. Fleischhacker WW et al. Effects of adjunctive treatment with aripiprazole on body weight and clinical efficacy in schizophrenia patients treated with clozapine: a randomized, double-blind, placebo-controlled trial. Int J Neuropsychopharmacol 2010; **13**:1115–1125.

15. Chen Y et al. Comparative effectiveness of switching antipsychotic drug treatment to aripiprazole or ziprasidone for improving metabolic profile and atherogenic dyslipidemia: a 12-month, prospective, open-label study. J Psychopharmacol 2012; **26**:1201–1210.

16. Lao KS et al. Tolerability and safety profile of cariprazine in treating psychotic disorders, bipolar disorder and major depressive disorder: a systematic review with meta-analysis of randomized controlled trials. CNS Drugs 2016; **30**:1043–1054.

17. Earley W et al. Tolerability of cariprazine in the treatment of acute bipolar I mania: a pooled post hoc analysis of 3 phase II/III studies. J Affect Disord 2017; **215**:205–212.

18. McEvoy J et al. Brexpiprazole for the treatment of schizophrenia: a review of this novel serotonin-dopamine activity modulator. Clin Schizophr Relat Psychoses 2016; **9**:177–186.

19. Correll CU et al. Efficacy and safety of brexpiprazole for the treatment of acute schizophrenia: a 6-week randomized, double-blind, placebo-controlled trial. Am J Psychiatry 2015; **172**:870–880.

20. Citrome L. Iloperidone: chemistry, pharmacodynamics, pharmacokinetics and metabolism, clinical efficacy, safety and tolerability, regulatory affairs, and an opinion. Expert Opin Drug Metab Toxicol 2010; **6**:1551–1564.

21. Cutler AJ et al. Long-term safety and tolerability of iloperidone: results from a 25-week, open-label extension trial. CNS Spectr 2013; **18**:43–54.

22. Sheitman BB et al. Olanzapine-induced elevation of plasma triglyceride levels. Am J Psychiatry 1999; 156:1471–1472.

23. Osser DN et al. Olanzapine increases weight and serum triglyceride levels. J Clin Psychiatry 1999; 60:767–770.

24. Meyer JM. Effects of atypical antipsychotics on weight and serum lipid levels. J Clin Psychiatry 2001; 62 Suppl 27:27–34.

25. Melkersson KI et al. Elevated levels of insulin, leptin, and blood lipids in olanzapine-treated patients with schizophrenia or related psychoses. J Clin Psychiatry 2000; 61:742–749.

26. Meyer JM. Novel antipsychotics and severe hyperlipidemia. J Clin Psychopharmacol 2001; 21:369–374.

27. Kinon BJ et al. Long-term olanzapine treatment: weight change and weight-related health factors in schizophrenia. J Clin Psychiatry 2001; 62:92–100.

28. Atmaca M et al. Serum leptin and triglyceride levels in patients on treatment with atypical antipsychotics. J Clin Psychiatry 2003; 64:598–604.

29. de Leon J et al. A clinical study of the association of antipsychotics with hyperlipidemia. Schizophr Res 2007; 92:95–102.

30. Koro CE et al. An assessment of the independent effects of olanzapine and risperidone exposure on the risk of hyperlipidemia in schizophrenic patients. Arch Gen Psychiatry 2002; 59:1021–1026.

31. Henderson DC et al. Clozapine, diabetes mellitus, weight gain, and lipid abnormalities: a five-year naturalistic study. Am J Psychiatry 2000; 157:975–981.

32. Ghaeli P et al. Serum triglyceride levels in patients treated with clozapine. Am J Health Syst Pharm 1996; 53:2079–2081.

33. Spivak B et al. Diminished suicidal and aggressive behavior, high plasma norepinephrine levels, and serum triglyceride levels in chronic neuroleptic-resistant schizophrenic patients maintained on clozapine. Clin Neuropharmacol 1998; 21:245–250.

34. Baptista T et al. Novel antipsychotics and severe hyperlipidemia: comments on the Meyer paper. J Clin Psychopharmacol 2002; 22:536–537.

35. Meyer JM et al. The effects of antipsychotic therapy on serum lipids: a comprehensive review. Schizophr Res 2004; 70:1–17.

36. Paton C et al. Obesity, dyslipidaemias and smoking in an inpatient population treated with antipsychotic drugs. Acta Psychiatr Scand 2004; 110:299–305.

37. De Hert M et al. The METEOR study of diabetes and other metabolic disorders in patients with schizophrenia treated with antipsychotic drugs. I. Methodology. Int J Methods Psychiatr Res 2010; 19:195–210.

38. Jin H et al. Comparison of longer-term safety and effectiveness of 4 atypical antipsychotics in patients over age 40: a trial using equipoise-stratified randomization. J Clin Psychiatry 2013; 74:10–18.

39. Barnes TR et al. Screening for the metabolic side effects of antipsychotic medication: findings of a 6-year quality improvement programme in the UK. BMJ Open 2015; 5:e007633.

40. National Institute for Health and Care Excellence. Psychosis and schizophrenia in adults: prevention and management Clinical Guideline 178, 2014. https://www.nice.org.uk/guidance/cg178

41. Birkenaes AB et al. Dyslipidemia independent of body mass in antipsychotic-treated patients under real-life conditions. J Clin Psychopharmacol 2008; 28:132–137.

42. Ghaeli P et al. Elevated serum triglycerides with clozapine resolved with risperidone in four patients. Pharmacotherapy 1999; 19:1099–1101.

43. Weiden PJ. Switching antipsychotics as a treatment strategy for antipsychotic-induced weight gain and dyslipidemia. J Clin Psychiatry 2007; 68 Suppl 4:34–39.

44. Newcomer JW et al. A multicenter, randomized, double-blind study of the effects of aripiprazole in overweight subjects with schizophrenia or schizoaffective disorder switched from olanzapine. J Clin Psychiatry 2008; 69:1046–1056.

45. Ojala K et al. Statins are effective in treating dyslipidemia among psychiatric patients using second-generation antipsychotic agents. J Psychopharmacol 2008; 22:33–38.

46. Cooper SJ et al. BAP guidelines on the management of weight gain, metabolic disturbances and cardiovascular risk associated with psychosis and antipsychotic drug treatment. J Psychopharmacol 2016; 30:717–748.

47. Tse L et al. Pharmacological treatment of antipsychotic-induced dyslipidemia and hypertension. Int Clin Psychopharmacol 2014; 29:125–137.

48. Heart Protection Study Collaborative Group. MRC/BHF Heart Protection Study of cholesterol lowering with simvastatin in 20,536 high-risk individuals: a randomised placebo-controlled trial. Lancet 2002; 360:7–22.

49. National Institute for Health and Care Excellence. Cardiovascular disease: risk assessment and reduction, including lipid modification. Clinical Guideline 181, 2016. http://www.nice.org.uk/Guidance/CG181.

50. Caniato RN et al. Effect of omega-3 fatty acids on the lipid profile of patients taking clozapine. Aust N Z J Psychiatry 2006; 40:691–697.

51. Freeman MP et al. Omega-3 fatty acids for atypical antipsychotic-associated hypertriglyceridemia. Ann Clin Psychiatry 2015; 27:197–202.

Diabetes and impaired glucose tolerance

Schizophrenia

Schizophrenia is associated with relatively high rates of insulin resistance and diabetes[1,2] – an observation that predates the discovery and widespread use of antipsychotics.[3-5] Lifestyle interventions (lower weight, more activity) are effective in preventing diabetes[6] and should be considered for all people with a diagnosis of schizophrenia.

Antipsychotics

Data relating to diabetes and antipsychotic use are numerous but less than perfect.[7-10] The main problem is that incidence and prevalence studies assume full or uniform screening for diabetes. Neither assumption is likely to be correct.[7] Many studies do not account for other factors affecting risk of diabetes.[10] Small differences between drugs are therefore difficult to substantiate but may in any case be ultimately unimportant: risk is probably increased for all those with schizophrenia receiving any antipsychotic.

The mechanisms involved in the development of antipsychotic-related diabetes are unclear, but may include $5\text{-HT}_{2A}/5\text{-HT}_{2C}$ antagonism, increased plasma lipids, weight gain and leptin resistance.[11] Insulin resistance may occur in the absence of weight gain.[12]

First-generation antipsychotics

Phenothiazine derivatives have long been associated with impaired glucose tolerance and diabetes.[13] Diabetes prevalence rates were reported to have increased substantially following the introduction and widespread use of FGA drugs.[14] The prevalence of impaired glucose tolerance seems to be higher with aliphatic phenothiazines than with fluphenazine or haloperidol.[15] Hyperglycaemia has also been reported with other FGAs, such as loxapine,[16] and other data confirm an association with haloperidol.[17] Some studies even suggest that FGAs are no different from SGAs in their propensity to cause diabetes,[18,19] whereas others suggest a modest but statistically significant excess incidence of diabetes with SGAs.[20]

Second-generation antipsychotics

Clozapine

Clozapine is strongly linked to hyperglycaemia, impaired glucose tolerance and diabetic ketoacidosis.[21] The risk of diabetes appears to be higher with clozapine than with other SGAs and conventional drugs, especially in younger patients,[22-25] although this is not a consistent finding.[26,27]

As many as a third of patients might develop diabetes after 5 years of treatment.[28] Many cases of diabetes are noted in the first 6 months of treatment and some occur within 1 month,[29] some only after many years.[27] Death from ketoacidosis has also been reported.[29] Diabetes associated with clozapine is not necessarily linked to obesity or to family history of diabetes,[21,30] although these factors greatly increase the risk of developing diabetes on clozapine.[31]

Clozapine appears to increase plasma levels of insulin in a clozapine level-dependent fashion.[32,33] It has been shown to be more likely than FGAs to increase plasma glucose and insulin following oral glucose challenge.[34] Testing for diabetes is essential given the high prevalence of diabetes in people receiving clozapine.[35]

Olanzapine

As with clozapine, olanzapine has been strongly linked to impaired glucose tolerance, diabetes and diabetic ketoacidosis.[36] Olanzapine and clozapine appear to directly induce insulin resistance.[37,38] Risk of diabetes has also been reported to be higher with olanzapine than with FGA drugs,[39] again with a particular risk in younger patients.[23] The time course of development of diabetes has not been established but impaired glucose tolerance seems to occur even in the absence of obesity and family history of diabetes.[21,30] Olanzapine is probably more diabetogenic than risperidone.[40–44] Olanzapine is also associated with plasma levels of glucose and insulin higher than those seen with FGAs (after oral glucose load).[34,45]

Risperidone

Risperidone has been linked, mainly in case reports, to impaired glucose tolerance,[46] diabetes[47] and ketoacidosis.[48] The number of reports of such adverse effects is substantially smaller than with either clozapine or olanzapine.[49] At least one study has suggested that changes in fasting glucose are significantly less common with risperidone than with olanzapine[40] but other studies have detected no difference.[50]

Risperidone seems no more likely than FGA drugs to be associated with diabetes,[23,39,41] although there may be an increased risk in patients under 40 years of age.[23] Risperidone has, however, been observed adversely to affect fasting glucose and plasma glucose (following glucose challenge) compared with levels seen in healthy volunteers (but not compared with patients taking conventional drugs).[34]

Quetiapine

Like risperidone, quetiapine has been linked to cases of new-onset diabetes and ketoacidosis.[51–53] Again, the number of reports is much lower than with olanzapine or clozapine. Quetiapine appears to be more likely than FGA drugs to be associated with diabetes.[23,54] Two studies showed quetiapine to be equal to olanzapine in incidence of diabetes.[50,55] Risk with quetiapine may be dose-related, with daily doses of 400 mg or more being clearly linked to changes in HbA_{1C}.[56]

Other SGAs

Amisulpride appears not to elevate plasma glucose[57] and seems not to be associated with diabetes.[58] There is one reported case of ketoacidosis occurring in a patient given the closely related sulpiride.[59] Data for aripiprazole[60–63] and ziprasidone[64,65] suggest that neither drug alters glucose homeostasis. Aripiprazole may even reverse diabetes caused by other drugs[66] (although ketoacidosis has been reported with aripiprazole[67–69]).

CHAPTER 1

A large case-control study has confirmed that neither amisulpride nor aripiprazole increase the risk of diabetes.[70] These three drugs (amisulpride, aripiprazole and ziprasidone) are recommended for those with a history of or predisposition to diabetes mellitus or as an alternative to other antipsychotics known to be diabetogenic. Data suggest neither lurasidone[71,72] nor asenapine[73,74] has any effect on glucose homeostasis. Likewise, initial data for brexpiprazole[75] and cariprazine[76,77] suggest minimal effects on glucose tolerance.

Predicting antipsychotic-related diabetes

Risk of diabetes is increased to a much greater extent in younger adults than in the elderly[78] (in whom antipsychotics may show no increased risk[79]). First-episode patients seem particularly prone to the development of diabetes when given a variety of antipsychotics.[80–82] During treatment, rapid weight gain and a rise in plasma triglycerides seem to predict the development of diabetes.[83]

Monitoring

Diabetes is a growing problem in Western society and has a strong association with obesity, (older) age, (lower) educational achievement and certain ethnic groups.[84,85] Diabetes markedly increases cardiovascular mortality, largely as a consequence of atherosclerosis.[86] Likewise, the use of antipsychotics also increases cardiovascular mortality.[87–89] Intervention to reduce plasma glucose levels and minimise other risk factors (obesity, hypercholesterolaemia) is therefore essential.[90]

There is no clear consensus on diabetes-monitoring practice for those receiving antipsychotics[91] and recommendations in formal guidelines vary considerably.[92] Given the previous known parlous state of testing for diabetes in the UK[7,93–95] and elsewhere,[96] arguments over precisely which tests are done and when seem to miss the point. There is an overwhelming need to improve monitoring by any means and so any tests for diabetes are supported – urine glucose and random plasma glucose included (Table 1.29).

Table 1.29 Recommended monitoring for diabetes in patients receiving antipsychotic drugs

	Ideally	Minimum
Baseline	OGTT or FPG HbA$_{1C}$ if fasting not possible	Urine glucose RPG
Continuation	All drugs: OGTT or FPG + HbA$_{1C}$ at 4–6 months then every 12 months For clozapine and olanzapine or if other risk factors present: OGTT or FPG after 1 month, then every 4–6 months For ongoing regular screening, HbA$_{1C}$ is a suitable test. Note that this test is not suitable for detecting short-term change	Urine glucose or RPG every 12 months, with symptom monitoring

FPG, fasting plasma glucose; OGTT, oral glucose tolerance tests; RPG, random plasma glucose.

Ideally, though, all patients should have oral glucose tolerance tests (OGTT) performed as this is the most sensitive method of detection.[97,98] Fasting plasma glucose (FPG) tests are less sensitive but recommended.[99] Any abnormality in FPG should provoke an OGTT. Fasting tests are often difficult to obtain in acutely ill, disorganised patients so measurement of random plasma glucose or glycosylated haemoglobin (HbA_{1C}) may also be used (fasting not required). HbA_{1C} is now recognised as a useful tool in detecting and monitoring diabetes.[100] Frequency of monitoring should then be determined by physical factors (e.g. weight gain) and known risk factors (e.g. family history of diabetes, lipid abnormalities, smoking status). The absolute minimum is yearly testing for diabetes for all patients. In addition, all patients should be asked to look out for and report signs and symptoms of diabetes (fatigue, candida infection, thirst polyuria).

Treatment of antipsychotic-related diabetes

Switching to a drug of low or minimal risk of diabetes is often effective in reversing changes in glucose tolerance. In this respect the most compelling evidence is for switching to aripiprazole[101,102] but also to ziprasidone[102] and perhaps lurasidone.[72] Standard antidiabetic treatments are otherwise recommended. Pioglitazone[103] may have particular benefit but note the hepatotoxic potential of this drug. GLP-1 agonists such as liraglutide are increasingly used.[104] The overall risk of impaired glucose tolerance and diabetes for different antipsychotics is summarised in Table 1.30.

Table 1.30 Antipsychotics – risk of diabetes and impaired glucose tolerance

Degree of risk	Antipsychotic drug
High	Clozapine, olanzapine
Moderate	Quetiapine, risperidone, phenothiazines
Low	High-potency FGAs (e.g. haloperidol)
Minimal	Aripiprazole, amisulpride, brexpiprazole, cariprazine, asenapine, lurasidone, ziprasidone

FGA, first-generation antipsychotic.

References

1. Schimmelbusch WH et al. The positive correlation between insulin resistance and duration of hospitalization in untreated schizophrenia. Br J Psychiatry 1971; 118:429–436.
2. Waitzkin L. A survey for unknown diabetics in a mental hospital. I. Men under age fifty. Diabetes 1966; 15:97–104.
3. Kasanin J. The blood sugar curve in mental disease. II. The schizophrenia (dementia praecox) groups. Arch Neurol Psychiatry 1926; 16:414–419.
4. Braceland FJ et al. Delayed action of insulin in schizophrenia. Am J Psychiatry 1945; 102:108–110.
5. Kohen D. Diabetes mellitus and schizophrenia: historical perspective. Br J Psychiatry Suppl 2004; 47:S64–S66.
6. Knowler WC et al. 10-year follow-up of diabetes incidence and weight loss in the Diabetes Prevention Program Outcomes Study. Lancet 2009; 374:1677–1686.
7. Taylor D et al. Testing for diabetes in hospitalised patients prescribed antipsychotic drugs. Br J Psychiatry 2004; 185:152–156.
8. Haddad PM. Antipsychotics and diabetes: review of non-prospective data. Br J Psychiatry Suppl 2004; 47:S80–S86.
9. Bushe C et al. Association between atypical antipsychotic agents and type 2 diabetes: review of prospective clinical data. Br J Psychiatry 2004; 184:S87–S93.

10. Gianfrancesco F et al. The influence of study design on the results of pharmacoepidemiologic studies of diabetes risk with antipsychotic therapy. Ann Clin Psychiatry 2006; 18:9–17.

11. Buchholz S et al. Atypical antipsychotic-induced diabetes mellitus: an update on epidemiology and postulated mechanisms. Intern Med J 2008; 38:602–606.

12. Teff KL et al. Antipsychotic-induced insulin resistance and postprandial hormonal dysregulation independent of weight gain or psychiatric disease. Diabetes 2013; 62:3232–3240.

13. Arneson GA. Phenothiazine derivatives and glucose metabolism. J Neuropsychiatr 1964; 5:181.

14. Lindenmayer JP et al. Hyperglycemia associated with the use of atypical antipsychotics. J Clin Psychiatry 2001; 62 Suppl 23:30–38.

15. Keskiner A et al. Psychotropic drugs, diabetes and chronic mental patients. Psychosomatics 1973; 14:176–181.

16. Tollefson G et al. Nonketotic hyperglycemia associated with loxapine and amoxapine: case report. J Clin Psychiatry 1983; 44:347–348.

17. Lindenmayer JP et al. Changes in glucose and cholesterol levels in patients with schizophrenia treated with typical or atypical antipsychotics. Am J Psychiatry 2003; 160:290–296.

18. Carlson C et al. Diabetes mellitus and antipsychotic treatment in the United Kingdom. Eur Neuropsychopharmacol 2006; 16:366–375.

19. Ostbye T et al. Atypical antipsychotic drugs and diabetes mellitus in a large outpatient population: a retrospective cohort study. Pharmacoepidemiol Drug Saf 2005; 14:407–415.

20. Smith M et al. First- v. second-generation antipsychotics and risk for diabetes in schizophrenia: systematic review and meta-analysis. Br J Psychiatry 2008; 192:406–411.

21. Mir S et al. Atypical antipsychotics and hyperglycaemia. Int Clin Psychopharmacol 2001; 16:63–74.

22. Lund BC et al. Clozapine use in patients with schizophrenia and the risk of diabetes, hyperlipidemia, and hypertension: a claims-based approach. Arch Gen Psychiatry 2001; 58:1172–1176.

23. Sernyak MJ et al. Association of diabetes mellitus with use of atypical neuroleptics in the treatment of schizophrenia. Am J Psychiatry 2002; 159:561–566.

24. Gianfrancesco FD et al. Differential effects of risperidone, olanzapine, clozapine, and conventional antipsychotics on type 2 diabetes: findings from a large health plan database. J Clin Psychiatry 2002; 63:920–930.

25. Guo JJ et al. Risk of diabetes mellitus associated with atypical antipsychotic use among patients with bipolar disorder: a retrospective, population-based, case-control study. J Clin Psychiatry 2006; 67:1055–1061.

26. Wang PS et al. Clozapine use and risk of diabetes mellitus. J Clin Psychopharmacol 2002; 22:236–243.

27. Sumiyoshi T et al. A comparison of incidence of diabetes mellitus between atypical antipsychotic drugs: a survey for clozapine, risperidone, olanzapine, and quetiapine (Letter). J Clin Psychopharmacol 2004; 24:345–348.

28. Henderson DC et al. Clozapine, diabetes mellitus, weight gain, and lipid abnormalities: a five-year naturalistic study. Am J Psychiatry 2000; 157:975–981.

29. Koller E et al. Clozapine-associated diabetes. Am J Med 2001; 111:716–723.

30. Sumiyoshi T et al. The effect of hypertension and obesity on the development of diabetes mellitus in patients treated with atypical antipsychotic drugs (Letter). J Clin Psychopharmacol 2004; 24:452–454.

31. Zhang R et al. The prevalence and clinical-demographic correlates of diabetes mellitus in chronic schizophrenic patients receiving clozapine. Hum Psychopharmacol 2011; 26:392–396.

32. Melkersson KI et al. Different influences of classical antipsychotics and clozapine on glucose-insulin homeostasis in patients with schizophrenia or related psychoses. J Clin Psychiatry 1999; 60:783–791.

33. Melkersson K. Clozapine and olanzapine, but not conventional antipsychotics, increase insulin release in vitro. Eur Neuropsychopharmacol 2004; 14:115–119.

34. Newcomer JW et al. Abnormalities in glucose regulation during antipsychotic treatment of schizophrenia. Arch Gen Psychiatry 2002; 59:337–345.

35. Lamberti JS et al. Diabetes mellitus among outpatients receiving clozapine: prevalence and clinical-demographic correlates. J Clin Psychiatry 2005; 66:900–906.

36. Wirshing DA et al. Novel antipsychotics and new onset diabetes. Biol Psychiatry 1998; 44:778–783.

37. Engl J et al. Olanzapine impairs glycogen synthesis and insulin signaling in L6 skeletal muscle cells. Mol Psychiatry 2005; 10:1089–1096.

38. Vestri HS et al. Atypical antipsychotic drugs directly impair insulin action in adipocytes: effects on glucose transport, lipogenesis, and antilipolysis. Neuropsychopharmacology 2007; 32:765–772.

39. Koro CE et al. Assessment of independent effect of olanzapine and risperidone on risk of diabetes among patients with schizophrenia: population based nested case-control study. BMJ 2002; 325:243.

40. Meyer JM. A retrospective comparison of weight, lipid, and glucose changes between risperidone- and olanzapine-treated inpatients: metabolic outcomes after 1 year. J Clin Psychiatry 2002; 63:425–433.

41. Gianfrancesco F et al. Antipsychotic-induced type 2 diabetes: evidence from a large health plan database. J Clin Psychopharmacol 2003; 23:328–335.

42. Leslie DL et al. Incidence of newly diagnosed diabetes attributable to atypical antipsychotic medications. Am J Psychiatry 2004; 161:1709–1711.

43. Duncan E et al. Relative risk of glucose elevation during antipsychotic exposure in a Veterans Administration population. Int Clin Psychopharmacol 2007; 22:1–11.

44. Meyer JM et al. Change in metabolic syndrome parameters with antipsychotic treatment in the CATIE Schizophrenia Trial: prospective data from phase 1. Schizophr Res 2008; 101:273–286.

45. Ebenbichler CF et al. Olanzapine induces insulin resistance: results from a prospective study. J Clin Psychiatry 2003; 64:1436–1439.

46. Mallya A et al. Resolution of hyperglycemia on risperidone discontinuation: a case report. J Clin Psychiatry 2002; 63:453–454.

47. Wirshing DA et al. Risperidone-associated new-onset diabetes. Biol Psychiatry 2001; 50:148–149.

48. Croarkin PE et al. Diabetic ketoacidosis associated with risperidone treatment? Psychosomatics 2000; 41:369–370.

49. Koller EA et al. Risperidone-associated diabetes mellitus: a pharmacovigilance study. Pharmacotherapy 2003; 23:735–744.

50. Lambert BL et al. Diabetes risk associated with use of olanzapine, quetiapine, and risperidone in veterans health administration patients with schizophrenia. Am J Epidemiol 2006; 164:672–681.

51. Henderson DC. Atypical antipsychotic-induced diabetes mellitus: how strong is the evidence? CNS Drugs 2002; 16:77–89.

52. Koller EA et al. A survey of reports of quetiapine-associated hyperglycemia and diabetes mellitus. J Clin Psychiatry 2004; 65:857–863.

53. Nanasawa H et al. Development of diabetes mellitus associated with quetiapine: a case series. Medicine (Baltimore) 2017; 96:e5900.

54. Citrome L et al. Relationship between antipsychotic medication treatment and new cases of diabetes among psychiatric inpatients. Psychiatr Serv 2004; 55:1006–1013.

55. Bushe C et al. Comparison of metabolic and prolactin variables from a six-month randomised trial of olanzapine and quetiapine in schizophrenia. J Psychopharmacol 2010; 24:1001–1009.

56. Guo Z et al. A real-world data analysis of dose effect of second-generation antipsychotic therapy on hemoglobin A1C level. Prog Neuropsychopharmacol Biol Psychiatry 2011; 35:1326–1332.

57. Vanelle JM et al. A double-blind randomised comparative trial of amisulpride versus olanzapine for 2 months in the treatment of subjects with schizophrenia and comorbid depression. Eur Psychiatry 2006; 21:523–530.

58. De Hert MA et al. Prevalence of the metabolic syndrome in patients with schizophrenia treated with antipsychotic medication. Schizophr Res 2006; 83:87–93.

59. Toprak O et al. New-onset type II diabetes mellitus, hyperosmolar non-ketotic coma, rhabdomyolysis and acute renal failure in a patient treated with sulpiride. Nephrol Dial Transplant 2005; 20:662–663.

60. Keck PE, Jr. et al. Aripiprazole: a partial dopamine D2 receptor agonist antipsychotic. Expert Opin Investig Drugs 2003; 12:655–662.

61. Pigott TA et al. Aripiprazole for the prevention of relapse in stabilized patients with chronic schizophrenia: a placebo-controlled 26-week study. J Clin Psychiatry 2003; 64:1048–1056.

62. van WR et al. Major changes in glucose metabolism, including new-onset diabetes, within 3 months after initiation of or switch to atypical antipsychotic medication in patients with schizophrenia and schizoaffective disorder. J Clin Psychiatry 2008; 69:472–479.

63. Baker RA et al. Atypical antipsychotic drugs and diabetes mellitus in the US Food and Drug Administration Adverse Event database: a systematic Bayesian signal detection analysis. Psychopharmacol Bull 2009; 42:11–31.

64. Simpson GM et al. Randomized, controlled, double-blind multicenter comparison of the efficacy and tolerability of ziprasidone and olanzapine in acutely ill inpatients with schizophrenia or schizoaffective disorder. Am J Psychiatry 2004; 161:1837–1847.

65. Sacher J et al. Effects of olanzapine and ziprasidone on glucose tolerance in healthy volunteers. Neuropsychopharmacology 2008; 33:1633–1641.

66. De Hert M et al. A case series: evaluation of the metabolic safety of aripiprazole. Schizophr Bull 2007; 33:823–830.

67. Church CO et al. Diabetic ketoacidosis associated with aripiprazole. Diabet Med 2005; 22:1440–1443.

68. Reddymasu S et al. Elevated lipase and diabetic ketoacidosis associated with aripiprazole. JOP 2006; 7:303–305.

69. Campanella LM et al. Severe hyperglycemic hyperosmolar nonketotic coma in a nondiabetic patient receiving aripiprazole. Ann Emerg Med 2009; 53:264–266.

70. Kessing LV et al. Treatment with antipsychotics and the risk of diabetes in clinical practice. Br J Psychiatry 2010; 197:266–271.

71. McEvoy JP et al. Effectiveness of lurasidone in patients with schizophrenia or schizoaffective disorder switched from other antipsychotics: a randomized, 6-week, open-label study. J Clin Psychiatry, 2013; 74:170–179.

72. Stahl SM et al. Effectiveness of lurasidone for patients with schizophrenia following 6 weeks of acute treatment with lurasidone, olanzapine, or placebo: a 6-month, open-label, extension study. J Clin Psychiatry 2013; 74:507–515.

73. McIntyre RS et al. Asenapine for long-term treatment of bipolar disorder: a double-blind 40-week extension study. J Affect Disord 2010; 126:358–365.

74. McIntyre RS et al. Asenapine versus olanzapine in acute mania: a double-blind extension study. Bipolar Disord 2009; 11:815–826.

75. Garnock-Jones KP. Brexpiprazole: a review in schizophrenia. CNS Drugs 2016; 30:335–342.

76. Lao KS et al. Tolerability and safety profile of cariprazine in treating psychotic disorders, bipolar disorder and major depressive disorder: a systematic review with meta-analysis of randomized controlled trials. CNS Drugs 2016; 30:1043–1054.

77. Earley W et al. Tolerability of cariprazine in the treatment of acute bipolar I mania: a pooled post hoc analysis of 3 phase II/III studies. J Affect Disord 2017; 215:205–212.

78. Hammerman A et al. Antipsychotics and diabetes: an age-related association. Ann Pharmacother 2008; 42:1316–1322.

79. Albert SG et al. Atypical antipsychotics and the risk of diabetes in an elderly population in long-term care: a retrospective nursing home chart review study. J Am Med Dir Assoc 2009; 10:115–119.

80. De Hert M et al. Typical and atypical antipsychotics differentially affect long-term incidence rates of the metabolic syndrome in first-episode patients with schizophrenia: a retrospective chart review. Schizophr Res 2008; 101:295–303.

81. Saddichha S et al. Metabolic syndrome in first episode schizophrenia – a randomized double-blind controlled, short-term prospective study. Schizophr Res 2008; 101:266–272.

82. Saddichha S et al. Diabetes and schizophrenia – effect of disease or drug? Results from a randomized, double-blind, controlled prospective study in first-episode schizophrenia. Acta Psychiatr Scand 2008; 117:342–347.

83. Reaven GM et al. In search of moderators and mediators of hyperglycemia with atypical antipsychotic treatment. J Psychiatr Res 2009; 43:997–1002.

84. Mokdad AH et al. The continuing increase of diabetes in the US. Diabetes Care 2001; **24**:412.

85. Mokdad AH et al. Diabetes trends in the US: 1990-1998. Diabetes Care 2000; **23**:1278–1283.

86. Beckman JA et al. Diabetes and atherosclerosis: epidemiology, pathophysiology, and management. JAMA 2002; **287**:2570–2581.

87. Henderson DC et al. Clozapine, diabetes mellitus, hyperlipidemia, and cardiovascular risks and mortality: results of a 10-year naturalistic study. J Clin Psychiatry 2005; **66**:1116–1121.

88. Lamberti JS et al. Prevalence of the metabolic syndrome among patients receiving clozapine. Am J Psychiatry 2006; **163**:1273–1276.

89. Goff DC et al. A comparison of ten-year cardiac risk estimates in schizophrenia patients from the CATIE study and matched controls. Schizophr Res 2005; **80**:45–53.

90. Haupt DW et al. Hyperglycemia and antipsychotic medications. J Clin Psychiatry 2001; **62 Suppl 27**:15–26.

91. Cohn TA et al. Metabolic monitoring for patients treated with antipsychotic medications. Can J Psychiatry 2006; **51**:492–501.

92. De Hert M et al. Guidelines for screening and monitoring of cardiometabolic risk in schizophrenia: systematic evaluation. Br J Psychiatry 2011; **199**:99–105.

93. Barnes TR et al. Screening for the metabolic syndrome in community psychiatric patients prescribed antipsychotics: a quality improvement programme. Acta Psychiatr Scand 2008; **118**:26–33.

94. Barnes TR et al. Screening for the metabolic side effects of antipsychotic medication: findings of a 6-year quality improvement programme in the UK. BMJ Open 2015; **5**:e007633.

95. Crawford MJ et al. Assessment and treatment of physical health problems among people with schizophrenia: national cross-sectional study. Br J Psychiatry 2014; **205**:473–477.

96. Morrato EH et al. Metabolic screening after the ADA's Consensus Statement on Antipsychotic Drugs and Diabetes. Diabetes Care 2009; **32**:1037–1042.

97. De Hert M et al. Oral glucose tolerance tests in treated patients with schizophrenia. Data to support an adaptation of the proposed guidelines for monitoring of patients on second generation antipsychotics? Eur Psychiatry 2006; **21**:224–226.

98. Pillinger T et al. Impaired glucose homeostasis in first-episode schizophrenia: a systematic review and meta-analysis. JAMA Psychiatry 2017; **74**:261–269.

99. Marder SR et al. Physical health monitoring of patients with schizophrenia. Am J Psychiatry 2004; **161**:1334–1349.

100. National Institute for Health and Care Excellence. Type 2 diabetes: The management of type 2 diabetes. Clinical guideline 87, 2009; last updatedDecember 2014. https://www.nice.org.uk/guidance/CG87

101. Stroup TS et al. Effects of switching from olanzapine, quetiapine, and risperidone to aripiprazole on 10-year coronary heart disease risk and metabolic syndrome status: results from a randomized controlled trial. Schizophr Res 2013; **146**:190–195.

102. Chen Y et al. Comparative effectiveness of switching antipsychotic drug treatment to aripiprazole or ziprasidone for improving metabolic profile and atherogenic dyslipidemia: a 12-month, prospective, open-label study. J Psychopharmacol 2012; **26**:1201–1210.

103. Smith RC et al. Effects of pioglitazone on metabolic abnormalities, psychopathology, and cognitive function in schizophrenic patients treated with antipsychotic medication: a randomized double-blind study. Schizophr Res 2013; **143**:18–24.

104. Larsen JR et al. Effect of liraglutide treatment on prediabetes and overweight or obesity in clozapine- or olanzapine-treated patients with schizophrenia spectrum disorder: a randomized clinical trial. JAMA Psychiatry 2017; **74**:719–728.

CHAPTER 1

Blood pressure changes

Orthostatic hypotension

Orthostatic hypotension is one of the most common cardiovascular adverse effects of antipsychotics and some antidepressants. Orthostatic hypotension generally presents acutely, during the initial dose titration period, but there is evidence to suggest it can also be a chronic problem.[1] Symptoms may include dizziness, light-headedness, asthenia, headache and visual disturbance. Patients may not be able to communicate the nature of these symptoms effectively and subjective reports of postural dizziness correlate weakly with the magnitude of measured postural hypotension.[2]

Factors increasing the risk for orthostatic hypertension[2] relate to:
- Treatment:
  - intramuscular administration route (as peak levels are achieved more rapidly)
  - rapid dose increases
  - antipsychotic polypharmacy
  - drug interactions (e.g. beta blockers and other antihypertensive drugs).
- Patient:
  - old age (young patients often develop sinus tachycardia with minimal changes in orthostatic blood pressure)
  - disease states associated with autonomic dysfunction (e.g. Parkinson's disease)
  - dehydration
  - cardiovascular disease.

Blood pressure monitoring is recommended in suspected cases to confirm orthostatic hypotension (defined as a ≥20 mmHg fall in systolic blood pressure or a ≥10 mmHg fall in diastolic blood pressure within 2–5 minutes of standing). Orthostatic hypotension may result in syncope and falls-related injuries. It has also been associated with an increased risk of coronary heart disease, heart failure and death.[3]

Slow dose titration is a commonly used and often effective strategy to avoid or minimise orthostatic hypotension. However, in some cases orthostasis may be a dose-limiting adverse effect, preventing optimal treatment. Potential management strategies are shown in Table 1.31.

Antipsychotics with a high affinity for postsynaptic α_1-adrenergic receptors are most frequently implicated. Among the SGAs, the reported incidence is highest with clozapine (24%), quetiapine (27%) and iloperidone (19.5%), and lowest with lurasidone (<2%) and asenapine (<2%).[2] There are limited quantitative data for FGAs, but low-potency phenothiazines (e.g. chlorpromazine) are considered most likely to cause orthostatic hypotension.[4] All reported frequencies are somewhat dependent on titration schedules used.

Hypertension

There are two ways in which antipsychotic drugs may be associated with the development or worsening of hypertension:

- **Slow steady rise in blood pressure over time.** This may be linked to weight gain. Being overweight increases the risk of developing hypertension. The magnitude of the effect

Table 1.31 Management of antipsychotic-induced orthostatic hypotension[2]

Minimise the risk of treatment	■ Limit initial doses and titrate slowly according to tolerability (most develop a tolerance to the hypotensive effect) ■ Consider a temporary dose reduction if hypotension develops ■ Avoid antipsychotics that are potent α_1-adrenergic receptor antagonists ■ Reduce peak plasma levels by using smaller and more frequent doses or by using modified-release preparations
Non-pharmacological therapies	■ Advice to patients, e.g. to sit on the edge of the bed for several minutes before attempting to stand in the morning and slowly rising from a seated position, may be helpful ■ Abdominal binders and compression stockings have been recommended in postural hypotension ■ Increasing fluid intake to 1.25–2.5 L/day is advisable for all patients who are not fluid restricted
Pharmacological therapies for patients with a compelling indication for treatment where alternatives are not suitable (e.g. clozapine) and management strategies have failed	■ Sodium chloride supplementation has been used to treat antidepressant-induced orthostatic hypotension ■ Fludrocortisone has been used to treat clozapine-induced orthostatic hypotension where other measures have failed (electrolyte and blood pressure monitoring essential) ■ A single case report describes the use of midodrine (an $\alpha1$-receptor agonist) for tricyclic antidepressant-induced orthostatic hypotension

has been modelled using the Framingham data: for every 30 people who gain 4 kg, one will develop hypertension over the next 10 years.[5] Note that this is a very modest weight gain; the majority of patients treated with some antipsychotics gain more than this, increasing further the risk of developing hypertension.

■ **Unpredictable rapid sharp increase in blood pressure on starting a new drug or increasing the dose.** Increases in blood pressure occur shortly after starting, ranging from within hours of the first dose to a month. The following information relates to the pharmacological mechanism behind this and the antipsychotic drugs that are most implicated.

Postural hypotension is commonly associated with antipsychotic drugs that are antagonists at postsynaptic α_1-adrenergic receptors. Some antipsychotics are also antagonists at presynaptic α_2-adrenergic receptors; this can lead to increased release of norepinephrine and vasoconstriction. As all antipsychotics that are antagonists at α_2 receptors are also antagonists at α_1 receptors, the end result for any given patient can be difficult to predict, but for a very small number the result can be hypertension. Some antipsychotics are more commonly implicated than others, but individual patient factors are undoubtedly also important.

Receptor binding studies have demonstrated that clozapine, olanzapine and risperidone have the highest affinity for α_2-adrenergic receptors[6] so it might be predicted that these drugs would be most likely to cause hypertension. Most case reports implicate clozapine,[7-17] with some clearly describing normal blood pressure before clozapine was introduced, a sharp rise during treatment and return to normal when clozapine was discontinued. Blood pressure has also been reported to rise again on re-challenge, and increased plasma catecholamines have been noted in some cases. Case reports also implicate aripiprazole,[18-23] sulpiride,[24,25] risperidone,[26] quetiapine[12] and ziprasidone.[27]

Data available through the UK Medicines and Healthcare Products Regulatory Agency (MHRA) yellow card system indicate that clozapine is the antipsychotic drug most associated with hypertension. There are a very small number of reports with aripiprazole, olanzapine, quetiapine and risperidone.[28] The timing of the onset of hypertension in these reports with respect to antipsychotic initiation is unknown, and likely to be variable.

In long-term treatment, hypertension is seen in around 30–40% of patients regardless of antipsychotic prescribed.[29] A cross-sectional study found an increased risk of hypertension only for perphenazine,[30] a finding not readily explained by its pharmacology.

No antipsychotic is contraindicated in essential hypertension but extreme care is needed when clozapine is prescribed. Concomitant treatment with SSRIs may increase risk of hypertension, possibly via inhibition of the metabolism of the antipsychotic.[12] It is also (theoretically) possible that α_2 antagonism may be at least partially responsible for clozapine-induced tachycardia and nausea.[31]

Treatment of antipsychotic-associated hypertension should follow standard protocols. There is specific evidence for the efficacy of valsartan and telmisartan in antipsychotic-related hypertension.[32]

References

1. Silver H et al. Postural hypotension in chronically medicated schizophrenics. J Clin Psychiatry 1990; 51:459–462.
2. Gugger JJ. Antipsychotic pharmacotherapy and orthostatic hypotension: identification and management. CNS Drugs 2011; 25:659–671.
3. Ricci F et al. Cardiovascular morbidity and mortality related to orthostatic hypotension: a meta-analysis of prospective observational studies. Eur Heart J 2015; 36:1609–1617.
4. Casey DE. The relationship of pharmacology to side effects. J Clin Psychiatry 1997; 58 Suppl 10:55–62.
5. Fontaine KR et al. Estimating the consequences of anti-psychotic induced weight gain on health and mortality rate. Psychiatry Res 2001; 101:277–288.
6. Abi-Dargham A et al. Mechanisms of action of second generation antipsychotic drugs in schizophrenia: insights from brain imaging studies. Eur Psychiatry 2005; 20:15–27.
7. Gupta S et al. Paradoxical hypertension associated with clozapine. Am J Psychiatry 1994; 151:148.
8. Krentz AJ et al. Drug points: pseudophaeochromocytoma syndrome associated with clozapine. BMJ 2001; 322:1213.
9. George TP et al. Hypertension after initiation of clozapine. Am J Psychiatry 1996; 153:1368–1369.
10. Prasad SE et al. Pseudophaeochromocytoma associated with clozapine treatment. Ir J Psychol Med 2003; 20:132–134.
11. Shiwach RS. Treatment of clozapine induced hypertension and possible mechanisms. Clin Neuropharmacol 1998; 21:139–140.
12. Coulter D. Atypical antipsychotics may cause hypertension. Prescriber Update 2003; 24:4.
13. Li JK et al. Clozapine: a mimicry of phaeochromocytoma. Aust N Z J Psychiatry 1997; 31:889–891.
14. Hoorn EJ et al. Hypokalemic hypertension related to clozapine: a case report. J Clin Psychopharmacol 2014; 34:390–392.
15. Sara J et al. Clozapine use presenting with pseudopheochromocytoma in a schizophrenic patient: a case report. Case Rep Endocrinol 2013; 2013:194927.
16. Sakalkale A et al. Pseudophaeochromocytoma: a clinical dilemma in clozapine therapy. Aust N Z J Psychiatry 2017; 51 (Suppl1).
17. Visscher AJ et al. Periorbital oedema and treatment-resistant hypertension as rare side effects of clozapine. Aust N Z J Psychiatry 2011; 45:1097–1098.
18. Borras L et al. Hypertension and aripiprazole. Am J Psychiatry 2005; 162:2392.
19. Hsiao YL et al. Aripiprazole augmentation induced hypertension in major depressive disorder: a case report. Prog Neuropsychopharmacol Biol Psychiatry 2011; 35:305–306.
20. Pitchot W et al. Aripiprazole, hypertension, and confusion. J Neuropsychiatry Clin Neurosci 2010; 22:123.
21. Yasui-Furukori N et al. Worsened hypertension control induced by aripiprazole. Neuropsychiatr Dis Treat 2013; 9:505–507.
22. Bat-Pitault F et al. Aripiprazole and hypertension in adolescents. J Child Adolesc Psychopharmacol 2009; 19:601–602.
23. Seven H et al. Aripiprazole-induced asymptomatic hypertension: a case report. Psychopharmacol Bull 2017; 47:53–56.
24. Mayer RD et al. Acute hypertensive episode induced by sulpiride – a case report. Hum Psychopharmacol 1989; 4:149–150.
25. Corvol P et al. [Hypertensive episodes initiated by sulpiride (Dogmatil)]. Ann Med Interne (Paris) 1973; 124:647–649.
26. Thomson SR et al. Risperidone induced hypertension in a young female: a case report. Adv Sci Lett 2017; 23:1980–1982.

27. Villanueva N et al. Probable association between ziprasidone and worsening hypertension. Pharmacotherapy 2006; **26**:1352–1357.

28. Medicines and Healthcare Products Regulatory Agency. Drug Analysis Profiles (iDAPs). 2017. https://www.gov.uk/drug-analysis-prints

29. Kelly AC et al. A naturalistic comparison of the long-term metabolic adverse effects of clozapine versus other antipsychotics for patients with psychotic illnesses. J Clin Psychopharmacol 2014; **34**:441–445.

30. Boden R et al. A comparison of cardiovascular risk factors for ten antipsychotic drugs in clinical practice. Neuropsychiatr Dis Treat 2013; **9**:371–377.

31. Pandharipande P et al. Alpha-2 agonists: can they modify the outcomes in the Postanesthesia Care Unit? Curr Drug Targets 2005; **6**:749–754.

32. Tse L et al. Pharmacological treatment of antipsychotic-induced dyslipidemia and hypertension. Int Clin Psychopharmacol 2014; **29**:125–137.

Hyponatraemia

Hyponatraemia can occur in the context of:

- **Water intoxication** where water consumption exceeds the maximal renal clearance capacity. Serum and urine osmolality are low. Cross-sectional studies of chronically ill, hospitalised psychiatric patients have found the prevalence of water intoxication to be approximately 5%.[1,2] A longitudinal study found that 10% of severely ill patients with a diagnosis of schizophrenia had episodic hyponatraemia secondary to fluid overload.[3] The primary aetiology is poorly understood. It has been postulated that it may be driven, at least in part, by an extreme compensatory response to the anticholinergic adverse effects of some antipsychotic drugs.[4]
- Drug-induced **syndrome of inappropriate antidiuretic hormone (SIADH)** where the kidney retains an excessive quantity of solute-free water. Serum osmolality is low and urine osmolality relatively high. The prevalence of SIADH has been estimated to be as high as 11% in acutely ill psychiatric patients.[5] Risk factors for antidepressant-induced SIADH (increasing age, female gender, medical co-morbidity and polypharmacy) seem to be less relevant in the population of patients treated with antipsychotic drugs.[6] SIADH usually develops in the first few weeks of treatment with the offending drug. Case reports and case series implicate phenothiazines, haloperidol, pimozide, risperidone, paliperidone, quetiapine, olanzapine, aripiprazole, cariprazine and clozapine.[6–15] A systematic review[16] and a case-control study[17] each suggested a clear increase in risk of hyponatraemia with antipsychotics. Another review[18] confirmed that drug-induced hyponatraemia is associated with concentrated urine and suggested that an antipsychotic was five times more likely than water intoxication to be the cause of hyponatraemia. Overall prevalence of antipsychotic-induced hyponatraemia has been estimated at 0.004%[19] and 26.1%[20] of patients. It is assumed that the true figure lies somewhere between these two extremes. Desmopressin use (for clozapine-induced enuresis) can also result in hyponatraemia.[21] Other drugs, including antidepressants and anticonvulsants (especially carbamazepine[22]), have also been implicated.[23]
- Severe **hyperlipidaemia** and/or **hyperglycaemia** lead to secondary increases in plasma volume and 'pseudohyponatraemia'.[4] Both are more common in people treated with antipsychotic drugs than in the general population and should be excluded as causes.

Mild to moderate hyponatraemia presents as confusion, nausea, headache and lethargy. As the plasma sodium falls, these symptoms become increasingly severe and seizures and coma can develop.

Monitoring of plasma sodium is desirable for all those receiving antipsychotics. Signs of confusion or lethargy should provoke thorough diagnostic analysis, including plasma sodium determination and urine osmolality.

Standard treatments for antipsychotic-induced hyponatraemia are summarised in Table 1.32. More recently introduced drugs such as tolvaptan,[32] a so-called 'vaptan' (non-peptide arginine-vasopressin antagonist – also known as aquaretics because they induce a highly hypotonic diuresis[33]), show promise in the treatment of hyponatraemia of varying aetiology, including that caused by drug-related SIADH.

Table 1.32 Treatment of antipsychotic-induced hyponatraemia

Cause of hyponatraemia	Antipsychotic drugs implicated	Treatment[4,5]
Water intoxication (serum and urine osmolality low)	Only very speculative evidence to support drugs as a cause Core part of illness in a minority of patients (e.g. psychotic polydipsia)	■ **Fluid restriction** with careful monitoring of serum sodium, particularly diurnal variation (Na drops as the day progresses). Refer to specialist medical care if Na <125 mmol/L. Note that the use of IV saline to correct hyponatraemia has been reported to precipitate rhabdomyolysis[24] ■ Consider treatment with **clozapine**: shown to increase plasma osmolality into the normal range and increase urine osmolality (not usually reaching the normal range).[25,26] These effects are consistent with reduced fluid intake. This effect is not clearly related to improvements in mental state[27] ■ There are both[6] positive and negative reports for olanzapine[28] and risperidone[29] and one positive case report for quetiapine.[30] Compared with clozapine, the evidence base is weak ■ There is no evidence that either reducing or increasing the dose of an antipsychotic results in improvements in serum sodium in water-intoxicated patients[31] ■ **Demeclocycline should not be used** (this exerts its effect by interfering with ADH and increasing water excretion, which is already at capacity in these patients)
SIADH (serum osmolality low; urine osmolality relatively high)	All antipsychotic drugs	■ If mild, **fluid restriction** with careful monitoring of serum sodium. Refer to specialist medical care if Na <125 mmol/L ■ **Switching to a different antipsychotic drug.** There are insufficient data available to guide choice. Be aware that cross-sensitivity may occur (the individual may be predisposed and the choice of drug relatively less important) ■ Consider **demeclocycline** (see formal prescribing instruction for details) ■ Lithium may be effective[6] but is a potentially toxic drug. Remember that hyponatraemia predisposes to lithium toxicity

ADH, antidiuretic hormone; IV, intravenous; SIADH, syndrome of inappropriate antidiuretic hormone.

References

1. de Leon J et al. Polydipsia and water intoxication in psychiatric patients: a review of the epidemiological literature. Biol Psychiatry 1994; 35:408–419.
2. Patel JK. Polydipsia, hyponatremia, and water intoxication among psychiatric patients. Hosp Community Psychiatry 1994; 45:1073–1074.
3. de Leon J. Polydipsia – a study in a long-term psychiatric unit. Eur Arch Psychiatry Clin Neurosci 2003; 253:37–39.
4. Siegel AJ et al. Primary and drug-induced disorders of water homeostasis in psychiatric patients: principles of diagnosis and management. Harv Rev Psychiatry 1998; 6:190–200.
5. Siegler EL et al. Risk factors for the development of hyponatremia in psychiatric inpatients. Arch Intern Med 1995; 155:953–957.
6. Madhusoodanan S et al. Hyponatraemia associated with psychotropic medications. A review of the literature and spontaneous reports. Adverse Drug React Toxicol Rev 2002; 21:17–29.
7. Bachu K et al. Aripiprazole-induced syndrome of inappropriate antidiuretic hormone secretion (SIADH). Am J Ther 2006; 13:370–372.
8. Dudeja SJ et al. Olanzapine induced hyponatraemia. Ulster Med J 2010; 79:104–105.
9. Yam FK et al. Syndrome of inappropriate antidiuretic hormone associated with aripiprazole. Am J Health Syst Pharm 2013; 70:2110–2114.
10. Kaur J et al. Paliperidone inducing concomitantly syndrome of inappropriate antidiuretic hormone, neuroleptic malignant syndrome, and rhabdomyolysis. Case Rep Crit Care 2016; 2016:2587963.

11. Lin MW et al. Aripiprazole-related hyponatremia and consequent valproic acid-related hyperammonemia in one patient. Aust N Z J Psychiatry 2017; **51**:296–297.

12. Koufakis T. Quetiapine-induced syndrome of inappropriate secretion of antidiuretic hormone. Case Rep Psychiatry 2016; **2016**:4803132.

13. Chen LC et al. Polydipsia, hyponatremia and rhabdomyolysis in schizophrenia: a case report. World J Psychiatry 2014; **4**:150–152.

14. Bakhla AK et al. A suspected case of olanzapine induced hyponatremia. Indian J Pharmacol 2014; **46**:441–442.

15. Kane JM et al. Efficacy and safety of cariprazine in acute exacerbation of schizophrenia: results from an international, phase III clinical trial. J Clin Psychopharmacol 2015; **35**:367–373.

16. Meulendijks D et al. Antipsychotic-induced hyponatraemia: a systematic review of the published evidence. Drug Saf 2010; **33**:101–114.

17. Mannesse CK et al. Hyponatraemia as an adverse drug reaction of antipsychotic drugs: a case-control study in VigiBase. Drug Saf 2010; **33**:569–578.

18. Atsariyasing W et al. A systematic review of the ability of urine concentration to distinguish antipsychotic- from psychosis-induced hyponatremia. Psychiatry Res 2014; **217**:129–133.

19. Letmaier M et al. Hyponatraemia during psychopharmacological treatment: results of a drug surveillance programme. Int J Neuropsychopharmacol 2012; **15**:739–748.

20. Serrano A et al. Safety of long-term clozapine administration. Frequency of cardiomyopathy and hyponatraemia: two cross-sectional, naturalistic studies. Aust N Z J Psychiatry 2014; **48**:183–192.

21. Sarma S et al. Severe hyponatraemia associated with desmopressin nasal spray to treat clozapine-induced nocturnal enuresis. Aust N Z J Psychiatry 2005; **39**:949.

22. Yang HJ et al. Antipsychotic use is a risk factor for hyponatremia in patients with schizophrenia: a 15-year follow-up study. Psychopharmacology (Berl) 2017; **234**:869–876.

23. Shepshelovich D et al. Medication-induced SIADH: distribution and characterization according to medication class. Br J Clin Pharmacol 2017; **83**:1801–1807.

24. Zaidi AN. Rhabdomyolysis after correction of hyponatremia in psychogenic polydipsia possibly complicated by ziprasidone. Ann Pharmacother 2005; **39**:1726–1731.

25. Canuso CM et al. Clozapine restores water balance in schizophrenic patients with polydipsia-hyponatremia syndrome. J Neuropsychiatry Clin Neurosci 1999; **11**:86–90.

26. Fujimoto M et al. Clozapine improved the syndrome of inappropriate antidiuretic hormone secretion in a patient with treatment-resistant schizophrenia. Psychiatry Clin Neurosci 2016; **70**:469.

27. Spears NM et al. Clozapine treatment in polydipsia and intermittent hyponatremia. J Clin Psychiatry 1996; **57**:123–128.

28. Littrell KH et al. Effects of olanzapine on polydipsia and intermittent hyponatremia. J Clin Psychiatry 1997; **58**:549.

29. Kawai N et al. Risperidone failed to improve polydipsia-hyponatremia of the schizophrenic patients. Psychiatry Clin Neurosci 2002; **56**:107–110.

30. Montgomery JH et al. Adjunctive quetiapine treatment of the polydipsia, intermittent hyponatremia, and psychosis syndrome: a case report. J Clin Psychiatry 2003; **64**:339–341.

31. Canuso CM et al. Does minimizing neuroleptic dosage influence hyponatremia? Psychiatry Res 1996; **63**:227–229.

32. Josiassen RC et al. Tolvaptan: a new tool for the effective treatment of hyponatremia in psychotic disorders. Expert Opin Pharmacother 2010; **11**:637–648.

33. Decaux G et al. Non-peptide arginine-vasopressin antagonists: the vaptans. Lancet 2008; **371**:1624–1632.

Further reading

Sailer C et al. Primary polydipsia in the medical and psychiatric patient: characteristics, complications and therapy. Swiss Med Wkly 2017; **147**:w14514.

Hyperprolactinaemia

Dopamine inhibits prolactin release and so dopamine antagonists can be expected to increase prolactin plasma levels. The degree of prolactin elevation is probably dose-related,[1] and for most antipsychotic medications the threshold activity (D_2 occupancy) for increased prolactin is very close to that of therapeutic efficacy.[2] Genetic differences may also play a part.[3] Table 1.33 groups individual antipsychotics according to their effect on prolactin concentrations.

Hyperprolactinaemia is often superficially asymptomatic (i.e. the patient does not spontaneously report problems) and there is some evidence that hyperprolactinaemia does not affect subjective quality of life.[10] Nonetheless, persistent elevation of plasma prolactin is associated with suppression of the hypothalamic–pituitary–gonadal axis.[11] Symptoms of this include sexual dysfunction[12] (but note that other pharmacological activities also give rise to sexual dysfunction[13]), menstrual disturbances,[4,14] breast growth and galactorrhoea,[14] and may include delusions of pregnancy.[15] Long-term adverse consequences are reductions in bone mineral density[16,17] and a possible increase in the risk of breast cancer.[18]

Prolactin can also be raised because of stress, pregnancy and lactation, seizures, renal impairment and other medical conditions,[7,19,20] including prolactinoma. When measuring prolactin, the sample should be taken early in the morning and stress during venepuncture should be minimised.[20]

Contraindications

Prolactin-elevating drugs with high risk should, if possible, be **avoided** in the following patient groups:

- patients under 25 years of age (i.e. before peak bone mass)
- patients with osteoporosis
- patients with a history of hormone-dependent breast cancer
- young women.

Table 1.33 Effects of antipsychotic medication on prolactin concentration[4-9]

Prolactin-sparing (prolactin increase very rare)	Prolactin-elevating (low risk; minor changes only)	Prolactin-elevating (high risk; major changes)
Aripiprazole	Lurasidone	Amisulpride
Asenapine	Olanzapine	Paliperidone
Brexpiprazole*	Ziprasidone	Risperidone
Cariprazine*		Sulpiride
Clozapine		FGAs (e.g. haloperidol and chlorpromazine)
Iloperidone*		
Quetiapine		

* Not available in the EU at the time of writing.
FGA, first-generation antipsychotic.

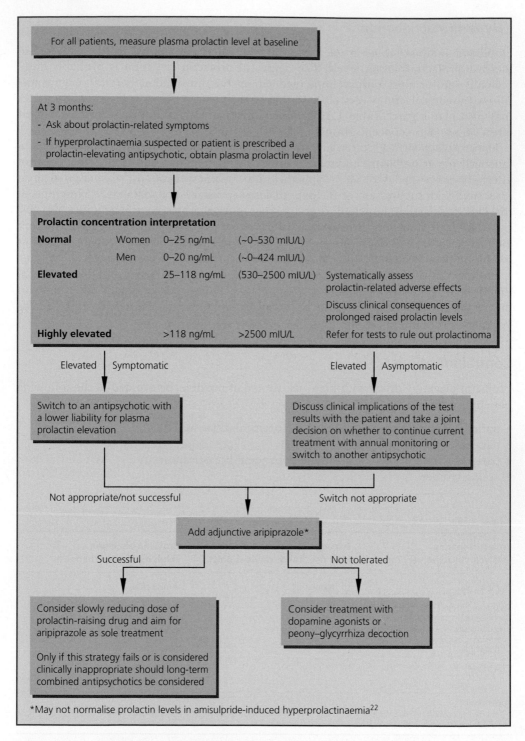

For all patients, measure plasma prolactin level at baseline

At 3 months:
- Ask about prolactin-related symptoms
- If hyperprolactinaemia suspected or patient is prescribed a prolactin-elevating antipsychotic, obtain plasma prolactin level

Prolactin concentration interpretation

Normal	Women	0–25 ng/mL	(~0–530 mIU/L)	
	Men	0–20 ng/mL	(~0–424 mIU/L)	
Elevated		25–118 ng/mL	(530–2500 mIU/L)	Systematically assess prolactin-related adverse effects
				Discuss clinical consequences of prolonged raised prolactin levels
Highly elevated		>118 ng/mL	>2500 mIU/L	Refer for tests to rule out prolactinoma

Elevated | Symptomatic   Elevated | Asymptomatic

Switch to an antipsychotic with a lower liability for plasma prolactin elevation

Discuss clinical implications of the test results with the patient and take a joint decision on whether to continue current treatment with annual monitoring or switch to another antipsychotic

Not appropriate/not successful   Switch not appropriate

Add adjunctive aripiprazole*

Successful   Not tolerated

Consider slowly reducing dose of prolactin-raising drug and aim for aripiprazole as sole treatment

Only if this strategy fails or is considered clinically inappropriate should long-term combined antipsychotics be considered

Consider treatment with dopamine agonists or peony–glycyrrhiza decoction

*May not normalise prolactin levels in amisulpride-induced hyperprolactinaemia[22]

Figure 1.6 Interpretation and management of antipsychotic-induced hyperprolactinaemia.[21]

Management

Treatment of hyperprolactinaemia depends more on symptoms and long-term risk than on the reported plasma prolactin level.

Figure 1.6 presents a suggested algorithm for managing antipsychotic-induced hyperprolactinaemia. If treatment of hyperprolactinaemia is required, switching to an antipsychotic with a lower liability for prolactin elevation is usually the first choice although switching always carries a risk of destabilising the illness and relapse.[23] An alternative is to add aripiprazole to existing treatment.[24] Aripiprazole lowers prolactin levels in a dose-dependent manner: 3 mg/day is effective but 6 mg/day more so. Higher doses appear unnecessary.[25] Other strategies to reduce long-term risk to bone mineral density should also be discussed (e.g. stopping smoking, increasing weight-bearing exercise, and ensuring adequate calcium and vitamin D_3 intake[16,26]).

For patients who need to remain on a prolactin-elevating antipsychotic medication and who cannot tolerate aripiprazole, dopamine agonists can be effective.[27–29] Amantadine, cabergoline and bromocriptine have all been used, but each has, theoretically at least, the potential to worsen psychosis (although this has not been reported in trials). A herbal remedy – peony–glycyrrhiza decoction – has also been shown to improve prolactin-related symptoms,[30,31] but the data are limited. A reduction in prolactin levels was also achieved by high daily doses (2.5–3 g) of metformin[32] in a study of diabetic women on antipsychotic medication.

Management of hyperprolactinaemia is summarised in Table 1.34.

Table 1.34 Summary of management of hyperprolactinaemia

First choice	Aripiprazole 5 mg/day
Second choice (in no particular order)	Dopamine agonists – cabergoline, bromocriptine, amantadine
	Peony–glycyrrhiza decoction
	Metformin 2.5–3 g/day

References

1. Suzuki Y et al. Differences in plasma prolactin levels in patients with schizophrenia treated on monotherapy with five second-generation antipsychotics. Schizophr Res 2013; **145**:116–119.

2. Tsuboi T et al. Hyperprolactinemia and estimated dopamine D2 receptor occupancy in patients with schizophrenia: analysis of the CATIE data. Prog Neuropsychopharmacol Biol Psychiatry 2013; **45**:178–182.

3. Young RM et al. Prolactin levels in antipsychotic treatment of patients with schizophrenia carrying the DRD2*A1 allele. Br J Psychiatry 2004; **185**:147–151.

4. Haddad PM et al. Antipsychotic-induced hyperprolactinaemia: mechanisms, clinical features and management. Drugs 2004; **64**:2291–2314.

5. Holt RI et al. Antipsychotics and hyperprolactinaemia: mechanisms, consequences and management. Clin Endocrinol (Oxf) 2011; **74**:141–147.

6. Leucht S et al. Comparative efficacy and tolerability of 15 antipsychotic drugs in schizophrenia: a multiple-treatments meta-analysis. Lancet 2013; **382**:951–962.

7. Peuskens J et al. The effects of novel and newly approved antipsychotics on serum prolactin levels: a comprehensive review. CNS Drugs 2014; **28**:421–453.

8. Citrome L. Cariprazine: chemistry, pharmacodynamics, pharmacokinetics, and metabolism, clinical efficacy, safety, and tolerability. Expert Opin Drug Metab Toxicol 2013; **9**:193–206.

9. Marder SR et al. Brexpiprazole in patients with schizophrenia: overview of short- and long-term phase 3 controlled studies. Acta Neuropsychiatr 2017; **29**:278–290.

10. Kaneda Y. The impact of prolactin elevation with antipsychotic medications on subjective quality of life in patients with schizophrenia. Clin Neuropharmacol 2003; 26:182–184.

11. Smith S et al. The effects of antipsychotic-induced hyperprolactinaemia on the hypothalamic-pituitary-gonadal axis. J Clin Psychopharmacol 2002; 22:109–114.

12. De Hert M et al. Second-generation and newly approved antipsychotics, serum prolactin levels and sexual dysfunctions: a critical literature review. Expert Opin Drug Saf 2014; 13:605–624.

13. Baldwin D et al. Sexual side-effects of antidepressant and antipsychotic drugs. Advances in Psychiatric Treatment 2003; 9:202–210.

14. Wieck A et al. Antipsychotic-induced hyperprolactinaemia in women: pathophysiology, severity and consequences. Selective literature review. Br J Psychiatry 2003; 182:199–204.

15. Ali JA et al. Delusions of pregnancy associated with increased prolactin concentrations produced by antipsychotic treatment. Int J Neuropsychopharmacol 2003; 6:111–115.

16. De Hert M et al. Relationship between antipsychotic medication, serum prolactin levels and osteoporosis/osteoporotic fractures in patients with schizophrenia: a critical literature review. Expert Opin Drug Saf 2016; 15:809–823.

17. Tseng PT et al. Bone mineral density in schizophrenia: an update of current meta-analysis and literature review under guideline of PRISMA. Medicine (Baltimore) 2015; 94:e1967.

18. De Hert M et al. Relationship between prolactin, breast cancer risk, and antipsychotics in patients with schizophrenia: a critical review. Acta Psychiatr Scand 2016; 133:5–22.

19. Holt RI. Medical causes and consequences of hyperprolactinaemia. A context for psychiatrists. J Psychopharmacol 2008; 22:28–37.

20. Melmed S et al. Diagnosis and treatment of hyperprolactinemia: an Endocrine Society clinical practice guideline. J Clin Endocrinol Metab 2011; 96:273–288.

21. Walters J et al. Clinical questions and uncertainty – prolactin measurement in patients with schizophrenia and bipolar disorder. J Psychopharmacol 2008; 22:82–89.

22. Chen CK et al. Differential add-on effects of aripiprazole in resolving hyperprolactinemia induced by risperidone in comparison to benzamide antipsychotics. Prog Neuropsychopharmacol Biol Psychiatry 2010; 34:1495–1499.

23. Montejo AL et al. Multidisciplinary consensus on the therapeutic recommendations for iatrogenic hyperprolactinemia secondary to antipsychotics. Front Neuroendocrinol 2017; 45:25–34.

24. Sá Esteves P et al. Low doses of adjunctive aripiprazole as treatment for antipsychotic-induced hyperprolactinemia: a literature review. Eur Psychiatry 2015; 30 Suppl1:393.

25. Yasui-Furukori N et al. Dose-dependent effects of adjunctive treatment with aripiprazole on hyperprolactinemia induced by risperidone in female patients with schizophrenia. J Clin Psychopharmacol 2010; 30:596–599.

26. Meaney AM et al. Bone mineral density changes over a year in young females with schizophrenia: relationship to medication and endocrine variables. Schizophr Res 2007; 93:136–143.

27. Hamner MB et al. Hyperprolactinaemia in antipsychotic-treated patients: guidelines for avoidance and management. CNS Drugs 1998; 10:209–222.

28. Duncan D et al. Treatment of psychotropic-induced hyperprolactinaemia. Psychiatr Bull 1995; 19:755–757.

29. Cavallaro R et al. Cabergoline treatment of risperidone-induced hyperprolactinemia: a pilot study. J Clin Psychiatry 2004; 65:187–190.

30. Yuan HN et al. A randomized, crossover comparison of herbal medicine and bromocriptine against risperidone-induced hyperprolactinemia in patients with schizophrenia. J Clin Psychopharmacol 2008; 28:264–370.

31. Man SC et al. Peony-glycyrrhiza decoction for antipsychotic-related hyperprolactinemia in women with schizophrenia: a randomized controlled trial. J Clin Psychopharmacol 2016; 36:572–579.

32. Krysiak R et al. The effect of metformin on prolactin levels in patients with drug-induced hyperprolactinemia. Eur J Intern Med 2016; 30:94–98.

CHAPTER 1

Sexual dysfunction

Primary sexual disorders are common, although reliable normative data are lacking.[1] Physical illness, psychiatric illness, substance misuse and prescribed drug treatment can all cause sexual dysfunction.[2] It has been estimated that 50–60% of people with schizophrenia have problems with sexual dysfunction compared with 30% of the general population,[3] but note that in both groups reported prevalence rates vary depending on the method of data collection (low numbers with spontaneous reports, increasing with confidential questionnaires and further still with direct questioning[2]). In one study of patients with psychosis, 37% spontaneously reported sexual problems but 46% were found to be experiencing difficulties when directly questioned.[4]

Baseline sexual functioning should be determined if possible (questionnaires may be useful) because sexual function can affect quality of life[5] and compliance with medication (sexual dysfunction is one of the major causes of treatment dropout).[6] Complaints of sexual dysfunction may also indicate progression or inadequate treatment of underlying medical or psychiatric conditions.[7,8] Sexual problems may also be caused by drug treatment where intervention may greatly improve quality of life.[9]

The human sexual response

There are four phases of the human sexual response, as detailed in Table 1.35.[2,10,11]

Effects of psychosis

Sexual dysfunction is a well-established phenomenon in first-episode schizophrenia[12] and up to 82% of men and 96% of women with established illness report problems, with associated reductions in quality of life.[5] Men[13] complain of reduced desire, inability to achieve an erection and premature ejaculation whereas women complain more generally about reduced enjoyment.[13,14] Women with psychosis are known to have reduced fertility.[15] People with psychosis are less able to develop good psychosexual relationships and, for some, treatment with an antipsychotic can improve sexual

Table 1.35 Phases of the human sexual response

1. Desire	▪ Related to testosterone levels in men ▪ Possibly increased by dopamine and decreased by prolactin ▪ Psychosocial context and conditioning significantly affect desire
2. Arousal	▪ Influenced by testosterone in men and oestrogen in women ▪ Other potential mechanisms include: central dopamine stimulation, modulation of the cholinergic/adrenergic balance, peripheral α_1 agonism and nitric oxide pathways ▪ Physical pathology such as hypertension or diabetes can have a significant effect
3. Orgasm	▪ May be related to oxytocin ▪ Inhibition of orgasm may be caused by an increase in serotonin activity and raised prolactin, as well as α_1 blockade
4. Resolution	▪ Occurs passively after orgasm

Note: Many other hormones and neurotransmitters may interact in a complex way at each phase.

functioning.[16] Assessment of sexual functioning can clearly be difficult in someone who is psychotic. The Arizona Sexual Experience Scale (ASEX) may be useful in this respect.[17]

Effects of antipsychotic medications

Sexual dysfunction has been reported as an adverse effect of all antipsychotics, and up to 45% of people taking older or conventional antipsychotics experience sexual dysfunction.[18] Individual susceptibility varies and all effects are reversible. Note though that physical illness and drugs other than antipsychotics can cause sexual dysfunction and many studies do not control for either, making the prevalence of sexual dysfunction with different antipsychotics difficult to compare.[19]

Antipsychotics decrease dopaminergic transmission, which in itself can decrease libido but may also increase prolactin levels via negative feedback. It has been estimated that prolactin elevation explains 40% of the sexual dysfunction that is associated with antipsychotic medication.[3] Hyperprolactinaemia can also cause amenorrhoea in women, and breast enlargement and galactorrhoea in both men and women.[20] Although it has been suggested that the overall propensity of an antipsychotic to cause sexual dysfunction is related to propensity to raise prolactin, i.e. risperidone > haloperidol > olanzapine > quetiapine > aripiprazole,[7,19,21] it should be noted that in the CUtLASS-1 study, FGAs (primarily sulpiride, but also other FGAs known to be associated with prolactin elevation) did not fare any worse than SGAs (70% of patients in this arm were prescribed an antipsychotic not associated with prolactin elevation) with respect to worsening sexual dysfunction. In fact, sexual functioning improved in both arms over the 1-year duration of the study.[16] Aripiprazole is relatively free of sexual adverse effects when used as monotherapy[22] and possibly also in combination with another antipsychotic.[23,24]

Anticholinergic effects can cause disorders of arousal,[25] and drugs that block peripheral α_1 receptors cause particular problems with erection and ejaculation in men.[9] Drugs that are antagonists at both peripheral α_1 receptors and cholinergic receptors can cause priapism.[26] Antipsychotic-induced sedation and weight gain may reduce sexual desire.[26] These principles can be used to predict the sexual adverse effects of different antipsychotic drugs (Table 1.36).

Treatment

Before attempting to treat sexual dysfunction, a thorough assessment is essential to determine the most likely cause. Assuming that physical pathology (diabetes, hypertension, cardiovascular disease, etc.) has been excluded, the following principles apply.

Spontaneous remission may occasionally occur.[26] The most obvious first step is to decrease the dose or discontinue the offending drug where appropriate. The next step is to switch to a different drug that is less likely to cause the specific sexual problem experienced (see Table 1.36). Another option is to add 5–10 mg aripiprazole – this can normalise prolactin and improve sexual function.[57–59] If this fails or is not practicable, 'antidote' drugs can be tried: for example, cyproheptadine (a 5-HT$_2$ antagonist at doses of 4–16 mg/day) has been used to treat SSRI-induced sexual dysfunction but sedation is a common adverse effect. There is some evidence that mirtazapine (also a 5-HT$_2$ antagonist as well as an α_2 antagonist) may relieve orgasmic dysfunction in FGA-treated

Table 1.36 Sexual adverse effects of antipsychotics

Drug	Type of problem
Aripiprazole	■ No effect on prolactin or α_1 receptors. No reported adverse effects on sexual function ■ Improves sexual function in those switched from other antipsychotics[22,24,27] ■ Case reports of aripiprazole-induced hypersexuality have been published[28,29]
Asenapine	■ Does not appear to significantly affect prolactin levels[30] ■ No reported cases of sexual dysfunction
Brexpiprazole	■ Similar mechanism of action to aripiprazole (5-HT$_{1A}$ agonist, 5-HT$_{2A}$ antagonist and partial D$_2$ agonist) ■ Causes negligible increases in prolactin[31] ■ No problems with sexual dysfunction reported in clinical trials[32]
Cariprazine	■ Similar mechanism of action to aripiprazole (5-HT$_{1A}$ agonist, 5-HT$_{2A}$ antagonist and partial D$_2$ agonist) ■ Not associated with hyperprolactinaemia[33] ■ No reported cases of sexual dysfunction
Clozapine	■ Significant α_1-adrenergic blockade and anticholinergic effects.[34] No effect on prolactin[35] ■ Probably fewer problems than with typical antipsychotics[36]
Haloperidol	■ Similar problems to the phenothiazines[37] but anticholinergic effects reduced[38] ■ Prevalence of sexual dysfunction reported to be up to 70%[39]
Lurasidone	■ Does not appear significantly to affect prolactin levels[40] ■ No reported cases of sexual dysfunction
Olanzapine	■ Possibly less sexual dysfunction due to relative lack of prolactin-related effects[37] ■ Priapism reported rarely[41,42] ■ Prevalence of sexual dysfunction reported to be >50%[39]
Paliperidone	■ Similar prolactin elevations to risperidone ■ One small study[43] and one case report[44] showing reduction in sexual dysfunction following switching from risperidone oral or depot to paliperidone depot
Phenothiazines (e.g. chlorpromazine)	■ Hyperprolactinaemia and anticholinergic effects. Reports of delayed orgasm at lower doses followed by normal orgasm but without ejaculation at higher doses[14] ■ Priapism has been reported with thioridazine, risperidone and chlorpromazine (probably due to α_1 blockade)[38,45,46]
Quetiapine	■ No effect on serum prolactin[47] ■ Possibly associated with low risk of sexual dysfunction,[48–51] but studies are conflicting[52,53]
Risperidone	■ Potent elevator of serum prolactin ■ Less anticholinergic ■ Specific peripheral α_1-adrenergic blockade leads to a moderately high reported incidence of ejaculatory problems such as retrograde ejaculation[54,55] ■ Priapism reported rarely[26] ■ Prevalence of sexual dysfunction reported to be 60–70%[39]
Sulpiride/amisulpride	■ Potent elevators of serum prolactin[18] but note that sulpiride (as the main FGA prescribed in the study) was not associated with greater sexual dysfunction than SGAs (with variable ability to raise prolactin) in the CUtLASS-1 study[16]
Thioxanthenes (e.g. flupentixol)	■ Arousal problems and anorgasmia[56]

FGA, first-generation antipsychotic; SGA, second-generation antipsychotic.

Table 1.37 Remedial treatments for psychotropic-induced sexual dysfunction

Drug	Pharmacology	Potential treatment for	Adverse effects
Alprostadil[1,11]	Prostaglandin	Erectile dysfunction	Pain, fibrosis, hypotension, priapism
Amantadine[1,61]	Dopamine agonist	Prolactin-induced reduction in desire and arousal (dopamine increases libido and facilitates ejaculation)	Return of psychotic symptoms, GI effects, nervousness, insomnia, rash
Bethanechol[62]	Cholinergic or cholinergic potentiation of adrenergic neurotransmission	Anticholinergic-induced arousal problems and anorgasmia (from TCAs, antipsychotics, etc.)	Nausea and vomiting, colic, bradycardia, blurred vision, sweating
Bromocriptine[9]	Dopamine agonist	Prolactin-induced reduction in desire and arousal	Return of psychotic symptoms, GI effects
Bupropion[63]	Noradrenaline and dopamine reuptake inhibitor	SSRI-induced sexual dysfunction (evidence poor)	Concentration problems, reduced sleep, tremor
Buspirone[64]	5-HT$_{1A}$ partial agonist	SSRI-induced sexual dysfunction, particularly decreased libido and anorgasmia	Nausea, dizziness, headache
Cyproheptadine[1,64,65]	5-HT$_2$ antagonist	Sexual dysfunction caused by increased serotonin transmission (e.g. SSRIs), particularly anorgasmia	Sedation and fatigue. Reversal of the therapeutic effect of antidepressants
Flibanserin (licensed in USA)[66]	5-HT$_{1A}$ agonist, 5-HT$_{2A}$ antagonist, dopamine antagonist	Lack or loss of sexual desire in premenopausal women	Hypotension, syncope, sedation, dizziness, nausea, dry mouth
Sildenafil[11,67–70] **Tadalafil**	Phosphodiesterase inhibitors	Erectile dysfunction of any aetiology. Anorgasmia in women. Effective when prolactin raised	Mild headaches, dizziness, nasal congestion
Yohimbine[1,11,71–73]	Central and peripheral α_2 adrenoceptor antagonist	SSRI-induced sexual dysfunction, particularly erectile dysfunction, decreased libido and anorgasmia (evidence poor)	Anxiety, nausea, fine tremor, increased BP, sweating, fatigue

Note: The use of the drugs listed above should ideally be under the care or supervision of a specialist in sexual dysfunction.
BP, blood pressure; GI, gastrointestinal; SSRI, selective serotonin reuptake inhibitor; TCA, tricyclic antidepressant.

patients.[60] Amantadine, bupropion, buspirone, bethanechol and yohimbine have all been used with varying degrees of success but have a number of unwanted adverse effects and interactions with other drugs (Table 1.37). Given that hyperprolactinaemia may contribute to sexual dysfunction, selegiline (enhances dopamine activity) has been tested in an RCT. This was negative.[74] Testosterone patches have been shown to increase libido in women, although be aware that breast cancer risk may be significantly increased.[75,76]

The evidence base supporting the use of 'antidotes' is poor.[26]

Drugs such as sildenafil (Viagra) or alprostadil (Caverject) are effective only in the treatment of erectile dysfunction (they have no effect on libido). Psychological approaches used by sexual dysfunction clinics may be difficult for clients with mental health problems to engage in.[9]

References

1. Baldwin DS et al. Effects of antidepressant drugs on sexual function. Int J Psychiatry Clin Pract 1997; 1:47–58.
2. Pollack MH et al. Genitourinary and sexual adverse effects of psychotropic medication. Int J Psychiatry Med 1992; 22:305–327.
3. Nunes LV et al. Strategies for the treatment of antipsychotic-induced sexual dysfunction and/or hyperprolactinemia among patients of the schizophrenia spectrum: a review. J Sex Marital Ther 2012; 38:281–301.
4. Montejo AL et al. Frequency of sexual dysfunction in patients with a psychotic disorder receiving antipsychotics. J Sex Med 2010; 7:3404–3413.
5. Olfson M et al. Male sexual dysfunction and quality of life in schizophrenia. J Clin Psychiatry 2005; 66:331–338.
6. Montejo AL et al. Incidence of sexual dysfunction associated with antidepressant agents: a prospective multicenter study of 1022 outpatients. Spanish Working Group for the Study of Psychotropic-Related Sexual Dysfunction. J Clin Psychiatry 2001; 62 Suppl 3:10–21.
7. Baggaley M. Sexual dysfunction in schizophrenia: focus on recent evidence. Hum Psychopharmacol 2008; 23:201–209.
8. Ucok A et al. Sexual dysfunction in patients with schizophrenia on antipsychotic medication. Eur Psychiatry 2007; 22:328–333.
9. Segraves RT. Effects of psychotropic drugs on human erection and ejaculation. Arch Gen Psychiatry 1989; 46:275–284.
10. Stahl SM. The psychopharmacology of sex, Part 1: Neurotransmitters and the 3 phases of the human sexual response. J Clin Psychiatry 2001; 62:80–81.
11. Garcia-Reboll L et al. Drugs for the treatment of impotence. Drugs Aging 1997; 11:140–151.
12. Bitter I et al. Antipsychotic treatment and sexual functioning in first-time neuroleptic-treated schizophrenic patients. Int Clin Psychopharmacol 2005; 20:19–21.
13. Macdonald S et al. Nithsdale Schizophrenia Surveys 24: sexual dysfunction. Case-control study. Br J Psychiatry 2003; 182:50–56.
14. Smith S. Effects of antipsychotics on sexual and endocrine function in women: implications for clinical practice. J Clin Psychopharmacol 2003; 23:S27–S32.
15. Howard LM et al. The general fertility rate in women with psychotic disorders. Am J Psychiatry 2002; 159:991–997.
16. Peluso MJ et al. Non-neurological and metabolic side effects in the Cost Utility of the Latest Antipsychotics in Schizophrenia Randomised Controlled Trial (CUtLASS-1). Schizophr Res 2013; 144:80–86.
17. Byerly MJ et al. An empirical evaluation of the Arizona sexual experience scale and a simple one-item screening test for assessing antipsychotic-related sexual dysfunction in outpatients with schizophrenia and schizoaffective disorder. Schizophr Res 2006; 81:311–316.
18. Smith SM et al. Sexual dysfunction in patients taking conventional antipsychotic medication. Br J Psychiatry 2002; 181:49–55.
19. Serretti A et al. A meta-analysis of sexual dysfunction in psychiatric patients taking antipsychotics. Int Clin Psychopharmacol 2011; 26:130–140.
20. Adverse effects of the atypical antipsychotics. Collaborative Working Group on Clinical Trial Evaluations. J Clin Psychiatry 1998; 59 Suppl 12:17–22.
21. Knegtering H et al. Are sexual side effects of prolactin-raising antipsychotics reducible to serum prolactin? Psychoneuroendocrinology 2008; 33:711–717.
22. Hanssens L et al. The effect of antipsychotic medication on sexual function and serum prolactin levels in community-treated schizophrenic patients: results from the Schizophrenia Trial of Aripiprazole (STAR) study (NCT00237913). BMC Psychiatry 2008; 8:95.
23. Mir A et al. Change in sexual dysfunction with aripiprazole: a switching or add-on study. J Psychopharm 2008; 22:244–253.
24. Byerly MJ et al. Effects of aripiprazole on prolactin levels in subjects with schizophrenia during cross-titration with risperidone or olanzapine: analysis of a randomized, open-label study. Schizophr Res 2009; 107:218–222.
25. Aldridge SA. Drug-induced sexual dysfunction. Clin Pharm 1982; 1:141–147.
26. Baldwin D et al. Sexual side-effects of antidepressant and antipsychotic drugs. Adv Psychiatr Treat 2003; 9:202–210.
27. Rykmans V et al. A comparision of switching strategies from risperidone to aripiprazole in patients with schizophrenia with insufficient efficacy/tolerability on risperidone (cn138-169). Eur Psychiatry 2008; 23:S111–S111.
28. Chen CY et al. Improvement of serum prolactin and sexual function after switching to aripiprazole from risperidone in schizophrenia: a case series. Psychiatry Clin Neurosci 2011; 65:95–97.
29. Vrignaud L et al. [Hypersexuality associated with aripiprazole: a new case and review of the literature]. Therapie 2014; 69:525–527.
30. Ajmal A et al. Psychotropic-induced hyperprolactinemia: a clinical review. Psychosomatics 2014; 55:29–36.
31. Kane JM et al. A multicenter, randomized, double-blind, controlled phase 3 trial of fixed-dose brexpiprazole for the treatment of adults with acute schizophrenia. Schizophr Res 2015; 164:127–135.

32. Citrome L. Brexpiprazole for schizophrenia and as adjunct for major depressive disorder: a systematic review of the efficacy and safety profile for this newly approved antipsychotic – what is the number needed to treat, number needed to harm and likelihood to be helped or harmed? Int J Clin Pract 2015; **69**:978–997.

33. Nasrallah HA et al. The safety and tolerability of cariprazine in long-term treatment of schizophrenia: a post hoc pooled analysis. BMC Psychiatry 2017; **17**:305.

34. Coward DM. General pharmacology of clozapine. Br J Psychiatry Suppl 1992; **160**:5–11.

35. Meltzer HY et al. Effect of clozapine on human serum prolactin levels. Am J Psychiatry 1979; **136**:1550–1555.

36. Aizenberg D et al. Comparison of sexual dysfunction in male schizophrenic patients maintained on treatment with classical antipsychotics versus clozapine. J Clin Psychiatry 2001; **62**:541–544.

37. Crawford AM et al. The acute and long-term effect of olanzapine compared with placebo and haloperidol on serum prolactin concentrations. Schizophr Res 1997; **26**:41–54.

38. Mitchell JE et al. Antipsychotic drug therapy and sexual dysfunction in men. Am J Psychiatry 1982; **139**:633–637.

39. Serretti A et al. Sexual side effects of pharmacological treatment of psychiatric diseases. Clin Pharmacol Ther 2011; **89**:142–147.

40. Citrome L et al. Long-term safety and tolerability of lurasidone in schizophrenia: a 12-month, double-blind, active-controlled study. Int Clin Psychopharmacol 2012; **27**:165–176.

41. Dossenbach M et al. Effects of atypical and typical antipsychotic treatments on sexual function in patients with schizophrenia: 12-month results from the Intercontinental Schizophrenia Outpatient Health Outcomes (IC-SOHO) study. Eur Psychiatry 2006; **21**:251–258.

42. Aurobindo Pharma – Milpharm Ltd. Summary of Product Characteristics. Olanzapine 10 mg tablets. 2013. http://www.medicines.org.uk/emc/medicine/27661/SPC/Olanzapine++10+mg+tablets/

43. Montalvo I et al. Changes in prolactin levels and sexual function in young psychotic patients after switching from long-acting injectable risperidone to paliperidone palmitate. Int Clin Psychopharmacol 2013; **28**:46–49.

44. Shiloh R et al. Risperidone-induced retrograde ejaculation. Am J Psychiatry 2001; **158**:650.

45. Loh C et al. Risperidone-induced retrograde ejaculation: case report and review of the literature. Int Clin Psychopharmacol 2004; **19**:111–112.

46. Thompson JW, Jr. et al. Psychotropic medication and priapism: a comprehensive review. J Clin Psychiatry 1990; **51**:430–433.

47. Peuskens J et al. A comparison of quetiapine and chlorpromazine in the treatment of schizophrenia. Acta Psychiatr Scand 1997; **96**:265–273.

48. Bobes J et al. Frequency of sexual dysfunction and other reproductive side-effects in patients with schizophrenia treated with risperidone, olanzapine, quetiapine, or haloperidol: the results of the EIRE study. J Sex Marital Ther 2003; **29**:125–147.

49. Byerly MJ et al. An open-label trial of quetiapine for antipsychotic-induced sexual dysfunction. J Sex Marital Ther 2004; **30**:325–332.

50. Knegtering R et al. A randomized open-label study of the impact of quetiapine versus risperidone on sexual functioning. J Clin Psychopharmacol 2004; **24**:56–61.

51. Montejo Gonzalez AL et al. A 6-month prospective observational study on the effects of quetiapine on sexual functioning. J Clin Psychopharmacol 2005; **25**:533–538.

52. Atmaca M et al. A new atypical antipsychotic: quetiapine-induced sexual dysfunctions. Int J Impot Res 2005; **17**:201–203.

53. Kelly DL et al. A randomized double-blind 12-week study of quetiapine, risperidone or fluphenazine on sexual functioning in people with schizophrenia. Psychoneuroendocrinology 2006; **31**:340–346.

54. Tran PV et al. Double-blind comparison of olanzapine versus risperidone in the treatment of schizophrenia and other psychotic disorders. J Clin Psychopharmacol 1997; **17**:407–418.

55. Raja M. Risperidone-induced absence of ejaculation. Int Clin Psychopharmacol 1999; **14**:317–319.

56. Aizenberg D et al. Sexual dysfunction in male schizophrenic patients. J Clin Psychiatry 1995; **56**:137–141.

57. Shim JC et al. Adjunctive treatment with a dopamine partial agonist, aripiprazole, for antipsychotic-induced hyperprolactinemia: a placebo-controlled trial. Am J Psychiatry 2007; **164**:1404–1410.

58. Yasui-Furukori N et al. Dose-dependent effects of adjunctive treatment with aripiprazole on hyperprolactinemia induced by risperidone in female patients with schizophrenia. J Clin Psychopharmacol 2010; **30**:596–599.

59. Trives MZ et al. Effect of the addition of aripiprazole on hyperprolactinemia associated with risperidone long-acting injection. J Clin Psychopharmacol 2013; **33**:538–541.

60. Terevnikov V et al. Add-on mirtazapine improves orgasmic functioning in patients with schizophrenia treated with first-generation antipsychotics. Nord J Psychiatry 2017; **71**:77–80.

61. Valevski A et al. Effect of amantadine on sexual dysfunction in neuroleptic-treated male schizophrenic patients. Clin Neuropharmacol 1998; **21**:355–357.

62. Gross MD. Reversal by bethanechol of sexual dysfunction caused by anticholinergic antidepressants. Am J Psychiatry 1982; **139**:1193–1194.

63. Masand PS et al. Sustained-release bupropion for selective serotonin reuptake inhibitor-induced sexual dysfunction: a randomized, double-blind, placebo-controlled, parallel-group study. Am J Psychiatry 2001; **158**:805–807.

64. Rothschild AJ. Sexual side effects of antidepressants. J Clin Psychiatry 2000; **61 Suppl 11**:28–36.

65. Lauerma H. Successful treatment of citalopram-induced anorgasmia by cyproheptadine. Acta Psychiatr Scand 1996; **93**:69–70.

66. Truven Health Analytics. Micromedix Software Product. 2018. http://truvenhealth.com/products/micromedex

67. Nurnberg HG et al. Sildenafil for women patients with antidepressant-induced sexual dysfunction. Psychiatr Serv 1999; **50**:1076–1078.

68. Salerian AJ et al. Sildenafil for psychotropic-induced sexual dysfunction in 31 women and 61 men. J Sex Marital Ther 2000; **26**:133–140.

69. Nurnberg HG et al. Treatment of antidepressant-associated sexual dysfunction with sildenafil: a randomized controlled trial. JAMA 2003; **289**:56–64.

70. Gopalakrishnan R et al. Sildenafil in the treatment of antipsychotic-induced erectile dysfunction: a randomized, double-blind, placebo-controlled, flexible-dose, two-way crossover trial. Am J Psychiatry 2006; **163**:494–499.

71. Jacobsen FM. Fluoxetine-induced sexual dysfunction and an open trial of yohimbine. J Clin Psychiatry 1992; **53**:119–122.

72. Michelson D et al. Mirtazapine, yohimbine or olanzapine augmentation therapy for serotonin reuptake-associated female sexual dysfunction: a randomized, placebo controlled trial. J Psychiatr Res 2002; **36**:147–152.

73. Woodrum ST et al. Management of SSRI-induced sexual dysfunction. Ann Pharmacother 1998; **32**:1209–1215.

74. Kodesh A et al. Selegiline in the treatment of sexual dysfunction in schizophrenic patients maintained on neuroleptics: a pilot study. Clin Neuropharmacol 2003; **26**:193–195.

75. Davis SR et al. Testosterone for low libido in postmenopausal women not taking estrogen. N Engl J Med 2008; **359**:2005–2017.

76. Schover LR. Androgen therapy for loss of desire in women: is the benefit worth the breast cancer risk? Fertil Steril 2008; **90**:129–140.

Further reading

Clayton AH et al. Sexual dysfunction due to psychotropic medications. Psychiatr Clin North Am 2016; **39**:427–463.

Pneumonia

Recent systematic reviews[1,2] have found that antipsychotic medication is associated with a 70–100% increase in risk of pneumonia in patients across a range of diagnoses. The risk was highest in the first week or first month of treatment and was seen with both SGAs and FGAs, with no difference between the two classes of antipsychotics.[2] The risk associated with clozapine persisted beyond 30 days in one study of people with schizophrenia, though effects estimates of risk were notably lower than in the first month of treatment.[3] A dose-related increase in risk has been reported, especially for clozapine[3–5] and other antipsychotics.[6] Polypharmacy involving FGAs and SGAs[3,5,7] and combinations involving a mood stabiliser[5] have been found to be associated with increased risk of pneumonia. In people with bipolar disorder, the risk with combinations involving all three classes of medication was higher than any other combinations.[5]

A study of bipolar patients found that clozapine, olanzapine and haloperidol were linked to increased rates of pneumonia while lithium was protective.[5] Another study suggests amisulpride is not linked to pneumonia.[3] Clozapine re-exposure was associated with a greater risk for recurrent pneumonia than the risk of baseline pneumonia with initial clozapine treatment in one study.[4] Schizophrenia itself seems to afford a higher risk of complications (e.g. admission to intensive care) in people diagnosed with pneumonia[8] though neither diagnosis nor age appears to modify the effect of antipsychotic use on pneumonia.[1] Likewise, risk of antipsychotic-associated pneumonia was increased in patients with Alzheimer's disease and those without.[9]

The mechanism by which antipsychotics increase the risk of pneumonia is not known. Possibilities include sedation (risk seems to be highest with drugs that show greatest H_1 antagonism[3,7]); dystonia or dyskinesia; dry mouth causing poor bolus transport and so increasing the risk of aspiration (hypersalivation in the case of clozapine); general poor physical health[3]; or perhaps some ill-defined effect on immune response.[7,10] Nevertheless, the fact that antipsychotics can increase the risk of aspiration pneumonia and not other pneumonia types offers support to this as a plausible (perhaps sole) mechanism.[11] With clozapine, pneumonia may also be secondary to constipation.[12]

An increased risk of pneumonia should be assumed for all patients (regardless of age) taking any antipsychotic for any period. All patients should be very carefully monitored for signs of chest infection and effective treatment started promptly. Extra vigilance should be taken when re-exposing to clozapine patients with previous history of clozapine-induced pneumonia. Early referral to general medical services should be considered where there is any doubt about the severity or type of chest infection.

Summary

- Assume the use of all antipsychotics will increase the risk of pneumonia.
- Monitor all patients for signs of chest infection and treat promptly.

References

1. Nose M et al. Antipsychotic drug exposure and risk of pneumonia: a systematic review and meta-analysis of observational studies. Pharmacoepidemiol Drug Saf 2015; **24**:812–820.
2. Dzahini O et al. Antipsychotics and risk of pneumonia. J Psychopharm 2018, submitted.

3. Kuo CJ et al. Second-generation antipsychotic medications and risk of pneumonia in schizophrenia. Schizophr Bull 2013; **39**:648–657.

4. Hung GC et al. Antipsychotic reexposure and recurrent pneumonia in schizophrenia: a nested case-control study. J Clin Psychiatry 2016; **77**:60–66.

5. Yang SY et al. Antipsychotic drugs, mood stabilizers, and risk of pneumonia in bipolar disorder: a nationwide case-control study. J Clin Psychiatry 2013; **74**:e79–e86.

6. Huybrechts KF et al. Comparative safety of antipsychotic medications in nursing home residents. J Am Geriatr Soc 2012; **60**:420–429.

7. Trifiro G et al. Association of community-acquired pneumonia with antipsychotic drug use in elderly patients: a nested case-control study. Ann Intern Med 2010; **152**:418–440.

8. Chen YH et al. Poor clinical outcomes among pneumonia patients with schizophrenia. Schizophr Bull 2011; **37**:1088–1094.

9. Tolppanen AM et al. Antipsychotic use and risk of hospitalization or death due to pneumonia in persons with and those without alzheimer disease. Chest 2016; **150**:1233–1241.

10. Knol W et al. Antipsychotic drug use and risk of pneumonia in elderly people. J Am Geriatr Soc 2008; **56**:661–666.

11. Herzig SJ et al. Antipsychotics and the risk of aspiration pneumonia in individuals hospitalized for nonpsychiatric conditions: a cohort study. J Am Geriatr Soc 2017; **65**:2580–2586.

12. Galappathie N et al. Clozapine-associated pneumonia and respiratory arrest secondary to severe constipation. Med Sci Law 2014; **54**:105–109.

Switching antipsychotics

General recommendations for switching antipsychotics because of poor tolerability are shown in Table 1.38.

Table 1.38 General recommendations for switching antipsychotic drugs

Adverse effect	Suggested drugs	Alternatives
Acute EPS[1–8] – dystonia, parkinsonism, bradykinesia	Aripiprazole Olanzapine Quetiapine	Brexpiprazole* Cariprazine* Clozapine Lurasidone Ziprasidone
Akathisia[2,9]	Olanzapine Quetiapine	Clozapine
Dyslipidaemia[7,8,10–15]	Amisulpride Aripiprazole† Lurasidone Ziprasidone*	Asenapine Brexpiprazole* Cariprazine*
Impaired glucose tolerance[7,8,14,16–19]	Amisulpride Aripiprazole† Lurasidone Ziprasidone*	Brexpiprazole* Cariprazine* Haloperidol
Hyperprolactinaemia[7,8,14,20–25]	Aripiprazole† Brexpiprazole* Cariprazine* Lurasidone Quetiapine	Clozapine Olanzapine Ziprasidone*
Postural hypotension[8,14,26]	Amisulpride Aripiprazole Lurasidone	Brexpiprazole* Cariprazine* Haloperidol Sulpiride Trifluoperazine
QT prolongation[25,27–33]	Brexpiprazole* Cariprazine* Lurasidone Paliperidone (all with ECG monitoring)	Low-dose monotherapy of any drug not formally contraindicated in QT prolongation (with ECG monitoring)
Sedation[7,8,25]	Amisulpride Aripiprazole Brexpiprazole* Cariprazine* Risperidone Sulpiride	Haloperidol Trifuoperazine Ziprasidone*
Sexual dysfunction[8,34–40]	Aripiprazole Lurasidone Quetiapine	Brexpiprazole* Cariprazine* Clozapine

Table 1.38 (*Continued*)

Adverse effect	Suggested drugs	Alternatives
Tardive dyskinesia[41–44]	Clozapine	Aripiprazole Olanzapine Quetiapine
Weight gain[15,32,45–52]	Amisulpride Aripiprazole[†] Haloperidol Lurasidone Ziprasidone*	Asenapine Brexpiprazole* Cariprazine* Trifluoperazine

*Not available in all countries; limited clinical experience with brexpiprazole and cariprazine.
[†] There is evidence that both switching to and co-prescription of aripiprazole are effective in reducing weight, prolactin and dyslipidaemia and in reversing impaired glucose tolerance.[53–55]
ECG, electrocardiogram; EPS, extrapyramidal symptoms.

References

1. Stanniland C et al. Tolerability of atypical antipsychotics. Drug Saf 2000; **22**:195–214.
2. Tarsy D et al. Effects of newer antipsychotics on extrapyramidal function. CNS Drugs 2002; **16**:23–45.
3. Caroff SN et al. Movement disorders associated with atypical antipsychotic drugs. J Clin Psychiatry 2002; 63 **Suppl 4**:12–19.
4. Lemmens P et al. A combined analysis of double-blind studies with risperidone vs. placebo and other antipsychotic agents: factors associated with extrapyramidal symptoms. Acta Psychiatr Scand 1999; **99**:160–170.
5. Taylor DM. Aripiprazole: a review of its pharmacology and clinical use. Int J Clin Pract 2003; **57**:49–54.
6. Meltzer HY et al. Lurasidone in the treatment of schizophrenia: a randomized, double-blind, placebo- and olanzapine-controlled study. Am J Psychiatry 2011; **168**:957–967.
7. Garnock-Jones KP. Cariprazine: a review in schizophrenia. CNS Drugs 2017; **31**:513–525.
8. Garnock-Jones KP. Brexpiprazole: a review in schizophrenia. CNS Drugs 2016; **30**:335–342.
9. Buckley PF. Efficacy of quetiapine for the treatment of schizophrenia: a combined analysis of three placebo-controlled trials. Curr Med Res Opin 2004; **20**:1357–1363.
10. Rettenbacher MA et al. Early changes of plasma lipids during treatment with atypical antipsychotics. Int Clin Psychopharmacol 2006; **21**:369–372.
11. Ball MP et al. Clozapine-induced hyperlipidemia resolved after switch to aripiprazole therapy. Ann Pharmacother 2005; **39**:1570–1572.
12. Chrzanowski WK et al. Effectiveness of long-term aripiprazole therapy in patients with acutely relapsing or chronic, stable schizophrenia: a 52-week, open-label comparison with olanzapine. Psychopharmacology (Berl) 2006; **189**:259–266.
13. De Hert M et al. A case series: evaluation of the metabolic safety of aripiprazole. Schizophr Bull 2007; **33**:823–830.
14. Citrome L et al. Long-term safety and tolerability of lurasidone in schizophrenia: a 12-month, double-blind, active-controlled study. Int Clin Psychopharmacol 2012; **27**:165–176.
15. Kemp DE et al. Weight change and metabolic effects of asenapine in patients with schizophrenia and bipolar disorder. J Clin Psychiatry 2014; **75**:238–245.
16. Haddad PM. Antipsychotics and diabetes: review of non-prospective data. Br J Psychiatry Suppl 2004; **47**:S80–S86.
17. Berry S et al. Improvement of insulin indices after switch from olanzapine to risperidone. Eur Neuropsychopharmacol 2002; **12**:316.
18. Gianfrancesco FD et al. Differential effects of risperidone, olanzapine, clozapine, and conventional antipsychotics on type 2 diabetes: findings from a large health plan database. J Clin Psychiatry 2002; **63**:920–930.
19. Mir S et al. Atypical antipsychotics and hyperglycaemia. Int Clin Psychopharmacol 2001; **16**:63–74.
20. Turrone P et al. Elevation of prolactin levels by atypical antipsychotics. Am J Psychiatry 2002; **159**:133–135.
21. David SR et al. The effects of olanzapine, risperidone, and haloperidol on plasma prolactin levels in patients with schizophrenia. Clin Ther 2000; **22**:1085–1096.
22. Hamner MB et al. Hyperprolactinaemia in antipsychotic-treated patients: guidelines for avoidance and management. CNS Drugs 1998; **10**:209–222.
23. Trives MZ et al. Effect of the addition of aripiprazole on hyperprolactinemia associated with risperidone long-acting injection. J Clin Psychopharmacol 2013; **33**:538–541.
24. Suzuki Y et al. Differences in plasma prolactin levels in patients with schizophrenia treated on monotherapy with five second-generation antipsychotics. Schizophr Res 2013; **145**:116–119.
25. Leucht S et al. Comparative efficacy and tolerability of 15 antipsychotic drugs in schizophrenia: a multiple-treatments meta-analysis. Lancet 2013; **382**:951–962.

26. Citrome L. Cariprazine: chemistry, pharmacodynamics, pharmacokinetics, and metabolism, clinical efficacy, safety, and tolerability. Expert Opin Drug Metab Toxicol 2013; 9:193–206.

27. Glassman AH et al. Antipsychotic drugs: prolonged QTc interval, torsade de pointes, and sudden death. Am J Psychiatry 2001; 158:1774–1782.

28. Taylor D. Antipsychotics and QT prolongation. Acta Psychiatr Scand 2003; 107:85–95.

29. Titier K et al. Atypical antipsychotics: from potassium channels to torsade de pointes and sudden death. Drug Saf 2005; 28:35–51.

30. Ray WA et al. Atypical antipsychotic drugs and the risk of sudden cardiac death. N Engl J Med 2009; 360:225–235.

31. Loebel A et al. Efficacy and safety of lurasidone 80 mg/day and 160 mg/day in the treatment of schizophrenia: a randomized, double-blind, placebo- and active-controlled trial. Schizophr Res 2013; 145:101–109.

32. Das S et al. Brexpiprazole: so far so good. Ther Adv Psychopharmacol 2016; 6:39–54.

33. Citrome L. Cariprazine for the treatment of schizophrenia: a review of this dopamine D3-preferring D3/D2 receptor partial agonist. Clin Schizophr Relat Psychoses 2016; 10:109–119.

34. Byerly MJ et al. An open-label trial of quetiapine for antipsychotic-induced sexual dysfunction. J Sex Marital Ther 2004; 30:325–332.

35. Byerly MJ et al. Sexual dysfunction associated with second-generation antipsychotics in outpatients with schizophrenia or schizoaffective disorder: an empirical evaluation of olanzapine, risperidone, and quetiapine. Schizophr Res 2006; 86:244–250.

36. Montejo Gonzalez AL et al. A 6-month prospective observational study on the effects of quetiapine on sexual functioning. J Clin Psychopharmacol 2005; 25:533–538.

37. Dossenbach M et al. Effects of atypical and typical antipsychotic treatments on sexual function in patients with schizophrenia: 12-month results from the Intercontinental Schizophrenia Outpatient Health Outcomes (IC-SOHO) study. Eur Psychiatry 2006; 21:251–258.

38. Kerwin R et al. A multicentre, randomized, naturalistic, open-label study between aripiprazole and standard of care in the management of community-treated schizophrenic patients Schizophrenia Trial of Aripiprazole: (STAR) study. Eur Psychiatry 2007; 22:433–443.

39. Hanssens L et al. The effect of antipsychotic medication on sexual function and serum prolactin levels in community-treated schizophrenic patients: results from the Schizophrenia Trial of Aripiprazole (STAR) study (NCT00237913). BMC Psychiatry 2008; 8:95.

40. Loebel A et al. Effectiveness of lurasidone vs. quetiapine XR for relapse prevention in schizophrenia: a 12-month, double-blind, noninferiority study. Schizophr Res 2013; 147:95–102.

41. Lieberman J et al. Clozapine pharmacology and tardive dyskinesia. Psychopharmacology (Berl) 1989; 99 Suppl 1:S54–S59.

42. O'Brien J et al. Marked improvement in tardive dyskinesia following treatment with olanzapine in an elderly subject. Br J Psychiatry 1998; 172:186.

43. Sacchetti E et al. Quetiapine, clozapine, and olanzapine in the treatment of tardive dyskinesia induced by first-generation antipsychotics: a 124-week case report. Int Clin Psychopharmacol 2003; 18:357–359.

44. Witschy JK et al. Improvement in tardive dyskinesia with aripiprazole use. Can J Psychiatry 2005; 50:188.

45. Taylor DM et al. Atypical antipsychotics and weight gain – a systematic review. Acta Psychiatr Scand 2000; 101:416–432.

46. Allison D et al. Antipsychotic-induced weight gain: a comprehensive research synthesis. Am J Psychiatry 1999; 156:1686–1696.

47. Brecher M et al. The long term effect of quetiapine (Seroquel™) monotherapy on weight in patients with schizophrenia. Int J Psychiatry Clin Pract 2000; 4:287–291.

48. Casey DE et al. Switching patients to aripiprazole from other antipsychotic agents: a multicenter randomized study. Psychopharmacology (Berl) 2003; 166:391–399.

49. Newcomer JW et al. A multicenter, randomized, double-blind study of the effects of aripiprazole in overweight subjects with schizophrenia or schizoaffective disorder switched from olanzapine. J Clin Psychiatry 2008; 69:1046–1056.

50. McEvoy JP et al. Effectiveness of lurasidone in patients with schizophrenia or schizoaffective disorder switched from other antipsychotics: a randomized, 6-week, open-label study. J Clin Psychiatry 2013; 74:170–179.

51. McEvoy JP et al. Effectiveness of paliperidone palmitate vs haloperidol decanoate for maintenance treatment of schizophrenia: a randomized clinical trial. JAMA 2014; 311:1978–1987.

52. Nasrallah HA et al. The safety and tolerability of cariprazine in long-term treatment of schizophrenia: a post hoc pooled analysis. BMC Psychiatry 2017; 17:305.

53. Shim JC et al. Adjunctive treatment with a dopamine partial agonist, aripiprazole, for antipsychotic-induced hyperprolactinemia: a placebo-controlled trial. Am J Psychiatry 2007; 164:1404–1410.

54. Fleischhacker WW et al. Weight change on aripiprazole-clozapine combination in schizophrenic patients with weight gain and suboptimal response on clozapine: 16-week double-blind study. Eur Psychiatry 2008; 23 Suppl 2:S114–S115.

55. Henderson DC et al. Aripiprazole added to overweight and obese olanzapine-treated schizophrenia patients. J Clin Psychopharmacol 2009; 29:165–169.

Venous thromboembolism

Evidence of an association

Antipsychotic treatment was first linked to an increased risk of thromboembolism in 1965.[1] Over a 10-year observation period, 3.1% of 1590 patients developed thromboembolism, of whom 9 (0.6%) died. However, the use of continuing antipsychotic medication is a proxy for severe mental illness and so observed associations with antipsychotics may reflect inherent pathological processes in the conditions for which they are prescribed. To some extent the relative contributions to risk of thromboembolism of antipsychotic treatment and the conditions they treat remain to be clearly defined.

In a landmark case-control study of nearly 30,000 patients[2] an attempt was made to control for age and gender (but not for diagnosed psychiatric conditions). Risk of thromboembolism was greatly increased overall in people prescribed antipsychotics compared with controls (odds ratio [OR] 7.1). The increased risk was driven by the effect of low-potency phenothiazines (thioridazine, chlorpromazine [OR 24.1]) and was seen chiefly in the first few weeks on treatment. Absolute risk of venous thromboembolism was very small – 0.14% of patients. A secondary analysis suggested no association with diagnosis (not all prescribing was for schizophrenia).

A later meta-analysis of seven case-control studies[3] confirmed an increased risk of thromboembolism with low-potency drugs (OR 2.91) and suggested lower but significantly increased risks with all types of antipsychotics. More recently a meta-analysis of 17 studies[4] reported a small increased risk of thromboembolism with antipsychotics as a whole (OR 1.54) and with FGAs (OR 1.74) and SGAs (OR 2.07) as individual groups. Risk of thromboembolism clearly decreased with age. The authors suggested that the best that could be said was that antipsychotics probably increased the risk by about 50% but that residual confounding could not be discounted (i.e. other factors may have accounted for the effect seen).

Since this time, several more case-control studies have confirmed both the slightly increased risk of thromboembolism and the small risk overall:[5-7] one study reported a risk for older people taking antipsychotics as 43 per 10,000 patient years.[7] Other noteworthy findings were a substantially increased association with thromboembolism for prochlorperazine, a drug not always (or even often) prescribed for psychotic disorders,[5] and an increased risk linked to antipsychotic dosage (risk was quadrupled in high-dose patients).[6] An association with prochlorperazine prescribing had previously been suggested by a UK study.[8] These findings add weight to the theory that antipsychotic medication (and not only the conditions it treats) is responsible for the increased hazard of thromboembolism. The highest risk of pathological blood clotting may be in the first 3 months or so of treatment.[9,10]

Mechanisms

Several mechanisms have been suggested to explain the association between antipsychotics and thromboembolism. These proposed mechanisms are outlined in Box 1.5.

CHAPTER 1

> **Box 1.5** Proposed mechanisms for antipsychotic-associated venous thromboembolism[9–11]
>
> - Sedation*
> - Obesity*
> - Hyperprolactinaemia*
> - Elevated phospholipid antibodies
> - Elevated platelet aggregation§
> - Elevated plasma homocysteine
>
> *Some evidence that these factors are not the mechanism for antipsychotic-induced thromboembolism.[12]
> §In vitro data suggest radically different effects on platelet aggregation for different antipsychotics.[10]

Outcomes

Increased risk of thromboembolism is reflected in numerous published reports of elevated incidence of pulmonary embolism,[13] stroke[14] and myocardial infarction.[15,16]

Summary

Antipsychotics are almost certainly associated with a small but important increased risk of venous thromboembolism and associated hazards of pulmonary embolism, stroke and myocardial infarction. Risk appears to be greatest during the early part of treatment and in younger people, and is probably dose-related.

Practice points

- Monitor closely all patients (but especially younger patients) starting antipsychotic treatment for signs of venous thromboembolism:
  - calf pain or swelling
  - sudden breathing difficulties
  - signs of myocardial infarction (chest pain, nausea, etc.)
  - signs of stroke (sudden unilateral weakness, etc.).
- Use the lowest therapeutic dose.
- Encourage good hydration and physical mobility.

References

1. Häfner H et al. Thromboembolic complications in neuroleptic treatment. Compr Psychiatry 1965; 6:25–34.
2. Zornberg GL et al. Antipsychotic drug use and risk of first-time idiopathic venous thromboembolism: a case-control study. Lancet 2000; 356:1219–1223.
3. Zhang R et al. Antipsychotics and venous thromboembolism risk: a meta-analysis. Pharmacopsychiatry 2011; 44:183–188.
4. Barbui C et al. Antipsychotic drug exposure and risk of venous thromboembolism: a systematic review and meta-analysis of observational studies. Drug Saf 2014; 37:79–90.
5. Ishiguro C et al. Antipsychotic drugs and risk of idiopathic venous thromboembolism: a nested case-control study using the CPRD. Pharmacoepidemiol Drug Saf 2014; 23:1168–1175.
6. Wang MT et al. Use of antipsychotics and risk of venous thromboembolism in postmenopausal women. A population-based nested case-control study. Thromb Haemost 2016; 115:1209–1219.
7. Letmaier M et al. Venous thromboembolism during treatment with antipsychotics: results of a drug surveillance programme. World J Biol Psychiatry 2017:1–12.
8. Parker C et al. Antipsychotic drugs and risk of venous thromboembolism: nested case-control study. BMJ 2010; 341:c4245.

9. Hagg S et al. Risk of venous thromboembolism due to antipsychotic drug therapy. Expert Opin Drug Saf 2009; 8:537–547.

10. Dietrich-Muszalska A et al. The first- and second-generation antipsychotic drugs affect ADP-induced platelet aggregation. World J Biol Psychiatry 2010; 11:268–275.

11. Tromeur C et al. Antipsychotic drugs and venous thromboembolism. Thromb Res 2012; 130:S29–S31.

12. Ferraris A et al. Antipsychotic use among adult outpatients and venous thromboembolic disease: a retrospective cohort study. J Clin Psychopharmacol 2017; 37:405–411.

13. Borras L et al. Pulmonary thromboembolism associated with olanzapine and risperidone. J Emerg Med 2008; 35:159–161.

14. Douglas IJ et al. Exposure to antipsychotics and risk of stroke: self controlled case series study. BMJ 2008; 337:a1227.

15. Brauer R et al. Antipsychotic drugs and risks of myocardial infarction: a self-controlled case series study. Eur Heart J 2015; 36:984–992.

16. Huang KL et al. Myocardial infarction risk and antipsychotics use revisited: a meta-analysis of 10 observational studies. J Psychopharmacol 2017; 31:1544–1555.

REFRACTORY SCHIZOPHRENIA AND CLOZAPINE

Clozapine initiation schedule

Clozapine – dosing regimen

Many of the adverse effects of clozapine are dose-dependent and associated with speed of titration. Adverse effects also tend to be more common and severe at the beginning of therapy. Standard maintenance doses may even prove fatal in clozapine-naïve subjects.[1] To minimise these problems it is important to start treatment at a low dose and to increase dosage slowly.

Clozapine should normally be started at a dose of 12.5 mg once a day, at night. Blood pressure should be monitored hourly for 6 hours because of the hypotensive effect of clozapine. This monitoring is not usually necessary if the first dose is given at night. On day 2, the dose can be increased to 12.5 mg twice daily. If the patient is tolerating

Table 1.39 Suggested starting regimen for clozapine (in-patients)

Day	Morning dose (mg)	Evening dose (mg)
1	–	12.5
2	12.5	12.5
3	25	25
4	25	25
5	25	50
6	25	50
7	50	50
8	50	75
9	75	75
10	75	100
11	100	100
12	100	125
13	125	125*
14	125	150
15	150	150
18	150	200†
21	200	200
28	200	250‡

*Target dose for female non-smokers (250 mg/day).
†Target dose for male non-smokers (350 mg/day).
‡Target dose for female smokers (450 mg/day).

clozapine, the dose can be increased by 25–50 mg a day, until a dose of 300 mg a day is reached. This can usually be achieved in 2–3 weeks. Further dosage increases should be made slowly in increments of 50–100 mg each week. A plasma level of 350 µg/L should be aimed for to ensure an adequate trial, but response may occur at a lower plasma level. The **average** (there is substantial variation) dose at which this plasma level is reached varies according to gender and smoking status. The range is approximately 250 mg/day (female non-smoker) to 550 mg/day (male smoker).[2] The total clozapine dose should be divided (usually twice daily) and, if sedation is a problem, the larger portion of the dose can be given at night.

Table 1.39 is a suggested starting regimen for clozapine. This is a cautious regimen – more rapid increases have been used. Slower titration may be necessary where sedation or other dose-related adverse effects are severe, in the elderly, the very young, those who are physically compromised or those who have poorly tolerated other antipsychotics. If the patient is not tolerating a particular dose, decrease to one that was previously tolerated. If the adverse effect resolves, increase the dose again but at a slower rate.

If for any reason a patient misses fewer than 2 days' clozapine, re-start at the dose prescribed before the event. Do not administer extra tablets to catch up. If more than 2 days are missed, re-start and increase slowly (but at a faster rate than in drug-naïve patients). Please see section on 'Re-starting clozapine after a break in treatment' in this chapter.

References

1. Stanworth D et al. Clozapine – a dangerous drug in a clozapine-naive subject. Forensic Sci Int 2011; **214**:e23–e25.
2. Rostami-Hodjegan A et al. Influence of dose, cigarette smoking, age, sex, and metabolic activity on plasma clozapine concentrations: a predictive model and nomograms to aid clozapine dose adjustment and to assess compliance in individual patients. J Clin Psychopharmacol 2004; **24**:70–78.

Optimising clozapine treatment

Using clozapine alone

Target dose

Note that dose is best adjusted according to patient tolerability and plasma level.

- The average dose in UK is around 450 mg/day.[1]
- Response usually seen in the range 150–900 mg/day.[2]
- Lower doses are required in the elderly, females and non-smokers, and in those pre-scribed certain enzyme inhibitors[3,4]: See Table 1.39.

Plasma levels

- Most studies indicate that the threshold for response is in the range 350–420 µg/L.[5,6] The threshold may be as high as 500 µg/L.[7]
- In male smokers who cannot achieve therapeutic plasma levels, metabolic inhibitors (fluvoxamine[8] or cimetidine[9] for example) can be co-prescribed but extreme caution is required.
- The importance of norclozapine levels has not been established but the clozapine/norclozapine ratio may aid assessment of recent compliance.

Clozapine augmentation

Clozapine 'augmentation' has become common practice because inadequate response to clozapine alone is a frequent clinical event. The evidence base supporting augmentation strategies is growing but remains insufficient to allow the development of any algorithm or schedule of treatment options. In practice, the result of clozapine augmentation is often disappointing and substantial changes in symptom severity are rarely observed. This clinical impression is supported by the equivocal results of many studies, which suggest a small effect size at best. Meta-analyses of antipsychotic augmentation suggest no effect,[10] a small effect in long-term studies[11] or, in the largest meta-analysis, a very small effect overall.[12] An update on this last study[13] confirmed this small effect size. Investigations into dopaminergic activity in refractory schizophrenia suggest there is no overproduction of dopamine.[14,15] Dopamine antagonists are thus unlikely to be effective.

It is recommended that all augmentation attempts are carefully monitored and, if no clear benefit is forthcoming, abandoned after 3–6 months. The addition of another drug to clozapine treatment must be expected to worsen overall adverse-effect burden and so continued ineffective treatment is not appropriate. In some cases, the addition of an augmenting agent may reduce the severity of some adverse effects (e.g. weight gain, dyslipidaemia – see Table 1.40) or allow a reduction in clozapine dose. The addition of aripiprazole to clozapine may be particularly effective in reversing metabolic effects.[16,17]

Table 1.40 shows suggested treatment options (in alphabetical order) where 3–6 months of optimised clozapine alone has not provided satisfactory benefit.

CHAPTER 1

Table 1.40 Suggested options for augmenting clozapine

Option	Comment
Add amisulpride[18–23] (400–800 mg/day)	■ Some evidence and experience suggests amisulpride augmentation may be worthwhile. Two small RCTs, one of which found an increased adverse-effect burden, including cardiac adverse effects.[24] May allow clozapine dose reduction[25]
Add aripiprazole[16,26–28] (15–30 mg/day)	■ Very limited evidence of therapeutic benefit, although a meta-analysis suggests some effect.[29] Reduces weight and LDL cholesterol[29]
Add haloperidol[28,30,31] (2–3 mg/day)	■ Modest evidence of benefit
Add lamotrigine[32–34] (25–300 mg/day)	■ May be useful in partial or non-responders. May reduce alcohol consumption.[35] Several equivocal reports[36–38] but meta-analyses suggest moderate effect size[39,40]
Add omega-3 triglycerides[41,42] (2–3 g EPA daily)	■ Modest, and somewhat contested, evidence to support efficacy in non- or partial responders to antipsychotics, including clozapine
Add risperidone[43,44] (2–6 mg/day)	■ Supported by an RCT but there are also two negative RCTs, each with minuscule response rates.[45,46] Small number of reports of increases in clozapine plasma levels. Long acting injection also an option[47]
Add sulpiride[48] (400 mg/day)	■ May be useful in partial or non-responders. Supported by a single randomised trial in English and three in Chinese.[49] Overall effect modest
Add topiramate[50–54] (50–300 mg/day)	■ Two positive RCTs, two negative. Can worsen psychosis in some.[33,55] Two meta-analyses including hitherto unknown Chinese data[40,56] suggested robust effect on positive and negative symptoms, substantial weight loss but with psychomotor slowing and attention difficulties
Add ziprasidone[57–60] (80–160 mg/day)	■ Supported by three RCTs.[60,61] Associated with QTc prolongation. Rarely used

Notes:
■ Always consider the use of mood stabilisers and/or antidepressants, especially where mood disturbance is thought to contribute to symptoms.[62–64]
■ Other options include adding **pimozide**, **olanzapine** or **sertindole**. None is recommended: pimozide and sertindole have important cardiac toxicity and the addition of olanzapine is poorly supported[65] and likely to exacerbate metabolic adverse effects. Studies of pimozide[66,67] and sertindole[68] have shown no effect. One small RCT supports the use of **Ginkgo biloba**,[69] another two support the use of **memantine**.[70,71] Another study suggests possible benefit of augmentation with **acetyl-L-carnitine**[72] and a case study reports good outcome with **thyroxine**.[73]
EPA, eicosapentaenoic acid; RCT, randomised controlled trial.

References

1. Taylor D et al. A prescription survey of the use of atypical antipsychotics for hospital inpatients in the United Kingdom. Int J Psychiatry Clin Pract 2000; **4**:41–46.
2. Murphy B et al. Maintenance doses for clozapine. Psychiatr Bull 1998; **22**:12–14.
3. Taylor D. Pharmacokinetic interactions involving clozapine. Br J Psychiatry 1997; **171**:109–112.
4. Lane HY et al. Effects of gender and age on plasma levels of clozapine and its metabolites: analyzed by critical statistics. J Clin Psychiatry 1999; **60**:36–40.
5. Taylor D et al. The use of clozapine plasma levels in optimising therapy. Psychiatr Bull 1995; **19**:753–755.

6. Spina E et al. Relationship between plasma concentrations of clozapine and norclozapine and therapeutic response in patients with schizophrenia resistant to conventional neuroleptics. Psychopharmacology (Berl) 2000; 148:83–89.

7. Perry PJ. Therapeutic drug monitoring of antipsychotics. Psychopharmacol Bull 2001; 35:19–29.

8. Papetti F et al. [Clozapine-resistant schizophrenia related to an increased metabolism and benefit of fluvoxamine: four case reports]. Encephale 2007; 33:811–818.

9. Watras M et al. A therapeutic interaction between cimetidine and clozapine: case study and review of the literature. Ther Adv Psychopharmacol 2013; 3:294–297.

10. Barbui C et al. Does the addition of a second antipsychotic drug improve clozapine treatment? Schizophr Bull 2009; 35:458–468.

11. Paton C et al. Augmentation with a second antipsychotic in patients with schizophrenia who partially respond to clozapine: a meta-analysis. J Clin Psychopharmacol 2007; 27:198–204.

12. Taylor DM et al. Augmentation of clozapine with a second antipsychotic – a meta-analysis of randomized, placebo-controlled studies. Acta Psychiatr Scand 2009; 119:419–425.

13. Taylor D et al. Augmentation of clozapine with a second antipsychotic. A meta analysis. Acta Psychiatr Scand 2012; 125:15–24.

14. Demjaha A et al. Dopamine synthesis capacity in patients with treatment-resistant schizophrenia. Am J Psychiatry 2012; 169:1203–1210.

15. Demjaha A et al. Antipsychotic treatment resistance in schizophrenia associated with elevated glutamate levels but normal dopamine function. Biol Psychiatry 2014; 75:e11–e13.

16. Fleischhacker WW et al. Effects of adjunctive treatment with aripiprazole on body weight and clinical efficacy in schizophrenia patients treated with clozapine: a randomized, double-blind, placebo-controlled trial. Int J Neuropsychopharmacol 2010; 13:1115–1125.

17. Correll CU et al. Selective effects of individual antipsychotic cotreatments on cardiometabolic and hormonal risk status: results from a systematic review and meta-analysis. Schizophr Bull 2013; 39 (Suppl 1):S29–S30.

18. Matthiasson P et al. Relationship between dopamine D2 receptor occupancy and clinical response in amisulpride augmentation of clozapine non-response. J Psychopharm 2001; 15:S41.

19. Munro J et al. Amisulpride augmentation of clozapine: an open non-randomized study in patients with schizophrenia partially responsive to clozapine. Acta Psychiatr Scand 2004; 110:292–298.

20. Zink M et al. Combination of clozapine and amisulpride in treatment-resistant schizophrenia – case reports and review of the literature. Pharmacopsychiatry 2004; 37:26–31.

21. Ziegenbein M et al. Augmentation of clozapine with amisulpride in patients with treatment-resistant schizophrenia. An open clinical study. German J Psychiatry 2006; 9:17–21.

22. Kampf P et al. Augmentation of clozapine with amisulpride: a promising therapeutic approach to refractory schizophrenic symptoms. Pharmacopsychiatry 2005; 38:39–40.

23. Assion HJ et al. Amisulpride augmentation in patients with schizophrenia partially responsive or unresponsive to clozapine. A randomized, double-blind, placebo-controlled trial. Pharmacopsychiatry 2008; 41:24–28.

24. Barnes TR et al. Amisulpride augmentation in clozapine-unresponsive schizophrenia (AMICUS): a double-blind, placebo-controlled, randomised trial of clinical effectiveness and cost-effectiveness. Health Technol Assess 2017; 21:1–56.

25. Croissant B et al. Reduction of side effects by combining clozapine with amisulpride: case report and short review of clozapine-induced hypersalivation – a case report. Pharmacopsychiatry 2005; 38:38–39.

26. Chang JS et al. Aripiprazole augmentation in clozapine-treated patients with refractory schizophrenia: an 8-week, randomized, double-blind, placebo-controlled trial. J Clin Psychiatry 2008; 69:720–731.

27. Muscatello MR et al. Effect of aripiprazole augmentation of clozapine in schizophrenia: a double-blind, placebo-controlled study. Schizophr Res 2011; 127:93–99.

28. Cipriani A et al. Aripiprazole versus haloperidol in combination with clozapine for treatment-resistant schizophrenia: a 12-month, randomized, naturalistic trial. J Clin Psychopharmacol 2013; 33:533–537.

29. Srisurapanont M et al. Efficacy and safety of aripiprazole augmentation of clozapine in schizophrenia: a systematic review and meta-analysis of randomized-controlled trials. J Psychiatr Res 2015; 62:38–47.

30. Rajarethinam R et al. Augmentation of clozapine partial responders with conventional antipsychotics. Schizophr Res 2003; 60:97–98.

31. Barbui C et al. Aripiprazole versus haloperidol in combination with clozapine for treatment-resistant schizophrenia in routine clinical care: a randomized, controlled trial. J Clin Psychopharmacol 2011; 31:266–273.

32. Dursun SM et al. Clozapine plus lamotrigine in treatment-resistant schizophrenia. Arch Gen Psychiatry 1999; 56:950.

33. Dursun SM et al. Augmenting antipsychotic treatment with lamotrigine or topiramate in patients with treatment-resistant schizophrenia: a naturalistic case-series outcome study. J Psychopharm 2001; 15:297–301.

34. Tiihonen J et al. Lamotrigine in treatment-resistant schizophrenia: a randomized placebo-controlled crossover trial. Biol Psychiatry 2003; 54:1241–1248.

35. Kalyoncu A et al. Use of lamotrigine to augment clozapine in patients with resistant schizophrenia and comorbid alcohol dependence: a potent anti-craving effect? J Psychopharmacol 2005; 19:301–305.

36. Goff DC et al. Lamotrigine as add-on therapy in schizophrenia: results of 2 placebo-controlled trials. J Clin Psychopharmacol 2007; 27:582–589.

37. Heck AH et al. Addition of lamotrigine to clozapine in inpatients with chronic psychosis. J Clin Psychiatry 2005; 66:1333.

38. Vayisoglu S et al. Lamotrigine augmentation in patients with schizophrenia who show partial response to clozapine treatment. Schizophr Res 2013; 143:207–214.

39. Tiihonen J et al. The efficacy of lamotrigine in clozapine-resistant schizophrenia: a systematic review and meta-analysis. Schizophr Res 2009; 109:10–14.

40. Zheng W et al. Clozapine augmentation with antiepileptic drugs for treatment-resistant schizophrenia: a meta-analysis of randomized controlled trials. J Clin Psychiatry 2017; 78:e498–e505.

41. Peet M et al. Double-blind placebo controlled trial of N-3 polyunsaturated fatty acids as an adjunct to neuroleptics. Schizophr Res 1998; 29:160–161.

42. Puri BK et al. Sustained remission of positive and negative symptoms of schizophrenia following treatment with eicosapentaenoic acid. Arch Gen Psychiatry 1998; 55:188–189.

43. Josiassen RC et al. Clozapine augmented with risperidone in the treatment of schizophrenia: a randomized, double-blind, placebo-controlled trial. Am J Psychiatry 2005; 162:130–136.

44. Raskin S et al. Clozapine and risperidone: combination/augmentation treatment of refractory schizophrenia: a preliminary observation. Acta Psychiatr Scand 2000; 101:334–336.

45. Anil Yagcioglu AE et al. A double-blind controlled study of adjunctive treatment with risperidone in schizophrenic patients partially responsive to clozapine: efficacy and safety. J Clin Psychiatry 2005; 66:63–72.

46. Honer WG et al. Clozapine alone versus clozapine and risperidone with refractory schizophrenia. N Engl J Med 2006; 354:472–482.

47. Se HK et al. The combined use of risperidone long-acting injection and clozapine in patients with schizophrenia non-adherent to clozapine: a case series. J Psychopharmacol 2010; 24:981–986.

48. Shiloh R et al. Sulpiride augmentation in people with schizophrenia partially responsive to clozapine. A double-blind, placebo-controlled study. Br J Psychiatry 1997; 171:569–573.

49. Wang J et al. Sulpiride augmentation for schizophrenia. Schizophr Bull 2010; 36:229–230.

50. Tiihonen J et al. Topiramate add-on in treatment-resistant schizophrenia: a randomized, double-blind, placebo-controlled, crossover trial. J Clin Psychiatry 2005; 66:1012–1015.

51. Afshar H et al. Topiramate add-on treatment in schizophrenia: a randomised, double-blind, placebo-controlled clinical trial. J Psychopharmacol 2009; 23:157–162.

52. Muscatello MR et al. Topiramate augmentation of clozapine in schizophrenia: a double-blind, placebo-controlled study. J Psychopharmacol 2011; 25:667–674.

53. Hahn MK et al. Topiramate augmentation in clozapine-treated patients with schizophrenia: clinical and metabolic effects. J Clin Psychopharmacol 2010; 30:706–710.

54. Behdani F et al. Effect of topiramate augmentation in chronic schizophrenia: a placebo-controlled trial. Arch Iran Med 2011; 14:270–275.

55. Millson RC et al. Topiramate for refractory schizophrenia. Am J Psychiatry 2002; 159:675.

56. Zheng W et al. Efficacy and safety of adjunctive topiramate for schizophrenia: a meta-analysis of randomized controlled trials. Acta Psychiatr Scand 2016; 134:385–398.

57. Zink M et al. Combination of ziprasidone and clozapine in treatment-resistant schizophrenia. Hum Psychopharmacol 2004; 19:271–273.

58. Ziegenbein M et al. Clozapine and ziprasidone: a useful combination in patients with treatment-resistant schizophrenia. J Neuropsychiatry Clin Neurosci 2006; 18:246–247.

59. Ziegenbein M et al. Combination of clozapine and ziprasidone in treatment-resistant schizophrenia: an open clinical study. Clin Neuropharmacol 2005; 28:220–224.

60. Zink M et al. Efficacy and tolerability of ziprasidone versus risperidone as augmentation in patients partially responsive to clozapine: a randomised controlled clinical trial. J Psychopharm 2009; 23:305–314.

61. Muscatello MR et al. Augmentation of clozapine with ziprasidone in refractory schizophrenia: a double-blind, placebo-controlled study. J Clin Psychopharmacol 2014; 34:129–133.

62. Citrome L. Schizophrenia and valproate. Psychopharmacol Bull 2003; 37 Suppl 2:74–88.

63. Tranulis C et al. Somatic augmentation strategies in clozapine resistance – what facts? Clin Neuropharmacol 2006; 29:34–44.

64. Suzuki T et al. Augmentation of atypical antipsychotics with valproic acid. An open-label study for most difficult patients with schizophrenia. Hum Psychopharmacol 2009; 24:628–638.

65. Gupta S et al. Olanzapine augmentation of clozapine. Ann Clin Psychiatry 1998; 10:113–115.

66. Friedman JI et al. Pimozide augmentation of clozapine inpatients with schizophrenia and schizoaffective disorder unresponsive to clozapine monotherapy. Neuropsychopharmacology 2011; 36:1289–1295.

67. Gunduz-Bruce H et al. Efficacy of pimozide augmentation for clozapine partial responders with schizophrenia. Schizophr Res 2013; 143:344–347.

68. Nielsen J et al. Augmenting clozapine with sertindole: a double-blind, randomized, placebo-controlled study. J Clin Psychopharmacol 2012; 32:173–178.

69. Doruk A et al. A placebo-controlled study of extract of ginkgo biloba added to clozapine in patients with treatment-resistant schizophrenia. Int Clin Psychopharmacol 2008; 23:223–227.

70. de Lucena D et al. Improvement of negative and positive symptoms in treatment-refractory schizophrenia: a double-blind, randomized, placebo-controlled trial with memantine as add-on therapy to clozapine. J Clin Psychiatry 2009; 70:1416–1423.

71. Veerman SR et al. Adjunctive memantine in clozapine-treated refractory schizophrenia: an open-label 1-year extension study. Psychol Med 2017; 47:363–375.

72. Bruno A et al. Acetyl-l-carnitine augmentation of clozapine in partial-responder schizophrenia: a 12-week, open-label uncontrolled preliminary study. Clin Neuropharmacol 2016; 39:277–280.

73. Seddigh R et al. Levothyroxine augmentation in clozapine resistant schizophrenia: a case report and review. Case Rep Psychiatry 2015; 2015:678040.

Alternatives to clozapine

Clozapine has the strongest evidence for efficacy for schizophrenia that has proved refractory to adequate trials of standard antipsychotic medication. Where treatment resistance has been established, clozapine treatment should not be delayed or withheld.[1,2] The practice of using successive antipsychotic medications (or the latest) instead of clozapine is widespread but not supported by research. Where clozapine cannot be used (because of toxicity or patient refusal to take the medication or comply with the mandatory monitoring tests), other drugs or drug combinations may be tried (see Table 1.41) but, in practice, outcome is usually disappointing. Long-term data on efficacy and safety/tolerability are generally lacking. The data that are available do not allow any distinction between treatment regimens to be drawn, particularly choice of antipsychotic medication,[3,4] but it seems wise to use single drugs before trying multiple drug options. Olanzapine is perhaps most often used as antipsychotic monotherapy, usually in dosage above the licensed range. If this fails, then the addition of a second antipsychotic (amisulpride, for example) is a possible next step, although the risk–benefit balance of combined antipsychotic medication regimens remains unclear.[5] Amongst unconventional agents, minocycline and ondansetron have the advantage of low toxicity and good tolerability. A depot/LAI antipsychotic preparation is an option where the avoidance of covert non-adherence is a clinical priority.

Many of the treatments listed in Table 1.41 are somewhat experimental and some of the compounds are difficult to obtain (e.g. glycine, D-serine, sarcosine, etc.).

Table 1.41 Alternatives to clozapine. Treatments are listed in alphabetical order: no preference is implied by position in table

Treatment	Comments
Allopurinol 300–600 mg/day **(+ antipsychotic)**[8–11]	Increases adenosinergic transmission which may reduce effects of dopamine. Three positive RCTs[8,9,11]
Amisulpride[12] (up to 1200 mg/day)	Single, small open study
Aripiprazole[13,14] (15–30 mg/day)	Single randomised controlled study indicating moderate effect in patients resistant to risperidone or olanzapine (+ others). Higher doses (60 mg/day) have been used[15]
Asenapine (+ antipsychotic)[16]	Two case reports
Bexarotene 75 mg/day[17] **(+ antipsychotic)**	Retinoid receptor agonist. One RCT (n=90) in non-refractory but suboptimally treated patients suggesting worthwhile effect on positive symptoms
Blonanserin (+ antipsychotic)[18]	Atypical antipsychotic licensed in Japan and Korea. One case series found it to be effective and well tolerated
CBT[19]	Non-drug therapies should always be considered
Celecoxib + risperidone[20] (400 mg + 6 mg/day)	COX-2 inhibitors modulate immune response and may prevent glutamate-related cell death. One RCT showed useful activity in all main symptom domains. Associated with increased cardiovascular mortality
Donepezil 5–10 mg/day **(+ antipsychotic)**[21–23]	Three RCTs, one negative,[22] two positive,[21,23] suggesting a small effect on cognitive and negative symptoms

Table 1.41 (*Continued*)

Treatment	Comments
D-alanine 100 mg/kg/day (+ antipsychotic)[24]	Glycine (NMDA) agonist. One positive RCT
D-serine 30 mg/kg/day (+ olanzapine)[25]	Glycine (NMDA) agonist. One positive RCT
D-serine up to 3 g as monotherapy[26]	Improved negative symptoms in one RCT, but inferior to high-dose olanzapine for treatment of positive symptoms
ECT[27]	Open studies suggest moderate effect, as does a retrospective study.[28] Often reserved for last-line treatment in practice but can be successful in the short[29] and long[30] term
Estradiol 100–200 μg transdermal/day (+ antipsychotic)[31]	Oestrogens may be psychoprotective and/or antipsychotic. RCT (n = 183) in women of child-bearing age suggested benefits on positive symptoms, especially at higher doses. Note contraindications include being post-menopausal, history of venous thromboembolism, stroke, breast cancer, migraine with aura. Unopposed estradiol over long periods increases the risk of endometrial hyperplasia and malignancy – consider consulting an endocrinologist. Evidence in men is lacking
Famotidine 100 mg bd + antipsychotic[32]	H_2 antagonist. One short (4-week) RCT suggested some benefit in overall PANSS and CGI scores
Ginkgo biloba (+ antipsychotic)[6,7]	Possibly effective in combination with haloperidol. Unlikely to give rise to additional adverse effects but clinical experience limited
Lurasidone up to 240 mg/day[33]	One RCT of high-dose lurasidone, full results not yet reported. Appears to be well tolerated, may be effective but no clozapine comparison arm included
Memantine 20 mg/day (+ antipsychotic)[34–36]	Memantine is an NMDA antagonist. Two RCTs. The larger of the two (n = 138) was negative. In the smaller (n = 21), memantine improved positive and negative symptoms when added to clozapine. In another study in non-refractory schizophrenia, memantine improved negative symptoms when added to risperidone
Mianserin + FGA 30 mg/day[32]	$5-HT_2$ antagonist. One, small positive RCT
Minocycline 200 mg/day (+ antipsychotic)[37,38]	May be anti-inflammatory and neuroprotective. One open study (n = 22) and one RCT (n = 54) suggest good effect on negative and cognitive symptoms. Also one RCT (n = 50) of augmentation of clozapine.[39] RCT evidence of neuroprotective effect in early psychosis[40]
Mirtazapine 30 mg/day (+ antipsychotic)[41–43]	$5-HT_2$ antagonist. Two RCTs, one negative,[42] one positive.[41] Effect seems to be mainly on positive symptoms
N-acetylcysteine 2 g/day (+ antipsychotic)[40]	One RCT suggests small benefits in negative symptoms and rates of akathisia. Another RCT showed benefits in chronic schizophrenia.[44] Case study of successful use of 600 mg a day.[45] Large RCT in progress[46]
Olanzapine[47–52] 5–25 mg/day	Supported by some well-conducted trials but clinical experience disappointing. Some patients show moderate response
Olanzapine[53–59] 30–60 mg/day	Contradictory findings in the literature but possibly effective. High-dose olanzapine is not atypical[60] and can be poorly tolerated[61] with gross metabolic changes[59]
Olanzapine + amisulpride[62] (up to 800 mg/day)	Small open study suggests benefit

(*Continued*)

Table 1.41 (*Continued*)

Treatment	Comments
Olanzapine + aripiprazole[63]	Single case report suggests benefit. Probably reduces metabolic toxicity
Olanzapine + glycine[64] (0.8 g/kg/day)	Small, double-blind crossover trial suggests clinically relevant improvement in negative symptoms
Olanzapine + lamotrigine[61,65] (up to 400 mg/day)	Reports contradictory and rather unconvincing. Reasonable theoretical basis for adding lamotrigine, which is usually well tolerated
Olanzapine + risperidone[66] (various doses)	Small study suggests some patients may benefit from combined therapy after sequential failure of each drug alone
Olanzapine + sulpiride[67] (600 mg/day)	Some evidence that this combination improves mood symptoms
Omega-3 triglycerides[68,69]	Suggested efficacy but data very limited
Ondansetron 8 mg/day (+ antipsychotic)[70–72]	Three RCTs. All show improvements in negative and cognitive symptoms
Propentofylline + risperidone[73] (900 mg + 6 mg/day)	One RCT suggests some activity against positive symptoms
Quetiapine[74–77]	Very limited evidence and clinical experience not encouraging. High doses (>1200 mg/day) have been used but are no more effective[78]
Quetiapine + amisulpride[79]	Single naturalistic observation of 19 patients suggested useful benefit. Doses averaged 700 mg quetiapine and 950 mg amisulpride
Quetiapine + haloperidol[80]	Two case reports
Raloxifene 60–120 mg/day (+ antipsychotic)[81]	Selective oestrogen receptor modulator; may offer benefits of estradiol without long-term risks. One case report[81] in post-menopausal treatment-resistant schizophrenia. Data in non-treatment resistance are rather conflicting, with two overlapping positive trials[82,83] and one negative trial.[84] One positive RCT in refractory women.[85] Evidence in men is lacking
Riluzole 100 mg/day + **risperidone** up to 6 mg/day[86]	Glutamate modulating agent. One RCT demonstrated improvement in negative symptoms
Risperidone[87–89] 4–8 mg/day	Doubtful efficacy in true treatment-refractory schziophrenia but some supporting evidence. May also be tried in combination with glycine[64] or lamotrigine[60] or indeed with other atypicals[90]
Risperidone LAI 50/100 mg 2/52[91]	One RCT showing good response for both doses in refractory schizophrenia. Plasma levels for 100 mg dose similar to 6–8 mg/day oral risperidone
Ritanserin + risperidone (12 mg + 6 mg/day)[92]	5-$HT_{2A/2C}$ antagonist. One RCT suggests small effect on negative symptoms
Sarcosine (2 g/day)[93,94] (+ antipsychotic)	Enhances glycine action. Supported by two RCTs
Sertindole[95] (12–24 mg/day)	One large RCT (conducted in 1996–1998 but published in 2011) suggested good effect and equivalence to risperidone. Around half of subjects responded. Another RCT[96] showed no effect at all when added to clozapine Little experience in practice
Topiramate (300 mg/day) (+ antipsychotic)[97]	Small effect shown in single RCT. Induces weight loss. Cognitive adverse effects likely

Table 1.41 (*Continued*)

Treatment	Comments
Transcranial magnetic stimulation[98–100]	Conflicting results
Valproate[101]	Doubtful effect but may be useful where there is a clear affective component
Yokukansan (+ antipsychotic)[102]	Japanese herbal medicine, partial agonist at D_2 and 5-HT_{1A}, antagonist at 5-HT_{2A} and glutamate receptors. Potential small benefit in excitement/hostility symptoms
Zotepine ≥ 300 mg/day[103]	One study showed that some patients do not deteriorate when switched from clozapine
Ziprasidone 80–160 mg/ day[104–106]	Two good RCTs. One[106] suggests superior efficacy to chlorpromazine in refractory schizophrenia, the other[104] suggests equivalence to clozapine in subjects with treatment intolerance/resistance. Disappointing results in practice, however. Supratherapeutic doses offer no advantage[107]

bd, *bis die* (twice a day); CBT, cognitive behavioural therapy; CGI, clinical global impression; COX, cyclo-oxgenase; ECT, electroconvulsive therapy; FGA, first-generation antipsychotic; LAI, long-acting injection; NMDA, N-methyl-D-aspartate; PANSS, positive and negative syndrome scale; RCT, randomised controlled trial.

Before using any of the regimens outlined, readers should consult the primary literature cited. Particular care should be taken to inform patients where prescribing is off-label and to ensure that they understand the potential adverse effects of the more experimental treatments.

Non-clozapine treatment of refractory schizophrenia is an area of active research. Glutamatergic drugs may hold promise (although bitopertin is inactive[6]), as may 5-HT_{2A} inverse agonists.[7]

References

1. Yoshimura B et al. The critical treatment window of clozapine in treatment-resistant schizophrenia: secondary analysis of an observational study. Psychiatry Res 2017; **250**:65–70.
2. Howes OD et al. Adherence to treatment guidelines in clinical practice: study of antipsychotic treatment prior to clozapine initiation. Br J Psychiatry 2012; **201**:481–485.
3. Molins C et al. Response to antipsychotic drugs in treatment-resistant schizophrenia: conclusions based on systematic review. Schizophr Res 2016; **178**:64–67.
4. Samara MT et al. Efficacy, acceptability, and tolerability of antipsychotics in treatment-resistant schizophrenia: a network meta-analysis. JAMA Psychiatry 2016; **73**:199–210.
5. Galling B et al. Antipsychotic augmentation vs. monotherapy in schizophrenia: systematic review, meta-analysis and meta-regression analysis. World Psychiatry 2017; **16**:77–89.
6. Bugarski-Kirola D et al. Efficacy and safety of adjunctive bitopertin versus placebo in patients with suboptimally controlled symptoms of schizophrenia treated with antipsychotics: results from three phase 3, randomised, double-blind, parallel-group, placebo-controlled, multi-centre studies in the SearchLyte clinical trial programme. Lancet Psychiatry 2016; **3**:1115–1128.
7. Garay RP et al. Potential serotonergic agents for the treatment of schizophrenia. Expert Opin Investig Drugs 2016; **25**:159–170.
8. Akhondzadeh S et al. Beneficial antipsychotic effects of allopurinol as add-on therapy for schizophrenia: a double blind, randomized and placebo controlled trial. Prog Neuropsychopharmacol Biol Psychiatry 2005; **29**:253–259.
9. Brunstein MG et al. A clinical trial of adjuvant allopurinol therapy for moderately refractory schizophrenia. J Clin Psychiatry 2005; **66**:213–219.
10. Buie LW et al. Allopurinol as adjuvant therapy in poorly responsive or treatment refractory schizophrenia. Ann Pharmacother 2006; **40**:2200–2204.
11. Dickerson FB et al. A double-blind trial of adjunctive allopurinol for schizophrenia. Schizophr Res 2009; **109**:66–69.

12. Kontaxakis VP et al. Switching to amisulpride monotherapy for treatment-resistant schizophrenia. Eur Psychiatry 2006; 21:214–217.
13. Kane JM et al. Aripiprazole for treatment-resistant schizophrenia: results of a multicenter, randomized, double-blind, comparison study versus perphenazine. J Clin Psychiatry 2007; 68:213–223.
14. Hsu WY et al. Aripiprazole in treatment-refractory schizophrenia. J Psychiatr Pract 2009; 15:221–226.
15. Crossman AM et al. Tolerability of high-dose aripiprazole in treatment-refractory schizophrenic patients. J Clin Psychiatry 2006; 67:1158–1159.
16. Smith EN et al. Asenapine augmentation and treatment-resistant schizophrenia in the high-secure hospital setting. Ther Adv Psychopharmacol 2014; 4:193–197.
17. Lerner V et al. The retinoid X receptor agonist bexarotene relieves positive symptoms of schizophrenia: a 6-week, randomized, double-blind, placebo-controlled multicenter trial. J Clin Psychiatry 2013; 74:1224–1232.
18. Tachibana M et al. Effectiveness of blonanserin for patients with drug treatment-resistant schizophrenia and dopamine supersensitivity: a retrospective analysis. Asian J Psychiatr 2016; 24:28–32.
19. Valmaggia LR et al. Cognitive-behavioural therapy for refractory psychotic symptoms of schizophrenia resistant to atypical antipsychotic medication. Randomised controlled trial. Br J Psychiatry 2005; 186:324–330.
20. Akhondzadeh S et al. Celecoxib as adjunctive therapy in schizophrenia: a double-blind, randomized and placebo-controlled trial. Schizophr Res 2007; 90:179–185.
21. Lee BJ et al. A 12-week, double-blind, placebo-controlled trial of donepezil as an adjunct to haloperidol for treating cognitive impairments in patients with chronic schizophrenia. J Psychopharmacol 2007; 21:421–427.
22. Keefe RSE et al. Efficacy and safety of donepezil in patients with schizophrenia or schizoaffective disorder: significant placebo/practice effects in a 12-week, randomized, double-blind, placebo-controlled trial. Neuropsychopharmacology 2007; 33:1217–1228.
23. Akhondzadeh S et al. A 12-week, double-blind, placebo-controlled trial of donepezil adjunctive treatment to risperidone in chronic and stable schizophrenia. Prog Neuropsychopharmacol Biol Psychiatry 2008; 32:1810–1815.
24. Tsai GE et al. D-alanine added to antipsychotics for the treatment of schizophrenia. Biol Psychiatry 2006; 59:230–234.
25. Heresco-Levy U et al. D-serine efficacy as add-on pharmacotherapy to risperidone and olanzapine for treatment-refractory schizophrenia. Biol Psychiatry 2005; 57:577–585.
26. Ermilov M et al. A pilot double-blind comparison of d-serine and high-dose olanzapine in treatment-resistant patients with schizophrenia. Schizophr Res 2013; 150:604–605.
27. Zheng W et al. Electroconvulsive therapy added to non-clozapine antipsychotic medication for treatment resistant schizophrenia: meta-analysis of randomized controlled trials. PLoS One 2016; 11:e0156510.
28. Grover S et al. Effectiveness of electroconvulsive therapy in patients with treatment resistant schizophrenia: a retrospective study. Psychiatry Res 2017; 249:349–353.
29. Chanpattana W et al. Electroconvulsive therapy in treatment-resistant schizophrenia: prediction of response and the nature of symptomatic improvement. J ECT 2010; 26:289–298.
30. Ravanic DB et al. Long-term efficacy of electroconvulsive therapy combined with different antipsychotic drugs in previously resistant schizophrenia. Psychiatr Danub 2009; 21:179–186.
31. Kulkarni J et al. Estradiol for treatment-resistant schizophrenia: a large-scale randomized-controlled trial in women of child-bearing age. Mol Psychiatry 2015; 20:695–702.
32. Meskanen K et al. A randomized clinical trial of histamine 2 receptor antagonism in treatment-resistant schizophrenia. J Clin Psychopharmacol 2013; 33:472–478.
33. Meltzer H et al. W162 - lurasidone is an effective treatment for treatment resistant schizophrenia. Neuropsychopharmacology 2015; 40 (Suppl 1):S546.
34. Lieberman JA et al. A randomized, placebo-controlled study of memantine as adjunctive treatment in patients with schizophrenia. Neuropsychopharmacology 2009; 34:1322–1329.
35. de Lucena D et al. Improvement of negative and positive symptoms in treatment-refractory schizophrenia: a double-blind, randomized, placebo-controlled trial with memantine as add-on therapy to clozapine. J Clin Psychiatry 2009; 70:1416–1423.
36. Rezaei F et al. Memantine add-on to risperidone for treatment of negative symptoms in patients with stable schizophrenia: randomized, double-blind, placebo-controlled study. J Clin Psychopharmacol 2013; 33:336–342.
37. Levkovitz Y et al. A double-blind, randomized study of minocycline for the treatment of negative and cognitive symptoms in early-phase schizophrenia. J Clin Psychiatry 2010; 71:138–149.
38. Miyaoka T et al. Minocycline as adjunctive therapy for schizophrenia: an open-label study. Clin Neuropharmacol 2008; 31:287–292.
39. Kelly DL et al. Adjunctive minocycline in clozapine-treated schizophrenia patients with persistent symptoms. J Clin Psychopharmacol 2015; 35:374–381.
40. Chaudhry IB et al. Minocycline benefits negative symptoms in early schizophrenia: a randomised double-blind placebo-controlled clinical trial in patients on standard treatment. J Psychopharmacol 2012; 26:1185–1193.
41. Joffe G et al. Add-on mirtazapine enhances antipsychotic effect of first generation antipsychotics in schizophrenia: a double-blind, randomized, placebo-controlled trial. Schizophr Res 2009; 108:245–251.
42. Berk M et al. Mirtazapine add-on therapy in the treatment of schizophrenia with atypical antipsychotics: a double-blind, randomised, placebo-controlled clinical trial. Hum Psychopharmacol 2009; 24:233–238.
43. Delle CR et al. Add-on mirtazapine enhances effects on cognition in schizophrenic patients under stabilized treatment with clozapine. Exp Clin Psychopharmacol 2007; 15:563–568.
44. Sepehrmanesh Z et al. Therapeutic effect of adjunctive N-acetyl cysteine (NAC) on symptoms of chronic schizophrenia: a double-blind, randomized clinical trial. Prog Neuropsychopharmacol Biol Psychiatry 2018; 82:289–296.

45. Bulut M et al. Beneficial effects of N-acetylcysteine in treatment resistant schizophrenia. World J Biol Psychiatry 2009; 10:626–628.

46. Rossell SL et al. N-acetylcysteine (NAC) in schizophrenia resistant to clozapine: a double blind randomised placebo controlled trial targeting negative symptoms. BMC Psychiatry 2016; 16:320.

47. Breier A et al. Comparative efficacy of olanzapine and haloperidol for patients with treatment-resistant schizophrenia. Biol Psychiatry 1999; 45:403–411.

48. Conley RR et al. Olanzapine compared with chlorpromazine in treatment-resistant schizophrenia. Am J Psychiatry 1998; 155:914–920.

49. Sanders RD et al. An open trial of olanzapine in patients with treatment-refractory psychoses. J Clin Psychopharmacol 1999; 19:62–66.

50. Taylor D et al. Olanzapine in practice: a prospective naturalistic study. Psychiatr Bull 1999; 23:178–180.

51. Bitter I et al. Olanzapine versus clozapine in treatment-resistant or treatment-intolerant schizophrenia. Prog Neuropsychopharmacol Biol Psychiatry 2004; 28:173–180.

52. Tollefson GD et al. Double-blind comparison of olanzapine versus clozapine in schizophrenic patients clinically eligible for treatment with clozapine. Biol Psychiatry 2001; 49:52–63.

53. Sheitman BB et al. High-dose olanzapine for treatment-refractory schizophrenia. Am J Psychiatry 1997; 154:1626.

54. Fanous A et al. Schizophrenia and schizoaffective disorder treated with high doses of olanzapine. J Clin Psychopharmacol 1999; 19:275–276.

55. Dursun SM et al. Olanzapine for patients with treatment-resistant schizophrenia: a naturalistic case-series outcome study. Can J Psychiatry 1999; 44:701–704.

56. Conley RR et al. The efficacy of high-dose olanzapine versus clozapine in treatment-resistant schizophrenia: a double-blind crossover study. J Clin Psychopharmacol 2003; 23:668–671.

57. Kumra S et al. Clozapine and "high-dose" olanzapine in refractory early-onset schizophrenia: a 12-week randomized and double-blind comparison. Biol Psychiatry 2008; 63:524–529.

58. Kumra S et al. Clozapine versus "high-dose" olanzapine in refractory early-onset schizophrenia: an open-label extension study. J Child Adolesc Psychopharmacol 2008; 18:307–316.

59. Meltzer HY et al. A randomized, double-blind comparison of clozapine and high-dose olanzapine in treatment-resistant patients with schizophrenia. J Clin Psychiatry 2008; 69:274–285.

60. Bronson BD et al. Adverse effects of high-dose olanzapine in treatment-refractory schizophrenia. J Clin Psychopharmacol 2000; 20:382–384.

61. Kelly DL et al. Adverse effects and laboratory parameters of high-dose olanzapine vs. clozapine in treatment-resistant schizophrenia. Ann Clin Psychiatry 2003; 15:181–186.

62. Zink M et al. Combination of amisulpride and olanzapine in treatment-resistant schizophrenic psychoses. Eur Psychiatry 2004; 19:56–58.

63. Duggal HS. Aripirazole-olanzapine combination for treatment of schizophrenia. Can J Psychiatry 2004; 49:151.

64. Heresco-Levy U et al. High-dose glycine added to olanzapine and risperidone for the treatment of schizophrenia. Biol Psychiatry 2004; 55:165–171.

65. Dursun SM et al. Augmenting antipsychotic treatment with lamotrigine or topiramate in patients with treatment-resistant schizophrenia: a naturalistic case-series outcome study. J Psychopharm 2001; 15:297–301.

66. Suzuki T et al. Effectiveness of antipsychotic polypharmacy for patients with treatment refractory schizophrenia: an open-label trial of olanzapine plus risperidone for those who failed to respond to a sequential treatment with olanzapine, quetiapine and risperidone. Hum Psychopharmacol 2008; 23:455–463.

67. Kotler M et al. Sulpiride augmentation of olanzapine in the management of treatment-resistant chronic schizophrenia: evidence for improvement of mood symptomatology. Int Clin Psychopharmacol 2004; 19:23–26.

68. Mellor JE et al. Omega-3 fatty acid supplementation in schizophrenic patients. Hum Psychopharmacol 1996; 11:39–46.

69. Puri BK et al. Sustained remission of positive and negative symptoms of schizophrenia following treatment with eicosapentaenoic acid. Arch Gen Psychiatry 1998; 55:188–189.

70. Zhang ZJ et al. Beneficial effects of ondansetron as an adjunct to haloperidol for chronic, treatment-resistant schizophrenia: a double-blind, randomized, placebo-controlled study. Schizophr Res 2006; 88:102–110.

71. Akhondzadeh S et al. Added ondansetron for stable schizophrenia: a double blind, placebo controlled trial. Schizophr Res 2009; 107:206–212.

72. Samadi R et al. Efficacy of risperidone augmentation with ondansetron in the treatment of negative and depressive symptoms in schizophrenia: a randomized clinical trial. Iran J Med Sci 2017; 42:14–23.

73. Salimi S et al. A placebo controlled study of the propentofylline added to risperidone in chronic schizophrenia. Prog Neuropsychopharmacol Biol Psychiatry 2008; 32:726–732.

74. Reznik I et al. Long-term efficacy and safety of quetiapine in treatment-refractory schizophrenia: a case report. Int J Psychiatry Clin Pract 2000; 4:77–80.

75. De Nayer A et al. Efficacy and tolerability of quetiapine in patients with schizophrenia switched from other antipsychotics. Int J Psychiatry Clin Pract 2003; 7:59–66.

76. Larmo I et al. Efficacy and tolerability of quetiapine in patients with schizophrenia who switched from haloperidol, olanzapine or risperidone. Hum Psychopharmacol 2005; 20:573–581.

77. Boggs DL et al. Quetiapine at high doses for the treatment of refractory schizophrenia. Schizophr Res 2008; 101:347–348.

78. Lindenmayer JP et al. A randomized, double-blind, parallel-group, fixed-dose, clinical trial of quetiapine at 600 versus 1200 mg/d for patients with treatment-resistant schizophrenia or schizoaffective disorder. J Clin Psychopharmacol 2011; 31:160–168.

79. Quintero J et al. The effectiveness of the combination therapy of amisulpride and quetiapine for managing treatment-resistant schizophrenia: a naturalistic study. J Clin Psychopharmacol 2011; 31:240–242.

80. Aziz MA et al. Remission of positive and negative symptoms in refractory schizophrenia with a combination of haloperidol and quetiapine: two case studies. J Psychiatr Pract 2006; 12:332–336.

81. Tharoor H et al. Raloxifene trial in postmenopausal woman with treatment-resistant schizophrenia. Arch Womens Ment Health 2015; 18:741–742.

82. Usall J et al. Raloxifene as an adjunctive treatment for postmenopausal women with schizophrenia: a 24-week double-blind, randomized, parallel, placebo-controlled trial. Schizophr Bull 2016; 42:309–317.

83. Usall J et al. Raloxifene as an adjunctive treatment for postmenopausal women with schizophrenia: a double-blind, randomized, placebo-controlled trial. J Clin Psychiatry 2011; 72:1552–1557.

84. Weiser M et al. Raloxifene plus antipsychotics versus placebo plus antipsychotics in severely ill decompensated postmenopausal women with schizophrenia or schizoaffective disorder: a randomized controlled trial. J Clin Psychiatry 2017; 78:e758–e765.

85. Kulkarni J et al. Effect of adjunctive raloxifene therapy on severity of refractory schizophrenia in women: a randomized clinical trial. JAMA Psychiatry 2016; 73:947–954.

86. Farokhnia M et al. A double-blind, placebo controlled, randomized trial of riluzole as an adjunct to risperidone for treatment of negative symptoms in patients with chronic schizophrenia. Psychopharmacology (Berl) 2014; 231:533–542.

87. Breier AF et al. Clozapine and risperidone in chronic schizophrenia: effects on symptoms, parkinsonian side effects, and neuroendocrine response. Am J Psychiatry 1999; 156:294–298.

88. Bondolfi G et al. Risperidone versus clozapine in treatment-resistant chronic schizophrenia: a randomized double-blind study. The Risperidone Study Group. Am J Psychiatry 1998; 155:499–504.

89. Conley RR et al. Risperidone, quetiapine, and fluphenazine in the treatment of patients with therapy-refractory schizophrenia. Clin Neuropharmacol 2005; 28:163–168.

90. Lerner V et al. Combination of "atypical" antipsychotic medication in the management of treatment-resistant schizophrenia and schizoaffective disorder. Prog Neuropsychopharmacol Biol Psychiatry 2004; 28:89–98.

91. Meltzer HY et al. A six month randomized controlled trial of long acting injectable risperidone 50 and 100 mg in treatment resistant schizophrenia. Schizophr Res 2014; 154:14–22.

92. Akhondzadeh S et al. Effect of ritanserin, a 5HT2A/2C antagonist, on negative symptoms of schizophrenia: a double-blind randomized placebo-controlled study. Prog Neuropsychopharmacol Biol Psychiatry 2008; 32:1879–1883.

93. Lane HY et al. Sarcosine or D-serine add-on treatment for acute exacerbation of schizophrenia: a randomized, double-blind, placebo-controlled study. Arch Gen Psychiatry 2005; 62:1196–1204.

94. Tsai G et al. Glycine transporter I inhibitor, N-methylglycine (sarcosine), added to antipsychotics for the treatment of schizophrenia. Biol Psychiatry 2004; 55:452–456.

95. Kane JM et al. A double-blind, randomized study comparing the efficacy and safety of sertindole and risperidone in patients with treatment-resistant schizophrenia. J Clin Psychiatry 2011; 72:194–204.

96. Nielsen J et al. Augmenting clozapine with sertindole: a double-blind, randomized, placebo-controlled study. J Clin Psychopharmacol 2012; 32:173–178.

97. Tiihonen J et al. Topiramate add-on in treatment-resistant schizophrenia: a randomized, double-blind, placebo-controlled, crossover trial. J Clin Psychiatry 2005; 66:1012–1015.

98. Franck N et al. Left temporoparietal transcranial magnetic stimulation in treatment-resistant schizophrenia with verbal hallucinations. Psychiatry Res 2003; 120:107–109.

99. Fitzgerald PB et al. A double-blind sham-controlled trial of repetitive transcranial magnetic stimulation in the treatment of refractory auditory hallucinations. J Clin Psychopharmacol 2005; 25:358–362.

100. Tuppurainen H et al. Repetitive navigated αTMS in treatment-resistant schizophrenia. Brain Stimulation 2017; 10:397–398.

101. Basan A et al. Valproate as an adjunct to antipsychotics for schizophrenia: a systematic review of randomized trials. Schizophr Res 2004; 70:33–37.

102. Miyaoka T et al. Efficacy and safety of yokukansan in treatment-resistant schizophrenia: a randomized, multicenter, double-blind, placebo-controlled trial. Evid Based Complement Alternat Med 2015; 2015:201592.

103. Lin CC et al. Switching from clozapine to zotepine in patients with schizophrenia: a 12-week prospective, randomized, rater blind, and parallel study. J Clin Psychopharmacol 2013; 33:211–214.

104. Sacchetti E et al. Ziprasidone vs clozapine in schizophrenia patients refractory to multiple antipsychotic treatments: the MOZART study. Schizophr Res 2009; 110:80–89.

105. Loebel AD et al. Ziprasidone in treatment-resistant schizophrenia: a 52-week, open-label continuation study. J Clin Psychiatry 2007; 68:1333–1338.

106. Kane JM et al. Efficacy and tolerability of ziprasidone in patients with treatment-resistant schizophrenia. Int Clin Psychopharmacol 2006; 21:21–28.

107. Goff DC et al. High-dose oral ziprasidone versus conventional dosing in schizophrenia patients with residual symptoms: the ZEBRAS study. J Clin Psychopharmacol 2013; 33:485–490.

Re-starting clozapine after a break in treatment

Re-titration of clozapine is somewhat constrained by the manufacturer's recommendation that re-titration should be the same as initial titration if clozapine has been missed for more than 48 hours. While somewhat arbitrary, this recommendation certainly recognises the dangers of giving clozapine to those who are intolerant of its effects (clozapine has been used in criminal poisonings[1]). However, there is evidence that faster titrations may be safe in both those naïve to clozapine[2] and those re-starting it.[3] It has been suggested that the starting dose of 12.5 mg or 25 mg can be seen as a pharmacological challenge test;[4] where this is well tolerated, rapid titration may be beneficial without an increased risk of problematic adverse effects. Nevertheless, more cautious dosage titration may still be suitable for certain patients, such as elderly patients, people with Parkinson's disease and out-patients starting clozapine who are uncertain about the potential benefits of the medication.[5]

Table 1.42 provides general advice on re-starting clozapine after gaps of various lengths. It takes account of the need to regain antipsychotic activity with clozapine while ensuring safety during titration. The key feature is **flexibility**: the dose prescribed for a patient depends upon their ability to tolerate previous doses.

Table 1.42 Re-starting clozapine

Time since last clozapine dose	Action to re-start
Up to 48 hours	**Re-start at previous dose** – no re-titration required
48–72 hours	**Begin rapid re-titration as soon as possible** On day 1, re-start with half of the previously prescribed total daily dose given in divided doses 12 hours apart. Then give 75% of previous daily dose on day 2 and, if prior doses have been tolerated, the whole of the previous daily dose in the normal dosing schedule on day 3
72 hours to 1 week	**Begin re-titration with 12.5 mg or 25 mg clozapine** Try a second dose 12 hours later if the first is well tolerated. Increase to 'normal' dose according to patient tolerability over at least 3 days
More than 1 week	**Re-titrate as if new patient** Aim to reach previously prescribed dose within 2–4 weeks. Increase according to tolerability

References

1. Shigeev SV et al. [Clozapine intoxication: theoretical aspects and forensic-medical examination]. Sud Med Ekspert 2013; 56:41–46.
2. Poyraz CA et al. Rapid clozapine titration in patients with treatment refractory schizophrenia. Psychiatr Q 2016; 87:315–322.
3. Ifteni P et al. Effectiveness and safety of rapid clozapine titration in schizophrenia. Acta Psychiatr Scand 2014: 130: 25–29.
4. Nielsen J et al. Reply to Comment on 'effectiveness and safety of rapid clozapine titration in schizophrenia' by Schulte P, Dijk D, Cohen D, Bogers J, Bakker B. Acta Psychiatr Scand 2014; 130:69–73.
5. Schulte PFJ et al. Comment on 'effectiveness and safety of rapid clozapine titration in schizophrenia'. Acta Psychiatr Scand 2014; 130:69–70.

Initiation of clozapine for community-based patients

Contraindications to community initiation

- History of seizures, significant cardiac disease, unstable diabetes, paralytic ileus, blood dyscrasia, NMS or other disorder that increases the risk of serious adverse effects (initiation with close monitoring in hospital may still be possible).
- Previous severe adverse effects on titration of clozapine or other antipsychotics.
- Unreliable or chaotic lifestyle that may affect adherence to the medication or the monitoring regimen.
- Significant abuse of alcohol or other drugs likely to increase the risk of adverse effects (e.g. cocaine).

Suitability for community initiation

All the answers should be yes.

- Is the patient likely to be adherent with oral medication and to monitoring requirements?
- Has the patient understood the need for regular physical monitoring and blood tests?
- Has the patient understood the possible adverse effects and what to do about them (particularly the rare but serious ones)?
- Is the patient readily contactable (e.g. in the event of a result that needs follow-up)?
- Is it possible for the patient to be seen every day during the early titration phase?
- Is the patient able to collect medication every week or can medication be delivered to their home?
- Is the patient likely to be able to seek help out of hours if they experience potentially serious adverse effects (e.g. indicators of myocarditis or infection such as fever, malaise, chest pain)?

Initial work-up

To screen for risk factors and provide a baseline:

- physical examination, full blood count, liver function tests, urea and electrolytes (U&Es), lipids, glucose/HbA$_{1C}$. Consider troponin, C-reactive protein (CRP), beta-natriuretic peptide, erythrocyte sedimentation rate (ESR) (as baseline for further tests)
- ECG – particularly to screen for evidence of past myocardial infarction or ventricular abnormality
- echocardiogram if clinically indicated.

Mandatory blood monitoring and registration

- Register with the relevant monitoring service.
- Perform baseline blood tests (white cell count and differential count) before starting clozapine.

- Further blood testing continues weekly for the first 18 weeks and then every 2 weeks for the remainder of the year. After that, the blood monitoring is usually done monthly.
- Inform the patient's GP.

Dosing

Starting clozapine in the community requires a slow and flexible titration schedule. Prior antipsychotics should be slowly discontinued during the titration phase (depots can usually be stopped at the start of titration). Clozapine can cause marked postural hypotension. The initial monitoring is partly aimed at detecting and managing this.

There are two basic methods for starting clozapine in the community. One is to give the first dose in the morning in clinic and then monitor the patient for at least 3 hours. If the dose is well tolerated, the patient is then allowed home with a dose to take before going to bed. This dosing schedule is described in Table 1.43. This is a very cautious schedule: most patients will tolerate faster titration. The second method involves giving the patient the first dose to take immediately before bed, so avoiding the need for close physical monitoring immediately after administration. Subsequent dosing and monitoring is as for the first method. All initiations should take place early in the week (e.g. on a Monday) so that adequate staffing and monitoring are assured.

Adverse effects

Sedation, hypersalivation and hypotension are common at the start of treatment. These effects can usually be managed (see section on 'Clozapine: common adverse effects' in this chapter) but require particular attention in community titration.

The formal carer (usually the Community Psychiatric Nurse) should inform the prescriber if:

- **temperature rises above 38 °C** (this is very common and is not a good reason, on its own, for stopping clozapine)
- **pulse is >100 bpm** (also common and not, on its own, a reason for stopping, but may sometimes be linked to myocarditis)
- **postural drop of >30 mmHg**
- **patient is clearly over-sedated**
- **any signs of constipation**
- **flu-like symptoms (malaise, fatigue, etc.)**
- **chest pain, dyspnoea, tachypnoea**
- **any other adverse effect that is intolerable.**

A doctor should see the patient at least once a week for the first month to assess mental and physical state.

Recommended additional monitoring

Recommended additional monitoring is summarised in Table 1.44.

Consider monitoring plasma troponin, beta-natriuretic peptide and CRP weekly in the first 6 weeks of treatment, particularly where there is any suspicion of myocarditis

Table 1.43 Suggested titration regimen for initiation of clozapine in the community. Note that much faster titrations can be undertaken in many patients where tolerability allows

Day	Day of the week	Morning dose (mg)	Evening dose (mg)	Monitoring	Percentage dose of previous antipsychotic
1	Monday	6.25	6.25	A	100
2	Tuesday	6.25	6.25	A	
3	Wednesday	6.25	6.25	A	
4	Thursday	6.25	12.5	A, B, FBC	
5	Friday	12.5	12.5	A Check results from day 4. Remind patient of out-of-hours arrangements for weekend	
6	Saturday	12.5	12.5	No routine monitoring unless clinically indicated	
7	Sunday	12.5	12.5	No routine monitoring unless clinically indicated	
8	Monday	12.5	25	A	75*
9	Tuesday	12.5	25	A	
10	Wednesday	25	25	A	
11	Thursday	25	37.5	A, B, FBC	
12	Friday	25	37.5	A Check results from day 1. Remind patient of out-of-hours arrangements for weekend	
13	Saturday	25	37.5	No routine monitoring unless clinically indicated	
14	Sunday	25	37.5	No routine monitoring unless clinically indicated	
15	Monday	37.5	37.5	A	50*
16	Tuesday	37.5	37.5	Not seen unless problems	
17	Wednesday	37.5	50	A	
18	Thursday	37.5	50	Not seen unless problems	
19	Friday	50	50	A, B, FBC	
20	Saturday	50	50	No routine monitoring unless clinically indicated	
21	Sunday	50	50	No routine monitoring unless clinically indicated	
22	Monday	50	75	A	25*
23	Tuesday	50	75	Not seen unless problems	
24	Wednesday	75	75	A	

Table 1.43 (Continued)

Day	Day of the week	Morning dose (mg)	Evening dose (mg)	Monitoring	Percentage dose of previous antipsychotic
25	Thursday	75	75	Not seen unless problems	
26	Friday	75	100	A, B, FBC	
27	Saturday	75	100	No routine monitoring unless clinically indicated	
28	Sunday	75	100	No routine monitoring unless clinically indicated	

Further increments should be 25–50 mg/day (generally 25 mg/day) until target dose is reached (use plasma levels). Beware sudden increase in plasma levels due to saturation of first-pass metabolism (watch for increase in sedation/ other adverse effects).

A. Pulse, postural blood pressure, temperature should be taken before the dose and, ideally, between 30 minutes and 6 hours after the dose. Enquire about adverse effects.
B. Mental state, weight, review and actively manage adverse effects (e.g. behavioural advice, slow clozapine titration or reduce dose of other antipsychotic, start adjunctive treatments – see sections on clozapine adverse effects in this chapter). Consider troponin, CRP, beta-natriuretic peptide.
* May need to be adjusted depending on adverse effects and mental state.

Table 1.44 Recommended additional monitoring

Baseline	1 month	3 months	4–6 months	12 months
Weight/BMI/waist	Weight/BMI/waist	Weight/BMI/waist	Weight/BMI/waist	Weight/BMI/waist
Plasma glucose and lipids	Plasma glucose and lipids		Plasma glucose and lipids	Plasma glucose and lipids
LFTs			LFTs	

BMI, body mass index; LFT, liver function test.

(see section on 'Clozapine: serious haematological and cardiovascular adverse effects' in this chapter).

Switching from other antipsychotics

- The switching regimen will be largely dependent on the patient's mental state.
- Consider potential additive adverse effects of antipsychotics (e.g. hypotension, sedation, effect on QTc interval).
- Consider drug interactions (e.g. some SSRIs may increase clozapine levels).
- All depots, sertindole, pimozide and ziprasidone should be stopped before clozapine is started.
- Other antipsychotics and clozapine may be cross-tapered with varying degrees of caution. ECG monitoring is prudent when clozapine is co-prescribed with other drugs known to affect QT interval.

Serious cardiac adverse effects

Patients should be closely observed for signs or symptoms of myocarditis, particularly during the first 2 months, and advised to inform staff if they experience these, and to seek out-of-hours review if necessary. These include persistent tachycardia (although commonly benign), palpitations, shortness of breath, fever, arrhythmia, symptoms mimicking myocardial infarction, chest pain and other unexplained symptoms of heart failure. (See section on 'Clozapine: serious haematological and cardiovascular adverse effects' in this chapter.)

Further reading

Beck K et al. The practical management of refractory schizophrenia – the Maudsley Treatment Review and Assessment Team service approach. Acta Psychiatr Scand 2014; 130:427–438.

Lovett L. Initiation of clozapine treatment at home. Prog Neurol Psychiatry 2004; 8:19–21.

O'Brien A. Starting clozapine in the community: a UK perspective. CNS Drugs 2004; 18:845–852.

CLOZAPINE ADVERSE EFFECTS

Clozapine: common adverse effects

Table 1.45 describes some more common adverse effects of clozapine (no particular frequency implied by order).

Table 1.45 Common adverse effects of clozapine

Adverse effect	Time course	Action
Sedation	First few months, may persist, but usually wears off to some extent	Give smaller dose in the morning Reduce dose if possible
Hypersalivation	First few months, may persist, but sometimes wears off Often very troublesome at night	Give hyoscine 300 μg sucked and swallowed up to three times a day. Many other options (see section on 'Clozapine-induced hypersalivation' in this chapter). Note anticholinergics worsen constipation and cognition
Constipation	First 4 months are the highest risk[1], usually persists	Advise patients of the risks before starting, screen regularly, ensure adequate fibre, fluid and exercise. Bulk-forming laxatives are usually first line, but have a low threshold for adding osmotic and/or stimulant laxatives early. Stop other medicines that may be contributing and reduce clozapine dose if possible. Effective treatment or prevention of constipation is essential as death may result.[1–5] See section on 'Clozapine-induced gastrointestinal hypomotility (CIGH)' in this chapter
Hypotension	First 4 weeks	Advise patient to take time when standing up Reduce dose or slow down rate of increase. Increase fluid intake to 2L daily.[6] If severe, consider moclobemide and Bovril,[7] or fludrocortisone. Over longer term, weight gain may lead to hypertension
Hypertension[8]	First 4 weeks, sometimes longer	Monitor closely and increase dose as slowly as is necessary. Hypotensive therapy is sometimes necessary[9]
Tachycardia	First 4 weeks, but sometimes persists	Very common in early stages of treatment but usually benign. May be dose-related.[10] Tachycardia, if persistent at rest and associated with fever, hypotension or chest pain, may indicate myocarditis[11,12] (see section on 'Clozapine: serious haematological and cardiovascular adverse effects' in this chapter). Referral to a cardiologist is advised. Clozapine should be stopped if tachycardia occurs in the context of chest pain or heart failure. Benign sinus tachycardia can be treated with bisoprolol or atenolol,[13] although evidence base is poor.[14] Ivabradine may be used if hypotension or contraindications limit the use of beta blockers.[15] Note that prolonged tachycardia can itself precipitate cardiomyopathy[16]
Weight gain	Usually during the first year of treatment, but may continue	Dietary counselling is essential. Advice may be more effective if given before weight gain occurs Weight gain is common and often profound (>10 lb). Many treatments available (see section on 'Weight gain' in this chapter)

(Continued)

CHAPTER 1

Table 1.45 (Continued)

Adverse effect	Time course	Action
Fever	First 4 weeks	Clozapine induces inflammatory response (increased CRP and interleukin-6).[17–19] Give paracetamol but check FBC for neutropenia. Reduce rate of dose titration.[20] This fever is not usually related to blood dyscrasias[21,22] but beware myocarditis and NMS
Seizures[23]	May occur at any time[24]	Related to dose, plasma level and rapid dose escalation.[25] Consider prophylactic topiramate, lamotrigine, gabapentin or valproate* if on high dose ($\geq$500 mg/day) or with high plasma level ($\geq$500 µg/L). Some suggest risk of seizures below 1300 µg/L (about 1 in 20 people) is not enough to support primary prophylaxis.[26] After a seizure: withhold clozapine for 1 day; re-start at half previous dose; give anticonvulsant.† EEG abnormalities are common in those on clozapine[27]
Nausea	First 6 weeks	May give anti-emetic. Avoid prochlorperazine and metoclopramide if previous EPS. Avoid domperidone if underlying cardiac risk or QTc prolongation. Ondansetron is a good choice, but it may worsen constipation
Nocturnal enuresis	May occur at any time	Try reducing the dose or manipulating dose schedule to avoid periods of deep sedation. Avoid fluids before bedtime. Consider scheduled night-time toileting. May resolve spontaneously[28] but may persist for months or years.[29] Seems to affect 1 in 5 people on clozapine.[30] In severe cases, desmopressin nasal spray (10–20 µg *nocte*) is usually effective[31] but is not without risk: hyponatraemia may result.[32] Anticholinergic agents may be effective[33] but support for this approach is weak and constipation and sedation may worsen. Ephedrine,[34] pseudoephedrine[35] and aripiprazole[36,37] have also been used
Neutropenia/ agranulocytosis	First 18 weeks (but may occur at any time)	Stop clozapine; admit to hospital if agranulocytosis confirmed
Gastro-oesophageal reflux disease (GORD)[38,39]	Any time	Proton pump inhibitors often prescribed but some are CYP1A2 inducers and possibly increase risk of neutropenia and agranulocytosis.[40,41] Reasons for GORD association unclear – clozapine is an H_2 antagonist[42]
Myoclonus[25,43–45]	During dose titration or plasma level increases	May precede full tonic-clonic seizure. Reduce dose. Anticonvulsants may help, and will reduce the likelihood of progression to seizures. Valproate is first choice; lamotrigine may worsen some types of myoclonus

* Usual dose is 1000–2000 mg/day. Plasma levels may be useful as a rough guide to dosing – aim for 50–100 mg/L. Use of modified-release preparation (Epilim Chrono) may aid compliance: can be given once-daily and may be better tolerated.
† Use valproate if schizoaffective; lamotrigine if poor response to clozapine or continued negative symptoms; topiramate if weight loss required (but beware cognitive adverse effects); gabapentin if other anticonvulsants are poorly tolerated.[25]
CRP, C-reactive protein; EEG, electroencephalogram; EPS, extrapyramidal symptoms; FBC, full blood count; NMS, neuroleptic malignant syndrome.

References

1. Palmer SE et al. Life-threatening clozapine-induced gastrointestinal hypomotility: an analysis of 102 cases. J Clin Psychiatry 2008; 69:759–768.

2. Townsend G et al. Case report: rapidly fatal bowel ischaemia on clozapine treatment. BMC Psychiatry 2006; 6:43.

3. Rege S et al. Life-threatening constipation associated with clozapine. Australas Psychiatry 2008; 16:216–219.

4. Leung JS et al. Rapidly fatal clozapine-induced intestinal obstruction without prior warning signs. Aust N Z J Psychiatry 2008; 42:1073–1074.

5. Flanagan RJ et al. Gastrointestinal hypomotility: an under-recognised life-threatening adverse effect of clozapine. Forensic Sci Int 2011; 206:e31–e36.

6. Ronaldson KJ. Cardiovascular disease in clozapine-treated patients: evidence, mechanisms and management. CNS Drugs 2017;31:777–95.

7. Taylor D et al. Clozapine-induced hypotension treated with moclobemide and Bovril. Br J Psychiatry 1995; 167:409–410.

8. Gonsai NH et al. Effects of dopamine receptor antagonist antipsychotic therapy on blood pressure. J Clin Pharm Ther 2018; 43:1–7.

9. Henderson DC et al. Clozapine and hypertension: a chart review of 82 patients. J Clin Psychiatry 2004; 65:686–689.

10. Nilsson BM et al. Tachycardia in patients treated with clozapine versus antipsychotic long-acting injections. Int Clin Psychopharmacol 2017; 32:219–224.

11. Committee on Safety of Medicines, and Medicines Control Agency. Clozapine and cardiac safety: updated advice for prescribers. Current Problems in Pharmacovigilance 2002; 28:8.

12. Hagg S et al. Myocarditis related to clozapine treatment. J Clin Psychopharmacol 2001; 21:382–388.

13. Stryjer R et al. Beta-adrenergic antagonists for the treatment of clozapine-induced sinus tachycardia: a retrospective study. Clin Neuropharmacol 2009; 32:290–292.

14. Lally J et al. Pharmacological interventions for clozapine-induced sinus tachycardia. Cochrane Database Syst Rev 2016; CD011566.

15. Lally J et al. Ivabradine, a novel treatment for clozapine-induced sinus tachycardia: a case series. Ther Adv Psychopharmacol 2014; 4:117–122.

16. Shinbane JS et al. Tachycardia-induced cardiomyopathy: a review of animal models and clinical studies. J Am Coll Cardiol 1997; 29:709–715.

17. Kohen I et al. Increases in C-reactive protein may predict recurrence of clozapine-induced fever. Ann Pharmacother 2009; 43:143–146.

18. Kluge M et al. Effects of clozapine and olanzapine on cytokine systems are closely linked to weight gain and drug-induced fever. Psychoneuroendocrinology 2009; 34:118–128.

19. Hung YP et al. Role of cytokine changes in clozapine-induced fever: a cohort prospective study. Psychiatry Clin Neurosci 2017; 71:395–402.

20. Pui-yin Chung J et al. The incidence and characteristics of clozapine- induced fever in a local psychiatric unit in Hong Kong. Can J Psychiatry 2008; 53:857–862.

21. Tham JC et al. Clozapine-induced fevers and 1-year clozapine discontinuation rate. J Clin Psychiatry 2002; 63:880–884.

22. Tremeau F et al. Spiking fevers with clozapine treatment. Clin Neuropharmacol 1997; 20:168–170.

23. Grover S et al. Association of clozapine with seizures: a brief report involving 222 patients prescribed clozapine. East Asian Arch Psychiatry 2015; 25:73–78.

24. Pacia SV et al. Clozapine-related seizures: experience with 5,629 patients. Neurology 1994; 44:2247–2249.

25. Varma S et al. Clozapine-related EEG changes and seizures: dose and plasma-level relationships. Ther Adv Psychopharmacol 2011; 1:47–66.

26. Caetano D. Use of anticonvulsants as prophylaxis for seizures in patients on clozapine. Australas Psychiatry 2014; 22:78–83.

27. Centorrino F et al. EEG abnormalities during treatment with typical and atypical antipsychotics. Am J Psychiatry 2002; 159:109–115.

28. Warner JP et al. Clozapine and urinary incontinence. Int Clin Psychopharmacol 1994; 9:207–209.

29. Jeong SH et al. A 2-year prospective follow-up study of lower urinary tract symptoms in patients treated with clozapine. J Clin Psychopharmacol 2008; 28:618–624.

30. Harrison-Woolrych M et al. Nocturnal enuresis in patients taking clozapine, risperidone, olanzapine and quetiapine: comparative cohort study. Br J Psychiatry 2011; 199:140–144.

31. Steingard S. Use of desmopressin to treat clozapine-induced nocturnal enuresis. J Clin Psychiatry 1994; 55:315–316.

32. Sarma S et al. Severe hyponatraemia associated with desmopressin nasal spray to treat clozapine-induced nocturnal enuresis. Aust N Z J Psychiatry 2005; 39:949.

33. Praharaj SK et al. Amitriptyline for clozapine-induced nocturnal enuresis and sialorrhoea. Br J Clin Pharmacol 2007; 63:128–129.

34. Fuller MA et al. Clozapine-induced urinary incontinence: incidence and treatment with ephedrine. J Clin Psychiatry 1996; 57:514–518.

35. Hanes A et al. Pseudoephedrine for the treatment of clozapine-induced incontinence. Innov Clin Neurosci 2013; 10:33–35.

36. Palaniappan P. Aripiprazole as a treatment option for clozapine-induced enuresis. Indian J Pharmacol 2015; 47:574–575.

37. Lee MJ et al. Use of aripiprazole in clozapine induced enuresis: report of two cases. J Korean Med Sci 2010; 25:333–335.

38. Taylor D et al. Use of antacid medication in patients receiving clozapine: a comparison with other second-generation antipsychotics. J Clin Psychopharmacol 2010; 30:460–461.

39. Van Veggel M et al. Clozapine and gastro-oesophageal reflux disease (GORD) – an investigation of temporal association. Acta Psychiatr Scand 2013; 127:69–77.

40. Wicinski M et al. Potential mechanisms of hematological adverse drug reactions in patients receiving clozapine in combination with proton pump inhibitors. J Psychiatr Pract 2017; 23:114–120.

41. Shuman MD et al. Exploring the potential effect of polypharmacy on the hematologic profiles of clozapine patients. J Psychiatr Pract 2014; 20:50–58.

42. Humbert-Claude M et al. Involvement of histamine receptors in the atypical antipsychotic profile of clozapine: a reassessment in vitro and in vivo. Psychopharmacology (Berl) 2011; 220:225–241.

43. Osborne IJ et al. Clozapine-induced myoclonus: a case report and review of the literature. Ther Adv Psychopharmacol 2015; 5:351–356.

44. Praharaj SK et al. Clozapine-induced myoclonus: a case study and brief review. Prog Neuropsychopharmacol Biol Psychiatry 2010; 34:242–243.

45. Sajatovic M et al. Clozapine-induced myoclonus and generalized seizures. Biol Psychiatry 1996; 39:367–370.

Further reading

Iqbal MM et al. Clozapine: a clinical review of adverse effects and management. Ann Clin Psychiatry 2003; 15:33–48.

Lieberman JA. Maximizing clozapine therapy: managing side effects. J Clin Psychiatry 1998; 59 (Suppl. 3):38–43.

Sagy R et al. Pharmacological and behavioral management of some often-overlooked clozapine-induced side effects. Int Clin Psychopharmacol 2014; 29:313–317.

Clozapine: uncommon or unusual adverse effects

Table 1.46 gives brief details (in alphabetical order) of unusual or uncommon adverse effects of clozapine.

Table 1.46 Uncommon or unusual adverse effects of clozapine

Adverse effect	Time course	Comment
Agranulocytosis/ neutropenia (delayed)[1–3]	Usually first 3 months but may occur at any time	Occasional reports of apparent clozapine-related blood dyscrasia even after 1 year of treatment. Risk may be elevated for up to 9 years.[4] It is possible that clozapine is not the causative agent in some cases.[5,6] See section on 'Clozapine: serious haematological and cardiovascular adverse effects' in this chapter
Colitis[7–11]	Any time	A few reports in the literature, but clear causative link to clozapine not determined. Any severe or chronic diarrhoea should prompt specialist referral as there is a substantial risk of death. Anticholinergic use probably increases risk of colitis and necrosis[12]
Delirium[13–15]	Any time	Reported to be fairly common, but rarely seen in practice if dose is titrated slowly and plasma level determinations are used
Eosinophilia[16–18]	First 4 weeks[19]	Reasonably common but significance unclear. Some suggestion that eosinophilia predicts neutropenia but this is disputed. May be associated with colitis and related symptoms.[20] Occasional reports linking eosinophilia with myocarditis[21] and interstitial nephritis.[22] Usually benign but investigate for signs of other organ damage.[23] Successful re-challenge in the absence of organ inflammation is possible.[24] Concomitant antidepressants may increase risk[25]
Heat stroke[26,27]	Any time	Occasional case reported. May be mistaken for NMS
Hepatic failure/enzyme abnormalities[28–34]	First few months	Benign changes in LFTs are common (up to 50% of patients) but worth monitoring because of the very small risk of fulminant hepatic failure.[35] Rash may be associated with clozapine-related hepatitis[36]
Interstitial nephritis[22,37–44]	Usually first 2 weeks, possibly up to 3 months[45]	A handful of reports implicating clozapine. Immune-mediated; may occur after only a few doses. Symptoms may include fever, skin rash and eosinophilia
Ocular effects	Any time	Single case report of ocular pigmentation.[46] Clozapine may cause dry eye syndrome[47]
Pancreatitis[48–55]	Usually first 6 weeks, possibly later in treatment[56]	Several reports of asymptomatic and symptomatic pancreatitis sometimes associated with eosinophilia. Some authors recommend monitoring serum amylase in all patients treated with clozapine. No cases of successful re-challenge after pancreatitis[51,57–59]
Parotid gland swelling[60–66]	Usually first few weeks, but may occur later[67]	Several case reports. Unclear mechanism, possibly immunological or thickening of saliva leading to calcium precipitation. May be recurrent. May resolve spontaneously.[68] Treatment of hypersalivation with terazosin in combination with benzatropine may be helpful
Pericardial effusion[69–75]	Any time	Several reports in the literature. Symptoms include fatigue, chest pain, dyspnoea and tachycardia, but may be asymptomatic.[76] Signs include raised inflammatory markers (specifically trop I) and proBNP levels. Use echocardiogram to confirm/rule out effusion. Successful re-challenge possible[77]

(Continued)

Table 1.46 *(Continued)*

Adverse effect	Time course	Comment
Pneumonia[78-85]	Usually early in treatment, but may be any time	May result from saliva aspiration (this may be why pneumonia sometimes appears to be dose-related[86,87]), very rarely constipation.[88] Pneumonia is a common cause of death in people on clozapine.[79] Infections in general may be more common in those on clozapine[89] and use of antibiotics is also increased.[90] Note that respiratory infections may give rise to elevated clozapine levels[91-94] (possibly an artefact: smoking usually ceases during an infection). Clozapine is often successfully continued after the pneumonia has resolved, but recurrence may be more likely[95-97]
Stuttering[98-106]	Any time	Case reports. May be a result of EPS or epileptiform activity. Check plasma levels, consider dose reduction and/or anticonvulsant – may be a warning sign for impending generalised seizures[107]
Thrombocytopenia[108-111]	First 3 months	Few data but apparently fairly common (incidence over 1 year of 3%[112]). Probably transient and clinically unimportant, but persistent in some cases.[113,114] Thrombocytosis also reported[115]
Skin reactions[116]	Any time	Presence of skin diseases in general is higher in those with schizophrenia.[117] Two reports of vasculitis[118,119] in which patients developed confluent erythematous rash on lower limbs. One report of Stevens–Johnson syndrome,[120] two reports of pityriasis rosea,[121,122] one report of a papular rash,[123] one report of exanthematic pustulosis[124] and one fatal case of Sweet's syndrome[125]
Thromboembolism[126-130]	Any time	Weight increase and sedation may contribute to risk of thromboembolism, but other mechanisms including increased platelet aggregation via 5-HT$_{2A}$ receptor activation may also be responsible.[131] Hyperprolactinaemia also increases the risk. Clozapine appears to increase risk of pulmonary thromboembolism by 28 times.[132] Threshold for prophylactic antithrombotic treatment where additional risk factors are present (surgery, immobility) should probably be low. Continuation of therapy after embolism may be possible[133] but consult haematologist as without prophylactic antithrombotic treatment recurrence is likely[134,135]

BNP, beta-natriuretic peptide; EPS, extrapyramidal symptoms; LFT, liver function test; NMS, neuroleptic malignant syndrome.

References

1. Thompson A et al. Late onset neutropenia with clozapine. Can J Psychiatry 2004; 49:647–648.
2. Bhanji NH et al. Late-onset agranulocytosis in a patient with schizophrenia after 17 months of clozapine treatment. J Clin Psychopharmacol 2003; 23:522–523.
3. Sedky K et al. Clozapine-induced agranulocytosis after 11 years of treatment (Letter). Am J Psychiatry 2005; 162:814.
4. Kang BJ et al. Long-term patient monitoring for clozapine-induced agranulocytosis and neutropenia in Korea: when is it safe to discontinue CPMS? Hum Psychopharmacol 2006; 21:387–391.
5. Panesar N et al. Late onset neutropenia with clozapine. Aust N Z J Psychiatry 2011; 45:684.
6. Tourian L et al. Late-onset agranulocytosis in a patient treated with clozapine and lamotrigine. J Clin Psychopharmacol 2011; 31:665–667.
7. Hawe R et al. Response to clozapine-induced microscopic colitis: a case report and review of the literature. J Clin Psychopharmacol 2008; 28:454–455.
8. Shah V et al. Clozapine-induced ischaemic colitis. BMJ Case Rep 2013; 2013.

9. Linsley KR et al. Clozapine-associated colitis: case report and review of the literature. J Clin Psychopharmacol 2012; 32:564–566.

10. Baptista T. A fatal case of ischemic colitis during clozapine administration. Rev Bras Psiquiatr 2014; 36:358.

11. Rodriguez-Sosa JT et al. Apropos of a case: relationship of ischemic colitis with clozapine. Actas Esp Psiquiatr 2014; 42:325–326.

12. Peyriere H et al. Antipsychotics-induced ischaemic colitis and gastrointestinal necrosis: a review of the French pharmacovigilance database. Pharmacoepidemiol Drug Saf 2009; 18:948–955.

13. Centorrino F et al. Delirium during clozapine treatment: incidence and associated risk factors. Pharmacopsychiatry 2003; 36:156–160.

14. Shankar BR. Clozapine-induced delirium. J Neuropsychiatry Clin Neurosci 2008; 20:239–240.

15. Khanra S et al. An unusual case of delirium after restarting clozapine. Clin Psychopharmacol Neurosci 2016; 14:107–108.

16. Hummer M et al. Does eosinophilia predict clozapine induced neutropenia? Psychopharmacology (Berl) 1996; 124:201–204.

17. Ames D et al. Predictive value of eosinophilia for neutropenia during clozapine treatment. J Clin Psychiatry 1996; 57:579–581.

18. Wysokinski A et al. Rapidly developing and self-limiting eosinophilia associated with clozapine. Psychiatry Clin Neurosci 2015; 69:122.

19. Aneja J et al. Eosinophilia induced by clozapine: a report of two cases and review of the literature. J Family Med Prim Care 2015; 4:127–129.

20. Karmacharya R et al. Clozapine-induced eosinophilic colitis (letter). Am J Psychiatry 2005; 162:1386–1387.

21. Chatterton R. Eosinophilia after commencement of clozapine treatment. Aust N Z J Psychiatry 1997; 31:874–876.

22. Chan SY et al. Clozapine-induced acute interstitial nephritis. Hong Kong Med J 2015; 21:372–374.

23. Marchel D et al. Multiorgan eosinophilic infiltration after initiation of clozapine therapy: a case report. BMC Res Notes 2017; 10:316.

24. McArdle PA et al. Successful rechallenge with clozapine after treatment associated eosinophilia. Australas Psychiatry 2016; 24:365–367.

25. Fabrazzo M et al. Clozapine versus other antipsychotics during the first 18 weeks of treatment: a retrospective study on risk factor increase of blood dyscrasias. Psychiatry Res 2017; 256:275–282.

26. Kerwin RW et al. Heat stroke in schizophrenia during clozapine treatment: rapid recognition and management. J Psychopharmacol 2004; 18:121–123.

27. Hoffmann MS et al. Heat stroke during long-term clozapine treatment: should we be concerned about hot weather? Trends Psychiatry Psychother 2016; 38:56–59.

28. Erdogan A et al. Management of marked liver enzyme increase during clozapine treatment: a case report and review of the literature. Int J Psychiatry Med 2004; 34:83–89.

29. Macfarlane B et al. Fatal acute fulminant liver failure due to clozapine: a case report and review of clozapine-induced hepatotoxicity. Gastroenterology 1997; 112:1707–1709.

30. Chang A et al. Clozapine-induced fatal fulminant hepatic failure: a case report. Can J Gastroenterol 2009; 23:376–378.

31. Chaplin AC et al. Re: Recent case report of clozapine-induced acute hepatic failure. Can J Gastroenterol 2010; 24:739–740.

32. Wu Chou AI et al. Hepatotoxicity induced by clozapine: a case report and review of literature. Neuropsychiatr Dis Treat 2014; 10:1585–1587.

33. Kane JP et al. Clozapine-induced liver injury and pleural effusion. Mental Illness 2014; 6:5403.

34. Douros A et al. Drug-induced liver injury: results from the hospital-based Berlin Case-Control Surveillance Study. Br J Clin Pharmacol 2015; 79:988–999.

35. Tucker P. Liver toxicity with clozapine. Aust N Z J Psychiatry 2013; 47:975–976.

36. Fong SY et al. Clozapine-induced toxic hepatitis with skin rash. J Psychopharmacol 2005; 19:107.

37. Hunter R et al. Clozapine-induced interstitial nephritis – a rare but important complication: a case report. J Med Case Rep 2009; 3:8574.

38. Elias TJ et al. Clozapine-induced acute interstitial nephritis. Lancet 1999; 354:1180–1181.

39. Parekh R et al. Clozapine induced tubulointerstitial nephritis in a patient with paranoid schizophrenia. BMJ Case Rep 2014; 2014.

40. An NY et al. A case of clozapine induced acute renal failure. Psychiatry Investig 2013; 10:92–94.

41. Kanofsky JD et al. A case of acute renal failure in a patient recently treated with clozapine and a review of previously reported cases. Prim Care Companion CNS Disord 2011; 13.

42. Au AF et al. Clozapine-induced acute interstitial nephritis. Am J Psychiatry 2004; 161:1501.

43. Southall KE A case of interstitial nephritis on clozapine. Aust N Z J Psychiatry 2000; 34:697–698.

44. Fraser D et al. An unexpected and serious complication of treatment with the atypical antipsychotic drug clozapine. Clin Nephrol 2000; 54:78–80.

45. Mohan T et al. Clozapine-induced nephritis and monitoring implications. Aust N Z J Psychiatry 2013; 47:586–587.

46. Borovik AM et al. Ocular pigmentation associated with clozapine. Med J Aust 2009; 190:210–211.

47. Ceylan E et al. The ocular surface side effects of an anti-psychotic drug, clozapine. Cutan Ocul Toxicol 2016; 35:62–66.

48. Bergemann N et al. Asymptomatic pancreatitis associated with clozapine. Pharmacopsychiatry 1999; 32:78–80.

49. Raja M et al. A case of clozapine-associated pancreatitis. Open Neuropsychopharmacol J 2011; 4:5–7.

50. Bayard JM et al. Case report: acute pancreatitis induced by clozapine. Acta Gastroenterol Belg 2005; 68:92–94.

51. Sani G et al. Development of asymptomatic pancreatitis with paradoxically high serum clozapine levels in a patient with schizophrenia and the CYP1A2*1F/1F genotype. J Clin Psychopharmacol 2010; 30:737–739.

52. Wehmeier PM et al. Pancreatitis followed by pericardial effusion in an adolescent treated with clozapine. J Clin Psychopharmacol 2003; 23:102–103.

53. Garlipp P et al. The development of a clinical syndrome of asymptomatic pancreatitis and eosinophilia after treatment with clozapine in schizophrenia: implications for clinical care, recognition and management. J Psychopharmacol 2002; 16:399–400.

54. Gatto EM et al. Clozapine and pancreatitis. Clin Neuropharmacol 1998; 21:203.

55. Martin A. Acute pancreatitis associated with clozapine use. Am J Psychiatry 1992; 149:714.

56. Cerulli TR. Clozapine-associated pancreatitis. Harv Rev Psychiatry 1999; 7:61–63.
57. Huang YJ et al. Recurrent pancreatitis without eosinophilia on clozapine rechallenge. Prog Neuropsychopharmacol Biol Psychiatry 2009; 33:1561–1562.
58. Chengappa KN et al. Recurrent pancreatitis on clozapine re-challenge. J Psychopharmacol 1995; 9:381–382.
59. Frankenburg FR et al. Eosinophilia, clozapine, and pancreatitis. Lancet 1992; 340:251.
60. Immadisetty V et al. A successful treatment strategy for clozapine-induced parotid swelling: a clinical case and systematic review. Ther Adv Psychopharmacol 2012; 2:235–239.
61. Gouzien C et al. [Clozapine-induced parotitis: a case study]. Encephale 2014; 40:81–85.
62. Saguem BN et al. Eosinophilia and parotitis occurring early in clozapine treatment. Int J Clin Pharm 2015; 37:992–995.
63. Vohra A. Clozapine-induced recurrent and transient parotid gland swelling. Afr J Psychiatry (Johannesbg) 2013; 16:236–238.
64. Acosta-Armas AJ. Two cases of parotid gland swelling in patients taking clozapine. Hosp Med 2001; 62:704–705.
65. Patkar AA et al. Parotid gland swelling with clozapine. J Clin Psychiatry 1996; 57:488.
66. Kathirvel N et al. Recurrent transient parotid gland swelling with clozapine therapy. Ir J Psychol Med 2014; 25:69–70.
67. Brodkin ES et al. Treatment of clozapine-induced parotid gland swelling. Am J Psychiatry 1996; 153:445.
68. Vasile JS et al. Clozapine and the development of salivary gland swelling: a case study. J Clin Psychiatry 1995; 56:511–513.
69. Raju P et al. Pericardial effusion in patients with schizophrenia: are they on clozapine? Emerg Med J 2008; 25:383–384.
70. Dauner DG et al. Clozapine-induced pericardial effusion. J Clin Psychopharmacol 2008; 28:455–456.
71. Markovic J et al. Clozapine-induced pericarditis. Afr J Psychiatry (Johannesbg) 2011; 14:236–238.
72. Bhatti MA et al. Clozapine-induced pericarditis, pericardial tamponade, polyserositis, and rash. J Clin Psychiatry 2005; 66:1490–1491.
73. Boot E et al. Pericardial and bilateral pleural effusion associated with clozapine treatment. Eur Psychiatry 2004; 19:65.
74. Murko A et al. Clozapine and pericarditis with pericardial effusion. Am J Psychiatry 2002; 159:494.
75. Paul I et al. Clozapine-induced pericarditis: an overlooked adverse effect. Clin Schizophr Relat Psychoses 2014; 8:133–134.
76. Prisco V et al. Brain natriuretic peptide as a biomarker of asymptomatic clozapine-related heart dysfunction: a criterion for a more cautious administration. Clin Schizophr Relat Psychoses 2016; [Epub ahead of print]
77. Crews MP et al. Clozapine rechallenge following clozapine-induced pericarditis. J Clin Psychiatry 2010; 71:959–961.
78. Hinkes R et al. Aspiration pneumonia possibly secondary to clozapine-induced sialorrhea. J Clin Psychopharmacol 1996; 16:462–463.
79. Taylor DM et al. Reasons for discontinuing clozapine: matched, case-control comparison with risperidone long-acting injection. Br J Psychiatry 2009; 194:165–167.
80. Stoecker ZR et al. Clozapine usage increases the incidence of pneumonia compared with risperidone and the general population: a retrospective comparison of clozapine, risperidone, and the general population in a single hospital over 25 months. Int Clin Psychopharmacol 2017; 32:155–160.
81. Kaplan J et al. Clozapine-associated aspiration pneumonia: case series and review of the literature. Psychosomatics 2017; doi: 10.1016/j.psym.2017.08.011. [Epub ahead of print]
82. Gurrera RJ et al. Aspiration pneumonia: an underappreciated risk of clozapine treatment. J Clin Psychopharmacol 2016; 36:174–176.
83. Aldridge G et al. Clozapine-induced pneumonitis. Aust N Z J Psychiatry 2013; 47:1215–1216.
84. Saenger RC et al. Aspiration pneumonia due to clozapine-induced sialorrhea. Clin Schizophr Relat Psychoses 2016; 9:170–172.
85. Patel SS et al. Physical complications in early clozapine treatment: a case report and implications for safe monitoring. Ther Adv Psychopharmacol 2011; 1:25–29.
86. Trigoboff E et al. Sialorrhea and aspiration pneumonia: a case study. Innov Clin Neurosci 2013; 10:20–27.
87. Kuo CJ et al. Second-generation antipsychotic medications and risk of pneumonia in schizophrenia. Schizophr Bull 2013; 39:648–657.
88. Galappathie N et al. Clozapine-associated pneumonia and respiratory arrest secondary to severe constipation. Med Sci Law 2014; 54:105–109.
89. Landry P et al. Increased use of antibiotics in clozapine-treated patients. Int Clin Psychopharmacol 2003; 18:297–298.
90. Nielsen J et al. Increased use of antibiotics in patients treated with clozapine. Eur Neuropsychopharmacol 2009; 19:483–486.
91. Raaska K et al. Bacterial pneumonia can increase serum concentration of clozapine. Eur J Clin Pharmacol 2002; 58:321–322.
92. de Leon J et al. Serious respiratory infections can increase clozapine levels and contribute to side effects: a case report. Prog Neuropsychopharmacol Biol Psychiatry 2003; 27:1059–1063.
93. Ruan CJ et al. Pneumonia can cause clozapine intoxication: a case report. Psychosomatics 2017; 58:652–656.
94. Leung JG et al. Necrotizing pneumonia in the setting of elevated clozapine levels. J Clin Psychopharmacol 2016; 36:176–178.
95. Hung GC et al. Antipsychotic reexposure and recurrent pneumonia in schizophrenia: a nested case-control study. J Clin Psychiatry 2016; 77:60–66.
96. Galappathie N et al. Clozapine re-trial in a patient with repeated life threatening pneumonias. Acta Biomed 2014; 85:175–179.
97. Schmidinger S et al. Pulmonary embolism and aspiration pneumonia after reexposure to clozapine: pulmonary adverse effects of clozapine. J Clin Psychopharmacol 2014; 34:385–387.
98. Kumar T et al. Dose dependent stuttering with clozapine: a case report. Asian J Psychiatr 2013; 6:178–179.
99. Grover S et al. Clozapine-induced stuttering: a case report and analysis of similar case reports in the literature. Gen Hosp Psychiatry 2012; 34:703–703.
100. Murphy R et al. Clozapine-induced stuttering: an estimate of prevalence in the west of Ireland. Ther Adv Psychopharmacol 2015; 5:232–236.
101. Rachamallu V et al. Clozapine-induced microseizures, orofacial dyskinesia, and speech dysfluency in an adolescent with treatment resistant early onset schizophrenia on concurrent lithium therapy. Case Rep Psychiatry 2017; 2017:7359095.

CHAPTER 1

102. Krishnakanth M et al. Clozapine-induced stuttering: a case series. Prim Care Companion J Clin Psychiatry 2008; **10**:333–334.

103. Begum M. Clozapine-induced stuttering, facial tics and myoclonic seizures: a case report. Aust N Z J Psychiatry 2005; **39**:202.

104. Bar KJ et al. Olanzapine- and clozapine-induced stuttering. A case series. Pharmacopsychiatry 2004; **37**:131–134.

105. Ebeling TA et al. Clozapine-induced stuttering. Am J Psychiatry 1997; **154**:1473.

106. Thomas P et al. Dose-dependent stuttering and dystonia in a patient taking clozapine. Am J Psychiatry 1994; **151**:1096a.

107. Duggal HS et al. Clozapine-induced stuttering and seizures. Am J Psychiatry 2002; **159**:315.

108. Jagadheesan K et al. Clozapine-induced thrombocytopenia: a pilot study. Hong Kong J Psychiatry 2003; **13**:12–15.

109. Mihaljevic-Peles A et al. Thrombocytopenia associated with clozapine and fluphenazine. Nord J Psychiatry 2001; **55**:449–450.

110. Rudolf J et al. Clozapine-induced agranulocytosis and thrombopenia in a patient with dopaminergic psychosis. J Neural Transm (Vienna) 1997; **104**:1305–1311.

111. Assion HJ et al. Lymphocytopenia and thrombocytopenia during treatment with risperidone or clozapine. Pharmacopsychiatry 1996; **29**:227–228.

112. Lee J et al. The effect of clozapine on hematological indices: a 1-year follow-up study. J Clin Psychopharmacol 2015; **35**:510–516.

113. Kate N et al. Clozapine associated thrombocytopenia. J Pharmacol Pharmacother 2013; **4**:149–151.

114. Gonzales MF et al. Evidence for immune etiology in clozapine-induced thrombocytopenia of 40 months' duration: a case report. CNS Spectr 2000; **5**:17–18.

115. Hampson ME. Clozapine-induced thrombocytosis. Br J Psychiatry 2000; **176**:400.

116. Warnock JK et al. Adverse cutaneous reactions to antipsychotics. Am J Clin Dermatol 2002; **3**:629–636.

117. Wu BY et al. Prevalence and associated factors of comorbid skin diseases in patients with schizophrenia: a clinical survey and national health database study. Gen Hosp Psychiatry 2014; **36**:415–421.

118. Voulgari C et al. Clozapine-induced late agranulocytosis and severe neutropenia complicated with streptococcus pneumonia, venous thromboembolism, and allergic vasculitis in treatment-resistant female psychosis. Case Rep Med 2015; **2015**:703218.

119. Penaskovic K et al. Clozapine-induced allergic vasculitis (letter). Am J Psychiatry 2005; **162**:1543–1542.

120. Wu MK et al. The severe complication of Stevens-Johnson syndrome induced by long-term clozapine treatment in a male schizophrenia patient: a case report. Neuropsychiatr Dis Treat 2015; **11**:1039–1041.

121. Lai YW et al. Pityriasis rosea-like eruption associated with clozapine: a case report. Gen Hosp Psychiatry 2012; **34**:703.e705–707.

122. Bhatia MS et al. Clozapine induced pityriasiform eruption. Indian J Dermatol 1997; **42**:245–246.

123. Stanislav SW et al. Papular rash and bilateral pleural effusion associated with clozapine. Ann Pharmacother 1999; **33**:1008–1009.

124. Bosonnet S et al. [Acute generalized exanthematic pustulosis after intake of clozapine (leponex). First case. Ann Dermatol Venereol 1997; **124**:547–548.

125. Kleinen JM et al. [Clozapine-induced agranulocytosis and Sweet's syndrome in a 74-year-old female patient. A case study]. Tijdschr Psychiatr 2008; **50**:119–123.

126. Chate S et al. Pulmonary thromboembolism associated with clozapine. J Neuropsychiatry Clin Neurosci 2013; **25**:E3–6.

127. Srinivasaraju R et al. Clozapine-associated cerebral venous thrombosis. J Clin Psychopharmacol 2010; **30**:335–336.

128. Werring D et al. Cerebral venous sinus thrombosis may be associated with clozapine. J Neuropsychiatry Clin Neurosci 2009; **21**:343–345.

129. Paciullo CA. Evaluating the association between clozapine and venous thromboembolism. Am J Health Syst Pharm 2008; **65**:1825–1829.

130. Yang TY et al. Massive pulmonary embolism in a young patient on clozapine therapy. J Emerg Med 2004; **27**:27–29.

131. Hagg S et al. Risk of venous thromboembolism due to antipsychotic drug therapy. Expert Opin Drug Saf 2009; **8**:537–547.

132. De Fazio P et al. Rare and very rare adverse effects of clozapine. Neuropsychiatr Dis Treat 2015; **11**:1995–2003.

133. Goh JG et al. A case report of clozapine continuation after pulmonary embolism in the context of other risk factors for thromboembolism. Aust N Z J Psychiatry 2016; **50**:1205–1206.

134. Munoli RN et al. Clozapine-induced recurrent pulmonary thromboembolism. J Neuropsychiatry Clin Neurosci 2013; **25**:E50–E51.

135. Selten JP et al. Clozapine and venous thromboembolism: further evidence. J Clin Psychiatry 2003; **64**:609.

Clozapine: serious haematological and cardiovascular adverse effects

Agranulocytosis, thromboembolism, cardiomyopathy and myocarditis

Clozapine is a somewhat toxic drug, but it may reduce overall mortality in schizophrenia, largely because of a reduction in the rate of suicide.[1,2] Clozapine can cause serious, life-threatening adverse effects, of which **agranulocytosis** is the best known. Early US data suggested a mortality rate of 12 in 99,502 (0.012%).[3] Risk is clearly well managed by the approved clozapine monitoring systems.

Thromboembolism

A possible association between clozapine and **thromboembolism** has been suggested.[4] Initially, Walker et al.[1] uncovered a risk of fatal pulmonary embolism of 1 in 4500 – about 20 times the risk in the population as a whole. Following a case report of non-fatal pulmonary embolism possibly related to clozapine,[5] data from the Swedish authorities were published.[6] Twelve cases of venous thromboembolism were described, of which five were fatal. The risk of thromboembolism was estimated to be 1 in 2000 to 1 in 6000 patients treated. Thromboembolism may be related to clozapine's observed effects on antiphospholipid antibodies[7] and platelet aggregation.[8] It seems most likely to occur in the first 3 months of treatment but can occur at any time. Other antipsychotic drugs are also strongly linked to thromboembolism[9–15] although clozapine appears to have the most reports.[16]

With all drugs, the causes of thromboembolism are probably multifactorial.[10] Sedation may lead to a reduction in movement and consequent venous stasis. Obesity, hyperprolactinaemia and smoking are additional independent risk factors for thromboembolism.[17,18] Encouraging exercise and ensuring good hydration are essential precautionary measures.[19]

Myocarditis and cardiomyopathy

Clozapine is associated with **myocarditis** and **cardiomyopathy**. Myocarditis is a hypersensitivity response to clozapine, resulting in inflammation of the myocardium. Some debate surrounds the prevalence of myocarditis, with several Australian studies finding it to occur in around 3% of patients.[20–22] Studies conducted elsewhere[23–25] have suggested a much lower incidence of 1% or less. The reason for such variation in reported incidence is unclear; some authors propose that a lack of robust monitoring leads to missed diagnoses in those countries reporting lower incidences.[26] Myocarditis is potentially fatal, and is most likely to occur in the first 6–8 weeks of starting clozapine treatment (median 3 weeks),[27] but may occur at any time.

Cardiomyopathy is usually diagnosed from echocardiography to establish left ventricular dilatation (resulting in a reduced ejection fraction) and/or hypertrophy. It may develop following myocarditis (if clozapine is not stopped), but other causative factors may include persistent tachycardia, obesity, diabetes, and previous personal or familial cardiac events.[26] Most incidence data originate from Australia and rates range from 0.02% to 5%.[22,28] Cardiomyopathy may occur later in treatment than myocarditis (median 9 months),[27] but as with myocarditis it may occur at any time.

Despite uncertainty over incidence, patients should be closely monitored for signs of myocarditis, especially in the first few months of treatment.[29] Symptoms include hypotension, tachycardia, fever, flu-like symptoms, fatigue, dyspnoea (with increased respiratory rate) and chest pain.[30] Signs include ECG changes (ST depression), enlarged heart on radiography/echocardiography and eosinophilia. Many of these symptoms occur in patients on clozapine not developing myocarditis[31] and, conversely, their absence does not rule out myocarditis.[32] Nonetheless, signs of heart failure should provoke immediate cessation of clozapine and referral to a cardiologist. Re-challenge has been successfully completed[33,34] (the use of beta blockers and angiotensin-converting enzyme [ACE] inhibitors may help[35,36]) but recurrence is also possible.[37–40] Use of echocardiography and measurement of CRP and troponin are essential in cases of re-challenge.[41–43]

Autopsy findings suggest that fatal myocarditis can occur in the absence of clear cardiac symptoms, although tachycardia and fever are usually present.[44] A group from Melbourne, Australia, has put forward a monitoring programme which is said to detect 100% of symptomatic cases of myocarditis[45] using measurement of troponin I or T and C-reactive protein (see Table 1.47). Echocardiography at baseline, 6 months and yearly thereafter is routine practice in Australia, although the benefit of this monitoring in the absence of other symptoms has recently been questioned.[47] The absence of resources to provide monitoring beyond routine blood tests (including CRP and troponin) and ECG should not be a barrier to prescribing for most patients.[25]

Factors that may increase the risk of developing myocarditis include rapid dose increases, concurrent use of sodium valproate, and older age (31% increased risk for each additional decade).[48] Other psychotropic drugs, including lithium, risperidone, haloperidol, chlorpromazine and fluphenazine, have also been associated with myocarditis.[49] It is probably preferable to avoid concomitant use of other medicines that may contribute to the risk, but this may be practically difficult. Any pre-existing cardiac disorder, previous cardiac event, use of illicit drugs[21] or family history of cardiac disease should provoke extra caution.

Cardiomyopathy should be suspected in any patient showing signs of heart failure, which should provoke immediate cessation of clozapine and referral. Presentation of cardiomyopathy varies somewhat[50,51] and is often asymptomatic in the early stages,[22] so any reported symptoms of palpitations, chest pain, syncope, sweating, decreased exercise capacity or breathing difficulties should be closely investigated. Successful re-challenge with rigorous cardiac monitoring (including echocardiography) may be possible.[52,53]

Note also that, despite an overall reduction in mortality, younger patients may have an increased risk of sudden death,[54] perhaps because of clozapine-induced ECG changes.[55] The overall picture remains very unclear but caution is required. There may, of course, be similar problems with other antipsychotics.[49,56,57]

Summary

- Overall mortality is lower for those on clozapine than in schizophrenia as a whole.
- Risk of fatal agranulocytosis is less than 1 in 8000 patients treated.
- Risk of fatal pulmonary embolism is estimated to be around 1 in 4500 patients treated.

- Risk of fatal myocarditis or cardiomyopathy may be as high as 1 in 1000 patients.
- Careful monitoring is essential during clozapine treatment, particularly during the first 3 months (see Table 1.47).

Table 1.47 Suggested monitoring for myocarditis[44–46]

Time/condition	Signs/symptoms to monitor
Baseline	Pulse, blood pressure, temperature, respiratory rate
	Full blood count (FBC)
	C-reactive protein (CRP)
	Troponin
	Echocardiography (if available)
	Electrocardiogram (ECG)
Daily, if possible	Pulse, blood pressure, temperature, respiratory rate
	Ask about: chest pain, fever, cough, shortness of breath, exercise capacity
On days 7, 14, 21, and 28	CRP
	Troponin
	FBC
	ECG if possible
If CRP >100 mg/L or troponin > twice upper limit of normal	Stop clozapine; repeat echo
If fever + tachycardia + raised CRP or troponin (but not as above)	Daily CRP and troponin measures

References

1. Walker AM et al. Mortality in current and former users of clozapine. Epidemiology 1997; 8:671–677.
2. Munro J et al. Active monitoring of 12760 clozapine recipients in the UK and Ireland. Br J Psychiatry 1999; 175:576–580.
3. Honigfeld G et al. Reducing clozapine-related morbidity and mortality: 5 years of experience with the Clozaril National Registry. J Clin Psychiatry 1998; 59 Suppl 3:3–7.
4. Paciullo CA. Evaluating the association between clozapine and venous thromboembolism. Am J Health Syst Pharm 2008; 65:1825–1829.
5. Lacika S et al. Pulmonary embolus possibly associated with clozapine treatment (Letter). Can J Psychiatry 1999; 44:396–397.
6. Hagg S et al. Association of venous thromboembolism and clozapine. Lancet 2000; 355:1155–1156.
7. Davis S et al. Antiphospholipid antibodies associated with clozapine treatment. Am J Hematol 1994; 46:166–167.
8. Axelsson S et al. In vitro effects of antipsychotics on human platelet adhesion and aggregation and plasma coagulation. Clin Exp Pharmacol Physiol 2007; 34:775–780.
9. Liperoti R et al. Venous thromboembolism among elderly patients treated with atypical and conventional antipsychotic agents. Arch Intern Med 2005; 165:2677–2682.
10. Lacut K. Association between antipsychotic drugs, antidepressant drugs, and venous thromboembolism. Clin Adv Hematol Oncol 2008; 6:887–890.
11. Borras L et al. Pulmonary thromboembolism associated with olanzapine and risperidone. J Emerg Med 2008; 35:159–161.
12. Maly R et al. Four cases of venous thromboembolism associated with olanzapine. Psychiatry Clin Neurosci 2009; 63:116–118.
13. Hagg S et al. Associations between venous thromboembolism and antipsychotics. A study of the WHO database of adverse drug reactions. Drug Saf 2008; 31:685–694.
14. Lacut K et al. Association between antipsychotic drugs, antidepressant drugs and venous thromboembolism: results from the EDITH case-control study. Fundam Clin Pharmacol 2007; 21:643–650.
15. Zink M et al. A case of pulmonary thromboembolism and rhabdomyolysis during therapy with mirtazapine and risperidone. J Clin Psychiatry 2006; 67:835.

16. Allenet B et al. Antipsychotic drugs and risk of pulmonary embolism. Pharmacoepidemiol Drug Saf 2012; 21:42–48.

17. Masopust J et al. Risk of venous thromboembolism during treatment with antipsychotic agents. Psychiatry Clin Neurosci 2012; 66:541–552.

18. Jonsson AK et al. Venous thromboembolism in recipients of antipsychotics: incidence, mechanisms and management. CNS Drugs 2012; 26:649–662.

19. Maly R et al. Assessment of risk of venous thromboembolism and its possible prevention in psychiatric patients. Psychiatry Clin Neurosci 2008; 62:3–8.

20. Ronaldson KJ. Cardiovascular disease in clozapine-treated patients: evidence, mechanisms and management. CNS Drugs 2017; 31:777–795.

21. Khan AA et al. Clozapine and incidence of myocarditis and sudden death – long term Australian experience. Int J Cardiol 2017; 238:136–139.

22. Youssef DL et al. Incidence and risk factors for clozapine-induced myocarditis and cardiomyopathy at a regional mental health service in Australia. Australas Psychiatry 2016; 24:176–180.

23. Cohen D et al. Beyond white blood cell monitoring: screening in the initial phase of clozapine therapy. J Clin Psychiatry 2012; 73:1307–1312.

24. Kilian JG et al. Myocarditis and cardiomyopathy associated with clozapine. Lancet 1999; 354:1841–1845.

25. Freudenreich O. Clozapine-induced myocarditis: prescribe safely but do prescribe. Acta Psychiatr Scand 2015; 132:240–241.

26. Ronaldson KJ et al. Clozapine-induced myocarditis, a widely overlooked adverse reaction. Acta Psychiatr Scand 2015; 132:231–240.

27. La Grenade L et al. Myocarditis and cardiomyopathy associated with clozapine use in the United States (Letter). N Engl J Med 2001; 345:224–225.

28. Curto M et al. Systematic review of clozapine cardiotoxicity. Curr Psychiatry Rep 2016; 18:68.

29. Marder SR et al. Physical health monitoring of patients with schizophrenia. Am J Psychiatry 2004; 161:1334–1349.

30. Annamraju S et al. Early recognition of clozapine-induced myocarditis. J Clin Psychopharmacol 2007; 27:479–483.

31. Wehmeier PM et al. Chart review for potential features of myocarditis, pericarditis, and cardiomyopathy in children and adolescents treated with clozapine. J Child Adolesc Psychopharmacol 2004; 14:267–271.

32. McNeil JJ et al. Clozapine-induced myocarditis: characterisation using case-control design. Eur Heart J 2013; 34 (Suppl 1):688.

33. Reinders J et al. Clozapine-related myocarditis and cardiomyopathy in an Australian metropolitan psychiatric service. Aust N Z J Psychiatry 2004; 38:915–922.

34. Manu P et al. When can patients with potentially life-threatening adverse effects be rechallenged with clozapine? A systematic review of the published literature. Schizophr Res 2012; 134:180–186.

35. Rostagno C et al. Beta-blocker and angiotensin-converting enzyme inhibitor may limit certain cardiac adverse effects of clozapine. Gen Hosp Psychiatry 2008; 30:280–283.

36. Floreani J et al. Successful re-challenge with clozapine following development of clozapine-induced cardiomyopathy. Aust N Z J Psychiatry 2008; 42:747–748.

37. Roh S et al. Cardiomyopathy associated with clozapine. Exp Clin Psychopharmacol 2006; 14:94–98.

38. Masopust J et al. Repeated occurrence of clozapine-induced myocarditis in a patient with schizoaffective disorder and comorbid Parkinson's disease. Neuro Endocrinol Lett 2009; 30:19–21.

39. Ronaldson KJ et al. Observations from 8 cases of clozapine rechallenge after development of myocarditis. J Clin Psychiatry 2012; 73:252–254.

40. Nielsen J et al. Termination of clozapine treatment due to medical reasons: when is it warranted and how can it be avoided? J Clin Psychiatry 2013; 74:603–613; quiz 613.

41. Hassan I et al. Monitoring in clozapine rechallenge after myocarditis. Australas Psychiatry 2011; 19:370–371.

42. Bray A et al. Successful clozapine rechallenge after acute myocarditis. Aust N Z J Psychiatry 2011; 45:90.

43. Rosenfeld AJ et al. Successful clozapine retrial after suspected myocarditis. Am J Psychiatry 2010; 167:350–351.

44. Ronaldson KJ et al. Clinical course and analysis of ten fatal cases of clozapine-induced myocarditis and comparison with 66 surviving cases. Schizophr Res 2011; 128:161–165.

45. Ronaldson KJ et al. A new monitoring protocol for clozapine-induced myocarditis based on an analysis of 75 cases and 94 controls. Aust N Z J Psychiatry 2011; 45:458–465.

46. Ronaldson KJ et al. Diagnostic characteristics of clozapine-induced myocarditis identified by an analysis of 38 cases and 47 controls. J Clin Psychiatry 2010; 71:976–981.

47. Robinson G et al. Echocardiography and clozapine: is current clinical practice inhibiting use of a potentially life-transforming therapy? Aust Fam Physician 2017; 46:169–170.

48. Ronaldson KJ et al. Rapid clozapine dose titration and concomitant sodium valproate increase the risk of myocarditis with clozapine: a case-control study. Schizophr Res 2012; 141:173–178.

49. Coulter DM et al. Antipsychotic drugs and heart muscle disorder in international pharmacovigilance: data mining study. BMJ 2001; 322:1207–1209.

50. Pastor CA et al. Masked clozapine-induced cardiomyopathy. J Am Board Fam Med 2008; 21:70–74.

51. Sagar R et al. Clozapine-induced cardiomyopathy presenting as panic attacks. J Psychiatr Pract 2008; 14:182–185.

52. Nederlof M et al. Clozapine re-exposure after dilated cardiomyopathy. BMJ Case Rep 2017; 2017.

53. Alawami M et al. A systematic review of clozapine induced cardiomyopathy. Int J Cardiol 2014; 176:315–320.

54. Modai I et al. Sudden death in patients receiving clozapine treatment: a preliminary investigation. J Clin Psychopharmacol 2000; 20:325–327.

55. Kang UG et al. Electrocardiographic abnormalities in patients treated with clozapine. J Clin Psychiatry 2000; **61**:441–446.
56. Thomassen R et al. Antipsychotic drugs and venous thromboembolism (Letter). Lancet 2000; **356**:252.
57. Hagg S et al. Antipsychotic-induced venous thromboembolism: a review of the evidence. CNS Drugs 2002; **16**:765–776.

Further reading

Caforio AL et al. Current state of knowledge on aetiology, diagnosis, management, and therapy of myocarditis: a position statement of the European Society of Cardiology Working Group on Myocardial and Pericardial Diseases. Eur Heart J 2013; **34**:2636–2648.
Joy G et al. Hearts and minds: real-life cardiotoxicity with clozapine in psychosis. J Clin Psychopharmacol 2017; **37**:708–712.
Razminia M et al. Clozapine induced myopericarditis: early recognition improves clinical outcome. Am J Ther 2006; **13**:274–276.
Wehmeier PM et al. Myocarditis, pericarditis and cardiomyopathy in patients treated with clozapine. J Clin Pharm Ther 2005; **30**:91–96.

Clozapine-induced hypersalivation

Clozapine is well known to be causally associated with hypersalivation (sialorrhoea), with excess salivary pooling in the mouth and drooling, particularly at night. The problem tends to occur in the early stages of treatment and is probably dose-related. Clinical observation suggests that hypersalivation reduces somewhat in severity over time (usually several months) but may persist. Clozapine-induced hypersalivation is socially embarrassing, has a negative impact on quality of life[1] and, given that it has been implicated as a contributory factor in the development of aspiration pneumonia, could be potentially life-threatening.[2–4] Treatment is therefore a matter of some urgency.

The pharmacological basis of clozapine-related hypersalivation remains unclear.[5] Suggested mechanisms include muscarinic M_4 agonism, adrenergic α_2 antagonism and inhibition of the swallowing reflex.[6,7] The last of these is supported by trials which suggest that saliva production is not increased in clozapine-treated patients,[8,9] although at least one study has observed marked increases in salivary flow in the first 3 weeks of treatment.[10]

Whatever the mechanism, drugs that reduce saliva production are likely to diminish the severity of this adverse effect. Non-drug treatments may be used if appropriate – these include chewing gum, elevating pillows and placing a towel on the pillow to prevent soaking of clothes.[5] Table 1.48 describes the pharmacological treatments so far examined.

Table 1.48 Clozapine-related hypersalivation

Treatment	Comments
Amisulpride 100–400 mg/day[11,12]	Supported by a positive RCT compared with placebo, one other in which it was compared with moclobemide and numerous case studies.[13–16] May allow dose reduction of clozapine
Amitriptyline 25–100 mg/day[17,18]	Limited literature support. Adverse effects may be troublesome. Worsens constipation
Atropine eye drops (1%) given sublingually[19–21] or as solution (1 mg/10 mL) used as a mouthwash	Limited literature support. Rarely used. Problems with administration have been reported[22]
Benzhexol (trihexyphenidyl) 5–15 mg/day[23]	Small, open study suggests useful activity. Used in some centres but may impair cognitive function. Lower doses (2 mg) may be effective[24]
Benzatropine 2 mg/day + **terazosin** 2 mg/day[25]	Combination shown to be better than either drug alone. Terazosin is an α_1 antagonist so may cause hypotension
Botulinum toxin[26–29] (Botox) bilateral parotid gland injections (150 IU into each gland)	Effective in treating sialorrhoea associated with neurological disorders. Six cases of successful treatment of clozapine-related hypersalivation in the literature
Bupropion 100–150 mg/day[30]	Single case report. May lower seizure threshold
Clonidine 0.1–0.2 mg patch weekly or 0.1 mg orally at night[31,32]	α_2 partial agonist. Limited literature support. May exacerbate psychosis and depression and cause hypotension

(Continued)

Table 1.48 (Continued)

Treatment	Comments
Glycopyrrolate 0.5–4 mg bd[33–36]	One RCT showed glycopyrrolate to be more effective than biperiden without worsening cognitive function while another found significant clinical improvement of 'nocturnal sialorrhoea' with 2 mg a day compared with placebo
Guanfacine 1 mg daily[37]	α_2 agonist. Single case report. May cause hypotension
Hyoscine 0.3 mg tablet sucked or chewed up to 3 times daily or 1.5 mg/72 h patch[38,39]	Peripheral and central anticholinergic. Very widely used but no published data available on oral treatment. May cause cognitive impairment and drowsiness and worsens constipation
Ipratropium nasal spray (0.03% or 0.06%) given sublingually up to two sprays three times a day of the 0.06% or intranasally, one spray into each nostril daily of the 0.03%[40,41]	Limited literature support. The only placebo-controlled RCT conducted was negative[42]
Lofexidine 0.2 mg twice daily[43]	α_2 agonist. Very few data. May exacerbate psychosis and depression and cause hypotension
Metoclopramide Starting dose of 10 mg a day[44]	Double-blind, placebo-controlled trial found metoclopramide was associated with a significant reduction in nocturnal hypersalivation and drooling
Moclobemide 150–300 mg/day[45]	Effective in 9 of 14 patients treated in one open study. Appears to be as effective as amisulpride (see above)
Oxybutynin 5 mg up to twice daily[46]	Single case report
Pirenzepine 50–150 mg/day[47–49]	Selective M_1, M_4 antagonist. Extensive clinical experience suggests efficacy in some but the only randomised trial suggested no effect. Still widely used. Does not have a UK licence for any indication. May cause constipation
Propantheline 7.5 mg at night[50]	Peripheral anticholinergic. No central effects. Two Chinese RCTs (one positive). May worsen constipation
Quetiapine[51]	May reduce hypersalivation by allowing lower doses of clozapine to be used
Sulpiride 150–300 mg/day[52,53]	Supported by one, small positive RCT and a Cochrane review of clozapine augmentation with sulpiride (at higher sulpiride doses). May allow dose reduction of clozapine

bd, *bis die* (twice a day); RCT, randomised controlled trial.

References

1. Maher S et al. Clozapine-induced hypersalivation: an estimate of prevalence, severity and impact on quality of life. Ther Adv Psychopharmacol 2016; 6:179–184.
2. Hinkes R et al. Aspiration pneumonia possibly secondary to clozapine-induced sialorrhea. J Clin Psychopharmacol 1996; 16:462–463.
3. Saenger RC et al. Aspiration pneumonia due to clozapine-induced sialorrhea. Clin Schizophr Relat Psychoses 2016; 9:170–172.
4. Gurrera RJ. Aspiration pneumonia: an underappreciated risk of clozapine treatment. J Clin Psychopharmacol 2016; 36:174–176.

5. Praharaj SK et al. Clozapine-induced sialorrhea: pathophysiology and management strategies. Psychopharmacology 2006; 185:265–273.

6. Davydov L et al. Clozapine-induced hypersalivation. Ann Pharmacother 2000; 34:662–665.

7. Rogers DP et al. Therapeutic options in the treatment of clozapine-induced sialorrhea. Pharmacotherapy 2000; 20:1092–1095.

8. Rabinowitz T et al. The effect of clozapine on saliva flow rate: a pilot study. Biol Psychiatry 1996; 40:1132–1134.

9. Ben Aryeh H et al. Salivary flow-rate and composition in schizophrenic patients on clozapine: subjective reports and laboratory data. Biol Psychiatry 1996; 39:946–949.

10. Praharaj SK et al. Salivary flow rate in patients with schizophrenia on clozapine. Clin Neuropharmacol 2010; 33:176–178.

11. Kreinin A et al. Amisulpride treatment of clozapine-induced hypersalivation in schizophrenia patients: a randomized, double-blind, placebo-controlled cross-over study. Int Clin Psychopharmacol 2006; 21:99–103.

12. Kreinin A et al. Amisulpride versus moclobemide in treatment of clozapine-induced hypersalivation. World J Biol Psychiatry 2010; 12:620–626.

13. Praharaj SK et al. Amisulpride treatment for clozapine-induced sialorrhea. J Clin Psychopharmacol 2009; 29:189–190.

14. Aggarwal A et al. Amisulpride for clozapine induced sialorrhea. Psychopharmacol Bull 2009; 42:69–71.

15. Praharaj SK et al. Amisulpride improved debilitating clozapine-induced sialorrhea. Am J Ther 2011; 18:e84–e85.

16. Kulkarni RR.Low-dose amisulpride for debilitating clozapine-induced sialorrhea: case series and review of literature. Indian J Psychol Med 2015; 37:446–448.

17. Copp P et al. Amitriptyline in clozapine-induced sialorrhoea. Br J Psychiatry 1991; 159:166.

18. Praharaj SK et al. Amitriptyline for clozapine-induced nocturnal enuresis and sialorrhea. Br J Clin Pharmacol 2007; 63:128–129.

19. Antonello C et al. Clozapine and sialorrhea: a new intervention for this bothersome and potentially dangerous side effect. J Psychiatry Neurosci 1999; 24:250.

20. Mustafa FA et al. Sublingual atropine for the treatment of severe and hyoscine-resistant clozapine-induced sialorrhea. Afr J Psychiatry (Johannesbg) 2013; 16:242.

21. Matos Santana TE et al. Sublingual atropine in the treatment of clozapine-induced sialorrhea. Schizophr Res 2017; 182:144–145.

22. Leung JG et al. Potential problems surrounding the use of sublingually administered ophthalmic atropine for sialorrhea. Schizophr Res 2017; 185:202–203.

23. Spivak B et al. Trihexyphenidyl treatment of clozapine-induced hypersalivation. Int Clin Psychopharmacol 1997; 12:213–215.

24. Praharaj SK et al. Complete resolution of clozapine-induced sialorrhea with low dose trihexyphenidyl. Psychopharmacol Bull 2010; 43:73–75.

25. Reinstein M et al. Comparative efficacy and tolerability of benzatropine and terazosin in the treatment of hypersalivation secondary to clozapine. Clin Drug Invest 1999; 17:97–102.

26. Kahl KG et al. Botulinum toxin as an effective treatment of clozapine-induced hypersalivation. Psychopharmacology 2004; 173:229–230.

27. Steinlechner S et al. Botulinum toxin B as an effective and safe treatment for neuroleptic-induced sialorrhea. Psychopharmacology (Berl) 2010; 207:593–597.

28. Kahl KG et al. [Pharmacological strategies for clozapine-induced hypersalivation: treatment with botulinum toxin B in one patient and review of the literature]. Nervenarzt 2005; 76:205–208.

29. Verma R et al. Botulinum toxin: a novel therapy for clozapine-induced sialorrhoea. Psychopharmacology (Berl) 2018; 235:369–371.

30. Stern RG et al. Clozapine-induced sialorrhea alleviated by bupropion – a case report. Prog Neuropsychopharmacol Biol Psychiatry 2009; 33:1578–1580.

31. Grabowski J. Clonidine treatment of clozapine-induced hypersalivation. J Clin Psychopharmacol 1992; 12:69–70.

32. Praharaj SK et al. Is clonidine useful for treatment of clozapine-induced sialorrhea? J Psychopharmacol 2005; 19:426–428.

33. Duggal HS. Glycopyrrolate for clozapine-induced sialorrhea. Prog Neuropsychopharmacol Biol Psychiatry 2007; 31:1546–1547.

34. Robb AS et al. Glycopyrrolate for treatment of clozapine-induced sialorrhea in three adolescents. J Child Adolesc Psychopharmacol 2008; 18:99–107.

35. Liang CS et al. Comparison of the efficacy and impact on cognition of glycopyrrolate and biperiden for clozapine-induced sialorrhea in schizophrenic patients: a randomized, double-blind, crossover study. Schizophr Res 2010; 119:138–144.

36. Man WH et al. The effect of glycopyrrolate on nocturnal sialorrhea in patients using clozapine: a randomized, crossover, double-blind, placebo-controlled trial. J Clin Psychopharmacol 2017; 37:155–161.

37. Webber MA et al. Guanfacine treatment of clozapine-induced sialorrhea. J Clin Psychopharmacol 2004; 24:675–676.

38. McKane JP et al. Hyoscine patches in clozapine-induced hypersalivation. Psychiatr Bull 2001; 25:277.

39. Gaftanyuk O et al. Scolpolamine patch for clozapine-induced sialorrhea. Psychiatr Serv 2004; 55:318.

40. Calderon J et al. Potential use of ipatropium bromide for the treatment of clozapine-induced hypersalivation: a preliminary report. Int Clin Psychopharmacol 2000; 15:49–52.

41. Freudenreich O et al. Clozapine-induced sialorrhea treated with sublingual ipratropium spray: a case series. J Clin Psychopharmacol 2004; 24:98–100.

42. Sockalingam S et al. Treatment of clozapine-induced hypersalivation with ipratropium bromide: a randomized, double-blind, placebo-controlled crossover study. J Clin Psychiatry 2009; 70:1114–1119.

43. Corrigan FM et al. Clozapine-induced hypersalivation and the alpha 2 adrenoceptor. Br J Psychiatry 1995; 167:412.

44. Kreinin A et al. Double-blind randomized, placebo-controlled trial of metoclopramide for hypersalivation associated with clozapine. J Clin Psychopharmacol 2016; 36:200–205.

45. Kreinin A et al. Moclobemide treatment of clozapine-induced hypersalivation: pilot open study. Clin Neuropharmacol 2009; 32:151–153.

46. Leung JG et al. Immediate-release oxybutynin for the treatment of clozapine-induced sialorrhea. Ann Pharmacother 2011; 45:e45.

47. Fritze J et al. Pirenzepine for clozapine-induced hypersalivation. Lancet 1995; 346:1034.
48. Bai YM et al. Therapeutic effect of pirenzepine for clozapine-induced hypersalivation: a randomized, double-blind, placebo-controlled, crossover study. J Clin Psychopharmacol 2001; 21:608–611.
49. Schneider B et al. Reduction of clozapine-induced hypersalivation by pirenzepine is safe. Pharmacopsychiatry 2004; 37:43–45.
50. Syed Sheriff RJ et al. Pharmacological interventions for clozapine-induced hypersalivation. Schizophr Bull 2008; 34:611–612.
51. Reinstein MJ et al. Use of quetiapine to manage patients who experienced adverse effects with clozapine. Clin Drug Invest 2003; 23:63–67.
52. Kreinin A et al. Sulpiride addition for the treatment of clozapine-induced hypersalivation: preliminary study. Isr J Psychiatry Relat Sci 2005; 42:61–63.
53. Wang J et al. Sulpiride augmentation for schizophrenia. Cochrane Database Syst Rev 2010; CD008125.

Further reading

Bird AM et al. Current treatment strategies for clozapine-induced sialorrhea. Ann Pharmacother 2011; 45:667–675.

Clozapine-induced gastrointestinal hypomotility (CIGH)

Constipation is a common adverse effect of clozapine treatment with a prevalence of more than 30%, three times that seen with other antipsychotics.[1] The mechanism of action is not completely understood but is thought to be a combination of the drug's anticholinergic[2,3] and antihistaminergic properties[4] which are further complicated by antagonism at 5-HT$_3$ receptors.[2,3,5] In addition, clozapine-induced sedation can result in a sedentary lifestyle which is itself a risk factor for constipation.[4] Clozapine causes constipation by slowing transit time through the gut. Mean transit times are four times longer than normal, and 80% of clozapine patients show reduced transit time.[6]

Clozapine-induced constipation is much more common than blood dyscrasias, and mortality rates are also higher.[4] When constipation is severe, the case fatality rate is around 20–30%.[4,7,8] The most recent (and largest) study[9] found an incidence of 37/10,000 cases of severe hypomotility and 7/10,000 constipation-related deaths. Case fatality was 18%. Enhanced monitoring of CIGH is clearly needed to reduce the likelihood of constipation-related fatality.

A gastrointestinal history and abdominal examination is recommended prior to starting treatment and, if the patient is constipated, clozapine should not be initiated until this has resolved.[8] CIGH is most severe during the first 4 months of treatment[8] but may occur at any time. Adopting the Rome III criteria[10] at routine FBCs might be a successful strategy to combat preventable deaths due to CIGH.

Opinions differ on the relationship between clozapine dose and constipation, and between clozapine plasma level and constipation.[8,11,12] However, patients who died as a result of CIGH had higher than average daily doses (mean 535 mg/day).[8] Median duration of clozapine treatment at the time of death is 2.5 years.[9]

The risk factors for developing clozapine-induced constipation are summarised in Box 1.6.

Box 1.6 Risk factors for developing clozapine-induced constipation[8,13–16]

- Increasing age
- Female sex
- Anticholinergic medication
- Higher clozapine dose/plasma level (consider the effect of interacting drugs or stopping smoking)
- Hypercalcaemia
- Gastrointestinal disease
- Obesity
- Diaphoresis
- Low-fibre diet
- Poor bowel habit
- Dehydration (exacerbated by hypersalivation)
- Diabetes
- Hypothyroidism
- Parkinson's disease
- Multiple sclerosis

CHAPTER 1

Prevention and simple management of CIGH

A slow clozapine titration may reduce the risk of developing constipation, with dose increments not exceeding 25 mg/day or 100 mg/week.[17] Increasing dietary fibre intake to at least 20–25 g/day can increase stool weight and decrease gut transit time.[16,18] If fibre intake is increased it is important that adequate fluid intake (1.5–2 L/day) is also maintained to avoid intestinal obstruction.[8,16,19] Daily food and fluid charts would be ideal to monitor fibre and fluid intake, especially during the titration phase of clozapine. Regular exercise (150 minutes/week)[20] in addition to a high-fibre diet and increased fluid intake also assist in the prevention of CIGH.[21,22]

Patients often do not self-report even life-threatening constipation.[8] Use of stool charts daily for the first 4 weeks, and weekly or monthly thereafter is recommended. If there is a change from usual baseline bowel habit or fewer than three bowel movements per week[10] an abdominal examination is indicated.[8] Where this excludes intestinal obstruction, both a stimulant and stool-softening laxative should be started (e.g. senna and docusate[8,23,24]). Bulk-forming laxatives are not effective in slow-transit constipation[2,25] and therefore should be avoided. There is some evidence that lactulose and polyethylene glycol (e.g. Movicol) are effective[2,26] and could be considered as second-line options or in addition to the stimulant and softener combination.[24] Choice of laxative should also be guided by the patient's previous response to certain agents in association with the required speed of action.[27] It would not be appropriate for example to start lactulose treatment (takes up to 72 hours of regular use to work[28]) for someone in need of urgent treatment. Stimulant laxatives are usually the fastest acting (6–10 hours).

Management of suspected acute CIGH

Signs and symptoms that warrant immediate medical attention are abdominal pain, distension, vomiting, overflow diarrhoea, absent bowel sounds, acute abdomen, feculent vomitus and symptoms of sepsis.[8,7,17,29–36] There have been case reports of fatalities occurring only hours after first symptoms present,[37] and this emphasises the urgency for prompt assessment and management. There should therefore be a low threshold for referral to a gastroenterologist and/or A&E when conservative management fails or constipation is severe and acute.[8,38]

Clozapine re-challenge following severe constipation

Some patients have been successfully re-challenged following severe cases of CIGH. However, this process does not come without risk. Prophylactic measures should therefore be considered for those with a history of CIGH or who are deemed at high risk of developing CIGH. Where conventional laxatives have not been tried in regular and adequate doses, this should be done. However, when this approach has previously failed, a number of more experimental options are available. Prescribers must familiarise themselves with the literature (at the very least by reading the SPC) before using any of these treatments.

The prostaglandin E1 analogue **lubiprostone** is licensed in the UK for the treatment of chronic idiopathic constipation and associated symptoms in adults, when response to diet and other non-pharmacological measures (e.g. educational measures, physical activity) are inappropriate.[39] The recommended dose for the licensed indication is 24 µg twice daily for a maximum of 2 weeks' duration.[39] Lubiprostone has been reported to be effective in obviating the need for other laxatives in a clozapine re-challenge following a severe case of CIGH[40] and is used in some centres for this indication.[40]

Orlistat, a drug used to aid weight loss, is also known to have a laxative effect, particularly when a high-fat diet is consumed. It was reported as being successfully used for three patients with severe constipation associated with opioid use (hypomotility-induced constipation).[41] A small, randomised, placebo-controlled study of orlistat for clozapine-induced constipation found a statistically significant favourable difference at study endpoint (week 16) for the prevalence of constipation, diarrhoea and normal stools for orlistat compared with placebo,[42] although 47 of the 54 participants required conventional laxatives. Note also that orlistat is known to reduce the absorption of some drugs from the gastrointestinal tract. It is therefore important to monitor plasma clozapine levels if starting treatment with orlistat. Orlistat may be particularly difficult to use outside clinical study settings as without adherence to a strict low-fat diet, gastric adverse effects can be unpleasant (specifically, oily rectal leakage).

Bethanechol, a cholinergic agonist, has been described as being effective in reducing the amount of laxatives and enemas required to maintain regular bowel movements for a patient diagnosed with clozapine-related CIGH.[43] Bethanechol in this case was used at a dose of 10 mg tds. Bethanechol should only ever be initiated after other options have failed and then in consultation with a gastroenterologist.[43]

References

1. Shirazi A et al. Prevalence and predictors of clozapine-associated constipation: a systematic review and meta-analysis. Int J Mol Sci 2016; **17**.
2. Hibbard KR et al. Fatalities associated with clozapine-related constipation and bowel obstruction: a literature review and two case reports. Psychosomatics 2009; **50**:416–419.
3. Rege S et al. Life-threatening constipation associated with clozapine. Australas Psychiatry 2008; **16**:216–219.
4. De Hert M et al. Second-generation antipsychotics and constipation: a review of the literature. Eur Psychiatry 2011; **26**:34–44.
5. Meltzer HY et al. Effects of antipsychotic drugs on serotonin receptors. Pharmacol Rev 1991; **43**:587–604.
6. Every-Palmer S et al. Clozapine-treated patients have marked gastrointestinal hypomotility, the probable basis of life-threatening gastrointestinal complications: a cross sectional study. EBioMedicine 2016; **5**:125–134.
7. Cohen D et al. Beyond white blood cell monitoring: screening in the initial phase of clozapine therapy. J Clin Psychiatry 2012; **73**:1307–1312.
8. Palmer SE et al. Life-threatening clozapine-induced gastrointestinal hypomotility: an analysis of 102 cases. J Clin Psychiatry 2008; **69**:759–768.
9. Every-Palmer S et al. Clozapine-induced gastrointestinal hypomotility: a 22-year bi-national pharmacovigilance study of serious or fatal 'slow gut' reactions, and comparison with international drug safety advice. CNS Drugs 2017; **31**:699–709.
10. Rome Foundation. Rome IV Disorders and Criteria. 2016. https://theromefoundation.org
11. Chengappa KN et al. Anticholinergic differences among patients receiving standard clinical doses of olanzapine or clozapine. J Clin Psychopharmacol 2000; **20**:311–316.
12. Vella-Brincat J et al. Clozapine-induced gastrointestinal hypomotility. Australas Psychiatry 2011; **19**:450–451.
13. Nielsen J et al. Termination of clozapine treatment due to medical reasons: when is it warranted and how can it be avoided? J Clin Psychiatry 2013; **74**:603–613; quiz 13.
14. Nielsen J et al. Risk factors for ileus in patients with schizophrenia. Schizophr Bull 2012; **38**:592–598.
15. Longmore M et al. *Oxford Handbook of Clinical Medicine*. Oxford: Oxford; 2010.
16. ZTAS. Zaponex Fact Sheet – Constipation. 2013. https://www.ztas.com/Manuals/ZFS_Constipation2.pdf
17. Hayes G et al. Clozapine-induced constipation. Am J Psychiatry 1995; **152**:298.
18. Muller-Lissner SA. Effect of wheat bran on weight of stool and gastrointestinal transit time: a meta analysis. Br Med J (Clin Res Ed) 1988; **296**:615–617.
19. National Prescribing Centre. The management of constipation. Med Rec Bulletin 2011; **21**:1–8.
20. NHS Choices. Physical activity guidelines for adults. 2013. http://www.nhs.uk/Livewell/fitness/Pages/physical-activity-guidelines-for-adults.aspx.

21. Fitzsimons J et al. A review of clozapine safety. Expert Opin Drug Saf 2005; 4:731–744.

22. Young CR et al. Management of the adverse effects of clozapine. Schizophr Bull 1998; 24:381–390.

23. Swegle JM et al. Management of common opioid-induced adverse effects. Am Fam Physician 2006; 74:1347–1354.

24. Every-Palmer S et al. The porirua protocol in the treatment of clozapine-induced gastrointestinal hypomotility and constipation: a pre- and post-treatment Study. CNS Drugs 2017; 31:75–85.

25. Voderholzer WA et al. Clinical response to dietary fiber treatment of chronic constipation. Am J Gastroenterol 1997; 92:95–98.

26. Brandt LJ et al. Systematic review on the management of chronic constipation in North America. Am J Gastroenterol 2005; 100 Suppl 1:S5–S21.

27. Bleakley S et al. *Clozapine Handbook*. Warwickshire, UK: Lloyd-Reinhold Communications LLP; 2013.

28. Intrapharm Laboratories Limited. Summary of Product Characteristics. Lactulose 10 g / 15 ml oral solution sachets. 2017. https://www.medicines.org.uk/emc/medicine/25597

29. Leong QM et al. Necrotising colitis related to clozapine? A rare but life threatening side effect. World J Emerg Surg 2007; 2:21.

30. Shammi CM et al. Clozapine-induced necrotizing colitis. J Clin Psychopharmacol 1997; 17:230–232.

31. Rondla S et al. A case of clozapine-induced paralytic ileus. Emerg Med J 2007; 24:e12.

32. Levin TT et al. Death from clozapine-induced constipation: case report and literature review. Psychosomatics 2002; 43:71–73.

33. Townsend G et al. Case report: rapidly fatal bowel ischaemia on clozapine treatment. BMC Psychiatry 2006; 6:43.

34. Karmacharya R et al. Clozapine-induced eosinophilic colitis. Am J Psychiatry 2005; 162:1386–1387.

35. Erickson B et al. Clozapine-associated postoperative ileus: case report and review of the literature. Arch Gen Psychiatry 1995; 52:508–509.

36. Schwartz BJ et al. A case report of clozapine-induced gastric outlet obstruction. Am J Psychiatry 1993; 150:1563.

37. Drew L et al. Clozapine and constipation: a serious issue. Aust N Z J Psychiatry 1997; 31:149.

38. Ikai S et al. Reintroduction of clozapine after perforation of the large intestine – a case report and review of the literature. Ann Pharmacother 2013; 47:e31.

39. Takeda UK Ltd. Summary of Product Characteristics. AMITIZA 24 microgram soft capsules. 2016. https://www.medicines.org.uk/emc/medicine/28268

40. Meyer JM et al. Lubiprostone for treatment-resistant constipation associated with clozapine use. Acta Psychiatr Scand 2014; 130:71–72.

41. Guarino AH. Treatment of intractable constipation with orlistat: a report of three cases. Pain Med 2005; 6:327–328.

42. Chukhin E et al. In a randomized placebo-controlled add-on study orlistat significantly reduced clozapine-induced constipation. Int Clin Psychopharmacol 2013; 28:67–70.

43. Poetter CE et al. Treatment of clozapine-induced constipation with bethanechol. J Clin Psychopharmacol 2013; 33:713–714.

Clozapine, neutropenia and lithium

Risk of clozapine-induced neutropenia and agranulocytosis

Around 2.7% of patients treated with clozapine develop neutropenia. Of these, half do so within the first 18 weeks of treatment and three-quarters by the end of the first year.[1] Risk factors include being Afro-Caribbean, younger age and having a low baseline white cell count (WCC).[1] Risk is not dose-related. The mechanism of clozapine-induced neutropenia/agranulocytosis is unclear; both immune-mediated and direct cytotoxic effects may be important. Furthermore, the mechanism may differ between individuals and also between mild and severe forms of marrow suppression.[2] One-third of patients who stop clozapine because they have developed neutropenia or agranulocytosis will develop a blood dyscrasia on re-challenge. Where the index dyscrasia was agranulocytosis, the second blood dyscrasia invariably occurs more rapidly and can be more severe and last longer,[3] although this is not necessarily the case where the index dyscrasia was neutropenia.[4]

Confusion arises because of the various possible reasons for a low neutrophil count in people taking clozapine. A single low count might just be a coincidental finding of no clinical relevance, as is common with all drugs. Several low counts (consecutive or intermittent) might be seen in people with benign ethnic neutropenia (BEN) or as a result of clozapine-associated bone marrow suppression (especially if consecutive and progressively falling). Full-blown agranulocytosis can probably always be interpreted as a result of severe bone marrow suppression caused by clozapine. The pattern of the results can be important. In non-BEN patients, agranulocytosis is normally preceded by normal neutrophil counts which are then followed by a precipitous fall in neutrophils (usually over a week or less) and a prolonged period of counts near to zero (assuming that it has not been treated). Neutrophil counts that do not follow this characteristic pattern are difficult to interpret. An Icelandic study found no difference in the risk of severe neutropenia between clozapine and non-clozapine antipsychotics, suggesting that many cases of neutropenia during clozapine treatment are probably not caused by clozapine.[5]

At least 0.8% of clozapine-treated patients develop agranulocytosis, which is potentially fatal. Over 80% of cases of agranulocytosis develop within the first 18 weeks of treatment.[1] Risk factors include increasing age and Asian ethnicity.[1] Some patients may be genetically predisposed.[6] Although the timescale and individual risk factors for the development of agranulocytosis are different from those associated with neutropenia, it is impossible to be certain in any given patient that neutropenia is not a precursor to agranulocytosis.

Haematological monitoring is mandatory to mitigate the haematological risk. However, worldwide, there are marked variations in the recommendations for monitoring frequency and the threshold for clozapine cessation,[7] reflecting, perhaps, the weak evidence on which they are based. In October 2015, the US FDA introduced changes to the clozapine monitoring system making only the absolute neutrophil count (ANC) mandatory and effectively lowering the threshold for cessation of clozapine treatment.[8] It is recommended that treatment with clozapine be stopped when neutrophils fall below 1000/mm³ (compared with UK recommendations for cessation if ANC is <1500/mm³).

There is evidence that clozapine is grossly under-utilised worldwide, with very wide variation in prescribing frequency from one country to another.[9] This may be explained at least in part by the stringent blood monitoring requirements. The new FDA regulations will undoubtedly improve clozapine use in the USA and may have implications internationally.

Benign ethnic neutropenia

Benign ethnic neutropenia (BEN) is a widely recognised hereditary condition in which the neutrophil count is relatively low. People of African or Middle Eastern descent have a higher prevalence. BEN is characterised by low WCCs which may frequently fall below the lower limit of normal. This pattern may be observed before, during and after the use of clozapine and very probably accounts for a proportion of observed or apparent clozapine-associated neutropenias and treatment cessation. Many countries allow registration of BEN status whereby different (lower) limits are set for neutrophil counts in these patients. While true clozapine-induced neutropenia can occur in the context of BEN, the current evidence suggests that BEN does not pose an increased risk of dyscrasias during clozapine treatment.[10,11]

Concurrent medications

Different classes of medicines associated with haematological adverse effects are co-prescribed with clozapine. These include other antipsychotics, anticonvulsants such as sodium valproate and carbamazepine, antibacterials and gastrointestinal agents such as proton-pump inhibitors. Many patients develop neutropenia on clozapine but not all cases are clozapine-related or even pathological. The possible contributory role of these agents should always be considered and these agents discontinued if clozapine re-challenge is attempted.[12]

Management options

Before treatment initiation, it is important to evaluate baseline haematological values. If a patient is suspected of having BEN, there should be a referral to a haematologist for confirmation.[13]

Distinguishing between true clozapine toxicity and neutropenia unrelated to clozapine is not possible with certainty but some factors are important. Consultation with a haematologist is advisable regarding BEN and to exclude any other co-prescribed medication that may be responsible. The use of iatrogenic agents to elevate WCC in patients with clear prior clozapine-induced neutropenia (i.e. certainty that clozapine was the cause) is not recommended. Lithium or other medicines should only be used to elevate WCC where it is strongly felt that prior neutropenic episodes were unrelated to clozapine. Patients who have had a previous episode of agranulocytosis that is attributable to clozapine should not be re-challenged.

Lithium

Lithium increases the neutrophil count and total WCC both acutely and chronically. The magnitude of this effect is poorly quantified, but a mean neutrophil count of $11.9 \times 10^9/L$ has been reported in lithium-treated patients and a mean rise in neutrophil count of 2×10^9/L was seen in clozapine-treated patients after the addition of lithium. This effect does not seem to be clearly dose-related although a minimum lithium serum level of 0.4 mmol/L may be required. The mechanism is not completely understood.[14]

Lithium has been used to increase the WCC in patients who have developed neutropenia while taking clozapine, allowing clozapine treatment to continue. Several case reports in adults[15–19] and in children[20,21] have been published. Almost all patients had serum lithium levels of >0.6 mmol/L. In a case series (n = 25) of patients who had stopped clozapine because of a blood dyscrasia and were re-challenged in the presence of lithium, only one developed a subsequent dyscrasia.[22] If considering lithium, discuss with the medical advisor at the relevant monitoring service to determine the optimum pharmacological strategy for the particular patient.

Lithium does not seem to protect against true clozapine-induced agranulocytosis: one case of fatal agranulocytosis has occurred with this combination[23] and a second case of agranulocytosis has been reported where the bone marrow was resistant to treatment with granulocyte colony-stimulating factor (G-CSF).[24]

Granulocyte colony-stimulating factor (G-CSF)

The use of G-CSF to facilitate uninterrupted clozapine therapy in patients with previous neutropenia is a strategy that is attracting increasing interest but is somewhat controversial. There are both successful[24–26] and unsuccessful[26,27] case reports of patients receiving regular long-term G-CSF to enable clozapine therapy. As well as the commonly reported adverse effects of bone pain[28] and neutrophil dysplasia,[29] the administration of G-CSF in the face of a low or declining neutrophil count may mask an impending neutropenia or agranulocytosis, leading to dire consequences. The long-term safety of G-CSF has not been determined; bone density and spleen size should probably be monitored.

'When required' G-CSF, to be administered if neutrophils drop below a defined threshold, may allow re-challenge with clozapine of patients in whom lithium is insufficient to prevent 'dipping' of WCC below the normal range. Again, this strategy risks masking a severe neutropenia or agranulocytosis. It is also likely to be practically difficult to manage outside a specialist unit, as frequent blood testing (twice to three times a week) is required, as well as immediate access to medical review and the G-CSF itself.

Consultation with a haematologist and discussion with the medical adviser at the clozapine monitoring service is essential before considering the use of G-CSF. A patient's individual clinical circumstances should be considered. In particular, patients should be considered to be very high risk for re-challenge with clozapine if the first episode of dyscrasia fulfilled any of the following criteria, all of which suggest that the low counts are clozapine-related:

- inconsistent with previous WCCs (i.e. not part of a pattern of repeated low WCCs)
- occurred within the first 18 weeks of treatment
- severe (neutrophils $<0.5 \times 10^9$/L), or
- prolonged.

While G-CSF has been reported as allowing successful re-challenge with clozapine in some people with previous episodes of clozapine-induced neutropenia,[30] the available evidence excludes this course of action for someone with a true clozapine-related agranulocytosis.[31]

CHAPTER 1

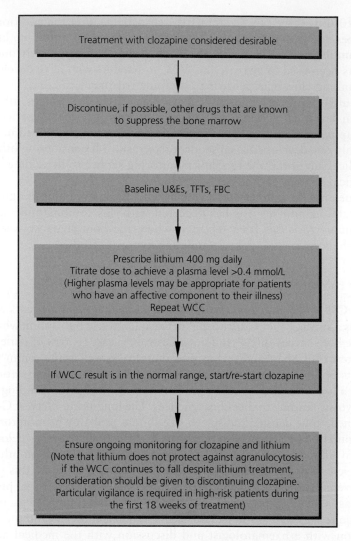

Figure 1.7 The use of lithium with clozapine. FBC, full blood count; TFTs, thyroid function tests; U&Es, urea and electrolytes; WCC, white cell count.

Management of patients with either of the following conditions is outlined in Figure 1.7.

- Low initial WCC ($<4 \times 10^9$/L) or neutrophils ($<2.5 \times 10^9$/L).
- Leucopenia (WCC $<3 \times 10^9$/L) or neutropenia (neutrophils $<1.5 \times 10^9$/L) thought to be linked to BEN. Such patients may be of African or Middle Eastern descent, have no history of susceptibility to infection and have morphologically normal white blood cells.[32]

References

1. Munro J et al. Active monitoring of 12760 clozapine recipients in the UK and Ireland. Br J Psychiatry 1999; **175**:576–580.

2. Whiskey E et al. Restarting clozapine after neutropenia: evaluating the possibilities and practicalities. CNS Drugs 2007; **21**:25–35.

3. Dunk LR et al. Rechallenge with clozapine following leucopenia or neutropenia during previous therapy. Br J Psychiatry 2006; **188**:255–263.

4. Prokopez CR et al. Clozapine rechallenge after neutropenia or leucopenia. J Clin Psychopharmacol 2016; **36**:377–380.

5. Ingimarsson O et al. Neutropenia and agranulocytosis during treatment of schizophrenia with clozapine versus other antipsychotics: an observational study in Iceland. BMC Psychiatry 2016; **16**:441.

6. Dettling M et al. Further evidence of human leukocyte antigen-encoded susceptibility to clozapine-induced agranulocytosis independent of ancestry. Pharmacogenetics 2001; **11**:135–141.

7. Nielsen J et al. Worldwide differences in regulations of clozapine use. CNS Drugs 2016; **30**:149–161.

8. FDA. FDA Drug Safety Communication: FDA modifies monitoring for neutropenia associated with schizophrenia medicine clozapine; approves new shared REMS program for all clozapine medicines. 2015. https://www.fda.gov/Drugs/DrugSafety/ucm461853.htm

9. Bachmann CJ et al. International trends in clozapine use: a study in 17 countries. Acta Psychiatr Scand 2017; **136**:37–51.

10. Manu P et al. Benign ethnic neutropenia and clozapine use: a systematic review of the evidence and treatment recommendations. J Clin Psychiatry 2016; **77**:e909–e916.

11. Richardson CM et al. Evaluation of the safety of clozapine use in patients with benign neutropenia. J Clin Psychiatry 2016; **77**:e1454–e1459.

12. Shuman MD et al. Exploring the potential effect of polypharmacy on the hematologic profiles of clozapine patients. J Psychiatr Pract 2014; **20**:50–58.

13. Whiskey E et al. The importance of the recognition of benign ethnic neutropenia in black patients during treatment with clozapine: case reports and database study. J Psychopharmacol 2011; **25**:842–845.

14. Paton C et al. Managing clozapine-induced neutropenia with lithium. Psychiatr Bull 2005; **29**:186–188.

15. Adityanjee A. Modification of clozapine-induced leukopenia and neutropenia with lithium carbonate. Am J Psychiatry 1995; **152**:648–649.

16. Silverstone PH. Prevention of clozapine-induced neutropenia by pretreatment with lithium. J Clin Psychopharmacol 1998; **18**:86–88.

17. Boshes RA et al. Initiation of clozapine therapy in a patient with preexisting leukopenia: a discussion of the rationale of current treatment options. Ann Clin Psychiatry 2001; **13**:233–237.

18. Papetti F et al. Treatment of clozapine-induced granulocytopenia with lithium (two observations). Encephale 2004; **30**:578–582.

19. Kutscher EC et al. Clozapine-induced leukopenia successfully treated with lithium. Am J Health Syst Pharm 2007; **64**:2027–2031.

20. Sporn A et al. Clozapine-induced neutropenia in children: management with lithium carbonate. J Child Adolesc Psychopharmacol 2003; **13**:401–404.

21. Mattai A et al. Adjunctive use of lithium carbonate for the management of neutropenia in clozapine-treated children. Hum Psychopharmacol 2009; **24**:584–589.

22. Kanaan RA et al. Lithium and clozapine rechallenge: a restrospective case analysis. J Clin Psychiatry 2006; **67**:756–760.

23. Valevski A et al. Clozapine-lithium combined treatment and agranulocytosis. Int Clin Psychopharmacol 1993; **8**:63–65.

24. Spencer BW et al. Granulocyte colony stimulating factor (G-CSF) can allow treatment with clozapine in a patient with severe benign ethnic neutropaenia (BEN): a case report. J Psychopharmacol 2012; **26**:1280–1282.

25. Hagg S et al. Long-term combination treatment with clozapine and filgrastim in patients with clozapine-induced agranulocytosis. Int Clin Psychopharmacol 2003; **18**:173–174.

26. Joffe G et al. Add-on filgrastim during clozapine rechallenge in patients with a history of clozapine-related granulocytopenia/agranulocytosis. Am J Psychiatry 2009; **166**:236.

27. Mathewson KA et al. Clozapine and granulocyte colony-stimulating factor: potential for long-term combination treatment for clozapine-induced neutropenia. J Clin Psychopharmacol 2007; **27**:714–715.

28. Puhalla S et al. Hematopoietic growth factors: personalization of risks and benefits. Mol Oncol 2012; **6**:237–241.

29. Bain BJ et al. Neutrophil dysplasia induced by granulocyte colony-stimulating factor. Am J Hematol 2010; **85**:354.

30. Myles N et al. Use of granulocyte-colony stimulating factor to prevent recurrent clozapine-induced neutropenia on drug rechallenge: a systematic review of the literature and clinical recommendations. Aust N Z J Psychiatry 2017; **51**:980–989.

31. Lally J et al. The use of granulocyte colony-stimulating factor in clozapine rechallenge: a systematic review. J Clin Psychopharmacol 2017; **37**:600–604.

32. Hsieh MM et al. Prevalence of neutropenia in the U.S. population: age, sex, smoking status, and ethnic differences. Ann Intern Med 2007; **146**:486–492.

CHAPTER 1

Clozapine and chemotherapy

The use of clozapine with agents that cause neutropenia is formally contraindicated. Most chemotherapy treatments cause significant bone marrow suppression. When the WCC drops below 3.0×10^9/L, clozapine is usually discontinued; this is an important safety precaution outlined in the formal licence/labelling. In many regimens it can be predicted that chemotherapy will reduce the WCC below this level, irrespective of the use of clozapine.

Where possible, clozapine should be discontinued before chemotherapy. However, this will place most patients at high risk of relapse or deterioration, which may then affect their capacity to consent to chemotherapy. This poses a therapeutic dilemma in patients prescribed clozapine and requiring chemotherapy. In practice, many patients, perhaps even a majority, continue clozapine during chemotherapy.

There are a number of case reports supporting continuing clozapine during chemotherapy,[1–18] but interpretation of this literature should take account of possible publication bias.[2] Before initiating chemotherapy in a patient receiving clozapine it is essential to put in place a treatment plan that is agreed with all relevant health-care staff involved and, of course, the patient and family members/carers; this will include the oncologist/physician, psychiatrist, pharmacist and the clozapine monitoring service. Plans should be made in advance for the action that should be taken when the WCC drops below the normally accepted minimum. This plan should cover the frequency of haematological monitoring, increased vigilance regarding the clinical consequences of neutropenia/agranulocytosis, if and when clozapine should be stopped, and the place of 'antidote' medication such as lithium and G-CSF.

In the UK, the clozapine monitoring service will normally ask for the psychiatrist to sign an 'unlicensed use' form and will request additional blood monitoring. Complications appear to be rare but there is one case report of neutropenia persisting for 6 months after doxorubicin, radiotherapy and clozapine.[8] G-CSF has been used to treat agranulocytosis associated with chemotherapy and clozapine in combination.[9,10,19] Risks of life-threatening blood dyscrasia are probably lowest in those who have received clozapine for longer than a year, in whom clozapine-induced neutropenia would be highly unusual.

Summary

- If possible, clozapine should be discontinued before starting chemotherapy. However, for most patients withdrawal is not possible or sensible.
- The risk of relapse or deterioration must be considered before discontinuing clozapine.
- If the patient's mental state deteriorates they may retract their consent for chemotherapy.
- When clozapine is continued during chemotherapy a collaborative approach between the oncologist, psychiatrist, pharmacy, patient and clozapine monitoring service is strongly recommended.

References

1. Wesson ML et al. Continuing clozapine despite neutropenia. Br J Psychiatry 1996; **168**:217–220.
2. Cunningham NT et al. Continuation of clozapine during chemotherapy: a case report and review of literature. Psychosomatics 2014; **55**:673–679.
3. Bareggi C et al. Clozapine and full-dose concomitant chemoradiation therapy in a schizophrenic patient with nasopharyngeal cancer. Tumori 2002; **88**:59–60.
4. Avnon M et al. Clozapine, cancer, and schizophrenia. Am J Psychiatry 1993; **150**:1562–1563.
5. Hundertmark J et al. Reintroduction of clozapine after diagnosis of lymphoma. Br J Psychiatry 2001; **178**:576.
6. McKenna RC et al. Clozapine and chemotherapy. Hosp Community Psychiatry 1994; **45**:831.
7. Haut FA. Clozapine and chemotherapy. J Drug Dev Clin Pract 1995; **7**:237–239.
8. Rosenstock J. Clozapine therapy during cancer treatment. Am J Psychiatry 2004; **161**:175.
9. Lee SY et al. Combined antitumor chemotherapy in a refractory schizophrenic receiving clozapine (Korean). J Korean Neuropsychiatr Assoc 2000; **39**:234–239.
10. Usta NG et al. Clozapine treatment of refractory schizophrenia during essential chemotherapy: a case study and mini review of a clinical dilemma. Ther Adv Psychopharmacol 2014; **4**:276–281.
11. Rosenberg I et al. Restarting clozapine treatment during ablation chemotherapy and stem cell transplant for Hodgkin's lymphoma. Am J Psychiatry 2007; **164**:1438–1439.
12. Goulet K et al. Case report: clozapine given in the context of chemotherapy for lung cancer. Psychooncology 2008; **17**:512–516.
13. Frieri T et al. Maintaining clozapine treatment during chemotherapy for non-Hodgkin's lymphoma. Prog Neuropsychopharmacol Biol Psychiatry 2008; **32**:1611–1612.
14. Sankaranarayanan A et al. Clozapine, cancer chemotherapy and neutropenia – dilemmas in management. Psychiatr Danub 2013; **25**:419–422.
15. De Berardis D et al. Safety and efficacy of combined clozapine-azathioprine treatment in a case of resistant schizophrenia associated with Behçet's disease: a 2-year follow-up. Gen Hosp Psychiatry 2013; **35**:213.
16. Deodhar JK et al. Clozapine and cancer treatment: adding to the experience and evidence. Indian J Psychiatry 2014; **56**:191–193.
17. Monga V et al. Clozapine and concomitant chemotherapy in a patient with schizophrenia and new onset esophageal cancer. Psychooncology 2015; **24**:971–972.
18. Overbeeke MR et al. Successful clozapine continuation during chemotherapy for the treatment of malignancy: a case report. Int J Clin Pharm 2016; **38**:199–202.
19. Kolli V et al. Treating chemotherapy induced agranulocytosis with granulocyte colony-stimulating factors in a patient on clozapine. Psychooncology 2013; **22**:1674–1675.

Chapter 2

Bipolar disorder

Lithium

Mechanism of action

Lithium is an element in the same group of the periodic table as sodium. The ubiquitous nature of sodium in the human body, its involvement in a wide range of biological processes and the potential for lithium to alter these processes (and lithium's multiplicity of other effects) have made it extremely difficult to ascertain the key mechanism(s) of action of lithium in regulating mood and behaviour. For example, there is some older evidence that people with bipolar illness have higher intracellular concentrations of sodium and calcium than controls and that lithium can reduce these. Glycogen synthase kinase 3 (GSK3), cAMP response element-binding protein (CREB) and Na^+/K^+-ATPase related mechanisms may be important for lithium's effects. For a recent review of lithium's potential mechanism(s) of action see Alda.[1] Lithium may have neuroprotective effects that preserve the function of neurones and neuronal circuits.[2] Lithium also promotes the creation of new neurones (neurogenesis) in the hippocampus, which is potentially important for learning, memory and stress responses.[3] Although the older literature pertaining to the possible neuroprotective effect of lithium consisted largely of either *in vitro* or animal studies, a recent meta-analysis suggests lithium may prevent transition to dementia.[4] Notably, however, both reversible and irreversible neurotoxicity related to lithium are recognised adverse effects.[5,6]

Clinical indications

Acute treatment of mania

Lithium is effective for the treatment of mania, at a plasma level of 0.8–1.0 mmol/L.[7] If a faster action is needed an adjunctive or single-agent antipsychotic with an evidence base for treating mania is recommended.[7] It can be difficult to achieve therapeutic plasma lithium levels rapidly and monitoring may be problematic if the patient is uncooperative.

The Maudsley Prescribing Guidelines in Psychiatry, Thirteenth Edition. David M. Taylor, Thomas R. E. Barnes and Allan H. Young.
© 2018 David M. Taylor. Published 2018 by John Wiley & Sons Ltd.

Treatment of acute mania in patients already on long-term lithium

British Association for Psychopharmacology (BAP) guidelines[7] suggest that in the event of relapse an urgent plasma lithium level should be obtained to indicate the level of compliance with lithium therapy and inform possible dose adjustment. If lithium level measurement indicates non-compliance, the reason should be ascertained. If the lithium level is confirmed to be optimal, but the control of mania is inadequate, then addition of a dopamine antagonist, dopamine partial agonist or valproate is recommended.[7]

Maintenance treatment of bipolar disorder

Aim for the highest tolerable lithium plasma level in the range 0.6–0.8 mmol/L[7] with the aim of complete remission of both manic and depressive episodes.[8] Lithium may be the best performing medicine for bipolar disorder in practice: Hayes et al.[9] prospectively analysed the progress of 5089 bipolar patients prescribed monotherapy maintenance treatment: lithium (n = 1505), olanzapine (n = 1366), valproate (n = 1173) and quetiapine (n = 1075). It was found that monotherapy failure in 75% of each cohort occurred by 2.05 years for lithium monotherapy, 1.13 years for olanzapine monotherapy, 0.98 years for valproate monotherapy, and 0.76 years for quetiapine monotherapy.[9]

Augmentation of antidepressants in unipolar depression

Approximately 30–50% of patients fail to respond to trials of first- or second-line antidepressants, and outcomes from 'treatment-resistant depression' are poor.[10] Providing evidence-based guidelines for treating depressive orders with antidepressants, Cleare et al.[11] suggest that either lithium or quetiapine are agents of first choice for augmenting the existing antidepressant and that lithium augmentation of selective serotonin reuptake inhibitors (SSRIs) or venlafaxine is most effective at a lithium plasma level of 0.6–1.0 mmol/L. To help determine which, if either, is the better of these two augmenting agents over a follow-up period of one year, a head-to-head, parallel group, open-label, multisite randomised pragmatic trial of lithium versus quetiapine augmentation in treatment-resistant depression (LQD) was initiated in England in 2017.[12] Clinical predictors associated with a better outcome in lithium augmentation for treatment-resistant depression included: more severe depressive symptomatology, psychomotor retardation, significant weight loss, a family history of major depression, and a personal experience of more than three episodes.[13] Of course, compliance with lithium augmentation should also be added to this list.

Prophylaxis of unipolar depression

The use of lithium for long-term treatment of unipolar depression has recently been reviewed.[14] Cipriani et al. (2006)[15] analysed eight randomised controlled trials (n = 475) and found lithium was significantly superior to antidepressants in preventing relapses that required hospitalisation with a relative risk of 0.34. Abou-Saleh et al. (2017)[16] proposed lithium prophylaxis in unipolar depression if a patient has suffered two depressive episodes in 5 years, or after one episode if the episode is severe and there is a strong suicide risk, with indefinite treatment if there is adherence and adverse events are not problematic, particularly if a bipolar background is suspected.

Other uses of lithium

Lithium is also used to treat aggressive and self-mutilating behaviour, and recent studies have confirmed benefits[17] to both prevent and treat steroid-induced psychosis[18] and to raise the white blood cell count in patients receiving clozapine.[19]

Lithium and suicide

It is estimated that 15% of people with bipolar disorder eventually take their own life.[20] A meta-analysis of clinical trials concluded that lithium reduced by 80% the risk of both attempted and completed suicide in patients with bipolar illness[21] and large database studies have shown that lithium-treated patients are less likely to complete suicide than patients treated with other mood-stabilising drugs.[22]

In patients with unipolar depression, lithium also seems to protect against suicide although the mechanism of this protective effect is unknown.[21]

Plasma levels

The minimum effective plasma level for prophylaxis is 0.4 mmol/L, with the optimal range being 0.6–1.2 mmol/L.[23] Levels above 0.75 mmol/L offer additional protection only against manic symptoms[24] so the target range for prophylaxis is effectively 0.6–0.75 mmol/L. Changes in plasma levels seem to worsen the risk of relapse.[24] The optimal plasma level range in patients who have unipolar depression is less clear and much research remains to be done in this area.[14]

Children and adolescents may require higher plasma levels than adults to ensure that an adequate concentration of lithium is present in the central nervous system (CNS).[25]

Lithium is rapidly absorbed from the gastrointestinal tract but has a long distribution phase. Blood samples for plasma lithium level estimations should be taken 10–14 (ideally 12) hours post dose in patients who are prescribed a single daily dose of a prolonged release preparation at bedtime.[7]

Formulations

There is no clinically significant difference in the pharmacokinetics of the two most widely prescribed brands of lithium in the UK: Priadel and Camcolit. Other preparations should not be assumed to be bioequivalent and should be prescribed by brand.

- Lithium carbonate 400 mg tablets each contain 10.8 mmol/lithium.
- Lithium citrate liquid is available in two strengths and should be administered twice daily:
  - 5.4 mmol/5 mL is equivalent to 200 mg lithium carbonate
  - 10.8 mmol/5 mL is equivalent to 400 mg lithium carbonate.

Lack of clarity over which liquid preparation is intended when prescribing can lead to the patient receiving a subtherapeutic or toxic dose.

CHAPTER 2

Adverse effects

Most adverse effects are dose and plasma level related. These include mild gastrointestinal upset, fine tremor, polyuria and polydipsia. Polyuria may occur more frequently with twice-daily dosing.[26,27] Propranolol can be useful in lithium-induced tremor. Some skin conditions such as psoriasis and acne can be aggravated by lithium therapy. Lithium can also cause a metallic taste in the mouth, ankle oedema and weight gain.

Lithium is often responsible for a reduction in urinary concentrating capacity – nephrogenic diabetes insipidus – hence the occurrence of thirst and polyuria. This effect is usually reversible in the short to medium term but may be irreversible after long-term treatment (>15 years).[28] Lithium treatment can also lead to a reduction in the glomerular filtration rate although the magnitude of the risk is uncertain.[28] Lithium levels of >0.8 mmol/L are associated with a higher risk of renal toxicity, and prolonged lithium treatment requires regular monitoring of kidney function.[29]

In the longer term, lithium increases the risk of hypothyroidism;[30] in middle-aged women, the risk may be up to 20%.[31] A case has been made for testing thyroid autoantibodies in this group before starting lithium (to better estimate risk) and for measuring thyroid function tests (TFTs) more frequently in the first year of treatment.[32] Hypothyroidism is easily treated with thyroxine. TFTs usually return to normal when lithium is discontinued. Lithium also increases the risk of hyperparathyroidism, and some recommend that calcium levels should be monitored in patients on long-term treatment.[33] Clinical consequences of chronically increased serum calcium include renal stones, osteoporosis, dyspepsia, hypertension and renal impairment. For a review of the toxicity profile of lithium, see McKnight et al.[33]

Lithium toxicity

Toxic effects reliably occur at levels >1.5 mmol/L and usually consist of gastrointestinal effects (increasing anorexia, nausea and diarrhoea) and CNS effects (muscle weakness, drowsiness, confusion, ataxia, coarse tremor and muscle twitching).[34] Above 2 mmol/L, increased disorientation and seizures usually occur, which can progress to coma, and ultimately death. In the presence of more severe symptoms, osmotic or forced alkaline diuresis should be used (NB **never** thiazide or loop diuretics). Above 3 mmol/L, peritoneal dialysis or haemodialysis is often used. These plasma levels are only a guide and individuals vary in their susceptibility to symptoms of toxicity. Neurotoxicity at normal plasma levels has also been described as brain lithium levels may not be reflected in the plasma.[35]

Most **risk factors for toxicity** involve changes in sodium levels or the way the body handles sodium, for example, low-salt diets, dehydration, drug interactions (see Table 2.2) and some uncommon physical illnesses such as Addison's disease.

Information relating to the symptoms of toxicity and the common risk factors should always be given to patients when treatment with lithium is initiated.[36] This information should be repeated at appropriate intervals to make sure that it is clearly understood.

Pre-treatment tests

Before prescribing lithium, renal, thyroid and cardiac function should be checked. As a minimum, eGFR[37] and TFTs should be checked. An ECG is also recommended in patients who have risk factors for, or existing cardiovascular disease. A baseline measure of weight is also desirable.

Lithium is a human teratogen. Women of child-bearing age should be advised to use a reliable form of contraception. See section on 'Drug choice in pregnancy' (Chapter 7).

On-treatment monitoring[7]

BAP guidelines recommend that before lithium is prescribed, baseline eGFR, thyroid function and calcium should be checked. Plasma lithium, eGFR and TFTs should be checked every 6 months. More frequent tests may be required in those who are prescribed interacting drugs, elderly or have established chronic kidney disease (CKD). A patient safety alert related to the importance of biochemical monitoring in patients prescribed lithium has been issued by the National Patient Safety Agency.[38] Weight (or BMI) should also be monitored. Lithium monitoring in clinical practice in the UK is known to be suboptimal,[39] although there has been a modest improvement over time.[40] The use of automated reminder systems has been shown to improve monitoring rates.[41]

Discontinuation

Intermittent treatment with lithium may worsen the natural course of bipolar illness. A much greater than expected incidence of manic relapse is seen in the first few months after abruptly discontinuing lithium,[42] even in patients who have been symptom free for as long as 5 years.[43] This has led to recommendations that lithium treatment should not be started unless there is a clear intention to continue it for at least 3 years.[44] This advice has obvious implications for initiating lithium treatment against a patient's will (or in a patient known to be non-compliant with medication) during a period of acute illness.

The risk of relapse **may** be reduced by decreasing the dose gradually over a period of at least a month[45] and avoiding decremental plasma level reductions of >0.2 mmol/L.[24] In contrast with these recommendations, a naturalistic study found that, in patients who had been in remission for at least 2 years and had discontinued lithium very slowly, the recurrence rate was at least three times greater than in patients who continued lithium; significant survival differences persisted for many years. Patients maintained on high lithium levels prior to discontinuation were particularly prone to relapse.[46]

One large US study based on prescription records found that half of those prescribed lithium took almost all of their prescribed doses, a quarter took between 50 and 80%, and the remaining quarter took less than 50%; in addition a third of patients took lithium for less than 6 months in total.[47] A large audit found that one in ten patients prescribed long-term lithium treatment had a plasma level below the therapeutic range.[48] It is clear that suboptimal adherence limits the effectiveness of lithium in clinical practice. One database study suggested that the extent to which lithium was taken was directly related to the risk of suicide (more prescriptions = lower suicide rate).[49]

Less convincing data support the emergence of depressive symptoms in bipolar patients after lithium discontinuation.[42] There are few data relating to patients with unipolar depression.

Prescribing and monitoring recommendations for lithium are summarised in Table 2.1.

Table 2.1 Lithium: prescribing and monitoring

Indications	Mania, hypomania, prophylaxis of bipolar affective disorder and recurrent depression. Reduces aggression and suicidality
Pre-lithium work-up	e-GRF and TFTs. ECG recommended in patients who have risk factors for, or existing cardiovascular disease. Baseline measure of weight and calcium desirable
Prescribing	Start at 400 mg at night (200 mg in the elderly). Plasma level after 7 days, then 7 days after every dose change until the desired level is reached (0.4 mmol/L may be effective in unipolar depression, 0.6–1.0 mmol/L in bipolar illness, slightly higher levels in difficult-to-treat mania). Blood should be taken 12 hours after the last dose. Take care when prescribing liquid preparations to clearly specify the strength required
Monitoring	Plasma lithium every 6 months (more frequent monitoring is necessary in those prescribed interacting drugs, the elderly and those with established renal impairment or other relevant physical illness). eGFR and TFTs every 6 months. Weight (or BMI) and calcium should also be monitored
Stopping	Reduce slowly over at least 1 month
	Avoid incremental reductions in plasma levels of >0.2 mmol/L

BMI, body mass index; ECG, electrocardiogram; eGFR, estimated glomerular filtration rate; TFT, thyroid function test.

Interactions with other drugs[50–52]

Because of lithium's relatively narrow therapeutic index, pharmacokinetic interactions with other drugs can precipitate lithium toxicity. Most clinically significant interactions are with drugs that alter renal sodium handling (Table 2.2).

Table 2.2 Lithium: clinically relevant drug interactions

Drug group	Magnitude of effect	Timescale of effect	Additional information
ACE inhibitors	▪ Unpredictable ▪ Up to 4-fold increases in [Li]	Develops over several weeks	▪ 7-fold increased risk of hospitalisation for lithium toxicity in the elderly ▪ **Angiotensin II receptor antagonists** may be associated with similar risk
Thiazide diuretics	▪ Unpredictable ▪ Up to 4-fold increases in [Li]	Usually apparent in first 10 days	▪ Loop diuretics are safer ▪ Any effect will be apparent in the first month
NSAIDs	▪ Unpredictable ▪ From 10% to >4-fold increases in [Li]	Variable; few days to several months	▪ NSAIDs are widely used on a prn basis ▪ Can be bought without a prescription

ACE, angiotensin converting enzyme; [Li], lithium; NSAIDs, non-steroidal anti-inflammatory drugs; prn, *pro re nata* (as required).

Angiotensin-converting enzyme (ACE) inhibitors

ACE inhibitors can (i) reduce thirst, which can lead to mild dehydration, and (ii) increase renal sodium loss leading to increased sodium re-absorption by the kidney, resulting in an increase in lithium plasma levels. The magnitude of this effect is variable, from no increase to a four-fold increase. The full effect can take several weeks to develop. The risk seems to be increased in patients with heart failure, dehydration and renal impairment (presumably because of changes in fluid balance/handling). In the elderly, ACE inhibitors increase seven-fold the risk of hospitalisation due to lithium toxicity. ACE inhibitors can also precipitate renal failure so, if co-prescribed with lithium, more frequent monitoring of eGFR and plasma lithium is required.

The following drugs are ACE inhibitors: captopril, cilazapril, enalapril, fosinopril, imidapril, lisinopril, moexipril, perindopril, quinapril, ramipril and trandolapril.

Care is also required with **angiotensin II receptor antagonists**: candesartan, eprosartan, irbesartan, losartan, olmesartan, telmisartan and valsartan.

Diuretics

Diuretics can reduce the renal clearance of lithium, the magnitude of this effect being greater with thiazide than loop diuretics. Lithium levels usually rise within 10 days of a **thiazide diuretic** being prescribed; the magnitude of the rise is unpredictable and can vary from an increase of 25 to 400%.

The following drugs are thiazide (or related) diuretics: bendroflumethiazide, chlortalidone, cyclopenthiazide, indapamide, metolazone and xipamide.

Although there are case reports of lithium toxicity induced by **loop diuretics**, many patients receive this combination of drugs without apparent problems. The risk of an interaction seems to be greatest in the first month after the loop diuretic has been prescribed and extra lithium plasma level monitoring during this time is recommended if these drugs are co-prescribed. Loop diuretics can increase sodium loss and subsequent re-absorption by the kidney. Patients taking loop diuretics may also have been advised to restrict their salt intake; this may contribute to the risk of lithium toxicity in these individuals.

The following drugs are loop diuretics: bumetanide, furosemide and torasemide.

Non-steroidal anti-inflammatory drugs (NSAIDs)

NSAIDs inhibit the synthesis of renal prostaglandins, thereby reducing renal blood flow and possibly increasing renal re-absorption of sodium and therefore lithium. The magnitude of the rise is unpredictable for any given patient; case reports vary from increases of around 10% to over 400%. The onset of effect also seems to be variable; from a few days to several months. Risk appears to be increased in those patients who have impaired renal function, renal artery stenosis or heart failure and who are dehydrated or on a low-salt diet. There are a number of case reports of an interaction between lithium and COX-2 inhibitors. NSAIDs do not appear to diminish the therapeutic effects of lithium,[53] as has previously been reported.

NSAIDs (or COX-2 inhibitors) can be combined with lithium but (i) they should be prescribed regularly, **not** prn, and (ii) more frequent plasma lithium monitoring is essential.

Some NSAIDs can be purchased without a prescription, so it is particularly important that patients are aware of the potential for interaction.

The following drugs are NSAIDs or COX-2 inhibitors: aceclofenac, acemetacin, celecoxib, dexibuprofen, dexketoprofen, diclofenac, diflunisal, etodolac, etoricoxib, fenbufen, fenoprofen, flurbiprofen, ibuprofen, indometacin, ketoprofen, lumiracoxib, mefenamic acid, meloxicam, nabumetone, naproxen, piroxicam, sulindac, tenoxicam and tiaprofenic acid.

Carbamazepine

There are rare reports of neurotoxicity when carbamazepine is combined with lithium. Most are old and in the context of treatment involving high plasma lithium levels. It is of note though that carbamazepine can cause hyponatraemia, which may in turn lead to lithium retention and toxicity. Similarly, rare reports of CNS toxicity implicate SSRIs, another group of drugs that can cause hyponatraemia.

References

1. Alda M. Lithium in the treatment of bipolar disorder: pharmacology and pharmacogenetics. Mol Psychiatry 2015; 20:661–670.
2. Jope RS, Nemeroff CB. Lithium to the Rescue. 2016. http://dana.org/Cerebrum/2016/Lithium_to_the_Rescue/.
3. Hanson ND et al. Lithium, but not fluoxetine or the corticotropin-releasing factor receptor 1 receptor antagonist R121919, increases cell proliferation in the adult dentate gyrus. J Pharmacol Exp Ther 2011; 337:180–186.
4. Matsunaga S et al. Lithium as a treatment for Alzheimer's disease: a systematic review and meta-analysis. J Alzheimers Dis 2015; 48:403–410.
5. Netto I et al. Reversible lithium neurotoxicity: review of the literature. Prim Care Companion CNS Disord 2012; 14: PCC.11r01197.
6. Adityanjee et al. The syndrome of irreversible lithium-effectuated neurotoxicity. Clin Neuropharmacol 2005; 28:38–49.
7. Goodwin GM et al. Evidence-based guidelines for treating bipolar disorder: revised third edition recommendations from the British Association for Psychopharmacology. J Psychopharmacol 2016; 30:495–553.
8. Severus E et al. Lithium for prevention of mood episodes in bipolar disorders: systematic review and meta-analysis. Int J Bipolar Disord 2014; 2:15.
9. Hayes JF et al. Lithium vs. valproate vs. olanzapine vs. quetiapine as maintenance monotherapy for bipolar disorder: a population-based UK cohort study using electronic health records. World Psychiatry 2016; 15:53–58.
10. Dunner DL et al. Prospective, long-term, multicenter study of the naturalistic outcomes of patients with treatment-resistant depression. J Clin Psychiatry 2006; 67:688–695.
11. Cleare A et al. Evidence-based guidelines for treating depressive disorders with antidepressants: a revision of the 2008 British Association for Psychopharmacology guidelines. J Psychopharmacol 2015; 29:459–525.
12. Marwood L et al. Study protocol for a randomised pragmatic trial comparing the clinical and cost effectiveness of lithium and quetiapine augmentation in treatment resistant depression (the LQD study). BMC Psychiatry 2017; 17:231.
13. Bauer M et al. Role of lithium augmentation in the management of major depressive disorder. CNS Drugs 2014; 28:331–342.
14. Young AH. Lithium for long-term treatment of unipolar depression. Lancet Psychiatry 2017; 4:511–512.
15. Cipriani A et al. Lithium versus antidepressants in the long-term treatment of unipolar affective disorder. Cochrane Database Syst Rev 2006:CD003492.
16. Abou-Saleh MT et al. Lithium in the episode and suicide prophylaxis and in augmenting strategies in patients with unipolar depression. Int J Bipolar Disord 2017; 5:11.
17. Correll CU et al. Biological treatment of acute agitation or aggression with schizophrenia or bipolar disorder in the inpatient setting. Ann Clin Psychiatry 2017; 29:92–107.
18. Sirois F. Steroid psychosis: a review. Gen Hosp Psychiatry 2003; 25:27–33.
19. Aydin M et al. Continuing clozapine treatment with lithium in schizophrenic patients with neutropenia or leukopenia: brief review of literature with case reports. Ther Adv Psychopharmacol 2016; 6:33–38.
20. Harris EC et al. Excess mortality of mental disorder. Br J Psychiatry 1998; 173:11–53.
21. Cipriani A et al. Lithium in the prevention of suicide in mood disorders: updated systematic review and meta-analysis. BMJ 2013; 346:f3646.
22. Hayes JF et al. Self-harm, unintentional injury, and suicide in bipolar disorder during maintenance mood stabilizer treatment: a UK population-based electronic health records study. JAMA Psychiatry 2016; 73:630–637.
23. Nolen WA et al. The association of the effect of lithium in the maintenance treatment of bipolar disorder with lithium plasma levels: a post hoc analysis of a double-blind study comparing switching to lithium or placebo in patients who responded to quetiapine (Trial 144). Bipolar Disord 2013; 15:100–109.

24. Severus WE et al. What is the optimal serum lithium level in the long-term treatment of bipolar disorder--a review? Bipolar Disord 2008; 10:231–237.

25. Moore CM et al. Brain-to-serum lithium ratio and age: an in vivo magnetic resonance spectroscopy study. Am J Psychiatry 2002; 159:1240–1242.

26. Bowen RC et al. Less frequent lithium administration and lower urine volume. Am J Psychiatry 1991; 148:189–192.

27. Ljubicic D et al. Lithium treatments: single and multiple daily dosing. Can J Psychiatry 2008; 53:323–331.

28. Gong R et al. What we need to know about the effect of lithium on the kidney. Am J Physiol Renal Physiol 2016; 311:F1168–f1171.

29. Aiff H et al. Effects of 10 to 30 years of lithium treatment on kidney function. J Psychopharmacol 2015; 29:608–614.

30. Frye MA et al. Depressive relapse during lithium treatment associated with increased serum thyroid-stimulating hormone: results from two placebo-controlled bipolar I maintenance studies. Acta Psychiatr Scand 2009; 120:10–13.

31. Johnston AM et al. Lithium-associated clinical hypothyroidism. Prevalence and risk factors. Br J Psychiatry 1999; 175:336–339.

32. Livingstone C et al. Lithium: a review of its metabolic adverse effects. J Psychopharmacol 2006; 20:347–355.

33. McKnight RF et al. Lithium toxicity profile: a systematic review and meta-analysis. Lancet 2012; 379:721–728.

34. Ott M et al. Lithium intoxication: incidence, clinical course and renal function – a population-based retrospective cohort study. J Psychopharmacol 2016; 30:1008–1019.

35. Bell AJ et al. Lithium neurotoxicity at normal therapeutic levels. Br J Psychiatry 1993; 162:689–692.

36. Gerrett D et al. Prescribing and monitoring lithium therapy: summary of a safety report from the National Patient Safety Agency. BMJ 2010; 341:c6258.

37. Morriss R et al. Lithium and eGFR: a new routinely available tool for the prevention of chronic kidney disease. Br J Psychiatry 2008; 193:93–95.

38. National Patient Safety Agency. Safer lithium therapy. NPSA/2009/PSA005. http://www.nrls.npsa.nhs.uk/2009.

39. Collins N et al. Standards of lithium monitoring in mental health trusts in the UK. BMC Psychiatry 2010; 10:80.

40. Paton C et al. Monitoring lithium therapy: the impact of a quality improvement programme in the UK. Bipolar Disord 2013; 15:865–875.

41. Kirkham E et al. Impact of active monitoring on lithium management in Norfolk. Ther Adv Psychopharmacol 2013; 3:260–265.

42. Cavanagh J et al. Relapse into mania or depression following lithium discontinuation: a 7-year follow-up. Acta Psychiatr Scand 2004; 109:91–95.

43. Yazici O et al. Controlled lithium discontinuation in bipolar patients with good response to long-term lithium prophylaxis. J Affect Disord 2004; 80:269–271.

44. Goodwin GM. Recurrence of mania after lithium withdrawal. Implications for the use of lithium in the treatment of bipolar affective disorder. Br J Psychiatry 1994; 164:149–152.

45. Baldessarini RJ et al. Effects of the rate of discontinuing lithium maintenance treatment in bipolar disorders. J Clin Psychiatry 1996; 57:441–448.

46. Biel MG et al. Continuation versus discontinuation of lithium in recurrent bipolar illness: a naturalistic study. Bipolar Disord 2007; 9:435–442.

47. Sajatovic M et al. Treatment adherence with lithium and anticonvulsant medications among patients with bipolar disorder. Psychiatr Serv 2007; 58:855–863.

48. Paton C et al. Lithium in bipolar and other affective disorders: prescribing practice in the UK. J Psychopharmacol 2010; 24:1739–1746.

49. Kessing LV et al. Suicide risk in patients treated with lithium. Arch Gen Psychiatry 2005; 62:860–866.

50. Medicines Complete. Stockley's Drug Interactions. 2017. https://www.medicinescomplete.com.

51. Juurlink DN et al. Drug-induced lithium toxicity in the elderly: a population-based study. J Am Geriatr Soc 2004; 52:794–798.

52. Finley PR. Drug Interactions with lithium: an update. Clin Pharmacokinet 2016; 55:925–941.

53. Kohler-Forsberg O et al. Nonsteroidal anti-inflammatory drugs (NSAIDs) and paracetamol do not affect 6-month mood-stabilizing treatment outcome among 482 patients with bipolar disorder. Depress Anxiety 2017; 34:281–290.

CHAPTER 2

Valproate

Mechanism of action[1]

Valproate is a simple branched-chain fatty acid. Its mechanism of action is complex and not fully understood. Valproate inhibits the catabolism of γ-aminobutyric acid (GABA), reduces the turnover of arachidonic acid, activates the extracellular signal-regulated kinase (ERK) pathway thus altering synaptic plasticity, interferes with intracellular signalling, promotes brain-derived neurotrophic factor (BDNF) expression and reduces levels of protein kinase C. Recent research has focused on the ability of valproate to alter the expression of multiple genes that are involved in transcription regulation, cytoskeletal modifications and ion homeostasis. Other mechanisms that have been proposed include depletion of inositol, and indirect effects on non-GABA pathways through inhibition of voltage-gated sodium channels.

There is a growing literature relating to the potential use of valproate as an adjunctive treatment in several types of cancer, the relevant mechanism of action being inhibition of histone deacetylase,[2-4] a property which may also confer some effects on neuroplasticity.[5]

Formulations

Valproate is available in the UK in three forms: sodium valproate and valproic acid (licensed for the treatment of epilepsy), and semi-sodium valproate, licensed for the treatment of acute mania. Both semi-sodium and sodium valproate are metabolised to valproic acid, which is responsible for the pharmacological activity of all three preparations.[6] Clinical studies of the treatment of affective disorders variably use sodium valproate, semi-sodium valproate, 'valproate' or valproic acid. The great majority have used semi-sodium valproate.

In the USA, valproic acid is widely used in the treatment of bipolar illness,[7] and in the UK sodium valproate is widely used. It is important to remember that doses of sodium valproate and semi-sodium valproate are not equivalent; a slightly higher (approximately 10%) dose is required if sodium valproate is used to allow for the extra sodium content.

It is unclear if there is any difference in efficacy between valproic acid, valproate semi-sodium and sodium valproate. One large US quasi-experimental study found that in-patients who initially received the semi-sodium preparation had a hospital stay that was a third longer than patients who initially received valproic acid.[8] Note that sodium valproate controlled release (Epilim Chrono) can be administered as a once-daily dose whereas other sodium and semi-sodium valproate preparations require at least twice-daily administration.

Indications

Randomised controlled trials (RCTs) have shown valproate to be effective in the treatment of **mania**,[9,10] with a response rate of 50% and a number needed to treat (NNT) of 2–4,[11] although large negative studies do exist.[12] One RCT found lithium to be more effective overall than valproate[10] but a large (n = 300) randomised open trial of 12 weeks duration found lithium and valproate to be equally effective in the treatment of acute mania.[13] Valproate may be effective in patients who have failed to respond to lithium; in a small placebo-controlled RCT (n = 36) in patients who had failed to respond to or could not tolerate lithium, the median decrease in Young Mania Rating Scale scores was 54% in the valproate group and 5% in the placebo group.[14] It may be less effective than olanzapine, both as monotherapy[15] **and** as an adjunctive treatment to lithium[12] in acute mania. A network meta-analysis reported that valproate was less effective but better tolerated than lithium.[16]

A meta-analysis of four small RCTs concluded that valproate is effective in **bipolar depression** with a small to medium effect size[17] although further data are required.[11]

Although open-label studies suggest that valproate is effective in the **prophylaxis** of bipolar affective disorder,[18] RCT data are limited.[19,20] Bowden et al.[21] found no difference between lithium, valproate and placebo in the primary outcome measure, time to any mood episode, although valproate was superior to lithium and placebo on some secondary outcome measures. This study can be criticised for including patients who were 'not ill enough' and for not lasting 'long enough' (1 year). In another RCT,[19] which lasted for 47 weeks, there was no difference in relapse rates between valproate and olanzapine. The study had no placebo arm and the attrition rate was high, so it is difficult to interpret. A *post hoc* analysis of data from this study found that patients with rapid cycling illness had a better very early response to valproate than to olanzapine but that this advantage was not maintained.[20] Outcomes with respect to manic symptoms for those who did not have a rapid cycling illness were better at 1 year with olanzapine than valproate. In a further 20-month RCT of lithium versus valproate in patients with rapid cycling illness, both the relapse and attrition rate were high, and no difference in efficacy between valproate and lithium was apparent.[22] More recently, the BALANCE study found lithium to be numerically superior to valproate, and the combination of lithium and valproate statistically superior to valproate alone.[23] Aripiprazole in combination with valproate is superior to valproate alone.[24]

NICE recommends valproate as a first-line option for the treatment of acute episodes of mania, in combination with an antidepressant for the treatment of acute episodes of depression, and for prophylaxis,[25] but importantly **not** in women of child-bearing potential.[25,26] Cochrane conclude that the evidence supporting the use of valproate as prophylaxis is limited,[27] yet use for this indication has substantially increased in recent years.[28]

Valproate is sometimes used to treat aggressive behaviours of variable aetiology.[29] One **very** small RCT (n = 16) failed to detect any advantage for risperidone augmented with valproate over risperidone alone in reducing hostility in patients with schizophrenia.[30] A mirror-image study found that, in patients with schizophrenia or bipolar disorder in a secure setting, valproate decreased agitation.[31]

There is a small positive placebo-controlled RCT of valproate in generalised anxiety disorder.[32]

Plasma levels

The pharmacokinetics of valproate are complex, following a three-compartmental model and showing protein-binding saturation. Plasma level monitoring is supposedly of more limited use than with lithium or carbamazepine.[33] There may be a linear association between valproate serum levels and response in acute mania, with serum levels <55 mg/L being no more effective than placebo and levels >94 mg/L being associated with the most robust response,[34] although these data are weak.[33] Note that this is the top of the reference range (for epilepsy) that is quoted on laboratory forms. Optimal serum levels during the maintenance phase are unknown, but are likely to be at least 50 mg/L.[35] Achieving therapeutic plasma levels rapidly using a loading dose regimen is generally well tolerated. Plasma levels can also be used to detect non-compliance or toxicity.

Adverse effects

Valproate can cause both gastric irritation and hyperammonaemia,[36] both of which can lead to nausea. Lethargy and confusion can occasionally occur with starting doses above 750 mg/day. Weight gain can be significant,[37] particularly when valproate is used in combination with clozapine. Valproate causes dose-related tremor in up to a quarter of patients.[38] In the majority of these patients it is intention/postural tremor that is problematic, but a very small proportion develop parkinsonism associated with cognitive decline; these symptoms are reversible when valproate is discontinued.[39]

Hair loss (with curly regrowth) and peripheral oedema can occur, as can thrombocytopenia, leucopenia, red cell hypoplasia and pancreatitis.[40] Valproate can cause hyperandrogenism in women[41] and has been linked with the development of polycystic ovaries; the evidence supporting this association is conflicting. Valproate is a major human teratogen (see section 'Drug choice in pregnancy' in Chapter 7). Valproate may very rarely cause fulminant hepatic failure. Young children receiving multiple anticonvulsants are most at risk. Any patient with raised liver function tests (LFTs) (common in early treatment[42]) should be evaluated clinically and other markers of hepatic function such as albumin and clotting time should be checked.

Many adverse effects of valproate are dose related (peak plasma level related) and increase in frequency and severity when the plasma level is >100 mg/L. The once-daily Chrono form of sodium valproate does not produce peak plasma levels as high as the conventional formulation, and so may be better tolerated.

Valproate and other anticonvulsant drugs have been associated with an increased risk of suicidal behaviour,[43] but this finding is not consistent across studies.[44] Patients with depression[45] or those who take another anticonvulsant drug that increases the risk of developing depression may be a sub-group at greater risk.[46]

Note that valproate is eliminated mainly through the kidneys, partly in the form of ketone bodies, and may give a false positive urine test for ketones.

Pre-treatment tests

Baseline full blood count (FBC), LFTs and weight or BMI are recommended by NICE.

On-treatment monitoring

NICE recommend that an FBC and LFTs should be repeated after 6 months, and that BMI should be monitored. Valproate summaries of product characteristics (SPCs) recommend more frequent LFTs during the first 6 months with albumin and clotting measured if enzyme levels are abnormal.

Discontinuation

It is unknown if abrupt discontinuation of valproate worsens the natural course of bipolar illness in the same way that discontinuation of lithium does. One small naturalistic retrospective study suggests that it might.[47] Until further data are available, if valproate is to be discontinued, it should be done slowly over at least a month.

Use in women of child-bearing age

Valproate is an established human teratogen. NICE recommend that alternative anticonvulsants are preferred in women with epilepsy[48] and that valproate should not be used to treat bipolar illness in women of child-bearing age.[25]

The SPCs for sodium valproate and semi-sodium valproate[49,50] state that:

- These drugs should not be initiated in women of child-bearing potential without specialist advice (from a neurologist or psychiatrist).
- Women who are trying to conceive and require valproate should be prescribed prophylactic folate.

Women who have mania are likely to be sexually disinhibited **when unwell**. The risk of unplanned pregnancy is likely to be above population norms (where 50% of pregnancies are unplanned).

The teratogenic potential of valproate is not widely appreciated and many women of child-bearing age are not advised of the need for contraception or prophylactic folate.[51,52] Valproate may also cause impaired cognitive function in children exposed *in utero*.[53] See section on 'Drug choice in pregnancy'. Most now agree that valproate should not be used in women under 50 years of age.

Interactions with other drugs

Valproate is highly protein bound and can be displaced by other protein-bound drugs such as aspirin leading to toxicity. Aspirin also inhibits the metabolism of valproate; a dose of at least 300 mg aspirin is required.[54] Other, less strongly protein-bound drugs such as warfarin can be displaced by valproate, leading to higher free levels and toxicity.

Valproate is hepatically metabolised; drugs that inhibit CYP enzymes can increase valproate levels (e.g. erythromycin, fluoxetine and cimetidine). Valproate can increase the plasma levels of some drugs by inhibition of glucuronidation. Examples include tricyclic antidepressants (TCAs) (particularly clomipramine[55]), lamotrigine,[56] quetiapine,[57] warfarin[58] and phenobarbital. Valproate may also significantly lower plasma olanzapine concentrations; the mechanism is unknown.[59]

Pharmacodynamic interactions also occur. The anticonvulsant effect of valproate is antagonised by drugs that lower the seizure threshold (e.g. antipsychotics). Weight gain can be exacerbated by other drugs such as clozapine and olanzapine.

The prescribing and monitoring of valproate are summarised in Table 2.3.

CHAPTER 2

Table 2.3 Valproate: prescribing and monitoring

Indications	Mania, hypomania, bipolar depression and prophylaxis of bipolar affective disorder. May reduce aggression in a range of psychiatric disorders (data weak)
	Note that sodium valproate is licensed only for epilepsy and semi-sodium valproate only for acute mania
Pre-valproate work-up	FBC and LFTs. Baseline measure of weight desirable
Prescribing	Titrate dose upwards against response and adverse effects. Loading doses can be used and are generally well tolerated
	Note that CR sodium valproate (Epilim Chrono) can be given once daily. All other formulations must be administered at least twice daily
	Plasma levels can be used to assure adequate dosing and treatment compliance. Blood should be taken immediately before the next dose
Monitoring	FBC and LFTs if clinically indicated
	Weight (or BMI)
Stopping	Reduce slowly over at least 1 month

BMI, body mass index; CR, controlled realease; FBC, full blood count; LFT, liver function test.

References

1. Rosenberg G. The mechanisms of action of valproate in neuropsychiatric disorders: can we see the forest for the trees? Cell Mol Life Sci 2007; 64:2090–2103.
2. Kuendgen A et al. Valproic acid for the treatment of myeloid malignancies. Cancer 2007; 110:943–954.
3. Atmaca A et al. Valproic acid (VPA) in patients with refractory advanced cancer: a dose escalating phase I clinical trial. Br J Cancer 2007; 97:177–182.
4. Hallas J et al. Cancer risk in long-term users of valproate: a population-based case-control study. Cancer Epidemiol Biomarkers Prev 2009; 18:1714–1719.
5. Gervain J et al. Valproate reopens critical-period learning of absolute pitch. Front Syst Neurosci 2013; 7:1–11.
6. Fisher C et al. Sodium valproate or valproate semisodium: is there a difference in the treatment of bipolar disorder? Psychiatr Bull 2003; 27:446–448.
7. Iqbal SU et al. Divalproex sodium vs. valproic acid: drug utilization patterns, persistence rates and predictors of hospitalization among VA patients diagnosed with bipolar disorder. J Clin Pharm Ther 2007; 32:625–632.
8. Wassef AA et al. Lower effectiveness of divalproex versus valproic acid in a prospective, quasi-experimental clinical trial involving 9,260 psychiatric admissions. Am J Psychiatry 2005; 162:330–339.
9. Bowden CL et al. Efficacy of divalproex vs lithium and placebo in the treatment of mania. The Depakote Mania Study Group. JAMA 1994; 271:918–924.
10. Freeman TW et al. A double-blind comparison of valproate and lithium in the treatment of acute mania. Am J Psychiatry 1992; 149:108–111.
11. Nasrallah HA et al. Carbamazepine and valproate for the treatment of bipolar disorder: a review of the literature. J Affect Disord 2006; 95:69–78.
12. Hirschfeld RM et al. A randomized, placebo-controlled, multicenter study of divalproex sodium extended-release in the acute treatment of mania. J Clin Psychiatry 2010; 71:426–432.
13. Bowden C et al. A 12-week, open, randomized trial comparing sodium valproate to lithium in patients with bipolar I disorder suffering from a manic episode. Int Clin Psychopharmacol 2008; 23:254–262.
14. Pope HG, Jr. et al. Valproate in the treatment of acute mania. A placebo-controlled study. Arch Gen Psychiatry 1991; 48:62–68.
15. Novick D et al. Translation of randomised controlled trial findings into clinical practice: comparison of olanzapine and valproate in the EMBLEM study. Pharmacopsychiatry 2009; 42:145–152.
16. Cipriani A et al. Comparative efficacy and acceptability of antimanic drugs in acute mania: a multiple-treatments meta-analysis. Lancet 2011; 378:1306–1315.
17. Smith LA et al. Valproate for the treatment of acute bipolar depression: systematic review and meta-analysis. J Affect Disord 2010; 122:1–9.

18. Calabrese JR et al. Spectrum of efficacy of valproate in 55 patients with rapid-cycling bipolar disorder. Am J Psychiatry 1990; **147**: 431–434.
19. Tohen M et al. Olanzapine versus divalproex sodium for the treatment of acute mania and maintenance of remission: a 47-week study. Am J Psychiatry 2003; **160**:1263–1271.
20. Suppes T et al. Rapid versus non-rapid cycling as a predictor of response to olanzapine and divalproex sodium for bipolar mania and maintenance of remission: post hoc analyses of 47-week data. J Affect Disord 2005; **89**:69–77.
21. Bowden CL et al. A randomized, placebo-controlled 12-month trial of divalproex and lithium in treatment of outpatients with bipolar I disorder. Divalproex Maintenance Study Group. Arch Gen Psychiatry 2000; **57**:481–489.
22. Calabrese JR et al. A 20-month, double-blind, maintenance trial of lithium versus divalproex in rapid-cycling bipolar disorder. Am J Psychiatry 2005; **162**:2152–2161.
23. Geddes JR et al. Lithium plus valproate combination therapy versus monotherapy for relapse prevention in bipolar I disorder (BALANCE): a randomised open-label trial. Lancet 2010; **375**:385–395.
24. Marcus R et al. Efficacy of aripiprazole adjunctive to lithium or valproate in the long-term treatment of patients with bipolar I disorder with an inadequate response to lithium or valproate monotherapy: a multicenter, double-blind, randomized study. Bipolar Disord 2011; **13**:133–144.
25. National Institute for Health and Care Excellence. Bipolar disorder: assessment and management: Clinical Guideline 185, 2014; last updated February 2016. https://www.nice.org.uk/guidance/cg185.
26. National Institute for Health and Care Excellence. Antenatal and postnatal mental health: clinical management and service guidance. Clinical Guideline 192, 2014; last updated August 2017. https://www.nice.org.uk/guidance/cg192.
27. Cipriani A et al. Valproic acid, valproate and divalproex in the maintenance treatment of bipolar disorder. Cochrane Database Syst Rev 2013; **10**:CD003196.
28. Hayes J et al. Prescribing trends in bipolar disorder: cohort study in the United Kingdom THIN primary care database 1995–2009. PLoSOne 2011; **6**:e28725.
29. Lindenmayer JP et al. Use of sodium valproate in violent and aggressive behaviors: a critical review. J Clin Psychiatry 2000; **61**:123–128.
30. Citrome L et al. Risperidone alone versus risperidone plus valproate in the treatment of patients with schizophrenia and hostility. Int Clin Psychopharmacol 2007; **22**:356–362.
31. Gobbi G et al. Efficacy of topiramate, valproate, and their combination on aggression/agitation behavior in patients with psychosis. J Clin Psychopharmacol 2006; **26**:467–473.
32. Aliyev NA et al. Valproate (depakine-chrono) in the acute treatment of outpatients with generalized anxiety disorder without psychiatric comorbidity: randomized, double-blind placebo-controlled study. Eur Psychiatry 2008; **23**:109–114.
33. Haymond J et al. Does valproic acid warrant therapeutic drug monitoring in bipolar affective disorder? Ther Drug Monit 2010; **32**:19–29.
34. Allen MH et al. Linear relationship of valproate serum concentration to response and optimal serum levels for acute mania. Am J Psychiatry 2006; **163**:272–275.
35. Taylor D et al. Doses of carbamazepine and valproate in bipolar affective disorder. Psychiatr Bull 1997; **21**:221–223.
36. Segura-Bruna N et al. Valproate-induced hyperammonemic encephalopathy. Acta Neurol Scand 2006; **114**:1–7.
37. El-Khatib F et al. Valproate, weight gain and carbohydrate craving: a gender study. Seizure 2007; **16**:226–232.
38. Zadikoff C et al. Movement disorders in patients taking anticonvulsants. J Neurol Neurosurg Psychiatry 2007; **78**:147–151.
39. Ristic AJ et al. The frequency of reversible parkinsonism and cognitive decline associated with valproate treatment: a study of 364 patients with different types of epilepsy. Epilepsia 2006; **47**:2183–2185.
40. Gerstner T et al. Valproic acid-induced pancreatitis: 16 new cases and a review of the literature. J Gastroenterol 2007; **42**:39–48.
41. Joffe H et al. Valproate is associated with new-onset oligoamenorrhea with hyperandrogenism in women with bipolar disorder. Biol Psychiatry 2006; **59**:1078–1086.
42. Bjornsson E. Hepatotoxicity associated with antiepileptic drugs. Acta Neurol Scand 2008; **118**:281–290.
43. Patorno E et al. Anticonvulsant medications and the risk of suicide, attempted suicide, or violent death. JAMA 2010; **303**:1401–1409.
44. Gibbons RD et al. Relationship between antiepileptic drugs and suicide attempts in patients with bipolar disorder. Arch Gen Psychiatry 2009; **66**:1354–1360.
45. Arana A et al. Suicide-related events in patients treated with antiepileptic drugs. N Engl J Med 2010; **363**:542–551.
46. Andersohn F et al. Use of antiepileptic drugs in epilepsy and the risk of self-harm or suicidal behavior. Neurology 2010; **75**:335–340.
47. Franks MA et al. Bouncing back: is the bipolar rebound phenomenon peculiar to lithium? A retrospective naturalistic study. J Psychopharmacol 2008; **22**:452–456.
48. National Institute for Health and Clinical Excellence. The epilepsies: the diagnosis and management of the epilepsies in adults and children in primary and secondary care. Clinical Guideline 137, 2012; last updated February 2016. https://www.nice.org.uk/guidance/cg137.
49. Sanofi. Summary of Product Characteristics. Epilim Chrono 500mg. 2017. https://www.medicines.org.uk/emc/medicine/6779.
50. Sanofi. Summary of Product Characteristics. Depakote 250mg Tablets. 2017. https://www.medicines.org.uk/emc/medicine/25929.
51. James L et al. Informing patients of the teratogenic potential of mood stabilising drugs; a case notes review of the practice of psychiatrists. J Psychopharmacol 2007; **21**:815–819.
52. James L et al. Mood stabilizers and teratogenicity – prescribing practice and awareness amongst practising psychiatrists. J Ment Health 2009; **18**:137–143.
53. Meador KJ et al. Cognitive function at 3 years of age after fetal exposure to antiepileptic drugs. N Engl J Med 2009; **360**:1597–1605.
54. Sandson NB et al. An interaction between aspirin and valproate: the relevance of plasma protein displacement drug-drug interactions. Am J Psychiatry 2006; **163**:1891–1896.

CHAPTER 2

55. Fehr C et al. Increase in serum clomipramine concentrations caused by valproate. J Clin Psychopharmacol 2000; 20:493–494.
56. Morris RG et al. Clinical study of lamotrigine and valproic acid in patients with epilepsy: using a drug interaction to advantage? Ther Drug Monit 2000; 22:656–660.
57. Aichhorn W et al. Influence of age, gender, body weight and valproate comedication on quetiapine plasma concentrations. Int Clin Psychopharmacol 2006; 21:81–85.
58. Gunes A et al. Inhibitory effect of valproic acid on cytochrome P450 2C9 activity in epilepsy patients. Basic Clin Pharmacol Toxicol 2007; 100:383–386.
59. Bergemann N et al. Valproate lowers plasma concentration of olanzapine. J Clin Psychopharmacol 2006; 26:432–434.

CHAPTER 2

Carbamazepine

Mechanism of action[1]

Carbamazepine blocks voltage-dependent sodium channels thus inhibiting repetitive neuronal firing. It reduces glutamate release and decreases the turnover of dopamine and noradrenaline. Carbamazepine has a similar molecular structure to TCAs.

As well as blocking voltage-dependent sodium channels, oxcarbazepine also increases potassium conductance and modulates high-voltage activated calcium channels.

Formulations

Carbamazepine is available as a liquid and chewable, immediate-release and controlled-release tablets. Conventional formulations generally have to be administered two to three times daily. The controlled-release preparation can be given once or twice daily, and the reduced fluctuation in serum levels usually leads to improved tolerability. This preparation has a lower bioavailability and an increase in dose of 10–15% may be required.

Indications

Carbamazepine is primarily used as an anticonvulsant in the treatment of grand mal and focal seizures. It is also used in the treatment of trigeminal neuralgia and, in the UK, is licensed for the treatment of bipolar illness in patients who do not respond to lithium.

With respect to the treatment of **mania**, two placebo-controlled randomised studies have found the extended-release formulation of carbamazepine to be effective; in both studies, the response rate in the carbamazepine arm was twice that in the placebo arm.[2,3] Carbamazepine was not particularly well tolerated; the incidence of dizziness, somnolence and nausea was high. Another study found carbamazepine alone to be as effective as carbamazepine plus olanzapine.[4] NICE does not recommend carbamazepine as a first-line treatment for mania.[5] A Cochrane review concluded that there were insufficient trials of adequate methodological quality on oxcarbazepine in the acute treatment of bipolar disorder to inform about its efficacy and acceptability.[6]

Open studies suggest that carbamazepine monotherapy has some efficacy in **bipolar depression**;[7] note that the evidence base supporting other strategies is stronger (see section on 'Bipolar depression'). Carbamazepine may also be useful in **unipolar depression**, either alone[8] or as an augmentation strategy.[9]

Carbamazepine is generally considered to be less effective than lithium in the **prophylaxis** of bipolar illness;[10] several published studies report a low response rate and high drop-out rate. A meta-analysis (n = 464) failed to find a significant difference in efficacy between lithium and carbamazepine, but those who received carbamazepine were more likely to drop out of treatment because of adverse effects.[11] Lithium is considered to be superior to carbamazepine in reducing suicidal behaviour,[12] although data are not consistent[13] and carbamazepine may have anti-suicidal properties.[14] NICE considers carbamazepine to be a third-line prophylactic agent[5] and data emerging since this guidance support this positioning.[15] Three small studies suggest the related oxcarbazepine may have some prophylactic efficacy when used in combination with other mood-stabilising drugs.[16–18]

There are data supporting the use of carbamazepine in the management of alcohol withdrawal symptoms,[19] although the high doses required initially are often poorly tolerated. Cochrane does not consider the evidence strong enough to support the use of carbamazepine for this indication.[20] Carbamazepine has also been used to manage aggressive behaviour in patients with schizophrenia;[21] the quality of data is weak and the mode of action unknown. There are a number of case reports and open case series that report on the use of carbamazepine in various psychiatric illnesses such as panic disorder, borderline personality disorder and episodic dyscontrol syndrome.

Plasma levels

When carbamazepine is used as an anticonvulsant, the therapeutic range is generally considered to be 4–12 mg/L, although the supporting evidence is not strong. In patients with affective illness, a dose of at least 600 mg/day and a plasma level of at least 7 mg/L may be required,[22] although this is not a consistent finding.[4,8,23] Levels above 12 mg/L are associated with a higher adverse effect burden.

Carbamazepine serum levels vary markedly within a dosage interval. It is therefore important to sample at a point in time where levels are likely to be reproducible for any given individual. The most appropriate way of monitoring is to take a trough level before the first dose of the day.

Carbamazepine is a hepatic enzyme inducer that induces its own metabolism as well as that of other drugs. An initial plasma half-life of around 30 hours is reduced to around 12 hours on chronic dosing. For this reason, plasma levels should be checked 2–4 weeks after an increase in dose to ensure that the desired level is still being obtained.

Most published clinical trials that demonstrate the efficacy of carbamazepine as a mood stabiliser use doses that are significantly higher (800–1200 mg/day) than those commonly prescribed in UK clinical practice.[24]

Adverse effects[1]

The main adverse effects associated with carbamazepine therapy are dizziness, diplopia, drowsiness, ataxia, nausea and headaches. They can sometimes be avoided by starting with a low dose and increasing slowly. Avoiding high peak blood levels by splitting the dose throughout the day or using a controlled-release formulation may also help. Dry mouth, oedema and hyponatraemia are also common. Sexual dysfunction can occur, probably mediated through reduced testosterone levels.[25] Around 3% of patients treated with carbamazepine develop a generalised erythematous rash. Serious exfoliative dermatological reactions can rarely occur; vulnerability is genetically determined,[26] and genetic testing of people of Han Chinese or Thai origin is recommended before carbamazepine is prescribed. Carbamazepine is a known human teratogen (see section on 'Drug choice in pregnancy' in Chapter 7).

Carbamazepine commonly causes a chronic low white blood cell (WBC) count. One patient in 20,000 develops agranulocytosis and/or aplastic anaemia.[27] Raised alkaline phosphatase (ALP) and γ-glutamyl transferase (GGT) are common (a GGT of 2–3 times normal is rarely a cause for concern[28]). A delayed multi-organ hypersensitivity reaction rarely occurs, mainly manifesting itself as various skin reactions, a low WBC count, and abnormal LFTs. Fatalities have been reported.[28,29] There is no clear timescale for these events.

Some anticonvulsant drugs have been associated with an increased risk of suicidal behaviour. Carbamazepine has not been implicated, either in general[30,31] or, more specifically, in those with bipolar illness.[32]

Pre-treatment tests

Baseline urea and electrolytes (U&Es), FBC and LFTs are recommended by NICE. A baseline measure of weight is also desirable.

On-treatment monitoring

NICE recommend that U&Es, FBC and LFTs should be repeated after 6 months, and that weight (or BMI) should also be monitored.

Discontinuation

It is not known if abrupt discontinuation of carbamazepine worsens the natural course of bipolar illness in the same way that abrupt cessation of lithium does. In one small case series (n = 6), one patient developed depression within a month of discontinuation,[33] while in another small case series (n = 4), 3 patients had a recurrence of their mood disorder within 3 months.[34] Until further data are available, if carbamazepine is to be discontinued, it should be done slowly (over at least a month).

Use in women of child-bearing age

Carbamazepine is an established human teratogen (see section on 'Drug choice in pregnancy' in Chapter 7).

Women who have mania are likely to be sexually disinhibited. The risk of unplanned pregnancy is likely to be above population norms (where 50% of pregnancies are unplanned). If carbamazepine cannot be avoided, adequate contraception should be ensured (note the interaction between carbamazepine and oral contraceptives outlined in the next paragraph) and prophylactic folate prescribed.

Interactions with other drugs[35–38]

Carbamazepine is a potent inducer of hepatic cytochrome enzymes and is metabolised by CYP3A4. Plasma levels of most **antidepressants**, most **antipsychotics, benzodiazepines, warfarin, zolpidem,** some **cholinesterase inhibitors, methadone, thyroxine, theophylline, oestrogens** and **other steroids** may be reduced by carbamazepine, resulting in treatment failure. Patients requiring contraception should either receive a preparation containing not less than 50 µg oestrogen or use a non-hormonal method. Drugs that inhibit CYP3A4 will increase carbamazepine plasma levels and may precipitate toxicity. Examples include **fluconazole, cimetidine, diltiazem, verapamil, erythromycin** and some **SSRIs.**

Pharmacodynamic interactions also occur. The anticonvulsant activity of carbamazepine is reduced by drugs that lower the seizure threshold (e.g. antipsychotics and antidepressants), the potential for carbamazepine to cause neutropenia may be increased by other drugs that have the potential to depress the bone marrow (e.g. clozapine), and the risk of hyponatraemia may be increased by other drugs that have the potential to deplete sodium (e.g. diuretics). Neurotoxicity has been reported when carbamazepine is used in combination with lithium. This is rare. For a full review of carbamazepine interactions see chapter 17 of *Applied Clinical Pharmacokinetics and Pharmacodynamics of Psychopharmacological Agents.*[39]

As carbamazepine is structurally similar to TCAs, in theory it should not be given within 14 days of discontinuing a monoamine oxidase inhibitor (MAOI).

The prescribing and monitoring of carbamazepine are summarised in Table 2.4.

Table 2.4 Carbamazepine: prescribing and monitoring

Indications	Mania (not first line), bipolar depression (evidence weak), unipolar depression (evidence weak) and prophylaxis of bipolar disorder (third line after antipsychotics and valproate). Alcohol withdrawal (may be poorly tolerated)
	Carbamazepine is licensed for the treatment of bipolar illness in patients who do not respond to lithium
Pre-carbamazepine work-up	U&Es, FBC and LFTs. Baseline measure of weight desirable
Prescribing	Titrate dose upwards against response and adverse effects; start with 100–200 mg bd and aim for 400 mg bd (some patients will require higher doses)
	Note that the modified-release formulation (Tegretol Retard) can be given once to twice daily, is associated with less severe fluctuations in serum levels and is generally better tolerated
	Plasma levels can be used to assure adequate dosing and treatment compliance. Blood should be taken immediately before the next dose. Carbamazepine induces its own metabolism; serum levels (if used) should be re-checked a month after an increase in dose
Monitoring	U&Es, FBC and LFTs if clinically indicated
	Weight (or BMI)
Stopping	Reduce slowly over at least 1 month

bd, *bis in die* (twice a day); BMI, body mass index; FBC, full blood count; LFT, liver function test, U&E, urea and electrolytes.

References

1. Novartis Pharmaceuticals UK Limited. Summary of Product Characteristics. Tegretol Tablets 100mg, 200mg, 400mg. 2017. https://www.medicines.org.uk/emc/medicine/1328.
2. Weisler RH et al. A multicenter, randomized, double-blind, placebo-controlled trial of extended-release carbamazepine capsules as monotherapy for bipolar disorder patients with manic or mixed episodes. J Clin Psychiatry 2004; 65:478–484.
3. Weisler RH et al. Extended-release carbamazepine capsules as monotherapy for acute mania in bipolar disorder: a multicenter, randomized, double-blind, placebo-controlled trial. J Clin Psychiatry 2005; 66:323–330.
4. Tohen M et al. Olanzapine plus carbamazepine v. carbamazepine alone in treating manic episodes. Br J Psychiatry 2008; 192:135–143.
5. National Institute for Health and Care Excellence. Bipolar disorder: assessment and management: Clinical Guideline 185, 2014; last updated February 2016 update. https://www.nice.org.uk/guidance/cg185.
6. Vasudev A et al. Oxcarbazepine for acute affective episodes in bipolar disorder. Cochrane Database Syst Rev 2011:CD004857.
7. Dilsaver SC et al. Treatment of bipolar depression with carbamazepine: results of an open study. Biol Psychiatry 1996; 40:935–937.
8. Zhang ZJ et al. The effectiveness of carbamazepine in unipolar depression: a double-blind, randomized, placebo-controlled study. J Affect Disord 2008; 109:91–97.
9. Kramlinger KG et al. The addition of lithium to carbamazepine. Antidepressant efficacy in treatment-resistant depression. Arch Gen Psychiatry 1989; 46:794–800.
10. Nasrallah HA et al. Carbamazepine and valproate for the treatment of bipolar disorder: a review of the literature. J Affect Disord 2006; 95:69–78.
11. Ceron-Litvoc D et al. Comparison of carbamazepine and lithium in treatment of bipolar disorder: a systematic review of randomized controlled trials. Hum Psychopharmacol 2009; 24:19–28.
12. Kleindienst N et al. Differential efficacy of lithium and carbamazepine in the prophylaxis of bipolar disorder: results of the MAP study. Neuropsychobiology 2000; 42 Suppl 1:2–10.
13. Yerevanian BI et al. Bipolar pharmacotherapy and suicidal behavior. Part I: Lithium, divalproex and carbamazepine. J Affect Disord 2007; 103:5–11.
14. Tsai CJ et al. The rapid suicide protection of mood stabilizers on patients with bipolar disorder: a nationwide observational cohort study in Taiwan. J Affect Disord 2016; 196:71–77.
15. Peselow ED et al. Prophylactic efficacy of lithium, valproic acid, and carbamazepine in the maintenance phase of bipolar disorder: a naturalistic study. Int Clin Psychopharmacol 2016; 31:218–223.
16. Vieta E et al. A double-blind, randomized, placebo-controlled prophylaxis trial of oxcarbazepine as adjunctive treatment to lithium in the long-term treatment of bipolar I and II disorder. Int J Neuropsychopharmacol 2008; 11:445–452.
17. Conway CR et al. An open-label trial of adjunctive oxcarbazepine for bipolar disorder. J Clin Psychopharmacol 2006; 26:95–97.
18. Juruena MF et al. Bipolar I and II disorder residual symptoms: oxcarbazepine and carbamazepine as add-on treatment to lithium in a double-blind, randomized trial. Prog Neuropsychopharmacol Biol Psychiatry 2009; 33:94–99.
19. Malcolm R et al. The effects of carbamazepine and lorazepam on single versus multiple previous alcohol withdrawals in an outpatient randomized trial. J Gen Intern Med 2002; 17:349–355.
20. Minozzi S et al. Anticonvulsants for alcohol withdrawal. Cochrane Database Syst Rev 2010:CD005064.
21. Brieden T et al. Psychopharmacological treatment of aggression in schizophrenic patients. Pharmacopsychiatry 2002; 35:83–89.
22. Taylor D et al. Doses of carbamazepine and valproate in bipolar affective disorder. Psychiatr Bull 1997; 21:221–223.
23. Simhandl C et al. The comparative efficacy of carbamazepine low and high serum level and lithium carbonate in the prophylaxis of affective disorders. J Affect Disord 1993; 28:221–231.
24. Taylor DM et al. Prescribing and monitoring of carbamazepine and valproate – a case note review. Psychiatr Bull 2000; 24:174–177.
25. Lossius MI et al. Reversible effects of antiepileptic drugs on reproductive endocrine function in men and women with epilepsy a prospective randomized double-blind withdrawal study. Epilepsia 2007; 48:1875–1882.
26. Hung SI et al. Genetic susceptibility to carbamazepine-induced cutaneous adverse drug reactions. Pharmacogenet Genomics 2006; 16:297–306.
27. Kaufman DW et al. Drugs in the aetiology of agranulocytosis and aplastic anaemia. Eur J Haematol Suppl 1996; 60:23–30.
28. Bjornsson E. Hepatotoxicity associated with antiepileptic drugs. Acta Neurol Scand 2008; 118:281290.
29. Ganeva M et al. Carbamazepine-induced drug reaction with eosinophilia and systemic symptoms (DRESS) syndrome: report of four cases and brief review. Int J Dermatol 2008; 47:853–860.
30. Patorno E et al. Anticonvulsant medications and the risk of suicide, attempted suicide, or violent death. JAMA 2010; 303:1401–1409.
31. Andersohn F et al. Use of antiepileptic drugs in epilepsy and the risk of self-harm or suicidal behavior. Neurology 2010; 75:335–340.
32. Gibbons RD et al. Relationship between antiepileptic drugs and suicide attempts in patients with bipolar disorder. Arch Gen Psychiatry 2009; 66:1354–1360.
33. Macritchie KA et al. Does 'rebound mania' occur after stopping carbamazepine? A pilot study. J Psychopharmacol 2000; 14:266–268.
34. Franks MA et al. Bouncing back: is the bipolar rebound phenomenon peculiar to lithium? A retrospective naturalistic study. J Psychopharmacol 2008; 22:452–456.
35. Spina E et al. Clinical significance of pharmacokinetic interactions between antiepileptic and psychotropic drugs. Epilepsia 2002; 43 Suppl 2:37–44.
36. Patsalos PN et al. The importance of drug interactions in epilepsy therapy. Epilepsia 2002; 43:365–385.
37. Crawford P. Interactions between antiepileptic drugs and hormonal contraception. CNS Drugs 2002; 16:263–272.
38. Citrome L et al. Pharmacokinetics of aripiprazole and concomitant carbamazepine. J Clin Psychopharmacol 2007; 27:279–283.
39. Taylor D et al. Clinically significant interactions with mood stabilisers. In: Jann M, Penzak S, Cohen L, eds. Applied Clinical Pharmacokinetics and Pharmacodynamics of Psychopharmacological Agents. Switzerland: ADIS; 2016, pp. 423–449.

Antipsychotic drugs in bipolar disorder

It is unhelpful to think of antipsychotic drugs as having only 'antipsychotic' actions. Individual antipsychotics variously possess sedative, anxiolytic, antimanic, mood-stabilising and antidepressant properties. Some antipsychotics (quetiapine and olanzapine) show all of these activities.[1]

First-generation antipsychotics (FGAs) have long been used in mania, and several studies support their use in a variety of hypomanic and manic presentations.[2,3] Their effectiveness is enhanced by the addition of a mood stabiliser.[4,5] In the longer-term treatment of bipolar disorder, FGAs are widely used (presumably as prophylaxis)[6] but robust supporting data are absent.[7] The observation that typical antipsychotic drugs are associated with both depression and tardive dyskinesia in bipolar patients militates against their long-term use.[7-9] Certainly the use of second-generation antipsychotics (SGAs) seems less likely to cause depression than treatment with haloperidol.[10] The use of FGA depots is common in practice but poorly supported and seems to be associated with a high risk of depression[11] (see section 'Antipsychotic long-acting injections in bipolar disorder').

Among newer antipsychotic drugs, olanzapine, risperidone, quetiapine, aripiprazole and asenapine have been most robustly evaluated and are licensed in many countries for the treatment of mania. Olanzapine is more effective than placebo in mania,[12,13] and at least as effective as valproate semi-sodium,[14,15] risperidone[16] and lithium.[17,18] As with FGAs, olanzapine is most effective when used in combination with a mood stabiliser[19,20] (although in one study olanzapine + carbamazepine was no better than carbamazepine alone[21]). Data suggest olanzapine may offer benefits in longer-term treatment;[22,23] it may be more effective than lithium,[24] and it is formally licensed as prophylaxis.

Data relating to quetiapine[25-27] suggest robust efficacy in all aspects of bipolar disorder including prevention of bipolar depression.[28] Aripiprazole is effective in mania both alone[29-31] and as an add-on agent,[32] and in long-term prophylaxis.[33,34] Clozapine seems to be effective in refractory bipolar conditions, including refractory mania.[35-38] Risperidone has shown efficacy in mania,[39] particularly in combination with a mood stabiliser.[40,41] Risperidone long-acting injection is also effective[42] (note though that the pharmacokinetics of this formulation generally render it an unsuitable choice for the acute treatment of mania). Aripiprazole long-acting injection is also effective for prophylaxis in bipolar 1 disorder with the effect predominantly on prevention of manic episodes.[43] There are few data for amisulpride,[44] rather more for ziprasidone[45] and effectively none for lurasidone (notwithstanding its effect as an acute treatment for bipolar depression[46,47]). Iloperidone may be effective in mixed episodes[48] but data are scant.

Asenapine is given by the sublingual route and is effective in mania.[49,50] Efficacy seems to be maintained in the longer term.[51] Asenapine is less sedative than olanzapine with a similar (low) propensity for akathisia and other movement disorders[50,51] and is less likely than olanzapine to cause weight gain and metabolic disturbance.[52] Cariprazine is efficacious for treating mania[53-55] and has a low propensity for weight gain.

Overall, antipsychotic drugs (particularly haloperidol, olanzapine and risperidone) may be more effective than traditional mood stabilisers in the treatment of mania, and quetiapine is similarly effective but better tolerated than aripiprazole or lithium.[2] Antipsychotic drugs are most often combined with mood stabilisers for optimal effect.[56] Limited data suggest that continuation of the antipsychotic drug beyond 24 weeks is unproductive.[16]

References

1. ECNP. Neuroscience based Nomenclature, 2nd edn. 2017. http://www.nbn2.com.
2. Cipriani A et al. Comparative efficacy and acceptability of antimanic drugs in acute mania: a multiple-treatments meta-analysis. Lancet 2011; **378**:130613–15.
3. Goodwin GM et al. Evidence-based guidelines for treating bipolar disorder: revised third edition recommendations from the British Association for Psychopharmacology. J Psychopharmacol 2016; **30**:495–553.
4. Chou JC et al. Acute mania: haloperidol dose and augmentation with lithium or lorazepam. J Clin Psychopharmacol 1999; **19**:500–505.
5. Small JG et al. A placebo-controlled study of lithium combined with neuroleptics in chronic schizophrenic patients. Am J Psychiatry 1975; **132**:1315–1317.
6. Soares JC et al. Adjunctive antipsychotic use in bipolar patients: an open 6-month prospective study following an acute episode. J Affect Disord 1999; **56**:1–8.
7. Keck PE, Jr. et al. Anticonvulsants and antipsychotics in the treatment of bipolar disorder. J Clin Psychiatry 1998; **59 Suppl 6**:74–81.
8. Tohen M et al. Antipsychotic agents and bipolar disorder. J Clin Psychiatry 1998; **59 Suppl 1**:38–48.
9. Zarate CA, Jr. et al. Double-blind comparison of the continued use of antipsychotic treatment versus its discontinuation in remitted manic patients. Am J Psychiatry 2004; **161**:169–171.
10. Goikolea JM et al. Lower rate of depressive switch following antimanic treatment with second-generation antipsychotics versus haloperidol. J Affect Disord 2013; **144**:191–198.
11. Gigante AD et al. Long-acting injectable antipsychotics for the maintenance treatment of bipolar disorder. CNS Drugs 2012; **26**:403–420.
12. Tohen M et al. Olanzapine versus placebo in the treatment of acute mania. Olanzapine HGEH Study Group. Am J Psychiatry 1999; **156**:702–709.
13. Tohen M et al. Efficacy of olanzapine in acute bipolar mania: a double-blind, placebo-controlled study. The Olanzipine HGGW Study Group. Arch Gen Psychiatry 2000; **57**:841–849.
14. Tohen M et al. Olanzapine versus divalproex in the treatment of acute mania. Am J Psychiatry 2002; **159**:1011–1017.
15. Tohen M et al. Olanzapine versus divalproex versus placebo in the treatment of mild to moderate mania: a randomized, 12-week, double-blind study. J Clin Psychiatry 2008; **69**:1776–1789.
16. Yatham LN et al. Optimal duration of risperidone or olanzapine adjunctive therapy to mood stabilizer following remission of a manic episode: a CANMAT randomized double-blind trial. Mol Psychiatry 2016; **21**:1050–1056.
17. Berk M et al. Olanzapine compared to lithium in mania: a double-blind randomized controlled trial. Int Clin Psychopharmacol 1999; **14**:339–343.
18. Niufan G et al. Olanzapine versus lithium in the acute treatment of bipolar mania: a double-blind, randomized, controlled trial. J Affect Disord 2008; **105**:101–108.
19. Tohen M et al. Efficacy of olanzapine in combination with valproate or lithium in the treatment of mania in patients partially nonresponsive to valproate or lithium monotherapy. Arch Gen Psychiatry 2002; **59**:62–69.
20. Tohen M et al. Relapse prevention in bipolar I disorder: 18-month comparison of olanzapine plus mood stabiliser v. mood stabiliser alone. Br J Psychiatry 2004; **184**:337–345.
21. Tohen M et al. Olanzapine plus carbamazepine v. carbamazepine alone in treating manic episodes. Br J Psychiatry 2008; **192**:135–143.
22. Sanger TM et al. Long-term olanzapine therapy in the treatment of bipolar I disorder: an open-label continuation phase study. J Clin Psychiatry 2001; **62**:273–281.
23. Vieta E et al. Olanzapine as long-term adjunctive therapy in treatment-resistant bipolar disorder. J Clin Psychopharmacol 2001; **21**:469–473.
24. Tohen M et al. Olanzapine versus lithium in the maintenance treatment of bipolar disorder: a 12-month, randomized, double-blind, controlled clinical trial. Am J Psychiatry 2005; **162**:1281–1290.
25. Ghaemi SN et al. The use of quetiapine for treatment-resistant bipolar disorder: a case series. Ann Clin Psychiatry 1999; **11**:137–140.
26. Sachs G et al. Quetiapine with lithium or divalproex for the treatment of bipolar mania: a randomized, double-blind, placebo-controlled study. Bipolar Disord 2004; **6**:213–223.
27. Altamura AC et al. Efficacy and tolerability of quetiapine in the treatment of bipolar disorder: preliminary evidence from a 12-month open label study. J Affect Disord 2003; **76**:267–271.
28. Young AH et al. A randomised, placebo-controlled 52-week trial of continued quetiapine treatment in recently depressed patients with bipolar I and bipolar II disorder. World J Biol Psychiatry 2014; **15**:96–112.
29. Sachs G et al. Aripiprazole in the treatment of acute manic or mixed episodes in patients with bipolar I disorder: a 3-week placebo-controlled study. J Psychopharmacol 2006; **20**:536–546.
30. Keck PE et al. Aripiprazole monotherapy in the treatment of acute bipolar I mania: a randomized, double-blind, placebo- and lithium-controlled study. J Affect Disord 2009; **112**:36–49.

31. Young AH et al. Aripiprazole monotherapy in acute mania: 12-week randomised placebo- and haloperidol-controlled study. Br J Psychiatry 2009; 194:40–48.

32. Vieta E et al. Efficacy of adjunctive aripiprazole to either valproate or lithium in bipolar mania patients partially nonresponsive to valproate/ lithium monotherapy: a placebo-controlled study. Am J Psychiatry 2008; 165:1316–1325.

33. Keck PE, Jr. et al. Aripiprazole monotherapy for maintenance therapy in bipolar I disorder: a 100-week, double-blind study versus placebo. J Clin Psychiatry 2007; 68:1480–1491.

34. Vieta E et al. Assessment of safety, tolerability and effectiveness of adjunctive aripiprazole to lithium/valproate in bipolar mania: a 46-week, open-label extension following a 6-week double-blind study. Curr Med Res Opin 2010; 26:1485–1496.

35. Calabrese JR et al. Clozapine for treatment-refractory mania. Am J Psychiatry 1996; 153:759–764.

36. Green AI et al. Clozapine in the treatment of refractory psychotic mania. Am J Psychiatry 2000; 157:982–986.

37. Kimmel SE et al. Clozapine in treatment-refractory mood disorders. J Clin Psychiatry 1994; 55 Suppl B:91–93.

38. Chang JS et al. The effects of long-term clozapine add-on therapy on the rehospitalization rate and the mood polarity patterns in bipolar disorders. J Clin Psychiatry 2006; 67:461–467.

39. Segal J et al. Risperidone compared with both lithium and haloperidol in mania: a double-blind randomized controlled trial. Clin Neuropharmacol 1998; 21:176–180.

40. Sachs GS et al. Combination of a mood stabilizer with risperidone or haloperidol for treatment of acute mania: a double-blind, placebo-controlled comparison of efficacy and safety. Am J Psychiatry 2002; 159:1146–1154.

41. Vieta E et al. Risperidone in the treatment of mania: efficacy and safety results from a large, multicentre, open study in Spain. J Affect Disord 2002; 72:15–19.

42. Quiroz JA et al. Risperidone long-acting injectable monotherapy in the maintenance treatment of bipolar I disorder. Biol Psychiatry 2010; 68:156–162.

43. Calabrese JR et al. Efficacy and safety of aripiprazole once-monthly in the maintenance treatment of bipolar I disorder: a double-blind, placebo-controlled, 52-week randomized withdrawal study. J Clin Psychiatry 2017; 78:324–331.

44. Vieta E et al. An open-label study of amisulpride in the treatment of mania. J Clin Psychiatry 2005; 66:575–578.

45. Vieta E et al. Ziprasidone in the treatment of acute mania: a 12-week, placebo-controlled, haloperidol-referenced study. J Psychopharm 2010; 24:547–558.

46. Loebel A et al. Lurasidone monotherapy in the treatment of bipolar I depression: a randomized, double-blind, placebo-controlled study. Am J Psychiatry 2014; 171:160–168.

47. Loebel A et al. Lurasidone as adjunctive therapy with lithium or valproate for the treatment of bipolar I depression: a randomized, double-blind, placebo-controlled study. Am J Psychiatry 2014; 171:169–177.

48. Singh V et al. An open trial of iloperidone for mixed episodes in bipolar disorder. J Clin Psychopharmacol 2017; 37:615–619.

49. McIntyre RS et al. Asenapine in the treatment of acute mania in bipolar I disorder: a randomized, double-blind, placebo-controlled trial. J Affect Disord 2010; 122:27–38.

50. McIntyre RS et al. Asenapine versus olanzapine in acute mania: a double-blind extension study. Bipolar Disord 2009; 11:815–826.

51. McIntyre RS et al. Asenapine for long-term treatment of bipolar disorder: a double-blind 40-week extension study. J Affect Disord 2010; 126:358–365.

52. Kemp DE et al. Weight change and metabolic effects of asenapine in patients with schizophrenia and bipolar disorder. J Clin Psychiatry 2014; 75:238–245.

53. Lao KS et al. Tolerability and safety profile of cariprazine in treating psychotic disorders, bipolar disorder and major depressive disorder: a systematic review with meta-analysis of randomized controlled trials. CNS Drugs 2016; 30:1043–1054.

54. Sachs GS et al. Cariprazine in the treatment of acute mania in bipolar I disorder: a double-blind, placebo-controlled, phase III trial. J Affect Disord 2015; 174:296–302.

55. Calabrese JR et al. Efficacy and safety of low- and high-dose cariprazine in acute and mixed mania associated with bipolar I disorder: a double-blind, placebo-controlled study. J Clin Psychiatry 2015; 76:284–292.

56. Nierenberg AA et al. Bipolar CHOICE (Clinical Health Outcomes Initiative in Comparative Effectiveness): a pragmatic 6-month trial of lithium versus quetiapine for bipolar disorder. J Clin Psychiatry 2016; 77:90–99.

Antipsychotic long-acting injections in bipolar disorder

Long-acting injections (LAIs) are widely used in bipolar disorder although none is formally licensed for this indication. Support for their use is rather limited: there have been approximately 20 open-label trials or case series published, but only five of these included more than a handful of subjects.[1–4] There have also been seven RCTs, five of which were arguably sufficiently powered to produce interpretable results (the remaining two trials included only 30 subjects in total[5,6]). These five RCTs represent, relatively speaking, the highest level of evidence for LAIs in bipolar disorder. Their details are set out in Table 2.5.

Few firm conclusions can be drawn from the RCTs outlined in Table 2.5. Risperidone LAI is clearly effective either as the sole treatment or as an adjunct but provides protection only against manic, hypomanic and mixed episodes and neither decreases nor increases the risk of depressive relapse. Risperidone LAI may be less effective than oral olanzapine. It might be tentatively assumed that paliperidone LAI has similar effects to risperidone LAI. Oral paliperidone prevents manic relapse in bipolar disorder[10] and case reports describe good outcomes with the LAI form.[11] Aripiprazole LAI also protects against manic relapse and does not affect risk of depression.

Data for FGAs in bipolar disorder are scarce and generally of low quality (open trials, case series and retrospective analyses). In these studies, FGA LAIs seem to reduce

Table 2.5 Randomised controlled trials of long-acting injections in bipolar disorder

Study	n	LAI	Comparator	Duration	Outcome
Ahlfors et al., 1981[7]	33 (19/14)	Flupentixol decanoate	Lithium	18 months	Neither treatment improved main outcome (number of mood episodes). No differences between treatments
Macfadden et al., 2009[8]*	124 (65/59)	Risperidone (adjunct)	Placebo (adjunct)	12 months	Risperidone LAI reduced rate of relapse compared with placebo (relative risk = 2.3)
Quiroz et al., 2010[9]*	303 (154/149)	Risperidone monotherapy	Placebo monotherapy	24 months	Overall relapse rate was 30% with risperidone, 56% with placebo. Risperidone did not protect against depressive relapse
Vieta et al., 2012*	398 (132/135/131)	Risperidone monotherapy	Placebo or oral olanzapine monotherapy	18 months	Recurrence of any mood episode: oral olanzapine 23.8%; risperidone LAI 38.9%; placebo 56.4%. Olanzapine and risperidone reduced risk of elevated mood episode but only olanzapine reduced risk of depression
Calabrese et al., 2017*	266 (133/133)	Aripiprazole monotherapy	Placebo monotherapy	12 months	Relapse to any mood episode 26.5% with aripiprazole, 51.1% with placebo. No effect on recurrence of depression

*Trial sponsored by manufacturer.
LAI, long-acting injection.

the risk of relapse compared with prior treatments. The largest (open) study[7] (n = 85) (note: reference 7 reports the results of two studies) suggested flupentixol decanoate (20 mg every 2–3 weeks) reduced recurrence risk of elevated mood episodes. Other reports describe similar effects for other FGA LAIs. The one RCT conducted with flupentixol LAI[7] showed no effect and no superiority over lithium.

Taking into account this RCT and all of the small and uncontrolled observations, there is very little evidence to support the often repeated lore that flupentixol LAI increases the risk of manic relapse and haloperidol LAI and fluphenazine LAI increase the risk of depressive relapse (or at least that FGAs provoke depression). It is notable that authors of systematic reviews[1,4] repeat this view, which seems to be based on the observed increase in depressive episodes in the open study conducted by Ahlfors and colleagues.[7] In fact, this increase occurred only in subjects whose lithium treatment had been stopped immediately before the study began. Nonetheless, oral haloperidol, when used for mania, is more likely than oral SGAs to cause a switch to depression[12] so some caution is clearly required.

We are not aware of any controlled comparisons of FGA and SGA LAIs. A Taiwanese retrospective cohort study[13] uncovered a higher risk of depressive episode recurrence and a higher likelihood of hospitalisation in those prescribed FGA LAIs (50% were prescribed flupentixol, 25% haloperidol, and 25% others) compared with those prescribed risperidone LAI. The hazard ratio for re-admission was 1.20 (95% confidence interval [CI] 1.04–1.38) – risperidone incident rate 0.42; FGAs 0.51. Of particular note was the substantial rate of treatment discontinuation. At one year only 7.2% of those initially prescribed risperidone and 2.2% of those initiated on FGA LAIs remained on the original treatment.

Conclusions

- Support for the use of FGA LAIs in bipolar disorder is weak.
- Very limited evidence suggests FGA LAIs may be effective in reducing recurrence of elevated mood but they do not prevent recurrence of depression and may increase the risk.
- Risperidone LAI and aripiprazole LAI are robustly associated with a reduced risk of recurrence of elevated mood compared with placebo.
- There is no evidence to suggest SGAs increase the risk of depression.
- Risperidone LAI and aripiprazole LAI have no effect on the risk of depressive recurrence.
- There is no evidence to support the benefit of LAIs over oral antipsychotic treatment in bipolar disorder.
- As with other conditions, the use of LAIs offers the advantage of transparency in respect to compliance: the LAI injection is either given or it is not.

References

1. Gigante AD et al. Long-acting injectable antipsychotics for the maintenance treatment of bipolar disorder. CNS Drugs 2012; **26**:403–420.

2. Samalin L et al. What is the evidence for the use of second-generation antipsychotic long-acting injectables as maintenance treatment in bipolar disorder? Nord J Psychiatry 2014; **68**:227–235.

3. Chou YH et al. A systemic review and experts' consensus for long-acting injectable antipsychotics in bipolar disorder. Clin Psychopharmacol Neurosci 2015; **13**:121–128.

4. Bond DJ et al. Depot antipsychotic medications in bipolar disorder: a review of the literature. Acta Psychiatr Scand Suppl 2007:3–16.

5. Esparon J et al. Comparison of the prophylactic action of flupenthixol with placebo in lithium treated manic-depressive patients. Br J Psychiatry 1986; **148**:723–725.

6. Yatham L et al. Randomised trial of oral vs. injectable antipsychotics in bipolar disorder. Presented at the 6th International Conference on Bipolar Disorder: June 16–18 2005: Pittsburgh, PA; 2005.

7. Ahlfors UG et al. Flupenthixol decanoate in recurrent manic-depressive illness. A comparison with lithium. Acta Psychiatr Scand 1981; **64**:226–237.

8. Macfadden W et al. A randomized, double-blind, placebo-controlled study of maintenance treatment with adjunctive risperidone long-acting therapy in patients with bipolar I disorder who relapse frequently. Bipolar Disord 2009; **11**:827–839.

9. Quiroz JA et al. Risperidone long-acting injectable monotherapy in the maintenance treatment of bipolar I disorder. Biol Psychiatry 2010; **68**:156–162.

10. Berwaerts J et al. A randomized, placebo- and active-controlled study of paliperidone extended-release as maintenance treatment in patients with bipolar I disorder after an acute manic or mixed episode. J Affect Disord 2012; **138**:247–258.

11. Buoli M et al. Paliperidone palmitate depot in the long-term treatment of psychotic bipolar disorder: a case series. Clin Neuropharmacol 2015; **38**:209–211.

12. Goikolea JM et al. Lower rate of depressive switch following antimanic treatment with second-generation antipsychotics versus haloperidol. J Affect Disord 2013; **144**:191–198.

13. Wu CS et al. Comparative effectiveness of long-acting injectable risperidone vs. long-acting injectable first-generation antipsychotics in bipolar disorder. J Affect Disord 2016; **197**:189–195.

CHAPTER 2

Physical monitoring for people with bipolar disorder (based on NICE Guidelines[1] and NPSA advice[2])

See Table 2.6.

Table 2.6 Physical monitoring for people with bipolar disorder

Test or measurement	Monitoring for all patients		Additional monitoring for specific drugs			
	Initial health check	Annual check-up	Antipsychotics	Lithium	Valproate	Carbamazepine
Thyroid function	Yes	Yes	—	At start and every 6 months; more often if evidence of deterioration		
Liver function	Yes	Yes	—		At start and periodically during treatment if clinically indicated	At start and periodically during treatment if clinically indicated
Renal function (eGFR)	Yes	Yes	—	At start and every 6 months; more often if there is evidence of deterioration or the patient starts taking interacting drugs		
Urea and electrolytes	Yes	Yes	—	At start and then every 6 months (include serum calcium)		Every 6 months. More often if clinically indicated
Full blood count	Yes	Yes	—	Only if clinically indicated	At start and at 6 months	At start and at 6 months
Blood (plasma) glucose	Yes	Yes, as part of a routine physical health check	At start and then every 4–6 months (and at 1 month if taking olanzapine); more often if evidence of elevated levels	—		
Lipid profile	Yes	Yes, as part of a routine physical health check	At start and at 3 months; more often initially if evidence of elevated levels	—		

References

Parameter					
Blood pressure	Yes	Yes, as part of a routine physical health check	During dosage titration if antipsychotic prescribed is associated with postural hypotension	—	
Prolactin	Children and adolescents only	—	At start and if symptoms of raised prolactin develop. Raised prolactin unlikely with quetiapine or aripiprazole. Very occasionally seen with olanzapine and asenapine. Very common with risperidone and FGAs		
ECG	If indicated by history or clinical picture	—	At start if there are risk factors for or existing cardiovascular disease (or haloperidol is prescribed). If relevant abnormalities are detected, as a minimum recheck after each dose increase	At start if risk factors for or existing cardiovascular disease. If relevant abnormalities are detected, as a minimum recheck after each dose increase	At start if risk factors for or existing cardiovascular disease. If relevant abnormalities are detected, as a minimum recheck after each dose increase
Weight (and height in adolescents only)	—	Yes, as part of a routine physical health check	At start then frequently for first 3 months then 3-monthly for first year. Thereafter, at least annually	At start, and when needed if the patient gains weight rapidly	At start and when needed if the patient gains weight rapidly
Plasma levels of drug	—	—	At least 3–4 days after initiation and 3–4 days after every dose change until levels stable, then **every 3 months** in the first year, then every 6 months for most patients (see NICE[1])	Titrate by effect and tolerability. Do not routinely measure unless there is evidence of lack of effectiveness, poor adherence or toxicity	Two weeks after initiation and two weeks after dose change. Thereafter, do not routinely measure unless there is evidence of lack of effectiveness, poor adherence or toxicity

For patients on **lamotrigine**, do an annual health check, but no special monitoring tests are needed although blood levels may indicate if high doses might be considered.

ECG, electrocardiogram; eGFR; estimated glomerular filtration rate; FGA, first-generation antipsychotic.

References

1. National Institute for Health and Care Excellence. Bipolar disorder: assessment and management. Clinical Guideline 185, 2014; last updated February 2016. https://www.nice.org.uk/guidance/cg185.
2. National Patient Safety Agency. Safer lithium therapy. NPSA/2009/PSA005. http://www.nrls.npsa.nhs.uk/2009.

Treatment of acute mania or hypomania

Drug treatment is the mainstay of therapy for mania and hypomania. Both antipsychotics and so-called 'mood stabilisers' are effective. Sedative and anxiolytic drugs (e.g. benzodiazepines) may add to the effects of these drugs. Drug choice is made difficult by the small number of direct comparisons and so no drug can be recommended over another on efficacy grounds. However, a multiple treatments meta-analysis[1] (which allows indirect comparison) suggested that olanzapine, risperidone, haloperidol and quetiapine had the best combination of efficacy and acceptability. The benefit of antipsychotic–mood stabiliser combinations (compared with mood stabiliser alone) is established for those relapsing while on mood stabilisers but unclear for those presenting on no treatment.[2–6]

CHAPTER 2

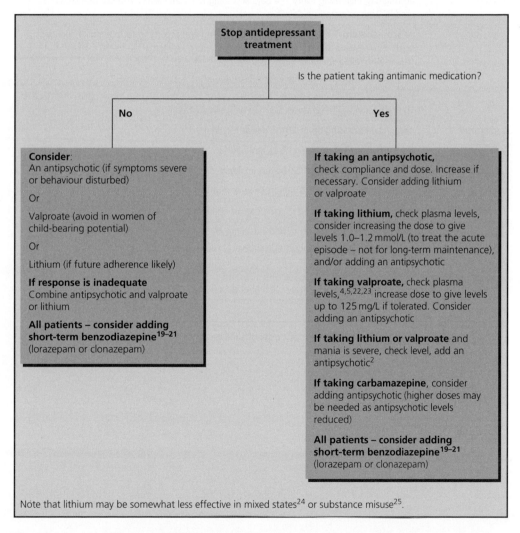

Figure 2.1 Treatment of acute mania or hypomania.[2–6,8–18]

Figure 2.1 outlines a treatment strategy for mania and hypomania. These recommendations are based on UK NICE guidelines,[3] BAP guidelines[7] and individual references cited. Where an antipsychotic is recommended, choose from those licensed for mania/bipolar disorder, that is, most conventional drugs (see individual labels/SPCs), aripiprazole, asenapine, olanzapine, risperidone and quetiapine. Suggested doses and alternative treatments are outlined in Tables 2.7 and 2.8 respectively.

Table 2.7 Drug treatment of mania: suggested doses

Drug	Dose
Lithium	400 mg/day, increasing every 3–4 days according to plasma levels. At least one study has used 800 mg as a starting dose[26]
Valproate	As **semi-sodium** – 250 mg three times daily increasing according to tolerability and plasma levels. Slow release semi-sodium valproate may also be effective (at 15–30 mg/kg)[27] but there is one failed study[28]
	As **sodium valproate** slow release – 500 mg/day increasing as above
	Higher, so-called 'loading' doses, have been used, both oral[29–31] and intravenous.[32,33] Dose is 20–30 mg/kg/day. These doses seem to be well tolerated
Aripiprazole	15 mg/day increasing up to 30 mg/day as required[34–36]
Asenapine	5 mg bd increasing to 10 mg bd as required
Cariprazine	3 mg/day increasing up to 12 mg/day as required[37]
Olanzapine	10 mg/day increasing to 15 mg or 20 mg as required
Risperidone	2 mg or 3 mg/day increased to 6 mg/day as required
Quetiapine	**IR** – 100 mg/day increasing to 800 mg as required. Higher starting doses have been used[38]
	XL – 300 mg/day increasing to 600 mg/day on day two
Haloperidol	5–10 mg/day increasing to 15 mg if required
Lorazepam[20,21]	Up to 4 mg/day (some centres use higher doses)
Clonazepam[19,21]	Up to 8 mg/day

bd, bis in die (twice a day); IR, immediate release; XL, extended release.

Table 2.8 Mania: other possible treatments. These are listed in alphabetical order – no preference is implied by the order in the table. Consult specialist and primary literature before using any treatment listed

Treatment	Comments
Allopurinol[39] (600 mg/day)	Clear therapeutic effect when added to lithium in one RCT (n = 120), and when added to valproate in another (n = 57)[40] but no effect in a smaller study[41]
Celecoxib (400 mg/day)[42]	Small RCT (n = 46) suggests benefit when used as adjunct to valproate
Clozapine[43–45]	Established treatment option for refractory mania/bipolar disorder. Rapid titration has been reported[46]
Gabapentin[47–49] (up to 2400 mg/day)	Probably only effective by virtue of an anxiolytic effect. Rarely used. Possibly useful as prophylaxis[50]
Lamotrigine[51,52] (up to 200 mg/day)	Possibly effective but better evidence for bipolar depression
Levetiracetam[53,54] (up to 4000 mg/day)	Possibly effective but controlled studies required. One case of levetiracetam causing mania[55]
Memantine[56] (10–30 mg/day)	Conflicting evidence[57,58]
Oxcarbazepine[59–65] (around 300–3000 mg/day)	Probably effective acutely and as prophylaxis although one controlled study conducted (in youths) was negative[66]
Phenytoin[67] (300–400 mg/day)	Rarely used. Limited data Complex kinetics with narrow therapeutic range
Ritanserin[68] (10 mg/day)	Supported by a single RCT. Well tolerated. May protect against EPS
Tamoxifen[69–72] (10–140 mg/day)	Possibly effective. Five small RCTs. Dose–response relationship unclear, but 80 mg/day effective when added to lithium. Evidence for efficacy as adjunct and monotherapy
Topiramate[73–76] (up to 300 mg/day)	Possibly effective. Causes weight loss but often poorly tolerated
Tryptophan depletion[77]	Supported by a small RCT
Ziprasidone[78–80]	Supported by three RCTs

EPS, extrapyramidal symptoms; RCT, randomised controlled trial.

References

1. Cipriani A et al. Comparative efficacy and acceptability of antimanic drugs in acute mania: a multiple-treatments meta-analysis. Lancet 2011; 378:1306–1315.
2. Smith LA et al. Acute bipolar mania: a systematic review and meta-analysis of co-therapy vs. monotherapy. Acta Psychiatr Scand 2007; 115:12–20.
3. National Institute for Health and Care Excellence. Bipolar disorder: assessment and management. Clinical Guideline 185, 2014; last updated February 2016. https://www.nice.org.uk/guidance/cg185.
4. Goodwin GM. Evidence-based guidelines for treating bipolar disorder: revised second edition – recommendations from the British Association for Psychopharmacology. J Psychopharmacol 2009; 23:346–388.
5. American Psychiatric Association. *Guideline Watch: Practice Guideline for the Treatment of Patients with Bipolar Disorder*, 2nd edn. Washington DC, USA: American Psychiatric Association. DOI: 10.1176/appi.books.9780890423363.148430; 2005.
6. Sachs GS. Decision tree for the treatment of bipolar disorder. J Clin Psychiatry 2003; 64 Suppl 8:35–40.
7. Goodwin GM et al. Evidence-based guidelines for treating bipolar disorder: Revised third edition recommendations from the British Association for Psychopharmacology. J Psychopharmacol 2016; 30:495–553.
8. Tohen M et al. A 12-week, double-blind comparison of olanzapine vs haloperidol in the treatment of acute mania. Arch Gen Psychiatry 2003; 60:1218–1226.
9. Baldessarini RJ et al. Olanzapine versus placebo in acute mania treatment responses in subgroups. J Clin Psychopharmacol 2003; 23:370–376.
10. Sachs G et al. Quetiapine with lithium or divalproex for the treatment of bipolar mania: a randomized, double-blind, placebo-controlled study. Bipolar Disord 2004; 6:213–223.
11. Yatham LN et al. Quetiapine versus placebo in combination with lithium or divalproex for the treatment of bipolar mania. J Clin Psychopharmacol 2004; 24:599–606.
12. Yatham LN et al. Risperidone plus lithium versus risperidone plus valproate in acute and continuation treatment of mania. Int Clin Psychopharmacol 2004; 19:103–109.
13. Bowden CL et al. Risperidone in combination with mood stabilizers: a 10-week continuation phase study in bipolar I disorder. J Clin Psychiatry 2004; 65:707–714.
14. Hirschfeld RM et al. Rapid antimanic effect of risperidone monotherapy: a 3-week multicenter, double-blind, placebo-controlled trial. Am J Psychiatry 2004; 161:1057–1065.
15. Bowden CL et al. A randomized, double-blind, placebo-controlled efficacy and safety study of quetiapine or lithium as monotherapy for mania in bipolar disorder. J Clin Psychiatry 2005; 66:111–121.
16. Khanna S et al. Risperidone in the treatment of acute mania: double-blind, placebo-controlled study. Br J Psychiatry 2005; 187:229–234.
17. Young RC et al. GERI-BD: A randomized double-blind controlled trial of lithium and divalproex in the treatment of mania in older patients with bipolar disorder. Am J Psychiatry 2017; 174:1086–1093.
18. Conus P et al. Olanzapine or chlorpromazine plus lithium in first episode psychotic mania: an 8-week randomised controlled trial. Eur Psychiatry 2015; 30:975–982.
19. Sachs GS et al. Adjunctive clonazepam for maintenance treatment of bipolar affective disorder. J Clin Psychopharmacol 1990; 10:42–47.
20. Modell JG et al. Inpatient clinical trial of lorazepam for the management of manic agitation. J Clin Psychopharmacol 1985; 5:109–113.
21. Curtin F et al. Clonazepam and lorazepam in acute mania: a Bayesian meta-analysis. J Affect Disord 2004; 78:201–208.
22. Taylor D et al. Doses of carbamazepine and valproate in bipolar affective disorder. Psychiatr Bull 1997; 21:221–223.
23. Allen MH et al. Linear relationship of valproate serum concentration to response and optimal serum levels for acute mania. Am J Psychiatry 2006; 163:272–275.
24. Swann AC et al. Lithium treatment of mania: clinical characteristics, specificity of symptom change, and outcome. Psychiatry Res 1986; 18:127–141.
25. Goldberg JF et al. A history of substance abuse complicates remission from acute mania in bipolar disorder. J Clin Psychiatry 1999; 60:733–740.
26. Bowden CL et al. Efficacy of valproate versus lithium in mania or mixed mania: a randomized, open 12-week trial. Int Clin Psychopharmacol 2010; 25:60–67.
27. McElroy SL et al. Randomized, double-blind, placebo-controlled study of divalproex extended release loading monotherapy in ambulatory bipolar spectrum disorder patients with moderate-to-severe hypomania or mild mania. J Clin Psychiatry 2010; 71:557–565.
28. Hirschfeld RM et al. A randomized, placebo-controlled, multicenter study of divalproex sodium extended-release in the acute treatment of mania. J Clin Psychiatry 2010; 71:426–432.
29. McElroy SL et al. A randomized comparison of divalproex oral loading versus haloperidol in the initial treatment of acute psychotic mania. J Clin Psychiatry 1996; 57:142–146.
30. Hirschfeld RM et al. Safety and tolerability of oral loading divalproex sodium in acutely manic bipolar patients. J Clin Psychiatry 1999; 60:815–818.
31. Hirschfeld RM et al. The safety and early efficacy of oral-loaded divalproex versus standard-titration divalproex, lithium, olanzapine, and placebo in the treatment of acute mania associated with bipolar disorder. J Clin Psychiatry 2003; 64:841–846.
32. Jagadheesan K et al. Acute antimanic efficacy and safety of intravenous valproate loading therapy: an open-label study. Neuropsychobiology 2003; 47:90–93.
33. Sekhar S et al. Efficacy of sodium valproate and haloperidol in the management of acute mania: a randomized open-label comparative study. J Clin Pharmacol 2010; 50:688–692.

34. Young AH et al. Aripiprazole monotherapy in acute mania: 12-week randomised placebo- and haloperidol-controlled study. Br J Psychiatry 2009; 194:40–48.

35. Keck PE et al. Aripiprazole monotherapy in the treatment of acute bipolar I mania: a randomized, double-blind, placebo- and lithium-controlled study. J Affect Disord 2009; 112:36–49.

36. Li DJ et al. Efficacy, safety and tolerability of aripiprazole in bipolar disorder: An updated systematic review and meta-analysis of randomized controlled trials. Prog Neuropsychopharmacol Biol Psychiatry 2017; 79:289–301.

37. Vieta E et al. Effect of cariprazine across the symptoms of mania in bipolar I disorder: Analyses of pooled data from phase II/III trials. Eur Neuropsychopharmacol 2015; 25:1882–1891.

38. Pajonk FG et al. Rapid dose titration of quetiapine for the treatment of acute schizophrenia and acute mania: a case series. J Psychopharmacol 2006; 20:119–124.

39. Machado-Vieira R et al. A double-blind, randomized, placebo-controlled 4-week study on the efficacy and safety of the purinergic agents allopurinol and dipyridamole adjunctive to lithium in acute bipolar mania. J Clin Psychiatry 2008; 69:1237–1245.

40. Jahangard L et al. In a double-blind, randomized and placebo-controlled trial, adjuvant allopurinol improved symptoms of mania in in-patients suffering from bipolar disorder. Eur Neuropsychopharmacol 2014; 24:1210–1221.

41. Fan A et al. Allopurinol augmentation in the outpatient treatment of bipolar mania: a pilot study. Bipolar Disord 2012; 14:206–210.

42. Arabzadeh S et al. Celecoxib adjunctive therapy for acute bipolar mania: a randomized, double-blind, placebo-controlled trial. Bipolar Disord 2015; 17:606–614.

43. Mahmood T et al. Clozapine in the management of bipolar and schizoaffective manic episodes resistant to standard treatment. Aust N Z J Psychiatry 1997; 31:424–426.

44. Green AI et al. Clozapine in the treatment of refractory psychotic mania. Am J Psychiatry 2000; 157:982–986.

45. Ifteni P et al. Switching bipolar disorder patients treated with clozapine to another antipsychotic medication: a mirror image study. Neuropsychiatr Dis Treat 2017; 13:201–204.

46. Aksoy Poyraz C et al. Effectiveness of ultra-rapid dose titration of clozapine for treatment-resistant bipolar mania: case series. Ther Adv Psychopharmacol 2015; 5:237–242.

47. Macdonald KJ et al. Newer antiepileptic drugs in bipolar disorder: rationale for use and role in therapy. CNS Drugs 2002; 16:549–562.

48. Cabras PL et al. Clinical experience with gabapentin in patients with bipolar or schizoaffective disorder: results of an open-label study. J Clin Psychiatry 1999; 60:245–248.

49. Pande AC et al. Gabapentin in bipolar disorder: a placebo-controlled trial of adjunctive therapy. Gabapentin Bipolar Disorder Study Group. Bipolar Disord 2000; 2 (3 Pt 2):249–255.

50. Vieta E et al. A double-blind, randomized, placebo-controlled, prophylaxis study of adjunctive gabapentin for bipolar disorder. J Clin Psychiatry 2006; 67:473–477.

51. Calabrese JR et al. Spectrum of activity of lamotrigine in treatment-refractory bipolar disorder. Am J Psychiatry 1999; 156:1019–1023.

52. Bowden CL et al. A placebo-controlled 18-month trial of lamotrigine and lithium maintenance treatment in recently manic or hypomanic patients with bipolar I disorder. Arch Gen Psychiatry 2003; 60:392–400.

53. Grunze H et al. Levetiracetam in the treatment of acute mania: an open add-on study with an on-off-on design. J Clin Psychiatry 2003; 64:781–784.

54. Goldberg JF et al. Levetiracetam for acute mania (Letter). Am J Psychiatry 2002; 159:148.

55. Park EM et al. Acute mania associated with levetiracetam treatment. Psychosomatics 2014; 55:98–100.

56. Koukopoulos A et al. Antimanic and mood-stabilizing effect of memantine as an augmenting agent in treatment-resistant bipolar disorder. Bipolar Disord 2010; 12:348–349.

57. Veronese N et al. Acetylcholinesterase inhibitors and memantine in bipolar disorder: a systematic review and best evidence synthesis of the efficacy and safety for multiple disease dimensions. J Affect Disord 2016; 197:268–280.

58. Serra G et al. Three-year, naturalistic, mirror-image assessment of adding memantine to the treatment of 30 treatment-resistant patients with bipolar disorder. J Clin Psychiatry 2015; 76:e91–97.

59. Benedetti A et al. Oxcarbazepine as add-on treatment in patients with bipolar manic, mixed or depressive episode. J Affect Disord 2004; 79:273–277.

60. Lande RG. Oxcarbazepine: efficacy, safety, and tolerability in the treatment of mania. Int J Psychiatry Clin Pract 2004; 8:37–40.

61. Ghaemi SN et al. Oxcarbazepine treatment of bipolar disorder. J Clin Psychiatry 2003; 64:943–945.

62. Pratoomsri W et al. Oxcarbazepine in the treatment of bipolar disorder: a review. Can J Psychiatry 2006; 51:540–545.

63. Juruena MF et al. Bipolar I and II disorder residual symptoms: oxcarbazepine and carbamazepine as add-on treatment to lithium in a double-blind, randomized trial. Prog Neuropsychopharmacol Biol Psychiatry 2009; 33:94–99.

64. Suppes T et al. Comparison of two anticonvulsants in a randomized, single-blind treatment of hypomanic symptoms in patients with bipolar disorder. Aust N Z J Psychiatry 2007; 41:397–402.

65. Vieta E et al. A double-blind, randomized, placebo-controlled prophylaxis trial of oxcarbazepine as adjunctive treatment to lithium in the long-term treatment of bipolar I and II disorder. Int J Neuropsychopharmacol 2008; 11:445–452.

66. Wagner KD et al. A double-blind, randomized, placebo-controlled trial of oxcarbazepine in the treatment of bipolar disorder in children and adolescents. Am J Psychiatry 2006; 163:1179–1186.

67. Mishory A et al. Phenytoin as an antimanic anticonvulsant: a controlled study. Am J Psychiatry 2000; 157:463–465.

68. Akhondzadeh S et al. Ritanserin as an adjunct to lithium and haloperidol for the treatment of medication-naive patients with acute mania: a double blind and placebo controlled trial. BMC Psychiatry 2003; 3:7.

CHAPTER 2

69. Zarate CA, Jr. et al. Efficacy of a protein kinase C inhibitor (tamoxifen) in the treatment of acute mania: a pilot study. Bipolar Disord 2007; 9:561–570.

70. Yildiz A et al. Protein kinase C inhibition in the treatment of mania: a double-blind, placebo-controlled trial of tamoxifen. Arch Gen Psychiatry 2008; 65:255–263.

71. Amrollahi Z et al. Double-blind, randomized, placebo-controlled 6-week study on the efficacy and safety of the tamoxifen adjunctive to lithium in acute bipolar mania. J Affect Disord 2011; 129:327–331.

72. Talaei A et al. Tamoxifen: a protein kinase C inhibitor to treat mania: a systematic review and meta-analysis of randomized, placebo-controlled trials. J Clin Psychopharmacol 2016; 36:272–275.

73. Grunze HC et al. Antimanic efficacy of topiramate in 11 patients in an open trial with an on-off-on design. J Clin Psychiatry 2001; 62:464–468.

74. Yatham LN et al. Third generation anticonvulsants in bipolar disorder: a review of efficacy and summary of clinical recommendations. J Clin Psychiatry 2002; 63:275–283.

75. Vieta E et al. 1-year follow-up of patients treated with risperidone and topiramate for a manic episode. J Clin Psychiatry 2003; 64:834–839.

76. Vieta E et al. Use of topiramate in treatment-resistant bipolar spectrum disorders. J Clin Psychopharmacol 2002; 22:431–435.

77. Applebaum J et al. Rapid tryptophan depletion as a treatment for acute mania: a double-blind, pilot-controlled study. Bipolar Disord 2007; 9:884–887.

78. Keck PE, Jr. et al. Ziprasidone in the treatment of acute bipolar mania: a three-week, placebo-controlled, double-blind, randomized trial. Am J Psychiatry 2003; 160:741–748.

79. Potkin SG et al. Ziprasidone in acute bipolar mania: a 21-day randomized, double-blind, placebo-controlled replication trial. J Clin Psychopharmacol 2005; 25:301–310.

80. Vieta E et al. Ziprasidone in the treatment of acute mania: a 12-week, placebo-controlled, haloperidol-referenced study. J Psychopharmacol 2010; 24:547–558.

Rapid-cycling bipolar disorder

Rapid cycling is usually defined as bipolar disorder in which four or more episodes of (hypo) mania or depression (or four clear switches in polarity) occur in a 12-month period. It is generally held to be less responsive to drug treatment than non-rapid-cycling bipolar illness[1,2] and entails considerable depressive morbidity and suicide risk.[3] Table 2.9 outlines a treatment strategy for rapid cycling based on rather limited data and very few direct comparisons of drugs.[4,5] This strategy is broadly in line with the findings of published systematic reviews.[5,6] NICE conclude that there is no evidence to support rapid-cycling illness being managed any differently from that with a more conventional course.[7] There is no formal first choice agent or combination – prescribing depends partly on what treatments have already been used in an attempt to prevent or treat mood episodes.

In practice, response to treatment is sometimes idiosyncratic: individuals may show significant response only to one or two drugs. Spontaneous or treatment-related remissions occur in around a third of rapid cyclers[8] and rapid cycling may come and go in many patients.[9] Non-drug methods may also be considered.[10,11]

Table 2.9 Recommended treatment strategy for rapid-cycling bipolar disorder

Step	Suggested treatment
1	**Withdraw antidepressants** in all patients[12–17] (some controversial evidence supports continuation of SSRIs[18,19])
2	**Evaluate possible precipitants** (e.g. alcohol, thyroid dysfunction, external stressors)[2]
3	**Optimise mood stabiliser treatment**[20–23] (using plasma levels), and **Consider combining mood stabilisers**, e.g. lithium + valproate; lithium + lamotrigine, or go to Step 4
4	**Consider other (usually adjunct) treatment options**: (alphabetical order; preferred treatment options in bold) **Aripiprazole**[24,25] (15–30 mg/day) Clozapine[26] (usual doses) Lamotrigine[27–29] (up to 225 mg/day) Levetiracetam[30] (up to 2000 mg/day) Nimodipine[31,32] (180 mg/day) **Olanzapine**[20] (usual doses) **Quetiapine**[33–36] (300–600 mg/day) Risperidone[37–39] (up to 6 mg/day) Thyroxine[40,41] (150–400 µg/day) Topiramate[42] (up to 300 mg/day)

Choice of drug is determined by patient factors – there are few comparative efficacy data to guide choice at the time of writing. **Quetiapine** probably has best supporting data[33–35] but there is no evidence of superiority over aripiprazole or olanzapine. Supporting data for levetiracetam, nimodipine, thyroxine and topiramate are rather limited.
SSRI, selective serotonin reuptake inhibitor.

References

1. Calabrese JR et al. Current research on rapid cycling bipolar disorder and its treatment. J Affect Disord 2001; 67:241–255.
2. Kupka RW et al. Rapid and non-rapid cycling bipolar disorder: a meta-analysis of clinical studies. J Clin Psychiatry 2003; 64:1483–1494.
3. Coryell W et al. The long-term course of rapid-cycling bipolar disorder. Arch Gen Psychiatry 2003; 60:914–920.
4. Tondo L et al. Rapid-cycling bipolar disorder: effects of long-term treatments. Acta Psychiatr Scand 2003; 108:4–14.
5. Fountoulakis KN et al. A systematic review of the evidence on the treatment of rapid cycling bipolar disorder. Bipolar Disord 2013; 15:115–137.
6. Fountoulakis KN et al. The International College of Neuro-Psychopharmacology (CINP) Treatment Guidelines for Bipolar Disorder in Adults (CINP-BD-2017), Part 2: Review, Grading of the Evidence, and a Precise Algorithm. Int J Neuropsychopharmacol 2017; 20:121–179.
7. National Institute for Health and Care Excellence. Bipolar disorder: assessment and management. Clinical Guideline 185, 2014; last updated February 2016. https://www.nice.org.uk/guidance/cg185.
8. Koukopoulos A et al. Duration and stability of the rapid-cycling course: a long-term personal follow-up of 109 patients. J Affect Disord 2003; 73:75–85.
9. Carvalho AF et al. Rapid cycling in bipolar disorder: a systematic review. J Clin Psychiatry 2014; 75:e578–586.
10. Dell'osso B et al. Augmentative transcranial magnetic stimulation (TMS) combined with brain navigation in drug-resistant rapid cycling bipolar depression: a case report of acute and maintenance efficacy. World J Biol Psychiatry 2009; 10:673–676.
11. Marangell LB et al. A 1-year pilot study of vagus nerve stimulation in treatment-resistant rapid-cycling bipolar disorder. J Clin Psychiatry 2008; 69:183–189.
12. Wehr TA et al. Can antidepressants cause mania and worsen the course of affective illness? Am J Psychiatry 1987; 144:1403–1411.
13. Altshuler LL et al. Antidepressant-induced mania and cycle acceleration: a controversy revisited. Am J Psychiatry 1995; 152:1130–1138.
14. American Psychiatric Association. Practice guideline for the treatment of patients with bipolar disorder. Am J Psychiatry 2002; 159 Suppl 4:1–50.
15. Ghaemi SN et al. Antidepressant discontinuation in bipolar depression: a Systematic Treatment Enhancement Program for Bipolar Disorder (STEP-BD) randomized clinical trial of long-term effectiveness and safety. J Clin Psychiatry 2010; 71:372–380.
16. Ghaemi SN. Treatment of rapid-cycling bipolar disorder: are antidepressants mood destabilizers? Am J Psychiatry 2008; 165:300–302.
17. El-Mallakh RS et al. Antidepressants worsen rapid-cycling course in bipolar depression: a STEP-BD randomized clinical trial. J Affect Disord 2015; 184:318–321.
18. Amsterdam JD et al. Efficacy and mood conversion rate during long-term fluoxetine v. lithium monotherapy in rapid- and non-rapid-cycling bipolar II disorder. Br J Psychiatry 2013; 202:301–306.
19. Amsterdam JD et al. Effectiveness and mood conversion rate of short-term fluoxetine monotherapy in patients with rapid cycling bipolar II depression versus patients with nonrapid cycling bipolar II depression. J Clin Psychopharmacol 2013; 33:420–424.
20. Sanger TM et al. Olanzapine in the acute treatment of bipolar I disorder with a history of rapid cycling. J Affect Disord 2003; 73:155–161.
21. Kemp DE et al. A 6-month, double-blind, maintenance trial of lithium monotherapy versus the combination of lithium and divalproex for rapid-cycling bipolar disorder and co-occurring substance abuse or dependence. J Clin Psychiatry 2009; 70:113–121.
22. da Rocha FF et al. Addition of lamotrigine to valproic acid: a successful outcome in a case of rapid-cycling bipolar affective disorder. Prog Neuropsychopharmacol Biol Psychiatry 2007; 31:1548–1549.
23. Woo YS et al. Lamotrigine added to valproate successfully treated a case of ultra-rapid cycling bipolar disorder. Psychiatry Clin Neurosci 2007; 61:130–131.
24. Suppes T et al. Efficacy and safety of aripiprazole in subpopulations with acute manic or mixed episodes of bipolar I disorder. J Affect Disord 2008; 107:145–154.
25. Muzina DJ et al. Aripiprazole monotherapy in patients with rapid-cycling bipolar I disorder: an analysis from a long-term, double-blind, placebo-controlled study. Int J Clin Pract 2008; 62:679–687.
26. Calabrese JR et al. Clozapine prophylaxis in rapid cycling bipolar disorder. J Clin Psychopharmacol 1991; 11:396–397.
27. Fatemi SH et al. Lamotrigine in rapid-cycling bipolar disorder. J Clin Psychiatry 1997; 58:522–527.
28. Calabrese JR et al. A double-blind, placebo-controlled, prophylaxis study of lamotrigine in rapid-cycling bipolar disorder. Lamictal 614 Study Group. J Clin Psychiatry 2000; 61:841–850.
29. Wang Z et al. Lamotrigine adjunctive therapy to lithium and divalproex in depressed patients with rapid cycling bipolar disorder and a recent substance use disorder: a 12-week, double-blind, placebo-controlled pilot study. Psychopharmacol Bull 2010; 43:5–21.
30. Braunig P et al. Levetiracetam in the treatment of rapid cycling bipolar disorder. J Psychopharmacol 2003; 17:239–241.
31. Goodnick PJ. Nimodipine treatment of rapid cycling bipolar disorder. J Clin Psychiatry 1995; 56:330.
32. Pazzaglia PJ et al. Preliminary controlled trial of nimodipine in ultra-rapid cycling affective dysregulation. Psychiatry Res 1993; 49:257–272.
33. Goldberg JF et al. Effectiveness of quetiapine in rapid cycling bipolar disorder: a preliminary study. J Affect Disord 2008; 105:305–310.
34. Vieta E et al. Quetiapine monotherapy in the treatment of patients with bipolar I or II depression and a rapid-cycling disease course: a randomized, double-blind, placebo-controlled study. Bipolar Disord 2007; 9:413–425.
35. Langosch JM et al. Efficacy of quetiapine monotherapy in rapid-cycling bipolar disorder in comparison with sodium valproate. J Clin Psychopharmacol 2008; 28:555–560.
36. Vieta E et al. Quetiapine in the treatment of rapid cycling bipolar disorder. Bipolar Disord 2002; 4:335–340.
37. Jacobsen FM. Risperidone in the treatment of affective illness and obsessive-compulsive disorder. J Clin Psychiatry 1995; 56:423–429.
38. Bobo WV et al. A randomized open comparison of long-acting injectable risperidone and treatment as usual for prevention of relapse, rehospitalization, and urgent care referral in community-treated patients with rapid cycling bipolar disorder. Clin Neuropharmacol 2011; 34:224–233.
39. Vieta E et al. Treatment of refractory rapid cycling bipolar disorder with risperidone. J Clin Psychopharmacol 1998; 18:172–174.
40. Weeston TF et al. High-dose T4 for rapid-cycling bipolar disorder. J Am Acad Child Adolesc Psychiatry 1996; 35:131–132.
41. Extein IL. High doses of levothyroxine for refractory rapid cycling. Am J Psychiatry 2000; 157:1704–1705.
42. Chen CK et al. Combination treatment of clozapine and topiramate in resistant rapid-cycling bipolar disorder. Clin Neuropharmacol 2005; 28:136–138.

Bipolar depression

Bipolar depression is a common and debilitating disorder which shares the same diagnostic criteria for a major depressive episode with unipolar disorder but may differ in severity, time course, liability to recurrence and response to drug treatment. Episodes of bipolar depression are, compared with unipolar depression, more rapid in onset, more frequent, more severe, shorter and more likely to involve delusions and reverse neuro-vegetative symptoms such as hyperphagia and hypersomnia.[1-3] Around 15% of people with bipolar disorder commit suicide,[4] a statistic which reflects the severity and frequency of depressive episodes. Bipolar depression affords greater socio-economic burden than either mania or unipolar depression[5] and represents the majority of symptomatic illness in bipolar disorder in respect to time.[6,7]

The drug treatment of bipolar depression is somewhat controversial for two reasons. First, until recently there were few well-conducted RCTs specifically in bipolar depression and, second, the condition entails consideration of the long-term outcome rather than only discrete episode response.[8] We have some knowledge of the therapeutic effects of drugs in bipolar depressive episodes but more limited awareness of the therapeutic or deleterious effects of drugs in the longer term. In the UK, NICE recommends the initial use of fluoxetine combined with olanzapine or quetiapine on its own (assuming an antipsychotic is not already prescribed).[9] Lamotrigine is considered to be second-line treatment. BAP guidelines[10] have lamotrigine as a first-line option, albeit with the caveat that a mood stabiliser or antipsychotic will be needed to protect against mania. Lurasidone is also a first-line option in the BAP guidelines. Tables 2.10, 2.11 and 2.12 give some broad guidance on treatment options in bipolar depression.

Meta-analysis in bipolar depression

Meta-analytic studies in bipolar depression are constrained by the variety of methods used to assess efficacy. This means that many scientifically robust studies cannot be included in some meta-analyses because their parameters (outcomes, duration, etc.) do not match, and so cannot be compared with other studies. Early lithium studies are an important example – their short duration and crossover design precludes their inclusion in meta-analysis. BAP guidelines are dismissive of network meta-analyses because outcome is heavily influenced by inclusion criteria and because findings often contradict direct comparisons.[10]

A meta-analysis of five trials (906 participants) revealed that antidepressants were no better than placebo in respect to response or remission, although results approached statistical significance.[85] Another analysis of trials not involving antidepressants[109] (7307 participants) found a statistical advantage over placebo for olanzapine + fluoxetine, valproate, quetiapine, lurasidone, olanzapine, aripiprazole and carbamazepine (in order of effect size, highest first).

The largest analysis is a multiple treatments or network meta-analysis of 29 studies including 8331 subjects.[110] Overall, olanzapine + fluoxetine, lurasidone, olanzapine, valproate, SSRIs and quetiapine were ranked highest in terms of effect size and response with olanzapine + fluoxetine ranked first for both.

Table 2.10 Established treatments for bipolar depression (listed in alphabetical order)

Drug/regime	Comments
Lamotrigine[1,11–17]	Lamotrigine appears to be effective both as a treatment for bipolar depression and as prophylaxis against further episodes. It does not induce switching or rapid cycling. It is as effective as citalopram and causes less weight gain than lithium. Overall, the effect of lamotrigine is modest, with numerous failed trials.[18,19] It may be useful as an adjunct to lithium[20] or as an alternative to it in pregnancy.[21] A recent trial[22] suggests robust efficacy when combined with quetiapine
	Treatment is somewhat complicated by the small risk of rash, which is associated with speed of dose titration. The necessity for titration may limit clinical utility
	A further complication is the question of dose: 50 mg/day has efficacy, but 200 mg/day is probably better. In the USA, doses of up to 1200 mg/day have been used (mean around 250 mg/day). Plasma concentrations (only the range for anticonvulsant effects is known) may guide the need for higher doses
Lithium[1,11,23–25]	Lithium is probably effective in treating bipolar depression but supporting data are methodologically questionable.[26] There is some evidence that lithium prevents depressive relapse but its effects on manic relapse are considered more robust. There is fairly strong support for lithium in reducing suicidality in bipolar disorder[27,28]
Lurasidone	Three RCTs show good effect for lurasidone either alone[29] or as an adjunct to mood stabilisers.[30,31] A further RCT reported good outcome in bipolar depression with sub-syndromal hypomanic symptoms.[32] Pooled analysis suggests response is dose-related.[33] Not licensed for bipolar depression in the UK (but is licensed in the USA) at the time of writing
Mood stabiliser + antidepressant[34–40]	Antidepressants are still widely used in bipolar depression, particularly for breakthrough episodes occurring in those on mood stabilisers. They have been assumed to be effective, although there is a risk of cycle acceleration and/or switching. Studies suggest mood stabilisers alone are just as effective as mood stabilisers/antidepressant combination although sub-analysis suggested higher doses of antidepressants may be effective.[41–43] Tricyclics and MAOIs are usually best avoided. SSRIs are generally recommended if an antidepressant is to be prescribed. Venlafaxine and bupropion (amfebutamone) have also been used. Venlafaxine may be more likely to induce a switch to mania[44,45]
	Continuing antidepressant treatment after resolution of symptoms may protect against depressive relapse,[46,47] although only in the absence of a mood stabiliser.[48] At the time of writing, there is no consensus on whether or not to continue antidepressants long term.[49] The most recent findings suggest that switch rates are no higher with sertraline alone than with lithium + sertraline[50]
Olanzapine +/– fluoxetine[11,26,51–54]	This combination (Symbyax®) is more effective than both placebo and olanzapine alone in treating bipolar depression. The dose is 6 and 25 mg or 12 and 50 mg/day (so presumably 5/20 mg and 10/40 mg are effective). May be more effective than lamotrigine. Reasonable evidence of prophylactic effect. Recommended as first-line treatment by NICE[9]
	Olanzapine alone is effective when compared with placebo,[55] but the combination with fluoxetine is more effective. (This is possibly the strongest evidence for a beneficial effect for an antidepressant in bipolar depression)
Quetiapine[56–60]	Five large RCTs have demonstrated clear efficacy for doses of 300 mg and 600 mg daily (as monotherapy) in bipolar I and bipolar II depression. A later study in Chinese patients demonstrated the efficacy of 300 mg/day[61] in bipolar I depression. May be superior to both lithium and paroxetine
	Quetiapine also prevents relapse into depression and mania[62,63] and so is one of the treatments of choice in bipolar depression. It appears not to be associated with switching to mania
Valproate[1,11,64–68]	Limited evidence of efficacy as monotherapy but recommended in some guidelines. Several very small RCTs but many negative, however meta-analyses do support antidepressant efficacy.[67] Probably protects against depressive relapse but database is small

MAOI, monoamine oxidase inhibitor; RCT, randomised controlled trial; SSRI, selective serotonin reuptake inhibitor.

Table 2.11 Alternative treatments for bipolar depression – refer to primary literature before using

Drug/regime	Comments
Antidepressants[69–77]	'Unopposed' antidepressants (i.e. without mood-stabiliser protection) are generally to be avoided in bipolar depression because of the risk of switching. There is also evidence that they are relatively less effective (perhaps not effective at all) in bipolar depression than in unipolar depression although dose may be critical.[43] Short-term use of fluoxetine, venlafaxine and moclobemide seems reasonably effective and safe even as monotherapy. A meta-analysis suggested a large effect size for tranylcypromine in the absence of any risk of switching.[78] Overall, however, unopposed antidepressant treatment should be avoided, especially in bipolar I disorder[49]
Carbamazepine[1,11,79]	Occasionally recommended but database is poor and effect modest. May have useful activity when added to other mood stabilisers
Cariprazine[80]	One RCT suggests that cariprazine at 1.5 mg/day is effective in bipolar I depression
Pramipexole[81,82]	Pramipexole is a dopamine agonist which is widely used in Parkinson's disease. Two small placebo-controlled trials suggest useful efficacy in bipolar depression. Effective dose averages around 1.7 mg/day. Both studies used pramipexole as an adjunct to existing mood-stabiliser treatment. Neither study detected an increased risk of switching to mania/hypomania (a theoretical consideration) but data are insufficient to exclude this possibility. Probably best reserved for specialist centres

RCT, randomised controlled trial.

Table 2.12 Other possible treatments for bipolar depression – seek specialist advice before using

Drug/regime	Comments
Aripiprazole[83–86]	Limited support from open studies as add-on treatment. RCT negative. Possibly not effective
Gabapentin[1,87,88]	Open studies suggest modest effect when added to mood stabilisers or antipsychotics. Doses average around 1750 mg/day. Anxiolytic effect may account for apparent effect in bipolar depression
Inositol[89]	Small, randomised, pilot study suggests that 12 g/day inositol is effective in bipolar depression
Ketamine[90–93]	A single IV dose of 0.5 mg/kg is effective in refractory bipolar depression. Very high response rate. Dissociative symptoms common but brief. Risk of ulcerative cystitis if repeatedly used
Mifepristone[94,95]	Some evidence of mood-elevating properties in bipolar depression. May also improve cognitive function. Dose is 600 mg/day
Modafinil[96,97]	One positive RCT as adjunct to mood stabiliser. Dose is 100–200 mg/day. Positive RCT with armodafinil 150 mg/day
Omega-3 fatty acids[98,99]	One positive RCT (1 g/2 g a day) and one negative (6 g a day)
Riluzole[100,101]	Riluzole shares some pharmacological characteristics with lamotrigine. Database is limited. The only RCT found no evidence of efficacy[102]
Thyroxine[103]	Limited evidence of efficacy as augmentation. Doses average around 300 µg/day. One failed RCT[104]
Zonisamide[105–108]	Supported by several open-label studies. Dose is 100–300 mg/day

IV, intravenous; RCT, randomised controlled trial.

Summary of drug choice

The combination of olanzapine + fluoxetine is probably the most effective treatment available for bipolar depression. Other SSRIs may be effective but should be avoided unless clear individual benefit is obvious.[49] Alternative first-line choices are quetiapine, olanzapine, lurasidone, lamotrigine and valproate. These drugs differ substantially in adverse effect profile, tolerability and cost, each of which needs to be considered when prescribing for an individual. Lithium is also effective but supporting evidence is relatively weak. Aripiprazole, risperidone, ziprasidone, tricyclics and MAOIs (with the possible exception of tranylcypromine) are probably not effective and should not be used routinely.[110]

References

1. Malhi GS et al. Bipolar depression: management options. CNS Drugs 2003; 17:9–25.
2. Perlis RH et al. Clinical features of bipolar depression versus major depressive disorder in large multicenter trials. Am J Psychiatry 2006; 163:225–231.
3. Mitchell PB et al. Comparison of depressive episodes in bipolar disorder and in major depressive disorder within bipolar disorder pedigrees. Br J Psychiatry 2011; 199:303–309.
4. Haddad P et al. Pharmacological management of bipolar depression. Acta Psychiatr Scand 2002; 105:401–403.
5. Hirschfeld RM. Bipolar depression: the real challenge. Eur Neuropsychopharmacol 2004; 14 Suppl 2:S83–S88.
6. Judd LL et al. The long-term natural history of the weekly symptomatic status of bipolar I disorder. Arch Gen Psychiatry 2002; 59:530–537.
7. Judd LL et al. A prospective investigation of the natural history of the long-term weekly symptomatic status of bipolar II disorder. Arch Gen Psychiatry 2003; 60:261–269.
8. Baldassano CF et al. Rethinking the treatment paradigm for bipolar depression: the importance of long-term management. CNS Spectr 2004; 9:11–18.
9. National Institute for Health and Care Excellence. Bipolar disorder: assessment and management. Clinical Guideline 185, 2014; last updated February 2016. https://www.nice.org.uk/guidance/cg185.
10. Goodwin GM et al. Evidence-based guidelines for treating bipolar disorder: Revised third edition recommendations from the British Association for Psychopharmacology. Psychopharmacol 2016; 30:495–553.
11. Yatham LN et al. Bipolar depression: criteria for treatment selection, definition of refractoriness, and treatment options. Bipolar Disord 2003; 5:85–97.
12. Calabrese JR et al. A double-blind placebo-controlled study of lamotrigine monotherapy in outpatients with bipolar I depression. Lamictal 602 Study Group. J Clin Psychiatry 1999; 60:79–88.
13. Bowden CL et al. Lamotrigine in the treatment of bipolar depression. Eur Neuropsychopharmacol 1999; 9 Suppl 4:S113–S117.
14. Marangell LB et al. Lamotrigine treatment of bipolar disorder: data from the first 500 patients in STEP-BD. Bipolar Disord 2004; 6:139–143.
15. Schaffer A et al. Randomized, double-blind pilot trial comparing lamotrigine versus citalopram for the treatment of bipolar depression. J Affect Disord 2006; 96:95–99.
16. Bowden CL et al. Impact of lamotrigine and lithium on weight in obese and nonobese patients with bipolar I disorder. Am J Psychiatry 2006; 163:1199–1201.
17. Suppes T et al. A single blind comparison of lithium and lamotrigine for the treatment of bipolar II depression. J Affect Disord 2008; 111:334–343.
18. Geddes JR et al. Lamotrigine for treatment of bipolar depression: independent meta-analysis and meta-regression of individual patient data from five randomised trials. Br J Psychiatry 2009; 194:4–9.
19. Calabrese JR et al. Lamotrigine in the acute treatment of bipolar depression: results of five double-blind, placebo-controlled clinical trials. Bipolar Disord 2008; 10:323–333.
20. van der Loos ML et al. Efficacy and safety of lamotrigine as add-on treatment to lithium in bipolar depression: a multicenter, double-blind, placebo-controlled trial. J Clin Psychiatry 2009; 70:223–231.
21. Newport DJ et al. Lamotrigine in bipolar disorder: efficacy during pregnancy. Bipolar Disord 2008; 10:432–436.
22. Geddes JR et al. Comparative evaluation of quetiapine plus lamotrigine combination versus quetiapine monotherapy (and folic acid versus placebo) in bipolar depression (CEQUEL): a 2 x 2 factorial randomised trial. Lancet Psychiatry 2016; 3:31–39.
23. Geddes JR et al. Long-term lithium therapy for bipolar disorder: systematic review and meta-analysis of randomized controlled trials. Am J Psychiatry 2004; 161:217–222.
24. Calabrese JR et al. A placebo-controlled 18-month trial of lamotrigine and lithium maintenance treatment in recently depressed patients with bipolar I disorder. J Clin Psychiatry 2003; 64:1013–1024.

25. Prien RF et al. Lithium carbonate and imipramine in prevention of affective episodes. A comparison in recurrent affective illness. Arch Gen Psychiatry 1973; 29:420–425.

26. Grunze H et al. The World Federation of Societies of Biological Psychiatry (WFSBP) Guidelines for the Biological Treatment of Bipolar Disorders: Update 2010 on the treatment of acute bipolar depression. World J Biol Psychiatry 2010; 11:81–109.

27. Goodwin FK et al. Suicide risk in bipolar disorder during treatment with lithium and divalproex. JAMA 2003; 290:1467–1473.

28. Kessing LV et al. Suicide risk in patients treated with lithium. Arch Gen Psychiatry 2005; 62:860–866.

29. Loebel A et al. Lurasidone monotherapy in the treatment of bipolar I depression: a randomized, double-blind, placebo-controlled study. Am J Psychiatry 2014; 171:160–168.

30. Loebel A et al. Lurasidone as adjunctive therapy with lithium or valproate for the treatment of bipolar I depression: a randomized, double-blind, placebo-controlled study. Am J Psychiatry 2014; 171:169–177.

31. Suppes T et al. Lurasidone adjunctive with lithium or valproate for bipolar depression: a placebo-controlled trial utilizing prospective and retrospective enrolment cohorts. J Psychiatr Res 2016; 78:86–93.

32. Suppes T et al. Lurasidone for the treatment of major depressive disorder with mixed features: a randomized, double-blind, placebo-controlled study. Am J Psychiatry 2016; 173:400–407.

33. Chapel S et al. Lurasidone dose response in bipolar depression: a population dose-response analysis. Clin Ther 2016; 38:4–15.

34. Calabrese JR et al. International Consensus Group on Bipolar I Depression Treatment Guidelines. J Clin Psychiatry 2004; 65:571–579.

35. Nemeroff CB et al. Double-blind, placebo-controlled comparison of imipramine and paroxetine in the treatment of bipolar depression. Am J Psychiatry 2001; 158:906–912.

36. Vieta E et al. A randomized trial comparing paroxetine and venlafaxine in the treatment of bipolar depressed patients taking mood stabilizers. J Clin Psychiatry 2002; 63:508–512.

37. Young LT et al. Double-blind comparison of addition of a second mood stabilizer versus an antidepressant to an initial mood stabilizer for treatment of patients with bipolar depression. Am J Psychiatry 2000; 157:124–126.

38. Fawcett JA. Lithium combinations in acute and maintenance treatment of unipolar and bipolar depression. J Clin Psychiatry 2003; 64 Suppl 5:32–37.

39. Altshuler L et al. The impact of antidepressant discontinuation versus antidepressant continuation on 1-year risk for relapse of bipolar depression: a retrospective chart review. J Clin Psychiatry 2001; 62:612–616.

40. Erfurth A et al. Bupropion as add-on strategy in difficult-to-treat bipolar depressive patients. Neuropsychobiology 2002; 45 Suppl 1:33–36.

41. Sachs GS et al. Effectiveness of adjunctive antidepressant treatment for bipolar depression. N Engl J Med 2007; 356:1711–1722.

42. Goldberg JF et al. Adjunctive antidepressant use and symptomatic recovery among bipolar depressed patients with concomitant manic symptoms: findings from the STEP-BD. Am J Psychiatry 2007; 164:1348–1355.

43. Tada M et al. Antidepressant dose and treatment response in bipolar depression: reanalysis of the Systematic Treatment Enhancement Program for Bipolar Disorder (STEP-BD) data. J Psychiatr Res 2015; 68:151–156.

44. Post RM et al. Mood switch in bipolar depression: comparison of adjunctive venlafaxine, bupropion and sertraline. Br J Psychiatry 2006; 189:124–131.

45. Leverich GS et al. Risk of switch in mood polarity to hypomania or mania in patients with bipolar depression during acute and continuation trials of venlafaxine, sertraline, and bupropion as adjuncts to mood stabilizers. Am J Psychiatry 2006; 163:232–239.

46. Salvi V et al. The use of antidepressants in bipolar disorder. J Clin Psychiatry 2008; 69:1307–1318.

47. Altshuler LL et al. Impact of antidepressant continuation after acute positive or partial treatment response for bipolar depression: a blinded, randomized study. J Clin Psychiatry 2009; 70:450–457.

48. Ghaemi SN et al. Long-term antidepressant treatment in bipolar disorder: meta-analyses of benefits and risks. Acta Psychiatr Scand 2008; 118:347–356.

49. Pacchiarotti I et al. The International Society for Bipolar Disorders (ISBD) task force report on antidepressant use in bipolar disorders. Am J Psychiatry 2013; 170:1249–1262.

50. Altshuler LL et al. Switch rates during acute treatment for bipolar II depression with lithium, sertraline, or the two combined: a randomized double-blind comparison. Am J Psychiatry 2017; 174:266–276.

51. Tohen M et al. Efficacy of olanzapine and olanzapine-fluoxetine combination in the treatment of bipolar I depression. Arch Gen Psychiatry 2003; 60:1079–1088.

52. Brown EB et al. A 7-week, randomized, double-blind trial of olanzapine/fluoxetine combination versus lamotrigine in the treatment of bipolar I depression. J Clin Psychiatry 2006; 67:1025–1033.

53. Corya SA et al. A 24-week open-label extension study of olanzapine-fluoxetine combination and olanzapine monotherapy in the treatment of bipolar depression. J Clin Psychiatry 2006; 67:798–806.

54. Dube S et al. Onset of antidepressant effect of olanzapine and olanzapine/fluoxetine combination in bipolar depression. Bipolar Disord 2007; 9:618–627.

55. Tohen M et al. Randomised, double-blind, placebo-controlled study of olanzapine in patients with bipolar I depression. Br J Psychiatry 2012; 201:376–382.

56. Calabrese JR et al. A randomized, double-blind, placebo-controlled trial of quetiapine in the treatment of bipolar I or II depression. Am J Psychiatry 2005; 162:1351–1360.

57. Thase ME et al. Efficacy of quetiapine monotherapy in bipolar I and II depression: a double-blind, placebo-controlled study (the BOLDER II study). J Clin Psychopharmacol 2006; 26:600–609.

58. Suppes T et al. Effectiveness of the extended release formulation of quetiapine as monotherapy for the treatment of acute bipolar depression. J Affect Disord 2010; 121:106–115.

59. Young AH et al. A double-blind, placebo-controlled study of quetiapine and lithium monotherapy in adults in the acute phase of bipolar depression (EMBOLDEN I). J Clin Psychiatry 2010; **71**:150–162.

60. McElroy SL et al. A double-blind, placebo-controlled study of quetiapine and paroxetine as monotherapy in adults with bipolar depression (EMBOLDEN II). J Clin Psychiatry 2010; **71**:163–174.

61. Li H et al. Efficacy and safety of quetiapine extended release monotherapy in bipolar depression: a multi-center, randomized, double-blind, placebo-controlled trial. Psychopharmacology (Berl) 2016; **233**:1289–1297.

62. Vieta E et al. Efficacy and safety of quetiapine in combination with lithium or divalproex for maintenance of patients with bipolar I disorder (international trial 126). J Affect Disord 2008; **109**:251–263.

63. Suppes T et al. Maintenance treatment for patients with bipolar I disorder: results from a north american study of quetiapine in combination with lithium or divalproex (trial 127). Am J Psychiatry 2009; **166**:476–488.

64. Goodwin GM. Evidence-based guidelines for treating bipolar disorder: revised second edition – recommendations from the British Association for Psychopharmacology. J Psychopharmacol 2009; **23**:346–388.

65. Davis LL et al. Divalproex in the treatment of bipolar depression: a placebo-controlled study. J Affect Disord 2005; **85**:259–266.

66. Ghaemi SN et al. Divalproex in the treatment of acute bipolar depression: a preliminary double-blind, randomized, placebo-controlled pilot study. J Clin Psychiatry 2007; **68**:1840–1844.

67. Smith LA et al. Valproate for the treatment of acute bipolar depression: systematic review and meta-analysis. J Affect Disord 2010; **122**:1–9.

68. Muzina DJ et al. Acute efficacy of divalproex sodium versus placebo in mood stabilizer-naive bipolar I or II depression: a double-blind, randomized, placebo-controlled trial. J Clin Psychiatry 2011; **72**:813–819.

69. Amsterdam JD et al. Short-term fluoxetine monotherapy for bipolar type II or bipolar NOS major depression – low manic switch rate. Bipolar Disord 2004; **6**:75–81.

70. Amsterdam JD et al. Efficacy and safety of fluoxetine in treating bipolar II major depressive episode. J Clin Psychopharmacol 1998; **18**:435–440.

71. Amsterdam J. Efficacy and safety of venlafaxine in the treatment of bipolar II major depressive episode. J Clin Psychopharmacol 1998; **18**:414–417.

72. Amsterdam JD et al. Venlafaxine monotherapy in women with bipolar II and unipolar major depression. J Affect Disord 2000; **59**:225–229.

73. Silverstone T. Moclobemide vs. imipramine in bipolar depression: a multicentre double-blind clinical trial. Acta Psychiatr Scand 2001; **104**:104–109.

74. Ghaemi SN et al. Antidepressant treatment in bipolar versus unipolar depression. Am J Psychiatry 2004; **161**:163–165.

75. Post RM et al. A re-evaluation of the role of antidepressants in the treatment of bipolar depression: data from the Stanley Foundation Bipolar Network. Bipolar Disord 2003; **5**:396–406.

76. Amsterdam JD et al. Comparison of fluoxetine, olanzapine, and combined fluoxetine plus olanzapine initial therapy of bipolar type I and type II major depression – lack of manic induction. J Affect Disord 2005; **87**:121–130.

77. Amsterdam JD et al. Fluoxetine monotherapy of bipolar type II and bipolar NOS major depression: a double-blind, placebo-substitution, continuation study. Int Clin Psychopharmacol 2005; **20**:257–264.

78. Heijnen WT et al. Efficacy of tranylcypromine in bipolar depression: a systematic review. J Clin Psychopharmacol 2015; **35**:700–705.

79. Dilsaver SC et al. Treatment of bipolar depression with carbamazepine: results of an open study. Biol Psychiatry 1996; **40**:935–937.

80. Durgam S et al. An 8-week randomized, double-blind, placebo-controlled evaluation of the safety and efficacy of cariprazine in patients with bipolar I depression. Am J Psychiatry 2016; **173**:271–281.

81. Goldberg JF et al. Preliminary randomized, double-blind, placebo-controlled trial of pramipexole added to mood stabilizers for treatment-resistant bipolar depression. Am J Psychiatry 2004; **161**:564–566.

82. Zarate CA, Jr. et al. Pramipexole for bipolar II depression: a placebo-controlled proof of concept study. Biol Psychiatry 2004; **56**:54–60.

83. Ketter TA et al. Adjunctive aripiprazole in treatment-resistant bipolar depression. Ann Clin Psychiatry 2006; **18**:169–172.

84. Mazza M et al. Beneficial acute antidepressant effects of aripiprazole as an adjunctive treatment or monotherapy in bipolar patients unresponsive to mood stabilizers: results from a 16-week open-label trial. Expert Opin Pharmacother 2008; **9**:3145–3149.

85. Sidor MM et al. Antidepressants for the acute treatment of bipolar depression: a systematic review and meta-analysis. J Clin Psychiatry 2011; **72**:156–167.

86. Cruz N et al. Efficacy of modern antipsychotics in placebo-controlled trials in bipolar depression: a meta-analysis. Int J Neuropsychopharmacol 2010; **13**:5–14.

87. Wang PW et al. Gabapentin augmentation therapy in bipolar depression. Bipolar Disord 2002; **4**:296–301.

88. Ashton H et al. GABA-ergic drugs: exit stage left, enter stage right. J Psychopharmacol 2003; **17**:174–178.

89. Chengappa KN et al. Inositol as an add-on treatment for bipolar depression. Bipolar Disord 2000; **2**:47–55.

90. Diazgranados N et al. A randomized add-on trial of an N-methyl-D-aspartate antagonist in treatment-resistant bipolar depression. Arch Gen Psychiatry 2010; **67**:793–802.

91. Shahani R et al. Ketamine-associated ulcerative cystitis: a new clinical entity. Urology 2007; **69**:810–812.

92. Zarate CA, Jr. et al. Replication of ketamine's antidepressant efficacy in bipolar depression: a randomized controlled add-on trial. Biol Psychiatry 2012; **71**:939–946.

93. Permoda-Osip A et al. Single ketamine infusion and neurocognitive performance in bipolar depression. Pharmacopsychiatry 2015; **48**:78–79.

94. Young AH et al. Improvements in neurocognitive function and mood following adjunctive treatment with mifepristone (RU-486) in bipolar disorder. Neuropsychopharmacology 2004; **29**:1538–1545.

CHAPTER 2

95. Watson S et al. A randomized trial to examine the effect of mifepristone on neuropsychological performance and mood in patients with bipolar depression. Biol Psychiatry 2012; **72**:943–949.

96. Frye MA et al. A placebo-controlled evaluation of adjunctive modafinil in the treatment of bipolar depression. Am J Psychiatry 2007; **164**:1242–1249.

97. Calabrese JR et al. Adjunctive armodafinil for major depressive episodes associated with bipolar I disorder: a randomized, multicenter, double-blind, placebo-controlled, proof-of-concept study. J Clin Psychiatry 2010; **71**:1363–1370.

98. Frangou S et al. Efficacy of ethyl-eicosapentaenoic acid in bipolar depression: randomised double-blind placebo-controlled study. Br J Psychiatry 2006; **188**:46–50.

99. Keck PE, Jr. et al. Double-blind, randomized, placebo-controlled trials of ethyl-eicosapentanoate in the treatment of bipolar depression and rapid cycling bipolar disorder. Biol Psychiatry 2006; **60**:1020–1022.

100. Singh J et al. Case report: successful riluzole augmentation therapy in treatment-resistant bipolar depression following the development of rash with lamotrigine. Psychopharmacology (Berl) 2004; **173**:227–228.

101. Brennan BP et al. Rapid enhancement of glutamatergic neurotransmission in bipolar depression following treatment with riluzole. Neuropsychopharmacology 2010; **35**:834–846.

102. Park LT et al. A double-blind, placebo-controlled, pilot study of riluzole monotherapy for acute bipolar depression. J Clin Psychopharmacol 2017; **37**:355–358.

103. Bauer M. Thyroid hormone augmentation with levothyroxine in bipolar depression. Bipolar Disord 2002; **4 Suppl 1**:109–110.

104. Stamm TJ et al. Supraphysiologic doses of levothyroxine as adjunctive therapy in bipolar depression: a randomized, double-blind, placebo-controlled study. J Clin Psychiatry 2014; **75**:162–168.

105. Ghaemi SN et al. An open prospective study of zonisamide in acute bipolar depression. J Clin Psychopharmacol 2006; **26**:385–388.

106. Anand A et al. A preliminary open-label study of zonisamide treatment for bipolar depression in 10 patients. J Clin Psychiatry 2005; **66**:195–198.

107. Wilson MS et al. Zonisamide for bipolar depression. Expert Opin Pharmacother 2007; **8**:111–113.

108. McElroy SL et al. Open-label adjunctive zonisamide in the treatment of bipolar disorders: a prospective trial. J Clin Psychiatry 2005; **66**:617–624.

109. Selle V et al. Treatments for acute bipolar depression: meta-analyses of placebo-controlled, monotherapy trials of anticonvulsants, lithium and antipsychotics. Pharmacopsychiatry 2014; **47**:43–52.

110. Taylor DM et al. Comparative efficacy and acceptability of drug treatments for bipolar depression: a multiple-treatments meta-analysis. Acta Psychiatr Scand 2014; **130**:452–469.

CHAPTER 2

Prophylaxis in bipolar disorder

The median duration of mood episodes in people with bipolar disorder has been reported to be 13 weeks, with a quarter of patients remaining unwell at 1 year.[1] Most people with bipolar disorder spend much more time depressed than manic,[2] and bipolar depression can be very difficult to treat. The suicide rate in bipolar illness is increased 25-fold over population norms and the vast majority of suicides occur during episodes of depression.[3] Mixed states are also common and present an increased risk of suicide.[4] The concept of mixed states has widened with the DSM mixed specifier but as yet there are very few studies which have used this.[5]

Residual symptoms after an acute episode are a strong predictor of recurrence.[1,6] Most evidence supports the efficacy of lithium[7–11] in preventing episodes of mania and depression.[12] Carbamazepine is somewhat less effective[11,13] and the long-term efficacy of valproate is uncertain,[9,10,14–16] although it too may protect against relapse both into depression and mania.[11,17] Lithium has the advantage of a proven anti-suicidal effect[18–21] but perhaps, relative to other mood stabilisers, the disadvantage of a worsened outcome following abrupt discontinuation.[22–25] Early use of lithium may increase likelihood of efficacy.[26]

The BALANCE study found that valproate as monotherapy was relatively less effective than lithium or the combination of lithium and valproate,[15] casting doubt on its use as a first-line single treatment. Also, a large observational study has shown that lithium is much more effective than valproate in preventing relapse to any condition and in preventing rehospitalisation.[27] Given this and the fact that valproate is not licensed for prophylaxis, it should now be best considered a second-line treatment.

Conventional antipsychotics have traditionally been used and are perceived to be effective although the objective evidence base is, again, weak.[28,29] FGA depots probably protect against mania but may worsen depression[30] (see section on 'Antipsychotic long-acting injections in bipolar disorder'). Evidence supports the efficacy of some SGAs, particularly olanzapine,[10,31] quetiapine,[32] aripiprazole[33] and risperidone.[34] Olanzapine, quetiapine and aripiprazole are licensed for prophylaxis and appear to protect against both mania and depression. Asenapine may also be effective.[35] Whether SGAs are more effective than FGAs or are truly associated with a reduced overall adverse-effect burden remains untested. There is likewise little to choose between individual SGAs.[36] Long-acting aripiprazole has been shown to delay the time to, and reduced the rate of recurrence of, manic episodes and was generally safe and well tolerated.[37] The use of risperidone LAI is well supported by RCTs[38] and naturalistic studies.[39]

NICE recommendations for prophylaxis of bipolar disorder are summarised in Box 2.1.

A significant proportion of patients with bipolar illness fail to be treated adequately with a single mood stabiliser,[15] so combinations of mood stabilisers[40,41] or a mood stabiliser and an antipsychotic[41,42] are commonly used.[43] Also, there is evidence that where combination treatments are effective in mania or depression, then continuation with the same combination provides optimal prophylaxis.[32,42] The use of polypharmacy needs to be balanced against the likely increased adverse-effect burden. Combinations of olanzapine, risperidone, quetiapine or haloperidol with lithium or valproate are recommended by NICE[31] and by the more recent BAP guidelines.[11] Alternative

> **Box 2.1** NICE recommendations for prophylaxis of bipolar disorder[31]
>
> - When planning long-term pharmacological interventions to prevent relapse, take into account drugs that have been effective during episodes of mania or bipolar depression. Discuss with the person whether they prefer to continue this treatment or switch to lithium, and explain that lithium is the most effective long-term treatment for bipolar disorder.
> - Offer lithium as a first-line, long-term pharmacological treatment for bipolar disorder and: if lithium is insufficiently effective, consider adding valproate; if lithium is poorly tolerated, consider valproate or olanzapine instead, or if it has been effective during an episode of mania or bipolar depression, quetiapine.
> - Do not offer valproate to women of child-bearing potential.
> - Discuss with the person the possible benefits and risks of each drug for them.
> - The secondary care team should maintain responsibility for monitoring the efficacy and tolerability of antipsychotic medication until the person's condition has stabilised.
> - Before stopping medication, discuss with the person how to recognise early signs of relapse and what to do if symptoms recur.
> - If stopping medication, do so gradually and monitor for signs of relapse.
> - Continue monitoring symptoms, mood and mental state for 2 years after stopping medication. This may be undertaken in primary care.

antipsychotics (e.g. aripiprazole) are also options in combinations with lithium or valproate, particularly if these have been found to be effective during the treatment of an acute episode of mania or depression.[32,44] Carbamazepine is considered to be third line. Lamotrigine may be useful in bipolar II disorder[31] but seems only to significantly prevent recurrence of depression.[45] Lurasidone may have broadly similar long-term efficacy, both as monotherapy and when combined with a mood stabiliser.[46,47] Extrapolation of currently available data suggests that lithium plus an SGA is probably the polypharmacy regime of choice.

A meta-analysis of long-term antidepressant treatment found that the number needed to treat to prevent a new episode of depression was larger than the number needed to harm related to precipitating a new episode of mania.[48] The STEP-BD study found no significant benefit for continuing (compared with discontinuing) an antidepressant and worse outcomes in those with rapid-cycling illness.[49] There is thus essentially no strong support for long-term use of antidepressants in bipolar illness although some bipolar patients may relapse into depression when antidepressants are discontinued.[25]

Substance misuse increases the risk of switching into mania.[50]

Box 2.2 summarises prophylaxis in bipolar disorder.

> **Box 2.2** Summary: prophylaxis in bipolar disorder
>
> **First line: lithium**
> Second line: *valproate, olanzapine, aripiprazole, risperidone or quetiapine
> Third line: alternative antipsychotic that has been effective during an acute episode, carbamazepine, lurasidone, lamotrigine
> - Always maintain successful acute treatment regimes (e.g. mood stabiliser + antipsychotic) as prophylaxis.
> - Avoid long-term antidepressants if possible.
>
> *Not in women of child bearing potential.

References

1. Solomon DA et al. Longitudinal course of bipolar I disorder: duration of mood episodes. Arch Gen Psychiatry 2010; 67:339–347.
2. Judd LL et al. A prospective investigation of the natural history of the long-term weekly symptomatic status of bipolar II disorder. Arch Gen Psychiatry 2003; 60:261–269.
3. Rihmer Z. Suicide and bipolar disorder. In: Zarate C, Jr., Manji HK, eds. *Bipolar Depression: Molecular Neurobiology, Clinical Diagnosis and Pharmacotherapy (Milestones in Drug Therapy)*. Switzerland: Birkhäuser Basel; 2009, pp. 47–58.
4. Houston JP et al. Reduced suicidal ideation in bipolar I disorder mixed-episode patients in a placebo-controlled trial of olanzapine combined with lithium or divalproex. J Clin Psychiatry 2006; 67:1246–1252.
5. American Psychiatric Association. *Diagnostic and Statistical Manual of Mental Disorders, Fifth Edition* (DSM-5). Arlington, VA: American Psychiatric Association; 2013.
6. Perlis RH et al. Predictors of recurrence in bipolar disorder: primary outcomes from the Systematic Treatment Enhancement Program for Bipolar Disorder (STEP-BD). Am J Psychiatry 2006; 163:217–224.
7. Young AH et al. Lithium in mood disorders: increasing evidence base, declining use? Br J Psychiatry 2007; 191:474–476.
8. Biel MG et al. Continuation versus discontinuation of lithium in recurrent bipolar illness: a naturalistic study. Bipolar Disord 2007; 9:435–442.
9. Bowden CL et al. A randomized, placebo-controlled 12-month trial of divalproex and lithium in treatment of outpatients with bipolar I disorder. Divalproex Maintenance Study Group. Arch Gen Psychiatry 2000; 57:481–489.
10. Tohen M et al. Olanzapine versus divalproex sodium for the treatment of acute mania and maintenance of remission: a 47-week study. Am J Psychiatry 2003; 160:1263–1271.
11. Goodwin GM et al. Evidence-based guidelines for treating bipolar disorder: revised third edition recommendations from the British Association for Psychopharmacology. J Psychopharmacol 2016; 30:495–553.
12. Sani G et al. Treatment of bipolar disorder in a lifetime perspective: is lithium still the best choice? Clin Drug Investig 2017; 37:713–727.
13. Hartong EG et al. Prophylactic efficacy of lithium versus carbamazepine in treatment-naive bipolar patients. J Clin Psychiatry 2003; 64:144–151.
14. Cipriani A et al. Valproic acid, valproate and divalproex in the maintenance treatment of bipolar disorder. Cochrane Database Syst Rev 2013; 10:CD003196.
15. Geddes JR et al. Lithium plus valproate combination therapy versus monotherapy for relapse prevention in bipolar I disorder (BALANCE): a randomised open-label trial. Lancet 2010; 375:385–395.
16. Kemp DE et al. A 6-month, double-blind, maintenance trial of lithium monotherapy versus the combination of lithium and divalproex for rapid-cycling bipolar disorder and co-occurring substance abuse or dependence. J Clin Psychiatry 2009; 70:113–121.
17. Smith LA et al. Effectiveness of mood stabilizers and antipsychotics in the maintenance phase of bipolar disorder: a systematic review of randomized controlled trials. Bipolar Disord 2007; 9:394–412.
18. Cipriani A et al. Lithium in the prevention of suicidal behavior and all-cause mortality in patients with mood disorders: a systematic review of randomized trials. Am J Psychiatry 2005; 162:1805–1819.
19. Kessing LV et al. Suicide risk in patients treated with lithium. Arch Gen Psychiatry 2005; 62:860–866.
20. Young AH et al. Lithium in maintenance therapy for bipolar disorder. J Psychopharmacol 2006; 20:17–22.
21. Song J et al. Suicidal behavior during lithium and valproate treatment: a within-individual 8-year prospective study of 50,000 patients with bipolar disorder. Am J Psychiatry 2017; 174:795–802.
22. Mander AJ et al. Rapid recurrence of mania following abrupt discontinuation of lithium. Lancet 1988; 2:15–17.
23. Faedda GL et al. Outcome after rapid vs gradual discontinuation of lithium treatment in bipolar disorders. Arch Gen Psychiatry 1993; 50:448–455.
24. Macritchie KA et al. Does 'rebound mania' occur after stopping carbamazepine? A pilot study. J Psychopharmacol 2000; 14:266–268.
25. Franks MA et al. Bouncing back: is the bipolar rebound phenomenon peculiar to lithium? A retrospective naturalistic study. J Psychopharmacol 2008; 22:452–456.
26. Kessing LV et al. Starting lithium prophylaxis early v. late in bipolar disorder. Br J Psychiatry 2014; 205:214–220.
27. Kessing LV et al. Valproate v. lithium in the treatment of bipolar disorder in clinical practice: observational nationwide register-based cohort study. Br J Psychiatry 2011; 199:57–63.
28. Gao K et al. Typical and atypical antipsychotics in bipolar depression. J Clin Psychiatry 2005; 66:1376–1385.
29. Hellewell JS. A review of the evidence for the use of antipsychotics in the maintenance treatment of bipolar disorders. J Psychopharmacol 2006; 20:39–45.
30. Gigante AD et al. Long-acting injectable antipsychotics for the maintenance treatment of bipolar disorder. CNS Drugs 2012; 26:403–420.
31. National Institute for Health and Care Excellence. Bipolar disorder: assessment and management. Clinical Guideline 185, 2014; last updated February 2016. https://www.nice.org.uk/guidance/cg185.
32. Vieta E et al. Efficacy and safety of quetiapine in combination with lithium or divalproex for maintenance of patients with bipolar I disorder (international trial 126). J Affect Disord 2008; 109:251–263.
33. McIntyre RS. Aripiprazole for the maintenance treatment of bipolar I disorder: a review. Clin Ther 2010; 32 Suppl 1:S32–S38.
34. Ghaemi SN et al. Long-term risperidone treatment in bipolar disorder: 6-month follow up. Int Clin Psychopharmacol 1997; 12:333–338.
35. Szegedi A et al. Randomized, double-blind, placebo-controlled trial of asenapine maintenance therapy in adults with an acute manic or mixed episode associated with bipolar I disorder. Am J Psychiatry 2018; 175:71–79.

36. Lindstrom L et al. Maintenance therapy with second generation antipsychotics for bipolar disorder – a systematic review and meta-analysis. J Affect Disord 2017; **213**:138–150.

37. Calabrese JR et al. Efficacy and safety of aripiprazole once-monthly in the maintenance treatment of bipolar I disorder: a double-blind, placebo-controlled, 52-week randomized withdrawal study. J Clin Psychiatry 2017; **78**:324–331.

38. Kishi T et al. Long-acting injectable antipsychotics for prevention of relapse in bipolar disorder: a systematic review and meta-analyses of randomized controlled trials. Int J Neuropsychopharmacol 2016; **19**.

39. Hsieh MH et al. Bipolar patients treated with long-acting injectable risperidone in Taiwan: a 1-year mirror-image study using a national claims database. J Affect Disord 2017; **218**:327–334.

40. Freeman MP et al. Mood stabilizer combinations: a review of safety and efficacy. Am J Psychiatry 1998; **155**:12–21.

41. Muzina DJ et al. Maintenance therapies in bipolar disorder: focus on randomized controlled trials. Aust N Z J Psychiatry 2005; **39**:652–661.

42. Tohen M et al. Relapse prevention in bipolar I disorder: 18-month comparison of olanzapine plus mood stabiliser v. mood stabiliser alone. Br J Psychiatry 2004; **184**:337–345.

43. Paton C et al. Lithium in bipolar and other affective disorders: prescribing practice in the UK. J Psychopharmacol 2010; **24**:1739–1746.

44. Marcus R et al. Efficacy of aripiprazole adjunctive to lithium or valproate in the long-term treatment of patients with bipolar I disorder with an inadequate response to lithium or valproate monotherapy: a multicenter, double-blind, randomized study. Bipolar Disord 2011; **13**:133–144.

45. Bowden CL et al. A placebo-controlled 18-month trial of lamotrigine and lithium maintenance treatment in recently manic or hypomanic patients with bipolar I disorder. Arch Gen Psychiatry 2003; **60**:392–400.

46. Pikalov A et al. Long-term use of lurasidone in patients with bipolar disorder: safety and effectiveness over 2 years of treatment. Int J Bipolar Disord 2017; **5**:9.

47. Calabrese JR et al. Lurasidone in combination with lithium or valproate for the maintenance treatment of bipolar I disorder. Eur Neuropsychopharmacol 2017; **27**:865–876.

48. Ghaemi SN et al. Long-term antidepressant treatment in bipolar disorder: meta-analyses of benefits and risks. Acta Psychiatr Scand 2008; **118**:347–356.

49. Ghaemi SN et al. Antidepressant discontinuation in bipolar depression: a Systematic Treatment Enhancement Program for Bipolar Disorder (STEP-BD) randomized clinical trial of long-term effectiveness and safety. J Clin Psychiatry 2010; **71**:372–380.

50. Ostacher MJ et al. Impact of substance use disorders on recovery from episodes of depression in bipolar disorder patients: prospective data from the Systematic Treatment Enhancement Program for Bipolar Disorder (STEP-BD). Am J Psychiatry 2010; **167**:289–297.

Chapter 3

Depression and anxiety disorders

Depression: introduction

Depression is, of course, widely recognised as a major public health problem around the world. The mainstay of treatment is the prescription of antidepressants although, of late, psychological treatments have found a place as an alternative to antidepressants in milder forms of depression.[1] Other methods of treating depression (vagal nerve stimulation [VNS],[2] repetitive transcranial magnetic stimulation [rTMS],[3] etc.) are also used but are not widely available.

   The basic principles of prescribing are described here, along with a summary of NICE guidance.

Basic principles of prescribing in depression

- Discuss with the patient choice of drug and utility/availability of other, non-pharmacological treatments.
- Discuss with the patient likely outcomes, such as gradual relief from depressive symptoms over several weeks.
- Prescribe a dose of antidepressant (after titration, if necessary) that is likely to be effective.
- For a single episode, continue treatment for at least 6–9 months after resolution of symptoms (multiple episodes may require longer).
- Withdraw antidepressants gradually; always inform patients of the risk and nature of discontinuation symptoms.

The Maudsley Prescribing Guidelines in Psychiatry, Thirteenth Edition. David M. Taylor, Thomas R. E. Barnes and Allan H. Young.
© 2018 David M. Taylor. Published 2018 by John Wiley & Sons Ltd.

Official guidance on the treatment of depression

NICE guidelines:[1] a summary

- Antidepressants are not recommended as a first-line treatment in recent-onset, mild depression – active monitoring, individual guided self-help, cognitive behavioural therapy (CBT) or exercise are preferred.
- Antidepressants are recommended for the treatment of moderate to severe depression and for dysthymia.
- When an antidepressant is prescribed, a generic selective serotonin reuptake inhibitor (SSRI) is recommended.
- All patients should be informed about the withdrawal (discontinuation) effects of antidepressants.
- For treatment-resistant depression, recommended strategies include augmentation with lithium or an antipsychotic or the addition of a second antidepressant (see section on 'Treatment of refractory depression' in this chapter).
- Patients with two prior episodes and functional impairment should be treated for at least 2 years.
- The use of electroconvulsive therapy (ECT) is supported in severe and treatment-resistant depression.

At the time of writing, new NICE Guidelines are available only in draft form.[4] Basic principles appear to be the same as in the earlier guideline but important differences are proposed for drug choice after first treatment failure (see Figure 3.1).

This chapter concentrates on the use of antidepressants and offers advice on drug choice, dosing, switching strategies and sequencing of treatments. The near exclusion of other treatment modalities does not imply any lack of confidence in their efficacy but simply reflects the need (in a prescribing guideline) to concentrate on medicines-related subjects.

References

1 National Institute for Health and Care Excellence. Depression in adults: recognition and management. Clinical guideline 90, 2009; last updated April 2016. https://www.nice.org.uk/guidance/cg90

2 George MS et al. Vagus nerve stimulation for the treatment of depression and other neuropsychiatric disorders. Expert Rev Neurother 2007; 7:63–74.

3 Loo CK et al. A review of the efficacy of transcranial magnetic stimulation (TMS) treatment for depression, and current and future strategies to optimize efficacy. J Affect Disord 2005; 88:255–267.

4 National Institute for Health and Care Excellence. Depression in adults: treatment and management. Full guideline (Draft for Consultation). 2017. https://www.nice.org.uk/guidance/GID-CGWAVE0725/documents/draft-guideline

Antidepressants: general overview

Effectiveness

The *severity* of depression at which antidepressants show consistent benefits over placebo is poorly defined. Although it is generally accepted that the more severe the symptoms, the greater the benefit from antidepressant treatment,[1-3] there is some evidence to support the view that response may be independent of symptom severity.[4] Antidepressants are normally recommended as first-line treatment in patients whose depression is of at least moderate severity. Of this patient group, approximately 20% will recover with no treatment at all, 30% will respond to placebo and 50% will respond to antidepressant drug treatment.[5] This gives a number needed to treat (NNT) of 3 for antidepressant over true no-treatment control and an NNT of 5 for antidepressant over placebo. Note though that response in clinical trials is generally defined as a 50% reduction in depression rating scale scores, a somewhat arbitrary dichotomy, and that change measured using continuous scales tends to show a relatively small mean difference between active treatment and placebo (which itself is an effective treatment for depression).

Drug–placebo differences have diminished over time, largely because of methodological changes.[6] Recent studies have reappraised drug–placebo differences. For example, Hieronymus et al.[7] undertook patient-level *post hoc* analyses of 18 industry-sponsored placebo-controlled trials of paroxetine, citalopram, sertraline or fluoxetine, including in total 6669 adults with major depression, the aim being to assess what the outcome would have been if the single-item depressed mood (rated 0–4) had been used as the measure of efficacy. In total, 32 drug–placebo comparisons were reassessed. While 18 out of 32 comparisons (56%) failed to separate active drug from placebo at week 6 with respect to reduction in Hamilton Depression Rating Scale (HDRS/HAM-D)-17 score, only 3 out of 32 comparisons (9%) were negative when depressed mood was used as an effect parameter (p = <0.001). Even when whole depression scales are used, a recent network meta-analysis showed robust superiority for antidepressants over placebo, with amitriptyline being the most efficacious.[8]

In patients with subsyndromal depression it is difficult to separate the response rate to antidepressants from that to placebo; antidepressant treatment is not indicated unless the patient has a history of severe depression (where less severe symptoms may indicate the onset of another episode) or symptoms persist. Patients with dysthymia (symptom *duration* of at least 2 years) benefit from antidepressant treatment; the minimum duration of symptoms associated with benefit is unknown. In other patients, the adverse effects associated with antidepressant treatment may outweigh any small benefit seen.

Onset of action

It is widely held that antidepressants do not exert their effects for 2–4 weeks. This is a myth. All antidepressants show a pattern of response in which the rate of improvement is highest during weeks 1–2 and lowest during weeks 4–6. Statistical separation from placebo is seen at 2–4 weeks in single trials (hence the idea of a lag effect) but

CHAPTER 3

after only 1–2 weeks in (statistically more powerful) meta-analyses.[9,10] Thus, where large numbers of patients are treated and detailed rating scales are used, an antidepressant effect is statistically evident at 1 week. In clinical practice using simple observations, an antidepressant effect in an individual is usually seen by 2 weeks.[11] It follows that in individuals where *no* antidepressant effect is evident after 3–4 weeks' treatment, a change in dose or drug should be considered. It is important, however, to be clear about what constitutes 'no effect'. Different patterns of response have been identified[12] and in some individuals response is slow to emerge. However, in those ultimately responsive to treatment, all will very probably have begun to show at least minor improvement at 3 weeks. Thus those showing no discernible improvement at this time will very probably never respond to the prescribed drug at that dose. In contrast, those showing small improvements at 3 weeks (that is, improvement not meeting criteria for 'response') may well go on to respond fully.[13] A recent 'mega-analysis'[14] has shown that if antidepressant (citalopram, paroxetine or sertraline specifically) trials are examined with regards to the effects on depressed mood alone (rather than the total HDRS score) then both a rapid effect and a dose–response relationship are evident.

Choice of antidepressant and relative adverse effects

Selective serotonin reuptake inhibitors (*SSRIs*) are well tolerated compared with the older tricyclic antidepressants (TCAs) and monoamine oxidase inhibitors (MAOIs), and are generally recommended as *first-line* pharmacological treatment for depression.[1] There is a suggestion from network meta-analyses[8,15] that some antidepressants may be more effective overall than others but this has not been consistently demonstrated in head-to-head studies and should therefore be treated with caution. Adverse-effect profiles of antidepressants do differ. For example, paroxetine has been associated with more weight gain and a higher incidence of sexual dysfunction, and sertraline with a higher incidence of diarrhoea than other SSRIs.[16] Dual reuptake inhibitors such as venlafaxine and duloxetine tend to be tolerated less well than SSRIs but better than TCAs. With all drugs there is marked inter-individual variation in tolerability which is not easily predicted by knowledge of a drug's likely adverse effects. A flexible approach is usually required to find the right drug for a particular patient.

As well as *headache* and *gastrointestinal (GI) symptoms*, SSRIs as a class are associated with a range of other adverse effects including *sexual dysfunction* (see section on 'Antidepressants and sexual dysfunction' in this chapter), *hyponatraemia* (see section on 'Antidepressant-induced hyponatraemia' in this chapter) and *GI bleeds* (see section on 'SSRIs and bleeding' in this chapter). TCAs have a number of *adverse cardiovascular effects* (hypotension, tachycardia and QTc prolongation), and are particularly *toxic in overdose*[17] (see section on 'Psychotropic drugs in overdose' in Chapter 13). The now rarely used *MAOIs* have the potential to interact with tyramine-containing foods to cause *hypertensive crisis*. All antidepressant drugs can cause *discontinuation symptoms*, with short half-life drugs probably being most problematic in this respect (see section on 'Antidepressant discontinuation symptoms' in this chapter). The rest of this section summarises the clinically relevant adverse effects of available antidepressant drugs.

Drug interactions

Some SSRIs are potent *inhibitors* of individual or multiple *hepatic cytochrome P450 (CYP)* pathways and the magnitude of these effects is dose-related. A number of clinically significant drug interactions can therefore be predicted. For example, fluvoxamine is a potent inhibitor of CYP1A2 which can result in increased theophylline serum levels, fluoxetine is a potent inhibitor of CYP2D6 which can result in increased seizure risk with clozapine, and paroxetine is a potent inhibitor of CYP2D6 which can result in treatment failure with tamoxifen (a prodrug), leading to increased mortality.[18]

Antidepressants can also cause pharmacodynamic interactions. For example, the cardiotoxicity of TCAs may be exacerbated by drugs such as diuretics that can cause electrolyte disturbances. A summary of clinically relevant drug interactions with antidepressants can be found in the section on 'Drug interactions with antidepressants' in this chapter.

Potential *pharmacokinetic* and *pharmacodynamic* interactions between antidepressants have to be considered when *switching* from one antidepressant to another (see section on 'Antidepressants: swapping and stopping' in this chapter).

Suicidality

Antidepressant treatment has been associated with an increased risk of suicidal thoughts and acts, particularly in adolescents and young adults,[19-22] leading to the recommendation that patients should be warned of this potential adverse effect during the early weeks of treatment and know how to seek help if required. Suicide and self-harm rates tend to be higher when antidepressants are started or stopped so the same care over risk assessment should be carried out when treatment is stopped as when it is started.[23] Furthermore, switching antidepressants may be a marker of increased risk of suicidal behaviours in those who initiate antidepressant treatment aged 75 years and over.[24]

All antidepressants have been implicated,[25] including those that are marketed for an indication other than depression (e.g. atomoxetine). It should be noted that: (i) although the relative risk may be elevated above placebo rates in some patient groups, the absolute risk remains very small; (ii) the most effective way to prevent suicidal thoughts and acts is to treat depression;[26-28] and (iii) antidepressant drugs are the most effective treatment currently available.[5,29] For the most part, suicidality is greatly reduced by the use of antidepressants.[30-32] Note, however, that those who experience treatment-emergent or worsening suicidal ideation with one antidepressant may be more likely to have a similar experience with subsequent treatments.[33] Worryingly, some data suggest that an increasing proportion of young women who later committed suicide had in the last few years been treated with antidepressants, prior to and at the time of the suicide.[34]

Toxicity in overdose varies both between and within groups of antidepressants.[35] See section on 'Psychotropics in overdose' in Chapter 13.

Duration of treatment

Antidepressants relieve the symptoms of depression but do not treat the underlying cause. They should therefore be taken **for 6–9 months after recovery from a single episode** (to cover the assumed duration of most single untreated episodes). In those patients who have had multiple episodes, there is evidence of benefit from maintenance treatment for at least 2 years; no upper duration of treatment has been identified (see section on 'Antidepressant prophylaxis' in this chapter). There are few data on which to base recommendations about the duration of treatment of augmentation regimens.

Next-step treatments

Approximately a third of patients do not respond to the first antidepressant that is prescribed. Options in this group include dose escalation, switching to a different drug and a number of augmentation strategies. The lessons from Sequenced Treatment Alternatives to Relieve Depression (STAR*D) are that a small proportion of non-responders will respond with each treatment change, but that **effect sizes are modest** and there is no clear difference in effectiveness between strategies. (See section on 'Treatment of refractory depression' in this chapter.)

Use of antidepressants in anxiety spectrum disorders

Antidepressants are first-line treatments in a number of anxiety spectrum disorders. (See section on 'Anxiety spectrum disorders' in this chapter.)

References

1 National Institute for Health and Care Excellence. Depression in adults: recognition and management. Clinical guideline 90, 2009; last updated April 2016. https://www.nice.org.uk/Guidance/cg90
2 Kirsch I et al. Initial severity and antidepressant benefits: a meta-analysis of data submitted to the Food and Drug Administration. PLoS Med 2008; 5:e45.
3 Fournier JC et al. Antidepressant drug effects and depression severity: a patient-level meta-analysis. JAMA 2010; 303:47–53.
4 Gibbons RD et al. Benefits from antidepressants: synthesis of 6-week patient-level outcomes from double-blind placebo-controlled randomized trials of fluoxetine and venlafaxine. Arch Gen Psychiatry 2012; 69:572–579.
5 Anderson IM et al. Evidence-based guidelines for treating depressive disorders with antidepressants: a revision of the 2000 British Association for Psychopharmacology guidelines. J Psychopharmacol 2008; 22:343–396.
6 Khan A et al. Why has the antidepressant-placebo difference in antidepressant clinical trials diminished over the past three decades? CNS Neurosci Ther 2010; 16:217–226.
7 Hieronymus F et al. Consistent superiority of selective serotonin reuptake inhibitors over placebo in reducing depressed mood in patients with major depression. Mol Psychiatry 2016; 21:523–530.
8 Cipriani A et al. Comparative efficacy and acceptability of 21 antidepressant drugs for the acute treatment of adults with major depressive disorder: a systematic review and network meta-analysis. Lancet 2018. doi: 10.1016/S0140-6736(17)32802-7. [Epub ahead of print]
9 Taylor MJ et al. Early onset of selective serotonin reuptake inhibitor antidepressant action: systematic review and meta-analysis. Arch Gen Psychiatry 2006; 63:1217–1223.
10 Papakostas GI et al. A meta-analysis of early sustained response rates between antidepressants and placebo for the treatment of major depressive disorder. J Clin Psychopharmacol 2006; 26:56–60.
11 Szegedi A et al. Early improvement in the first 2 weeks as a predictor of treatment outcome in patients with major depressive disorder: a meta-analysis including 6562 patients. J Clin Psychiatry 2009; 70:344–353.
12 Uher R et al. Early and delayed onset of response to antidepressants in individual trajectories of change during treatment of major depression: a secondary analysis of data from the Genome-Based Therapeutic Drugs for Depression (GENDEP) study. J Clin Psychiatry 2011; 72:1478–1484.
13 Posternak MA et al. Response rates to fluoxetine in subjects who initially show no improvement. J Clin Psychiatry 2011; 72:949–954.
14 Hieronymus F et al. A mega-analysis of fixed-dose trials reveals dose-dependency and a rapid onset of action for the antidepressant effect of three selective serotonin reuptake inhibitors. Transl Psychiatry 2016; 6:e834.
15 Cipriani A et al. Comparative efficacy and acceptability of 12 new-generation antidepressants: a multiple-treatments meta-analysis. Lancet 2009; 373:746–758.
16 Gartlehner G et al. Comparative benefits and harms of second-generation antidepressants: background paper for the American College of Physicians. Ann Intern Med 2008; 149:734–750.
17 Flanagan RJ. Fatal toxicity of drugs used in psychiatry. Hum Psychopharmacol 2008; 23 Suppl 1:43–51.

18 Kelly CM et al. Selective serotonin reuptake inhibitors and breast cancer mortality in women receiving tamoxifen: a population based cohort study. BMJ 2010; 340:c693.

19 Stone M et al. Risk of suicidality in clinical trials of antidepressants in adults: analysis of proprietary data submitted to US Food and Drug Administration. BMJ 2009; 339:b2880.

20 Carpenter DJ et al. Meta-analysis of efficacy and treatment-emergent suicidality in adults by psychiatric indication and age subgroup following initiation of paroxetine therapy: a complete set of randomized placebo-controlled trials. J Clin Psychiatry 2011; 72:1503–1514.

21 Barbui C et al. Selective serotonin reuptake inhibitors and risk of suicide: a systematic review of observational studies. CMAJ 2009; 180: 291–297.

22 Umetsu R et al. Association between selective serotonin reuptake inhibitor therapy and suicidality: analysis of U.S. Food and Drug Administration adverse event reporting system data. Biol Pharm Bull 2015; 38:1689–1699.

23 Coupland C et al. Antidepressant use and risk of suicide and attempted suicide or self harm in people aged 20 to 64: cohort study using a primary care database. BMJ 2015; 350:h517.

24 Hedna K et al. Antidepressants and suicidal behaviour in late life: a prospective population-based study of use patterns in new users aged 75 and above. Eur J Clin Pharmacol 2018; 74:201–208.

25 Schneeweiss S et al. Variation in the risk of suicide attempts and completed suicides by antidepressant agent in adults: a propensity score-adjusted analysis of 9 years' data. Arch Gen Psychiatry 2010; 67:497–506.

26 Isacsson G et al. The increased use of antidepressants has contributed to the worldwide reduction in suicide rates. Br J Psychiatry 2010; 196:429–433.

27 Gibbons RD et al. Suicidal thoughts and behavior with antidepressant treatment: reanalysis of the randomized placebo-controlled studies of fluoxetine and venlafaxine. Arch Gen Psychiatry 2012; 69:580–587.

28 Lu CY et al. Changes in antidepressant use by young people and suicidal behavior after FDA warnings and media coverage: quasi-experimental study. BMJ 2014; 348:g3596.

29 Isacsson G et al. Antidepressant medication prevents suicide in depression. Acta Psychiatr Scand 2010; 122:454–460.

30 Simon GE et al. Suicide risk during antidepressant treatment. Am J Psychiatry 2006; 163:41–47.

31 Mulder RT et al. Antidepressant treatment is associated with a reduction in suicidal ideation and suicide attempts. Acta Psychiatr Scand 2008; 118:116–122.

32 Tondo L et al. Suicidal status during antidepressant treatment in 789 Sardinian patients with major affective disorder. Acta Psychiatr Scand 2008; 118:106–115.

33 Perlis RH et al. Do suicidal thoughts or behaviors recur during a second antidepressant treatment trial? J Clin Psychiatry 2012; 73: 1439–1442.

34 Larsson J. Antidepressants and suicide among young women in Sweden 1999-2013. Int J Risk Saf Med 2017; 29:101–106.

35 Hawton K et al. Toxicity of antidepressants: rates of suicide relative to prescribing and non-fatal overdose. Br J Psychiatry 2010; 196:354–358.

CHAPTER 3

Recognised minimum effective doses of antidepressants

The recommended minimum effective doses of antidepressants are summarised in Table 3.1.

Table 3.1 The recommended minimum effective doses of antidepressants

Antidepressant	Dose
Tricyclics	Unclear; at least 75–100 mg/day,[1] possibly 125 mg/day[2]
Lofepramine	140 mg/day[3]
SSRIs	
Citalopram	20 mg/day[4]
Escitalopram	10 mg/day[5]
Fluoxetine	20 mg/day[6]
Fluvoxamine	50 mg/day[7]
Paroxetine	20 mg/day[8]
Sertraline	50 mg/day[9]
Others	
Agomelatine	25 mg/day[10]
Desvenlafaxine	50 mg/day[11]
Duloxetine	60 mg/day[12,13]
Levomilnacipran	40 mg/day[14]
Mirtazapine	30 mg/day[15]
Moclobemide	300 mg/day[16]
Reboxetine	8 mg/day[17]
Trazodone	150 mg/day[18]
Venlafaxine	75 mg/day[19]
Vilazodone	20 mg/day[14]
Vortioxetine	10 mg/day[14]

References

1 Furukawa TA et al. Meta-analysis of effects and side effects of low dosage tricyclic antidepressants in depression: systematic review. BMJ 2002; 325:991.
2 Donoghue J et al. Suboptimal use of antidepressants in the treatment of depression. CNS Drugs 2000; 13:365–368.
3 Lancaster SG et al. Lofepramine. A review of its pharmacodynamic and pharmacokinetic properties, and therapeutic efficacy in depressive illness. Drugs 1989; 37:123–140.
4 Montgomery SA et al. The optimal dosing regimen for citalopram – a meta-analysis of nine placebo-controlled studies. Int Clin Psychopharmacol 1994; 9 Suppl 1:35–40.
5 Burke WJ et al. Fixed-dose trial of the single isomer SSRI escitalopram in depressed outpatients. J Clin Psychiatry 2002; 63:331–336.
6 Altamura AC et al. The evidence for 20 mg a day of fluoxetine as the optimal dose in the treatment of depression. Br J Psychiatry Suppl 1988:109–112.

7 Walczak DD et al. The oral dose-effect relationship for fluvoxamine: a fixed-dose comparison against placebo in depressed outpatients. Ann Clin Psychiatry 1996; 8:139–151.

8 Dunner DL et al. Optimal dose regimen for paroxetine. J Clin Psychiatry 1992; 53 Suppl:21–26.

9 Moon CAL et al. A double-blind comparison of sertraline and clomipramine in the treatment of major depressive disorder and associative anxiety in general practice. J Psychopharm 1994; 8:171–176.

10 Loo H et al. Determination of the dose of agomelatine, a melatoninergic agonist and selective 5-HT(2C) antagonist, in the treatment of major depressive disorder: a placebo-controlled dose range study. Int Clin Psychopharmacol 2002; 17:239–247.

11 Kornstein SG et al. The effect of desvenlafaxine 50 mg/day on a subpopulation of anxious/depressed patients: a pooled analysis of seven randomized, placebo-controlled studies. Hum Psychopharmacol 2014; 29:492–501.

12 Goldstein DJ et al. Duloxetine in the treatment of depression: a double-blind placebo-controlled comparison with paroxetine. J Clin Psychopharmacol 2004; 24:389–399.

13 Detke MJ et al. Duloxetine, 60 mg once daily, for major depressive disorder: a randomized double-blind placebo-controlled trial. J Clin Psychiatry 2002; 63:308–315.

14 He H et al. Efficacy and tolerability of different doses of three new antidepressants for treating major depressive disorder: a PRISMA-compliant meta-analysis. J Psychiatr Res 2018; 96:247–259.

15 van Moffaert M et al. Mirtazapine is more effective than trazodone: a double-blind controlled study in hospitalized patients with major depression. Int Clin Psychopharmacol 1995; 10:3–9.

16 Priest RG et al. Moclobemide in the treatment of depression. Rev Contemp Pharmacother 1994; 5:35–43.

17 Schatzberg AF. Clinical efficacy of reboxetine in major depression. J Clin Psychiatry 2000; 61 Suppl 10:31–38.

18 Brogden RN et al. Trazodone: a review of its pharmacological properties and therapeutic use in depression and anxiety. Drugs 1981; 21:401–429.

19 Feighner JP et al. Efficacy of once-daily venlafaxine extended release (XR) for symptoms of anxiety in depressed outpatients. J Affect Disord 1998; 47:55–62.

CHAPTER 3

Drug treatment of depression

The drug treatment of depression is summarised in Figure 3.1.

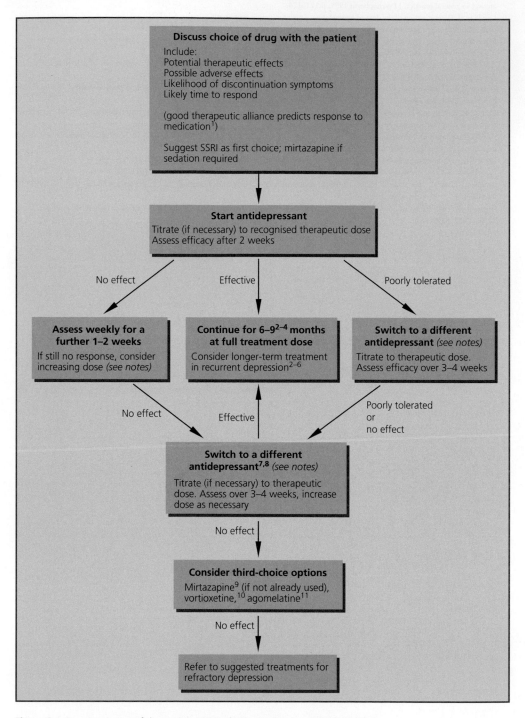

Figure 3.1 Drug treatment of depression. SSRI, selective serotonin reuptake inhibitor.

Notes for Figure 3.1

- Tools such as the Montgomery–Asberg Depression Rating Scale (MADRS)[12] and the HDRS[13] are used in trials to assess drug effect. The HDRS is now somewhat anachronistic and few clinicians are familiar with the MADRS (although it is probably the best scale to measure severity and change). The Patient Health Questionnaire-9 (PHQ-9)[14] is simple to use and is recommended for assessing symptom change in depression (although it better measures frequency rather than severity of symptoms).

- Switching between drug classes in cases of poor tolerability is not clearly supported by published studies but has a strong theoretical basis. Having said that, in practice, many patients who cannot tolerate one SSRI will readily tolerate another.

- In cases of non-response, there is some evidence that switching within a drug class is effective,[8,15–18] but switching between classes is, in practice, the most common option and is supported by some analyses.[19] The American Psychological Association (APA) recommend both options.[2] The 2017 NICE draft guidelines[20] noted (p. 439 et seq.) that there is little cogent evidence for switching between antidepressants (a suggestion supported by another analysis[21]) and that combining antidepressants or adding a second-generation antipsychotic (SGA) are better supported options. The strongest evidence in support of switching after the failure of one treatment is probably for vortioxetine.[10]

- There is minimal evidence to recommend increasing the dose of most SSRIs in depression, at least when severity is measured using total rating scale scores.[22] Examining only the mood item on the HDRS suggests some dose–response relationship for SSRIs.[23] Other evidence suggests that increasing the dose of venlafaxine, escitalopram and tricyclics may be helpful.[3]

- Switch treatments early (e.g. after a week or two) if adverse effects are intolerable or if no improvement at all is seen by 3–4 weeks. Opinions on when to switch vary somewhat but it is clear that antidepressants have a fairly prompt onset of action[24–26] and that non-response at 2–6 weeks is a good predictor of overall non-response.[27–29] The absence of any improvement at all at 3–4 weeks should normally provoke a change in treatment (British Association for Psychopharmacology [BAP] guidelines suggest 4 weeks[3]). If there is some improvement at this time, continue and assess for a further 2–3 weeks (see section on 'Antidepressants: general overview' in this chapter).

References

1 Leuchter AF et al. Role of pill-taking, expectation and therapeutic alliance in the placebo response in clinical trials for major depression. Br J Psychiatry 2014; 205:443–449.

2 American Psychiatric Association. Practice Guideline for the Treatment of Patients with Major Depressive Disorder, 3rd edn. Washington, DC: American Psychiatric Association.doi: 10.1176/appi.books.9780890423387.654001, 2010.

3 Anderson IM et al. Evidence-based guidelines for treating depressive disorders with antidepressants: a revision of the 2000 British Association for Psychopharmacology guidelines. J Psychopharmacol 2008; 22:343–396.

4 Crismon ML et al. The Texas Medication Algorithm Project: report of the Texas Consensus Conference Panel on Medication Treatment of Major Depressive Disorder. J Clin Psychiatry 1999; 60:142–156.

5 Kocsis JH et al. Maintenance therapy for chronic depression. A controlled clinical trial of desipramine. Arch Gen Psychiatry 1996; 53:769–774.

6 Dekker J et al. The use of antidepressants after recovery from depression. Eur J Psychiatry 2000; 14:207–212.

7 Nelson JC. Treatment of antidepressant nonresponders: augmentation or switch? J Clin Psychiatry 1998; 59 Suppl 15:35–41.

8 Joffe RT. Substitution therapy in patients with major depression. CNS Drugs 1999; 11:175–180.

9 National Institute for Health and Care Excellence. Depression in adults: recognition and management. Clinical Guideline 90, 2009; last updated April 2016. http://www.nice.org.uk/Guidance/cg90

10 Montgomery SA et al. A randomised, double-blind study in adults with major depressive disorder with an inadequate response to a single course of selective serotonin reuptake inhibitor or serotonin-noradrenaline reuptake inhibitor treatment switched to vortioxetine or agomelatine. Hum Psychopharmacol 2014; 29:470–482.

11 Sparshatt A et al. A naturalistic evaluation and audit database of agomelatine: clinical outcome at 12 weeks. Acta Psychiatr Scand 2013; 128:203–211.

12 Montgomery SA et al. A new depression scale designed to be sensitive to change. Br J Psychiatry 1979; 134:382–389.

13 Hamilton M. Development of a rating scale for primary depressive illness. Br J Soc Clin Psychol 1967; 6:278–296.

14 Kroenke K et al. The PHQ-9: validity of a brief depression severity measure. J Gen Intern Med 2001; 16:606–613.

15 Thase ME et al. Citalopram treatment of fluoxetine nonresponders. J Clin Psychiatry 2001; 62:683–687.

16 Rush AJ et al. Bupropion-SR, sertraline, or venlafaxine-XR after failure of SSRIs for depression. N Engl J Med 2006; 354:1231–1242.

17 Ruhe HG et al. Switching antidepressants after a first selective serotonin reuptake inhibitor in major depressive disorder: a systematic review. J Clin Psychiatry 2006; 67:1836–1855.

18 Brent D et al. Switching to another SSRI or to venlafaxine with or without cognitive behavioral therapy for adolescents with SSRI-resistant depression: The TORDIA Randomized Controlled Trial. JAMA 2008; 299:901–913.

19 Papakostas GI et al. Treatment of SSRI-resistant depression: a meta-analysis comparing within- versus across-class switches. Biol Psychiatry 2008; 63:699–704.

20 National Institute for Health and Care Excellence. Depression in adults: treatment and management. Full guideline (Draft for Consultation). 2017. https://www.nice.org.uk/guidance/GID-CGWAVE0725/documents/draft-guideline

21 Bschor T et al. Switching the antidepressant after nonresponse in adults with major depression: a systematic literature search and meta-analysis. J Clin Psychiatry 2018; 79.

22 Adli M et al. Is dose escalation of antidepressants a rational strategy after a medium-dose treatment has failed? A systematic review. Eur Arch Psychiatry Clin Neurosci 2005; 255:387–400.

23 Hieronymus F et al. A mega-analysis of fixed-dose trials reveals dose-dependency and a rapid onset of action for the antidepressant effect of three selective serotonin reuptake inhibitors. Transl Psychiatry 2016; 6:e834.

24 Papakostas GI et al. A meta-analysis of early sustained response rates between antidepressants and placebo for the treatment of major depressive disorder. J Clin Psychopharmacol 2006; 26:56–60.

25 Taylor MJ et al. Early onset of selective serotonin reuptake inhibitor antidepressant action: systematic review and meta-analysis. Arch Gen Psychiatry 2006; 63:1217–1223.

26 Posternak MA et al. Is there a delay in the antidepressant effect? A meta-analysis. J Clin Psychiatry 2005; 66:148–158.

27 Szegedi A et al. Early improvement in the first 2 weeks as a predictor of treatment outcome in patients with major depressive disorder: a meta-analysis including 6562 patients. J Clin Psychiatry 2009; 70:344–353.

28 Baldwin DS et al. How long should a trial of escitalopram treatment be in patients with major depressive disorder, generalised anxiety disorder or social anxiety disorder? An exploration of the randomised controlled trial database. Hum Psychopharmacol 2009; 24:269–275.

29 Nierenberg AA et al. Early nonresponse to fluoxetine as a predictor of poor 8-week outcome. Am J Psychiatry 1995; 152:1500–1503.

Further reading

Barbui C et al. Amitriptyline v. the rest: still the leading antidepressant after 40 years of randomised controlled trials. Br J Psychiatry 2001; 178:129–144.

Rubinow DR. Treatment strategies after SSRI failure – good news and bad news. N Engl J Med 2006; 354:1305–1307.

Smith D et al. Efficacy and tolerability of venlafaxine compared with selective serotonin reuptake inhibitors and other antidepressants: a meta-analysis. Br J Psychiatry 2002; 180:396–404.

Treatment of refractory depression: first choice

Refractory depression is difficult to treat successfully and outcomes are often poor,[1–3] especially if evidence-based protocols are not followed.[4] Refractory depression is not a uniform entity but a complex spectrum of severity which can be graded[5] and in which outcome is closely linked to grading.[6] A significant minority of apparently resistant unipolar depression may in fact be bipolar-type depression[7,8] which is often unresponsive to standard antidepressants[9,10] (see section on 'Bipolar depression' in Chapter 2).

Treatment of refractory depression is to some extent still informed by results of the Sequenced Treatment Alternatives to Relieve Depression (STAR*D) programme. This was a pragmatic effectiveness study that used remission of symptoms as its main outcome. At stage 1,[11] 2786 subjects received citalopram (mean dose 41.8 mg/day) for 14 weeks; remission was seen in 28% (response [50% reduction in symptoms score] in 47%). Subjects who failed to remit were entered into the continued study of sequential treatments.[12–16] Remission rates are given in Figure 3.2. Very few statistically significant

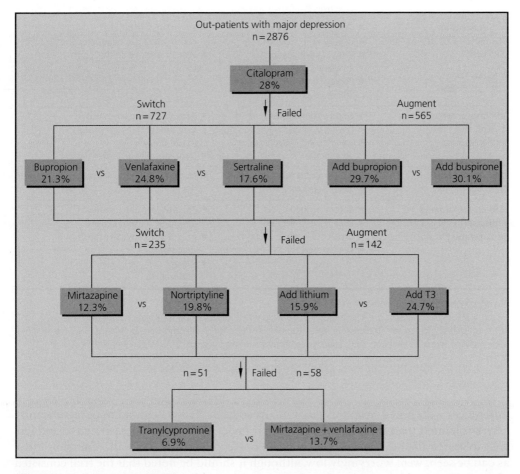

Figure 3.2 Remission rates in STAR*D.

Table 3.2 Refractory depression: first choice. Commonly used treatments generally well supported by published literature (no preference implied by order)

Treatment	Advantages	Disadvantages	Refs
Add **lithium** Aim for plasma level of 0.4–0.8 mmol/L initially, increasing to up to 1.0 mmol/L if suboptimal response	■ Well established ■ Well supported in the literature ■ Recommended by NICE[17]	■ Sometimes poorly tolerated at higher plasma levels ■ Potentially toxic ■ Usually needs specialist referral ■ Plasma level monitoring is essential (and TFTs, e-GFR) ■ May not be effective in patients refractory to multiple treatments	15,18–21
Combine **olanzapine** and **fluoxetine** (6.25–12.5 mg + 25–50 mg daily US licensed dose)*	■ Well researched ■ Usually well tolerated ■ Olanzapine + TCA may also be effective[22] ■ Olanzapine alone may be effective[23,24]	■ Risk of weight gain ■ Limited clinical experience outside USA ■ Most data relate to bipolar depression	25
Add **quetiapine** (150 mg or 300 mg a day) to SSRI/SNRI	■ Good evidence base ■ Usually well tolerated ■ Plausible explanation for antidepressant effect ■ Possibly more effective than lithium	■ Dry mouth, sedation, constipation can be problematic ■ Weight gain risk in the longer term	26–31
Add **aripiprazole** (2–20 mg/day) to antidepressant	■ Good evidence base ■ Usually well tolerated and safe ■ Low doses (2–10 mg/day) may be effective	■ Akathisia and restlessness common at standard doses (≥10 mg/day) ■ Insomnia may be problematic	32–39
SSRI + bupropion Up to 400 mg/day	■ Supported by STAR*D ■ Well tolerated	■ Not licensed for depression in the UK	13,40–45
SSRI or **venlafaxine** + **mianserin** (30 mg/day) or **mirtazapine** (30–45 mg/day)	■ Recommended by NICE ■ Usually well tolerated ■ Excellent literature support ■ Widely used	■ Theoretical risk of serotonin syndrome (inform patient) ■ Risk of blood dyscrasia with mianserin ■ Weight gain and sedation with mirtazapine	16,45–48

Always consider non-drug approaches (e.g. CBT).
* 5 mg + 20 mg rising to 10 mg + 40 mg seems reasonable where combination formulations not available.
eGFR, estimated glomerular filtration rate; NICE, National Institute for Health and Care Excellence; SNRI, serotonin–noradrenaline reuptake inhibitor; SSRI, selective serotonin reuptake inhibitor; STAR*D, Sequenced Treatment Alternatives to Relieve Depression; TCA, tricyclic antidepressant; TFT, thyroid function test.

differences were noted from this point on. At stage 3,[15] T3 was found to be significantly better tolerated than lithium. At stage 4,[16] tranylcypromine was less effective and less well tolerated than the mirtazapine/venlafaxine combination. Overall, remission rates, as can be seen, were worryingly low, although it should be noted that the trial consisted of participants with long histories of recurrent depression.

STAR*D demonstrated that the treatment of refractory depression requires a flexible approach and that response to a particular treatment option is not readily predicted by pharmacology or previous treatments. The programme established bupropion and bus-pirone augmentation as worthwhile options and resurrected from some obscurity the use of T3 augmentation and of nortriptyline. It also, to some extent, confirmed the safety and (to a lesser extent) efficacy of the combination of mirtazapine and venlafaxine.

The treatments commonly used in the treatment of refractory depression, with generally good evidence from the literature, are shown in Table 3.2.

References

1 Dunner DL et al. Prospective, long-term, multicenter study of the naturalistic outcomes of patients with treatment-resistant depression. J Clin Psychiatry 2006; 67:688–695.

2 Wooderson SC et al. Prospective evaluation of specialist inpatient treatment for refractory affective disorders. J Affect Disord 2011; 131:92–103.

3 Fekadu A et al. What happens to patients with treatment-resistant depression? A systematic review of medium to long term outcome studies. J Affect Disord 2009; 116:4–11.

4 Trivedi MH et al. Clinical results for patients with major depressive disorder in the Texas Medication Algorithm Project. Arch Gen Psychiatry 2004; 61:669–680.

5 Fekadu A et al. A multidimensional tool to quantify treatment resistance in depression: the Maudsley staging method. J Clin Psychiatry 2009; 70:177–184.

6 Fekadu A et al. The Maudsley Staging Method for treatment-resistant depression: prediction of longer-term outcome and persistence of symptoms. J Clin Psychiatry 2009; 70:952–957.

7 Angst J et al. Toward a re-definition of subthreshold bipolarity: epidemiology and proposed criteria for bipolar-II, minor bipolar disorders and hypomania. J Affect Disord 2003; 73:133–146.

8 Smith DJ et al. Unrecognised bipolar disorder in primary care patients with depression. Br J Psychiatry 2011; 199:49–56.

9 Sidor MM et al. Antidepressants for the acute treatment of bipolar depression: a systematic review and meta-analysis. J Clin Psychiatry 2011; 72:156–167.

10 Taylor DM et al. Comparative efficacy and acceptability of drug treatments for bipolar depression: a multiple-treatments meta-analysis. Acta Psychiatr Scand 2014; 130:452–469.

11 Trivedi MH et al. Evaluation of outcomes with citalopram for depression using measurement-based care in STAR*D: implications for clinical practice. Am J Psychiatry 2006; 163:28–40.

12 Rush AJ et al. Bupropion-SR, sertraline, or venlafaxine-XR after failure of SSRIs for depression. N Engl J Med 2006; 354:1231–1242.

13 Trivedi MH et al. Medication augmentation after the failure of SSRIs for depression. N Engl J Med 2006; 354:1243–1252.

14 Fava M et al. A comparison of mirtazapine and nortriptyline following two consecutive failed medication treatments for depressed outpatients: a STAR*D report. Am J Psychiatry 2006; 163:1161–1172.

15 Nierenberg AA et al. A comparison of lithium and T(3) augmentation following two failed medication treatments for depression: a STAR*D report. Am J Psychiatry 2006; 163:1519–1530.

16 McGrath PJ et al. Tranylcypromine versus venlafaxine plus mirtazapine following three failed antidepressant medication trials for depression: a STAR*D report. Am J Psychiatry 2006; 163:1531–1541.

17 National Institute for Health and Care Excellence. Depression in adults: recognition and management. Clinical Guideline 90, 2009; last updated April 2016. https://www.nice.org.uk/guidance/cg90

18 Fava M et al. Lithium and tricyclic augmentation of fluoxetine treatment for resistant major depression: a double-blind, controlled study. Am J Psychiatry 1994; 151:1372–1374.

19 Bauer M et al. Lithium augmentation in treatment-resistant depression: meta-analysis of placebo-controlled studies. J Clin Psychopharmacol 1999; 19:427–434.

20 Crossley NA et al. Acceleration and augmentation of antidepressants with lithium for depressive disorders: two meta-analyses of randomized, placebo-controlled trials. J Clin Psychiatry 2007; 68:935–940.

21 Nierenberg AA et al. Lithium augmentation of nortriptyline for subjects resistant to multiple antidepressants. J Clin Psychopharmacol 2003; 23:92–95.

22 Takahashi H et al. Augmentation with olanzapine in TCA-refractory depression with melancholic features: a consecutive case series. Hum Psychopharmacol 2008; 23:217–220.

23 Corya SA et al. A randomized, double-blind comparison of olanzapine/fluoxetine combination, olanzapine, fluoxetine, and venlafaxine in treatment-resistant depression. Depress Anxiety 2006; 23:364–372.

24 Thase ME et al. A randomized, double-blind comparison of olanzapine/fluoxetine combination, olanzapine, and fluoxetine in treatment-resistant major depressive disorder. J Clin Psychiatry 2007; 68:224–236.

25 Luan S et al. Efficacy and safety of olanzapine/fluoxetine combination in the treatment of treatment-resistant depression: a meta analysis of randomized controlled trials. Neuropsychiatr Dis Treat 2017; 13:609–620.

CHAPTER 3

26 Jensen NH et al. N-desalkylquetiapine, a potent norepinephrine reuptake inhibitor and partial 5-HT1A agonist, as a putative mediator of quetiapine's antidepressant activity. Neuropsychopharmacology 2008; 33:2303–2312.

27 El-Khalili N et al. Extended-release quetiapine fumarate (quetiapine XR) as adjunctive therapy in major depressive disorder (MDD) in patients with an inadequate response to ongoing antidepressant treatment: a multicentre, randomized, double-blind, placebo-controlled study. Int J Neuropsychopharmacol 2010; 13:917–932.

28 Bauer M et al. Extended-release quetiapine as adjunct to an antidepressant in patients with major depressive disorder: results of a randomized, placebo-controlled, double-blind study. J Clin Psychiatry 2009; 70:540–549.

29 Bauer M et al. A pooled analysis of two randomised, placebo-controlled studies of extended release quetiapine fumarate adjunctive to antidepressant therapy in patients with major depressive disorder. J Affect Disord 2010; 127:19–30.

30 Montgomery S et al. P01-75 – Quetiapine XR or lithium combination with antidepressants in treatment resistant depression. Eur Psychiatry 2010; 25:296.

31 Doree JP et al. Quetiapine augmentation of treatment-resistant depression: a comparison with lithium. Curr Med Res Opin 2007; 23:333–341.

32 Marcus RN et al. The efficacy and safety of aripiprazole as adjunctive therapy in major depressive disorder: a second multicenter, randomized, double-blind, placebo-controlled study. J Clin Psychopharmacol 2008; 28:156–165.

33 Hellerstein DJ et al. Aripiprazole as an adjunctive treatment for refractory unipolar depression. Prog Neuropsychopharmacol Biol Psychiatry 2008; 32:744–750.

34 Simon JS et al. Aripiprazole augmentation of antidepressants for the treatment of partially responding and nonresponding patients with major depressive disorder. J Clin Psychiatry 2005; 66:1216–1220.

35 Papakostas GI et al. Aripiprazole augmentation of selective serotonin reuptake inhibitors for treatment-resistant major depressive disorder. J Clin Psychiatry 2005; 66:1326–1330.

36 Berman RM et al. Aripiprazole augmentation in major depressive disorder: a double-blind, placebo-controlled study in patients with inadequate response to antidepressants. CNS Spectr 2009; 14:197–206.

37 Fava M et al. A double-blind, placebo-controlled study of aripiprazole adjunctive to antidepressant therapy among depressed outpatients with inadequate response to prior antidepressant therapy (ADAPT-A Study). Psychother Psychosom 2012; 81:87–97.

38 Jon DI et al. Augmentation of aripiprazole for depressed patients with an inadequate response to antidepressant treatment: a 6-week prospective, open-label, multicenter study. Clin Neuropharmacol 2013; 36:157–161.

39 Yoshimura R et al. Comparison of the efficacy between paroxetine and sertraline augmented with aripiprazole in patients with refractory major depressive disorder. Prog Neuropsychopharmacol Biol Psychiatry 2012; 39:355–357.

40 Zisook S et al. Use of bupropion in combination with serotonin reuptake inhibitors. Biol Psychiatry 2006; 59:203–210.

41 Fatemi SH et al. Venlafaxine and bupropion combination therapy in a case of treatment-resistant depression. Ann Pharmacother 1999; 33:701–703.

42 Pierre JM et al. Bupropion-tranylcypromine combination for treatment-refractory depression. J Clin Psychiatry 2000; 61:450–451.

43 Lam RW et al. Citalopram and bupropion-SR: combining versus switching in patients with treatment-resistant depression. J Clin Psychiatry 2004; 65:337–340.

44 Papakostas GI et al. The combination of duloxetine and bupropion for treatment-resistant major depressive disorder. Depress Anxiety 2006; 23:178–181.

45 Henssler J et al. Combining antidepressants in acute treatment of depression: a meta-analysis of 38 studies including 4511 patients. Can J Psychiatry 2016; 61:29–43.

46 Carpenter LL et al. A double-blind, placebo-controlled study of antidepressant augmentation with mirtazapine. Biol Psychiatry 2002; 51:183–188.

47 Carpenter LL et al. Mirtazapine augmentation in the treatment of refractory depression. J Clin Psychiatry 1999; 60:45–49.

48 Ferreri M et al. Benefits from mianserin augmentation of fluoxetine in patients with major depression non-responders to fluoxetine alone. Acta Psychiatr Scand 2001; 103:66–72.

Treatment of refractory depression: second choice

Treatments that may be used in the treatment of refractory depression, although less commonly and with less support from published evaluations, are shown in Table 3.3.

Table 3.3 Second choice: less commonly used, variably supported by published evaluations (no preference implied by order)

Treatment	Advantages	Disadvantages	Refs
Add **ketamine** (0.5 mg/kg IV over 40 minutes) Intranasal **esketamine** may become available and supplant the intravenous form[1]	▪ Very rapid response (within hours) ▪ High remission rate ▪ Some evidence of maintained response if repeated doses given ▪ Usually well tolerated at this sub-anaesthetic dose	▪ IV needs to be administered in hospital ▪ Cognitive effects (confusion, dissociation, etc.) do occasionally occur ▪ Associated with transient increase in BP, tachycardia and arrhythmias. Pre-treatment ECG required with IV form[2] ▪ Adverse effects may have been underestimated[3] ▪ Repeated treatment necessary to maintain effect ▪ Not widely available	4–9
Add **lamotrigine** (100 mg, 200 mg and 400 mg a day have been used)	▪ Reasonably well researched ▪ Quite widely used ▪ Probably best tolerated augmentation strategy[10]	▪ Slow titration ▪ Risk of rash ▪ Appropriate dosing unclear ▪ Two failed RCTs	11–15
SSRI + buspirone Up to 60 mg/day	▪ Supported by STAR*D	▪ Higher doses required ▪ Poorly tolerated (dizziness common) ▪ Not widely used	16,17
High-dose **venlafaxine** (>200 mg/day)	▪ Usually well tolerated ▪ Can be initiated in primary care ▪ Recommended by NICE[18] ▪ Supported by STAR*D	▪ Limited support in literature ▪ Nausea and vomiting more common ▪ Discontinuation reactions common ▪ Can increase BP. Blood pressure monitoring essential	19–22
ECT	▪ Well established ▪ Effective ▪ Well supported in the literature	▪ Poor reputation in public domain ▪ Necessitates general anaesthetic ▪ Needs specialist referral ▪ Usually reserved for last-line treatment or if rapid response needed ▪ Usually combined with other treatments	23–25
Add **tri-iodothyronine** (20–50 µg/day) Higher doses have been safely used	▪ Usually well tolerated ▪ Reasonable literature support ▪ May be effective in bipolar depression	▪ Clinical and biochemical TFT monitoring required ▪ Usually needs specialist referral ▪ Some negative studies ▪ No advantage over antidepressant alone in non-refractory illness[26] ▪ Manufacturer monopoly may provoke high purchase cost in some countries	27–33
Add **risperidone** (0.5–3 mg/day) to antidepressant	▪ Small evidence base ▪ Usually well tolerated	▪ Hypotension ▪ Hyperprolactinaemia ▪ Generally less robust RCT support than for other SGAs	34–39

BP, blood pressure; ECG, electrocardiogram; ECT, electroconvulsive therapy; IV, intravenous; NICE, National Institute for Health and Care Excellence; RCT, randomised controlled trial; SGA, second-generation antipsychotic; STAR*D, Sequenced Treatment Alternatives to Relieve Depression; TFT, thyroid function test.

References

1 Daly EJ et al. Efficacy and safety of intranasal esketamine adjunctive to oral antidepressant therapy in treatment-resistant depression: a randomized clinical trial. JAMA Psychiatry 2018; 75:139–148.

2 aan het Rot M et al. Safety and efficacy of repeated-dose intravenous ketamine for treatment-resistant depression. Biol Psychiatry 2010; 67:139–145.

3 Short B et al. Side-effects associated with ketamine use in depression: a systematic review. Lancet Psychiatry 2018; 5:65–78.

4 Ibrahim L et al. Course of improvement in depressive symptoms to a single intravenous infusion of ketamine vs add-on riluzole: results from a 4-week, double-blind, placebo-controlled study. Neuropsychopharmacology 2012; 37:1526–1533.

5 Murrough JW et al. Rapid and longer-term antidepressant effects of repeated ketamine infusions in treatment-resistant major depression. Biol Psychiatry 2013; 74:250–256.

6 Murrough JW et al. Antidepressant efficacy of ketamine in treatment-resistant major depression: a two-site randomized controlled trial. Am J Psychiatry 2013; 170:1134–1142.

7 Segmiller F et al. Repeated S-ketamine infusions in therapy resistant depression: a case series. J Clin Pharmacol 2013; 53:996–998.

8 Diamond PR et al. Ketamine infusions for treatment resistant depression: a series of 28 patients treated weekly or twice weekly in an ECT clinic. J Psychopharmacol 2014; 28:536–544.

9 Singh JB et al. a double-blind, randomized, placebo-controlled, dose-frequency study of intravenous ketamine in patients with treatment-resistant depression. Am J Psychiatry 2016; 173:816–826.

10 Papadimitropoulou K et al. Comparative efficacy and tolerability of pharmacological and somatic interventions in adult patients with treatment-resistant depression: a systematic review and network meta-analysis. Curr Med Res Opin 2017; 33:701–711.

11 Normann C et al. Lamotrigine as adjunct to paroxetine in acute depression: a placebo-controlled, double-blind study. J Clin Psychiatry 2002; 63:337–344.

12 Barbosa L et al. A double-blind, randomized, placebo-controlled trial of augmentation with lamotrigine or placebo in patients concomitantly treated with fluoxetine for resistant major depressive episodes. J Clin Psychiatry 2003; 64:403–407.

13 Santos MA et al. Efficacy and safety of antidepressant augmentation with lamotrigine in patients with treatment-resistant depression: a randomized, placebo-controlled, double-blind study. Prim Care Companion J Clin Psychiatry 2008; 10:187–190.

14 Barbee JG et al. Lamotrigine as an augmentation agent in treatment-resistant depression. J Clin Psychiatry 2002; 63:737–741.

15 Barbee JG et al. A double-blind placebo-controlled trial of lamotrigine as an antidepressant augmentation agent in treatment-refractory unipolar depression. J Clin Psychiatry 2011; 72:1405–1412.

16 Trivedi MH et al. Medication augmentation after the failure of SSRIs for depression. N Engl J Med 2006; 354:1243–1252.

17 Appelberg BG et al. Patients with severe depression may benefit from buspirone augmentation of selective serotonin reuptake inhibitors: results from a placebo-controlled, randomized, double-blind, placebo wash-in study. J Clin Psychiatry 2001; 62:448–452.

18 National Institute for Health and Care Excellence. Depression in adults: recognition and management. Clinical Guideline 90; last updated April 2016. https://www.nice.org.uk/guidance/cg90

19 Poirier MF et al. Venlafaxine and paroxetine in treatment-resistant depression. Double-blind, randomised comparison. Br J Psychiatry 1999; 175:12–16.

20 Nierenberg AA et al. Venlafaxine for treatment-resistant unipolar depression. J Clin Psychopharmacol 1994; 14:419–423.

21 Smith D et al. Efficacy and tolerability of venlafaxine compared with selective serotonin reuptake inhibitors and other antidepressants: a meta-analysis. Br J Psychiatry 2002; 180:396–404.

22 Rush AJ et al. Bupropion-SR, sertraline, or venlafaxine-XR after failure of SSRIs for depression. N Engl J Med 2006; 354:1231–1242.

23 Folkerts HW et al. Electroconvulsive therapy vs. paroxetine in treatment-resistant depression – a randomized study. Acta Psychiatr Scand 1997; 96:334–342.

24 Gonzalez-Pinto A et al. Efficacy and safety of venlafaxine-ECT combination in treatment-resistant depression. J Neuropsychiatry Clin Neurosci 2002; 14:206–209.

25 Eranti S et al. A randomized, controlled trial with 6-month follow-up of repetitive transcranial magnetic stimulation and electroconvulsive therapy for severe depression. Am J Psychiatry 2007; 164:73–81.

26 Garlow SJ et al. The combination of triiodothyronine (T3) and sertraline is not superior to sertraline monotherapy in the treatment of major depressive disorder. J Psychiatr Res 2012; 46:1406–1413.

27 Joffe RT et al. A comparison of triiodothyronine and thyroxine in the potentiation of tricyclic antidepressants. Psychiatry Res 1990; 32:241–251.

28 Anderson IM. Drug treatment of depression: reflections on the evidence. Adv Psychiatr Treat 2003; 9:11–20.

29 Nierenberg AA et al. A comparison of lithium and T(3) augmentation following two failed medication treatments for depression: a STAR*D report. Am J Psychiatry 2006; 163:1519–1530.

30 Iosifescu DV et al. An open study of triiodothyronine augmentation of selective serotonin reuptake inhibitors in treatment-resistant major depressive disorder. J Clin Psychiatry 2005; 66:1038–1042.

31 Abraham G et al. T3 augmentation of SSRI resistant depression. J Affect Disord 2006; 91:211–215.

32 Kelly TF et al. Long term augmentation with T3 in refractory major depression. J Affect Disord 2009; 115:230–233.

33 Parmentier T et al. The use of triiodothyronine (T3) in the treatment of bipolar depression: a review of the literature. J Affect Disord 2018; 229:410–414.

34 Yoshimura R et al. Addition of risperidone to sertraline improves sertraline-resistant refractory depression without influencing plasma concentrations of sertraline and desmethylsertraline. Hum Psychopharmacol 2008; 23:707–713.

35 Mahmoud RA et al. Risperidone for treatment-refractory major depressive disorder: a randomized trial. Ann Intern Med 2007; **147**: 593–602.

36 Ostroff RB et al. Risperidone augmentation of selective serotonin reuptake inhibitors in major depression. J Clin Psychiatry 1999; **60**: 256–259.

37 Rapaport MH et al. Effects of risperidone augmentation in patients with treatment-resistant depression: results of open-label treatment followed by double-blind continuation. Neuropsychopharmacology 2006; **31**:2505–2513.

38 Stoll AL et al. Tranylcypromine plus risperidone for treatment-refractory major depression. J Clin Psychopharmacol 2000; **20**:495–496.

39 Keitner GI et al. A randomized, placebo-controlled trial of risperidone augmentation for patients with difficult-to-treat unipolar, non-psychotic major depression. J Psychiatr Res 2009; **43**:205–214.

Treatment of refractory depression: other reported treatments

Other pharmacological treatments have been reported in the literature, but the evidence is sparse (Table 3.4). Prescribers *must* familiarise themselves with the primary literature before using these strategies.

Table 3.4 Other reported treatments (alphabetical order – no preference implied)

Treatment	Comments	References
Add amantadine (up to 300 mg/day)	Limited data	1
Buprenorphine	Reasonable evidence but obvious contraindications	2
Add cabergoline 2 mg/day	Very limited data	3
Add D-cycloserine (1000 mg/day)	One small RCT showing useful effect	4
Add mecamylamine (up to 10 mg/day)	One pilot study of 21 patients	5,6
Add pindolol (5 mg tds or 7.5 mg once daily)	Well tolerated, can be initiated in primary care, reasonably well researched, but data mainly relate to acceleration of response. Refractory data somewhat contradictory	7–12
Add tianeptine (25–50 mg/day)	Tiny database. Tianeptine not available in many countries	13,14
Add tryptophan 2–3 g tds	Long history of successful use	15–18
Add zinc (25 mg Zn+/day)	One RCT (n = 60) showed good results in refractory illness	19
Add ziprasidone Up to 160 mg/day	Poorly supported. Probably has no antidepressant effects	20–22
Combine MAOI and TCA e.g. trimipramine and phenelzine	Formerly very widely used, but great care needed	23–25
Dexamethasone 3–4 mg/day	Use for 4 days only. Limited data	26,27
Hyoscine (scopolomine) (4 µg/kg IV)	Growing evidence base of prompt and sizeable effect	28
Ketoconazole 400–800 mg/day	Rarely used. Risk of hepatotoxicity	29
Modafinil 100–400 mg/day	Data mainly relate to non-refractory illness. Usually added to antidepressant treatment. May worsen anxiety (see section on 'Stimulants in depression' in this chapter)	12,30–33
Nemifitide (40–240 mg/day SC)	One pilot study in 25 patients	34
Nortriptyline ± lithium	Re-emergent treatment option	35–38

Table 3.4 (*Continued*)

Treatment	Comments	References
Oestrogens (various regimens)	Limited data	39
Omega-3 triglycerides EPA 1–2 g/day	Usually added to antidepressant treatment	40,41
Pramipexole 0.125–5 mg/day	One good RCT showing clear effect	42,43
Riluzole 100–200 mg/day	Very limited data. Costly	44
S-adenosyl-L-methionine 400 mg/day IM; 1600 mg/day oral	Limited data in refractory depression Use weakly supported by a Cochrane review[45]	46–48
SSRI+TCA	Formerly widely used	49
Stimulants: amfetamine; methylphenidate	Varied outcomes	See section on 'Stimulants in depression' in this chapter
TCA – high dose	Formerly widely used. Cardiac monitoring essential	50
Testosterone gel	Effective in those with low testosterone levels	12,51
Venlafaxine – very high dose (up to 600 mg/day)	Cardiac monitoring essential	52
Venlafaxine+IV clomipramine	Cardiac monitoring essential	53

Note: Other non-drug treatments are available, including various psychological approaches, repetitive transcranial magnetic stimulation (rTMS), vagus nerve stimulation, deep brain stimulation and psychosurgery. Discussion of these is beyond the scope of the book.

EPA, eicosapentanoic acid; IM, intramuscular; IV, intravenous; MAOI, monoamine oxidase inhibitor; RCT, randomised controlled trial; SC, subcutaneous; SSRI, selective serotonin reuptake inhibitor; TCA, tricyclic antidepressant; tds, three times a day.

References

1 Stryjer R et al. Amantadine as augmentation therapy in the management of treatment-resistant depression. Int Clin Psychopharmacol 2003; **18**:93–96.

2 Stanciu CN et al. Use of buprenorphine in treatment of refractory depression – a review of current literature. Asian J Psychiatr 2017; **26**:94–98.

3 Takahashi H et al. Addition of a dopamine agonist, cabergoline, to a serotonin-noradrenalin reuptake inhibitor, milnacipran as a therapeutic option in the treatment of refractory depression: two case reports. Clin Neuropharmacol 2003; **26**:230–232.

4 Heresco-Levy U et al. A randomized add-on trial of high-dose D-cycloserine for treatment-resistant depression. Int J Neuropsychopharmacol 2013; **16**:501–506.

5 George TP et al. Nicotinic antagonist augmentation of selective serotonin reuptake inhibitor-refractory major depressive disorder: a preliminary study. J Clin Psychopharmacol 2008; **28**:340–344.

6 Bacher I et al. Mecamylamine – a nicotinic acetylcholine receptor antagonist with potential for the treatment of neuropsychiatric disorders. Expert Opin Pharmacother 2009; **10**:2709–2721.

7 McAskill R et al. Pindolol augmentation of antidepressant therapy. Br J Psychiatry 1998; **173**:203–208.

8 Rasanen P et al. Mitchell B. Balter Award – 1998. Pindolol and major affective disorders: a three-year follow-up study of 30,485 patients. J Clin Psychopharmacol 1999; **19**:297–302.

9 Perry EB et al. Pindolol augmentation in depressed patients resistant to selective serotonin reuptake inhibitors: a double-blind, randomized, controlled trial. J Clin Psychiatry 2004; **65**:238–243.

10 Sokolski KN et al. Once-daily high-dose pindolol for SSRI-refractory depression. Psychiatry Res 2004; **125**:81–86.

11 Whale R et al. Pindolol augmentation of serotonin reuptake inhibitors for the treatment of depressive disorder: a systematic review. J Psychopharmacol 2010; **24**:513–520.

12 Kleeblatt J et al. Efficacy of off-label augmentation in unipolar depression: a systematic review of the evidence. Eur Neuropsychopharmacol 2017; **27**:423–441.

13 Tobe EH et al. Possible usefulness of tianeptine in treatment-resistant depression. Int J Psychiatry Clin Pract 2013; **17**:313–316.

14 Woo YS et al. Tianeptine combination for partial or non-response to selective serotonin re-uptake inhibitor monotherapy. Psychiatry Clin Neurosci 2013; **67**:219–227.

15 Angst J et al. The treatment of depression with L-5-hydroxytryptophan versus imipramine. Results of two open and one double-blind study. Arch Psychiatr Nervenkr 1977; **224**:175–186.

16 Alino JJ et al. 5-Hydroxytryptophan (5-HTP) and a MAOI (nialamide) in the treatment of depressions. A double-blind controlled study. Int Pharmacopsychiatry 1976; **11**:8–15.

17 Hale AS et al. Clomipramine, tryptophan and lithium in combination for resistant endogenous depression: seven case studies. Br J Psychiatry 1987; **151**:213–217.

18 Young SN. Use of tryptophan in combination with other antidepressant treatments: a review. J Psychiatry Neurosci 1991; **16**:241–246.

19 Siwek M et al. Zinc supplementation augments efficacy of imipramine in treatment resistant patients: a double blind, placebo-controlled study. J Affect Disord 2009; **118**:187–195.

20 Papakostas GI et al. Ziprasidone augmentation of selective serotonin reuptake inhibitors (SSRIs) for SSRI-resistant major depressive disorder. J Clin Psychiatry 2004; **65**:217–221.

21 Dunner DL et al. Efficacy and tolerability of adjunctive ziprasidone in treatment-resistant depression: a randomized, open-label, pilot study. J Clin Psychiatry 2007; **68**:1071–1077.

22 Papakostas GI et al. A 12-week, randomized, double-blind, placebo-controlled, sequential parallel comparison trial of ziprasidone as monotherapy for major depressive disorder. J Clin Psychiatry 2012; **73**:1541–1547.

23 White K et al. The combined use of MAOIs and tricyclics. J Clin Psychiatry 1984; **45**:67–69.

24 Kennedy N et al. Treatment and response in refractory depression: results from a specialist affective disorders service. J Affect Disord 2004; **81**:49–53.

25 Connolly KR et al. If at first you don't succeed: a review of the evidence for antidepressant augmentation, combination and switching strategies. Drugs 2011; **71**:43–64.

26 Dinan TG et al. Dexamethasone augmentation in treatment-resistant depression. Acta Psychiatr Scand 1997; **95**:58–61.

27 Bodani M et al. The use of dexamethasone in elderly patients with antidepressant-resistant depressive illness. J Psychopharmacol 1999; **13**:196–197.

28 Drevets WC et al. Antidepressant effects of the muscarinic cholinergic receptor antagonist scopolamine: a review. Biol Psychiatry 2013; **73**:1156–1163.

29 Wolkowitz OM et al. Antiglucocorticoid treatment of depression: double-blind ketoconazole. Biol Psychiatry 1999; **45**:1070–1074.

30 DeBattista C et al. A prospective trial of modafinil as an adjunctive treatment of major depression. J Clin Psychopharmacol 2004; **24**:87–90.

31 Ninan PT et al. Adjunctive modafinil at initiation of treatment with a selective serotonin reuptake inhibitor enhances the degree and onset of therapeutic effects in patients with major depressive disorder and fatigue. J Clin Psychiatry 2004; **65**:414–420.

32 Menza MA et al. Modafinil augmentation of antidepressant treatment in depression. J Clin Psychiatry 2000; **61**:378–381.

33 Taneja I et al. A randomized, double-blind, crossover trial of modafinil on mood. J Clin Psychopharmacol 2007; **27**:76–78.

34 Feighner JP et al. Clinical effect of nemifitide, a novel pentapeptide antidepressant, in the treatment of severely depressed refractory patients. Int Clin Psychopharmacol 2008; **23**:29–35.

35 Nierenberg AA et al. Nortriptyline for treatment-resistant depression. J Clin Psychiatry 2003; **64**:35–39.

36 Nierenberg AA et al. Lithium augmentation of nortriptyline for subjects resistant to multiple antidepressants. J Clin Psychopharmacol 2003; **23**:92–95.

37 Fava M et al. A comparison of mirtazapine and nortriptyline following two consecutive failed medication treatments for depressed outpatients: a STAR*D report. Am J Psychiatry 2006; **163**:1161–1172.

38 Shelton RC et al. Olanzapine/fluoxetine combination for treatment-resistant depression: a controlled study of SSRI and nortriptyline resistance. J Clin Psychiatry 2005; **66**:1289–1297.

39 Stahl SM. Basic psychopharmacology of antidepressants, part 2: oestrogen as an adjunct to antidepressant treatment. J Clin Psychiatry 1998; **59 Suppl 4**:15–24.

40 Nemets B et al. Addition of omega-3 fatty acid to maintenance medication treatment for recurrent unipolar depressive disorder. Am J Psychiatry 2002; **159**:477–479.

41 Appleton KM et al. Updated systematic review and meta-analysis of the effects of n-3 long-chain polyunsaturated fatty acids on depressed mood. Am J Clin Nutr 2010; **91**:757–770.

42 Whiskey E et al. Pramipexole in unipolar and bipolar depression. Psychiatr Bull 2004; **28**:438–440.

43 Cusin C et al. A randomized, double-blind, placebo-controlled trial of pramipexole augmentation in treatment-resistant major depressive disorder. J Clin Psychiatry 2013; **74**:e636–641.

44 Zarate CA, Jr. et al. An open-label trial of riluzole in patients with treatment-resistant major depression. Am J Psychiatry 2004; **161**:171–174.

45 Galizia I et al. S-adenosyl methionine (SAMe) for depression in adults. Cochrane Database Syst Rev 2016; **10**:CD011286.

46 Pancheri P et al. A double-blind, randomized parallel-group, efficacy and safety study of intramuscular S-adenosyl-L-methionine 1,4-butan-edisulphonate (SAMe) versus imipramine in patients with major depressive disorder. Int J Neuropsychopharmacol 2002; 5:287–294.

47 Alpert JE et al. S-adenosyl-L-methionine (SAMe) as an adjunct for resistant major depressive disorder: an open trial following partial or nonresponse to selective serotonin reuptake inhibitors or venlafaxine. J Clin Psychopharmacol 2004; 24:661–664.

48 Sharma A et al. S-Adenosylmethionine (SAMe) for neuropsychiatric disorders: a clinician-oriented review of research. J Clin Psychiatry 2017; 78:e656–e667.

49 Taylor D. Selective serotonin reuptake inhibitors and tricyclic antidepressants in combination – interactions and therapeutic uses. Br J Psychiatry 1995; 167:575–580.

50 Malhi GS et al. Management of resistant depression. Int J Psychiatry Clin Pract 1997; 1:269–276.

51 Pope HG, Jr et al. Testosterone gel supplementation for men with refractory depression: a randomized, placebo-controlled trial. Am J Psychiatry 2003; 160:105–111.

52 Harrison CL et al. Tolerability of high-dose venlafaxine in depressed patients. J Psychopharmacol 2004; 18:200–204.

53 Fountoulakis KN et al. Combined oral venlafaxine and intravenous clomipramine-A: successful temporary response in a patient with extremely refractory depression. Can J Psychiatry 2004; 49:73—74.

CHAPTER 3

Psychotic depression

Although psychotic symptoms can occur across the whole spectrum of depression severity,[1] those patients who have psychotic symptoms are generally more severely unwell than those who do not have psychotic symptoms.[2] Combined treatment with an antidepressant and antipsychotic is often recommended first line[3] but until fairly recently the data underpinning this practice have been weak.[4,5]

When given in adequate doses, TCAs are probably more effective than newer antidepressants in the treatment of psychotic depression.[4,6,7] Prior failure to respond to previous adequate treatment predicts reduced chance of response to subsequent treatment.[8]

There are few studies of newer antidepressants and atypical antipsychotics, either alone or in combination, specifically for psychotic depression. One large RCT showed response rates of 64% for combined olanzapine and fluoxetine compared with 35% for olanzapine alone and 28% for placebo.[9] Another showed a remission rate of 42% with olanzapine plus sertraline compared with 24% with olanzapine alone.[10] There was no antidepressant-alone group in either study. Small open studies have found quetiapine,[11] aripiprazole[12] and amisulpride[13] augmentation of an antidepressant to be effective and relatively well tolerated, but again there were no data available for antidepressant treatment alone. One RCT (n = 122)[7] found venlafaxine plus quetiapine to be more effective than venlafaxine alone but not more effective than imipramine alone. These findings could be interpreted as supporting the increased efficacy of a TCA over venlafaxine, and supporting combined antidepressant–antipsychotic treatment over an antidepressant drug alone.

A review of all combination studies concluded that the combination of an antipsychotic and antidepressant was superior to either alone (four of nine studies showed some advantage for combination[14]). A meta-analysis concluded that a combination of an antipsychotic and an antidepressant is more effective than either an antipsychotic alone (NNT 5) or an antidepressant alone (NNT 7).[15] NICE[16] recommends that consideration should be given to augmenting an antidepressant with an antipsychotic in the treatment of an acute episode of psychotic depression. Cochrane is in agreement but with reservations regarding the number and quality of trials.[17] Note that these data relate to acute treatment. Virtually nothing is known of the optimum duration of treatment with a combination of an antidepressant and antipsychotic. NICE recommends augmentation of an antidepressant with an antipsychotic in non-psychotic depression that does not respond adequately to an antidepressant alone and states that if one agent is to be stopped during the maintenance phase it should usually be the augmenting agent. It would seem reasonable to use the same approach in psychotic depression, although supporting data are lacking.

In clinical practice, at least until recent years, only a small proportion of patients with psychotic depression received an antipsychotic drug,[18] perhaps reflecting clinicians' uncertainty regarding the risk–benefit ratio of this treatment strategy and the lack of consensus across published guidelines.[19] Under-diagnosis (and hence inadequacy of treatment) of psychotic symptoms in depression is also a significant problem.[20] Nonetheless, some antipsychotic drugs such as quetiapine and olanzapine have useful antidepressant effects (as well as being antipsychotic) and so there is an empiric basis (in addition to the trial outcomes mentioned previously) for their use as additive agents to antidepressant treatment.

Long-term outcome is generally poorer for psychotic than non-psychotic depression.[21,22] Patients with psychotic depression may also have a poorer response to combined pharmacological and psychological treatment than those with non-psychotic depression.[23] People with psychotic depression are much more likely than those with non-psychotic depression to attempt and complete suicide.[24]

Psychotic depression is one of the indications for ECT. Not only is ECT effective, it may also be more protective against relapse in psychotic depression than in non-psychotic depression.[25] One small RCT demonstrated superiority of maintenance ECT plus nortriptyline over nortriptyline alone at 2 years.[26]

Novel approaches being developed include those based on antiglucocorticoid strategies, since hypothalamic-pituitary-adrenal (HPA) axis hyperactivity is more common in psychotic depression. One small open study found rapid effects of the glucocorticoid receptor antagonist mifepristone,[27] although these findings have been criticised.[28] Response may be related to mifepristone plasma levels (>1800 ng/mL).[29] Another analysis suggested that a plasma concentration of above 1637 ng/mL was robustly associated with response,[30] albeit in a trial that stopped early because of lack of efficacy of mifepristone.

There is an anecdotal report of the successful use of methylphenidate in a patient who did not respond to robust doses of an antidepressant and antipsychotic combined.[31] Other case reports describe successful outcome with lamotrigine[32] and a combination of phenelzine, aripiprazole and quetiapine.[33] Minocycline has also shown good effect in an open study.[34]

Ketamine may also be effective in psychotic depression. One report[35] describes successful use of intravenous ketamine (0.5 mg/kg) in two patients unresponsive to standard treatments (one of the two patients had a diagnosis of schizoaffective disorder). Another[36] outlines rapid response to esketamine (0.5 mg/kg given intravenously or subcutaneously) in four patients, two of whom had a primary diagnosis of unipolar depression.

There is no specific indication for other therapies or augmentation strategies in psychotic depression over and above that for resistant depression or psychosis described elsewhere.

Summary

- TCAs are probably drugs of first choice in psychotic depression.
- SSRIs/SNRIs are a second-line alternative when TCAs are poorly tolerated.
- Augmentation of an antidepressant with olanzapine or quetiapine is recommended.
- The optimum dose and duration of antipsychotic augmentation are unknown. If one treatment is to be stopped during the maintenance phase, this should usually be the antipsychotic.
- ECT should always be considered where a rapid response is required or where other treatments have failed.

References

1 Forty L et al. Is depression severity the sole cause of psychotic symptoms during an episode of unipolar major depression? A study both between and within subjects. J Affect Disord 2009; **114**:103–109.
2 Gaudiano BA et al. Depressive symptom profiles and severity patterns in outpatients with psychotic vs nonpsychotic major depression. Compr Psychiatry 2008; **49**:421–429.

3 Cleare A et al. Evidence-based guidelines for treating depressive disorders with antidepressants: a revision of the 2008 British Association for Psychopharmacology guidelines. J Psychopharmacol 2015; 29:459–525.

4 Wijkstra J et al. Pharmacological treatment for unipolar psychotic depression: systematic review and meta-analysis. Br J Psychiatry 2006; 188:410–415.

5 Mulsant BH et al. A double-blind randomized comparison of nortriptyline plus perphenazine versus nortriptyline plus placebo in the treatment of psychotic depression in late life. J Clin Psychiatry 2001; 62:597–604.

6 Birkenhager TK et al. Efficacy of imipramine in psychotic versus nonpsychotic depression. J Clin Psychopharmacol 2008; 28:166–170.

7 Wijkstra J et al. Treatment of unipolar psychotic depression: a randomized, double-blind study comparing imipramine, venlafaxine, and venlafaxine plus quetiapine. Acta Psychiatr Scand 2010; 121:190–200.

8 Blumberger DM et al. Impact of prior pharmacotherapy on remission of psychotic depression in a randomized controlled trial. J Psychiatr Res 2011; 45:896–901.

9 Rothschild AJ et al. A double-blind, randomized study of olanzapine and olanzapine/fluoxetine combination for major depression with psychotic features. J Clin Psychopharmacol 2004; 24:365–373.

10 Meyers BS et al. A double-blind randomized controlled trial of olanzapine plus sertraline vs olanzapine plus placebo for psychotic depression: the study of pharmacotherapy of psychotic depression (STOP-PD). Arch Gen Psychiatry 2009; 66:838–847.

11 Konstantinidis A et al. Quetiapine in combination with citalopram in patients with unipolar psychotic depression. Prog Neuropsychopharmacol Biol Psychiatry 2007; 31:242–247.

12 Matthews JD et al. An open study of aripiprazole and escitalopram for psychotic major depressive disorder. J Clin Psychopharmacol 2009; 29:73–76.

13 Politis AM et al. Combination therapy with amisulpride and antidepressants: clinical observations in case series of elderly patients with psychotic depression. Prog Neuropsychopharmacol Biol Psychiatry 2008; 32:1227–1230.

14 Rothschild AJ. Challenges in the treatment of major depressive disorder with psychotic features. Schizophr Bull 2013; 39:787–796.

15 Farahani A et al. Are antipsychotics or antidepressants needed for psychotic depression? A systematic review and meta-analysis of trials comparing antidepressant or antipsychotic monotherapy with combination treatment. J Clin Psychiatry 2012; 73:486–496.

16 National Institute of Health and Care Excellence. Depression in adults: recognition and management. Clinical Guideline 90, 2009; last updated April 2016. https://www.nice.org.uk/Guidance/cg90

17 Wijkstra J et al. Pharmacological treatment for psychotic depression. Cochrane Database Syst Rev 2015:CD004044.

18 Andreescu C et al. Persisting low use of antipsychotics in the treatment of major depressive disorder with psychotic features. J Clin Psychiatry 2007; 68:194–200.

19 Leadholm AK et al. The treatment of psychotic depression: is there consensus among guidelines and psychiatrists? J Affect Disord 2013; 145:214–220.

20 Rothschild AJ et al. Missed diagnosis of psychotic depression at 4 academic medical centers. J Clin Psychiatry 2008; 69:1293–1296.

21 Flint AJ et al. Two-year outcome of psychotic depression in late life. Am J Psychiatry 1998; 155:178–183.

22 Maj M et al. Phenomenology and prognostic significance of delusions in major depressive disorder: a 10-year prospective follow-up study. J Clin Psychiatry 2007; 68:1411–1417.

23 Gaudiano BA et al. Differential response to combined treatment in patients with psychotic versus nonpsychotic major depression. J Nerv Ment Dis 2005; 193:625–628.

24 Gournellis R et al. Psychotic (delusional) depression and suicidal attempts: a systematic review and meta-analysis. Acta Psychiatr Scand 2018; 137:18–29.

25 Birkenhager TK et al. One-year outcome of psychotic depression after successful electroconvulsive therapy. J ECT 2005; 21:221–226.

26 Navarro V et al. Continuation/maintenance treatment with nortriptyline versus combined nortriptyline and ECT in late-life psychotic depression: a two-year randomized study. Am J Geriatr Psychiatry 2008; 16:498–505.

27 Belanoff JK et al. An open label trial of C-1073 (mifepristone) for psychotic major depression. Biol Psychiatry 2002; 52:386–392.

28 Rubin RT. Dr. Rubin replies (Letter). Am J Psychiatry 2004; 161:1722.

29 Blasey CM et al. A multisite trial of mifepristone for the treatment of psychotic depression: a site-by-treatment interaction. Contemp Clin Trials 2009; 30:284–288.

30 Block T et al. Mifepristone plasma level and glucocorticoid receptor antagonism associated with response in patients with psychotic depression. J Clin Psychopharmacol 2017; 37:505–511.

31 Huang CC et al. Adjunctive use of methylphenidate in the treatment of psychotic unipolar depression. Clin Neuropharmacol 2008; 31:245–247.

32 Kajiya T et al. Effect of lamotrigine in the treatment of bipolar depression with psychotic features: a case report. Ann Gen Psychiatry 2017; 16:31.

33 Meyer JM et al. Augmentation of phenelzine with aripiprazole and quetiapine in a treatment-resistant patient with psychotic unipolar depression: case report and literature review. CNS Spectr 2017; 22:391–396.

34 Miyaoka T et al. Minocycline as adjunctive therapy for patients with unipolar psychotic depression: an open-label study. Prog Neuropsychopharmacol Biol Psychiatry 2012; 37:222–226.

35 Ribeiro CM et al. the use of ketamine for the treatment of depression in the context of psychotic symptoms: To the Editor. Biol Psychiatry 2016; 79:e65–e66.

36 Ajub E et al. Efficacy of esketamine in the treatment of depression with psychotic features: a case series. Biol Psychiatry 2018; 83:e15–e16.

Electroconvulsive therapy and psychotropic drugs

Psychotropic drugs are often continued during ECT, and some agents (particularly anti-depressants[1,2]) enhance its efficacy.

Table 3.5 summarises the effect of various psychotropics on seizure duration during ECT. Note that there are few well-controlled studies in this area and so recommendations should be viewed with this in mind. Note also that choice of anaesthetic agent profoundly affects seizure duration,[3–8] post-ictal confusion and ECT efficacy.[9,10] The use of ketamine as an anaesthetic does not improve outcome with ECT.[11,12] Aside from concurrent medication, there are many factors that influence seizure threshold and duration.[13]

Table 3.5 Effect of psychotropic drugs on seizure duration in ECT

Drug	Effect on ECT seizure duration	Comments[14–19]
Benzodiazepines[20]	Reduced	All may raise seizure threshold and so should be avoided where possible. Many are long-acting and may need to be discontinued some days before ECT. Benzodiazepines may also complicate anaesthesia and may reduce efficacy of ECT
		If sedation is required, consider hydroxyzine. If benzodiazepine use is very long term and essential, continue and use higher stimulus, bilaterally
SSRIs[2,21–24]	Minimal effect; small increase possible	Generally considered safe to use during ECT. Beware complex pharmacokinetic interactions with anaesthetic agents
Venlafaxine[25]	Minimal effect at standard doses	Limited data suggest no effect on seizure duration but possibility of increased risk of asystole with doses above 300 mg/day.[26] Clearly epileptogenic in higher doses. ECG advised
Mirtazapine[2,27]	Minimal effect – small increase	Apparently safe in ECT and, like other antidepressants, may enhance ECT efficacy. May reduce post-ECT nausea and headache
Duloxetine[28,29]	Not known	One case report suggests duloxetine does not complicate ECT. Another links its use to ventricular tachycardia
TCAs[2,22,30]	Possibly increased	Few data relevant to ECT but many TCAs lower seizure threshold. TCAs are associated with arrhythmia following ECT and should be avoided in elderly patients and those with cardiac disease. In others, it is preferable to continue TCA treatment during ECT. Close monitoring is essential. Beware hypotension and risk of prolonged seizures
MAOIs[31]	Minimal effect	Data relating to ECT very limited but long history of ECT use during MAOI therapy
		MAOIs probably do not affect seizure duration but interactions with sympathomimetics occasionally used in anaesthesia are possible and may lead to hypertensive crisis. Transdermal selegiline seems safe[32]
		MAOIs may be continued during ECT but the anaesthetist must be informed. Beware hypotension

(Continued)

CHAPTER 3

Table 3.5 (Continued)

Drug	Effect on ECT seizure duration	Comments[14–19]
Lithium[33–35]	Possibly increased	Conflicting data on lithium and ECT. The combination may be more likely to lead to delirium and confusion, and some authorities suggest discontinuing lithium 48 hours before ECT. In the UK, ECT is often used during lithium therapy but starting with a low stimulus and with very close monitoring. The combination is generally well tolerated.[36] Note that lithium potentiates the effects of non-depolarising neuromuscular blockers such as suxamethonium. Concomitant use of thiopentone or propofol with lithium treatment lowers seizure threshold[37]
Antipsychotics[38–42]	Variable – increased with phenothiazines and clozapine Others – no obvious effect reported	Few published data but widely used. Phenothiazines and clozapine are perhaps most likely to prolong seizures, and some suggest withdrawal before ECT. However, safe concurrent use has been reported (particularly with clozapine[43,44] which is now usually continued). ECT is effective in clozapine non-response[45]
		ECT and antipsychotics appear generally to be a safe combination. Few data on aripiprazole, quetiapine and ziprasidone, but they too appear to be safe. One case series[46] suggests antipsychotics increase post-ictal cognitive dysfunction
Anticonvulsants[47–50]	Reduced	If used as a mood stabiliser, continue but be prepared to use higher energy stimulus (not always required). If used for epilepsy, their effect is to normalise seizure threshold. Interactions are possible. Valproate may prolong the effect of thiopental; carbamazepine may inhibit neuromuscular blockade. Lamotrigine is reported to cause no problems
Barbiturates	Reduced	All barbiturates reduce seizure duration in ECT but are widely used as sedative anaesthetic agents
		Thiopental and methohexital may be associated with cardiac arrhythmia

ECG, electrocardiogram; ECT, electroconvulsive therapy; MAOI, monoamine oxidase inhibitor; SSRI, selective serotonin reuptake inhibitor; TCA, tricyclic antidepressant.

For drugs known to lower seizure threshold, treatment is best begun with a low-energy stimulus (50 mC). Staff should be alerted to the possibility of prolonged seizures and IV diazepam should be available. With drugs known to elevate seizure threshold, higher stimuli may, of course, be required. Methods are available to lower seizure threshold or prolong seizures,[51] but discussion of these is beyond the scope of this book.

ECT frequently causes confusion and disorientation; more rarely, it causes delirium. There have also been two case reports of serotonin syndrome; one occurred after ECT in a patient on combination of trazodone, bupropion and quetiapine[52] and the other after combination of lithium and ECT therapy.[53] Close observation is essential. Very limited data support the use of thiamine (200 mg daily) in reducing post-ECT confusion.[54] Nortriptyline seems to enhance ECT efficacy and reduce cognitive adverse effects.[1] Donepezil has been shown to improve recovery time post ECT (and appears to be safe).[55] Ibuprofen may be used to prevent headache,[56] and intranasal sumatriptan[57] can be used to treat it.

References

1 Sackeim HA et al. Effect of concomitant pharmacotherapy on electroconvulsive therapy outcomes: short-term efficacy and adverse effects. Arch Gen Psychiatry 2009; 66:729–737.

2 Baghai TC et al. The influence of concomitant antidepressant medication on safety, tolerability and clinical effectiveness of electroconvulsive therapy. World J Biol Psychiatry 2006; 7:82–90.

3 Avramov MN et al. The comparative effects of methohexital, propofol, and etomidate for electroconvulsive therapy. Anesth Analg 1995; 81:596–602.

4 Stadtland C et al. A switch from propofol to etomidate during an ECT course increases EEG and motor seizure duration. J ECT 2002; 18:22–25.

5 Gazdag G et al. Etomidate versus propofol for electroconvulsive therapy in patients with schizophrenia. J ECT 2004; 20:225–229.

6 Conca A et al. Etomidate vs. thiopentone in electroconvulsive therapy. An interdisciplinary challenge for anesthesiology and psychiatry. Pharmacopsychiatry 2003; 36:94–97.

7 Rasmussen KG et al. Seizure length with sevoflurane and thiopental for induction of general anesthesia in electroconvulsive therapy: a randomized double-blind trial. J ECT 2006; 22:240–242.

8 Bundy BD et al. Influence of anesthetic drugs and concurrent psychiatric medication on seizure adequacy during electroconvulsive therapy. J Clin Psychiatry 2010; 71:775–777.

9 Stripp TK et al. Anaesthesia for electroconvulsive therapy – new tricks for old drugs: a systematic review. Acta Neuropsychiatr 2017:1–9.

10 Eser D et al. The influence of anaesthetic medication on safety, tolerability and clinical effectiveness of electroconvulsive therapy. World J Biol Psychiatry 2010; 11:447–456.

11 McGirr A et al. Adjunctive ketamine in electroconvulsive therapy: updated systematic review and meta-analysis. Br J Psychiatry 2017; 210:403–407.

12 Fernie G et al. Ketamine as the anaesthetic for electroconvulsive therapy: the KANECT randomised controlled trial. Br J Psychiatry 2017; 210:422–428.

13 van Waarde JA et al. Clinical predictors of seizure threshold in electroconvulsive therapy: a prospective study. Eur Arch Psychiatry Clin Neurosci 2013; 263:167–175.

14 Royal College of Psychiatrists. *The ECT Handbook – Council Report 176*, 3rd edn. London: RCPsych Publications, 2013.

15 Kellner CH et al. ECT–drug interactions: a review. Psychopharmacol Bull 1991; 27:595–609.

16 Creelman W et al. Electroconvulsive therapy. In: Ciraulo DA, Shader RI, Greenblatt DJ et al., eds. *Drug Interactions in Psychiatry*, 3rd edn. Philidelphia: Lippincott Williams and Wilkins; 2005, 337–389.

17 Naguib M et al. Interactions between psychotropics, anaesthetics and electroconvulsive therapy: implications for drug choice and patient management. CNS Drugs 2002; 16:229–247.

18 Maidment I. The interaction between psychiatric medicines and ECT. Hosp Pharm 1997; 4:102–105.

19 Chi SH et al. Effects of psychotropic drugs on seizure threshold during electroconvulsive therapy. Psychiatry Investig 2017; 14:647–655.

20 Tang VM et al. Should benzodiazepines and anticonvulsants be used during electroconvulsive therapy?: a case study and literature review. J ECT 2017; 33:237–242.

21 Masdrakis VG et al. The safety of the electroconvulsive therapy-escitalopram combination. J ECT 2008; 24:289–291.

22 Dursun SM et al. Effects of antidepressant treatments on first-ECT seizure duration in depression. Prog Neuropsychopharmacol Biol Psychiatry 2001; 25:437–443.

23 Jarvis MR et al. Novel antidepressants and maintenance electroconvulsive therapy: a review. Ann Clin Psychiatry 1992; 4:275–284.

24 Papakostas YG et al. Administration of citalopram before ECT: seizure duration and hormone responses. J ECT 2000; 16:356–360.

25 Gonzalez-Pinto A et al. Efficacy and safety of venlafaxine-ECT combination in treatment-resistant depression. J Neuropsychiatry Clin Neurosci 2002; 14:206–209.

26 Kranaster L et al. Venlafaxine-associated post-ictal asystole during electroconvulsive therapy. Pharmacopsychiatry 2012; 45:122–124.

27 Li TC et al. Mirtazapine relieves post-electroconvulsive therapy headaches and nausea: a case series and review of the literature. J ECT 2011; 27:165–167.

28 Hanretta AT et al. Combined use of ECT with duloxetine and olanzapine: a case report. J ECT 2006; 22:139–141.

29 Heinz B et al. Postictal ventricular tachycardia after electroconvulsive therapy treatment associated with a lithium-duloxetine combination. J ECT 2013; 29:e33–e35.

30 Birkenhager TK et al. Possible synergy between electroconvulsive therapy and imipramine: a case report. J Psychiatr Pract 2016; 22:478–480.

31 Dolenc TJ et al. Electroconvulsive therapy in patients taking monoamine oxidase inhibitors. J ECT 2004; 20:258–261.

32 Horn PJ et al. Transdermal selegiline in patients receiving electroconvulsive therapy. Psychosomatics 2010; 51:176–178.

33 Jha AK et al. Negative interaction between lithium and electroconvulsive therapy – a case-control study. Br J Psychiatry 1996; 168:241–243.

34 Rucker J et al. A case of prolonged seizure after ECT in a patient treated with clomipramine, lithium, L-tryptophan, quetiapine, and thyroxine for major depression. J ECT 2008; 24:272–274.

35 Dolenc TJ et al. The safety of electroconvulsive therapy and lithium in combination: a case series and review of the literature. J ECT 2005; 21:165–170.

36 Thirthalli J et al. A prospective comparative study of interaction between lithium and modified electroconvulsive therapy. World J Biol Psychiatry 2011; 12:149–155.

37 Galvez V et al. Predictors of seizure threshold in right unilateral ultrabrief electroconvulsive therapy: role of concomitant medications and anaesthesia used. Brain Stimul 2015; 8:486–492.

CHAPTER 3

38 Havaki-Kontaxaki BJ et al. Concurrent administration of clozapine and electroconvulsive therapy in clozapine-resistant schizophrenia. Clin Neuropharmacol 2006; 29:52–56.

39 Nothdurfter C et al. The influence of concomitant neuroleptic medication on safety, tolerability and clinical effectiveness of electroconvulsive therapy. World J Biol Psychiatry 2006; 7:162–170.

40 Gazdag G et al. The impact of neuroleptic medication on seizure threshold and duration in electroconvulsive therapy. Ideggyogy Sz 2004; 57:385–390.

41 Masdrakis VG et al. The safety of the electroconvulsive therapy-aripiprazole combination: four case reports. J ECT 2008; 24:236–238.

42 Oulis P et al. Corrected QT interval changes during electroconvulsive therapy-antidepressants-atypical antipsychotics coadministration: safety issues. J ECT 2011; 27:e4–e6.

43 Grover S et al. Combined use of clozapine and ECT: a review. Acta Neuropsychiatr 2015; 27:131–142.

44 Flamarique I et al. Electroconvulsive therapy and clozapine in adolescents with schizophrenia spectrum disorders: is it a safe and effective combination? J Clin Psychopharmacol 2012; 32:756–766.

45 Arumugham SS et al. Efficacy and safety of combining clozapine with electrical or magnetic brain stimulation in treatment-refractory schizophrenia. Expert Rev Clin Pharmacol 2016; 9:1245–1252.

46 van Waarde JA et al. Patient, treatment, and anatomical predictors of outcome in electroconvulsive therapy: a prospective study. J ECT 2013; 29: 113–121.

47 Penland HR et al. Combined use of lamotrigine and electroconvulsive therapy in bipolar depression: a case series. J ECT 2006; 22:142–147.

48 Zarate CA, Jr. et al. Combined valproate or carbamazepine and electroconvulsive therapy. Ann Clin Psychiatry 1997; 9:19–25.

49 Sienaert P et al. Concurrent use of lamotrigine and electroconvulsive therapy. J ECT 2011; 27:148–152.

50 Jahangard L et al. Comparing efficacy of ECT with and without concurrent sodium valproate therapy in manic patients. J ECT 2012; 28:118–123.

51 Datto C et al. Augmentation of seizure induction in electroconvulsive therapy: a clinical reappraisal. J ECT 2002; 18:118–125.

52 Cheng YC et al. Serotonin syndrome after electroconvulsive therapy in a patient on trazodone, bupropion, and quetiapine: a case report. Clin Neuropharmacol 2015; 38:112–113.

53 Deuschle M et al. Electroconvulsive therapy induces transient sensitivity for a serotonin syndrome: a case report. Pharmacopsychiatry 2017; 50:41–42.

54 Linton CR et al. Using thiamine to reduce post-ECT confusion. Int J Geriatr Psychiatry 2002; 17:189–192.

55 Prakash J et al. Therapeutic and prophylactic utility of the memory-enhancing drug donepezil hydrochloride on cognition of patients undergoing electroconvulsive therapy: a randomized controlled trial. J ECT 2006; 22:163–168.

56 Leung M et al. Pretreatment with ibuprofen to prevent electroconvulsive therapy-induced headache. J Clin Psychiatry 2003; 64:551–553.

57 Markowitz JS et al. Intranasal sumatriptan in post-ECT headache: results of an open-label trial. J ECT 2001; 17:280–283.

Stimulants in depression

Psychostimulants reduce fatigue, promote wakefulness and are mood elevating (as distinct from antidepressants). Amfetamines have been used as treatments for depression since the 1930s[1] and more recently modafinil has been evaluated as an adjunct to standard antidepressants.[2] Amfetamines are now rarely used in depression because of their propensity for the development of tolerance and dependence. Prolonged use of high doses is associated with paranoid psychosis.[3] Methylphenidate is now more widely used but may have similar shortcomings. Modafinil seems not to induce tolerance, dependence or psychosis but lacks the marked euphoric effects of amfetamines. Armodafinil, the longer-acting isomer of modafinil, is available in some countries.

Psychostimulants differ importantly from standard antidepressants in that their mood-elevating effects are usually seen within a few hours, but their antidepressant action may be short-lived. Amfetamines and methylphenidate may thus be useful where a prompt effect is required and where dependence would not be problematic (e.g. in depression associated with terminal illness) although ketamine might also be considered (if available). Their use might also be justified in severe, prolonged depression unresponsive to standard treatments (e.g. in those considered for psychosurgery). Modafinil might justifiably be used as an adjunct to antidepressants in a wider range of patients and as a specific treatment for hypersomnia and fatigue.[4]

Table 3.6 outlines support (or the absence of it) for the use of psychostimulants in various clinical situations. Generally speaking, data relating to stimulants in depression are rather poor and inconclusive.[5-7] Careful consideration should be given to any use of any psychostimulant in depression since their short- and long-term safety have not been clearly established. Inclusion of individual drugs in Table 3.6 should not in itself be considered a recommendation for their use.

CHAPTER 3

Table 3.6 Stimulants in depression

Clinical use	Regimens evaluated	Comments	Recommendations
Monotherapy in uncomplicated depression	Modafinil 100–200 mg/day[8,9]	Case reports only – efficacy unproven	Standard antidepressants preferred. Avoid psychostimulants as monotherapy in uncomplicated depression[12]
	Methylphenidate 20–40 mg/day[10,11]	Minimal efficacy	
	Dexamfetamine 20 mg/day[10]	Minimal efficacy	
Adjunctive therapy to accelerate or improve response	SSRI + methylphenidate 10–20 mg/day[13,14]	No clear effect on time to response	Psychostimulants in general not recommended, but modafinil may be useful
	SSRI + modafinil 400 mg/day[15]	Improved response over SSRI alone	
	Tricyclic + methylphenidate 5–15 mg/day[16]	Single open-label trial suggests faster response	
	SSRI or SNRI + lisdexamfetamine 20–70 mg/day[17]	No superiority over placebo	
Adjunctive treatment of depression with fatigue and hypersomnia	SSRI + modafinil 200 mg/day[18,19]	Beneficial effect only on hypersomnia. Modafinil may induce suicidal ideation	Possible effect on fatigue, but weak evidence base. An option where fatigue is prominent and otherwise unresponsive
	SSRI + methylphenidate 10–40 mg/day[20]	Clear effect on fatigue in hospice patients	
Adjunctive therapy in refractory depression	SSRI + modafinil 100–400 mg/day[21–26]	Effect mainly on fatigue and daytime sleepiness	Data limited. Modafinil may be useful for fatigue
	MAOI + dexamfetamine 7.5–40 mg/day[27] or lisdexamfetamine 50 mg/day[28]	Support from single case series and one case report	Stimulants an option in refractory illness but other options better supported
	Methylphenidate or dexamfetamine ± antidepressant[29]	Large case series (n = 50) suggests benefit in the majority	
	Lisdexamfetamine + escitalopram 20–50 mg/day[30]	RCT shows significant effect on depression	
	Lisdexamfetamine + antidepressant 20–30 mg/day[31]	RCT shows significant benefit on executive functioning and depression	
Adjunctive treatment in bipolar depression[32]	Mood stabiliser and/or antidepressants + modafinil 100–200 mg/day[33]	Significantly superior to placebo	Possible treatment option where other standard treatments fail
	Mood stabiliser + armodafinil 150–200 mg/day[35–39]	Superior to placebo on some measures	No evidence of treatment-emergent mania[34]
	Mood stabiliser + methylphenidate 10–40 mg/day[40]	Mixed results, mainly positive	
	Mood stabiliser and/or antipsychotic + lisdexamfetamine 20–70 mg/day[41]	Greater rates of improvement compared to placebo on patient-rated measures	

Table 3.6 (*Continued*)

Clinical use	Regimens evaluated	Comments	Recommendations
Monotherapy or add-on treatment in late-stage terminal cancer	Methylphenidate 5–30 mg/day[42–46]	Case series and open prospective studies	Useful treatment options in those expected to live only for a few weeks
	Dexamfetamine 2.5–20 mg/day[47,48]	Beneficial effects seen on mood, fatigue and pain	
	Methylphenidate 20 mg/day + mirtazapine 30 mg/day[49]	RCT shows benefit for combination from third day of treatment	
	Methylphenidate 20 mg/day + SSRI[50]	RCT failed to show benefit for combination	
	Modafinil 200 mg/day[51]	Benefit to depression scores only in those also experiencing severe cancer-related fatigue	
Monotherapy or add-on treatment for depression in the elderly	Methylphenidate 1.25–20 mg/day[52,53]	Use supported by two placebo-controlled studies. Rapid effect observed on mood and activity	Recommended only where patients fail to tolerate standard antidepressants or where contraindications apply
	Methylphenidate 5–40 mg + citalopram 20–60 mg/day[54]	One placebo-controlled study. Faster rate of response with combination compared to monotherapy with either drug	Monitor for increased heart rate – significant increase seen in one trial[54]
Monotherapy in post-stroke depression	Methylphenidate 5–40 mg/day[55–58]	Variable support but including two placebo-controlled trials.[55,58] Effect on mood evident after a few days	Standard antidepressants preferred. Further investigation required: stimulants may improve cognition and motor function
	Modafinil 100 mg/day[59]	Single case report	
Monotherapy in depression secondary to medical illness	Methylphenidate 5–20 mg/day[60] Dexamfetamine 2.5–30 mg/day[61,62]	Limited data	Psychostimulants not appropriate therapy. Standard antidepressant preferred
Monotherapy in depression and fatigue associated with HIV	Dexamfetamine 2.5–40 mg/day[63,64]	Supported by one good, controlled study[64] Beneficial effect on mood and fatigue	Possible treatment option where fatigue is not responsive to standard antidepressants

HIV, human immunodeficiency virus; MAOI, monoamine oxidase inhibitor; RCT, randomised controlled trial; SNRI, serotonin–noradrenaline reuptake inhibitor; SSRI, selective serotonin reuptake inhibitor.

CHAPTER 3

References

1   Satel SL et al. Stimulants in the treatment of depression: a critical overview. J Clin Psychiatry 1989; 50:241–249.

2   Menza MA et al. Modafinil augmentation of antidepressant treatment in depression. J Clin Psychiatry 2000; 61:378–381.

3   Warneke L. Psychostimulants in psychiatry. Can J Psychiatry 1990; 35:3–10.

4   Goss AJ et al. Modafinil augmentation therapy in unipolar and bipolar depression: a systematic review and meta-analysis of randomized controlled trials. J Clin Psychiatry 2013; 74:1101–1107.

5   Candy M et al. Psychostimulants for depression. Cochrane Database Syst Rev 2008:CD006722.

6   Hardy SE. Methylphenidate for the treatment of depressive symptoms, including fatigue and apathy, in medically ill older adults and terminally ill adults. Am J Geriatr Pharmacother 2009; 7:34–59.

7   McIntyre RS et al. The efficacy of psychostimulants in major depressive episodes: a systematic review and meta-analysis. J Clin Psychopharmacol 2017; 37:412–418.

8   Lundt L. Modafinil treatment in patients with seasonal affective disorder/winter depression: an open-label pilot study. J Affect Disord 2004; 81:173–178.

9   Kaufman KR et al. Modafinil monotherapy in depression. Eur Psychiatry 2002; 17:167–169.

10 Little KY. d-Amphetamine versus methylphenidate effects in depressed inpatients. J Clin Psychiatry 1993; 54:349–355.

11 Robin AA et al. A controlled trial of methylphenidate (ritalin) in the treatment of depressive states. J Neurol Neurosurg Psychiatry 1958; 21:55–57.

12 Hegerl U et al. Why do stimulants not work in typical depression? Aust N Z J Psychiatry 2017; 51:20–22.

13 Lavretsky H et al. Combined treatment with methylphenidate and citalopram for accelerated response in the elderly: an open trial. J Clin Psychiatry 2003; 64:1410–1414.

14 Postolache TT et al. Early augmentation of sertraline with methylphenidate. J Clin Psychiatry 1999; 60:123–124.

15 Abolfazli R et al. Double-blind randomized parallel-group clinical trial of efficacy of the combination fluoxetine plus modafinil versus fluoxetine plus placebo in the treatment of major depression. Depress Anxiety 2011; 28:297–302.

16 Gwirtsman HE et al. The antidepressant response to tricyclics in major depressives is accelerated with adjunctive use of methylphenidate. Psychopharmacol Bull 1994; 30:157–164.

17 Giacobbe P et al. Efficacy and tolerability of lisdexamfetamine as an antidepressant augmentation strategy: a meta-analysis of randomized controlled trials. J Affect Disord 2018; 226:294–300.

18 Dunlop BW et al. Coadministration of modafinil and a selective serotonin reuptake inhibitor from the initiation of treatment of major depressive disorder with fatigue and sleepiness: a double-blind, placebo-controlled study. J Clin Psychopharmacol 2007; 27:614–619.

19 Fava M et al. Modafinil augmentation of selective serotonin reuptake inhibitor therapy in MDD partial responders with persistent fatigue and sleepiness. Ann Clin Psychiatry 2007; 19:153–159.

20 Kerr CW et al. Effects of methylphenidate on fatigue and depression: a randomized, double-blind, placebo-controlled trial. J Pain Symptom Manage 2012; 43:68–77.

21 DeBattista C et al. Adjunct modafinil for the short-term treatment of fatigue and sleepiness in patients with major depressive disorder: a preliminary double-blind, placebo-controlled study. J Clin Psychiatry 2003; 64:1057–1064.

22 Fava M et al. A multicenter, placebo-controlled study of modafinil augmentation in partial responders to selective serotonin reuptake inhibitors with persistent fatigue and sleepiness. J Clin Psychiatry 2005; 66:85–93.

23 Rasmussen NA et al. Modafinil augmentation in depressed patients with partial response to antidepressants: a pilot study on self-reported symptoms covered by the major depression inventory (MDI) and the symptom checklist (SCL-92). Nord J Psychiatry 2005; 59:173–178.

24 DeBattista C et al. A prospective trial of modafinil as an adjunctive treatment of major depression. J Clin Psychopharmacol 2004; 24:87–90.

25 Markovitz PJ et al. An open-label trial of modafinil augmentation in patients with partial response to antidepressant therapy. J Clin Psychopharmacol 2003; 23:207–209.

26 Ravindran AV et al. Osmotic-release oral system methylphenidate augmentation of antidepressant monotherapy in major depressive disorder: results of a double-blind, randomized, placebo-controlled trial. J Clin Psychiatry 2008; 69:87–94.

27 Fawcett J et al. CNS stimulant potentiation of monoamine oxidase inhibitors in treatment refractory depression. J Clin Psychopharmacol 1991; 11:127–132.

28 Israel JA. Combining stimulants and monoamine oxidase inhibitors: a reexamination of the literature and a report of a new treatment combination. Prim Care Companion CNS Disord 2015; 17.

29 Parker G et al. Do the old psychostimulant drugs have a role in managing treatment-resistant depression? Acta Psychiatr Scand 2010; 121:308–314.

30 Trivedi MH et al. A randomized controlled trial of the efficacy and safety of lisdexamfetamine dimesylate as augmentation therapy in adults with residual symptoms of major depressive disorder after treatment with escitalopram. J Clin Psychiatry 2013; 74:802–809.

31 Madhoo M et al. Lisdexamfetamine dimesylate augmentation in adults with persistent executive dysfunction after partial or full remission of major depressive disorder. Neuropsychopharmacology 2014; 39:1388–1398.

32 Perugi G et al. Use of stimulants in bipolar disorder. Curr Psychiatry Rep 2017; 19:7.

33 Frye MA et al. A placebo-controlled evaluation of adjunctive modafinil in the treatment of bipolar depression. Am J Psychiatry 2007; 164:1242–1249.

34 Szmulewicz AG et al. Dopaminergic agents in the treatment of bipolar depression: a systematic review and meta-analysis. Acta Psychiatr Scand 2017; 135:527–538.

35 Calabrese JR et al. Adjunctive armodafinil for major depressive episodes associated with bipolar I disorder: a randomized, multicenter, double-blind, placebo-controlled, proof-of-concept study. J Clin Psychiatry 2010; 71:1363–1370.

36 Ketter TA et al. Long-term safety and efficacy of armodafinil in bipolar depression: a 6-month open-label extension study. J Affect Disord 2016; 197:51–57.

37 Ketter TA et al. Adjunctive armodafinil for major depressive episodes associated with bipolar I disorder. J Affect Disord 2015; 181:87–91.

38 Frye MA et al. Randomized, placebo-controlled, adjunctive study of armodafinil for bipolar I depression: implications of novel drug design and heterogeneity of concurrent bipolar maintenance treatments. Int J Bipolar Disord 2015; 3:34.

39 Calabrese JR et al. Efficacy and safety of adjunctive armodafinil in adults with major depressive episodes associated with bipolar I disorder: a randomized, double-blind, placebo-controlled, multicenter trial. J Clin Psychiatry 2014; 75:1054–1061.

40 Dell'Osso B et al. Assessing the roles of stimulants/stimulant-like drugs and dopamine-agonists in the treatment of bipolar depression. Curr Psychiatry Rep 2013; 15:378.

41 McElroy SL et al. Adjunctive lisdexamfetamine in bipolar depression: a preliminary randomized, placebo-controlled trial. Int Clin Psychopharmacol 2015; 30:6–13.

42 Fernandez F et al. Methylphenidate for depressive disorders in cancer patients. Psychosomatics 1987; 28:455–461.

43 Macleod AD. Methylphenidate in terminal depression. J Pain Symptom Manage 1998; 16:193–198.

44 Homsi J et al. Methylphenidate for depression in hospice practice. Am J Hosp Palliat Care 2000; 17:393–398.

45 Sarhill N et al. Methylphenidate for fatigue in advanced cancer: a prospective open-label pilot study. Am J Hosp Palliat Care 2001; 18:187–192.

46 Homsi J et al. A phase II study of methylphenidate for depression in advanced cancer. Am J Hosp Palliat Care 2001; 18:403–407.

47 Burns MM et al. Dextroamphetamine treatment for depression in terminally ill patients. Psychosomatics 1994; 35:80–83.

48 Olin J et al. Psychostimulants for depression in hospitalized cancer patients. Psychosomatics 1996; 37:57–62.

49 Ng CG et al. Rapid response to methylphenidate as an add-on therapy to mirtazapine in the treatment of major depressive disorder in terminally ill cancer patients: a four-week, randomized, double-blinded, placebo-controlled study. Eur Neuropsychopharmacol 2014; 24:491–498.

50 Sullivan DR et al. Randomized, double-blind, placebo-controlled study of methylphenidate for the treatment of depression in SSRI-treated cancer patients receiving palliative care. Psychooncology 2017; 26:1763–1769.

51 Conley CC et al. Modafinil moderates the relationship between cancer-related fatigue and depression in 541 patients receiving chemotherapy. J Clin Psychopharmacol 2016; 36:82–85.

52 Kaplitz SE. Withdrawn, apathetic geriatric patients responsive to methylphenidate. J Am Geriatr Soc 1975; 23:271–276.

53 Wallace AE et al. Double-blind, placebo-controlled trial of methylphenidate in older, depressed, medically ill patients. Am J Psychiatry 1995; 152:929–931.

54 Lavretsky H et al. Citalopram, methylphenidate, or their combination in geriatric depression: a randomized, double-blind, placebo-controlled trial. Am J Psychiatry 2015; 172:561–569.

55 Grade C et al. Methylphenidate in early poststroke recovery: a double-blind, placebo-controlled study. Arch Phys Med Rehabil 1998; 79:1047–1050.

56 Lazarus LW et al. Efficacy and side effects of methylphenidate for poststroke depression. J Clin Psychiatry 1992; 53:447–449.

57 Lingam VR et al. Methylphenidate in treating poststroke depression. J Clin Psychiatry 1988; 49:151–153.

58 Delbari A et al. Effect of methylphenidate and/or levodopa combined with physiotherapy on mood and cognition after stroke: a randomized, double-blind, placebo-controlled trial. Eur Neurol 2011; 66:7–13.

59 Sugden SG et al. Modafinil monotherapy in poststroke depression. Psychosomatics 2004; 45:80–81.

60 Rosenberg PB et al. Methylphenidate in depressed medically ill patients. J Clin Psychiatry 1991; 52:263–267.

61 Woods SW et al. Psychostimulant treatment of depressive disorders secondary to medical illness. J Clin Psychiatry 1986; 47:12–15.

62 Kaufmann MW et al. The use of d-amphetamine in medically ill depressed patients. J Clin Psychiatry 1982; 43:463–464.

63 Wagner GJ et al. Dexamphetamine as a treatment for depression and low energy in AIDS patients: a pilot study. J Psychosom Res 1997; 42:407–411.

64 Wagner GJ et al. Effects of dextroamphetamine on depression and fatigue in men with HIV: a double-blind, placebo-controlled trial. J Clin Psychiatry 2000; 61:436–440.

CHAPTER 3

Post-stroke depression

Depression itself is a well-established risk factor for stroke.[1–3] In addition, depression is seen in at least 30–40% of survivors of stroke[4,5] and post-stroke depression is known to slow functional rehabilitation.[6] Antidepressants may reduce depressive symptoms[7] and thereby facilitate faster rehabilitation.[8] They may also improve global cognitive functioning,[9,10] enhance motor recovery[11,12] and even reduce mortality.[13] Despite these benefits, post-stroke depression often goes untreated.[14]

Prophylaxis

The high incidence of depression after stroke makes prophylaxis worthy of consideration. Pooled data suggest a robust prophylactic effect for antidepressants.[15] Nortriptyline, fluoxetine, escitalopram, duloxetine and sertraline appear to prevent post-stroke depression.[16–20] Mirtazapine may both protect against depressive episodes and treat them.[21] Note, though, that a large cohort study that examined adverse outcomes in elderly patients treated with antidepressants reported that mirtazapine (and venlafaxine) may be associated with an increased risk of a new stroke compared with SSRIs or TCAs.[22] Mianserin seems ineffective in the treatment of post-stroke depression.[23] Amitriptyline is effective in treating central post-stroke pain.[24]

Treatment

Treatment is complicated by medical co-morbidity and by the potential for interaction with other co-prescribed drugs (especially warfarin, as described later in this section). Contraindication to antidepressant treatment is more likely with tricyclics than with SSRIs.[25] Fluoxetine,[11,26,27] citalopram[9,28,29] and nortriptyline[30,31] are probably the most studied[32] and seem to be effective and safe.[33] SSRIs and nortriptyline are widely recommended for post-stroke depression. Reboxetine (which does not affect platelet activity) may also be effective and well tolerated[34] although its effects overall are doubtful.[35] Vortioxetine may be of particular interest owing to its additional benefits on cognition (independent of effects on depressive symptoms). It also does not appear to adversely affect cardiovascular parameters or interact with warfarin or aspirin, but there are currently no data to support its use specifically in post-stroke depression.

Despite fears, SSRIs seem not to increase risk of stroke[36] (post-stroke), although some doubt remains.[37,38] (Stroke can be embolic or haemorrhagic; SSRIs may protect against the former and provoke the latter[39,40] although the evidence base for this is rather weak[41] – see section on 'SSRIs and bleeding' in this chapter).

Antidepressants are clearly effective in post-stroke depression[33,42] and treatment should not usually be withheld (even though Cochrane [albeit in 2008] was rather lukewarm about the benefits of antidepressants[43]). Two recent multiple-treatments meta-analyses suggested that paroxetine might be the drug of choice when considering both efficacy and tolerability post stroke, although small sample sizes and a lack of high-quality studies in this area limit the strength of this recommendation.[44,45]

Post-stroke depression: recommended drugs

- SSRIs* – paroxetine may be first choice.
- Nortriptyline.

*Caution is clearly required if the index stroke was known to be haemorrhagic because SSRIs increase the risk of *de novo* haemorrhagic stroke (although absolute risk is low), especially when combined with warfarin or other antiplatelet drugs.[46] If the patient is taking warfarin, suggest citalopram or escitalopram (probably lowest interaction potential[47]). Little is known of the pharmacokinetic interaction potential with direct-acting oral anticoagulants (DOACs). Citalopram or escitalopram may again be preferred as neither drug affects enzymes associated with DOAC metabolism.[48]

Where SSRIs are given in any anticoagulated or aspirin-treated patient, consideration should be given to the prescription of a proton pump inhibitor for gastric protection. Nortriptyline, which does not appear to increase risk of bleeding, is an alternative.

References

1 Pan A et al. Depression and risk of stroke morbidity and mortality: a meta-analysis and systematic review. JAMA 2011; **306**:1241–1249.

2 Pequignot R et al. Depressive symptoms, antidepressants and disability and future coronary heart disease and stroke events in older adults: the Three City Study. Eur J Epidemiol 2013; **28**:249–256.

3 Li CT et al. Major depressive disorder and stroke risks: a 9-year follow-up population-based, matched cohort study. PLoS One 2012; **7**:e46818.

4 Gainotti G et al. Relation between depression after stroke, antidepressant therapy, and functional recovery. J Neurol Neurosurg Psychiatry 2001; **71**:258–261.

5 Hayee MA et al. Depression after stroke-analysis of 297 stroke patients. Bangladesh Med Res Counc Bull 2001; **27**:96–102.

6 Paolucci S et al. Post-stroke depression, antidepressant treatment and rehabilitation results. A case-control study. Cerebrovasc Dis 2001; **12**:264–271.

7 Xu XM et al. Efficacy and feasibility of antidepressant treatment in patients with post-stroke depression. Medicine (Baltimore) 2016; **95**:e5349.

8 Gainotti G et al. Determinants and consequences of post-stroke depression. Curr Opin Neurol 2002; **15**:85–89.

9 Jorge RE et al. Escitalopram and enhancement of cognitive recovery following stroke. Arch Gen Psychiatry 2010; **67**:187–196.

10 Gu SC et al. Early selective serotonin reuptake inhibitors for recovery after stroke: a meta-analysis and trial sequential analysis. J Stroke Cerebrovasc Dis 2017; doi: 10.1016/j.jstrokecerebrovasdis.2017.11.031. [Epub ahead of print]

11 Chollet F et al. Fluoxetine for motor recovery after acute ischaemic stroke (FLAME): a randomised placebo-controlled trial. Lancet Neurol 2011; **10**:123–130.

12 Thilarajah S et al. Factors associated with post-stroke physical activity: a systematic review and meta-analysis. Arch Phys Med Rehabil 2017; doi: 10.1016/j.apmr.2017.09.117. [Epub ahead of print]

13 Krivoy A et al. Low adherence to antidepressants is associated with increased mortality following stroke: a large nationally representative cohort study. Eur Neuropsychopharmacol 2017; **27**:970–976.

14 El Husseini N et al. Depression and antidepressant use after stroke and transient ischemic attack. Stroke 2012; **43**:1609–1616.

15 Chen Y et al. Antidepressant prophylaxis for poststroke depression: a meta-analysis. Int Clin Psychopharmacol 2007; **22**:159–166.

16 Narushima K et al. Preventing poststroke depression: a 12-week double-blind randomized treatment trial and 21-month follow-up. J Nerv Ment Dis 2002; **190**:296–303.

17 Rasmussen A et al. A double-blind, placebo-controlled study of sertraline in the prevention of depression in stroke patients. Psychosomatics 2003; **44**:216–221.

18 Robinson RG et al. Escitalopram and problem-solving therapy for prevention of poststroke depression: a randomized controlled trial. JAMA 2008; **299**:2391–2400.

19 Almeida OP et al. Preventing depression after stroke: results from a randomized placebo-controlled trial. J Clin Psychiatry 2006; **67**:1104–1109.

20 Zhang LS et al. Prophylactic effects of duloxetine on post-stroke depression symptoms: an open single-blind trial. Eur Neurol 2013; **69**:336–343.

21 Niedermaier N et al. Prevention and treatment of poststroke depression with mirtazapine in patients with acute stroke. J Clin Psychiatry 2004; **65**:1619–1623.

22 Coupland C et al. Antidepressant use and risk of adverse outcomes in older people: population based cohort study. BMJ 2011; **343**:d4551.

CHAPTER 3

23 Palomaki H et al. Prevention of poststroke depression: 1 year randomised placebo controlled double blind trial of mianserin with 6 month follow up after therapy. J Neurol Neurosurg Psychiatry 1999; 66:490–494.

24 Lampl C et al. Amitriptyline in the prophylaxis of central poststroke pain. Preliminary results of 39 patients in a placebo-controlled, long-term study. Stroke 2002; 33:3030–3032.

25 Cole MG et al. Feasibility and effectiveness of treatments for post-stroke depression in elderly inpatients: systematic review. J Geriatr Psychiatry Neurol 2001; 14:37–41.

26 Wiart L et al. Fluoxetine in early poststroke depression: a double-blind placebo-controlled study. Stroke 2000; 31:1829–1832.

27 Choi-Kwon S et al. Fluoxetine improves the quality of life in patients with poststroke emotional disturbances. Cerebrovasc Dis 2008; 26:266–271.

28 Andersen G et al. Effective treatment of poststroke depression with the selective serotonin reuptake inhibitor citalopram. Stroke 1994; 25:1099–1104.

29 Tan S et al. Efficacy and safety of citalopram in treating post-stroke depression: a meta-analysis. Eur Neurol 2015; 74:188–201.

30 Robinson RG et al. Nortriptyline versus fluoxetine in the treatment of depression and in short-term recovery after stroke: a placebo-controlled, double-blind study. Am J Psychiatry 2000; 157:351–359.

31 Zhang WH et al. Nortriptyline protects mitochondria and reduces cerebral ischemia/hypoxia injury. Stroke 2008; 39:455–462.

32 Starkstein SE et al. Antidepressant therapy in post-stroke depression. Expert Opin Pharmacother 2008; 9:1291–1298.

33 Mead GE et al. Selective serotonin reuptake inhibitors for stroke recovery. JAMA 2013; 310:1066–1067.

34 Rampello L et al. An evaluation of efficacy and safety of reboxetine in elderly patients affected by 'retarded' post-stroke depression. A random, placebo-controlled study. Arch Gerontol Geriatr 2005; 40:275–285.

35 Eyding D et al. Reboxetine for acute treatment of major depression: systematic review and meta-analysis of published and unpublished placebo and selective serotonin reuptake inhibitor controlled trials. BMJ 2010; 341:c4737.

36 Douglas I et al. The use of antidepressants and the risk of haemorrhagic stroke: a nested case control study. Br J Clin Pharmacol 2011; 71:116–120.

37 Ramasubbu R. SSRI treatment-associated stroke: causality assessment in two cases. Ann Pharmacother 2004; 38:1197–1201.

38 Hackam DG et al. Selective serotonin reuptake inhibitors and brain hemorrhage: a meta-analysis. Neurology 2012; 79:1862–1865.

39 Trifiro G et al. Risk of ischemic stroke associated with antidepressant drug use in elderly persons. J Clin Psychopharmacol 2010; 30:252–258.

40 Wu CS et al. Association of cerebrovascular events with antidepressant use: a case-crossover study. Am J Psychiatry 2011; 168:511–521.

41 Mortensen JK et al. Safety of selective serotonin reuptake inhibitor treatment in recovering stroke patients. Expert Opin Drug Saf 2015; 14:911–919.

42 Chen Y et al. Treatment effects of antidepressants in patients with post-stroke depression: a meta-analysis. Ann Pharmacother 2006; 40:2115–2122.

43 Hackett ML et al. Interventions for treating depression after stroke. Cochrane Database Syst Rev 2008:CD003437.

44 Sun Y et al. Comparative efficacy and acceptability of antidepressant treatment in poststroke depression: a multiple-treatments meta-analysis. BMJ Open 2017; 7:e016499.

45 Deng L et al. Interventions for management of post-stroke depression: a Bayesian network meta-analysis of 23 randomized controlled trials. Sci Rep 2017; 7:16466.

46 Quinn GR et al. Effect of selective serotonin reuptake inhibitors on bleeding risk in patients with atrial fibrillation taking warfarin. Am J Cardiol 2014; 114:583–586.

47 Sayal KS et al. Psychotropic interactions with warfarin. Acta Psychiatr Scand 2000; 102:250–255.

48 Fitzgerald JL et al. Drug interactions of direct-acting oral anticoagulants. Drug Saf 2016; 39:841–845.

Further reading

Paolucci S. Advances in antidepressants for treating post-stroke depression. Expert Opin Pharmacother 2017; 18:1011–1017.

Treatment of depression in the elderly

The prevalence of most physical illnesses increases with age. Many physical problems such as cardiovascular disease, chronic pain, diabetes and Parkinson's disease are associated with a high risk of depressive illness.[1,2] The morbidity and mortality associated with depression are increased in the elderly[3] as they are more likely to be physically frail and therefore vulnerable to serious consequences from self-neglect (e.g. life-threatening dehydration or hypothermia) and immobility (e.g. venous stasis). Almost 20% of completed suicides occur in the elderly.[4] Mortality is reduced by effective treatment of depression.

In common with placebo-controlled studies in younger adults, at least some adequately powered studies in elderly patients have failed to find 'active' antidepressants to be more effective than placebo,[5–8] although it is commonly perceived that the elderly may take longer to respond to antidepressants than younger adults.[9] Nonetheless, even in the elderly, it may still be possible to identify non-responders as early as 4 weeks into treatment.[10]

Two studies have found that in elderly people who had recovered from an episode of depression and had received antidepressants for 2 years, 60% relapsed within 2 years if antidepressant treatment was withdrawn.[11,12] This finding held true for first-episode patients. Lower doses of antidepressants may be effective as prophylaxis. Dothiepin (dosulepin) 75 mg/day has been shown to be effective in this regard.[13] Note that NICE recommend that dosulepin should not be used as it is particularly cardiotoxic in overdose.[14] There is no evidence to suggest that the response to antidepressants is reduced in the physically ill,[15] although outcome in the elderly in general is sometimes suboptimal[16–18] (this may not always be the case[19]).

There is no ideal antidepressant in the elderly. All are associated with problems. SSRIs are generally better tolerated than TCAs;[20] they do, however, increase the risk of gastrointestinal bleeds, particularly in the very elderly and those with established risk factors such as a history of bleeds or treatment with a non-steroidal anti-inflammatory drug (NSAID), steroid or warfarin. The risk of other types of bleed such as haemorrhagic stroke may also be increased[21,22] (see section on 'SSRIs and bleeding' in this chapter). The elderly are also particularly prone to develop hyponatraemia[23] with SSRIs (see section on 'Antidepressant-induced hyponatraemia' in this chapter), as well as postural hypotension and falls (the clinical consequences of which may be increased by SSRI-induced osteopenia[24]).

Agomelatine is effective in older patients, is well tolerated and has not been linked to hyponatraemia.[25,26] Its use is limited by the need for frequent blood sampling to check liver function tests (LFTs). Vortioxetine and duloxetine have also been shown to be effective and reasonably well tolerated in the elderly[27] but caveats related to SSRIs, described previously, are relevant here. A general practice database study found that, compared with SSRIs, 'other antidepressants' (venlafaxine, mirtazapine, etc.) were associated with a greater risk of a number of potentially serious adverse effects in the elderly (stroke/transient ischaemic attack [TIA], fracture, seizures, attempted suicide/self-harm) as well as increased all-cause mortality);[23] the study was observational and so could not separate the effect of antidepressants from any increased risk inherent in the group of patients treated with these antidepressants. Polyunsaturated fatty acids (fish oils) are probably not effective.[28]

CHAPTER 3

Table 3.7 Antidepressants and the elderly

Drug	Anticholinergic adverse effect (urinary retention, dry mouth, blurred vision, constipation)	Postural hypotension	Sedation	Weight gain	Safety in overdose	Other adverse effects	Drug interactions
Older tricyclics[32]	Variable: moderate with nortriptyline, imipramine and dosulepin (dothiepin) Marked with others	All can cause postural hypotension Dosage titration is required	Variable: from minimal with imipramine to profound with trimipramine	All tricyclics can cause weight gain	Dothiepin and amitriptyline are the most toxic (seizures and cardiac arrhythmia)	Seizures, anticholinergic-induced cognitive impairment Increased risk of bleeds with serotonergic drugs	Mainly pharmacodynamic: increased sedation with benzodiazepines, increased hypotension with diuretics, increased constipation with other anticholinergic drugs, etc.
Lofepramine	Moderate, although constipation/sweating can be severe	Can be a problem but generally better tolerated than the older tricyclics	Minimal	Few data, but lack of spontaneous reports may indicate less potential than the older tricyclics	Relatively safe	Raised LFTs	
SSRIs[32,33]	Dry mouth can be a problem with paroxetine	Much less of a problem, but an increased risk of falls is documented with SSRIs	Can be a problem with paroxetine and fluvoxamine Unlikely with the other SSRIs	Paroxetine and possibly citalopram may cause weight gain Others are weight neutral	Safe with the possible exception of citalopram; one minor metabolite can cause QTc prolongation. Significance unknown	GI effects and headaches, hyponatraemia, increased risk of bleeds in the elderly (add gastroprotection if also on an NSAID or aspirin), orofacial dyskinesia with paroxetine, cognitive impairment,[29] interstitial lung disease[34]	Fluvoxamine, fluoxetine and paroxetine are potent inhibitors of several hepatic cytochrome enzymes (see section on 'Drug interactions with antidepressants' in this chapter). Sertraline is safer and citalopram, escitalopram and vortioxetine are safest

(Continued)

Table 3.7 (Continued)

Others[35,36]	Minimal with mirtazapine and venlafaxine* Can rarely be a problem with reboxetine* Duloxetine* – few effects Very low incidence with agomelatine	Venlafaxine can cause hypotension at lower doses, but it can increase BP at higher doses, as can duloxetine Dizziness common with agomelatine	Mirtazapine, mianserin and trazodone are sedative Venlafaxine, duloxetine – neutral effects Agomelatine aids sleep	Greatest problem is with mirtazapine, although the elderly are not particularly prone to weight gain Low incidence with agomelatine	Venlafaxine is more toxic in overdose than SSRIs, but safer than TCAs Others are relatively safe	Insomnia and hypokalaemia with reboxetine Nausea with venlafaxine, duloxetine Weight loss and nausea with duloxetine Possibly hepatotoxicity with agomelatine. Monitor LFTs Cognitive impairment with trazodone[29] Interstitial lung disease with SNRIs[34]	Duloxetine inhibits CYP2D6 Moclobemide and venlafaxine inhibit CYP450 enzymes. Check for potential interactions Reboxetine is safe Agomelatine should be avoided in patients who take potent CYP1A2 inhibitors

*Noradrenergic drugs may produce 'anticholinergic' effects via norepinephrine reuptake inhibition.

BP, blood pressure; GI, gastrointestinal; LFT, liver function test; NSAID, non-steroidal anti-inflammatory drug; SNRI, serotonin–noradrenaline reuptake inhibitor; SSRI, selective serotonin reuptake inhibitor; TCA, tricyclic antidepressant.

The effect of antidepressants on cognition in later life is still debated – some studies find antidepressants to worsen cognitive outcomes,[29] others find no effect.[30] The choice of antidepressant may affect the risk; highly anticholinergic medicines are known to increase the likelihood of developing dementia.[31]

Ultimately, choice is determined by the individual clinical circumstances of each patient, particularly physical co-morbidity and concomitant medication (both prescribed and 'over the counter'). (See section on 'Drug interactions with antidepressants' in this chapter.)

The selection of antidepressants for elderly patients is summarised in Table 3.7.

References

1 Katona C et al. Impact of screening old people with physical illness for depression? Lancet 2000; 356:91–92.
2 Lyketsos CG. Depression and diabetes: more on what the relationship might be. Am J Psychiatry 2010; 167:496–497.
3 Gallo JJ et al. Long term effect of depression care management on mortality in older adults: follow-up of cluster randomized clinical trial in primary care. BMJ 2013; 346:f2570.
4 Cattell H et al. One hundred cases of suicide in elderly people. Br J Psychiatry 1995; 166:451–457.
5 Schatzberg A et al. A double-blind, placebo-controlled study of venlafaxine and fluoxetine in geriatric outpatients with major depression. Am J Geriatr Psychiatry 2006; 14:361–370.
6 Wilson K et al. Antidepressant versus placebo for depressed elderly. Cochrane Database Syst Rev 2001:CD000561.
7 O'Connor CM et al. Safety and efficacy of sertraline for depression in patients with heart failure: results of the SADHART-CHF (Sertraline Against Depression and Heart Disease in Chronic Heart Failure) trial. J Am Coll Cardiol 2010; 56:692–699.
8 Seitz DP et al. Citalopram versus other antidepressants for late-life depression: a systematic review and meta-analysis. Int J Geriatr Psychiatry 2010; 25:1296–1305.
9 Paykel ES et al. Residual symptoms after partial remission: an important outcome in depression. Psychol Med 1995; 25:1171–1180.
10 Mulsant BH et al. What is the optimal duration of a short-term antidepressant trial when treating geriatric depression? J Clin Psychopharmacol 2006; 26:113–120.
11 Flint AJ et al. Recurrence of first-episode geriatric depression after discontinuation of maintenance antidepressants. Am J Psychiatry 1999; 156:943–945.
12 Reynolds CF, III et al. Maintenance treatment of major depression in old age. N Engl J Med 2006; 354:1130–1138.
13 Old Age Depression Interest Group. How long should the elderly take antidepressants? A double-blind placebo-controlled study of continuation/prophylaxis therapy with dothiepin. Br J Psychiatry 1993; 162:175–182.
14 National Institute for Health and Care Excellence. Depression in adults: recognition and management. Clinical guideline 90, 2009; last updated April 2016. https://www.nice.org.uk/Guidance/cg90
15 Evans M et al. Placebo-controlled treatment trial of depression in elderly physically ill patients. Int J Geriatr Psychiatry 1997; 12:817–824.
16 Calati R et al. Antidepressants in elderly: metaregression of double-blind, randomized clinical trials. J Affect Disord 2013; 147:1–8.
17 Tedeschini E et al. Efficacy of antidepressants for late-life depression: a meta-analysis and meta-regression of placebo-controlled randomized trials. J Clin Psychiatry 2011; 72:1660–1668.
18 Dong L et al. Model-based comparing efficacy of fluoxetine between elderly and non-elderly participants with major depressive disorder. J Affect Disord 2018; 229:224–230.
19 Steiner AJ et al. Quality of life, functioning, and depressive symptom severity in older adults with major depressive disorder treated with citalopram in the STAR*D Study. J Clin Psychiatry 2017; 78:897–903.
20 Mottram P et al. Antidepressants for depressed elderly. Cochrane Database Syst Rev 2006:CD003491.
21 Smoller JW et al. Antidepressant use and risk of incident cardiovascular morbidity and mortality among postmenopausal women in the Women's Health Initiative study. Arch Intern Med 2009; 169:2128–2139.
22 Laporte S et al. Bleeding risk under selective serotonin reuptake inhibitor (SSRI) antidepressants: a meta-analysis of observational studies. Pharmacol Res 2017; 118:19–32.
23 Coupland C et al. Antidepressant use and risk of adverse outcomes in older people: population based cohort study. BMJ 2011; 343:d4551.
24 Williams LJ et al. Selective serotonin reuptake inhibitor use and bone mineral density in women with a history of depression. Int Clin Psychopharmacol 2008; 23:84–87.
25 Heun R et al. The efficacy of agomelatine in elderly patients with recurrent major depressive disorder: a placebo-controlled study. J Clin Psychiatry 2013; 74:587–594.
26 Laux G. The antidepressant efficacy of agomelatine in daily practice: results of the non-interventional study VIVALDI. Eur Psychiatry 2011; 26 Suppl 1:647.
27 Katona C et al. A randomized, double-blind, placebo-controlled, duloxetine-referenced, fixed-dose study comparing the efficacy and safety of Lu AA21004 in elderly patients with major depressive disorder. Int Clin Psychopharmacol 2012; 27:215–223.
28 Sinn N et al. Effects of n-3 fatty acids, EPA v. DHA, on depressive symptoms, quality of life, memory and executive function in older adults with mild cognitive impairment: a 6-month randomised controlled trial. Br J Nutr 2012; 107:1682–1693.

29 Leng Y et al. Antidepressant use and cognitive outcomes in very old women. J Gerontol A Biol Sci Med Sci 2017; doi: 10.1093/gerona/glx226. [Epub ahead of print]

30 Carriere I et al. Antidepressant use and cognitive decline in community-dwelling elderly people – The Three-City Cohort. BMC Med 2017; 15:81.

31 Heser K et al. Potentially inappropriate medication: association between the use of antidepressant drugs and the subsequent risk for dementia. J Affect Disord 2018; 226:28–35.

32 Draper B et al. Tolerability of selective serotonin reuptake inhibitors: issues relevant to the elderly. Drugs Aging 2008; 25:501–519.

33 Bose A et al. Escitalopram in the acute treatment of depressed patients aged 60 years or older. Am J Geriatr Psychiatry 2008; 16:14–20.

34 Rosenberg T et al. The relationship of SSRI and SNRI usage with interstitial lung disease and bronchiectasis in an elderly population: a case-control study. Clin Interv Aging 2017; 12:1977–1984.

35 Raskin J et al. Safety and tolerability of duloxetine at 60 mg once daily in elderly patients with major depressive disorder. J Clin Psychopharmacol 2008; 28:32–38.

36 Johnson EM et al. Cardiovascular changes associated with venlafaxine in the treatment of late-life depression. Am J Geriatr Psychiatry 2006; 14:796–802.

Further reading

Kok RM et al. Management of depression in older adults: a Review. JAMA 2017; 317:2114–2122.

National Institute for Health and Care Excellence. Depression in adults with a chronic physical health problem: recognition and management. Clinical Guideline 91, 2009. https://www.nice.org.uk/guidance/CG91

Pinquart M et al. Treatments for later-life depressive conditions: a meta-analytic comparison of pharmacotherapy and psychotherapy. Am J Psychiatry 2006; 163:1493–1501.

Van der Wurff FB et al. Electroconvulsive therapy for the depressed elderly. Cochrane Database Syst Rev 2003:CD003593

Wilkinson P et al. Continuation and maintenance treatments for depression in older people. Cochrane Database Syst Rev 2016; 9:CD006727.

CHAPTER 3

CHAPTER 3

Antidepressants: alternative routes of administration

In rare cases, patients may be unable or unwilling to take antidepressants orally, and alternative treatments including psychological interventions and ECT are either impractical or contraindicated.

One such scenario is depression in the medically ill,[1] particularly those who have undergone surgical resection procedures affecting the gastrointestinal tract. Where the intra-gastric (IG) route is used, antidepressants can usually be crushed and administered. If an intra-jejunal (IJ) tube is used then more care is required because of changes in pharmacokinetics; there are few data on the exact site of absorption for the majority of antidepressants. In clinical practice it is often assumed (perhaps wrongly) that administration via the IJ route is likely to result in the same absorption characteristics as via the oral or IG route.

Very few non-oral formulations are available as commercial products. Most formulations do not have UK licences and may be very difficult to obtain, being available only through pharmaceutical importers or from Specials manufacturers. In addition, the use of these preparations beyond their licence or in an absence of a licence usually means that accountability for adverse effects lies with the prescriber. As a consequence, non-oral administration of antidepressants should be undertaken only when absolutely necessary. Table 3.8 shows possible alternative formulations and routes of administration. This table includes case reports not otherwise mentioned elsewhere in the text.

Alternative antidepressant delivery methods

Sublingual

There are a small number of case reports supporting the effectiveness of **fluoxetine** liquid used sublingually in depressed, medically compromised patients.[2] In these reports doses of 20 mg a day produced plasma fluoxetine and norfluoxetine levels towards the lower end of the proposed therapeutic range.[2] If other antidepressants were to be used then it would be advisable to conduct plasma level monitoring of the antidepressant to assess the extent of sublingual absorption.

Buccal

Currently, there are no commercially available antidepressant buccal formulations.[3] A study of orally disintegrating high-dose selegiline for buccal absorption confirmed significant inhibition of brain MAO-A and antidepressant activity.[4] Various studies have investigated development of a buccal-adhesive delivery system for doxepin.[5,6]

Intravenous and intramuscular injections

Intravenous **citalopram** followed by maintenance oral citalopram is a clinically useful treatment strategy for severely depressed, hospitalised patients.[7] Better efficacy and faster response (compared with oral doses) have also been demonstrated when using IV citalopram in treating symptoms of obsessive compulsive disorder.[8] The IV preparation

Table 3.8 Alternative formulations and routes of administration of antidepressants

Drug name and route	Dosing information	Manufacturer	Notes
Sublingual fluoxetine	20 mg/day	Use liquid fluoxetine preparation	Plasma levels may be slightly lower compared with oral dosing
Buccal selegiline	10 mg for 28 days (loses MAO-B selectivity and significantly inhibits brain MAO-A)	Cephalon UK Limited	Orally disintegrating freeze-dried formulation (Zelapar® using the Zydis® fast-dissolving technology) for the treatment of Parkinson's
Buccal amitriptyline	Initiated at 25 mg nocte and titrated up to 125 mg daily	Generic amitriptyline	Tablets were crushed and allowed to dissolve in patient's mouth to promote buccal absorption. Authors report a decrease in the patient's depression[53]
Buccal bupropion[54]	No detailed information available	Clinical trial use only	Bupropion content in bilayer film was 121 mg/9 cm^2. Smoking cessation
Buccal doxepin	No detailed information available	Clinical trial use only	A mucoadhesive paste Orabase® used as a doxepin platform, containing permeation enhancers M (5%) and T (10%); provides sustained release of doxepin and extends contact time with tissue
Intravenous amitriptyline	25–100 mg given in 250 mL NaCl 0.9% by slow infusion over 120 minutes	Contact local importer	Adverse effects tend to be dose related and are largely similar to the oral formulation. At higher doses drowsiness and dizziness occur Bradycardia may occur with doses around 100 mg. ECG monitoring recommended
Intravenous clomipramine	25 mg/2 mL injection Starting dose is 25 mg diluted in 500 mL NaCl 0.9% by slow infusion over 90 minutes. Increased to 250–300 mg in increments of 25 mg/day over 10–14 days[55,56]	Novartis Defiante	The most common reported adverse effects are similar to the oral formulation, which included nausea, sweating, restlessness, flushing, drowsiness, fatigue, abdominal distress and nervousness. ECG monitoring recommended
	Another report used starting dose of 50 mg IV per day and titrated up to a maximum dose of 225 mg/day over 5–7 days[57]		Reduction of symptoms was detected after 1 week of the first IV dose

(Continued)

Table 3.8 (*Continued*)

Drug name and route	Dosing information	Manufacturer	Notes
Intravenous citalopram	40 mg/mL injection Doses from 20 to 40 mg in 250 mL NaCl 0.9% or glucose 5% Doses up to 80 mg have been used for OCD Rate of infusion is 20 mg/hour	Lundbeck – available in some countries. Not licensed in the UK. Check specialist importers or contact Lundbeck for possible supply on a named-patient basis	The most commonly reported adverse effects are nausea, headache, tremor and somnolence, similar to adverse effects of the oral preparation. A case of acute hyperkinetic delirium has also been reported. Used for depression and OCD. ECG monitoring recommended
Intravenous escitalopram	10 mg slow infusion over 60 minutes	Lundbeck – not marketed anywhere in the world	Studies to date have only looked at pharmacokinetic profile. ECG monitoring recommended
Intravenous mirtazapine	6 mg/2 mL infusion solution 15 mg/5 mL infusion solution Dose 15 mg in glucose 5% over 60 minutes	Contact local importer	The most common reported adverse effects are nausea, sedation and dizziness, similar to adverse effects of the oral preparation
Intravenous trazodone[58]	25–100 mg in 250 mL of saline daily for 1 week, lasting approximately 1.5 hours. IV doses were decided according to the severity of depressive symptoms	Available only in Italy	Trazodone showed a significant improvement of symptoms only after 1 week of IV treatment and was better tolerated than clomipramine
Intramuscular flupentixol decanoate depot[59]	5–10 mg/2 weeks	Lundbeck Mylan	IM flupentixol has a mood-elevating effect and is well tolerated at these doses. Extrapyramidal symptoms are rarely seen. Adverse effects reported include dry mouth, dizziness and drowsiness. Flupentixol may be useful in patients for whom tricyclic antidepressants are contraindicated
Amitriptyline gel	50 mmol/L or 100 mmol/L gel 5% amitriptyline, 5% lidocaine gel	Prepared by manufacturing pharmacies	No data on plasma amitriptyline levels This preparation has been used for pain relief rather than antidepressant activity
Amitriptyline 4% and ketamine 2% cream[60]	4 mL cream twice daily	Maxim Pharmaceuticals Entering phase 3 trials	AmiKet™ is an analgesic cream used to relieve pain of peripheral neuropathies. Minimal systemic absorption. Significant sleep improvements in diabetic peripheral neuropathy. Unlikely to have antidepressant effects

Table 3.8 (*Continued*)

Drug name and route	Dosing information	Manufacturer	Notes
Nortriptyline patches	25–75 mg per 24-hour patch	Clinical trial use only	This preparation has been used for smoking cessation rather than antidepressant activity
Imipramine or doxepin nanoemulsion	Unknown. Antidepressant concentration 3% (w/w)	Clinical trial use only	Formulated for potential analgesic therapy rather than antidepressant activity
Transdermal selegiline	6 mg/24 hours, 9 mg/24 hours, 12 mg/24 hours Starting dose is 6 mg/24 hours. Titration to higher doses in 3 mg/24 hour increments at ≥2-week intervals, up to a maximum dose of 12 mg/24 hours[44]	Bristol Myers Squib	The 6 mg/24 hour dose does not require a tyramine-restricted diet At higher doses, although no hypertensive crisis reactions have been reported, the manufacturer recommends avoiding food substances with high tyramine content Application site reactions and insomnia are the most common reported adverse effects
Rectal amitriptyline	Doses up to 50 mg bd	Suppositories have been manufactured by pharmacies	Very little information on rectal administration Largely in the form of case reports
Rectal clomipramine	No detailed information available		
Rectal imipramine	No detailed information available		
Rectal doxepin	No detailed information available	Capsules have been used rectally	
Rectal sertraline	Starting dose: a 25 mg tablet was placed inside the rectal chamber daily. This was titrated up at 3-day intervals to a maximal dose of 100 mg on day 10	Tablets have been used rectally	Levels at the 100 mg steady-state dose revealed detectable serum levels of sertraline, but not the metabolite. The levels fell within the reported range of levels for orally administered sertraline. No adverse effects were recorded
Rectal trazodone	No detailed information available	Suppositories have been manufactured by pharmacies	Trazodone in the rectal formulation has been used for post-operative or cancer pain control rather than antidepressant activity

Note: Availability of all preparations listed varies over time and from country to country.
bd, twice a day; ECG, electrocardiogram; IM, intramuscular; MAO, monoamine oxidase; OCD, obsessive compulsive disorder.

CHAPTER 3

appears to be well tolerated with the most common adverse events being nausea, headache, tremor and somnolence – similar to oral administration.[9,10] A case report of a 65-year-old man describes acute hyperkinetic delirium associated with IV citalopram.[11] Intravenous **escitalopram** also exists although studies reported to date are pharmacokinetic studies.[12] Note that oral citalopram is associated with a higher risk of QTc prolongation than other SSRIs; if used IV in a medically compromised patient, ECG monitoring is recommended.

Mirtazapine is also available as an intravenous preparation. It has been administered by slow infusion at a dose of 15 mg/day for 14 days in two studies and was well tolerated in depressed patients.[13,14] There are reports of IV mirtazapine 6–30 mg/day being used to treat hyperemesis gravidarum.[15,16]

Amitriptyline was once available as both an IV and IM injection (IM injection has been given IV) and both routes have been used in the treatment of post-operative pain and depression.[17] The concentration of the IM preparation (10 mg/mL) necessitated a high volume injection to achieve antidepressant doses; this clearly discourages its use intramuscularly.[18] It is no longer available in most parts of the world. **Clomipramine** is probably the most widely studied IV antidepressant. Pulse loading doses of intravenous clomipramine have been shown to produce a larger, more rapid decrease in obsessive compulsive disorder symptoms compared with oral doses.[19,20] The potential for serious cardiac adverse effects when using any tricyclic antidepressant intravenously necessitates monitoring of pulse, blood pressure and ECG.

The primary rationale for IV administration of antidepressants is the more rapid onset of antidepressant action. However, most trials have generally not supported this rationale.[21] Intravenous formulations also avoid the first-pass effect, leading to higher drug plasma levels[19,22] and perhaps greater response.[22,23] However negative reports also exist.[7,23,24] The placebo effect associated with IV administration is known to be large.[25] Note that calculating the correct parenteral dose of antidepressants is difficult given the variable first-pass effect to which oral drugs are usually subjected. Parenteral doses can be expected to be much lower than oral doses and give the same effect.

Extensive studies of IV **ketamine**, a glutamate N-methyl-D-aspartate (NMDA) receptor antagonist, have demonstrated rapid, albeit short-lived antidepressant effects; however more information is required on safety, dosing, duration of response and most suitable route of administration before implementation into clinical practice.[26] Ketamine has also been delivered via intranasal,[27] IM and subcutaneous routes,[28] sublingually[29] and via transmucosal routes.[30] IV **hyoscine (scopolamine)** as an antidepressant has also been investigated and has produced rapid antidepressant effects within 72 hours in both unipolar and bipolar depression.[31–33] Again, further investigation is needed before use in clinical practice.

Transdermal

Amitriptyline, usually in the form of a gel preparation, is used in pain clinics as an adjuvant in the treatment of a variety of chronic pain conditions.[34,35] It is usually prepared as a 50 mmol/L or 100 mmol/L gel with or without lidocaine. Although it has proven analgesic activity, there are no published data on the plasma levels attained via this route. **Nortriptyline** hydrochloride has been formulated as a transdermal patch for use in smoking cessation.[36] Nanoemulsion formulations of **imipramine** and of **doxepin** have also been formulated for transdermal delivery for use as analgesics.[37] At the time of writing there are no published studies on nortriptyline patches or imipramine or doxepin nanoemulsions in depression.

Oral selegiline at doses greater than 20 mg/day may be an effective antidepressant but enzyme selectivity is lost at these doses, necessitating a tyramine-restricted diet.[38,39] **Selegiline** can be administered transdermally; it is efficacious and tolerable and delivers 25–30% of the selegiline content over 24 hours. Steady-state plasma concentrations are achieved within 5 days of daily dosing.[40] This route bypasses first-pass metabolism, thereby providing a higher, more sustained, plasma concentration of selegiline while being relatively sparing of the gastrointestinal MAO-A system.[41,42] There seems to be no need for tyramine restriction when the lower-dose patch (6 mg/24 hour) is used and there have been no reports of hypertensive reactions even with the higher-dose patch. However, because safety experience with the higher selegiline transdermal system (STS) doses (9 mg/24 hour and 12 mg/24 hour) is more limited, it is recommended that patients using these patches should avoid food substances with very high tyramine content.[43] Age and gender do not affect the pharmacokinetics of the STS.[44,45] When selegiline is administered transdermally, application site reactions and insomnia are the two most commonly reported adverse effects; both are dose related, usually mild or moderate in intensity, and do not lead to dropout from treatment.[43,44,46,47] There appear to be no clinically significant effects of the STS on sexual function or weight gain.[44,47] Advantages of the STS include once-daily dosing, a visual indicator of adherence and its potential in dysphagic patients.[45]

Rectal

The rectal mucosa lacks the extensive villi and microvilli of other parts of the gastrointestinal tract, limiting its surface area. Therefore rectal agents need to be in a formulation that maximises the extent of contact the active ingredient will have with the mucosa. There are no readily available antidepressant suppositories, but extemporaneous preparation is possible. For example, **amitriptyline** (in cocoa butter) suppositories have been manufactured by a hospital pharmacy and administered in a dose of 50 mg twice daily with some subjective success.[48,49] **Doxepin** capsules have been administered via the rectal route directly in the treatment of cancer-related pain (without a special formulation) and produced plasma concentrations within the supposed therapeutic range.[50] Similarly it has been reported that extemporaneously manufactured **imipramine** and **clomipramine** suppositories produced plasma levels comparable with the oral route of administration.[51] **Trazodone** has also been successfully administered in a suppository formulation post-operatively for a patient who was stable on the oral formulation prior to surgery.[49,50] Sertraline tablets administered rectally have also been used with success in a critically ill patient with bowel compromise.[52]

References

1 Cipriani A et al. Metareview on short term effectiveness and safety of antidepressants for depression: an evidence-based approach to inform clinical practice. Can J Psychiatry 2007; 52:553–562.
2 Pakyurek M et al. Sublingually administered fluoxetine for major depression in medically compromised patients. Am J Psychiatry 1999; 156:1833–1834.

CHAPTER 3

3 Kaminsky BM et al. Alternate routes of administration of antidepressant and antipsychotic medications. Ann Pharmacother 2015; 49:808–817.

4 Fowler JS et al. Evidence that formulations of the selective MAO-B inhibitor, selegiline, which bypass first-pass metabolism, also inhibit MAO-A in the human brain. Neuropsychopharmacology 2015; 40:650–657.

5 Laffleur F et al. Modified biomolecule as potential vehicle for buccal delivery of doxepin. Ther Deliv 2016; 7:683–689.

6 Sanz R et al. Development of a buccal doxepin platform for pain in oral mucositis derived from head and neck cancer treatment. Eur J Pharm Biopharm 2017; 117:203–211.

7 Baumann P et al. A double-blind double-dummy study of citalopram comparing infusion versus oral administration. J Affect Disord 1998; 49:203–210.

8 Bhikram TP et al. The effect of intravenous citalopram on the neural substrates of obsessive-compulsive disorder. J Neuropsychiatry Clin Neurosci 2016; 28:243–247.

9 Guelfi JD et al. Efficacy of intravenous citalopram compared with oral citalopram for severe depression. Safety and efficacy data from a double-blind, double-dummy trial. J Affect Disord 2000; 58:201–209.

10 Kasper S et al. Intravenous antidepressant treatment: focus on citalopram. Eur Arch Psychiatry Clin Neurosci 2002; 252:105–109.

11 Delic M et al. Delirium during i.v. citalopram treatment: a case report. Pharmacopsychiatry 2013; 46:37–38.

12 Sogaard B et al. The pharmacokinetics of escitalopram after oral and intravenous administration of single and multiple doses to healthy subjects. J Clin Pharmacol 2005; 45:1400–1406.

13 Konstantinidis A et al. Intravenous mirtazapine in the treatment of depressed inpatients. Eur Neuropsychopharmacol 2002; 12:57–60.

14 Muhlbacher M et al. Intravenous mirtazapine is safe and effective in the treatment of depressed inpatients. Neuropsychobiology 2006; 53:83–87.

15 Guclu S et al. Mirtazapine use in resistant hyperemesis gravidarum: report of three cases and review of the literature. Arch Gynecol Obstet 2005; 272:298–300.

16 Schwarzer V et al. Treatment resistant hyperemesis gravidarum in a patient with type 1 diabetes mellitus: neonatal withdrawal symptoms after successful antiemetic therapy with mirtazapine. Arch Gynecol Obstet 2008; 277:67–69.

17 Collins JJ et al. Intravenous amitriptyline in pediatrics. J Pain Symptom Manage 1995; 10:471–475.

18 RX List. Elavil. 2018. https://www.rxlist.com

19 Deisenhammer EA et al. Intravenous versus oral administration of amitriptyline in patients with major depression. J Clin Psychopharmacol 2000; 20:417–422.

20 Koran LM et al. Pulse loading versus gradual dosing of intravenous clomipramine in obsessive-compulsive disorder. Eur Neuropsychopharmacol 1998; 8:121–126.

21 Moukaddam NJ et al. Intravenous antidepressants: a review. Depress Anxiety 2004; 19:1–9.

22 Koran LM et al. Rapid benefit of intravenous pulse loading of clomipramine in obsessive-compulsive disorder. Am J Psychiatry 1997; 154:396–401.

23 Svestka J et al. [Citalopram (Seropram) in tablet and infusion forms in the treatment of major depression]. Cesk Psychiatr 1993; 89:331–339.

24 Pollock BG et al. Acute antidepressant effect following pulse loading with intravenous and oral clomipramine. Arch Gen Psychiatry 1989; 46:29–35.

25 Sallee FR et al. Pulse intravenous clomipramine for depressed adolescents: double-blind, controlled trial. Am J Psychiatry 1997; 154:668–673.

26 Murrough JW et al. Antidepressant efficacy of ketamine in treatment-resistant major depression: a two-site randomized controlled trial. Am J Psychiatry 2013; 170:1134–1142.

27 Lapidus KA et al. A randomized controlled trial of intranasal ketamine in major depressive disorder. Biol Psychiatry 2014; 76:970–976.

28 Loo CK et al. Placebo-controlled pilot trial testing dose titration and intravenous, intramuscular and subcutaneous routes for ketamine in depression. Acta Psychiatr Scand 2016; 134:48–56.

29 Lara DR et al. Antidepressant, mood stabilizing and procognitive effects of very low dose sublingual ketamine in refractory unipolar and bipolar depression. Int J Neuropsychopharmacol 2013; 16:2111–2117.

30 Nguyen L et al. Off-label use of transmucosal ketamine as a rapid-acting antidepressant: a retrospective chart review. Neuropsychiatr Dis Treat 2015; 11:2667–2673.

31 Jaffe RJ et al. Scopolamine as an antidepressant: a systematic review. Clin Neuropharmacol 2013; 36:24–26.

32 Furey ML et al. Pulsed intravenous administration of scopolamine produces rapid antidepressant effects and modest side effects. J Clin Psychiatry 2013; 74:850–851.

33 Drevets WC et al. Replication of scopolamine's antidepressant efficacy in major depressive disorder: a randomized, placebo-controlled clinical trial. Biol Psychiatry 2010; 67:432–438.

34 Gerner P et al. Topical amitriptyline in healthy volunteers. Reg Anesth Pain Med 2003; 28:289–293.

35 Ho KY et al. Topical amitriptyline versus lidocaine in the treatment of neuropathic pain. Clin J Pain 2008; 24:51–55.

36 Melero A et al. Nortriptyline for smoking cessation: release and human skin diffusion from patches. Int J Pharm 2009; 378:101–107.

37 Sandig AG et al. Transdermal delivery of imipramine and doxepin from newly oil-in-water nanoemulsions for an analgesic and anti-allodynic activity: development, characterization and in vivo evaluation. Colloids Surf B Biointerfaces 2013; 103:558–565.

38 Sunderland T et al. High-dose selegiline in treatment-resistant older depressive patients. Arch Gen Psychiatry 1994; 51:607–615.

39 Mann JJ et al. A controlled study of the antidepressant efficacy and side effects of (–)-deprenyl. A selective monoamine oxidase inhibitor. Arch Gen Psychiatry 1989; 46:45–50.

40 Mylan Specialty L.P. Prescribing Information and Medication Guide EMSAM. 2015. https://www.emsam.com/en/prescribing-information

41 Wecker L et al. Transdermal selegiline: targeted effects on monoamine oxidases in the brain. Biol Psychiatry 2003; 54:1099–1104.

42 Azzaro AJ et al. Pharmacokinetics and absolute bioavailability of selegiline following treatment of healthy subjects with the selegiline transdermal system (6 mg/24 h): a comparison with oral selegiline capsules. J Clin Pharmacol 2007; 47:1256–1267.

43 Amsterdam JD et al. Selegiline transdermal system in the prevention of relapse of major depressive disorder: a 52-week, double-blind, placebo-substitution, parallel-group clinical trial. J Clin Psychopharmacol 2006; 26:579–586.

44 Nandagopal JJ et al. Selegiline transdermal system: a novel treatment option for major depressive disorder. Expert Opin Pharmacother 2009; 10:1665–1673.

45 VanDenBerg CM. The transdermal delivery system of monoamine oxidase inhibitors. J Clin Psychiatry 2012; 73 Suppl 1:25–30.

46 Robinson DS et al. The selegiline transdermal system in major depressive disorder: a systematic review of safety and tolerability. J Affect Disord 2008; 105:15–23.

47 Citrome L et al. Placing transdermal selegiline for major depressive disorder into clinical context: number needed to treat, number needed to harm, and likelihood to be helped or harmed. J Affect Disord 2013; 151:409–417.

48 Adams S. Amitriptyline suppositories. N Engl J Med 1982; 306:996.

49 Mirassou MM. Rectal antidepressant medication in the treatment of depression. J Clin Psychiatry 1998; 59:29.

50 Storey P et al. Rectal doxepin and carbamazepine therapy in patients with cancer. N Engl J Med 1992; 327:1318–1319.

51 Chaumeil JC et al. Formulation of suppositories containing imipramine and clomipramine chlorhydrates. Drug Dev Ind Pharm 1988; 15-17:2225–2239.

52 Leung JG et al. Rectal bioavailability of sertraline tablets in a critically ill patient with bowel compromise. J Clin Psychopharmacol 2017; 37:372–373.

53 Robbins B et al. Amitriptyline absorption in a patient with short bowel syndrome. Am J Gastroenterol 1999; 94:2302–2304.

54 Almeida N et al. A novel dosage form for buccal administration of bupropion. Brazilian Journal of Pharmaceutical Sciences 2015; 51:91–100.

55 Lopes R et al. The utility of intravenous clomipramine in a case of Cotard's syndrome. Rev Bras Psiquiatr 2013; 35:212–213.

56 Fallon BA et al. Intravenous clomipramine for obsessive-compulsive disorder refractory to oral clomipramine: a placebo-controlled study. Arch Gen Psychiatry 1998; 55:918–924.

57 Karameh WK et al. Intravenous clomipramine for treatment-resistant obsessive-compulsive disorder. Int J Neuropsychopharmacol 2015; 19:pyv084.

58 Buoli M et al. Is trazodone more effective than clomipramine in major depressed outpatients? A single-blind study with intravenous and oral administration. CNS Spectr 2017:1–7.

59 Maragakis BP. A double-blind comparison of oral amitriptyline and low-dose intramuscular flupenthixol decanoate in depressive illness. Curr Med Res Opin 1990; 12:51–57.

60 Sawynok J et al. Topical amitriptyline and ketamine for post-herpetic neuralgia and other forms of neuropathic pain. Expert Opin Pharmacother 2016; 17:601–609.

CHAPTER 3

Antidepressant prophylaxis

First episode

A single episode of depression should be treated for at least 6–9 months after full remission.[1] If antidepressant therapy is stopped immediately on recovery, 50% of patients experience a return of their depressive symptoms within 3–6 months.[1,2] Even non-continuous use of antidepressants during the first 6 months of treatment predicts higher rates of relapse.[3]

Recurrent depression

Of those patients who have one episode of major depression, 50–85% will go on to have a second episode, and 80–90% of those who have a second episode will go on to have a third.[4] Many factors are known to increase the risk of recurrence, including a family history of depression, recurrent dysthymia, concurrent non-affective psychiatric illness, female gender, long episode duration, degree of treatment resistance,[5] chronic medical illness and social factors (e.g. lack of confiding relationships and psychosocial stressors). Some prescription drugs may precipitate depression.[5,6]

Figure 3.3 outlines the risk of recurrence for multiple-episode patients: those recruited to the study had already experienced at least three episodes of depression, with 3 years or less between episodes.[7,8] People with depression are at increased risk of cardiovascular disease.[9] Suicide mortality is significantly increased over population norms.

A meta-analysis of antidepressant continuation studies[10] concluded that continuing treatment with antidepressants reduces the odds of depressive relapse by around two-thirds, which is approximately equal to halving the absolute risk. A later meta-analysis of 54 studies produced almost exactly the same results: odds of relapse were reduced by 65%.[11] The risk of relapse is greatest in the first few months after discontinuation; this holds true irrespective of the duration of prior treatment.[12] Benefits persist at 36 months and beyond and seem to be similar across heterogeneous patient groups (first episode, multiple episode and chronic), although none of the studies included first-episode patients only. Specific studies in first-episode patients are required to confirm that treatment beyond 6–9 months confers additional benefit in this patient group. Most data are for adults. Vortioxetine (a relatively new antidepressant) has been shown to be safe and effective over 52 weeks.[13]

An RCT of maintenance treatment in elderly patients, many of whom were first episode, found continuation treatment with antidepressants beneficial over 2 years with a similar effect size to that seen in adults.[14] One small RCT (n = 22) demonstrated benefit from prophylactic antidepressants in adolescents.[15]

Many patients who might benefit from maintenance treatment with antidepressants do not receive them.[16] Assuring optimal management of long-term depression vastly reduces mortality associated with the condition.[17]

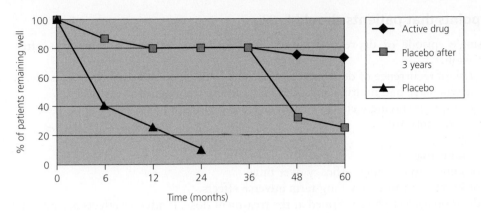

Figure 3.3 The risk of recurrence of depression in multi-episode patients. Patients had experienced at least three episodes of depression with 3 years or less between episodes.

Potential disadvantages of long-term antidepressants include an increased risk of GI and cerebral haemorrhage (see section on 'SSRIs and bleeding' in this chapter) and an additional risk of interaction with co-prescribed drugs likely to increase risk of bleeding or hyponatraemia.

NICE recommends that:[18]

- Patients who have had two or more episodes of depression in the recent past, and who have experienced significant functional impairment during these episodes, should be advised to continue antidepressants for at least 2 years.
- Patients on maintenance treatment should be re-evaluated, taking into account age, co-morbid conditions and other risk factors in the decision to continue maintenance treatment beyond 2 years.

Dose for prophylaxis

Adults should receive the same dose as used for acute treatment.[1] There is some evidence to support the use of lower doses in elderly patients: dosulepin 75 mg/day offers effective prophylaxis[19] but is now rarely used. There is no evidence to support the use of lower than standard doses of SSRIs.[20]

Relapse rates after ECT are similar to those after stopping antidepressants.[21] Antidepressant prophylaxis will be required, ideally with a different drug from the one that failed to get the patient well in the first instance, although good data in this area are lacking.

Lithium also has some efficacy in the prophylaxis of unipolar depression; efficacy relative to antidepressants is unknown.[22] However, lithium treatment has been shown to be associated with the best outcomes of any treatment for unipolar depression.[23] NICE recommends that lithium should not be used as the sole prophylactic drug in unipolar depression.[18] There is some support for the use of a combination of lithium and nortriptyline.[24]

Maintenance treatment with lithium protects against suicide.[1]

CHAPTER 3

Key points that patients should know

- A single episode of depression should be treated for at least 6–9 months after remission.
- The risk of recurrence of depressive illness is high and increases with each episode.
- Those who have had multiple episodes may require treatment for many years.
- The chances of staying well are greatly increased by taking antidepressants.
- Antidepressants are:
  - effective
  - not addictive
  - not known to lose their efficacy over time
  - not known to cause new long-term adverse effects.
- Medication needs to be continued at the treatment dose. If adverse effects are intolerable, it may be possible to find a more suitable alternative.
- If patients decide to stop their medication, this must not be done abruptly, as it may lead to unpleasant discontinuation effects (see section on 'Antidepressant discontinuation symptoms' in this chapter) and confers a higher risk of relapse.[25] The medication needs to be reduced slowly under the supervision of a doctor.

References

1 Anderson IM et al. Evidence-based guidelines for treating depressive disorders with antidepressants: a revision of the 2000 British Association for Psychopharmacology guidelines. J Psychopharmacol 2008; **22**:343–396.

2 Reimherr FW et al. Optimal length of continuation therapy in depression: a prospective assessment during long-term fluoxetine treatment. Am J Psychiatry 1998; **155**:1247–1253.

3 Kim KH et al. The effects of continuous antidepressant treatment during the first 6 months on relapse or recurrence of depression. J Affect Disord 2011; **132**:121–129.

4 Forshall S et al. Maintenance pharmacotherapy of unipolar depression. Psychiatr Bull 1999; **23**:370–373.

5 National Institute for Health and Care Excellence. Depression in adults with a chronic physical health problem: recognition and management. Clinical Guideline 91, 2009. http://www.nice.org.uk/CG91.

6 Patten SB et al. Drug-induced depression. Psychother Psychosom 1997; **66**:63–73.

7 Frank E et al. Three-year outcomes for maintenance therapies in recurrent depression. Arch Gen Psychiatry 1990; **47**:1093–1099.

8 Kupfer DJ et al. Five-year outcome for maintenance therapies in recurrent depression. Arch Gen Psychiatry 1992; **49**:769–773.

9 Taylor D. Antidepressant drugs and cardiovascular pathology: a clinical overview of effectiveness and safety. Acta Psychiatr Scand 2008; **118**:434–442.

10 Geddes JR et al. Relapse prevention with antidepressant drug treatment in depressive disorders: a systematic review. Lancet 2003; **361**:653–661.

11 Glue P et al. Meta-analysis of relapse prevention antidepressant trials in depressive disorders. Aust N Z J Psychiatry 2010; **44**:697–705.

12 Keller MB et al. The prevention of recurrent episodes of depression with venlafaxine for two years (PREVENT) study: outcomes from the 2-year and combined maintenance phases. J Clin Psychiatry 2007; **68**:1246–1256.

13 Vieta E et al. Effectiveness of long-term vortioxetine treatment of patients with major depressive disorder. Eur Neuropsychopharmacol 2017; **27**:877–884.

14 Reynolds CF, III et al. Maintenance treatment of major depression in old age. N Engl J Med 2006; **354**:1130–1138.

15 Cheung A et al. Maintenance study for adolescent depression. J Child Adolesc Psychopharmacol 2008; **18**:389–394.

16 Holma IA et al. Maintenance pharmacotherapy for recurrent major depressive disorder: 5-year follow-up study. Br J Psychiatry 2008; **193**:163–164.

17 Gallo JJ et al. Long term effect of depression care management on mortality in older adults: follow-up of cluster randomized clinical trial in primary care. BMJ 2013; **346**:f2570.

18 National Institute for Health and Care Excellence. Depression in adults: recognition and management. Clinical Guideline 90, 2009; last updated April 2016. https://www.nice.org.uk/guidance/cg90.

19 How long should the elderly take antidepressants? A double-blind placebo-controlled study of continuation/prophylaxis therapy with dothiepin. Old Age Depression Interest Group. Br J Psychiatry 1993; **162**:175–182.

20 Franchini L et al. Dose-response efficacy of paroxetine in preventing depressive recurrences: a randomized, double-blind study. J Clin Psychiatry 1998; **59**:229–232.

21 Nobler MS et al. *Refractory Depression and Electroconvulsive Therapy*. Chichester: John Wiley & Sons Ltd, 1994.

22 Cipriani A et al. Lithium versus antidepressants in the long-term treatment of unipolar affective disorder. Cochrane Database Syst Rev 2006:CD003492.

23 Young AH. Lithium for long-term treatment of unipolar depression. Lancet Psychiatry 2017; **4**:511–512.

24 Sackeim HA et al. Continuation pharmacotherapy in the prevention of relapse following electroconvulsive therapy: a randomized controlled trial. JAMA 2001; **285**:1299–1307.

25 Baldessarini RJ et al. Illness risk following rapid versus gradual discontinuation of antidepressants. Am J Psychiatry 2010; **167**:934–941.

Antidepressant discontinuation symptoms

What are discontinuation symptoms?

The term 'discontinuation symptoms' is used to describe symptoms experienced on stopping prescribed drugs that are not drugs of dependence. There is an important semantic difference between 'discontinuation' and 'withdrawal' symptoms – the latter implies addiction, the former does not. While this distinction is important for precise medical terminology, it may be irrelevant to patient experience. Discontinuation symptoms may occur after stopping many drugs, including antidepressants, and can sometimes be explained in the context of 'receptor rebound'[1,2] – e.g. an antidepressant with potent anticholinergic adverse effects may be associated with diarrhoea on discontinuation.

Discontinuation symptoms may be entirely new or similar to some of the original symptoms of the illness, and so cannot be attributed to other causes. They are also more likely to have an earlier onset, whilst recurrent symptoms of the original illness generally present with a gradual return.[3] They can be broadly divided into six categories: affective (e.g. irritability); gastrointestinal (e.g. nausea); neuromotor (e.g. ataxia); vasomotor (e.g. diaphoresis); neurosensory (e.g. paraesthesia); and other neurological (e.g. increased dreaming).[2] Rarely, mania may occur.[4] The reported prevalence of discontinuation symptoms varies widely,[3] but symptoms are probably experienced by at least a third of patients[5-8] and are seen to some extent with all antidepressants,[3,9] with the possible exceptions of agomelatine[10] and vortioxetine.[11]

The onset of symptoms is usually within a few days of stopping treatment (depending on the half-life of the antidepressant) or occasionally during taper or after missed doses[3] (short half-life drugs only). Symptoms can vary in duration, form and intensity and occur in any combination.[3] They are usually mild and self-limiting[12] but can occasionally be severe and prolonged. The perception of symptom severity is probably made worse by the absence of forewarnings. Some symptoms are more likely with individual drugs (Table 3.9). Symptoms can be quantified using the Discontinuation–Emergent Signs and Symptoms (DESS) scale.[3]

Agomelatine seems to be associated with a very low, if any, risk of discontinuation symptoms.[10] Mirtazapine discontinuation symptoms seem to be characterised by anxiety, panic attacks, insomnia, irritability and nausea.[15] Bupropion discontinuation symptoms are documented in few case reports but appear broadly similar to those seen with SSRIs.[16,17] Vortioxetine has shown placebo level discontinuation symptoms on abrupt withdrawal in RCTs, possibly because of its relatively long half-life.[11] The summary of product characteristics (SPC) in the UK suggests abrupt withdrawal is possible[18] whilst US prescribing information recommends reducing higher doses to 10 mg/day for a week before stopping.[19]

Clinical relevance[20,21]

The symptoms of a discontinuation reaction may be mistaken for a relapse of illness or the emergence of a new physical illness,[22] leading to unnecessary investigations or reintroduction of the antidepressant. Symptoms may be severe enough to interfere with

Table 3.9 Antidepressant discontinuation symptoms

	MAOIs	TCAs	SSRIs and related
Symptoms	Common	Common	Common
	Agitation, irritability, ataxia, movement disorders, insomnia, somnolence, vivid dreams, cognitive impairment, slowed speech, pressured speech	Flu-like symptoms (chills, myalgia, excessive sweating, headache, nausea), insomnia, excessive dreaming	Flu-like symptoms, 'shock-like' sensations, dizziness exacerbated by movement, insomnia, excessive (vivid) dreaming, irritability, crying spells
	Occasionally	Occasionally	Occasionally
	Hallucinations, paranoid delusions	Movement disorders, mania, cardiac arrhythmia	Movement disorders, problems with concentration and memory
Drugs most commonly associated with discontinuation symptoms	All	Amitriptyline Imipramine	Paroxetine Venlafaxine
	Tranylcypromine may have amfetamine-like properties at higher doses[13] and therefore could be associated with a true 'withdrawal syndrome'. Delirium may occur[14]		

MAOI, monoamine oxidase inhibitor; SSRI, selective serotonin reuptake inhibitor; TCA, tricyclic antidepressant.

daily functioning and those who have experienced discontinuation symptoms may reason (perhaps appropriately) that antidepressants are 'addictive' and not wish to accept treatment. There is also evidence of emergent suicidal thoughts on discontinuation with paroxetine.[7]

Who is most at risk?[20–23]

Although anyone can experience discontinuation symptoms, the risk is increased in those prescribed short half-life drugs[3] (e.g. paroxetine, venlafaxine), particularly if they do not take them regularly. Two-thirds of patients prescribed antidepressants skip a few doses from time to time,[24] and many patients stop their antidepressant abruptly.[5] The risk is also increased in those who have been taking antidepressants for 8 weeks or longer,[25] those taking antidepressants at higher doses, those who have developed anxiety symptoms at the start of antidepressant therapy (particularly with SSRIs), those receiving other centrally acting medication (e.g. antihypertensives, antihistamines, antipsychotics), children and adolescents,[3] and those who have experienced discontinuation symptoms before.

Antidepressant discontinuation symptoms are common in neonates born to women taking antidepressants (see section on 'Drug choice in pregnancy' in Chapter 7).

CHAPTER 3

How to avoid[20–23]

Generally, antidepressant therapy should be discontinued over at least a 4-week period (this is not required with fluoxetine).[12] The shorter the half-life of the drug, the more important it is that this rule is followed. The end of the taper may need to be slower, as symptoms may not appear until the reduction in the total daily dosage of the antidepressant is (proportionately) substantial. Patients receiving MAOIs may need to be tapered over a longer period. Tranylcypromine may be particularly difficult to stop.[14] At-risk patients (see earlier in this section) may need a slower taper. Agomelatine and vortioxetine can probably be stopped abruptly.

Many people suffer symptoms despite slow withdrawal and even if they have received adequate education regarding discontinuation symptoms.[3,7] For these patients the option of abrupt withdrawal should be discussed. Some may prefer to face a week or two of intense symptoms rather than months of less severe discontinuation effects. Of note, although tapering as a standard approach makes intuitive sense, a significant advantage for gradual tapering in comparison to abrupt discontinuation did not emerge in a systematic review of existing literature.[3]

How to treat[20–22,26]

There are few systematic studies in this area. Treatment is pragmatic. If symptoms are mild, reassure the patient that these symptoms are common after discontinuing an antidepressant and will pass in a few days. If symptoms are severe, reintroduce the original antidepressant (or another with a longer half-life from the same class) and taper gradually while monitoring for symptoms.[12]

Some evidence supports the use of anticholinergic agents in tricyclic withdrawal[27] and fluoxetine for symptoms associated with stopping paroxetine,[28] sertraline,[28] clomipramine[29] or venlafaxine[30] – fluoxetine, having a longer plasma half-life, seems to be associated with a lower incidence of discontinuation symptoms than other similar drugs.[3]

Key points that patients should know

- Antidepressants are not addictive (patients' most frequently mentioned reason for a negative opinion on antidepressants is addiction,[31] and a survey of 1946 people across the UK conducted in 1997 found that 74% thought that antidepressants were addictive[32]). Note, however, that the semantic and categorical distinctions between addiction and the withdrawal symptoms seen with antidepressants may be unimportant to patients.
- Patients should be informed that they may experience discontinuation symptoms (and the most likely symptoms associated with the drug that they are taking) when they stop their antidepressant.
- Short half-life antidepressants should not generally be stopped abruptly, although some patients may prefer to risk a short period of intense symptoms rather than a prolonged period of milder symptoms.
- Discontinuation symptoms can occur after missed doses if the antidepressant prescribed has a short half-life. A very few patients experience pre-dose discontinuation symptoms which provoke the taking of the antidepressant at an earlier time each day.

References

1 Blier P et al. Physiologic mechanisms underlying the antidepressant discontinuation syndrome. J Clin Psychiatry 2006; 67 Suppl 4:8–13.

2 Delgado PL. Monoamine depletion studies: implications for antidepressant discontinuation syndrome. J Clin Psychiatry 2006; 67 Suppl 4:22–26.

3 Fava GA et al. Withdrawal symptoms after selective serotonin reuptake inhibitor discontinuation: a systematic review. Psychother Psychosom 2015; 84:72–81.

4 Narayan V et al. Antidepressant discontinuation manic states: a critical review of the literature and suggested diagnostic criteria. J Psychopharmacol 2011; 25:306–313.

5 van Geffen EC et al. Discontinuation symptoms in users of selective serotonin reuptake inhibitors in clinical practice: tapering versus abrupt discontinuation. Eur J Clin Pharmacol 2005; 61:303–307.

6 Perahia DG et al. Symptoms following abrupt discontinuation of duloxetine treatment in patients with major depressive disorder. J Affect Disord 2005; 89:207–212.

7 Tint A et al. The effect of rate of antidepressant tapering on the incidence of discontinuation symptoms: a randomised study. J Psychopharmacol 2008; 22:330–332.

8 Fava GA et al. Effects of gradual discontinuation of selective serotonin reuptake inhibitors in panic disorder with agoraphobia. Int J Neuropsychopharmacol 2007; 10:835–838.

9 Taylor D et al. Antidepressant withdrawal symptoms-telephone calls to a national medication helpline. J Affect Disord 2006; 95:129–133.

10 Goodwin GM et al. Agomelatine prevents relapse in patients with major depressive disorder without evidence of a discontinuation syndrome: a 24-week randomized, double-blind, placebo-controlled trial. J Clin Psychiatry 2009; 70:1128–1137.

11 Baldwin DS et al. The safety and tolerability of vortioxetine: analysis of data from randomized placebo-controlled trials and open-label extension studies. J Psychopharmacol 2016; 30:242–252.

12 National Institute for Health and Care Excellence. Depression in adults: recognition and management. Clinical guideline CG90, 2009; last updated April 2016. https://www.nice.org.uk/Guidance/cg90

13 Ricken R et al. Tranylcypromine in mind (Part II): review of clinical pharmacology and meta-analysis of controlled studies in depression. Eur Neuropsychopharmacol 2017; 27:714–731.

14 Gahr M et al. Withdrawal and discontinuation phenomena associated with tranylcypromine: a systematic review. Pharmacopsychiatry 2013; 46:123–129.

15 Cosci F. Withdrawal symptoms after discontinuation of a noradrenergic and specific serotonergic antidepressant: a case report and review of the literature. Personalized Medicine in Psychiatry 2017; 1-2:81–84.

16 Berigan TR et al. Bupropion-associated withdrawal symptoms: a case report. Prim Care Companion J Clin Psychiatry 1999; 1:50–51.

17 Berigan TR. Bupropion-associated withdrawal symptoms revisited: a case report. Prim Care Companion J Clin Psychiatry 2002; 4:78.

18 Lundbeck Limited. Summary of Product Characteristics. Brintellix (vortioxetine) tablets 5, 10 and 20mg. 2017. https://www.medicines.org.uk/emc/medicine/30904

19 Takeda Pharmaceuticals USA. Highlights of Prescribing Information – TRINTELLIX (vortioxetine) tablets. 2017. http://www.us.trintellix.com

20 Lejoyeux M et al. Antidepressant withdrawal syndrome: recognition, prevention and management. CNS Drugs 1996; 5:278–292.

21 Haddad PM et al. Recognising and managing antidepressant discontinuation symptoms. Adv Psychiatr Treat 2007; 13:447–457.

22 Haddad PM. Antidepressant discontinuation syndromes. Drug Saf 2001; 24:183–197.

23 Ogle NR et al. Guidance for the discontinuation or switching of antidepressant therapies in adults. J Pharm Pract 2013; 26:389–396.

24 Meijer WE et al. Spontaneous lapses in dosing during chronic treatment with selective serotonin reuptake inhibitors. Br J Psychiatry 2001; 179:519–522.

25 Kramer JC et al. Withdrawal symptoms following discontinuation of imipramine therapy. Am J Psychiatry 1961; 118:549–550.

26 Wilson E et al. A review of the management of antidepressant discontinuation symptoms. Ther Adv Psychopharmacol 2015; 5:357–368.

27 Dilsaver SC et al. Antidepressant withdrawal symptoms treated with anticholinergic agents. Am J Psychiatry 1983; 140:249–251.

28 Benazzi F. Re: Selective serotonin reuptake inhibitor discontinuation syndrome: putative mechanisms and prevention strategies. Can J Psychiatry 1999; 44:95–96.

29 Benazzi F. Fluoxetine for clomipramine withdrawal symptoms. Am J Psychiatry 1999; 156:661–662.

30 Giakas WJ et al. Intractable withdrawal from venlafaxine treated with fluoxetine. Psychiatric Annals 1997; 27:85–93.

31 Gibson K et al. Patient-centered perspectives on antidepressant use. Int J Ment Health 2014; 43:81–99.

32 Paykel ES et al. Changes in public attitudes to depression during the Defeat Depression Campaign. Br J Psychiatry 1998; 173:519–522.

Further reading

Fava GA et al. Withdrawal symptoms after selective serotonin reuptake inhibitor discontinuation: a systematic review. Psychother Psychosom 2015; 84:72–81.

Haddad PM et al. Recognising and managing antidepressant discontinuation symptoms. Adv Psychiatr Treat 2007; 13:447–457.

Schatzberg AF et al. Antidepressant discontinuation syndrome: consensus panel recommendations for clinical management and additional research. J Clin Psychiatry 2006; 67 Suppl 4:27–30.

Shelton RC. The nature of the discontinuation syndrome associated with antidepressant drugs. J Clin Psychiatry 2006; 67 Suppl 4:3–7.

CHAPTER 3

Antidepressants: swapping and stopping

General guidelines

- All antidepressants have the potential to cause withdrawal phenomena.[1] When taken continuously *for 6 weeks or longer*, antidepressants should not be stopped abruptly unless a serious adverse event has occurred (e.g. cardiac arrhythmia with a tricyclic). (See section on 'Antidepressant discontinuation symptoms' in this chapter.)
- All patients should be informed of the risk of discontinuation symptoms with all antidepressants, particularly with drugs with a reported greater likelihood of causing such symptoms such as paroxetine and venlafaxine.[2]
- Discontinuation symptoms can last between 1 and 2 weeks, are usually mild and rapidly disappear upon readministration of the drug[3] but many variations are possible, including late onset and/or longer persistence.[4] These differences can sometimes be explained by drug pharmacokinetics but this is not always the case.
- Although abrupt cessation is generally not recommended, slow tapering may not always reduce the incidence or severity of discontinuation reactions.[5] Some patients may therefore prefer abrupt cessation and a shorter discontinuation syndrome. However, abrupt stopping of antidepressants probably increases the risk of relapse.[6]
- When changing from one antidepressant to another, abrupt withdrawal should usually be avoided. Cross-tapering is preferred, in which the dose of the ineffective or poorly tolerated drug is slowly reduced while the new drug is slowly introduced. See Table 3.10 for an example.
- The speed of cross-tapering is best judged by monitoring patient tolerability. Few studies have been done, so caution is required.
- Note that the co-administration of some antidepressants, even when cross-tapering, is absolutely contraindicated. In other cases, theoretical risks or lack of experience preclude recommending cross-tapering.
- The switching strategy depends not only on the reason for switching – inadequate or non-response, poor tolerability or adverse effects, but also on the pharmacokinetic and pharmacodynamic properties of the antidepressants involved.[7–9]

Table 3.10 Changing from citalopram to mirtazapine

Example		Week 1	Week 2	Week 3	Week 4
Withdrawing citalopram	40 mg od	20 mg od	10 mg od	Nil	Nil
Introducing mirtazapine	Nil	15 mg od	30 mg od	30 mg od	45 mg od (if required)

od, once a day.

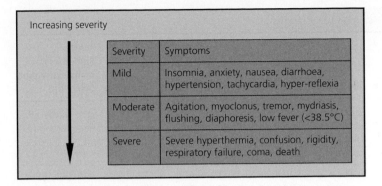

Figure 3.4 Serotonin syndrome – symptoms.[11]

CHAPTER 3

- In some cases cross-tapering may not be necessary. An example is when switching from one SSRI to another: their effects are so similar that administration of the second drug is likely to ameliorate withdrawal effects of the first. In fact, the use of fluoxetine has been advocated as an abrupt switch treatment for SSRI discontinuation symptoms.[10] Abrupt cessation may also be acceptable when switching to a drug with a similar, but not identical, mode of action.[11] Thus, in some cases, abruptly stopping one antidepressant and starting another antidepressant at the usual dose may not only be well tolerated but may also reduce the risk and severity of discontinuation symptoms.
- Potential dangers of simultaneously administering two antidepressants include pharmacodynamic interactions (serotonin syndrome, hypotension, drowsiness; depending on the drugs involved) and pharmacokinetic interactions (e.g. elevation of tricyclic plasma levels by some SSRIs).
- Agomelatine should be stopped completely before beginning another antidepressant. It does not seem to be associated with a discontinuation syndrome,[12] but slow withdrawal is nonetheless recommended. Given agomelatine's mode of action (melatonin agonism; 5-HT_{2C} antagonism), it is not expected to mitigate discontinuation reactions of other antidepressants. There is no theoretical basis to suggest that interactions might occur between agomelatine and other co-administered antidepressants, but caution is advised in the absence of useful data.
- Serotonin syndrome (Figure 3.4) can occur with a single serotonergic drug at a therapeutic dose or more frequently with a combination of serotonergic drugs or in overdose. Most severe cases of serotonin syndrome involve an MAOI (including moclobemide) plus an SSRI.[13,14] Caution is advised when switching strategies call for the combining of serotonergic drugs.

The advice given in Table 3.11 should be treated with caution and patients should be very carefully monitored when switching.

Table 3.11 Antidepressants – swapping and stopping[*]

From	Agomelatine	Bupropion	Clomipramine	Fluoxetine	Fluvoxamine	MAOIs Phenelzine Tranylcypromine Selegiline
Agomelatine[a]		Stop agomelatine then start bupropion	Stop agomelatine then start clomipramine	Stop agomelatine then start fluoxetine	Stop agomelatine then start fluvoxamine	Stop agomelatine then start MAOIs
Bupropion[b]	Cross-taper cautiously		Cross-taper cautiously with low-dose clomipramine	Cross-taper cautiously	Cross-taper cautiously	Taper and stop then wait for 2 weeks then start MAOIs
Clomipramine	Cross-taper cautiously	Cross-taper cautiously		Taper and stop then start fluoxetine at 10 mg/day	Taper and stop then start low-dose fluvoxamine	Taper and stop then wait for 3 weeks then start MAOIs
Fluoxetine[c]	Cross-taper cautiously	Stop fluoxetine. Wait 4–7 days then start bupropion	Stop fluoxetine. Wait 2 weeks then start low-dose clomipramine		Stop fluoxetine. Wait 4–7 days then start fluvoxamine	Stop fluoxetine then wait for 5–6 weeks then start MAOIs
Fluvoxamine[d]	Taper and stop then wait for 4 days	Direct switch possible	Taper and stop then start low-dose clomipramine	Direct switch possible		Taper and stop then wait for 1 week then start MAOIs
MAOIs Phenelzine Tranylcypromine Selegiline	Cross-taper cautiously	Taper and stop then wait for 2 weeks	Taper and stop then wait for 3 weeks	Taper and stop then wait for 2 weeks	Taper and stop then wait for 2 weeks	Taper and stop then wait for 2 weeks
Moclobemide	Taper and stop then wait 24 hours	Taper and stop then wait 24 hours	Taper and stop then wait 24 hours	Taper and stop then wait 24 hours	Taper and stop then wait 24 hours	Taper and stop, wait 24 hours then start MAOIs
Mirtazapine	Cross-taper cautiously	Cross-taper cautiously	Cross-taper cautiously	Cross-taper cautiously	Cross-taper cautiously	Taper and stop then wait for 2 weeks
Reboxetine[e]	Cross-taper cautiously	Direct switch possible	Cross-taper cautiously	Cross-taper cautiously	Cross-taper cautiously	Taper and stop then wait for 1 week then start MAOIs

To Moclobemide	Mirtazapine	Reboxetine	Trazodone	Other SSRIs[f], vortioxetine	SNRI Duloxetine Venlafaxine Desvenlafaxine	TCAs (except clomipramine)
Stop agomelatine then start moclobemide	Stop agomelatine then start mirtazapine	Stop agomelatine then start reboxetine	Stop agomelatine then start trazodone	Stop agomelatine then start SSRI	Stop agomelatine then start SNRI	Stop agomelatine then start TCA
Taper and stop then start moclobemide	Cross-taper cautiously	Cross-taper cautiously	Cross-taper cautiously	Cross-taper cautiously	Cross-taper cautiously	Cross-taper cautiously with low-dose TCA
Taper and stop then wait for 1 week then start moclobemide	Cross-taper cautiously	Cross-taper cautiously	Cross-taper cautiously	Taper and stop then start low dose	Taper and stop. Start low-dose SNRI	Cross-taper cautiously
Stop fluoxetine then wait for 5–6 weeks then start moclobemide	Cross-taper cautiously	Cross-taper cautiously	Cross-taper cautiously	Stop fluoxetine. Wait 4–7 days then start low dose	Stop fluoxetine. Wait 4–7 days then start SNRI	Stop fluoxetine. Wait 4–7 days then start low-dose TCA
Taper and stop then wait for 1 week then start moclobemide	Cross-taper cautiously. Start mirtazapine at 15 mg	Cross-taper cautiously	Cross-taper cautiously	Direct switch possible	Direct switch possible	Cross-taper cautiously with low-dose TCA
Taper and stop then wait for 2 weeks then start moclobemide	Taper and stop then wait for 2 weeks	Taper and stop then wait for 2 weeks	Taper and stop then wait for 2 weeks	Taper and stop then wait for 2 weeks	Taper and stop then wait for 2 weeks	Taper and stop then wait for 2 weeks[j]
	Taper and stop then wait 24 hours	Taper and stop then wait 24 hours	Taper and stop then wait 24 hours	Taper and stop then wait 24 hours	Taper and stop then wait 24 hours	Taper and stop then wait 24 hours
Taper and stop then wait for 1 week then start moclobemide		Cross-taper cautiously	Cross-taper cautiously	Cross-taper cautiously	Cross-taper cautiously	Cross-taper cautiously
Taper and stop then wait for 1 week then start moclobemide	Cross-taper cautiously		Cross-taper cautiously	Cross-taper cautiously	Cross-taper cautiously	Cross-taper cautiously

(Continued)

Table 3.11 (*Continued*)

From	Agomelatine	Bupropion	Clomipramine	Fluoxetine	Fluvoxamine	MAOIs Phenelzine Tranylcypromine Selegiline
Trazodone	Cross-taper cautiously	Cross-taper cautiously	Cross-taper cautiously with low-dose clomipramine	Cross-taper cautiously	Cross-taper cautiously	Taper and stop then wait for 1 week
Other SSRIs,[f] vortioxetine[g,l]	Cross-taper cautiously	Direct switch possible	Taper and stop then start low-dose clomipramine	Direct switch possible	Direct switch possible	Taper and stop then wait for 1 week[h]
SNRI Duloxetine[i] Venlafaxine Desvenlafaxine	Cross-taper cautiously	Cross-taper cautiously	Taper and stop then start low-dose clomipramine	Direct switch possible	Direct switch possible	Taper and stop then wait for 1 week
Tricyclics	Cross-taper cautiously	Halve dose and add bupropion and then slow withdrawal	Direct switch possible	Halve dose and add fluoxetine and then slow withdrawal	Cross-taper cautiously	Taper and stop then wait for 2 weeks[j]
Stopping[k]	Can be stopped abruptly	Reduce over 4 weeks	Reduce over 4 weeks	At 20 mg/ day just stop. At higher doses reduce over 2 weeks	Reduce over 4 weeks	Reduce over 4 weeks or longer if necessary

Notes

*Advice given in this table is partly derived from manufacturers' information and available published data and partly theoretical. There are several factors that affect individual drug handling and caution is required in every instance.

Cross taper cautiously – usually over 1–2 weeks as per example.

Direct switch – stopping the standard dose of one antidepressant, e.g. citalopram 20 mg and starting the standard dose of another, e.g. duloxetine 60 mg

[a] Agomelatine has no effect on monoamine uptake and no affinity for α, β adrenergic, histaminergic, cholinergic, dopaminergic and benzodiazepine receptors. The potential for interactions between agomelatine and other antidepressants is low and it is not expected to mitigate discontinuation reactions of other antidepressants.

[b] Bupropion is licensed for smoking cessation but unlicensed for the treatment of depression in the UK. It is a CYP2D6 inhibitor and particular caution is required when cross-tapering with drugs metabolised by this enzyme.

[c] Beware: interactions with fluoxetine may still occur for 5 weeks after stopping fluoxetine because of its long half-life.

[d] Fluvoxamine is a potent inhibitor of CYP1A2, and to a lesser extent of CYP2C and CYP3A4, and has a high potential for interactions hence extra caution is required.

[e] Switching to reboxetine as antidepressant monotherapy is no longer recommended.

[f] Citalopram, escitalopram, paroxetine and sertraline.

[g] Limited experience with vortioxetine and extra caution required. Particular care when switching to or from bupropion and other CYP2D6 inhibitors such as fluoxetine and paroxetine.[15]

[h] Wait 3 weeks in the case of vortioxetine.[16]

[i] Abrupt switch from SSRIs and venlafaxine to duloxetine is possible starting at 60 mg/day.[11]

[j] Wait 3 weeks in the case of imipramine.

[k] See general guidance at the beginning of this section.

[l] Vortioxetine - Reduce over 1 week to 10 mg/day, then stop.

MAOI, monoamine oxidase inhibitor; SNRI, serotonin–noradrenaline reuptake inhibitor; SSRI, selective serotonin reuptake inhibitor; TCA, tricyclic antidepressant.

To Moclobemide	Mirtazapine	Reboxetine	Trazodone	Other SSRIs[f], vortioxetine	SNRI Duloxetine Venlafaxine Desvenlafaxine	TCAs (except clomipramine)
Taper and stop then wait for 1 week then start moclobemide	Cross-taper cautiously	Cross-taper cautiously		Cross-taper cautiously	Cross-taper cautiously	Cross-taper cautiously with low-dose TCA
Taper and stop then wait for 1 week then start moclobemide	Cross-taper cautiously	Cross-taper cautiously	Cross-taper cautiously	Direct switch possible	Direct switch possible	Cross-taper cautiously with low-dose TCA
Taper and stop then wait for 1 week then start moclobemide	Cross-taper cautiously	Cross-taper cautiously	Cross-taper cautiously	Direct switch possible	Direct switch possible	Cross-taper cautiously with low-dose TCA
Taper and stop then wait for 1 week then start moclobemide	Cross-taper cautiously	Cross-taper cautiously	Halve dose and add trazodone and then slow withdrawal	Halve dose and add SSRI then slow withdrawal	Cross-taper cautiously starting with low-dose SNRI	Direct switch possible
Reduce over 4 weeks	Reduce over 4 weeks	Reduce over 4 weeks	Reduce over 4 weeks	Reduce over 4 weeks or longer if necessary[i]	Reduce over 4 weeks or longer if necessary	Reduce over 4 weeks

References

1 Taylor D et al. Antidepressant withdrawal symptoms-telephone calls to a national medication helpline. J Affect Disord 2006; **95**:129–133.
2 National Institute for Health and Care Excellence. Depression in adults: recognition and management. Clinical Guideline 90, 2009; last updated April 2016. https://www.nice.org.uk/guidance/cg90
3 Wilson E et al. A review of the management of antidepressant discontinuation symptoms. Ther Adv Psychopharmacol 2015; **5**:357–368.
4 Fava GA et al. Withdrawal symptoms after selective serotonin reuptake inhibitor discontinuation: a systematic review. Psychother Psychosom 2015; **84**:72–81.
5 Tint A et al. The effect of rate of antidepressant tapering on the incidence of discontinuation symptoms: a randomised study. J Psychopharmacol 2008; **22**:330–332.
6 Baldessarini RJ et al. Illness risk following rapid versus gradual discontinuation of antidepressants. Am J Psychiatry 2010; **167**:934–941.
7 Cleare A et al. Evidence-based guidelines for treating depressive disorders with antidepressants: a revision of the 2008 British Association for Psychopharmacology guidelines. J Psychopharmacol 2015; **29**:459–525.
8 Harvey BH et al. New insights on the antidepressant discontinuation syndrome. Hum Psychopharmacol 2014; **29**:503–516.
9 Malhi GS et al. Royal Australian and New Zealand College of Psychiatrists clinical practice guidelines for mood disorders. Aust N Z J Psychiatry 2015; **49**:1087–1206.
10 Benazzi F. Fluoxetine for the treatment of SSRI discontinuation syndrome. Int J Neuropsychopharmacol 2008; **11**:725–726.
11 Perahia DG et al. Switching to duloxetine from selective serotonin reuptake inhibitor antidepressants: a multicenter trial comparing 2 switching techniques. J Clin Psychiatry 2008; **69**:95–105.
12 Goodwin GM et al. Agomelatine prevents relapse in patients with major depressive disorder without evidence of a discontinuation syndrome: a 24-week randomized, double-blind, placebo-controlled trial. J Clin Psychiatry 2009; **70**:1128–1137.
13 Buckley NA et al. Serotonin syndrome. BMJ 2014; **348**:g1626.
14 Abadie D et al. Serotonin syndrome: analysis of cases registered in the french pharmacovigilance database. J Clin Psychopharmacol 2015; **35**:382–388.
15 Chen G et al. Pharmacokinetic drug interactions involving vortioxetine (Lu AA21004), a multimodal antidepressant. Clin Drug Investig 2013; **33**:727–736.
16 Citrome L. Vortioxetine for major depressive disorder: a systematic review of the efficacy and safety profile for this newly approved antidepressant – what is the number needed to treat, number needed to harm and likelihood to be helped or harmed? Int J Clin Pract 2014; **68**:60–82.

Drug interactions with antidepressants

Drugs can interact with each other in two different ways:

- **Pharmacokinetic interactions** where one drug interferes with the absorption, distribution, metabolism or elimination of another drug. This may result in a subtherapeutic effect or toxicity. The largest group of pharmacokinetic interactions involves drugs that inhibit or induce hepatic CYP450 enzymes (see Tables 3.12 and 11.8). Other enzyme systems include FMO[10] and UGT.[11] While both of these latter enzyme systems are involved in the metabolism of psychotropic drugs, the potential for drugs to inhibit or induce these enzyme systems has been less well studied.

   The clinical consequences of pharmacokinetic interactions in an individual patient can be difficult to predict. Some are highly clinically significant; for example, when paroxetine is taken with tamoxifen, up to 1 extra woman in 20 will die within 5 years of stopping tamoxifen.[1] The following factors affect outcome of interactions: the degree of enzyme inhibition or induction, the pharmacokinetic properties of the affected drug and other co-administered drugs, the relationship between plasma level and pharmacodynamic effect for the affected drug, and patient-specific factors such as variability in the role of primary and secondary metabolic pathways and the presence of co-morbid physical illness.[12]

- **Pharmacodynamic interactions** where the effects of one drug are altered by another drug via physiological mechanisms such as direct competition at receptor sites (e.g. dopamine agonists with dopamine blockers may negate any therapeutic effect), augmentation of the same neurotransmitter pathway (e.g. fluoxetine with tramadol or a triptan can lead to serotonin syndrome) or an effect on the physiological functioning of an organ/organ system in different ways (e.g. SSRIs impair clotting and NSAIDs irritate the gastic mucosa; when these drugs are used together, the risk of gastrointestinal bleeds is increased). Most of these interactions can be easily predicted by a sound knowledge of pharmacology, but up-to-date interaction tables are readily available online and most known interactions are described in an individual product's literature/labelling.

Pharmacodynamic interactions

Tricyclic antidepressants:[13,14]

- are H_1 blockers (sedative). This effect can be exacerbated by other sedative drugs or alcohol. Beware respiratory depression
- are anticholinergic (dry mouth, blurred vision, constipation). This effect can be exacerbated by other anticholinergic drugs such as antihistamines or antipsychotics. Beware cognitive impairment and gastrointestinal obstruction
- are adrenergic α_1 blockers (postural hypotension). This effect can be exacerbated by other drugs that block α_1 receptors and by antihypertensive drugs in general. Beware falls. Adrenaline in combination with α_1 blockers can lead to hypertension
- are arrhythmogenic. Caution is required with other drugs that can alter cardiac conduction directly (e.g. antiarrhythmics or phenothiazines) or indirectly through a potential to cause electrolyte disturbance (e.g. diuretics)

Table 3.12 Pharmacokinetic interactions[1–9]

p4501A2	p4502C	p4502D6	p4503A
Genetic polymorphism Ultra-rapid metabolisers occur	5–10% of Caucasians poor metabolisers	3–5% of Caucasians poor metabolisers	60% p450 content
Induced by:	*Induced by:*	*Induced by:*	*Induced by:*
carbamazepine charcoal cooking cigarette smoke omeprazole phenobarbital phenytoin	phenytoin rifampicin	carbamazepine phenytoin	carbamazepine phenytoin prednisolone rifampicin
Inhibited by:	*Inhibited by:*	*Inhibited by:*	*Inhibited by:*
cimetidine ciprofloxacin erythromycin fluvoxamine	cimetidine fluoxetine fluvoxamine moclobemide sertraline	chlorpromazine bupropion duloxetine fluoxetine fluphenazine haloperidol paroxetine sertraline tricyclics	erythromycin fluoxetine fluvoxamine grapefruit juice ketoconazole norfluoxetine paroxetine sertraline tricyclics
Metabolises:	*Metabolises:*	*Metabolises:*	*Metabolises:*
agomelatine benzodiazepines caffeine clozapine duloxetine haloperidol mirtazapine olanzapine ramelteon theophylline tricyclics warfarin	agomelatine bupropion citalopram diazepam omeprazole phenytoin tricyclics warfarin	clozapine codeine donepezil duloxetine haloperidol phenothiazines risperidone tamoxifen tricyclics tramadol trazodone venlafaxine vortioxetine	calcium blockers carbamazepine clozapine donepezil erythromycin galantamine methadone levomilnacipran mirtazapine reboxetine risperidone statins tricyclics valproate venlafaxine vilazodone vortioxetine Z-hypnotics

- lower the seizure threshold. Caution is required with other proconvulsive drugs (e.g. antipsychotics) and particularly if the patient is being treated for epilepsy (higher doses of anticonvulsants may be required)
- may be serotonergic (e.g. amitriptyline, imipramine, clomipramine). There is the potential for these drugs to interact with other serotonergic drugs (e.g. tramadol, SSRIs, selegiline, triptans) to cause serotonin syndrome.

SSRIs/SNRIs:[2,15–19]

- increase serotonergic neurotransmission. The main concern when co-prescribed with other serotonergic drugs is serotonin syndrome
- inhibit platelet aggregation and increase the risk of bleeding, particularly of the upper gastrointestinal tract. This effect is exacerbated by aspirin and NSAIDs (see section on 'SSRIs and bleeding' in this chapter)
- may be more likely than other antidepressants to cause hyponatraemia (see section on 'Antidepressant-induced hyponatraemia' in this chapter). This may exacerbate electrolyte disturbances caused by other drugs such as diuretics
- may cause osteopenia. This adds to the negative effects prolactin-elevating drugs have on bone mineral density and increases the risks of clinical harm should the patient have a fall.

MAOIs:[20,21]

- prevent the destruction of monoamine neurotransmitters. Sympathomimetic and dopaminergic drugs can lead to monoamine overload and hypertensive crisis. Pethidine and fermented foods can have the same effect
- can interact with serotonergic drugs to cause serotonin syndrome.

Avoid/minimise problems by:

- where antidepressant polypharmacy is used, select drugs that are safer to use together and monitor carefully for adverse effects when the second antidepressant is initiated (see sections on 'Treatment of refractory depression' in this chapter)
- avoiding the co-prescription of other drugs with a similar pharmacology but not marketed as antidepressants (e.g. atomoxetine, bupropion)
- knowing your pharmacology (most interactions can be easily predicted).

References

1 Kelly CM et al. Selective serotonin reuptake inhibitors and breast cancer mortality in women receiving tamoxifen: a population based cohort study. BMJ 2010; 340:c693.

2 Mitchell PB. Drug interactions of clinical significance with selective serotonin reuptake inhibitors. Drug Saf 1997; 17:390–406.

3 Lin JH et al. Inhibition and induction of cytochrome P450 and the clinical implications. Clin Pharmacokinet 1998; 35:361–390.

4 Richelson E. Pharmacokinetic interactions of antidepressants. J Clin Psychiatry 1998; 59 Suppl 10:22–26.

5 Greenblatt DJ et al. Drug interactions with newer antidepressants: role of human cytochrome P450. J Clin Psychiatry 1998; 59 Suppl 15:19–27.

6 Taylor D. Pharmacokinetic interactions involving clozapine. Br J Psychiatry 1997; 171:109–112.

7 Chen G et al. Vortioxetine: clinical pharmacokinetics and drug interactions. Clin Pharmacokinet 2017; doi: 10.1007/s40262-017-0612-7. [Epub ahead of print]

8 Spina E et al. Clinically significant drug interactions with newer antidepressants. CNS Drugs 2012; 26:39–67.

9 Bruno A et al. The role of levomilnacipran in the management of major depressive disorder: a comprehensive review. Curr Neuropharmacol 2016; 14:191–199.

10 Cashman JR. Human flavin-containing monooxygenase: substrate specificity and role in drug metabolism. Curr Drug Metab 2000; 1:181–191.

11 Anderson GD. A mechanistic approach to antiepileptic drug interactions. Ann Pharmacother 1998; 32:554–563.

12 Devane CL. Antidepressant-drug interactions are potentially but rarely clinically significant. Neuropsychopharmacology 2006; 31:1594–1604.

13 Watsky EJ et al. Psychotropic drug interactions. Hosp Community Psychiatry 1991; 42:247–256

14 British Medical Association, et al. British National Formulary – 74th edn. London: BMJ Group and Pharmaceutical Press, 2017.

15 Edwards JG et al. Systematic review and guide to selection of selective serotonin reuptake inhibitors. Drugs 1999; 57:507–533.

CHAPTER 3

CHAPTER 3

16 Loke YK et al. Meta-analysis: gastrointestinal bleeding due to interaction between selective serotonin uptake inhibitors and non-steroidal anti-inflammatory drugs. Aliment Pharmacol Ther 2008; 27:31–40.

17 Williams LJ et al. Selective serotonin reuptake inhibitor use and bone mineral density in women with a history of depression. Int Clin Psychopharmacol 2008; 23:84–87.

18 Spina E et al. Clinically relevant pharmacokinetic drug interactions with second-generation antidepressants: an update. Clin Ther 2008; 30:1206–1227.

19 Montastruc F et al. The importance of drug-drug interactions as a cause of adverse drug reactions: a pharmacovigilance study of serotoninergic reuptake inhibitors in France. Eur J Clin Pharmacol 2012; 68:767–775.

20 Livingston MG et al. Monoamine oxidase inhibitors. An update on drug interactions. Drug Saf 1996; 14:219–227.

21 Wimbiscus M et al. MAO inhibitors: risks, benefits, and lore. Cleve Clin J Med 2010; 77:859–882.

Cardiac effects of antidepressants

The cardiac effects of antidepressants are summarised in Table 3.13.

SSRIs are generally recommended in cardiac disease but beware antiplatelet activity and cytochrome-mediated interactions with co-administered cardiac drugs. Mirtazapine has been suggested as a suitable alternative[28] but recent data analysis suggests that it too is associated with bleeding disorders.[57]

SSRIs may protect against myocardial infarction (MI),[58,59] and untreated depression worsens prognosis in cardiovascular disease.[60] Post MI, SSRIs and mirtazapine have either a neutral or beneficial effect on mortality.[61] Treatment of depression with SSRIs should not therefore be withheld post MI. Protective effects of treatment of depression post MI appear to relate to antidepressant administration, possibly because of an anticoagulant effect or because of indirect reduction in arrhythmia frequency.[41,62] CBT may be ineffective in this respect.[63] Note that the antiplatelet effect of SSRIs may have adverse consequences too: upper gastrointestinal bleeding is more common in those taking SSRIs.[64]

References

1 Dolder CR et al. Agomelatine treatment of major depressive disorder. Ann Pharmacother 2008; **42**:1822–1831.
2 Kozian R et al. [QTc prolongation during treatment with agomelatine]. Psychiatr Prax 2010; **37**:405–407.
3 Roose SP et al. Pharmacologic treatment of depression in patients with heart disease. Psychosom Med 2005; **67** Suppl 1:S54–S57.
4 Dwoskin LP et al. Review of the pharmacology and clinical profile of bupropion, an antidepressant and tobacco use cessation agent. CNS Drug Rev 2006; **12**:178–207.
5 Castro VM et al. QT interval and antidepressant use: a cross sectional study of electronic health records. BMJ 2013; **346**:f288.
6 Eisenberg MJ et al. Bupropion for smoking cessation in patients hospitalized with acute myocardial infarction: a randomized, placebo-controlled trial. J Am Coll Cardiol 2013; **61**:524–532.
7 Rasmussen SL et al. Cardiac safety of citalopram: prospective trials and retrospective analyses. J Clin Psychopharmacol 1999; **19**:407–415.
8 Catalano G et al. QTc interval prolongation associated with citalopram overdose: a case report and literature review. Clin Neuropharmacol 2001; **24**:158–162.
9 Lesperance F et al. Effects of citalopram and interpersonal psychotherapy on depression in patients with coronary artery disease: the Canadian Cardiac Randomized Evaluation of Antidepressant and Psychotherapy Efficacy (CREATE) trial. JAMA 2007; **297**:367–379.
10 Astrom-Lilja C et al. Drug-induced torsades de pointes: a review of the Swedish pharmacovigilance database. Pharmacoepidemiol Drug Saf 2008; **17**:587–592.
11 Zivin K et al. Evaluation of the FDA warning against prescribing citalopram at doses exceeding 40 mg. Am J Psychiatry 2013; **170**:642–650.
12 Sharma A et al. Pharmacokinetics and safety of duloxetine, a dual-serotonin and norepinephrine reuptake inhibitor. J Clin Pharmacol 2000; **40**:161–167.
13 Schatzberg AF. Efficacy and tolerability of duloxetine, a novel dual reuptake inhibitor, in the treatment of major depressive disorder. J Clin Psychiatry 2003; **64** Suppl 13:30–37.
14 Detke MJ et al. Duloxetine, 60 mg once daily, for major depressive disorder: a randomized double-blind placebo-controlled trial. J Clin Psychiatry 2002; **63**:308–315.
15 Colucci VJ et al. Heart failure worsening and exacerbation after venlafaxine and duloxetine therapy. Ann Pharmacother 2008; **42**:882–887.
16 Stuhec M. Duloxetine-induced life-threatening long QT syndrome. Wien Klin Wochenschr 2013; **125**:165–166.
17 Orozco BS et al. Duloxetine: an uncommon cause of fatal ventricular arrhythmia. Clin Toxicol 2014; **51**:672–672.
18 Fisch C. Effect of fluoxetine on the electrocardiogram. J Clin Psychiatry 1985; **46**:42–44.
19 Ellison JM et al. Fluoxetine-induced bradycardia and syncope in two patients. J Clin Psychiatry 1990; **51**:385–386.
20 Roose SP et al. Cardiovascular effects of fluoxetine in depressed patients with heart disease. Am J Psychiatry 1998; **155**:660–665.
21 Strik JJ et al. Efficacy and safety of fluoxetine in the treatment of patients with major depression after first myocardial infarction: findings from a double-blind, placebo-controlled trial. Psychosom Med 2000; **62**:783–789.
22 Strik JJ et al. Cardiac side-effects of two selective serotonin reuptake inhibitors in middle-aged and elderly depressed patients. Int Clin Psychopharmacol 1998; **13**:263–267.
23 Stirnimann G et al. Brugada syndrome ECG provoked by the selective serotonin reuptake inhibitor fluvoxamine. Europace 2010; **12**:282–283.
24 Warrington SJ et al. The cardiovascular effects of antidepressants. Psychol Med Monogr Suppl 1989; **16**:i–40.

Table 3.13 Cardiac effects of antidepressants

Drug	Heart rate	Blood pressure	QTc	Arrhythmia	Conduction disturbance	Licensed restrictions post MI	Comments
Agomelatine[1,2]	No changes reported	No changes reported	Single case of QTc prolongation	No arrhythmia reported	Unclear	No specific contraindication	Cautiously recommended
Bupropion[3–6]	Slight increase	Slight increases in blood pressure but can sometimes be significant. Rarely postural hypotension	QTc shortening, but prolongation has been reported in cases of overdose	No effect. Rare reports in overdose	None	Well tolerated for smoking cessation in post-MI patients	Be aware of interaction potential. Monitor blood pressure
Citalopram[7–11] (assume same for escitalopram)	Small decrease in heart rate	Slight drop in systolic blood pressure	Dose-related increase in QTc	Torsades de pointes reported, mainly in overdose	None	Caution but some evidence of safety in CVD	Minor metabolite which increases QTc interval. No clear evidence of increased risk of arrhythmia at any licensed dose
Duloxetine[12–17]	Slight increase	Important effect (see SPC). Caution in hypertension	Isolated reports of QT prolongation	Isolated reports of toxicity	Isolated reports of toxicity	Caution in patients with recent MI	Limited clinical experience – not recommended
Fluoxetine[18–21]	Small decrease in mean heart rate	Minimal effect on blood pressure	No effect on QTc interval	None	None	Caution. Clinical experience is limited	Evidence of safety post MI
Fluvoxamine[22,23]	Minimal effect on heart rate	Small drop in systolic blood pressure	No significant effect on QTc	None	None	Caution	Limited changes in ECG have been observed
Lofepramine[24,25]	Modest increase in heart rate	Less decrease in postural blood pressure compared with other TCAs	Can possibly prolong QTc interval at higher doses	May occur at higher doses, but rare	Unclear	CI in patients with recent MI	Less cardiotoxic than other TCAs. Reasons unclear
MAOIs[24,26]	Decrease in heart rate	Postural hypotension. Risk of hypertensive crisis	Unclear but may shorten QTc interval	May cause arrhythmia and decrease LVF	No clear effect on cardiac conduction	Use with caution in patients with CVD	Not recommended in CVD
Mirtazapine[27,28]	Minimal change in heart rate	Minimal effect on blood pressure	No effect on QTc	None	None	Caution in patients with recent MI	Evidence of safety post MI. Good alternative to SSRIs

(Continued)

Table 3.13 (Continued)

Drug	Heart rate	Blood pressure	ECG (QTc interval)	Arrhythmia	Conduction	CI	Comments
Moclobemide[29-31]	Marginal decrease in heart rate	Minimal effect on blood pressure. Isolated cases of hypertensive episodes	No effect on QTc interval in normal doses. Prolongation in overdose	None	None	None	Possibly arrhythmogenic in overdose
Paroxetine[32,33]	Small decrease in mean heart rate	Minimal effect on blood pressure	No effect on QTc interval	None	None	General caution in cardiac patients	Probably safe post MI
Reboxetine[34-36]	Significant increase in heart rate	Marginal increase in both systolic and diastolic blood pressure. Postural decrease at higher doses	No effect on QTc	Rhythm abnormalities may occur	Atrial and ventricular ectopic beats, especially in the elderly	Caution in patient with cardiac disease	Probably best avoided in coronary disease
Sertraline[37-41]	Minimal effect on heart rate	Minimal effect on blood pressure	No effect on QTc interval	None	None	None – drug of choice	Safe post MI and in heart failure
Trazodone[24,42,43]	Decrease in heart rate more common, although increase can also occur	Can cause significant postural hypotension	Can prolong QTc interval	Several case reports of prolonged QT and arrhythmia	Unclear	Care in patients with severe cardiac disease	May be arrhythmogenic in patients with pre-existing cardiac disease
Tricyclics[24,44-46]	Increase in heart rate	Postural hypotension	Prolongation of QTc interval and QRS interval	Ventricular arrhythmia common in overdose. Torsades de pointes reported	Slows cardiac conduction – blocks cardiac Na/K channels	Contraindicated in patients with recent MI	TCAs affect cardiac contractility. Some TCAs linked to ischaemic heart disease and sudden cardiac death. Avoid in coronary artery disease
Venlafaxine[15,47-50] (assume same for desvenlafaxine)	Marginally increased	Some increase in postural blood pressure. At higher doses increase in blood pressure	Possible prolongation in overdose, but very rare	Rare reports of cardiac arrhythmia in overdose	Rare reports of conduction abnormalities	Has not been evaluated in post-MI patients. Avoid	Evidence for arrhythmogenic potential is slim, but avoid in coronary disease
Vilazodone[51-53]	Increased in overdose	Increased in overdose	No effect, even in overdose	No reports, even in overdose	No effect	No specific contraindication	Probably no effect on CV function in clinical doses
Vortioxetine[54-56]	No effect	No effect	No effect	No effect	No effect	No specific contraindication	Trial data suggest no effect on QTc or on coagulation parameters

CI, contraindicated; CV, cardiovascular; CVD, cardiovascular disease; ECG, electrocardiogram; LVF, left ventricular fraction; MAOI, monoamine oxidase inhibitor; MI, myocardial infarction; SPC, summary of product characteristics; SSRI, selective serotonin reuptake inhibitor; TCA, tricyclic antidepressant.

25 Stern H et al. Cardiovascular effects of single doses of the antidepressants amitriptyline and lofepramine in healthy subjects. Pharmacopsychiatry 1985; **18**:272–277.

26 Waring WS et al. Acute myocarditis after massive phenelzine overdose. Eur J Clin Pharmacol 2007; **63**:1007–1009.

27 Montgomery SA. Safety of mirtazapine: a review. Int Clin Psychopharmacol 1995; **10** Suppl 4:37–45.

28 Honig A et al. Treatment of post-myocardial infarction depressive disorder: a randomized, placebo-controlled trial with mirtazapine. Psychosom Med 2007; **69**:606–613.

29 Moll E et al. Safety and efficacy during long-term treatment with moclobemide. Clin Neuropharmacol 1994; **17** Suppl 1:S74–S87.

30 Hilton S et al. Moclobemide safety: monitoring a newly developed product in the 1990s. J Clin Psychopharmacol 1995; **15**:76S–83S.

31 Downes MA et al. QTc abnormalities in deliberate self-poisoning with moclobemide. Intern Med J 2005; **35**:388–391.

32 Kuhs H et al. Cardiovascular effects of paroxetine. Psychopharmacology (Berl) 1990; **102**:379–382.

33 Roose SP et al. Comparison of paroxetine and nortriptyline in depressed patients with ischemic heart disease. JAMA 1998; **279**:287–291.

34 Mucci M. Reboxetine: a review of antidepressant tolerability. J Psychopharmacol 1997; **11**:S33–S37.

35 Holm KJ et al. Reboxetine: a review of its use in depression. CNS Drugs 1999; **12**:65–83.

36 Fleishaker JC et al. Lack of effect of reboxetine on cardiac repolarization. Clin Pharmacol Ther 2001; **70**:261–269.

37 Shapiro PA et al. An open-label preliminary trial of sertraline for treatment of major depression after acute myocardial infarction (the SADHAT Trial). Sertraline Anti-Depressant Heart Attack Trial. Am Heart J 1999; **137**:1100–1106.

38 Glassman AH et al. Sertraline treatment of major depression in patients with acute MI or unstable angina. JAMA 2002; **288**:701–709.

39 Winkler D et al. Trazodone-induced cardiac arrhythmias: a report of two cases. Hum Psychopharmacol 2006; **21**:61–62.

40 Jiang W et al. Safety and efficacy of sertraline for depression in patients with CHF (SADHART-CHF): a randomized, double-blind, placebo-controlled trial of sertraline for major depression with congestive heart failure. Am Heart J 2008; **156**:437–444.

41 Leftheriotis D et al. The role of the selective serotonin re-uptake inhibitor sertraline in nondepressive patients with chronic ischemic heart failure: a preliminary study. Pacing Clin Electrophysiol 2010; **33**:1217–1223.

42 Service JA et al. QT prolongation and delayed atrioventricular conduction caused by acute ingestion of trazodone. Clin Toxicol (Phila) 2008; **46**:71–73.

43 Dattilo PB et al. Prolonged QT associated with an overdose of trazodone. J Clin Psychiatry 2007; **68**:1309–1310.

44 Hippisley-Cox J et al. Antidepressants as risk factor for ischaemic heart disease: case-control study in primary care. BMJ 2001; **323**:666–669.

45 Whyte IM et al. Relative toxicity of venlafaxine and selective serotonin reuptake inhibitors in overdose compared to tricyclic antidepressants. QJM 2003; **96**:369–374.

46 van Noord C et al. Psychotropic drugs associated with corrected QT interval prolongation. J Clin Psychopharmacol 2009; **29**:9–15.

47 Khawaja IS et al. Cardiovascular effects of selective serotonin reuptake inhibitors and other novel antidepressants. Heart Dis 2003; **5**:153–160.

48 Pfizer Limited. Summary of Product Characteristics. Efexor XL 75 mg hard prolonged release capsules. 2018. https://www.medicines.org.uk/emc/product/5474.

49 Letsas K et al. QT interval prolongation associated with venlafaxine administration. Int J Cardiol 2006; **109**:116–117.

50 Taylor D et al. Volte-face on venlafaxine – reasons and reflections. J Psychopharmacol 2006; **20**:597–601.

51 Edwards J et al. Vilazodone lacks proarrhythmogenic potential in healthy participants: a thorough ECG study. Int J Clin Pharmacol Ther 2013; **51**:456–465.

52 Heise CW et al. A review of vilazodone exposures with focus on serotonin syndrome effects. Clin Toxicol (Phila) 2017; **55**:1004–1007.

53 Gaw CE et al. Evaluation of dose and outcomes for pediatric vilazodone ingestions. Clin Toxicol (Phila) 2018; **56**:113–119.

54 Citrome L. Vortioxetine for major depressive disorder: a systematic review of the efficacy and safety profile for this newly approved antidepressant – what is the number needed to treat, number needed to harm and likelihood to be helped or harmed? Int J Clin Pract 2014; **68**:60–82.

55 Takeda Pharmaceuticals America Inc. Highlights of Prescribing Information. BRINTELLIX (vortioxetine) tablets. 2018. http://www.us.brintellix.com/

56 Baldwin DS et al. The safety and tolerability of vortioxetine: analysis of data from randomized placebo-controlled trials and open-label extension studies. J Psychopharmacol 2016; **30**:242–252.

57 Na K-S et al. Can we recommend mirtazapine and bupropion for patients at risk for bleeding?: a systematic review and meta-analysis. J Affect Disord 2018; **225**:221–226.

58 Sauer WH et al. Selective serotonin reuptake inhibitors and myocardial infarction. Circulation 2001; **104**:1894–1898.

59 Sauer WH et al. Effect of antidepressants and their relative affinity for the serotonin transporter on the risk of myocardial infarction. Circulation 2003; **108**:32–36.

60 Davies SJ et al. Treatment of anxiety and depressive disorders in patients with cardiovascular disease. BMJ 2004; **328**:939–943.

61 Taylor D et al. Pharmacological interventions for people with depression and chronic physical health problems: systematic review and meta-analyses of safety and efficacy. Br J Psychiatry 2011; **198**:179–188.

62 Chen S et al. Serotonin and catecholaminergic polymorphic ventricular tachycardia: a possible therapeutic role for SSRIs? Cardiovasc J Afr 2010; **21**:225–228.

63 Berkman LF et al. Effects of treating depression and low perceived social support on clinical events after myocardial infarction: the Enhancing Recovery in Coronary Heart Disease Patients (ENRICHD) Randomized Trial. JAMA 2003; **289**:3106–3116.

64 Dalton SO et al. Use of selective serotonin reuptake inhibitors and risk of upper gastrointestinal tract bleeding: a population-based cohort study. Arch Intern Med 2003; **163**:59–64.

Antidepressant-induced arrhythmia

Depression confers an increased of risk of cardiovascular disease[1] and sudden cardiac death,[2] perhaps because of platelet activation,[3] decreased heart rate variability,[4] reduced physical activity,[5] an association with an increased risk of diabetes and/or other factors.

Tricyclic antidepressants (TCAs) have established arrhythmogenic activity which arises as a result of potent blockade of cardiac sodium channels and variable activity at potassium channels.[6] ECG changes produced include PR, QRS and QT prolongation and the Brugada syndrome.[7] Normal clinical use of nortriptyline has been associated in one study with an increased risk of cardiac arrest[8] although a large cohort study did not confirm this finding.[9] In patients taking TCAs, ECG monitoring is a more meaningful and useful measure of toxicity than plasma level monitoring. **Lofepramine**, for reasons unknown, seems to lack the overdose arrhythmogenicity of other TCAs, despite its major metabolite, desipramine, being a potent potassium channel blocker.[10] Oddly, in one study,[11] clinical use of lofepramine was associated with an increased risk of myocardial infarction whereas other antidepressants were not.

There is limited evidence that **venlafaxine** is a sodium channel antagonist[12] and a weak antagonist at hERG potassium channels. Arrhythmia is a rare occurrence even after massive overdose[13–16] and ECG changes no more common than with SSRIs.[17] No ECG changes are seen in therapeutic dosing[18] and sudden cardiac death in clinical use is no more common than with fluoxetine or citalopram.[9,19] **Moclobemide**,[20] **citalopram**,[21,22] **escitalopram**,[23] **bupropion** (amfebutamone),[24] **trazodone**[25,26] and **sertraline**,[27] amongst others,[1] have been reported to prolong the QTc interval in overdose but the clinical consequences of this are uncertain. QT changes are not usually seen at normal clinical doses.[28,29] Nonetheless an association between SSRIs (as a group) and QT changes in normal dosing can be shown[30] but this seems largely to be driven by the effects of citalopram and escitalopram.[31] The effect is dose-related[31] but modest.[30] Neither a large database study[9] nor a large cohort study[32] found any association between citalopram treatment and arrhythmia or cardiac mortality in routine clinical practice; in fact higher doses of citalopram (>40 mg) were associated with fewer adverse outcomes than were lower doses.[32] The most recent study found no excess risk of cardiac arrest and sudden death for citalopram or escitalopram.[33] **Vortioxetine** seems to have no effect on QT;[34–36] similarly, **agomelatine** has no effect, even at supratherapeutic doses.[37] **Vilazodone** has no effect on cardiac conduction.[38]

Use in at-risk patients

There is clear evidence for the safety of sertraline[39] and mirtazapine[40] (and to a lesser extent citalopram,[40] fluoxetine[41] and bupropion[42]) in subjects at risk of arrhythmia due to recent myocardial infarction. Another study supports the safety of citalopram in patients with coronary artery disease[43] (although citalopram is linked to a risk of torsades de pointes[44]). Escitalopram did not affect mortality in a trial in patients with heart failure.[45] Sertraline may help improve cardiovascular risk factors.[46]

CHAPTER 3

Relative cardiotoxicity

Relative cardiotoxicity of antidepressants is difficult to establish with any precision. Yellow Card (ADROIT) data suggest that all marketed antidepressants are associated with arrhythmia (ranging from clinically insignificant to life threatening) and sudden cardiac death. For a substantial proportion of drugs these figures are more likely to reflect coincidence rather than causation. The Fatal Toxicity Index (FTI) may provide some means for comparison. This is a measure of the number of overdose deaths per million (FP10) prescriptions issued. FTI figures suggest high toxicity for tricyclic drugs (especially dosulepin but not lofepramine), medium toxicity for venlafaxine and moclobemide, and low toxicity for SSRIs, mirtazapine and reboxetine.[47–51] However, the FTI does not necessarily reflect only cardiotoxicity (antidepressants variously cause serotonin syndrome, seizures and coma) and is, in any case, open to other influences. This is best evidenced in the change in FTI over time. A good example here is nortriptyline, the FTI of which has been estimated at 0.6[16] and 39.2[12] and several values in between.[47,48,50] This change probably reflects changes in the type of patient prescribed nortriptyline, but 'double-counting' (nortriptyline is a metabolite of amitriptyline) at post mortem also plays a part. There is good evidence that venlafaxine is relatively more often prescribed to patients with more severe depression and who are relatively more likely to attempt suicide.[52–54] This is likely to inflate venlafaxine's FTI and erroneously suggest greater inherent toxicity. Drugs with a consistently low FTI can probably be assumed to have very low risk of arrhythmias.

Citalopram and escitalopram have very low overdose toxicity despite QT prolongation occurring in about one-third of reported overdoses.[55] Standard doses of citalopram may be linked to an increased risk of cardiac arrest[8] but, as mentioned earlier, other data suggest no increased risk of arrhythmia or death with standard and higher licensed doses of citalopram and escitalopram.[32] Citalopram and escitalopram are probably the most cardiotoxic of the SSRIs but their toxicity is modest at worst, and possibly insignificant.

Summary

- Tricyclics (but not lofepramine) have an established link to ion channel blockade and cardiac arrhythmia.
- Non-tricyclics generally have a very low risk of inducing arrhythmia.
- Sertraline is recommended post MI, but other SSRIs and mirtazapine are also likely to be safe.
- Bupropion, citalopram, escitalopram, moclobemide, lofepramine and venlafaxine should be used with caution or avoided in those at risk of serious arrhythmia (those with heart failure, left ventricular hypertrophy, previous arrhythmia or MI). An ECG should be performed at baseline and 1 week after every increase in dose if any of these drugs are used in at-risk patients.
- TCAs (with the exception of lofepramine) are best avoided completely in patients at risk of serious arrhythmia. If use of a TCA cannot be avoided, an ECG should be performed at baseline, 1 week after each increase in dose and periodically throughout treatment. Frequency will be determined by the stability of the cardiac disorder and the TCA (and dose) being used; advice from cardiology should be sought.

- The arrhythmogenic potential of TCAs and other antidepressants is dose-related. Consideration should be given to ECG monitoring of all patients prescribed doses towards the top of the licensed range and those who are prescribed other drugs that through pharmacokinetic (e.g. fluoxetine) or pharmacodynamic (e.g. diuretics) mechanisms may add to the risk posed by the TCA.

References

1 Taylor D. Antidepressant drugs and cardiovascular pathology: a clinical overview of effectiveness and safety. Acta Psychiatr Scand 2008; 118:434–442.

2 Whang W et al. Depression and risk of sudden cardiac death and coronary heart disease in women: results from the Nurses' Health Study. J Am Coll Cardiol 2009; 53:950–958.

3 Ziegelstein RC et al. Platelet function in patients with major depression. Intern Med J 2009; 39:38–43.

4 Glassman AH et al. Heart rate variability in acute coronary syndrome patients with major depression: influence of sertraline and mood improvement. Arch Gen Psychiatry 2007; 64:1025–1031.

5 Whooley MA et al. Depressive symptoms, health behaviors, and risk of cardiovascular events in patients with coronary heart disease. JAMA 2008; 300:2379–2388.

6 Thanacoody HK et al. Tricyclic antidepressant poisoning: cardiovascular toxicity. Toxicol Rev 2005; 24:205–214.

7 Sicouri S et al. Sudden cardiac death secondary to antidepressant and antipsychotic drugs. Expert Opin Drug Saf 2008; 7:181–194.

8 Weeke P et al. Antidepressant use and risk of out-of-hospital cardiac arrest: a nationwide case-time-control study. Clin Pharmacol Ther 2012; 92:72–79.

9 Leonard CE et al. Antidepressants and the risk of sudden cardiac death and ventricular arrhythmia. Pharmacoepidemiol Drug Saf 2011; 20:903–913.

10 Hong HK et al. Block of the human ether-a-go-go-related gene (hERG) K+ channel by the antidepressant desipramine. Biochem Biophys Res Commun 2010; 394:536–541.

11 Coupland C et al. Antidepressant use and risk of cardiovascular outcomes in people aged 20 to 64: cohort study using primary care database. BMJ 2016; 352:i1350.

12 Khalifa M et al. Mechanism of sodium channel block by venlafaxine in guinea pig ventricular myocytes. J Pharmacol Exp Ther 1999; 291:280–284.

13 Colbridge MG et al. Venlafaxine in overdose – experience of the National Poisons Information Service (London centre). J Toxicol Clin Toxicol 1999; 37:383.

14 Blythe D et al. Cardiovascular and neurological toxicity of venlafaxine. Hum Exp Toxicol 1999; 18:309–313.

15 Combes A et al. Conduction disturbances associated with venlafaxine. Ann Intern Med 2001; 134:166–167.

16 Isbister GK. Electrocardiogram changes and arrhythmias in venlafaxine overdose. Br J Clin Pharmacol 2009; 67:572–576.

17 Whyte IM et al. Relative toxicity of venlafaxine and selective serotonin reuptake inhibitors in overdose compared to tricyclic antidepressants. QJM 2003; 96:369–374.

18 Feighner JP. Cardiovascular safety in depressed patients: focus on venlafaxine. J Clin Psychiatry 1995; 56:574–579.

19 Martinez C et al. Use of venlafaxine compared with other antidepressants and the risk of sudden cardiac death or near death: a nested case-control study. BMJ 2010; 340:c249.

20 Downes MA et al. QTc abnormalities in deliberate self-poisoning with moclobemide. Intern Med J 2005; 35:388–391.

21 Kelly CA et al. Comparative toxicity of citalopram and the newer antidepressants after overdose. J Toxicol Clin Toxicol 2004; 42:67–71.

22 Grundemar L et al. Symptoms and signs of severe citalopram overdose. Lancet 1997; 349:1602.

23 Mohammed R et al. Prolonged QTc interval due to escitalopram overdose. J Miss State Med Assoc 2010; 51:350–353.

24 Isbister GK et al. Bupropion overdose: QTc prolongation and its clinical significance. Ann Pharmacother 2003; 37:999–1002.

25 Service JA et al. QT Prolongation and delayed atrioventricular conduction caused by acute ingestion of trazodone. Clin Toxicol (Phila) 2008; 46:71–73.

26 Dattilo PB et al. Prolonged QT associated with an overdose of trazodone. J Clin Psychiatry 2007; 68:1309–1310.

27 de Boer RA et al. QT interval prolongation after sertraline overdose: a case report. BMC Emerg Med 2005; 5:5.

28 van Noord C et al. Psychotropic drugs associated with corrected QT interval prolongation. J Clin Psychopharmacol 2009; 29:9–15.

29 van Haelst IM et al. QT interval prolongation in users of selective serotonin reuptake inhibitors in an elderly surgical population: a cross-sectional study. J Clin Psychiatry 2014; 75:15–21.

30 Beach SR et al. Meta-analysis of selective serotonin reuptake inhibitor-associated QTc prolongation. J Clin Psychiatry 2014; 75:e441–449.

31 Castro VM et al. QT interval and antidepressant use: a cross sectional study of electronic health records. BMJ 2013; 346:f288.

32 Zivin K et al. Evaluation of the FDA warning against prescribing citalopram at doses exceeding 40mg. Am J Psychiatry 2013; 170:642–650.

33 Ray WA et al. High-dose citalopram and escitalopram and the risk of out-of-hospital death. J Clin Psychiatry 2017; 78:190–195.

34 Dubovsky SL. Pharmacokinetic evaluation of vortioxetine for the treatment of major depressive disorder. Expert Opin Drug Metab Toxicol 2014; 10:759–766.

35 Alam MY et al. Safety, tolerability, and efficacy of vortioxetine (Lu AA21004) in major depressive disorder: results of an open-label, flexible-dose, 52-week extension study. Int Clin Psychopharmacol 2014; 29:36–44.

36 Wang Y et al. Effect of vortioxetine on cardiac repolarization in healthy adult male subjects: results of a thorough QT/QTc study. Clin Pharmacol Drug Dev 2013; 2:298–309.

37 Donazzolo Y et al. Evaluation of the effects of therapeutic and supra-therapeutic doses of agomelatine on the QT/QTc interval – a phase I, randomised, double-blind, placebo-controlled and positive-controlled, crossover thorough QT/QTc study conducted in healthy volunteers. J Cardiovasc Pharmacol 2014; 64:440–451.

38 Edwards J et al. Vilazodone lacks proarrhythmogenic potential in healthy participants: a thorough ECG study. Int J Clin Pharmacol Ther 2013; 51:456–465.

39 Glassman AH et al. Sertraline treatment of major depression in patients with acute MI or unstable angina. JAMA 2002; 288:701–709.

40 van Melle JP et al. Effects of antidepressant treatment following myocardial infarction. Br J Psychiatry 2007; 190:460–466.

41 Strik JJ et al. Efficacy and safety of fluoxetine in the treatment of patients with major depression after first myocardial infarction: findings from a double-blind, placebo-controlled trial. Psychosom Med 2000; 62:783–789.

42 Rigotti NA et al. Bupropion for smokers hospitalized with acute cardiovascular disease. Am J Med 2006; 119:1080–1087.

43 Lesperance F et al. Effects of citalopram and interpersonal psychotherapy on depression in patients with coronary artery disease: the Canadian Cardiac Randomized Evaluation of Antidepressant and Psychotherapy Efficacy (CREATE) trial. JAMA 2007; 297:367–379.

44 Astrom-Lilja C et al. Drug-induced torsades de pointes: a review of the Swedish pharmacovigilance database. Pharmacoepidemiol Drug Saf 2008; 17:587–592.

45 Angermann CE et al. Effect of escitalopram on all-cause mortality and hospitalization in patients with heart failure and depression: the MOOD-HF randomized clinical trial. JAMA 2016; 315:2683–2693.

46 Sherwood A et al. Effects of exercise and sertraline on measures of coronary heart disease risk in patients with major depression: results from the SMILE-II randomized clinical trial. Psychosom Med 2016; 78:602–609.

47 Crome P. The toxicity of drugs used for suicide. Acta Psychiatr Scand Suppl 1993; 371:33–37.

48 Cheeta S et al. Antidepressant-related deaths and antidepressant prescriptions in England and Wales, 1998-2000. Br J Psychiatry 2004; 184:41–47.

49 Buckley NA et al. Fatal toxicity of serotoninergic and other antidepressant drugs: analysis of United Kingdom mortality data. BMJ 2002; 325:1332–1333.

50 Buckley NA et al. Greater toxicity in overdose of dothiepin than of other tricyclic antidepressants. Lancet 1994; 343:159–162.

51 Morgan O et al. Fatal toxicity of antidepressants in England and Wales, 1993-2002. Health Stat Q 2004:18–24.

52 Egberts ACG et al. Channeling of three newly introduced antidepressants to patients not responding satisfactorily to previous treatment. J Clin Psychopharmacol 1997; 17:149–155.

53 Mines D et al. Prevalence of risk factors for suicide in patients prescribed venlafaxine, fluoxetine, and citalopram. Pharmacoepidemiol Drug Saf 2005; 14:367–372.

54 Chan AN et al. A comparison of venlafaxine and SSRIs in deliberate self-poisoning. J Med Toxicol 2010; 6:116–121.

55 Hasnain M et al. Escitalopram and QTc prolongation. J Psychiatry Neurosci 2013; 38:E11.

Antidepressant-induced hyponatraemia

Most antidepressants have been associated with hyponatraemia. The onset is usually within 30 days of starting treatment (median 11 days).[1–3] The effect appears not to be dose-related.[1,4] The most likely mechanism of this adverse effect is the syndrome of inappropriate secretion of antidiuretic hormone (SIADH). Risk of hospitalisation with hyponatraemia is elevated from 1 in 1600 in the general population to 1 in 300 for those on any antidepressant.[5] Hyponatraemia is a potentially serious adverse effect of antidepressants that demands careful monitoring,[6] particularly in those patients at greatest risk. Hyponatraemia of all severities is associated with increased mortality.[7]

Antidepressants

No antidepressant has been definitively shown *not* to be associated with hyponatraemia and almost all have a reported association.[8] It has been suggested that serotonergic drugs are relatively more likely than noradrenergic drugs to cause hyponatraemia,[9,10] although this is disputed.[11] One review of the literature suggests that SSRIs are more likely to cause hyponatraemia than TCAs or mirtazapine,[12] and that older women who are co-prescribed other medication known to reduce plasma sodium are at the greatest risk.[13] None of the more recently introduced serotonergic drugs is free of this effect: cases of hyponatraemia have been described with mirtazapine[14–16] (although the reported incidence overall is very low[13]), escitalopram[17,18] and duloxetine.[4] Vortioxetine has also been linked to hyponatraemia,[19] as has desvenlafaxine.[20] Noradrenergic antidepressants are also clearly linked to hyponatraemia[21–27] (albeit at a lower frequency than SSRIs). There are notably few reports for MAOIs,[28,29] and none for agomelatine.

CYP2D6 poor metabolisers may be at increased risk[30] of antidepressant-induced hyponatraemia although evidence is somewhat inconsistent.[31]

Table 3.14 summarises the risk of hyponatraemia with antidepressants.

Table 3.14 Summary of risk of hyponatraemia with antidepressants[5,12,32]

Drug/drug group	Risk of ↓Na	Level of supporting evidence
SSRIs	High	Strong
SNRIs	High	Strong
Tricyclics	Moderate	Strong
MAOIs	Low	Weak
NaSSAs (mirtazapine, mianserin)	Low	Strong
Bupropion	Low	Moderate
Agomelatine	Low	Weak

MAOI, monoamine oxidase inhibitor; NaSSA, noradrenergic and specific serotonergic antidepressant; SNRI, serotonin–noradrenaline reuptake inhibitor; SSRI, selective serotonin reuptake inhibitor.

Monitoring[1,12,13,33–37]

All patients taking antidepressants should be informed about and observed for signs of hyponatraemia (dizziness, nausea, lethargy, confusion, cramps, seizures). Serum sodium should be determined (at baseline and 2 and 4 weeks, and then 3-monthly[38]) for those at high risk of drug-induced hyponatraemia. High-risk factors are as follows:

- older age
- female gender
- major surgery
- history of hyponatraemia or a low baseline Na concentration
- co-therapy with other drugs known to be associated with hyponatraemia (e.g. diuretics, NSAIDs, antipsychotics, carbamazepine, cancer chemotherapy, calcium antagonists, angiotensin-converting enzyme [ACE] inhibitors and laxatives)
- reduced renal function (glomerular filtration rate [GFR] <50 mL/min)
- medical co-morbidity (e.g. hypothyroidism, diabetes, chronic obstructive pulmonary disease [COPD], hypertension, head injury, congestive cardiac failure [CCF], cerebrovascular accident [CVA], various cancers)
- low body weight.

Age is perhaps the most important risk factor so for older people monitoring is essential.[13,39,40]

Treatment[40]

It may be possible to manage mild hyponatraemia with fluid restriction.[34] Some suggest increasing sodium intake,[4] although this is likely to be impractical. If symptoms persist, the antidepressant should be discontinued.

- The normal range for serum sodium is 136–145 mmol/L.
- If serum sodium is >125 mmol/L, monitor sodium daily until normal. Symptoms include headache, nausea, vomiting, muscle cramps, restlessness, lethargy, confusion and disorientation. Consider withdrawing the offending antidepressant.
- If serum sodium is <125 mmol/L, refer to specialist medical care. There is an increased risk of life-threatening symptoms such as seizures, coma and respiratory arrest. The antidepressant should be discontinuted immediately. (Note risk of discontinuation symptoms which may complicate the clinical picture.) Note also that rapid correction of hyponatraemia may be harmful.[16]

Re-starting treatment

- For those who develop hyponatraemia with an SSRI, there are many case reports of recurrent hyponatraemia on rechallenge with the same, or a different SSRI, and relatively fewer reports of recurrence occurring with an antidepressant from another class.[13,14] There are also a handful of case reports of successful rechallenge.[1]
- Consider withdrawing other drugs associated with hyponatraemia (risk increases exponentially when antidepressants are combined with diuretics, etc.[3]).

- Prescribe a drug from a different class. Consider noradrenergic drugs such as nortriptyline and lofepramine, mirtazapine or an MAOI such as moclobemide. Agomelatine or bupropion might also be considered. Begin with a low dose, increasing slowly, and monitor closely. If hyponatraemia recurs and continued antidepressant use is essential, consider water restriction and/or careful use of demeclocycline.
- Consider ECT.

Other prescribed drugs

Carbamazepine has a well-known association with SIADH. Note also that antipsychotic use has been linked to hyponatraemia[41–43] (see section on 'Hyponatraemia' in Chapter 1). Other commonly prescribed drugs such as thiazide diuretics, opiates, NSAIDs, tramadol, cytotoxics, omeprazole and trimethoprim can also cause hyponatraemia.[2,35,44]

References

1 Egger C et al. A review on hyponatremia associated with SSRIs, reboxetine and venlafaxine. Int J Psychiatry Clin Pract 2006; 10:17–26.
2 Liamis G et al. A review of drug-induced hyponatremia. Am J Kidney Dis 2008; 52:144–153.
3 Letmaier M et al. Hyponatraemia during psychopharmacological treatment: results of a drug surveillance programme. Int J Neuropsychopharmacol 2012; 15:739–748.
4 Kruger S et al. Duloxetine and hyponatremia: a report of 5 cases. J Clin Psychopharmacol 2007; 27:101–104.
5 Gandhi S et al. Second-generation antidepressants and hyponatremia risk: a population-based cohort study of older adults. Am J Kidney Dis 2017; 69:87–96.
6 Mohan S et al. Prevalence of hyponatremia and association with mortality: results from NHANES. Am J Med 2013; 126:1127–1137.e1121.
7 Selmer C et al. Hyponatremia, all-cause mortality, and risk of cancer diagnoses in the primary care setting: a large population study. Eur J Intern Med 2016; 36:36–43.
8 Thomas A et al. Hyponatraemia and the syndrome of inappropriate antidiuretic hormone secretion associated with drug therapy in psychiatric patients. CNS Drugs 1995; 5:357–369.
9 Movig KL et al. Serotonergic antidepressants associated with an increased risk for hyponatraemia in the elderly. Eur J Clin Pharmacol 2002; 58:143–148.
10 Movig KL et al. Association between antidepressant drug use and hyponatraemia: a case-control study. Br J Clin Pharmacol 2002; 53:363–369.
11 Kirby D et al. Hyponatraemia and selective serotonin re-uptake inhibitors in elderly patients. Int J Geriatr Psychiatry 2001; 16:484–493.
12 De Picker L et al. Antidepressants and the risk of hyponatremia: a class-by-class review of literature. Psychosomatics 2014; 55:536–547.
13 Dirks AC et al. Recurrent hyponatremia after substitution of citalopram with duloxetine. J Clin Psychopharmacol 2007; 27:313.
14 Bavbek N et al. Recurrent hyponatremia associated with citalopram and mirtazapine. Am J Kidney Dis 2006; 48:e61–e62.
15 Ladino M et al. Mirtazapine-induced hyponatremia in an elderly hospice patient. J Palliat Med 2006; 9:258–260.
16 Cheah CY et al. Mirtazapine associated with profound hyponatremia: two case reports. Am J Geriatr Pharmacother 2008; 6:91–95.
17 Grover S et al. Escitalopram-associated hyponatremia. Psychiatry Clin Neurosci 2007; 61:132–133.
18 Covyeou JA et al. Hyponatremia associated with escitalopram. N Engl J Med 2007; 356:94–95.
19 Lundbeck Limited. Summary of Product Characteristics. Brintellix (vortioxetine) tablets 5, 10 and 20mg. 2017. https://www.medicines.org.uk/emc/medicine/30904
20 Lee G et al. Syndrome of inappropriate secretion of antidiuretic hormone due to desvenlafaxine. Gen Hosp Psychiatry 2013; 35:574.e571–573.
21 O'Sullivan D et al. Hyponatraemia and lofepramine. Br J Psychiatry 1987; 150:720–721.
22 Wylie KR et al. Lofepramine-induced hyponatraemia. Br J Psychiatry 1989; 154:419–420.
23 Ranieri P et al. Reboxetine and hyponatremia. N Engl J Med 2000; 342:215–216.
24 Miller MG. Tricyclics as a possible cause of hyponatremia in psychiatric patients. Am J Psychiatry 1989; 146:807.
25 Colgate R. Hyponatraemia and inappropriate secretion of antidiuretic hormone associated with the use of imipramine. Br J Psychiatry 1993; 163:819–822.
26 Koelkebeck K et al. A case of non-SIADH-induced hyponatremia in depression after treatment with reboxetine. World J Biol Psychiatry 2009; 10:609–611.
27 Kate N et al. Bupropion-induced hyponatremia. Gen Hosp Psychiatry 2013; 35:681.e611–682.
28 Mercier S et al. Severe hyponatremia induced by moclobemide (in French). Therapie 1997; 52:82–83.
29 Peterson JC et al. Inappropriate antidiuretic hormone secondary to a monamine oxidase inhibitor. JAMA 1978; 239:1422–1423.

30 Kwadijk-de GS et al. Variation in the CYP2D6 gene is associated with a lower serum sodium concentration in patients on antidepressants. Br J Clin Pharmacol 2009; 68:221–225.

31 Stedman CA et al. Cytochrome P450 2D6 genotype does not predict SSRI (fluoxetine or paroxetine) induced hyponatraemia. Hum Psychopharmacol 2002; 17:187–190.

32 Leth-Moller KB et al. Antidepressants and the risk of hyponatremia: a Danish register-based population study. BMJ Open 2016; 6:e011200.

33 Jacob S et al. Hyponatremia associated with selective serotonin-reuptake inhibitors in older adults. Ann Pharmacother 2006; 40: 1618–1622.

34 Roxanas M et al. Venlafaxine hyponatraemia: incidence, mechanism and management. Aust N Z J Psychiatry 2007; 41:411–418.

35 Reddy P et al. Diagnosis and management of hyponatraemia in hospitalised patients. Int J Clin Pract 2009; 63:1494–1508.

36 Siegler EL et al. Risk factors for the development of hyponatremia in psychiatric inpatients. Arch Intern Med 1995; 155:953–957.

37 Mannesse CK et al. Characteristics, prevalence, risk factors, and underlying mechanism of hyponatremia in elderly patients treated with antidepressants: a cross-sectional study. Maturitas 2013; 76:357–363.

38 Arinzon ZH et al. Delayed recurrent SIADH associated with SSRIs. Ann Pharmacother 2002; 36:1175–1177.

39 Fabian TJ et al. Paroxetine-induced hyponatremia in the elderly due to the syndrome of inappropriate secretion of antidiuretic hormone (SIADH). J Geriatr Psychiatry Neurol 2003; 16:160–164.

40 Sharma H et al. Antidepressant-induced hyponatraemia in the aged. Avoidance and management strategies. Drugs Aging 1996; 8:430–435.

41 Ohsawa H et al. An epidemiological study on hyponatremia in psychiatric patients in mental hospitals in Nara Prefecture. Jpn J Psychiatry Neurol 1992; 46:883–889.

42 Leadbetter RA et al. Differential effects of neuroleptic and clozapine on polydipsia and intermittent hyponatremia. J Clin Psychiatry 1994; 55 Suppl B:110–113.

43 Collins A. SIADH induced by two atypical antipsychotics. Int J Geriatr Psychiatry 2000; 15:282–283.

44 Shepshelovich D et al. Medication-induced SIADH: distribution and characterization according to medication class. Br J Clin Pharmacol 2017; 83:1801–1807.

Antidepressants and hyperprolactinaemia

Prolactin release is controlled by endogenous dopamine but is also indirectly modulated by serotonin via stimulation of 5-HT_{1C} and 5-HT_2 receptors.[1,2] Long-standing increased plasma prolactin (with or without symptoms) is very occasionally seen with antidepressant use.[3] Where antidepressant-induced hyperprolactinaemia does occur, rises in prolactin are usually small and short-lived[4] and so symptoms are very rare. There is no association between SSRI use and breast cancer.[5] Routine monitoring of prolactin is not recommended but where symptoms suggest the possibility of hyperprolactinaemia then measurement of plasma prolactin is essential. Where symptomatic hyperprolactinaemia is confirmed, a switch to mirtazapine is recommended, although there is also evidence that switching to an alternative SSRI can resolve symptoms.[6,7]

Some details of associations between antidepressants and increased prolactin are given in Table 3.15.

Table 3.15 Reported associations between antidepressants and increased prolactin

Drug/group	Prospective studies	Case reports/series
Agomelatine	No mention of prolactin changes in clinical trials[8] Melatonin itself may inhibit prolactin production[9]	None
Bupropion (amfebutamone)	Single doses of up to 100mg seem not to affect prolactin[10]	None
MAOIs	Small mean changes observed with phenelzine[11] and tranylcypromine[12]	None
Mirtazapine	Strong evidence that mirtazapine has no effect on prolactin[13–15]	None
Reboxetine	Small, transient elevation of prolactin observed after reboxetine administration[16]	None
SNRIs	Clear association observed between venlafaxine and prolactin elevation[17]	Galactorrhoea reported with venlafaxine[18,19] and duloxetine[20,21]
SSRIs	Prospective studies generally show no change in prolactin.[22–24] Some evidence from prescription event monitoring that SSRIs are associated with higher risk of non-puerperal lactation.[25] In a French study, 1.6% of adverse event reports for SSRIs were of hyperprolactinaemia.[3]	Galactorrhoea reported with fluoxetine[6,26] and paroxetine[27,28] Euprolactinaemic galactorrhoea reported with escitalopram[29] and fluvoxamine[30] Hyperprolactinaemia reported with sertraline[7]
Tricyclics	Small mean changes seen in some studies[11,31,32] but no changes in others[11,33]	Symptomatic hyperprolactinaemia reported with imipramine,[29] dosulepin[34] and clomipramine[35,36] Galactorrhoea reported with nortriptyline[37] and when trazodone was added to citalopram[38]
Vortioxetine	No mention of prolactin changes in clinical trials, e.g.[39,40]	None, although clinical experience is limited

MAOI, monoamine oxidase inhibitor; SNRI, serotonin–noradrenaline reuptake inhibitor; SSRI, selective serotonin reuptake inhibitor.

References

1 Emiliano AB et al. From galactorrhea to osteopenia: rethinking serotonin-prolactin interactions. Neuropsychopharmacology 2004; 29:833–846.

2 Rittenhouse PA et al. Neurons in the hypothalamic paraventricular nucleus mediate the serotonergic stimulation of prolactin secretion via 5-HT1c/2 receptors. Endocrinology 1993; 133:661–667.

3 Trenque T et al. Serotonin reuptake inhibitors and hyperprolactinaemia: a case/non-case study in the French pharmacovigilance database. Drug Saf 2011; 34:1161–1166.

4 Voicu V et al. Drug-induced hypo- and hyperprolactinemia: mechanisms, clinical and therapeutic consequences. Expert Opin Drug Metab Toxicol 2013; 9:955–968.

5 Ashbury JE et al. Selective serotonin reuptake inhibitor (SSRI) antidepressants, prolactin and breast cancer. Front Oncol 2012; 2:177.

6 Mondal S et al. A new logical insight and putative mechanism behind fluoxetine-induced amenorrhea, hyperprolactinemia and galactorrhea in a case series. Ther Adv Psychopharmacol 2013; 3:322–334.

7 Strzelecki D et al. Hyperprolactinemia and bleeding following use of sertraline but not use of citalopram and paroxetine: a case report. Arch Psychiatry Psychother 2012; 1:45–48.

8 Taylor D et al. Antidepressant efficacy of agomelatine: meta-analysis of published and unpublished studies. BMJ 2014; 348:g1888.

9 Chu YS et al. Stimulatory and entraining effect of melatonin on tuberoinfundibular dopaminergic neuron activity and inhibition on prolactin secretion. J Pineal Res 2000; 28:219–226.

10 Whiteman PD et al. Bupropion fails to affect plasma prolactin and growth hormone in normal subjects. Br J Clin Pharmacol 1982; 13:745.

11 Meltzer HY et al. Effect of antidepressants on neuroendocrine axis in humans. Adv Biochem Psychopharmacol 1982; 32:303–316.

12 Price LH et al. Effects of tranylcypromine treatment on neuroendocrine, behavioral, and autonomic responses to tryptophan in depressed patients. Life Sci 1985; 37:809–818.

13 Laakmann G et al. Effects of mirtazapine on growth hormone, prolactin, and cortisol secretion in healthy male subjects. Psychoneuroendocrinology 1999; 24:769–784.

14 Laakmann G et al. Mirtazapine: an inhibitor of cortisol secretion that does not influence growth hormone and prolactin secretion. J Clin Psychopharmacol 2000; 20:101–103.

15 Schule C et al. The influence of mirtazapine on anterior pituitary hormone secretion in healthy male subjects. Psychopharmacology (Berl) 2002; 163:95–101.

16 Schule C et al. Reboxetine acutely stimulates cortisol, ACTH, growth hormone and prolactin secretion in healthy male subjects. Psychoneuroendocrinology 2004; 29:185–200.

17 Daffner-Bugia C et al. The neuroendocrine effects of venlafaxine in healthy subjects. Hum Psychopharmacol 1996; 11:1–9.

18 Sternbach H. Venlafaxine-induced galactorrhea. J Clin Psychopharmacol 2003; 23:109–110.

19 Demir EY et al. Hyperprolactinemia connected with venlafaxine: a case report. Anadolu Psikiyatri Derg 2014; 15:S10–S14.

20 Ashton AK et al. Hyperprolactinemia and galactorrhea induced by serotonin and norepinephrine reuptake inhibiting antidepressants. Am J Psychiatry 2007; 164:1121–1122.

21 Korkmaz S et al. Galactorrhea during duloxetine treatment: a case report. Turk Psikiyatri Derg 2011; 22:200–201.

22 Sagud M et al. Effects of sertraline treatment on plasma cortisol, prolactin and thyroid hormones in female depressed patients. Neuropsychobiology 2002; 45:139–143.

23 Schlosser R et al. Effects of subchronic paroxetine administration on night-time endocrinological profiles in healthy male volunteers. Psychoneuroendocrinology 2000; 25:377–388.

24 Nadeem HS et al. Comparison of the effects of citalopram and escitalopram on 5-HT-mediated neuroendocrine responses. Neuropsychopharmacology 2004; 29:1699–1703.

25 Egberts AC et al. Non-puerperal lactation associated with antidepressant drug use. Br J Clin Pharmacol 1997; 44:277–281.

26 Peterson MC. Reversible galactorrhea and prolactin elevation related to fluoxetine use. Mayo Clin Proc 2001; 76:215–216.

27 Morrison J et al. Galactorrhea induced by paroxetine. Can J Psychiatry 2001; 46:88–89.

28 Evrensel A et al. A case of galactorrhea during paroxetine treatment. Int J Psychiatry Med 2016; 51:302–305.

29 Mahasuar R et al. Euprolactinemic galactorrhea associated with use of imipramine and escitalopram in a postmenopausal woman. Gen Hosp Psychiatry 2010; 32:341–343.

30 Vispute C et al. Fluvoxamine-induced reversible euprolactinemic galactorrhea in a case of obsessive-compulsive disorder. Ann Indian Psychiatry 2017; 1:127–128.

31 Fava GA et al. Prolactin, cortisol, and antidepressant treatment. Am J Psychiatry 1988; 145:358–360.

32 Orlander H et al. Imipramine induced elevation of prolactin levels in patients with HIV/AIDS improved their immune status. West Indian Med J 2009; 58:207–213.

33 Meltzer HY et al. Lack of effect of tricyclic antidepressants on serum prolactin levels. Psychopharmacology (Berl) 1977; 51:185–187.

34 Gadd EM et al. Antidepressants and galactorrhoea. Int Clin Psychopharmacol 1987; 2:361–363.

35 Anand VS. Clomipramine – induced galactorrhoea and amenorrhoea. Br J Psychiatry 1985; 147:87–88.

36 Fowlie S et al. Hyperprolactinaemia and nonpuerperal lactation associated with clomipramine. Scott Med J 1987; 32:52.

37 Kukreti P et al. Rising trend of use of antidepressants induced non-puerperal lactation: a case report. J Clin Diagn Res 2016; 10: VD01–VD02.

38 Arslan FC et al. Trazodone induced galactorrhea: a case report. Gen Hosp Psychiatry 2015; 37:373.e371–372.

39 Mahableshwarkar AR et al. A randomized, double-blind, fixed-dose study comparing the efficacy and tolerability of vortioxetine 2.5 and 10 mg in acute treatment of adults with generalized anxiety disorder. Hum Psychopharmacol 2014; 29:64–72.

40 Baldwin DS et al. Vortioxetine (Lu AA21004) in the long-term open-label treatment of major depressive disorder. Curr Med Res Opin 2012; 28:1717–1724.

Further reading

Coker F et al. Antidepressant-induced hyperprolactinaemia: incidence, mechanisms and management. CNS Drugs 2010; 24:563–574.

Antidepressants and diabetes mellitus

Depression and diabetes

There is an established link between diabetes and depression.[1] Prevalence rates of co-morbid depressive symptoms in diabetic patients have been reported to range from 9% to 60% depending on the study design and screening method used.[2] Moreover, having diabetes doubles the odds of co-morbid depression[2] and a diagnosis of diabetes is linked to an increased likelihood of antidepressant prescription.[3,4] Patients with depression and diabetes have a high number of cardiovascular risk factors and 50% increased

Table 3.16 Effect of antidepressants on glucose homeostasis and weight

Antidepressant class	Effect on glucose homeostasis and weight
SSRIs[8–23]	■ Studies indicate that SSRIs have a favourable effect on diabetic parameters in patients with type 2 diabetes. Insulin requirements may be decreased ■ Fluoxetine has been associated with improvement in HbA$_{1c}$ levels, reduced insulin requirements, weight loss and enhanced insulin sensitivity. Its effect on insulin sensitivity is independent of its effect on weight loss. Sertraline may also reduce HbA$_{1c}$ ■ Escitalopram also seems to improve glycaemic control ■ Some evidence that long-term SSRIs may increase the risk of diabetes to a modest extent but also evidence of no effect
TCAs[14,16, 24–26]	■ TCAs are associated with increased appetite, weight gain and hyperglycaemia ■ Nortriptyline improved depression but worsened glycaemic control in diabetic patients in one study. Overall improvement in depression had a beneficial effect on HbA$_{1c}$. ■ Clomipramine has been reported to precipitate diabetes ■ Long-term use of TCAs seems to increase risk of diabetes
MAOIs[27,28]	■ Irreversible MAOIs have a tendency to cause extreme hypoglycaemic episodes and weight gain ■ No known effects with moclobemide
SNRIs[25,29,30]	■ SNRIs do not appear to disrupt glycaemic control and have minimal impact on weight ■ Studies of duloxetine in the treatment of diabetic neuropathy show that it has little influence on glycaemic control. No data in depression and diabetes ■ Limited data on venlafaxine
Mirtazapine[31,32]	■ Mirtazapine does not appear to impair glucose tolerance in non-diabetic depressed patients ■ Improvement in HBA$_{1c}$ was seen with short-term use but HbA$_{1c}$ worsened during a 1-year follow-up ■ Mirtazapine was associated with an increase in body mass index (BMI) in diabetic patients both in the short and long term
Agomelatine[22,23,33,34]	■ A few studies suggest agomelatine is effective with some improvement or no worsening of glycaemic parameters ■ Agomelatine also demonstrated a minimum effect on body weight
Reboxetine, trazodone and vortioxetine	■ No data in patients with diabetes

MAOI, monoamine oxidase inhibitor; SNRI, serotonin–noradrenaline reuptake inhibitor; SSRI, selective serotonin reuptake inhibitor; TCA, tricyclic antidepressant.

risk of mortality.[5,6] The presence of depression has a negative impact on metabolic control and likewise poor metabolic control may worsen depression.[7] Considering all of this, the treatment of co-morbid depression in patients with diabetes is of vital importance and drug choice should take into account likely effects on metabolic control (see Table 3.16). Cochrane[35] suggests that antidepressants are effective and moderately improve glycaemic control. Be aware, however, that the prescribing of antidepressants may be associated with reduced adherence to antidiabetic medication.[36]

Recommendation: **all patients with a diagnosis of depression should be screened for diabetes.** In those who are diabetic:

- Use SSRIs first line; data support sertraline, escitalopram and fluoxetine.
- SNRIs are also likely to be safe but there are fewer supporting data.
- Agomelatine seems promising with limited data available.
- Avoid TCAs and MAOIs if possible due to their effects on weight and glucose homeostasis.
- Monitor blood glucose and HbA_{1c} carefully when antidepressant treatment is initiated, when the dose is changed and after discontinuation.

References

1 Katon WJ. The comorbidity of diabetes mellitus and depression. Am J Med 2008; **121** Suppl 2:S8–S15.

2 Anderson RJ et al. The prevalence of comorbid depression in adults with diabetes: a meta-analysis. Diabetes Care 2001; **24**:1069–1078.

3 Musselman DL et al. Relationship of depression to diabetes types 1 and 2: epidemiology, biology, and treatment. Biol Psychiatry 2003; **54**:317–329.

4 Knol MJ et al. Antidepressant use before and after initiation of diabetes mellitus treatment. Diabetologia 2009; **52**:425–432.

5 Katon WJ et al. Cardiac risk factors in patients with diabetes mellitus and major depression. J Gen Intern Med 2004; **19**:1192–1199.

6 van Dooren FE et al. Depression and risk of mortality in people with diabetes mellitus: a systematic review and meta-analysis. PLoS One 2013; **8**:e57058.

7 Lustman PJ et al. Depression in diabetic patients: the relationship between mood and glycemic control. J Diabetes Complications 2005; **19**:113–122.

8 Maheux P et al. Fluoxetine improves insulin sensitivity in obese patients with non-insulin-dependent diabetes mellitus independently of weight loss. Int J Obes Relat Metab Disord 1997; **21**:97–102.

9 Gulseren L et al. Comparison of fluoxetine and paroxetine in type II diabetes mellitus patients. Arch Med Res 2005; **36**:159–165.

10 Lustman PJ et al. Sertraline for prevention of depression recurrence in diabetes mellitus: a randomized, double-blind, placebo-controlled trial. Arch Gen Psychiatry 2006; **63**:521–529.

11 Gray DS et al. A randomized double-blind clinical trial of fluoxetine in obese diabetics. Int J Obes Relat Metab Disord 1992; **16** Suppl 4:S67–S72.

12 Knol MJ et al. Influence of antidepressants on glycaemic control in patients with diabetes mellitus. Pharmacoepidemiol Drug Saf 2008; **17**:577–586.

13 Briscoe VJ et al. Effects of a selective serotonin reuptake inhibitor, fluoxetine, on counterregulatory responses to hypoglycemia in healthy individuals. Diabetes 2008; **57**:2453–2460.

14 Andersohn F et al. Long-term use of antidepressants for depressive disorders and the risk of diabetes mellitus. Am J Psychiatry 2009; **166**:591–598.

15 Derijks HJ et al. Influence of antidepressant use on glycemic control in patients with diabetes mellitus: an open-label comparative study. J Clin Psychopharmacol 2009; **29**:405–408.

16 Kivimaki M et al. Antidepressant medication use, weight gain, and risk of type 2 diabetes: a population-based study. Diabetes Care 2010; **33**:2611–2616.

17 Rubin RR et al. Antidepressant medicine use and risk of developing diabetes during the diabetes prevention program and diabetes prevention program outcomes study. Diabetes Care 2010; **33**:2549–2551.

18 Echeverry D et al. Effect of pharmacological treatment of depression on A1C and quality of life in low-income Hispanics and African Americans with diabetes: a randomized, double-blind, placebo-controlled trial. Diabetes Care 2009; **32**:2156–2160.

19 Gehlawat P et al. Diabetes with comorbid depression: role of SSRI in better glycemic control. Asian J Psychiatr 2013; **6**:364–368.

20 Dhavale HS et al. Depression and diabetes: impact of antidepressant medications on glycaemic control. J Assoc Physicians India 2013; **61**:896–899.

21 Mojtabai R. Antidepressant use and glycemic control. Psychopharmacology (Berl) 2013; **227**:467–477.

22 Salman MT et al. Comparative effect of agomelatine versus escitalopram on glycemic control and symptoms of depression in patients with type 2 diabetes mellitus and depression. Int J Pharm Sci Res 2015; 6:4304–4309.

23 Kang R et al. Comparison of paroxetine and agomelatine in depressed type 2 diabetes mellitus patients: a double-blind, randomized, clinical trial. Neuropsychiatr Dis Treat 2015; 11:1307–1311.

24 Lustman PJ et al. Effects of nortriptyline on depression and glycemic control in diabetes: results of a double-blind, placebo-controlled trial. Psychosom Med 1997; 59:241–250.

25 McIntyre RS et al. The effect of antidepressants on glucose homeostasis and insulin sensitivity: synthesis and mechanisms. Expert Opin Drug Saf 2006; 5:157–168.

26 Mumoli N et al. Clomipramine-induced diabetes. Ann Intern Med 2008; 149:595–596.

27 Goodnick PJ. Use of antidepressants in treatment of comorbid diabetes mellitus and depression as well as in diabetic neuropathy. Ann Clin Psychiatry 2001; 13:31–41.

28 McIntyre RS et al. Mood and psychotic disorders and type 2 diabetes: a metabolic triad. Can J Diabetes 2005; 29:122–132.

29 Raskin J et al. Duloxetine versus routine care in the long-term management of diabetic peripheral neuropathic pain. J Palliat Med 2006; 9:29–40.

30 Crucitti A et al. Duloxetine treatment and glycemic controls in patients with diagnoses other than diabetic peripheral neuropathic pain: a meta-analysis. Curr Med Res Opin 2010; 26:2579–2588.

31 Song HR et al. Does mirtazapine interfere with naturalistic diabetes treatment? J Clin Psychopharmacol 2014; 34:588–594.

32 Song HR et al. Effects of mirtazapine on patients undergoing naturalistic diabetes treatment: a follow-up study extended from 6 to 12 months. J Clin Psychopharmacol 2015; 35:730–731.

33 Karaiskos D et al. Agomelatine and sertraline for the treatment of depression in type 2 diabetes mellitus. Int J Clin Pract 2013; 67:257–260.

34 Vasile D et al. P.2.c.002 Agomelatine versus selective serotoninergic reuptake inhibitors in major depressive disorder and comorbid diabetes mellitus. Eur Neuropsychopharmacol 2011; 21:S383–S384.

35 Baumeister H et al. Psychological and pharmacological interventions for depression in patients with diabetes mellitus and depression. Cochrane Database Syst Rev 2012; 12:Cd008381.

36 Lunghi C et al. The association between depression and medication nonpersistence in new users of antidiabetic drugs. Value Health 2017; 20:728–735.

Antidepressants and sexual dysfunction

Sexual dysfunction is common in the general population, although reliable normative data are lacking.[1] Reported prevalence rates vary depending on how sexual dysfunction is defined and assessed and also on the method of data collection.[1] Physical illness, psychiatric illness, substance misuse and prescribed drug treatment can all cause sexual dysfunction.[2] People with depression are more likely to be obese,[3] have diabetes,[4] and have cardiovascular disease[5] than the general population, making them more likely to suffer sexual dysfunction.

Baseline sexual functioning should be determined, if possible, because treatment-emergent sexual dysfunction adversely affects quality of life and may contribute to reduced compliance.[6] Questionnaires or rating scales may be useful (for example, the Arizona Sexual Experience Scale[7]). If scales are not used then direct questioning should be, since it is much more effective than relying on patient report.[8] Complaints of sexual dysfunction may also indicate progression or inadequate treatment of underlying medical or psychiatric conditions. It may also be the result of drug treatment, and intervention may greatly improve quality of life.[6]

Effects of depression

Both depression and the drugs used to treat it can cause disorders of desire, arousal and orgasm. The precise nature of the sexual dysfunction may indicate whether depression or treatment is the more likely cause. For example, 40–50% of people with depression report diminished libido and problems regarding sexual arousal in the month before diagnosis, but only 15–20% experience orgasm problems before taking an antidepressant.[9] The prevalence for loss of libido appears to correlate with depression severity.[10]

Although many patients experience treatment-emergent sexual dysfunction whilst taking antidepressants, in others the reduction in depressive symptoms can be accompanied by improvements in sexual desire and satisfaction.[6] Improvements appear more commonly among those who respond to antidepressant treatment.[6] For example, a *post hoc* analysis of data from the STAR*D study revealed that sexual dysfunction was problematic in 21% of patients whose depression remitted with citalopram treatment compared with 61% of those whose depression did not remit.[11]

Effects of antidepressant drugs

Antidepressants can cause sedation, hormonal changes, disturbance of cholinergic/adrenergic balance, peripheral α-adrenergic agonism, inhibition of nitric oxide and increased serotonin neurotransmission, all of which can result in sexual dysfunction. Sexual dysfunction has been reported as an adverse effect of all antidepressants, although rates vary (see Table 3.17). Individual susceptibility also varies and may be at least partially genetically determined.[12] Sexual dysfunction with antidepressants is likely to be both dose-dependent and fully reversible.[12]

Not all of the sexual adverse effects of antidepressants are undesirable: serotonergic antidepressants including clomipramine are effective in the treatment of premature ejaculation[6] and may also be beneficial in paraphilias. The short-acting SSRI dapoxetine

Table 3.17 Relative frequency sexual dysfunction (SD) with antidepressants[10,12–14]

| Antidepressant | Impact on sexual response | | | Comments[12] |
	Sexual desire*	Sexual arousal[†]	Orgasm[‡]	
Agomelatine	−	−	−	Rates of SD may be similar to placebo[6]
Bupropion	−	+/−	−	Low rates of SD compared to some other antidepressants.[15] Overall, considerable evidence that SD occurs at or below the rate of placebo
Duloxetine	++	+	++	Rate of SD similar to some SSRIs and venlafaxine in one meta-analysis[15]
Levomilnacipran	?	++	++	Limited comparative studies with other antidepressants[16] so relative frequency of SD is uncertain. Erectile dysfunction and disorders of ejaculation shown in RCTs against placebo
MAOIs	++	++	++	Limited evidence though reported incidence of SD ranges from 20% to 42%. Rates of SD with transdermal selegiline are comparable to placebo
Mirtazapine	+	−	−	Causes less SD than SSRIs[17]
Moclobemide	−	−	−	Consistently shown to have a low risk of SD
Reboxetine	−	−	−	Probably causes less SD than SSRIs/SNRIs though efficacy has been questioned[18]
SSRIs	++	++	++	Overall evidence suggests relatively high rates of SD across all the SSRIs (although reported incidence varies widely)[12]
Trazodone	−	+	+	Priapism reported in case studies; however, overall reports of SD seem to be low. Earlier case reports document increased sexual desire
Tricyclics	++	++	++	SD more common with clomipramine (particularly anorgasmia), amitriptyline and imipramine. Less common with secondary amine TCAs (desipramine, nortriptyline)
Venlafaxine	++	++	++	High rates of SD. Isolated case reports of increased libido, orgasm and spontaneous erections
Vilazodone	+	+	+	Rates of SD possibly lower than citalopram and similar to placebo in RCTs. However, a clear advantage over other antidepressants remains uncertain[16]
Vortioxetine	−	+	+	Incidence of SD reportedly similar to placebo at doses 10 mg/day or less;[18,19] however, a clear advantage over other antidepressants remains uncertain[16,20]

++, common; +, may occur; −, absent or rare; ?, unknown/insufficient information.
*Or sex drive.
[†] Ease of arousal and ability to achieve lubrication or erections.
[‡] Ease of reaching orgasm and orgasm satisfaction.
MAOI, monoamine oxidase inhibitor; RCT, randomised controlled trial; SD, sexual dysfunction; SNRI, serotonin–noradrenaline reuptake inhibitor; SSRI, selective serotonin reuptake inhibitor; TCA, tricyclic antidepressant.

Table 3.18 Management of sexual adverse effects

Strategy	Details
1. Rule out other possible causes[23]	■ Depressive symptoms are associated with impaired sexual functioning. Compare sexual functioning on antidepressants with sexual functioning before antidepressants, not before the onset of depressive illness ■ Consider other possible contributing causes, e.g. alcohol/substance misuse, diabetes, atherosclerosis, cardiac disease and central and peripheral nervous system conditions
2. Switch to a lower-risk antidepressant[18]	■ Lower-risk antidepressants include agomelatine, bupropion, mirtazapine, vilazodone, vortioxetine and moclobemide.[12] Of these, agomelatine, bupropion and vortioxetine have the best evidence supporting a more favourable sexual adverse-effect profile[12]
Non-pharmacological treatment strategies	■ **Waiting for spontaneous remission:** may occur in a small number of people (5–10%) but can take up to 4–6 months[12] ■ **Dose reduction:** can be considered in patients who have achieved full remission on an antidepressant[6] ■ **Drug holidays:** intermittently missing one or two doses prior to planned sexual activity may possibly help but risks discontinuation symptoms.[12] Not an effective strategy with fluoxetine due to its long half-life[12]
Pharmacological treatments	■ **Phosphodiesterase inhibitors:** both sildenafil and tadalafil have been shown to improve sexual functioning in men with antidepressant-related erectile dysfunction.[18,24] Limited evidence in women though one RCT found benefits[18] ■ **Bupropion:** may be useful in women at higher doses (300 mg/day).[24] Lower doses appear to be ineffective.[18] A positive RCT in men[25] was later retracted ■ **Mirtazapine:** evidence is mixed. Open studies suggest some benefit for antidepressant-induced SD, but negative results were found in one RCT[23] ■ **Transdermal testosterone:** RCTs provide evidence of possible efficacy in women with SSRI/SNRI-emergent loss of libido[26] and in men who continue to take serotonergic antidepressants with low or low-normal testosterone levels[27] ■ **Others:**[12] many other agents have been studied; however, some of these have little or no evidence of effectiveness. **Buspirone** was effective in one study for citalopram- or paroxetine-induced SD, but ineffective in another study with fluoxetine. **Cyproheptadine** has been used successfully in case reports of SSRI-induced SD in men, and for anorgasmia in women. **Loratadine** was effective in a small open study for men with SSRI-induced erectile dysfunction. **Amantadine** was effective in earlier studies for SSRI-induced SD, but recent results have been negative. **Yohimbine** may be more effective for medication-induced SD and improvements were reported by patients in two small studies (although results were non-significant). **Bethanechol** appears to help with TCA-induced SD when taken before sexual activity. **Granisetron** has been evaluated but the existing data are not definitive

RCT, randomised controlled trial; SD, sexual dysfunction; SNRI, serotonin–noradrenaline reuptake inhibitor; SSRI, selective serotonin reuptake inhibitor; TCA, tricyclic antidepressant.

is an effective treatment for premature ejaculation and is licensed for this indication in many countries.[6,21] A systematic review of RCTs with trazodone showed benefit for reducing 'psychogenic erectile dysfunction'.[6]

Sexual adverse effects can be minimised by careful selection of the antidepressant drug – see Table 3.17. Note that the assessment of sexual adverse effects in clinical trials is generally inadequate (relying on spontaneous reports rather than using validated questionnaires, and lacking positive controls).[22] Where possible, information has been obtained from studies where sexual adverse effects are purposefully and directly investigated. Management strategies for people who do develop sexual dysfunction on antidepressants are summarised in Table 3.18. No single approach can be considered 'ideal'[6] so individual assessment on a case-by-case basis is recommended.

References

1 McCabe MP et al. Incidence and prevalence of sexual dysfunction in women and men: a consensus statement from the Fourth International Consultation on Sexual Medicine 2015. J Sex Med 2016; 13:144–152.
2 Chokka PR et al. Assessment and management of sexual dysfunction in the context of depression. Ther Adv Psychopharmacol 2018; 8:13–23.
3 Pereira-Miranda E et al. Overweight and obesity associated with higher depression prevalence in adults: a systematic review and meta-analysis. J Am Coll Nutr 2017; 36:223–233.
4 Semenkovich K et al. Depression in type 2 diabetes mellitus: prevalence, impact, and treatment. Drugs 2015; 75:577–587.
5 Cohen BE et al. State of the art review: depression, stress, anxiety, and cardiovascular disease. Am J Hypertens 2015; 28:1295–1302.
6 Montejo AL et al. The impact of severe mental disorders and psychotropic medications on sexual health and its implications for clinical management. World Psychiatry 2018; 17:3–11.
7 McGahuey CA et al. The Arizona Sexual Experience Scale (ASEX): reliability and validity. J Sex Marital Ther 2000; 26:25–40.
8 Papakostas GI. Identifying patients who need a change in depression treatment and implementing that change. J Clin Psychiatry 2016; 77:e1009.
9 Kennedy SH et al. Sexual dysfunction before antidepressant therapy in major depression. J Affect Disord 1999; 56:201–208.
10 Clayton AH et al. Antidepressants and sexual dysfunction: mechanisms and clinical implications. Postgrad Med 2014; 126:91–99.
11 Ishak WW et al. Sexual satisfaction and quality of life in major depressive disorder before and after treatment with citalopram in the STAR*D study. J Clin Psychiatry 2013; 74:256–261.
12 Clayton AH et al. Sexual dysfunction due to psychotropic medications. Psychiatr Clin North Am 2016; 39:427–463.
13 Serretti A et al. Treatment-emergent sexual dysfunction related to antidepressants: a meta-analysis. J Clin Psychopharmacol 2009; 29:259–266.
14 Chiesa A et al. Antidepressants and sexual dysfunction: epidemiology, mechanisms and management. J Psychopathol 2010; 16:104–113.
15 Reichenpfader U et al. Sexual dysfunction associated with second-generation antidepressants in patients with major depressive disorder: results from a systematic review with network meta-analysis. Drug Saf 2014; 37:19–31.
16 Wagner G et al. Efficacy and safety of levomilnacipran, vilazodone and vortioxetine compared with other second-generation antidepressants for major depressive disorder in adults: a systematic review and network meta-analysis. J Affect Disord 2018; 228:1–12.
17 Watanabe N et al. Mirtazapine versus other antidepressive agents for depression. Cochrane Database Syst Rev 2011:CD006528.
18 Cleare A et al. Evidence-based guidelines for treating depressive disorders with antidepressants: a revision of the 2008 British Association for Psychopharmacology guidelines. J Psychopharmacol 2015; 29:459–525.
19 Jacobsen PL et al. Treatment-emergent sexual dysfunction in randomized trials of vortioxetine for major depressive disorder or generalized anxiety disorder: a pooled analysis. CNS Spectr 2016; 21:367–378.
20 Koesters M et al. Vortioxetine for depression in adults. Cochrane Database Syst Rev 2017; 7:CD011520.
21 McMahon CG. Dapoxetine: a new option in the medical management of premature ejaculation. Ther Adv Urol 2012; 4:233–251.
22 Khin NA et al. Regulatory and scientific issues in studies to evaluate sexual dysfunction in antidepressant drug trials. J Clin Psychiatry 2015; 76:1060–1063.
23 Francois D et al. Antidepressant-induced sexual side effects: incidence, assessment, clinical implications, and management. Psychiatric Annals 2017; 47:154–160.
24 Taylor MJ et al. Strategies for managing sexual dysfunction induced by antidepressant medication. Cochrane Database Syst Rev 2013; 5:CD003382.
25 Safarinejad MR. The effects of the adjunctive bupropion on male sexual dysfunction induced by a selective serotonin reuptake inhibitor: a double-blind placebo-controlled and randomized study. BJU Int 2010; 106:840–847.
26 Montejo AL et al. Sexual side-effects of antidepressant and antipsychotic drugs. Curr Opin Psychiatry 2015; 28:418–423.
27 Amiaz R et al. Testosterone gel replacement improves sexual function in depressed men taking serotonergic antidepressants: a randomized, placebo-controlled clinical trial. J Sex Marital Ther 2011; 37:243–254.

Further reading

Williams VS et al. Prevalence and impact of antidepressant-associated sexual dysfunction in three European countries: replication in a cross-sectional patient survey. J Psychopharmacology 2010; 24:489–496.

SSRIs and bleeding

Serotonin is released from platelets in response to vascular injury, promoting vasoconstriction and morphological changes in platelets that lead to aggregation.[1] Selective serotonin reuptake inhibitors (SSRIs) inhibit the serotonin transporter, which is responsible for the uptake of serotonin into platelets. It might thus be predicted that SSRIs will deplete platelet serotonin, leading to a reduced ability to form clots and a subsequent increase in the risk of bleeding.[2] SSRIs may also increase gastric acid secretion and therefore may be indirectly irritant to the gastric mucosa.[3] Use of SSRIs certainly seems to increase the risk of peptic ulcer.[4] The risk of abnormal bleeding (of any kind) with SSRIs is highest during the first 30 days of commencing treatment.[5,6] Effect on bleeding is probably related to the affinity of individual SSRIs for the serotonin transporter[7,8] (see Table 3.19).

Risk factors for bleeding with SSRIs

- Age, particularly >65 years.
- Alcohol misuse.
- Coronary artery disease.
- Drug misuse.
- Hypertension.
- History of gastrointestinal bleed.
- History of stroke.
- History of major bleeding or predisposition to bleeding.
- Liver disease.
- Labile international normalised ratio (INR).
- Medication usage predisposing to bleeding.
- Peptic ulcer.
- Renal disease.
- Smoking.

Caution should be exercised when prescribing serotonergic antidepressants for people with medical conditions such as gout, asthma, COPD, lupus, psoriasis, interferon-induced depression in hepatitis C patients,[10] and arthritis, when patients might also be taking corticosteroids, aspirin or NSAIDs.

Table 3.19 Antidepressants and degree of serotonin reuptake inhibition[6,9]

Degree of serotonin reuptake inhibition	Antidepressant (SSRI)
Strong inhibition	Sertraline, paroxetine, fluoxetine, duloxetine, clomipramine
Intermediate inhibition	Citalopram, escitalopram, fluvoxamine, vilazodone, vortioxetine, venlafaxine, amitriptyline, imipramine
Weak or no inhibition	Agomelatine, dosulepin, doxepin, lofepramine, mirtazapine, moclobemide, nortriptyline, reboxetine, mianserin

Gastrointestinal (GI) bleeding

The use of serotonergic antidepressants is an independent risk factor for bleeding events. A population-based study revealed that SSRIs increase the rate of upper gastrointestinal bleeding (UGIB), with hazard ratio (HR) of 1.97, and lower gastrointestinal bleeding (LGIB) (HR 2.96) after adjusting for all relevant risk factors.[11] In absolute terms, it is likely that SSRIs are responsible for an additional three episodes of bleeding in every 1000 patient years of treatment over the normal background incidence[7,12] but this figure masks large variations in risk. For example 1 in 85 patients with a history of GI bleed will have a further bleed attributable to treatment with an SSRI.[13] One database study suggests that gastroprotective drugs (proton pump inhibitors; PPIs) decrease the risk of GI bleeds associated with SSRIs (alone or in combination with NSAIDs) although not quite to control levels.[14]

Other database studies have found that patients who take SSRIs are at significantly increased risk of being admitted to hospital with an upper GI bleed (UGIB) compared with age- and sex-matched controls.[7,14–16] This association holds when age, gender, and the effects of other drugs such as aspirin and NSAIDs are controlled for.[2]

A meta-analysis of 22 studies concluded that current users of SSRIs are 55% more at risk of UGIB compared with those who do not take SSRIs. This risk was significantly and further increased by concurrent use of antiplatelet drugs or NSAIDs.[5]

Co-prescription of low-dose aspirin at least doubles the risk of GI bleeding associated with SSRIs alone, and co-prescription of NSAIDs approximately quadruples risk.[17] Combined need for SSRIs and NSAIDs greatly increases the use of anti-acid drugs.[18] The elderly and those with a history of GI bleeding are at greatest risk.[13,14,16]

Some early studies found that in patients who take warfarin, SSRIs increase the risk of a non-GI bleed two- to three-fold (similar to the effect size of NSAIDs) but do not seem to increase the risk of a GI bleed.[19,20] A more recent study[11] has shown an increased risk of UGIB and LGIB in concomitant users of warfarin and a serotonergic antidepressant (see Table 3.20). This effect does not seem to be associated with any change in

Table 3.20 Approximate absolute risk of gastrointestinal bleeding with concomitant use of SSRIs (YL Cheng, personal communication 2017)

Drug	Absolute risk of UGIB	Absolute risk of LGIB
Aspirin + SSRI	6%	3%
Warfarin + SSRI	4%	3%
NSAID + SSRI	3%	1%
SSRI alone	2%	1%

Percentage figures rounded to nearest integer.
LGIB, lower gastrointestinal bleeding; NSAID, non-steroidal anti-inflammatory drug; SSRI, selective serotonin reuptake inhibitor; UGIB, upper gastrointestinal bleeding.

INR, making it difficult to identify those at highest risk.[20] In keeping with these findings, SSRI use in anticoagulated patients being treated for acute coronary syndromes may decrease the risk of minor cardiac events at the expense of an increased risk of a bleed.[21] Thus the increased risk of UGIB associated with SSRIs may be balanced by a decreased risk of embolic events. One database study failed to find a reduction in the risk of a first myocardial infarction (MI) in SSRI treated-patients compared with controls[22] while another[23] found a reduction in the risk of being admitted to hospital with a first MI in smokers on SSRIs. The effect size in the second study was large: approximately 1 in 10 hospitalisations were avoided in SSRI-treated patients.[23] This is similar to the effect size of other antiplatelet therapies such as aspirin.[24]

Many studies do not state changes in absolute risk of intestinal bleeding. Table 3.20 shows approximate absolute risks derived from a single study[11] and directly communicated (YL Cheng, personal communication 2017).

Risk decreases to the same level as controls in past users of SSRIs, indicating that bleeding is likely to be associated with treatment itself rather than some inherent characteristic of the patients being treated.[7] It also means that the effect of SSRIs disappears after their withdrawal.

The excess risk of bleeding is not confined to UGIB (see Table 3.20). The risk of LGIB may also be increased[25] and an increased risk of uterine bleeding (see later in this section) has also been reported.[12]

Intracranial haemorrhage (ICH)

There is a clear association between the use of SSRIs and ICH, and risk is further increased by concomitant use of NSAIDs and anticoagulants.

In early research, three large database studies failed to find either a reduction in the risk of an ischaemic stroke or increase in the risk of haemorrhagic stroke in SSRI users.[26–28] One cohort study reported an increased risk of haemorrhagic stroke.[29] The absolute risk was small. A further nested case-control study showed an 11% increased odds of haemorrhagic stroke in people on SSRIs[30] (absolute risk 1:10,000 patient years of treatment).

Elevated risk of ICH has now been observed across all classes of antidepressants with serotonergic activity. In a cohort study of 1,363,990 users of antidepressants,[6] the overall rate of ICH was 3.8 per 10,000 patient years. Current use of an SSRI increased the risk of ICH (relative risk [RR] 1.17) compared with a TCA with an absolute adjusted rate difference of 6.7 per 100,000 persons per year. Amongst the SSRI group the risk of ICH was 25% greater in those who used strong inhibitors of the serotonin reuptake system than in users of weak inhibitors (see Table 3.19). This correlates to an absolute adjusted rate difference of 9.5 events per 100,000 persons per year. Overall risk was highest during the first 30 days of use.

A recent database study[31] also identified an increased risk of ICH in those who have been taking SSRIs alone or in combination with NSAIDs. This and other studies providing data on absolute risk are summarised in Table 3.21.

Table 3.21 gives estimates of absolute risk of ICH derived from three studies.

Table 3.21 Absolute risk of intracranial haemorrhage with SSRI with or without anticoagulant or NSAIDs

Study	Risk with SSRI alone	Risk with SSRI+NSAID	Risk with antidepressant+ anticoagulant
Shin et al. 2015[31]	1 in 632*(0.16%)	1 in 175*(0.57%)	–
Renoux et al. 2017[6]	1 in 450[†] (0.22%)	–	1 in 260[†] (0.38%)
Smoller et al. 2009[29]	1 in 240[§] (0.42%)	–	–

*Within 30 days of taking antidepressant.
[†] Incident users (no time limit).
[§] Annual risk (older patients).
NSAID, non-steroidal anti-inflammatory drug; SSRI, selective serotonin reuptake inhibitor.

Gynaecological and obstetrical haemorrhage

A multicentre cross-sectional study[32] found an association between the use of antidepressants and menstruation disorders (unusual or excess bleeding, irregular menstruation, menorrhagia, etc.). This study found that the prevalence of menstrual disorder in the study group who were taking SSRIs, venlafaxine or mirtazapine combined with SSRIs or mirtazapine was significantly higher (24.6%) than in the control group (12.2%) who did not take any antidepressants. Cases of abnormal vaginal bleeding associated with SSRIs have been reported in a young woman,[33] a postmenopausal woman[34] and a pre-adolescent girl aged 11.[35]

Post-partum haemorrhage (PPH)

Whilst one study[36] could not find an increased risk of PPH with the use of SSRI or non-SSRI antidepressants, a large cohort study[37] found an association between PPH and all classes of antidepressants, with a number needed to harm of 80 for current users of SSRIs and 97 for those on other antidepressants. One hospital-based cohort study[38] found an absolute risk of PPH of 18% and an absolute risk of post-partum anaemia of 12.8% after a non-surgical vaginal delivery in women who were current users of SSRIs. The absolute risk of both PPH and post-partum anaemia for those without any exposure to antidepressants was 8.7%. The blood loss during delivery was also higher for those who had SSRI exposure (484 mL) compared with those who did not take antidepressants (398 mL). The length of hospital stay was also significantly increased for those who had been taking an SSRI. The most recent population study[39] identified that the use of serotonergic medications was associated with a 1.5 times increased risk of PPH compared with those who did not take any psychoactive medications. This study highlighted that women who had been taking other psychoactive medications such as antipsychotics and mood stabilisers were at three times greater risk of PPH compared to mothers who did not take any medications, suggesting that the occurrence of PPH might not be entirely due to serotonergic activity and that further research is needed to investigate other mechanisms.

Surgical and post-operative bleeding (see Table 3.22)

Use of SSRIs in the pre-operative period has been associated with a 20% increase in in-patient mortality (absolute risk 1 in 1000), although patient factors rather than drug factors could not be excluded as the cause.[41] One study[42] found that patients prescribed SSRIs who underwent orthopaedic surgery had an almost four-fold risk of requiring a blood transfusion. This equated to one additional patient requiring transfusion for every 10 SSRI patients undergoing surgery and was double the risk of patients who were taking NSAIDs alone. It should be noted in this context that treatment with SSRIs has been associated with a 2.4-fold increase in the risk of hip fracture[43] and a two-fold increase of fracture in old age.[44] (Mirtazapine[45] and TCAs[43] also increase the risk of hip fracture.) One recent study recognised pre-operative treatment with SSRIs, other antidepressants or antipsychotics as independent risk factors for blood transfusion in elective fast-track hip and knee arthroplasty.[46]

The combination of advanced age, SSRI treatment, orthopaedic surgery and NSAIDs clearly presents a very high risk. However, there does not seem to be an increased risk of bleeding in patients who undergo coronary artery bypass surgery.[47]

During a 10-year review of women who underwent cosmetic breast surgery procedures, the use of SSRIs increased the risk of post-operative bleeding by a factor of 4.14 compared with those who did not take SSRIs. The authors emphasised the importance of balancing the risks and benefits of stopping antidepressants prior to elective surgeries, particularly in psychologically vulnerable patients.[48]

A review of 13 studies found an increased odds ratio (1.21–4.14) of peri-operative bleeding with SSRIs.[49] One study noted an increased risk of bleeding in women undergoing breast surgery[50] and the authors suggest withholding SSRIs for 2 weeks prior to such planned surgery. Others conclude that there is insufficient evidence to support routine discontinuation of SSRIs prior to surgery and call for RCTs to be conducted in this area of care.[51] Venlafaxine may have similar effects[49] but duloxetine may not affect bleeding risk.[52]

Table 3.22 Risk of peri-operative blood loss and blood transfusion in SSRI users compared with non-SSRI users[40]

Surgical procedure	Need for reoperation due to bleeding event in users of SADs versus non-users	Need for blood product or red blood cell transfusion in users of SADs versus non-users	Increased risk of mortality in users of SADs versus non-users
Coronary artery bypass graft	OR 1.07 (0.66–1.74)	OR 1.06 (0.90–1.24)	OR 1.53 (1.15–2.04)
Breast cancer directed surgery	OR 2.7 (1.6–4.56)	–	–
Orthopaedic surgery	–	OR 1.61 (0.97–2.68)	OR 0.83 (0.69–1.00)
Major surgery	–	OR 1.19 (1.15–1.23)	OR 1.19 (1.03–1.37)

OR, odds ratio; SADs, serotonergic antidepressants.

Overall

Serotonergic antidepressants increase the risk of various types of bleeding. Evidence is strongest for SSRIs and it is likely that risk of bleeding is related to affinity for the serotonin transporter (although there is limited evidence that bleeding risk with mirtazapine and bupropion is similar to that of SSRIs[53]). SSRIs increase the risk of GI bleeding, haemorrhagic stroke, peri-operative bleeding, post-partum haemorrhage and uterine bleeding. Their effect is exacerbated by co-prescription with aspirin, anticoagulants and NSAIDs. In most cases the use of SSRIs increases the risk of an event by a clinically meaningful extent, but especially when co-prescribed with other drugs which affect clotting.

Summary

- SSRIs increase the risk of GI, uterine, cerebral and peri-operative bleeding.
- Risk is increased still further in those also receiving aspirin, NSAIDs or oral anticoagulants.
- Try to avoid SSRIs in patients receiving NSAIDs, aspirin or oral anticoagulants or in those with a history of cerebral or GI bleeds.
- If SSRI use cannot be avoided, monitor closely and prescribe gastroprotective proton pump inhibitors.
- Limited evidence suggests risks may be lower with less potent serotonin reuptake inhibitors.

References

1　Skop BP et al. Potential vascular and bleeding complications of treatment with selective serotonin reuptake inhibitors. Psychosomatics 1996; 37:12–16.

2　Laporte S et al. Bleeding risk under selective serotonin reuptake inhibitor (SSRI) antidepressants: a meta-analysis of observational studies. Pharmacol Res 2017; 118:19–32.

3　Andrade C et al. Serotonin reuptake inhibitor antidepressants and abnormal bleeding: a review for clinicians and a reconsideration of mechanisms. J Clin Psychiatry 2010; 71:1565–1575.

4　Dall M et al. There is an association between selective serotonin reuptake inhibitor use and uncomplicated peptic ulcers: a population-based case-control study. Aliment Pharmacol Ther 2010; 32:1383–1391.

5　Jiang HY et al. Use of selective serotonin reuptake inhibitors and risk of upper gastrointestinal bleeding: a systematic review and meta-analysis. Clin Gastroenterol Hepatol 2015; 13:42–50.

6　Renoux C et al. Association of selective serotonin reuptake inhibitors with the risk for spontaneous intracranial hemorrhage. JAMA Neurol 2017; 74:173–180.

7　Dalton SO et al. Use of selective serotonin reuptake inhibitors and risk of upper gastrointestinal tract bleeding: a population-based cohort study. Arch Intern Med 2003; 163:59–64.

8　Verdel BM et al. Use of serotonergic drugs and the risk of bleeding. Clin Pharmacol Ther 2011; 89:89–96.

9　Tatsumi M et al. Pharmacological profile of antidepressants and related compounds at human monoamine transporters. Eur J Pharmacol 1997; 340:249–258.

10　Weinrieb RM et al. A critical review of selective serotonin reuptake inhibitor-associated bleeding: balancing the risk of treating hepatitis C-infected patients. J Clin Psychiatry 2003; 64:1502–1510.

11　Cheng YL et al. Use of SSRI, but not SNRI, increased upper and lower gastrointestinal bleeding: a nationwide population-based cohort study in Taiwan. Medicine (Baltimore) 2015; 94:e2022.

12　Meijer WE et al. Association of risk of abnormal bleeding with degree of serotonin reuptake inhibition by antidepressants. Arch Intern Med 2004; 164:2367–2370.

13　van Walraven C et al. Inhibition of serotonin reuptake by antidepressants and upper gastrointestinal bleeding in elderly patients: retrospective cohort study. BMJ 2001; 323:655–658.

14　de Abajo FJ et al. Risk of upper gastrointestinal tract bleeding associated with selective serotonin reuptake inhibitors and venlafaxine therapy: interaction with nonsteroidal anti-inflammatory drugs and effect of acid-suppressing agents. Arch Gen Psychiatry 2008; 65:795–803.

15 de Abajo FJ et al. Association between selective serotonin reuptake inhibitors and upper gastrointestinal bleeding: population based case-control study. BMJ 1999; **319**:1106–1109.

16 Lewis JD et al. Moderate and high affinity serotonin reuptake inhibitors increase the risk of upper gastrointestinal toxicity. Pharmacoepidemiol Drug Saf 2008; **17**:328–335.

17 Paton C et al. SSRIs and gastrointestinal bleeding. BMJ 2005; **331**:529–530.

18 de Jong JC et al. Combined use of SSRIs and NSAIDs increases the risk of gastrointestinal adverse effects. Br J Clin Pharmacol 2003; **55**:591–595.

19 Schalekamp T et al. Increased bleeding risk with concurrent use of selective serotonin reuptake inhibitors and coumarins. Arch Intern Med 2008; **168**:180–185.

20 Wallerstedt SM et al. Risk of clinically relevant bleeding in warfarin-treated patients – influence of SSRI treatment. Pharmacoepidemiol Drug Saf 2009; **18**:412–416.

21 Ziegelstein RC et al. Selective serotonin reuptake inhibitor use by patients with acute coronary syndromes. Am J Med 2007; **120**:525–530.

22 Meier CR et al. Use of selective serotonin reuptake inhibitors and risk of developing first-time acute myocardial infarction. Br J Clin Pharmacol 2001; **52**:179–184.

23 Sauer WH et al. Selective serotonin reuptake inhibitors and myocardial infarction. Circulation 2001; **104**:1894–1898.

24 Antiplatelet Trialists' Collaboration. Collaborative overview of randomised trials of antiplatelet therapy – I: Prevention of death, myocardial infarction, and stroke by prolonged antiplatelet therapy in various categories of patients. BMJ 1994; **308**:81–106.

25 Wessinger S et al. Increased use of selective serotonin reuptake inhibitors in patients admitted with gastrointestinal haemorrhage: a multicentre retrospective analysis. Aliment Pharmacol Ther 2006; **23**:937–944.

26 Bak S et al. Selective serotonin reuptake inhibitors and the risk of stroke: a population-based case-control study. Stroke 2002; **33**:1465–1473.

27 Barbui C et al. Past use of selective serotonin reuptake inhibitors and the risk of cerebrovascular events in the elderly. Int Clin Psychopharmacol 2005; **20**:169–171.

28 Kharofa J et al. Selective serotonin reuptake inhibitors and risk of hemorrhagic stroke. Stroke 2007; **38**:3049–3051.

29 Smoller JW et al. Antidepressant use and risk of incident cardiovascular morbidity and mortality among postmenopausal women in the Women's Health Initiative study. Arch Intern Med 2009; **169**:2128–2139.

30 Douglas I et al. The use of antidepressants and the risk of haemorrhagic stroke: a nested case control study. Br J Clin Pharmacol 2011; **71**:116–120.

31 Shin JY et al. Risk of intracranial haemorrhage in antidepressant users with concurrent use of non-steroidal anti-inflammatory drugs: nationwide propensity score matched study. BMJ 2015; **351**:h3517.

32 Uguz F et al. Antidepressants and menstruation disorders in women: a cross-sectional study in three centers. Gen Hosp Psychiatry 2012; **34**:529–533.

33 Andersohn F et al. Citalopram-induced bleeding due to severe thrombocytopenia. Psychosomatics 2009; **50**:297–298.

34 Durmaz O et al. Vaginal bleeding associated with antidepressants. Int J Gynaecol Obstet 2015; **130**:284.

35 Turkoglu S et al. Vaginal bleeding and hemorrhagic prepatellar bursitis in a preadolescent girl, possibly related to fluoxetine. J Child Adolesc Psychopharmacol 2015; **25**:186–187.

36 Salkeld E et al. The risk of postpartum hemorrhage with selective serotonin reuptake inhibitors and other antidepressants. J Clin Psychopharmacol 2008; **28**:230–234.

37 Palmsten K et al. Use of antidepressants near delivery and risk of postpartum hemorrhage: cohort study of low income women in the United States. BMJ 2013; **347**:f4877.

38 Lindqvist PG et al. Selective serotonin reuptake inhibitor use during pregnancy increases the risk of postpartum hemorrhage and anemia: a hospital-based cohort study. J Thromb Haemost 2014; **12**:1986–1992.

39 Heller HM et al. Increased postpartum haemorrhage, the possible relation with serotonergic and other psychopharmacological drugs: a matched cohort study. BMC Pregnancy Childbirth 2017; **17**:166.

40 Singh I et al. Influence of pre-operative use of serotonergic antidepressants (SADs) on the risk of bleeding in patients undergoing different surgical interventions: a meta-analysis. Pharmacoepidemiol Drug Saf 2015; **24**:237–245.

41 Auerbach AD et al. Perioperative use of selective serotonin reuptake inhibitors and risks for adverse outcomes of surgery. JAMA Intern Med 2013; **173**:1075–1081.

42 Movig KL et al. Relationship of serotonergic antidepressants and need for blood transfusion in orthopedic surgical patients. Arch Intern Med 2003; **163**:2354–2358.

43 Liu B et al. Use of selective serotonin-reuptake inhibitors of tricyclic antidepressants and risk of hip fractures in elderly people. Lancet 1998; **351**:1303–1307.

44 Richards JB et al. Effect of selective serotonin reuptake inhibitors on the risk of fracture. Arch Intern Med 2007; **167**:188–194.

45 Leach MJ et al. The risk of hip fracture due to mirtazapine exposure when switching antidepressants or using other antidepressants as add-on therapy. Drugs Real World Outcomes 2017; **4**:247–255.

46 Gylvin SH et al. Psychopharmacologic treatment and blood transfusion in fast-track total hip and knee arthroplasty. Transfusion (Paris) 2017; **57**:971–976.

47 Andreasen JJ et al. Effect of selective serotonin reuptake inhibitors on requirement for allogeneic red blood cell transfusion following coronary artery bypass surgery. Am J Cardiovasc Drugs 2006; **6**:243–250.

48 Basile FV et al. Use of selective serotonin reuptake inhibitors antidepressants and bleeding risk in breast cosmetic surgery. Aesthetic Plast Surg 2013; **37**:561–566.

CHAPTER 3

49 Mahdanian AA et al. Serotonergic antidepressants and perioperative bleeding risk: a systematic review. Expert Opin Drug Saf 2014; 13:695–704.

50 Jeong BO et al. Use of serotonergic antidepressants and bleeding risk in patients undergoing surgery. Psychosomatics 2014; 55:213–220.

51 Mrkobrada M et al. Selective serotonin reuptake inhibitors and surgery: to hold or not to hold, that is the question: comment on "Perioperative use of selective serotonin reuptake inhibitors and risks for adverse outcomes of surgery". JAMA Intern Med 2013; 173: 1082–1083.

52 Perahia DG et al. The risk of bleeding with duloxetine treatment in patients who use nonsteroidal anti-inflammatory drugs (NSAIDs): analysis of placebo-controlled trials and post-marketing adverse event reports. Drug Healthc Patient Saf 2013; 5:211–219.

53 Na K-S et al. Can we recommend mirtazapine and bupropion for patients at risk for bleeding?: A systematic review and meta-analysis. J Affect Disord 2018; 225:221–226.

St John's wort

St John's wort (SJW) is the popular name for the plant *Hypericum perforatum*. It contains a combination of at least 10 different compounds, including hypericin, hyperforin and flavonoids.[1] Preparations of SJW are often unstandardised and this has complicated the interpretation of clinical trials. The active ingredient(s) and mechanism(s) of action of SJW are unclear.[1] Constituents of SJW may inhibit MAO, inhibit the reuptake of noradrenaline and serotonin, upregulate serotonin receptors and decrease serotonin receptor expression.[1]

Some preparations of SJW have been granted a traditional herbal registration certificate; note that this is based on traditional use rather than proven efficacy and tolerability. SJW is licensed in Germany for the treatment of depression.

Evidence for SJW in the treatment of depression

A number of trials have examined the efficacy of SJW in the treatment of depression. They have been extensively reviewed[2–5] and most authors conclude that SJW is likely to be effective in the treatment of mild–moderate depression,[2,4,5] for example Cochrane concludes that SJW is more effective than placebo in the treatment of mild–moderate depression, and is as effective as, and better tolerated than, standard antidepressants.[3] The supporting evidence is not without several limitations. Studies in German-speaking countries showed more favourable results than studies elsewhere.[3] Concerns have also been raised about the inadequate dosing of SSRIs in comparative studies.[6,7] In two reanalyses of data from a large negative randomised controlled trial (RCT) of SJW, both participant and clinician beliefs about treatment assignment were more strongly associated with clinical outcomes than the actual treatment received: those who guessed randomisation to active treatment fared better than those who guessed randomisation to placebo.[8,9] Efficacy in severe depression remains uncertain.[3–5]

It should be noted that:

- The active component of SJW for treating depression has not yet been determined. Trials used different preparations of SJW, most of which were standardised according to their total content of hypericins. However, evidence suggests that hypericins alone do not treat depression.[4]
- Published studies are generally acute treatment studies. There are only preliminary data to support the effectiveness of SJW in the medium term; longer-term and relapse prevention data are lacking.[10]

On balance, SJW should not be prescribed: we lack understanding of what the active ingredient is or what constitutes a therapeutic dose. Most preparations of SJW are unlicensed.

Adverse effects

St John's wort (SJW) appears to be well tolerated.[4,5] In a systematic review of existing studies, adverse effects were significantly less than with older antidepressants, slightly less than SSRIs and similar to placebo.[5] The most common, if infrequent, adverse effects are nausea, rash, fatigue, restlessness and photosensitivity.[11] Although severe photo-toxic reactions seem to be rare, patients should be informed that SJW can increase light sensitivity.[11] SJW may also share the propensity of SSRIs to increase the risk of bleeding; a case report describes prolonged epistaxis after nasal insertion of SJW.[12] In common with other antidepressant drugs, SJW has been known to precipitate hypomania in people with bipolar affective disorder.[13]

Drug interactions

St John's wort (SJW) is a potent inducer of intestinal and hepatic CYP3A4, CYP2C9, CYP2c39, CYP2E1 and intestinal p-glycoprotein.[11,14,15] Hyperforin is responsible for this effect.[16] The hyperforin content of SJW preparations varies 50-fold, which will result in a different propensity for drug interactions between brands. Preparations providing a daily dose of <1 mg hyperforin are less likely to induce CYP enzymes.[16] CYP3A4 activity is induced over 1–2 weeks and returns to normal approximately 7 days after SJW is discontinued.[17]

Studies have shown that SJW significantly reduces plasma concentrations of warfarin,[18] hormonal contraceptives,[19] digoxin and indinavir[11] (a drug used in the treatment of HIV). According to case reports, SJW has lowered the plasma concentrations of clozapine,[20] theophylline, ciclosporin, gliclazide and statins.[11,15,21] There is a theoretical risk that SJW may interact with some anticonvulsant drugs.[22] It has also been reported that SJW can increase the effects of clopidogrel (a prodrug).[23] Serotonin syndrome has been reported when SJW was taken together with sertraline, paroxetine, nefazodone and the triptans[22,24] (a group of serotonin agonists used to treat migraine). SJW should not be taken with any drugs that have a predominantly serotonergic action.

Many people regard herbal remedies as 'natural' and therefore harmless.[25] Many are not aware of the potential of such remedies for causing adverse effects or interacting with other drugs. A large study from Germany (n = 588), where SJW is a licensed antidepressant, found that for every prescription written for SJW, one person purchased SJW without seeking the advice of a doctor.[26] Many of these people had severe or persistent depression but few told their doctor that they took SJW. A small US study (n = 22) found that people tend to take SJW because it is easy to obtain alternative medicines

---

Box 3.1 St John's wort: key points that patients should know

- Evidence suggests that SJW may be effective in the treatment of mild to moderate depression, but we do not know enough about how much should be taken or what the adverse effects are. There is less evidence of benefit in severe depression.
- SJW is not a licensed medicine.
- SJW can interact with other medicines, resulting in serious adverse effects. Some important drugs may be metabolised more rapidly and therefore become ineffective with serious consequences (e.g. increased viral load in HIV, failure of oral contraceptives leading to unwanted pregnancy, reduced anticoagulant effect with warfarin leading to thrombosis).
- The symptoms of depression can sometimes be caused by other physical or mental illness. It is important that these possible causes are investigated.
- It is always best to consult the doctor if any herbal or natural remedy is being taken or the patient is thinking of taking one.

and also because they perceive herbal medicines as being purer and safer than prescription medicines. Few would discuss this medication with their conventional health-care provider.[27] Clinicians need to be proactive in asking patients if they use such treatments and try to dispel the myth that natural is the same as safe. Box 3.1 lists information that should be given to patients.

References

1 Velingkar VS et al. A current update on phytochemistry, pharmacology and herb–drug interactions of *Hypericum perforatum*. Phytochem Rev 2017; **16**:725–744.

2 National Institute for Health and Care Excellence. Depression in adults: recognition and management. Clinical Guideline 90, 2009; last updated April 2016. https://www.nice.org.uk/guidance/cg90

3 Linde K et al. St John's Wort for major depression. Cochrane Database Syst Rev 2008:CD000448.

4 Ng QX et al. Clinical use of Hypericum perforatum (St John's wort) in depression: a meta-analysis. J Affect Disord 2017; **210**:211–221.

5 Apaydin EA et al. A systematic review of St. John's wort for major depressive disorder. Syst Rev 2016; **5**:148.

6 Asher GN et al. Comparative benefits and harms of complementary and alternative medicine therapies for initial treatment of major depressive disorder: systematic review and meta-analysis. J Altern Complement Med 2017; **23**:907–919.

7 Gartlehner G et al. Pharmacological and non-pharmacological treatments for major depressive disorder: review of systematic reviews. BMJ Open 2017; **7**:e014912.

8 Chen JA et al. Association between patient beliefs regarding assigned treatment and clinical response: reanalysis of data from the Hypericum Depression Trial Study Group. J Clin Psychiatry 2011; **72**:1669–1676.

9 Chen JA et al. Association between physician beliefs regarding assigned treatment and clinical response: re-analysis of data from the Hypericum Depression Trial Study Group. Asian J Psychiatr 2015; **13**:23–29.

10 Cleare A et al. Evidence-based guidelines for treating depressive disorders with antidepressants: a revision of the 2008 British Association for Psychopharmacology guidelines. J Psychopharmacol 2015; **29**:459–525.

11 Russo E et al. Hypericum perforatum: pharmacokinetic, mechanism of action, tolerability, and clinical drug-drug interactions. Phytother Res 2014; **28**:643–655.

12 Crampsey DP et al. Nasal insertion of St John's wort: an unusual cause of epistaxis. J Laryngol Otol 2007; **121**:279–280.

13 Nierenberg AA et al. Mania associated with St. John's wort. Biol Psychiatry 1999; **46**:1707–1708.

14 Rahimi R et al. An update on the ability of St. John's wort to affect the metabolism of other drugs. Expert Opin Drug Metab Toxicol 2012; **8**:691–708.

15 Xu H et al. Effects of St John's wort and CYP2C9 genotype on the pharmacokinetics and pharmacodynamics of gliclazide. Br J Pharmacol 2008; **153**:1579–1586.

16 Chrubasik-Hausmann S et al. Understanding drug interactions with St John's wort (Hypericum perforatum L.): impact of hyperforin content. J Pharm Pharmacol 2018; doi: 10.1111/jphp.12858. [Epub ahead of print]

17 Imai H et al. The recovery time-course of CYP3A after induction by St John's wort administration. Br J Clin Pharmacol 2008; **65**:701–707.

18 Choi S et al. A systematic review of the pharmacokinetic and pharmacodynamic interactions of herbal medicine with warfarin. PLoS One 2017; **12**:e0182794.

19 Berry-Bibee EN et al. Co-administration of St. John's wort and hormonal contraceptives: a systematic review. Contraception 2016; **94**:668–677.

20 Van Strater AC et al. Interaction of St John's wort (Hypericum perforatum) with clozapine. Int Clin Psychopharmacol 2012; **27**:121–124.

21 Andren L et al. Interaction between a commercially available St. John's wort product (Movina) and atorvastatin in patients with hypercholesterolemia. Eur J Clin Pharmacol 2007; **63**:913–916.

22 Anon. Reminder: St John's Wort (*Hypericum perforatum*) interactions. Curr Probl Pharmacovigilance 2000; **26**:6–7.

23 Lau WC et al. The effect of St. John's Wort on the pharmacodynamic response of clopidogrel in hyporesponsive volunteers and patients: increased platelet inhibition by enhancement of CYP 3A4 metabolic activity. J Cardiovasc Pharmacol 2011; **57**:86–93.

24 Lantz MS et al. St. John's wort and antidepressant drug interactions in the elderly. J Geriatr Psychiatry Neurol 1999; **12**:7–10.

25 Barnes J et al. Different standards for reporting ADRs to herbal remedies and conventional OTC medicines: face-to-face interviews with 515 users of herbal remedies. Br J Clin Pharmacol 1998; **45**:496–500.

26 Linden M et al. Self medication with St. John's wort in depressive disorders: an observational study in community pharmacies. J Affect Disord 2008; **107**:205–210.

27 Wagner PJ et al. Taking the edge off: why patients choose St. John's Wort. J Fam Pract 1999; **48**:615–619.

Antidepressants: relative adverse effects – a rough guide

Table 3.23 gives a very approximate view of the absolute and relative risk of a small range of adverse effects associated with antidepressants. In some cases further details can be found in specific sections in this chapter.

Table 3.23 Common adverse effects of antidepressants

Drug	Sedation	Postural hypotension	Cardiac conduction disturbance	Anticholinergic effects	Nausea/ vomiting	Sexual dysfunction
Tricyclics						
Amitriptyline	+++	+++	+++	+++	+	+++
Clomipramine	++	+++	+++	++	++	+++
Dosulepin	+++	+++	+++	++	+	+
Doxepin	+++	++	+++	+++	+	+
Imipramine	++	+++	+++	+++	+	+
Lofepramine	+	+	+	++	+	+
Nortriptyline	+	++	++	+	+	+
Trimipramine	+++	+++	++	++	+	+
Other antidepressants						
Agomelatine	+	–	–	–	–	–
Duloxetine (SNRI)	–	–*	–	–	++	++
Levomilnacipran (SNRI)	–	–*	–	–	++	++
Mianserin	++	–	–	–	–	–
Mirtazapine	+++	+	–	+	+	–
Reboxetine	+	–	–	+	+	+
Trazodone	+++	+	+	+	+	+
Venlafaxine (SNRI)	–	–*	+	–	+++	+++
Selective serotonin reuptake inhibitors (SSRIs)						
Citalopram	–	–	+	–	++	+++
Escitalopram	–	–	+	–	++	+++
Fluoxetine	–	–	–	–	++	+++
Fluvoxamine	+	–	–	–	+++	+++
Paroxetine	+	–	–	+	++	+++
Sertraline	–	–	–	–	++	+++
Vilazodone	–	–	–?	–	++	++
Vortioxetine	–	+	–	–	++	+

Table 3.23 (*Continued*)

Drug	Sedation	Postural hypotension	Cardiac conduction disturbance	Anticholinergic effects	Nausea/ vomiting	Sexual dysfunction
Monoamine oxidase inhibitors (MAOIs)						
Isocarboxazid	+	++	+	++	+	+
Phenelzine	+	+	+	+	+	+
Tranylcypromine	–	+	+	+	+	+
Reversible inhibitor of monoamine oxidase A (RIMA)						
Moclobemide	–	–	–	–	+	+

+++, high incidence/severity; ++, moderate; +, low; – very low/none.
*Hypertension reported.

Anxiety spectrum disorders

Anxiety is a normal emotion that is experienced by everyone at some time. Symptoms can be psychological, physical or a mixture of both. Intervention is required when symptoms become excessively distressing or disabling, or reduce quality of life, in the context of the absence of any clear external threat.

There are several disorders within the overall spectrum of anxiety disorders, each with its own characteristic symptoms. These are outlined briefly in Boxes 3.2, 3.3, 3.4, 3.5 and 3.6 at the end of this section.

Anxiety disorders can occur on their own, be co-morbid with other psychiatric disorders (particularly depression), be a consequence of physical illness such as thyrotoxicosis

---

Box 3.2 Generalised anxiety disorder

Clinical presentation
- Excessive and uncontrollable worry
- Motor tension, restlessness, irritability
- Somatic symptoms (e.g. hyperventilation, tachycardia and sweating)
- GAD is often co-morbid with major depression, panic disorder or OCD
- 12-month prevalence 1.7–3.4%

Drug	Comment
Crisis management	
Benzodiazepines	Normally for short-term use only: max. 2–4 weeks, although some are of the opinion that risks are overstated[35]
First-line drug treatment (in order of preference)[25]	
SSRIs (up to maximum licensed dose)	May initially exacerbate symptoms. A lower starting dose is recommended. Fluoxetine and sertraline are preferred options[11]
SNRIs (up to maximum licensed dose)	May initially exacerbate symptoms. A lower starting dose is recommended
Pregabalin 150–600 mg/day in divided doses	Response may be seen in the first week of treatment[36]
Second-line drug treatment (less well tolerated or weak evidence base, no order of preference)	
Agomelatine 10–50 mg/day[37,38]	10 mg tablets are not available in the UK. Agomelatine has been shown to prevent relapse over a 6-month period[39]
Beta blockers Propranolol 40–120 mg/day in divided doses	Initiate at 40 mg and titrate dose up to effect if needed. Useful for somatic symptoms, particularly tachycardia[40]
Buspirone 15–60 mg/day in divided doses	Has a delayed onset of action, takes up to 6 weeks to show equal efficacy with benzodiazepines[41]
Hydroxyzine 50–100 mg/day in divided doses	It is unclear whether hydroxyzine's efficacy is due to an anxiolytic effect or a sedative effect[42]
Quetiapine (MR, 50–300 mg)	Recommended as monotherapy. Probably not effective as adjunctive therapy to SSRI/SNRI in treatment resistance[43]

Box 3.2 (*Continued*)

Drug	Comment
Tricyclic antidepressants Clomipramine 50–250 mg/day[44–46] Imipramine 75–200 mg/day in divided doses[47]	Initiate clomipramine at 10 mg/day and increase the dose gradually Initiate imipramine 25 mg every 4 days; when at 100 mg can increase in 50 mg increments[9]
MAOI Phenelzine 45–90 mg/day in divided doses[48]	For mixed anxiety and depressive states. Patients need to avoid food high in tyramine
Mirtazapine 15–30 mg nocte[49,50]	
Vortioxetine 2.5–10 mg[51]	Standardised mean difference = −0.118, i.e. small effect size. Greater benefit for patients with severe GAD, HAMA ≥25
Experimental	
Chamomile 220–1500 mg/day	Two RCTs, one positive, one negative, using standardised doses of chamomile and placebo[52]
Gingko biloba 240–480 mg/day	One positive RCT using two standardised doses of *Gingko biloba* and placebo[53]
Lavender oil preparation 80–160 mg/day	One positive RCT using standardised doses of lavender oil compared to placebo and paroxetine[54]
Riluzole 50–100 mg/day doses[55]	Liver function monitoring required
Non-drug treatments[25,56]	

- Applied relaxation
- CBT
- Exercise

CBT, cognitive behavioural therapy; GAD, generalised anxiety disorder; HAMA, Hamilton Anxiety Rating Scale; MAOI, monoamine oxidase inhibitor; MR, modified release; RCT, randomised controlled trial; SNRI, serotonin–noradrenaline reuptake inhibitor; SSRI, selective serotonin reuptake inhibitor; TCA, tricyclic antidepressant.

or be drug induced (e.g. by caffeine). Co-morbidity with other psychiatric disorders is very common.

Anxiety spectrum disorders tend to be chronic and treatment is often only partially successful. People with anxiety disorders may be especially prone to adverse effects.[1] High initial doses of SSRIs in particular may be poorly tolerated.

Benzodiazepines

Benzodiazepines provide rapid symptomatic relief from acute anxiety states.[2] All guidelines and consensus statements recommend that this group of drugs should be used only to treat anxiety that is severe, disabling or subjecting the individual to extreme distress. Because of their potential to cause physical dependence and withdrawal symptoms,

Box 3.3 Panic disorder

Clinical presentation
- Sudden unpredictable episodes of severe anxiety, usually 30–45 minutes in duration
- Shortness of breath and other autonomic symptoms
- Fear of suffocation/dying
- Urgent desire to flee
- 12-month prevalence 1.8%

Drug	Comment
Crisis management	
Benzodiazepines	Rapid effect although panic symptoms return quickly if the drug is withdrawn.[57] NICE does not recommend[5]
First-line drug treatment (in order of preference)[5,58]	
SSRIs (up to maximum licensed dose)	Therapeutic effect can be delayed (this applies to all antidepressants[59]) and patients can experience an initial exacerbation of panic symptoms[5]
Venlafaxine MR 75–225 mg[58]	Initiate at 37.5 mg for 7 days
Second-line treatment (less well tolerated or weak evidence base, no order of preference)	
Mirtazapine 15–60 mg/day[60]	A meta-analysis suggests that mirtazapine does not help with panic symptoms but with the anxiety associated with this disorder[58]
Moclobemide 300–600 mg/day[61]	One fixed dose study of 450 mg and one flexible dose study suggest efficacy[61,62]
MAOIs Phenelzine 10–60 mg/day[59]	No long-term studies, reserve for treatment-resistant cases due to poor tolerability[59]
Tricyclic antidepressants Clomipramine 25–250 mg/day[59] Desipramine 50–300 mg/day[63] Imipramine 25–300 mg/day[59] Lofepramine 70–140 mg/day in divided doses[64]	Start with a low dose and increase dose according to response and tolerability
Experimental	
D-cycloserine 50 mg/day	A DB-RCT suggests acceleration of treatment response to CBT but this advantage is lost at follow-up[65]
Gabapentin 600–3600 mg/day	One DB-RCT showed no difference between gabapentin and placebo. However, significant improvement was demonstrated in the more severely ill[66]
Inositol 12 g/day[67]	One positive DB-PCT in 21 patients
Pindolol 7.5 mg/day	Efficacy suggested in a small 21-patient DB-PCT where pindolol 2.5 mg tds was used to augment fluoxetine in treatment-resistant panic disorder[68]
Valproate 500–2250 mg/day	Two very small positive open studies[69,70]
Non-drug treatments	

- CBT
- Anxiety management, including relaxation training

CBT, cognitive behavioural therapy; DB-PCT, double-blinded placebo controlled trial; DB-RCT, double-blinded randomised controlled trial; MAOI, monoamine oxidase inhibitor; MR, modified release; tds, *ter die sumendum* (three times a day).

Box 3.4 Post-traumatic stress disorder

Clinical presentation
- Exposure to a traumatic event
- Emotional numbness or detachment
- Intrusive flashbacks or vivid dreams
- Disabling fear of re-exposure causing avoidance of perceived similar situations
- 12-month prevalence 1.1–2.9%

Drug	Comment
First-line drug treatment (in order of preference)	
SSRIs (up to maximum licensed doses)	Paroxetine, sertraline or fluoxetine are the preferred SSRIs[71,72]
Venlafaxine modified release 37.5–300 mg[73]	
Second-line treatment (less well tolerated or weak evidence base, no order of preference)	
Antipsychotics Olanzapine 5–20 mg	Antipsychotics have been found to be effective for the intrusion symptoms (flashbacks and nightmares) but not the avoidance and hyperarousal symptoms of PTSD. Studies done as monotherapy or as adjunctive treatment.[74] Most studies done with risperidone, which suggest lower doses of risperidone are effective
Risperidone 0.5–6 mg	
Quetiapine 50–800 mg[75]	
Mirtazapine 15–45 mg/day[76]	Mirtazapine is recommended by NICE[77]
MAOI Phenelzine 15–75 mg/day[78]	Phenelzine is recommended by NICE[77]
Prazosin 2–15 mg nocte[79]	For nightmares and sleep disturbances. Initiate at 1 mg nocte and titrate dose gradually to reduce the risk of hypotension
Tricyclic antidepressants Amitriptyline 50–300 mg/day[80] Imipramine 50–300 mg/day	Amitriptyline is recommended by NICE.[77] For all TCAs start at a low dose and increase dose according to tolerability
Experimental	
Duloxetine 60–120 mg	Two small open studies suggest efficacy. Start at 30 mg for 1 week[81,82]
Lamotrigine up to 500 mg/day	Small double-blind study in 15 patients[83]
Phenytoin plasma concentration 10–20 ng/mL[84]	Open-label study in 12 patients
Valproate up to 2.5 g[85]	A meta-analysis conducted by Adamou et al. found no DB-RCT for valproate in PTSD
IV Ketamine[86]	Rapid reduction in symptom severity suggested
Non-drug treatments	

- Eye movement desensitisation and reprocessing (EMDR)
- Trauma-focused CBT

CBT, cognitive behavioural therapy; DB-RCT, double-blinded randomised controlled trial; IV, intravenous; PTSD, post-traumatic stress disorder; SSRI, selective serotonin reuptake inhibitor; TCA, tricyclic antidepressant.

CHAPTER 3

Box 3.5 Obsessive compulsive disorder

Clinical presentation
- Obsessional thinking (e.g. constantly thinking the door has been left unlocked)
- Compulsive behaviour (e.g. constantly going back to check)
- 12-month prevalence 0.7%

Drug	Comments
First-line drug treatment (in order of preference)	
Any SSRI[32] (up to maximum licensed dose)	If the first SSRI is not tolerated or has a poor response an alternative SSRI may be tried[25]
Clomipramine (up to 250 mg)	Owing to poorer tolerability it is recommended to try at least one SSRI first[25]
Second-line drug treatment (unlicensed and weak evidence base)	
Add antipsychotic to SSRI (low to moderate doses of antipsychotics used in studies)[87,88]	Most evidence supports the use of aripiprazole or risperidone.[87] Some evidence for haloperidol[88]
Citalopram 40 mg with clomipramine 150 mg	Based on small randomised open-label study.[89] Recommended by NICE.[25] ECG monitoring required
Acetylcysteine up to 2400 mg/day added to SSRI or clomipramine	Two positive studies and one negative.[90–92] Gastrointestinal adverse effects may be problematic
Lamotrigine 100 mg added to SSRI[93]	Lamotrigine dose must be titrated up gradually as indicated in the SPC
Topiramate up to 400 mg added to SSRI[94,95]	Topiramate is not well tolerated. There are suggested benefits to compulsion but not obsessions.[94] One trial found topiramate ineffective[96]
Experimental	
High-dose SSRI (above UK SPC doses) Escitalopram 25–50 mg[97] Sertraline 250–400 mg[98]	Dose titrated up gradually according to tolerability. ECG monitoring recommended
Memantine 20 mg with fluvoxamine 200 mg[99]	One small double-blind randomised trial done over 8 weeks
SNRIs Venlafaxine up to 375 mg[100] Duloxetine 60 mg[101]	
Mirtazapine 30–60 mg[102]	Small trial in 30 patients
5-HT$_3$ antagonists Granisetron 1 mg with fluvoxamine 200 mg[103] Ondansetron 4 mg with fluoxetine 20 mg[104]	Small double-blind placebo-controlled trial for each drug Unpublished studies suggest no effect

Box 3.5 (Continued)	

Drug	Comments
Riluzole 50 mg bd added to existing drug treatment[105]	Open-label trial in 13 patients
Anti-androgen Triptorelin 3.75 mg IM every 4 weeks added to existing drug treatment[106]	Open-label study done in 6 men
IV treatment	Quicker onset of action suggested compared with oral treatments
Clomipramine IV[107]	One study suggests clomipramine IV efficacy after failure with oral clomipramine
Ketamine IV[108,109]	One positive and one negative small study
Once-weekly morphine 15–45 mg added to existing drug treatment[110]	Small study involving 23 treatment-resistant patients. Positive effects were transient
Non-drug treatments	

- CBT
- Exposure and response prevention therapy
- Surgery

bd, *bis die* (twice a day); CBT, cognitive behavioural therapy; ECG, electrocardiogram; IM, intramuscular; IV, intravenous; NICE, National Institute for Health and Care Excellence; SPC, summary of product characteristics; SSRI, selective serotonin reuptake inhibitor.

these drugs should be used at the lowest effective dose for the shortest period of time (maximum 4 weeks), while medium-/long-term treatment strategies are put in place and with caution in patients with substance misuse. For the majority of patients these recommendations are sensible and should be adhered to. A very small number of patients with severely disabling anxiety may benefit from long-term treatment with a benzodiazepine and these patients should not be denied treatment. Benzodiazepines are, however, known to be over-prescribed in the long term for treatment of both anxiety[3] and depression,[4] usually in place of more appropriate treatment.

NICE recommends that benzodiazepines should not be used to treat panic disorder.[5] In other countries, alprazolam is widely used for this indication. Benzodiazepines should be used with care in post-traumatic stress disorder (PTSD).[6]

SSRIs/SNRIs

When used to treat **generalised anxiety disorder (GAD)**, SSRIs should initially be prescribed at half the normal starting dose for the treatment of depression and the dose titrated upwards into the normal antidepressant dosage range as tolerated (initial worsening of anxiety may be seen when treatment is started[7]). The same advice applies to the use of venlafaxine and duloxetine. Modest benefit is usually seen within 6 weeks and

Box 3.6 Social phobia (also known as social anxiety disorder)

Clinical presentation
- Extreme fear of social situations, e.g. eating in public or public speaking
- Fear of humiliation or embarrassment
- Avoidant behaviour, e.g. never eating in restaurants
- Anxious anticipation, e.g. feeling sick on entering a restaurant
- 12-month prevalence 2.3%

Drug	Comments
First-line drug treatment[111] (in order of preference)	
SSRIs (up to maximum licensed dose)	If no response to the first SSRI, try an alternative SSRI
Venlafaxine modified release 75–225 mg/day	
Second-line drug treatment (less well tolerated or weak evidence base, no order of preference)	
Atypical antipsychotics Olanzapine 5–20 mg[112]	Few studies with antipsychotics. Most evidence with olanzapine
Beta blockers Atenolol 25–100 mg/day	Reduces autonomic symptoms in performance situations[112]
Benzodiazepines Clonazepam 0.3–6 mg/day[112]	Benzodiazepines are helpful on a prn basis. Most evidence for treatment found with clonazepam and bromazepam
Sertraline plus clonazepam up to 3 mg/day[113]	Switching an SSRI to venlafaxine no more effective than adding clonazepam to SSRI[113]
Gabapentin 900–3600 mg/day[112]	
Levetiracetam 300–3000 mg/day in divided doses[114]	
Moclobemide 600 mg/day in divided doses	Initiate at 300 mg/day in divided doses. Moclobemide has a UK licence for social phobia. Recommended by NICE[111]
Phenelzine 15–90 mg/day[115]	Avoidance of tyramine-rich food important Recommended by NICE[111]
Pregabalin 150–600 mg/day[112]	600 mg/day found to be superior to placebo[112]
Experimental	
Topiramate 25–400 mg/day[116]	Small open-label study of 23 patients suggests efficacy but poorly tolerated
Valproate 500–2500 mg/day[117]	Small open-label study of 17 patients suggests efficacy
Non-drug treatments	
- CBT - Exposure therapy	

CBT, cognitive behavioural therapy; NICE, National Institute for Health and Care Excellence; prn, *pro re nata* (as required); SSRI, selective serotonin reuptake inhibitor.

continues to increase over time.[8] The optimal duration of treatment has not been determined but should be at least 1 year.[9,10] Effective treatment of GAD may prevent the development of major depression.[9] Fluoxetine is probably the most effective SSRI in GAD, and sertraline the best tolerated.[11]

When used to treat **panic disorder**, the same starting dose and dosage titration as in GAD should be used. Doses of clomipramine,[12] citalopram[13] and sertraline[14] towards the bottom of the antidepressant range give the best balance between efficacy and adverse effects, whereas higher doses of paroxetine (40 mg and above) may be required.[15] Higher doses of all drugs may be effective when standard doses have failed. Onset of action may be as long as 6 weeks. Women may respond better than men to SSRIs.[16] There is some evidence that augmentation with clonazepam leads to a more rapid response (but not a greater magnitude of response overall).[15] The optimal duration of treatment is unknown, but should be at least 8 months.[17] A large naturalistic study showed convincing evidence of benefit for at least 3 years.[18] Less than half are likely to remain well after medication is withdrawn.[19]

Lower starting doses are also required in **PTSD**, although high doses (e.g. fluoxetine 60 mg) are usually required for full effect. Response is usually seen within 8 weeks, but can take up to 12 weeks.[19] Treatment should be continued for at least 6 months and probably longer.[10,20,21]

Although the doses of SSRIs licensed for the treatment of **obsessive compulsive disorder (OCD)** are higher than those licensed for the treatment of depression (e.g. fluoxetine 60 mg, paroxetine 40–60 mg), lower (standard antidepressant) doses may be effective, particularly for maintenance treatment.[22] Initial response is usually slower to emerge than in depression (can take 10–12 weeks). The dose should be increased to gain maximal benefit. Treatment should continue for at least 1 year.[10] The relapse rate in those who continue treatment for 2 years is half that of those who stop treatment after initial response (25–40% vs 80%).[23] In most people with OCD, the condition is persistent and symptom severity fluctuates over time.[24] Second-line treatment is usually the addition of either risperidone or aripiprazole.

Body dysmorphic disorder (BDD) should be treated initially with CBT. If symptoms are moderate to severe, adding an SSRI may improve outcome.[25] Buspirone may usefully augment the SSRI,[25] although no RCT has been conducted.

Standard antidepressant starting doses are well tolerated in **social phobia**.[26,27] Dosage titration may benefit some patients but is not always required. Some benefit is usually seen within 8 weeks and treatment should be continued for at least a year and probably longer.[27]

NICE recommends CBT as first-line treatment for social anxiety.[28]

All patients treated with SSRIs should be monitored for the development of akathisia, increased anxiety and the emergence of suicidal ideation; the risk is thought to be greatest in those <30 years, those with co-morbid depression and those already known to be at higher risk of suicide.[25,29]

SSRIs should not be stopped abruptly as patients with anxiety spectrum disorders are particularly sensitive to discontinuation symptoms (see section on 'Antidepressant discontinuation symptoms' in this chapter). The dose should be reduced slowly as tolerated over several weeks to months.

CHAPTER 3

Pregabalin

Pregabalin is licensed for the treatment of GAD. Several large RCTs have demonstrated its efficacy and tolerability and comparable speed of onset of action to a benzodiazepine.[30] The dose of pregabalin in GAD is initially 150 mg, increased gradually to a maximum of 600 mg in 2–3 divided doses. Pregabalin should not be stopped abruptly as it may precipitate seizures.

Psychological approaches

There is good evidence to support the efficacy of some psychological interventions in anxiety spectrum disorders.[10,31] Examples include exposure therapy in OCD and social phobia. Initial drug therapy may be required to help the patient become more receptive to psychological input although evidence to support this assumption is slim. Some studies suggest that optimal outcome is achieved by combining psychological and drug therapies,[5,32] but negative studies also exist.[33,34] Combined treatment should not be withheld, however, in severe and disabling conditions.

A discussion of the evidence base for psychological interventions is outside the scope of these guidelines. It is recognised that for many patients psychological therapies are an appropriate first-line treatment, and indeed this is supported by NICE.[5]

Summary of NICE guidelines for the treatment of generalised anxiety disorder,[5] panic disorder[5] and OCD[25]

- A 'stepped care' approach is recommended to help in choosing the most effective intervention.
- A comprehensive assessment is recommended that considers the degree of distress and functional impairment; the effect of any co-morbid mental illness, substance misuse or medical condition; and past response to treatment.
- Treat the primary disorder first.
- Psychological therapy is more effective than pharmacological therapy and should be used as first line where possible. Details of the types of therapy recommended and their duration can be found in the NICE guidelines.
- Pharmacological therapy is also effective. Most evidence supports the use of the SSRIs (sertraline as first line).
- Provide verbal and written information on the likely benefits and disadvantages of each mode of treatment.
- Consider combination therapy for complex anxiety disorders that are refractory to treatment.

Panic disorder

- Benzodiazepines should not be used.
- An SSRI should be used as first line. If SSRIs are contraindicated or there is no response, imipramine or clomipramine can be used.
- Self-help (based on CBT principles) should be encouraged, as should formal CBT.

Generalised anxiety disorder

- Benzodiazepines should not be used beyond 2–4 weeks.
- An SSRI should be used as first-line treatment.
- SNRIs and pregabalin are alternative choices.
- High-intensity psychological intervention and self-help (based on CBT principles) should be encouraged.

OCD (where there is moderate or severe functional impairment)

- Use an SSRI or intensive CBT.
- Combine the SSRI and CBT if response to a single strategy is suboptimal.
- Use clomipramine if SSRIs fail.
- If response is still suboptimal, add an antipsychotic or combine clomipramine and citalopram.

References

1 Nash JR et al. Pharmacotherapy of anxiety. Handb Exp Pharmacol 2005:469–501.
2 Martin JL et al. Benzodiazepines in generalized anxiety disorder: heterogeneity of outcomes based on a systematic review and meta-analysis of clinical trials. J Psychopharmacol 2007; **21**:774–782.
3 Benitez CI et al. Use of benzodiazepines and selective serotonin reuptake inhibitors in middle-aged and older adults with anxiety disorders: a longitudinal and prospective study. Am J Geriatr Psychiatry 2008; **16**:5–13.
4 Demyttenaere K et al. Clinical factors influencing the prescription of antidepressants and benzodiazepines: results from the European study of the epidemiology of mental disorders (ESEMeD). J Affect Disord 2008; **110**:84–93.
5 National Institute for Health and Care Excellence. Generalised anxiety disorder and panic disorder in adults: management. Clinical Guideline **113**, 2011. http://guidance.nice.org.uk/CG113
6 Davidson JR. Use of benzodiazepines in social anxiety disorder, generalized anxiety disorder, and posttraumatic stress disorder. J Clin Psychiatry 2004; **65** Suppl 5:29–33.
7 Scott A et al. Antidepressant drugs in the treatment of anxiety disorders. Adv Psychiatr Treat 2001; **7**:275–282.
8 Ballenger JC. Remission rates in patients with anxiety disorders treated with paroxetine. J Clin Psychiatry 2004; **65**:1696–1707.
9 Davidson JR et al. A psychopharmacological treatment algorithm for generalised anxiety disorder (GAD). J Psychopharmacol 2010; **24**:3–26.
10 Baldwin DS et al. Evidence-based pharmacological treatment of anxiety disorders, post-traumatic stress disorder and obsessive-compulsive disorder: a revision of the 2005 guidelines from the British Association for Psychopharmacology. J Psychopharmacol 2014; **28**:403–439.
11 Baldwin D et al. Efficacy of drug treatments for generalised anxiety disorder: systematic review and meta-analysis. BMJ 2011; **342**:d1199.
12 Caillard V et al. Comparative effects of low and high doses of clomipramine and placebo in panic disorder: a double-blind controlled study. French University Antidepressant Group. Acta Psychiatr Scand 1999; **99**:51–58.
13 Wade AG et al. The effect of citalopram in panic disorder. Br J Psychiatry 1997; **170**:549–553.
14 Londborg PD et al. Sertraline in the treatment of panic disorder. A multi-site, double-blind, placebo-controlled, fixed-dose investigation. Br J Psychiatry 1998; **173**:54–60.
15 Pollack MH et al. Combined paroxetine and clonazepam treatment strategies compared to paroxetine monotherapy for panic disorder. J Psychopharmacol 2003; **17**:276–282.
16 Clayton AH et al. Sex differences in clinical presentation and response in panic disorder: pooled data from sertraline treatment studies. Arch Womens Ment Health 2006; **9**:151–157.
17 Rickels K et al. Panic disorder: long-term pharmacotherapy and discontinuation. J Clin Psychopharmacol 1998; **18**:12S–18S.
18 Choy Y et al. Three-year medication prophylaxis in panic disorder: to continue or discontinue? A naturalistic study. Compr Psychiatry 2007; **48**:419–425.
19 Michelson D et al. Continuing treatment of panic disorder after acute response: randomised, placebo-controlled trial with fluoxetine. The Fluoxetine Panic Disorder Study Group. Br J Psychiatry 1999; **174**:213–218.
20 Davidson J et al. Efficacy of sertraline in preventing relapse of posttraumatic stress disorder: results of a 28-week double-blind, placebo-controlled study. Am J Psychiatry 2001; **158**:1974–1981.
21 Stein DJ et al. Pharmacotherapy for post traumatic stress disorder (PTSD). Cochrane Database Syst Rev 2006:CD002795.
22 Martenyi F et al. Fluoxetine v. placebo in prevention of relapse in post-traumatic stress disorder. Br J Psychiatry 2002; **181**:315–320.
23 The Expert Consensus Panel for obsessive-compulsive disorder. Treatment of obsessive-compulsive disorder. J Clin Psychiatry 1997; **58** Suppl 4:2–72.

CHAPTER 3

24 Catapano F et al. Obsessive-compulsive disorder: a 3-year prospective follow-up study of patients treated with serotonin reuptake inhibitors OCD follow-up study. J Psychiatr Res 2006; 40:502–510.

25 National Institute for Health and Care Excellence. Obsessive-compulsive disorder and body dysmorphic disorder: treatment. Clinical Guideline 31, 2005. https://www.nice.org.uk/guidance/cg31

26 Blomhoff S et al. Randomised controlled general practice trial of sertraline, exposure therapy and combined treatment in generalised social phobia. Br J Psychiatry 2001; 179:23–30.

27 Hood SD, Nutt DJ. Psychopharmacological treatments: an overview. In: Crozier WR, ed. *International Handbook of Social Anxiety Concepts, Research and Interventions Relating to the Self and Shyness*. Oxford: John Wiley and Sons Ltd; 2001.

28 Mayo-Wilson E et al. Psychological and pharmacological interventions for social anxiety disorder in adults: a systematic review and network meta-analysis. Lancet Psychiatry 2014; 1:368–376.

29 National Institute for Health and Care Excellence. Depression in adults: recognition and management. Clinical Guideline 90, 2009; last updated April 2016. https://www.nice.org.uk/guidance/cg90

30 Pollack MH. Refractory generalized anxiety disorder. J Clin Psychiatry 2009; 70 Suppl 2:32–38.

31 Roberts NP et al. Early psychological interventions to treat acute traumatic stress symptoms. Cochrane Database Syst Rev 2010:CD007944.

32 Skapinakis P et al. Pharmacological and psychotherapeutic interventions for management of obsessive-compulsive disorder in adults: a systematic review and network meta-analysis. Lancet Psychiatry 2016; 3:730–739.

33 van Apeldoorn FJ et al. Is a combined therapy more effective than either CBT or SSRI alone? Results of a multicenter trial on panic disorder with or without agoraphobia. Acta Psychiatr Scand 2008; 117:260–270.

34 Marcus SM et al. A comparison of medication side effect reports by panic disorder patients with and without concomitant cognitive behavior therapy. Am J Psychiatry 2007; 164:273–275.

35 Offidani E et al. Efficacy and tolerability of benzodiazepines versus antidepressants in anxiety disorders: a systematic review and meta-analysis. Psychother Psychosom 2013; 82:355–362.

36 Generoso MB et al. Pregabalin for generalized anxiety disorder: an updated systematic review and meta-analysis. Int Clin Psychopharmacol 2017; 32:49–55.

37 Stein DJ et al. Efficacy and safety of agomelatine (10 or 25 mg/day) in non-depressed out-patients with generalized anxiety disorder: a 12-week, double-blind, placebo-controlled study. Eur Neuropsychopharmacol 2017; 27:526–537.

38 Stein DJ et al. Agomelatine in generalized anxiety disorder: an active comparator and placebo-controlled study. J Clin Psychiatry 2014; 75:362–368.

39 Stein DJ et al. Agomelatine prevents relapse in generalized anxiety disorder: a 6-month randomized, double-blind, placebo-controlled discontinuation study. J Clin Psychiatry 2012; 73:1002–1008.

40 Hayes PE et al. Beta-blockers in anxiety disorders. J Affect Disord 1987; 13:119–130.

41 Chessick CA et al. Azapirones for generalized anxiety disorder. Cochrane Database Syst Rev 2006:CD006115.

42 Guaiana G et al. Hydroxyzine for generalised anxiety disorder. Cochrane Database Syst Rev 2010:CD006815.

43 Khan A et al. Extended-release quetiapine fumarate (quetiapine XR) as adjunctive therapy in patients with generalized anxiety disorder and a history of inadequate treatment response: a randomized, double-blind study. Ann Clin Psychiatry 2014; 26:3–18.

44 Wingerson D et al. Clomipramine treatment for generalized anxiety disorder. J Clin Psychopharmacol 1992; 12:214–215.

45 den Boer JA et al. Effect of serotonin uptake inhibitors in anxiety disorders; a double-blind comparison of clomipramine and fluvoxamine. Int Clin Psychopharmacol 1987; 2:21–32.

46 Kahn RS et al. Effect of a serotonin precursor and uptake inhibitor in anxiety disorders; a double-blind comparison of 5-hydroxytryptophan, clomipramine and placebo. Int Clin Psychopharmacol 1987; 2:33–45.

47 Rickels K et al. Antidepressants for the treatment of generalized anxiety disorder. A placebo-controlled comparison of imipramine, trazodone, and diazepam. Arch Gen Psychiatry 1993; 50:884–895.

48 Robinson DS et al. The monoamine oxidase inhibitor, phenelzine, in the treatment of depressive-anxiety states. A controlled clinical trial. Arch Gen Psychiatry 1973; 29:407–413.

49 Gambi F et al. Mirtazapine treatment of generalized anxiety disorder: a fixed dose, open label study. J Psychopharmacol 2005; 19:483–487.

50 Sitsen JMA et al. Mirtazapine, a novel antidepressant, in the treatment of anxiety symptoms. Drug Invest 1994; 8:339–344.

51 Pae CU et al. Vortioxetine, a multimodal antidepressant for generalized anxiety disorder: a systematic review and meta-analysis. J Psychiatr Res 2015; 64:88–98.

52 Amsterdam JD et al. A randomized, double-blind, placebo-controlled trial of oral Matricaria recutita (chamomile) extract therapy for generalized anxiety disorder. J Clin Psychopharmacol 2009; 29:378–382.

53 Woelk H et al. Ginkgo biloba special extract EGb 761 in generalized anxiety disorder and adjustment disorder with anxious mood: a randomized, double-blind, placebo-controlled trial. J Psychiatr Res 2007; 41:472–480.

54 Kasper S et al. Lavender oil preparation Silexan is effective in generalized anxiety disorder – a randomized, double-blind comparison to placebo and paroxetine. Int J Neuropsychopharmacol 2014; 17:859–869.

55 Mathew SJ et al. Open-label trial of riluzole in generalized anxiety disorder. Am J Psychiatry 2005; 162:2379–2381.

56 Jayakody K et al. Exercise for anxiety disorders: systematic review. Br J Sports Med 2014; 48:187–196.

57 Otto MW et al. Discontinuation of benzodiazepine treatment: efficacy of cognitive-behavioral therapy for patients with panic disorder. Am J Psychiatry 1993; 150:1485–1490.

58 Andrisano C et al. Newer antidepressants and panic disorder: a meta-analysis. Int Clin Psychopharmacol 2013; 28:33–45.

59 Batelaan NM et al. Evidence-based pharmacotherapy of panic disorder: an update. Int J Neuropsychopharmacol 2012; 15:403–415.

60 Boshuisen ML et al. The effect of mirtazapine in panic disorder: an open label pilot study with a single-blind placebo run-in period. Int Clin Psychopharmacol 2001; 16:363–368.

61 Tiller JW et al. Moclobemide for anxiety disorders: a focus on moclobemide for panic disorder. Int Clin Psychopharmacol 1997; **12** Suppl 6:S27–S30.

62 Kruger MB et al. The efficacy and safety of moclobemide compared to clomipramine in the treatment of panic disorder. Eur Arch Psychiatry Clin Neurosci 1999; **249** Suppl 1:S19–S24.

63 Kalus O et al. Desipramine treatment in panic disorder. J Affect Disord 1991; **21**:239–244.

64 Fahy TJ et al. The Galway Study of Panic Disorder. I: Clomipramine and lofepramine in DSM III-R panic disorder: a placebo controlled trial. J Affect Disord 1992; **25**:63–75.

65 Otto MW et al. Randomized trial of D-cycloserine enhancement of cognitive-behavioral therapy for panic disorder. Depress Anxiety 2016; **33**:737–745.

66 Pande AC et al. Placebo-controlled study of gabapentin treatment of panic disorder. J Clin Psychopharmacol 2000; **20**:467–471.

67 Benjamin J et al. Double-blind, placebo-controlled, crossover trial of inositol treatment for panic disorder. Am J Psychiatry 1995; **152**:1084–1086.

68 Hirschmann S, et al. Pindolol augmentation in patients with treatment-resistant panic disorder: a double-blind, placebo-controlled trial. J Clin Psychopharmacol 2000; **20**:556–559.

69 Woodman CL et al. Panic disorder: treatment with valproate. J Clin Psychiatry 1994; **55**:134–136.

70 Primeau F et al. Valproic acid and panic disorder. Can J Psychiatry 1990; **35**:248–250.

71 Hoskins M et al. Pharmacotherapy for post-traumatic stress disorder: systematic review and meta-analysis. Br J Psychiatry 2015; **206**:93–100.

72 Lee DJ et al. Psychotherapy versus pharmacotherapy for posttraumatic stress disorder: systematic review and meta-analyses to determine first-line treatments. Depress Anxiety 2016; **33**:792–806.

73 Davidson J et al. Treatment of posttraumatic stress disorder with venlafaxine extended release: a 6-month randomized controlled trial. Arch Gen Psychiatry 2006; **63**:1158–1165.

74 Han C et al. The potential role of atypical antipsychotics for the treatment of posttraumatic stress disorder. J Psychiatr Res 2014; **56**:72–81.

75 Villarreal G et al. Efficacy of quetiapine monotherapy in posttraumatic stress disorder: a randomized, placebo-controlled trial. Am J Psychiatry 2016; **173**:1205–1212.

76 Davidson JR et al. Mirtazapine vs. placebo in posttraumatic stress disorder: a pilot trial. Biol Psychiatry 2003; **53**:188–191.

77 National Institute for Health and Care Excellence. Post-traumatic stress disorder: management. Clinical guideline 26, 2005. http://www.nice.org.uk/guidance/CG26

78 Kosten TR et al. Pharmacotherapy for posttraumatic stress disorder using phenelzine or imipramine. J Nerv Ment Dis 1991; **179**:366–370.

79 George KC et al. Meta-analysis of the efficacy and safety of prazosin versus placebo for the treatment of nightmares and sleep disturbances in adults with posttraumatic stress disorder. J Trauma Dissociation 2016; **17**:494–510.

80 Davidson J et al. Treatment of posttraumatic stress disorder with amitriptyline and placebo. Arch Gen Psychiatry 1990; **47**:259–266.

81 Walderhaug E et al. Effects of duloxetine in treatment-refractory men with posttraumatic stress disorder. Pharmacopsychiatry 2010; **43**:45–49.

82 Villarreal G et al. Duloxetine in military posttraumatic stress disorder. Psychopharmacol Bull 2010; **43**:26–34.

83 Hertzberg MA et al. A preliminary study of lamotrigine for the treatment of posttraumatic stress disorder. Biol Psychiatry 1999; **45**:1226–1229.

84 Bremner DJ et al. Treatment of posttraumatic stress disorder with phenytoin: an open-label pilot study. J Clin Psychiatry 2004; **65**:1559–1564.

85 Adamou M et al. Valproate in the treatment of PTSD: systematic review and meta analysis. Curr Med Res Opin 2007; **23**:1285–1291.

86 Feder A et al. Efficacy of intravenous ketamine for treatment of chronic posttraumatic stress disorder: a randomized clinical trial. JAMA Psychiatry 2014; **71**:681–688.

87 Veale D et al. Atypical antipsychotic augmentation in SSRI treatment refractory obsessive-compulsive disorder: a systematic review and meta-analysis. BMC Psychiatry 2014; **14**:317.

88 Dold M et al. Antipsychotic augmentation of serotonin reuptake inhibitors in treatment-resistant obsessive-compulsive disorder: an update meta-analysis of double-blind, randomized, placebo-controlled trials. Int J Neuropsychopharmacol 2015; **18**.

89 Pallanti S et al. Citalopram for treatment-resistant obsessive-compulsive disorder. Eur Psychiatry 1999; **14**:101–106.

90 Afshar H et al. N-acetylcysteine add-on treatment in refractory obsessive-compulsive disorder: a randomized, double-blind, placebo-controlled trial. J Clin Psychopharmacol 2012; **32**:797–803.

91 Ghanizadeh A et al. Efficacy of N-acetylcysteine augmentation on obsessive compulsive disorder: a multicenter randomized double blind placebo controlled clinical trial. Iran J Psychiatry 2017; **12**:134–141.

92 Costa DLC et al. Randomized, double-blind, placebo-controlled trial of N-acetylcysteine augmentation for treatment-resistant obsessive-compulsive disorder. J Clin Psychiatry 2017; **78**:e766–e773.

93 Bruno A et al. Lamotrigine augmentation of serotonin reuptake inhibitors in treatment-resistant obsessive-compulsive disorder: a double-blind, placebo-controlled study. J Psychopharmacol 2012; **26**:1456–1462.

94 Berlin HA et al. Double-blind, placebo-controlled trial of topiramate augmentation in treatment-resistant obsessive-compulsive disorder. J Clin Psychiatry 2011; **72**:716–721.

95 Mowla A et al. Topiramate augmentation in resistant OCD: a double-blind placebo-controlled clinical trial. CNS Spectr 2010; **15**:613–617.

96 Afshar H et al. Topiramate augmentation in refractory obsessive-compulsive disorder: a randomized, double-blind, placebo-controlled trial. J Res Med Sci 2014; **19**:976–981.

97 Rabinowitz I et al. High-dose escitalopram for the treatment of obsessive-compulsive disorder. Int Clin Psychopharmacol 2008; **23**:49–53.

98 Ninan PT et al. High-dose sertraline strategy for nonresponders to acute treatment for obsessive-compulsive disorder: a multicenter double-blind trial. J Clin Psychiatry 2006; **67**:15–22.

CHAPTER 3

99 Ghaleiha A et al. Memantine add-on in moderate to severe obsessive-compulsive disorder: randomized double-blind placebo-controlled study. J Psychiatr Res 2013; **47**:175–180.

100 Dell'Osso B et al. Serotonin-norepinephrine reuptake inhibitors in the treatment of obsessive-compulsive disorder: a critical review. J Clin Psychiatry 2006; **67**:600–610.

101 Mowla A et al. Duloxetine augmentation in resistant obsessive-compulsive disorder: a double-blind controlled clinical trial. J Clin Psychopharmacol 2016; **36**:720–723.

102 Koran LM et al. Mirtazapine for obsessive-compulsive disorder: an open trial followed by double-blind discontinuation. J Clin Psychiatry 2005; **66**:515–520.

103 Askari N et al. Granisetron adjunct to fluvoxamine for moderate to severe obsessive-compulsive disorder: a randomized, double-blind, placebo-controlled trial. CNS Drugs 2012; **26**:883–892.

104 Soltani F et al. A double-blind, placebo-controlled pilot study of ondansetron for patients with obsessive-compulsive disorder. Hum Psychopharmacol 2010; **25**:509–513.

105 Coric V et al. Riluzole augmentation in treatment-resistant obsessive-compulsive disorder: an open-label trial. Biol Psychiatry 2005; **58**:424–428.

106 Eriksson T. Anti-androgenic treatment of obsessive-compulsive disorder: an open-label clinical trial of the long-acting gonadotropin-releasing hormone analogue triptorelin. Int Clin Psychopharmacol 2007; **22**:57–61.

107 Fallon BA et al. Intravenous clomipramine for obsessive-compulsive disorder refractory to oral clomipramine: a placebo-controlled study. Arch Gen Psychiatry 1998; **55**:918–924.

108 Rodriguez CI et al. Randomized controlled crossover trial of ketamine in obsessive-compulsive disorder: proof-of-concept. Neuropsychopharmacology 2013; **38**:2475–2483.

109 Bloch MH et al. Effects of ketamine in treatment-refractory obsessive-compulsive disorder. Biol Psychiatry 2012; **72**:964–970.

110 Koran LM et al. Double-blind treatment with oral morphine in treatment-resistant obsessive-compulsive disorder. J Clin Psychiatry 2005; **66**:353–359.

111 National Institute for Health and Care Excellence. Social anxiety disorder: recognition, assessment and treatment. Clinical Guideline **159**, 2013. https://www.nice.org.uk/guidance/cg159

112 Blanco C et al. The evidence-based pharmacotherapy of social anxiety disorder. Int J Neuropsychopharmacol 2013; **16**:235–249.

113 Pollack MH et al. A double-blind randomized controlled trial of augmentation and switch strategies for refractory social anxiety disorder. Am J Psychiatry 2014; **171**:44–53.

114 Simon NM et al. An open-label study of levetiracetam for the treatment of social anxiety disorder. J Clin Psychiatry 2004; **65**:1219–1222.

115 Blanco C et al. A placebo-controlled trial of phenelzine, cognitive behavioral group therapy, and their combination for social anxiety disorder. Arch Gen Psychiatry 2010; **67**:286–295.

116 Van Ameringen M et al. An open trial of topiramate in the treatment of generalized social phobia. J Clin Psychiatry 2004; **65**:1674–1678.

117 Kinrys G et al. Valproic acid for the treatment of social anxiety disorder. Int Clin Psychopharmacol 2003; **18**:169–172.

CHAPTER 3

Benzodiazepines in the treatment of psychiatric disorders

Benzodiazepines are normally divided into two groups depending on their half-life: hypnotics (short half-life) or anxiolytics (long half-life). Although benzodiazepines have a place in the treatment of some forms of epilepsy and severe muscle spasm, and as premedicants in some surgical procedures, the vast majority of prescriptions are written for their hypnotic and anxiolytic effects. Benzodiazepines are also used for rapid tranquillisation (see section on 'Acutely disturbed or violent behaviour' in Chapter 1) and, as adjuncts, in the treatment of depression and schizophrenia.

Benzodiazepines are commonly prescribed; a European study found that almost 10% of adults had taken a benzodiazepine over the course of a year.[1]

Anxiolytic effect

Benzodiazepines reduce pathological anxiety, agitation and tension. Although useful in the short-term management of generalised anxiety disorder,[2] either alone or to augment SSRIs, benzodiazepines are clearly addictive; many patients continue to take these drugs for years[3] with unknown benefits and many likely harms. If a benzodiazepine is prescribed, this should not routinely be for longer than 1 month.

NICE recommends that benzodiazepines should not be routinely used in patients with generalised anxiety disorder except as a short-term measure during crisis.[4] Evidence is mixed in other anxiety disorders, and potential benefits should be viewed in the context of the known risks associated with benzodiazepine use. A small number of trials report the efficacy of benzodiazepines in social anxiety disorder.[5] Benzodiazepines may be useful in panic disorders,[6] but further studies are needed to draw reliable conclusions about their efficacy and safety with long-term use.[6,7] Benzodiazepines are ineffective or even potentially harmful for the treatment of PTSD[8] or phobias.[9]

Repeat prescriptions should be avoided in those with major personality problems whose difficulties are unlikely ever to resolve. Benzodiazepines should also be avoided, if possible, in those with a history of substance misuse.

Hypnotic effect

Benzodiazepines inhibit rapid eye movement (REM) sleep and a rebound increase is seen when they are discontinued.[9] There is a debate over the clinical significance of this property.[10]

Benzodiazepines are effective hypnotics, at least in the short term.[11] RCTs support the effectiveness of Z-hypnotics over a period of at least 6 months.[11,12] It is unclear if this holds true for benzodiazepine hypnotics.

Physical causes (pain, dyspnoea, etc.) or substance misuse (most commonly high caffeine consumption) should always be excluded before a hypnotic drug is prescribed. Where possible, behavioural therapies (e.g. CBT for insomnia) should be offered before prescribing hypnotics.[12,13] A high proportion of hospitalised patients are prescribed hypnotics.[14] Care should be taken to avoid using hypnotics regularly or for long periods of time.

Be particularly careful to avoid routinely prescribing hypnotics on discharge from hospital, as this may result in iatrogenic dependence.

CHAPTER 3

Use in depression

Benzodiazepines are not a treatment for major depressive illness. In the UK, the National Service Framework for Mental Health[15] at one time emphasised this point by including a requirement that GPs audit the ratio of benzodiazepines to antidepressants prescribed in their practice. NICE suggests that a benzodiazepine may be helpful for up to 2 weeks early in treatment, particularly in combination with an SSRI (to help with sleep and the management of SSRI-induced agitation).[4] Use beyond this timeframe is discouraged. Limiting initial supply quantities to short periods (1–7 days) may reduce the risk of patients becoming long-term users of benzodiazepines.[16]

Use in psychosis

Benzodiazepines are commonly used for rapid tranquillisation, either alone or in combination with an antipsychotic.[17] However, a Cochrane review concluded that there is no convincing evidence that combining an antipsychotic and a benzodiazepine offers any advantage over the use of antipsychotics or benzodiazepines alone.[18]

A further Cochrane review in schizophrenia concluded that there are no proven benefits, outside short-term sedation.[19] In contrast, another systematic review using different outcome measures found superiority over placebo for global, psychiatric and behavioural outcomes, but inferiority to antipsychotics on longer-term global outcomes.[20] A significant minority of patients with established psychotic illness fail to respond adequately to antipsychotics alone, and this can result in benzodiazepines being prescribed on a chronic basis.[21] There is, however, no evidence to support benzodiazepine augmentation of antipsychotics in schizophrenia, and use should be reserved for the short-term sedation of acutely agitated patients.[22]

Adverse effects

Headaches, confusion, ataxia, dysarthria, blurred vision, gastrointestinal disturbances, jaundice and paradoxical excitement are all possible adverse effects. Benzodiazepines impair cognition, and long-term use has been associated with a range of cognitive deficits (e.g. memory, attention and processing speed) which may even persist after withdrawal.[23] The use of benzodiazepines has been associated with at least a 50% increase in the risk of hip fracture in the elderly.[24] This is probably because benzodiazepines increase the risk of falls.[25] Patients newly prescribed a benzodiazepine have the highest risk.[24] High doses are particularly problematic.[25] This would seem to be a class effect (short-half-life drugs still increase the risk[25]). Benzodiazepines often cause anterograde amnesia and can adversely affect driving performance.[26,27] Benzodiazepines can also cause disinhibition; this seems to be more common with short-acting drugs. Benzodiazepines have been linked to aggressive behaviour, though the association is modest and possibly related to dose or personality factors.[28]

Epidemiologic research has recently linked benzodiazepine exposure to other serious medical conditions including dementia, infections and cancer.[29] However, a causal relationship has not been established and some evidence is conflicting.[29] For example, although benzodiazepine use has been associated with dementia, the absence of a dose–response association argues against a causal link.[30]

Respiratory depression is rare with oral therapy but is possible when the IV route is used. A specific benzodiazepine antagonist, flumazenil, is available. The use of flumazenil is not without risk (e.g. convulsions, particularly in mixed overdoses with TCAs) so selective use is recommended.[31] Flumazenil has a much shorter half-life than diazepam, making close observation of the patient essential for several hours after administration.

IV injections can be painful and lead to thrombophlebitis because of the low water solubility of benzodiazepines. It is therefore necessary to use solvents in the preparation of injectable forms. Diazepam is available in emulsion form (Diazemuls) to overcome these problems.

Drug interactions

Benzodiazepines do not induce microsomal enzymes and so do not frequently precipitate pharmacokinetic interactions with any other drugs. Most benzodiazepines are metabolised by CYP3A4, which is inhibited by erythromycin, several SSRIs and ketoconazole. It is theoretically possible that co-administration of these drugs will result in higher serum levels of benzodiazepines. Pharmacodynamic interactions (usually increased sedation) can occur. Benzodiazepines are associated with an important interaction with methadone (see Chapter 5) and should be used with caution in patients prescribed clozapine (increased risk of cardio-pulmonary depression).

References

1 Demyttenaere K et al. Clinical factors influencing the prescription of antidepressants and benzodiazepines: results from the European study of the epidemiology of mental disorders (ESEMeD). J Affect Disord 2008; 110:84–93.
2 Baldwin DS et al. Evidence-based pharmacological treatment of anxiety disorders, post-traumatic stress disorder and obsessive-compulsive disorder: revision of the 2005 guidelines from the British Association for Psychopharmacology. J Psychopharmacol 2014; 28:403–439.
3 Kurko TA et al. Long-term use of benzodiazepines: definitions, prevalence and usage patterns – a systematic review of register-based studies. Eur Psychiatry 2015; 30:1037–1047.
4 National Institute for Health and Care Excellence. Generalised anxiety disorder and panic disorder in adults: management. Clinical Guideline 113, 2011. http://www.nice.org.uk/cg113
5 Williams T et al. Pharmacotherapy for social anxiety disorder (SAnD). Cochrane Database Syst Rev 2017; 10:CD001206.
6 Perna G et al. Long-term pharmacological treatments of anxiety disorders: an updated systematic review. Curr Psychiatry Rep 2016; 18:23.
7 Bighelli I et al. Antidepressants and benzodiazepines for panic disorder in adults. Cochrane Database Syst Rev 2016; 9:CD011567.
8 Guina J et al. Benzodiazepines for PTSD: a systematic review and meta-analysis. J Psychiatr Pract 2015; 21:281–303.
9 Guina J et al. Benzodiazepines I: upping the care on downers: the evidence of risks, benefits and alternatives. J Clin Med 2018; 7.
10 Roehrs T et al. Drug-related sleep stage changes: functional significance and clinical relevance. Sleep Med Clin 2010; 5:559–570.
11 Winkler A et al. Drug treatment of primary insomnia: a meta-analysis of polysomnographic randomized controlled trials. CNS Drugs 2014; 28:799–816.
12 Riemann D et al. European guideline for the diagnosis and treatment of insomnia. J Sleep Res 2017; 26:675–700.
13 Qaseem A et al. Management of chronic insomnia disorder in adults: a clinical practice guideline from the American College of Physicians. Ann Intern Med 2016; 165:125–133.
14 Mahomed R et al. Prescribing hypnotics in a mental health trust: what consultants say and what they do. Pharm J 2002; 268:657–659.
15 Department of Health. National Service Framework for Mental Health: Modern Standards and Service Models. London: Department of Health; 1999.
16 Bushnell GA et al. Simultaneous antidepressant and benzodiazepine new use and subsequent long-term benzodiazepine use in adults with depression, United States, 2001-2014. JAMA Psychiatry 2017; 74:747–755.
17 Baldwin DS et al. Benzodiazepines: risks and benefits. A reconsideration. J Psychopharmacol 2013; 27:967–971.
18 Zaman H et al. Benzodiazepines for psychosis-induced aggression or agitation. Cochrane Database Syst Rev 2017; 12:CD003079.
19 Dold M et al. Benzodiazepines for schizophrenia. Cochrane Database Syst Rev 2012; 11:CD006391.
20 Sim F et al. Re-examining the role of benzodiazepines in the treatment of schizophrenia: a systematic review. J Psychopharmacol 2015; 29:212–223.
21 Paton C et al. Benzodiazepines in schizophrenia. Is there a trend towards long-term prescribing? Psychiatr Bull 2000; 24:113–115.

22 Dold M et al. Benzodiazepine augmentation of antipsychotic drugs in schizophrenia: a meta-analysis and Cochrane review of randomized controlled trials. Eur Neuropsychopharmacol 2013; **23**:1023–1033.

23 Crowe SF et al. The residual medium and long-term cognitive effects of benzodiazepine use: an updated meta-analysis. Arch Clin Neuropsychol 2017; doi: 10.1093/arclin/acx120. [Epub ahead of print]

24 Donnelly K et al. Benzodiazepines, Z-drugs and the risk of hip fracture: a systematic review and meta-analysis. PLoS One 2017; **12**:e0174730.

25 Diaz-Gutierrez MJ et al. Relationship between the use of benzodiazepines and falls in older adults: a systematic review. Maturitas 2017; **101**:17–22.

26 Barbone F et al. Association of road-traffic accidents with benzodiazepine use. Lancet 1998; **352**:1331–1336.

27 Rudisill TM et al. Medication use and the risk of motor vehicle collisions among licensed drivers: a systematic review. Accid Anal Prev 2016; **96**:255–270.

28 Albrecht B et al. Benzodiazepine use and aggressive behaviour: a systematic review. Aust N Z J Psychiatry 2014; **48**:1096–1114.

29 Brandt J et al. Benzodiazepines and Z-drugs: an updated review of major adverse outcomes reported on in epidemiologic research. Drugs R D 2017; **17**:493–507.

30 Gray SL et al. Benzodiazepine use and risk of incident dementia or cognitive decline: prospective population based study. BMJ 2016; **352**:i90.

31 Penninga EI et al. Adverse events associated with flumazenil treatment for the management of suspected benzodiazepine intoxication – a systematic review with meta-analyses of randomised trials. Basic Clin Pharmacol Toxicol 2016; **118**:37–44.

Further reading

Chouinard G. Issues in the clinical use of benzodiazepines: potency, withdrawal, and rebound. J Clin Psychiatry 2004; **65** Suppl 5:7–12.

CHAPTER 3

Benzodiazepines: dependence and detoxification

Benzodiazepines are widely acknowledged to be addictive, and withdrawal symptoms can occur after 4–6 weeks of continuous use (Box 3.7). Long-term use remains common in the UK.[1] At least a third of long-term users experience problems on dosage reduction or withdrawal.[2] Short-acting drugs such as lorazepam are associated with more severe problems on withdrawal than longer-acting drugs such as diazepam.[2,3] To avoid or reduce the severity of these problems, good practice dictates that benzodiazepines should not be prescribed as hypnotics or anxiolytics for longer than 4 weeks.[4,5] Intermittent use (i.e. not every day) may also help avoid dependence and tolerance.

In the majority, symptoms last no longer than a few weeks, although a minority experience disabling symptoms for much longer.[2] Minimal intervention strategies, for example simply sending the patient a letter advising them to stop taking benzodiazepine,[6] increase the odds of successfully stopping at least three-fold.[8,9] A cluster randomised trial supports the effectiveness of a face-to-face educational intervention.[10] Continuing support can be required (e.g. psychological therapies or self-help groups).

If clinically indicated and assuming the patient is in agreement, benzodiazepines should be withdrawn in line with the following considerations.

Confirming use

If benzodiazepines are not prescribed and patients are obtaining their own supply, use should be confirmed by urine screening (a negative urine screen in combination with an absence of benzodiazepine withdrawal rules out physical dependence). Very short-acting benzodiazepines may not give a positive urine screen despite daily use.

Tolerance test

This will be required if the patient has been obtaining illicit supplies. No benzodiazepines or alcohol should be consumed for 12 hours before the test. A test dose of 10 mg diazepam should be administered (20 mg if consumption of >50 mg daily is claimed or suspected) and the patient observed for 2–3 hours. If there are no signs of sedation, it is

---

Box 3.7 Problems on withdrawal from benzodiazepines[6,7]

Physical	Psychological
▪ Stiffness	▪ Anxiety/insomnia
▪ Weakness	▪ Nightmares
▪ Gastrointestinal disturbance	▪ Depersonalisation
▪ Paraesthesia	▪ Decreased memory and concentration
▪ Flu-like symptoms	▪ Delusions and hallucinations
▪ Visual disturbances	▪ Depression
▪ Convulsions	▪ Psychosis
▪ Cognitive impairment	

CHAPTER 3

generally safe to prescribe the same dose as the test dose three times a day. Some patients may require much higher doses. In-patient assessment may be desirable in these cases.

Switching to diazepam

Patients who take short- or intermediate-acting benzodiazepines should be offered an equivalent dose of diazepam (which has a long half-life and therefore probably provokes less severe withdrawal).[2,7] Note that Cochrane was lukewarm about this approach.[11] Approximate 'diazepam equivalent'[2] doses are shown in Table 3.24.

The half-lives of benzodiazepines vary greatly. The degree of sedation that they induce also varies, making it difficult to determine exact equivalents. Table 3.24 is an approximate guide only. Extra precautions apply in patients with hepatic dysfunction, as diazepam and other longer-acting drugs may accumulate to toxic levels. Diazepam substitution may not be appropriate in this group of patients.

Dosage reduction

Systematic reduction strategies are twice as likely to lead to abstinence than simply advising the patient to stop.[8] Although gradual withdrawal is more acceptable to patients than abrupt withdrawal,[11] there is no evidence to support the differential efficacy of different tapering schedules, be they fixed dose or symptom guided.[8] Nonetheless it should be remembered that benzodiazepine withdrawal has potentially fatal consequences. The following is a suggested taper schedule; some patients may tolerate more rapid reduction and others may require a slower taper. A fixed schedule with a precise duration of withdrawal treatment is recommended.[7]

- Reduce by 10 mg/day every 1–2 weeks, down to a daily dose of 50 mg.
- Reduce by 5 mg/day every 1–2 weeks, down to a daily dose of 30 mg.
- Reduce by 2 mg/day every 1–2 weeks, down to a daily dose of 20 mg.
- Reduce by 1 mg/day every 1–2 weeks until stopped.

Table 3.24 Switching from benzodiazepines to diazepam: doses

Benzodiazepine	Approximate dose (mg) equivalent to 10 mg diazepam
Chlordiazepoxide	25 mg
Clonazepam	1–2 mg
Lorazepam	1 mg
Lormetazepam	1 mg
Nitrazepam	10 mg
Oxazepam	30 mg
Temazepam	20 mg

For out-patients, usually no more than 1 week's supply (prescribe the exact number of tablets) should be issued at any one time.

Gradual dose reduction accompanied by psychological interventions (relaxation, CBT) is more likely to be successful than supervised dose reduction alone[12] or psychological interventions alone.[13]

Anticipating problems[2,6,14]

Problematic withdrawal can be anticipated if previous attempts have been unsuccessful, the patient lacks social support, there is a history of alcohol/polydrug abuse or withdrawal seizures, the patient is elderly, or there is concomitant severe physical/psychiatric disorder or personality disorder. The acceptable rate of withdrawal may inevitably be slower in these patients. Some may never succeed. Risk–benefit analysis may conclude that maintenance treatment with benzodiazepines is appropriate, and there is support for a RCT examining the benefits and risks of this strategy.[15] The main risk is that benzodiazepines permanently impair cognitive function.[16] Some patients may need interventions for underlying disorders masked by benzodiazepine dependence. If the patient is indifferent to withdrawal (i.e. is not motivated to stop), success is unlikely.

Too rapid withdrawal may be risky; a case report describes a fatal outcome.[17] Those withdrawing from daily doses of >100 mg diazepam should probably withdraw as in-patients.[7]

Adjunctive treatments

There is some evidence to support the use of antidepressant and mood-stabilising drugs as adjuncts during benzodiazepine withdrawal.[2,8,11,18–21] The best evidence is probably for carbamazepine.[22] Low-dose slow flumazenil infusion can safely and successfully detoxify patients when anticonvulsant prophylaxis is used.[23] There is more limited evidence to support the use of pregabalin,[24] but more patients who take very high daily doses of benzodiazepines.[25–27] People with insomnia may benefit from adjunctive treatment with melatonin, and those with panic disorder may benefit from CBT during the taper period.[7,8,22]

References

1 Davies J et al. Long-term benzodiazepine and Z-drugs use in the UK: a survey of general practice. Br J Gen Pract 2017; 67:e609–e613.

2 Schweizer E et al. Benzodiazepine dependence and withdrawal: a review of the syndrome and its clinical management. Acta Psychiatr Scand 1998; 98 Suppl 393:95–101.

3 Uhlenhuth EH et al. International study of expert judgment on therapeutic use of benzodiazepines and other psychotherapeutic medications: IV. Therapeutic dose dependence and abuse liability of benzodiazepines in the long-term treatment of anxiety disorders. J Clin Psychopharmacol 1999; 19:23S–29S.

4 British Medical Association and Royal Pharmaceutical Society of Great Britain. British National Formulary, 66th edn. London: BMJ Group and Pharmaceutical Press; 2013.

5 The Committee on Safety of Medicines. Benzodiazepines, dependence and withdrawal symptoms. Curr Probl 1988; 21:1–2.

6 Petursson H. The benzodiazepine withdrawal syndrome. Addiction 1994; 89:1455–1459.

7 Soyka M. Treatment of benzodiazepine dependence. N Engl J Med 2017; 376:1147–1157.

8 Voshaar RCO et al. Strategies for discontinuing long-term benzodiazepine use: meta-analysis. Br J Psychiatry 2006; 189:213–220.

9 Salonoja M et al. One-time counselling decreases the use of benzodiazepines and related drugs among community-dwelling older persons. Age Ageing 2010; 39:313–319.

CHAPTER 3

10 Tannenbaum C et al. Reduction of inappropriate benzodiazepine prescriptions among older adults through direct patient education: the EMPOWER cluster randomized trial. JAMA Intern Med 2014; **174**:890–898.

11 Denis C et al. Pharmacological interventions for benzodiazepine mono-dependence management in outpatient settings. Cochrane Database Syst Rev 2006:CD005194.

12 Parr JM et al. Effectiveness of current treatment approaches for benzodiazepine discontinuation: a meta-analysis. Addiction 2009; **104**: 13–24.

13 Gould RL et al. Interventions for reducing benzodiazepine use in older people: meta-analysis of randomised controlled trials. Br J Psychiatry 2014; **204**:98–107.

14 Tyrer P. Risks of dependence on benzodiazepine drugs: the importance of patient selection. BMJ 1989; **298**:102–105.

15 Tyrer P. Benzodiazepine substitution for dependent patients-going with the flow. Addiction 2010; **105**:1875–1876.

16 Crowe SF et al. The residual medium and long-term cognitive effects of benzodiazepine use: an updated meta-analysis. Arch Clin Neuropsychol 2017; doi: 10.1093/arclin/acx120. [Epub ahead of print]

17 Lann MA et al. A fatal case of benzodiazepine withdrawal. Am J Forensic Med Pathol 2009; **30**:177–179.

18 Rickels K et al. Imipramine and buspirone in treatment of patients with generalized anxiety disorder who are discontinuing long-term benzodiazepine therapy. Am J Psychiatry 2000; **157**:1973–1979.

19 Tyrer P et al. A controlled trial of dothiepin and placebo in treating benzodiazepine withdrawal symptoms. Br J Psychiatry 1996; **168**:457–461.

20 Schweizer E et al. Carbamazepine treatment in patients discontinuing long-term benzodiazepine therapy. Effects on withdrawal severity and outcome. Arch Gen Psychiatry 1991; **48**:448–452.

21 Zitman FG et al. Chronic benzodiazepine use in general practice patients with depression: an evaluation of controlled treatment and taper-off: report on behalf of the Dutch Chronic Benzodiazepine Working Group. Br J Psychiatry 2001; **178**:317–324.

22 Fluyau D et al. Challenges of the pharmacological management of benzodiazepine withdrawal, dependence, and discontinuation. Ther Adv Psychopharmacol 2018; 0:2045125317753340.

23 Tamburin S et al. Low risk of seizures with slow flumazenil infusion and routine anticonvulsant prophylaxis for high-dose benzodiazepine dependence. J Psychopharmacol 2017; **31**:1369–1373.

24 Caniff K et al. Pregabalin as adjunctive therapy in benzodiazepine discontinuation. Am J Health Syst Pharm 2018; **75**:67–71.

25 Oulis P et al. Pregabalin in the discontinuation of long-term benzodiazepines' use. Hum Psychopharmacol 2008; **23**:337–340.

26 Oulis P et al. Pregabalin in the discontinuation of long-term benzodiazepine use: a case-series. Int Clin Psychopharmacol 2008; **23**: 110–112.

27 Oulis P et al. Pregabalin in the treatment of alcohol and benzodiazepines dependence. CNS Neurosci Ther 2010; **16**:45–50.

Further reading

Ahmed M et al. A self-help handout for benzodiazepine discontinuation using cognitive behavioral therapy. Cogn Behav Pract 2008; **15**:317–324.

Heberlein A et al. Neuroendocrine pathways in benzodiazepine dependence: new targets for research and therapy. Hum Psychopharmacol 2008; **23**:171–181.

Benzodiazepines and disinhibition

Unexpected increases in aggressive or impulsive behaviour secondary to drug treatment are usually called disinhibitory or paradoxical reactions.[1] These reactions may include acute excitement, hyperactivity, increased anxiety, vivid dreams, sexual disinhibition, aggression, hostility and rage. It is possible for a drug to have the potential both to decrease and increase aggressive behaviour. Examples of causative agents include amfetamines, methylphenidate, benzodiazepines and alcohol.

How common are disinhibitory reactions with benzodiazepines?

The incidence of disinhibitory reactions varies widely depending on the population studied (see 'Who is at risk?' later in this section). For example, a meta-analysis of benzodiazepine RCTs that included many hundreds of patients with a wide range of diagnoses reported an incidence of less than 1% (similar to placebo).[2] A Norwegian study that reported on 415 cases of 'driving under the influence', in which flunitrazepam was the sole substance implicated, found that 6% of adverse effects could be described as disinhibitory reactions.[3] An RCT that recruited patients with panic disorder reported an incidence of disinhibition of 13%.[4] Authors of case series (often describing use in high-risk patients) reported rates of 10–20%,[2] and an RCT that included patients with borderline personality disorder reported a rate of 58%.[5]

Disinhibition is rather problematic to define and so incidence rates are correspondingly difficult to determine. Aggression may be considered to be a disinhibition reaction but not defined as disinhibition per se. It is robustly linked to benzodiazepine use, both in the long term and after exposure to a single dose.[6,7]

Other GABA agonists, particularly zolpidem, have also been linked to disinhibition associated with somnambulism, automatism and amnesia.[8–10]

Who is at risk?

Those who have a learning disability, neurological disorder or central nervous system (CNS) degenerative disease,[11] are young (child or adolescent) or elderly,[11–13] or have a history of aggression or poor impulse control[5,14] are at increased risk of experiencing a disinhibitory reaction. The risk is further increased if the benzodiazepine is a high-potency drug, has a short half-life, is given in a high dose or is administered intravenously (so provoking high and rapidly fluctuating plasma levels).[11,15–17] Some people may be genetically predisposed to disinhibition reactions.[18]

Combinations of risk factors are clearly important: low-risk long-acting benzodiazepines may cause disinhibition in high-risk populations such as children;[13] higher-risk short-acting drugs are extremely likely to cause disinhibition in personality disorder.

What is the mechanism?[15,19–21]

Various theories of the mechanism have been proposed. First, the anxiolytic and amnesic properties of benzodiazepines may lead to a loss of the restraint that governs normal social behaviour. Second, the sedative and amnesic properties of benzodiazepines may lead to a reduced ability to concentrate on the external social cues that guide appropriate behaviour. Lastly, benzodiazepine-mediated increases in GABA neurotransmission may lead to a reduction in the restraining influence of the cortex, resulting in untrammelled excitement, anxiety and hostility.

Subjective reports

People who take benzodiazepines rate themselves as being more tolerant and friendly, but respond more to provocation, than placebo-treated patients.[22] People with impulse control problems who take benzodiazepines may self-report feelings of power and overwhelming self-esteem.[14] Psychology rating scales demonstrate increased suggestibility, failure to recognise anger in others and reduced ability to recognise social cues. The experience of this author (DT, having once been given intravenous midazolam for a pre-surgical procedure) is that the patient may be completely unaware that their bizarre behaviour is a result of drug-induced disinhibition.

Clinical implications

Benzodiazepines are frequently used in rapid tranquillisation and the short-term management of disturbed behaviour. In the vast majority of treatment episodes, benzodiazepines produce sedation, reductions in anxiety and aggression. It is important to be aware, nonetheless, of their propensity to cause paradoxical disinhibitory reactions.

Paradoxical disinhibitory/aggressive outbursts in the context of benzodiazepine use:

- are rare in the general population but more frequent in people with impulse control problems or CNS damage and in the very young or very old
- are most often associated with high doses of high-potency drugs that are administered parenterally
- usually occur in response to (often very mild) provocation, the exact nature of which is not always obvious to others
- are recognised by others but often not by the sufferer, who often believes that he is friendly and tolerant.

Suspected paradoxical reactions should be clearly documented in the clinical notes. In extreme cases, flumazenil can be used to reverse the reaction. If the benzodiazepine was prescribed to control acute behavioural disturbance, future episodes should be managed with antipsychotic drugs[1] or other non-benzodiazepine sedatives.

References

1 Paton C. Benzodiazepines and disinhibition: a review. Psychiatr Bull 2002; 26:460–462.
2 Dietch JT et al. Aggressive dyscontrol in patients treated with benzodiazepines. J Clin Psychiatry 1988; 49:184–188.
3 Bramness JG et al. Flunitrazepam: psychomotor impairment, agitation and paradoxical reactions. Forensic Sci Int 2006; 159:83–91.
4 O'Sullivan GH et al. Safety and side-effects of alprazolam. Controlled study in agoraphobia with panic disorder. Br J Psychiatry 1994; 165:79–86.
5 Gardner DL et al. Alprazolam-induced dyscontrol in borderline personality disorder. Am J Psychiatry 1985; 142:98–100.
6 Albrecht B et al. Motivational drive and alprazolam misuse: a recipe for aggression? Psychiatry Res 2016; 240:381–389.
7 Albrecht B et al. Benzodiazepine use and aggressive behaviour: a systematic review. Aust N Z J Psychiatry 2014; 48:1096–1114.
8 Poceta JS. Zolpidem ingestion, automatisms, and sleep driving: a clinical and legal case series. J Clin Sleep Med 2011; 7:632–638.

9   Pressman MR. Sleep driving: sleepwalking variant or misuse of z-drugs? Sleep Med Rev 2011; 15:285–292.

10 Daley C et al. "I did what?" Zolpidem and the courts. J Am Acad Psychiatry Law 2011; 39:535–542.

11 Bond AJ. Drug-induced behavioural disinhibition incidence, mechanisms and therapeutic implications. CNS Drugs 1998; 9:41—57.

12 Hawkridge SM et al. A risk-benefit assessment of pharmacotherapy for anxiety disorders in children and adolescents. Drug Saf 1998; 19:283–297.

13 Kandemir H et al. Behavioral disinhibition, suicidal ideation, and self-mutilation related to clonazepam. J Child Adolesc Psychopharmacol 2008; 18:409.

14 Daderman AM et al. Flunitrazepam (rohypnol) abuse in combination with alcohol causes premeditated, grievous violence in male juvenile offenders. J Am Acad Psychiatry Law 1999; 27:83–99.

15 van der Bijl P et al. Disinhibitory reactions to benzodiazepines: a review. J Oral Maxillofac Surg 1991; 49:519–523.

16 McKenzie WS et al. Paradoxical reaction following administration of a benzodiazepine. J Oral Maxillofac Surg 2010; 68:3034–3036.

17 Wilson KE et al. Complications associated with intravenous midazolam sedation in anxious dental patients. Prim Dent Care 2011; 18:161–166.

18 Short TG et al. Paradoxical reactions to benzodiazepines – a genetically determined phenomenon? Anaesth Intensive Care 1987; 15:330–331.

19 Weisman AM et al. Effects of clorazepate, diazepam, and oxazepam on a laboratory measurement of aggression in men. Int Clin Psychopharmacol 1998; 13:183–188.

20 Blair RJ et al. Selective impairment in the recognition of anger induced by diazepam. Psychopharmacology (Berl) 1999; 147:335–338.

21 Wallace PS et al. Reduction of appeasement-related affect as a concomitant of diazepam-induced aggression: evidence for a link between aggression and the expression of self-conscious emotions. Aggress Behav 2009; 35:203–212.

22 Bond AJ et al. Behavioural aggression in panic disorder after 8 weeks' treatment with alprazolam. J Affect Disord 1995; 35:117–123.

CHAPTER 3

Chapter 4

Addictions and substance misuse

Introduction

Mental and behavioural problems due to psychoactive substance use are common. The World Health Organization (WHO) in the International Classification of Diseases 10 (ICD-10)[1] identifies acute intoxication, harmful use, dependence syndrome, withdrawal state, withdrawal state with delirium, psychotic disorder, amnesic syndrome, residual and late-onset psychotic disorder, other mental and behavioural disorders and unspecified mental and behavioural disorders as substance-related disorders. A wide range of psychoactive substances may be problematic including alcohol, opioids, benzodiazepines, γ-hydroxybutyrate (GHB)/γ-butaryl-lactone (GBL), stimulants, new psychoactive substances (NPS) and tobacco.

Substance misuse is frequently seen in people with severe mental illness (so-called 'dual diagnosis') and personality disorder. In many adult psychiatry settings, dual diagnosis is the norm rather than the exception. Bizarrely, substance misuse services are commissioned and provided separately from psychiatric services. The model of care in most addiction services means that patients who are not motivated to engage will not be assertively treated and followed up. Dual diagnosis teams are not universally available resulting in sub-optimal treatment for substance misuse related problems for many patients with mental illness.[2]

According to ICD-10, dependence syndrome is 'A cluster of cognitive, behavioural, cognitive, physiological phenomena that develop after repeated substance use and that typically include a strong desire to take the drug, difficulties in controlling its use, persisting in its use despite harmful consequences, a higher priority given to drug use than to other activities and obligations, increased tolerance, and sometimes a physical withdrawal state'. A definite diagnosis of dependence should only be made if at least three of the following have been present together in the last year:

- compulsion to take substance
- difficulties controlling substance-taking behaviour

The Maudsley Prescribing Guidelines in Psychiatry, Thirteenth Edition. David M. Taylor,
Thomas R. E. Barnes and Allan H. Young.
© 2018 David M. Taylor. Published 2018 by John Wiley & Sons Ltd.

- physiological withdrawal state
- evidence of tolerance
- neglect of alternative interests
- persistent use despite harm.

Substance use disorders should generally be treated with a combination of psychosocial and pharmacological interventions. This chapter will concentrate on pharmacological interventions for alcohol, opioids and nicotine use. Treatments for people misusing benzodiazepines, GHB/GBL, stimulants, NPS (including cathinones, synthetic cannabinoids and phenylethylamines), khat, nitrates, hallucinogens and anabolic steroids will be discussed briefly. Note that various National Institute for Health and Care Excellence (NICE) guidelines and technology appraisals (see relevant sections), Department of Health Substance Misuse Guidelines[3] and Public Health England[2] also provide a comprehensive overview of treatment approaches, as does the most recent British Association for Psychopharmacology consensus guideline.[4]

References

1. World Health Organization. International Statistical Classification of Diseases and Related Health Problems. Online version, 2016. http://apps. who.int/classifications/icd10/browse/2016/en.
2. Public Health England. Better care for people with co-occurring mental health and alcohol/drug use conditions. A guide for commissioners and service providers. 2017. https://www.gov.uk/government/uploads/system/uploads/attachment_data/file/625809/Co-occurring_mental_health_ and_alcohol_drug_use_conditions.pdf.
3. Department of Health. Drug misuse and dependence: UK guidelines on clinical management. 2017. https://www.gov.uk/government/ publications/drug-misuse-and-dependence-uk-guidelines-on-clinical-management.
4. Lingford-Hughes AR et al. BAP updated guidelines: evidence-based guidelines for the pharmacological management of substance abuse, harmful use, addiction and comorbidity: recommendations from BAP. J Psychopharmacol 2012; 26:899–952.

Alcohol dependence

Alcohol

What is a unit of alcohol?

One unit = 10 mL of ethanol or 1L of 1% alcohol. For example, 250 mL of wine that is 10% alcohol contains 2.5 units.

How much alcohol is too much?

The UK Department of Health in 2016 gave the following advice and recommendations to minimise the health risks from alcohol consumption:[1]

- No more than 14 units should be consumed per week on a regular basis. This applies to both men and women.
- Harm is minimised when these units are spread across 3 or more days.
- Heavy single-occasion drinking is associated with risk of harm, injury and accidents.
- The consumption of any volume of alcohol is still associated with a number of illnesses such as cancers of the throat, mouth and breast.
- There are no completely safe levels of drinking during pregnancy and precautionary avoidance of alcohol is recommended to reduce risk of harm to the baby.

Assessment and brief structured intervention

The UK NICE guideline on the diagnosis, assessment and management of harmful drinking and alcohol dependence recommends that staff working in services which might encounter problem drinkers should be competent in identifying and assessing harmful drinking and alcohol dependence.[2] The NICE public health guideline on reducing harmful drinking[3] recommends a session of brief structured advice based on FRAMES principles (feedback, responsibility, advice, menu, empathy, self-efficacy) as a useful intervention for everyone at increased risk of alcohol-related problems.

Where consumption above recommended levels has been identified, a more detailed clinical assessment is required. Depending on the context, this could include the following:

- history of alcohol use, including daily consumption and recent patterns of drinking
- history of previous episodes of alcohol withdrawal
- time of most recent drink
- collateral history from a family member or carer
- other drug (illicit and prescribed) use
- severity of dependence and of withdrawal symptoms
- co-existing medical and psychiatric problems
- physical examination including cognitive function
- breathalyser: absolute breath alcohol level and whether rising or falling (take at least 20 minutes after last drink to avoid falsely high readings from the mouth, and 1 hour later)

CHAPTER 4

- laboratory investigations: full blood count (FBC), urea and electrolytes (U&E), liver function tests (LFTs), international normalised ratio (INR), prothrombin time (PT) and urinary drug screen.

The following structured assessment tools are recommended:[2]

- The **Alcohol Use Disorders Identification Test (AUDIT)**[4] questionnaire, a 10-item questionnaire which is useful as a screening tool in those identified as being at increasing risk. Questions 1–3 address the quantity of alcohol consumed, 4–6 the signs and symptoms of dependence and 7–10 the behaviours and symptoms associated with harmful alcohol use. Each question is scored 0–4, giving a maximum total score of 40. A score of 8 or more is suggestive of hazardous or harmful alcohol use. Hazardous drinking = consumption of alcohol likely to cause harm. Harmful drinking = consumption already causing mental or physical health problems.
- The **Severity of Alcohol Dependence Questionnaire (SADQ)**[5] is a more detailed 20-item questionnaire with the score on each item ranging from 0 to 3, giving a maximum total score of 60 (Box 4.1).

Box 4.1   Severity of alcohol dependence
Mild   = SADQ score of 15 or less Moderate = SADQ score 15–30 Severe   = SADQ score >30

Alcohol withdrawal

In alcohol-dependent drinkers, the central nervous system has adjusted to the constant presence of alcohol in the body (neuro-adaptation). When the blood alcohol concentration (BAC) is suddenly lowered, the brain remains in a hyper-excited state, resulting in the withdrawal syndrome (Table 4.1).

Table 4.1 Manifestations and complications of mild and severe alcohol withdrawal

Mild alcohol withdrawal

Manifestations	Usual timing of onset after the last drink	Other information
- Agitation/anxiety/irritability - Tremor of hands, tongue, eyelids - Sweating - Nausea/vomiting/diarrhoea - Fever - Tachycardia - Systolic hypertension - General malaise	Onset at 3–12 hours Peak at 24–48 hours Duration up to 14 days	- Symptoms are non-specific - Absence does not exclude withdrawal - May commence before blood alcohol levels reach zero

Management
May be self-limiting, but mitigated with adequate benzodiazepine cover and supportive treatment.
*See below for the various benzodiazepine regimes recommended.

Table 4.1 (*Continued*)

Severe alcohol withdrawal

Complications	Usual timing of onset after the last drink	Other information
Generalised seizures	12–18 hours	■ May commence before blood alcohol levels reach zero

Management
- The occurrence of a first seizure during medically assisted withdrawal requires investigation to rule out organic disease or idiopathic epilepsy.
- A meta-analysis of trials assessing the efficacy of drugs in preventing alcohol withdrawal seizures demonstrated that benzodiazepines, particularly long-acting preparations such as diazepam, significantly reduced seizures *de novo*.[6]
- Long-acting benzodiazepines are recommended as prophylaxis in those with a previous history of seizures.[7]
- Some anticonvulsants are as effective as benzodiazepines, with some units recommending carbamazepine loading in patients with untreated epilepsy, or where seizures have occurred despite adequate benzodiazepine loading.[6]
- Phenytoin does not prevent alcohol withdrawal related seizures when used on its own or in combination with benzodiazepines.[8]
- There is no need to continue anticonvulsants long term when used to prevent seizures in alcohol withdrawal.[8]

Complications	Usual timing of onset after the last drink	Other information and management
Delirium tremens ■ Clouding of consciousness/confusion ■ Vivid hallucinations, particularly visual and tactile ■ Marked tremor	3–4 days (72–96 hours)	■ Develops in 5% ■ Mortality 10–20% if untreated
Other clinical features also include: autonomic hyperactivity (tachycardia, hypertension, sweating and fever), paranoid delusions, agitation and insomnia		
Prodromal symptoms include: night-time insomnia, restlessness, fear and confusion		
Risk factors: severe alcohol dependence, self-detoxification without medical input, multiple previous admissions for alcohol withdrawal, concurrent medical illness, previous history of delirium tremens and alcohol withdrawal seizures		

Management
- This is a medical emergency and requires prompt transfer to a general medical setting.
- Intravenous (IV) benzodiazepines, i.e. diazepam.
- IV Pabrinex.
- Supportive management such as IV fluids and correction of electrolyte imbalance.
- Antipsychotics such as haloperidol are useful in managing hallucinations and agitation. However be mindful of the risk of hypotension, QTc prolongation, and reduced seizure threshold. Have parenteral procyclidine available in case of dystonic reactions.
- Full delirium screen investigations to rule out other organic causes of delirium.

CHAPTER 4

Pharmacologically assisted withdrawal (alcohol detoxification)

Alcohol withdrawal is associated with significant morbidity and mortality when improperly managed.

Pharmacologically assisted withdrawal is likely to be needed when:

- Regular consumption of >15 units/day.
- AUDIT score >20.
- There is a history of significant withdrawal symptoms.

Symptom scales can be helpful in determining the amount of pharmacological support required to manage withdrawal symptoms. The Clinical Institute Withdrawal Assessment of Alcohol Scale Revised (CIWA-Ar; Figure 4.1)[9] and Short Alcohol Withdrawal Scale (SAWS; Table 4.2)[10] are both 10-item scales that can be completed in around 5 minutes. The CIWA-Ar is an objective scale and the SAWS is a self-complete tool. A CIWA-Ar score >10 or a SAWS score >12 should prompt assisted withdrawal.

Community detoxification is usually possible when:

- There is a supervising carer, ideally 24 hours a day throughout the duration of the detoxification process.
- The treatment plan has been agreed with the patient, their carer and their GP.
- A contingency plan has been agreed with the patient, their carer and their GP.
- The patient is able to pick up medication daily and be reviewed by professionals regularly throughout the process.
- Outpatient/community-based programmes including psychosocial support are available.

Community detoxification should be stopped if the patient resumes drinking or fails to engage with the agreed treatment plan.

Inpatient detoxification is likely to be required if:

- Regular consumption of >30 units/day.
- SADQ >30 (severe dependence).
- There is a history of seizures or delirium tremens.
- The patient is very young or old.
- There is current benzodiazepine use in combination with alcohol.
- Substances other than alcohol are also being misused/abused.
- There is co-morbid mental or physical illness, learning disability or cognitive impairment.
- The patient is pregnant.
- The patient is homeless or has no social support.
- There is a history of failed community detoxification.

In certain situations, there may be a clinical justification for undertaking a community detoxification in these patients, however the reasons must be clear and the decision made by an experienced clinician.

Withdrawal treatment interventions are summarised in Table 4.3.

Benzodiazepines are the treatment of choice for alcohol withdrawal. They exhibit cross-tolerance with alcohol and have anticonvulsant properties. Use is supported by NICE guidelines;[2,11] a Cochrane systematic review;[12] and the British Association for

Patient: _____ Date: _____
Time: _____ (24 hour clock, midnight = 00:00)

Pulse or heart rate, taken for 1 minute: _____
Blood pressure: _____

NAUSEA AND VOMITING – Ask 'Do you feel sick to your stomach? Have you vomited?' Observation.
0 no nausea and no vomiting
1 mild nausea with no vomiting
2
3
4 intermittent nausea with dry heaves
5
6
7 constant nausea, frequent dry heaves and vomiting

TREMOR – Arms extended and fingers spread apart. Observation.
0 no tremor
1 not visible, but can be felt fingertip to fingertip
2
3
4 moderate, with patient's arms extended
5
6
7 severe, even with arms not extended

PAROXYSMAL SWEATS – Observation.
0 no sweat visible
1 barely perceptible sweating, palms moist
2
3
4 beads of sweat obvious on forehead
5
6
7 drenching sweats

ANXIETY – Ask 'Do you feel nervous?' Observation.
0 no anxiety, at ease
1 mildly anxious
2
3
4 moderately anxious, or guarded, so anxiety is inferred
5
6
7 equivalent to acute panic states as seen in severe delirium or acute schizophrenic reactions

AGITATION – Observation.
0 normal activity
1 somewhat more than normal activity
2
3
4 moderately fidgety and restless
5
6
7 paces back and forth during most of the interview, or constantly thrashes about
Scores
≤ 10 – mild withdrawal (do not need additional medication)
≤ 15 – moderate withdrawal
> 15 – severe withdrawal

TACTILE DISTURBANCES – Ask 'Have you any itching, pins and needles sensations, any burning, any numbness, or do you feel bugs crawling on or under your skin?' Observation.
0 none
1 very mild itching, pins and needles, burning or numbness
2 mild itching, pins and needles, burning or numbness
3 moderate itching, pins and needles, burning or numbness
4 moderately severe hallucinations
5 severe hallucinations
6 extremely severe hallucinations
7 continuous hallucinations

AUDITORY DISTURBANCES – Ask 'Are you more aware of sounds around you? Are they harsh? Do they frighten you? Are you hearing anything that is disturbing to you? Are you hearing things you know are not there?' Observation.
0 not present
1 very mild harshness or ability to frighten
2 mild harshness or ability to frighten
3 moderate harshness or ability to frighten
4 moderately severe hallucinations
5 severe hallucinations
6 extremely severe hallucinations
7 continuous hallucinations

VISUAL DISTURBANCES – Ask 'Does the light appear to be too bright? Is its colour different? Does it hurt your eyes? Are you seeing anything that is disturbing to you? Are you seeing things you know are not there?' Observation.
0 not present
1 very mild sensitivity
2 mild sensitivity
3 moderate sensitivity
4 moderately severe hallucinations
5 severe hallucinations
6 extremely severe hallucinations
7 continuous hallucinations

HEADACHE, FULLNESS IN HEAD – Ask 'Does your head feel different? Does it feel like there is a band around your head?' Do not rate for dizziness or light-headedness. Otherwise, rate severity.
0 not present
1 very mild
2 mild
3 moderate
4 moderately severe
5 severe
6 very severe
7 extremely severe

ORIENTATION AND CLOUDING OF SENSORIUM – Ask 'What day is this? Where are you? Who am I?'
0 oriented and can do serial additions
1 cannot do serial additions or is uncertain about date
2 disoriented for date by no more than 2 calendar days
3 disoriented for date by more than 2 calendar days
4 disoriented for place or person

Total **CIWA-Ar** Score_____
Rater's initials _____
Maximum possible score 67

CHAPTER 4

Figure 4.1 Clinical Institute Withdrawal Assessment of Alcohol Scale, Revised.[9] The CIWA-Ar is not copyrighted and may be reproduced freely.

Table 4.2 Short Alcohol Withdrawal Scale (SAWS).[10]

	None (0)	Mild (1)	Moderate (2)	Severe (3)
Anxious				
Sleep disturbance				
Problems with memory				
Nausea				
Restless				
Tremor (shakes)				
Feeling confused				
Sweating				
Miserable				
Heart pounding				

The SAWS is a self-completion questionnaire. SAWS is not copyrighted and may be reproduced freely. Symptoms cover the previous 24-hour period

Table 4.3 Alcohol withdrawal treatment interventions – summary

Severity	Supportive/ medical care	Pharmacotherapy for neuro-adaptation reversal	Thiamine supplementation	Setting
Mild CIWA-Ar ≤10	Moderate-to-high level supportive care; little, if any, medical care required	Little to none required. Simple remedies only (see below)	Oral likely to be sufficient if patient is well nourished	Home
Moderate CIWA-Ar ≤15	Moderate-to-high level supportive care; little medical care required	Little to none required. Symptomatic treatment only	Intramuscular Pabrinex should be offered if the patient is malnourished followed by oral supplementation	Home or community team
Severe CIWA-Ar >15	High level supportive care plus medical monitoring	Symptomatic and substitution treatment (chlordiazepoxide) probably required	Intramuscular Pabrinex should be offered followed by oral supplementation	Community team or hospital
CIWA-Ar >10 plus co-morbid alcohol-related medical problems	High level supportive care plus specialist medical care	Symptomatic and substitution treatments usually required	Intramuscular Pabrinex followed by oral supplementation	Hospital

Psychopharmacology guidelines.[8] **Parenteral thiamine (vitamin B₁)**, and other vitamin replacement is an important adjunctive treatment for the prophylaxis and/or treatment of Wernicke–Korsakoff syndrome and other vitamin-related neuropsychiatric conditions.

In the UK, chlordiazepoxide is the benzodiazepine used for most patients in most centres as it is considered to have a relatively low dependence-forming potential. Some centres use diazepam. A short-acting benzodiazepine such as oxazepam or lorazepam may be used in individuals with impaired liver function.

There are three types of assisted withdrawal regimes: **fixed dose reduction** (the most common in non-specialist settings), **variable dose reduction** (usually results in less benzodiazepine being administered but best reserved for settings where staff have specialist skills in managing alcohol withdrawal), and finally **front-loading** (infrequently used).[2,8] Assisted withdrawal regimes should never be started if the blood alcohol concentration is very high or is still rising.

Fixed dose reduction regime

Fixed dose regimes can be used in community or non-specialist inpatient/residential settings for uncomplicated patients. Patients should be started on a dose of benzodiazepine selected after an assessment of the severity of alcohol dependence (clinical history, number of units per drinking day and score on the SADQ). With respect to chlordiazepoxide, a general rule of thumb is that the starting dose can be estimated from current alcohol consumption. For example, if 20 units/day are being consumed, the starting dose should be 20 mg four times a day. The dose is then tapered to zero over 5–10 days. Alcohol withdrawal symptoms should be monitored using a validated instrument such as the CIWA-Ar[9] or the Short Alcohol Withdrawal Scale (SAWS).[10]

Mild alcohol dependence usually requires very small doses of chlordiazepoxide or else may be managed without medication.

For **moderate alcohol dependence**, a typical regime might be 10–20 mg chlordiazepoxide four times a day, reducing gradually over 5–7 days (see Table 4.4). Note that 5–7 days' treatment is adequate and longer treatment is rarely helpful or necessary. It is advisable to monitor withdrawal and BAC daily before providing the days medication. This may mean that community pharmacologically assisted alcohol withdrawals should start on a Monday and last 5 days.

Table 4.4 Moderate alcohol dependence: example of a fixed dose chlordiazepoxide treatment regime

		Total daily dose (mg)
Day 1	20 mg qds	80
Day 2	15 mg qds	60
Day 3	10 mg qds	40
Day 4	5 mg qds	20
Day 5	5 mg bd	10

bd, *bis die* (twice a day); qds, *quarter die sumendum* (four times a day).

Severe alcohol dependence usually requires inpatient treatment for assisted withdrawal because of the significant risk of life-threatening complications. However, there are rare occasions when a pragmatic community approach is required. In such situations, the decision to undertake a community-assisted withdrawal must be made clear by an experienced clinician. Intensive daily monitoring is advised for the first 2–3 days. This may require special arrangements over a weekend.

Prescribing should not start if the patient is intoxicated. In such circumstances the patient should be reviewed at the earliest opportunity when not intoxicated. The dose of benzodiazepine may need to be reduced over a 7- to 10-day period in this group (occasionally longer if dependence is very severe or there is a history of complications during previous detoxifications) (see Table 4.5).

Table 4.5 Severe alcohol dependence: example of a fixed dose chlordiazepoxide regime

		Total daily dose (mg)
Day 1 (first 24 hours)	40 mg qds + 40 mg prn	200
Day 2	40 mg qds	160
Day 3	30 mg qds	120
Day 4	25 mg qds	100
Day 5	20 mg qds	80
Day 6	15 mg qds	60
Day 7	10 mg qds	40
Day 8	10 mg tds	30
Day 9	5 mg qds	20
Day 10	10 mg nocte	10

bd, *bis die* (twice a day); nocte, at night; prn, *pro re nata* (as required); qds, *quarter die sumendum* (four times a day); tds, *ter die sumendum* (three times a day).

Symptom-triggered regime

This should be reserved for managing assisted withdrawal in specialist alcohol inpatient or residential settings. Regular monitoring is required, for example pulse, blood pressure, temperature and level of consciousness. Medication is only given when withdrawal symptoms are observed as determined using CIWA-Ar, SAWS or an alternative validated measure. Symptom-triggered therapy is generally used in patients without a history of complications. A typical symptom-triggered regime would be chlordiazepoxide 20–30 mg hourly as needed (see Table 4.6). Note that the total dose given each day

Table 4.6 Example of a symptom-triggered chlordiazepoxide regime[2]

Day 1–5	20–30 mg chlordiazepoxide as needed, up to hourly, based on symptoms

would be expected to decrease from day 2 onwards. It is common for symptom-triggered treatment to last only 24–48 hours before switching to an individualised fixed dose reducing schedule. Occasionally (e.g. in delirium tremens) the flexible regime may need to be prolonged beyond the first 24 hours.

Wernicke's encephalopathy

Wernicke's encephalopathy is an acute neuropsychiatric condition caused by thiamine deficiency. In alcohol dependence, thiamine deficiency is secondary to both reduced dietary intake and reduced absorption.

Risk factors for Wernicke's encephalopathy in alcohol dependence[11]

- Acute withdrawal.
- Malnourishment.
- Decompensated liver disease.
- Emergency department attendance.
- Hospitalisation for co-morbidity.
- Homelessness.

Presentation

The 'classical' triad of ophthalmoplegia, ataxia and confusion is rarely present in Wernicke's encephalopathy, and the syndrome is much more common than is perceived. A presumptive diagnosis of Wernicke's encephalopathy should therefore be made in any patient undergoing detoxification who experiences any of the following signs:

- ataxia
- hypothermia
- hypotension
- confusion
- ophthalmoplegia/nystagmus
- memory disturbance
- unconsciousness/coma.

Any history of malnutrition, recent weight loss, vomiting or diarrhoea or peripheral neuropathy should also be noted.[13]

Prophylactic thiamine

Low-risk drinkers without neuropsychiatric complications and with an adequate diet should be offered oral thiamine: a minimum of 300 mg daily during assisted alcohol withdrawal and periods of continued alcohol intake.[8]

Thiamine is required to utilise glucose. A glucose load in a thiamine-deficient patient can precipitate Wernicke's encephalopathy.

Parenteral B complex (Pabrinex) must be administered *before* glucose is administered in all patients presenting with altered mental status.

It is generally advised that patients undergoing in-patient detoxification should be given parenteral thiamine as **prophylaxis**[2,8,11,14,15] although there is insufficient evidence from randomised controlled trials (RCTs) as to the best dose, frequency or duration of use. Guidance is based on 'expert opinion'[8] and the standard advice is **one pair of Pabrinex IMHP daily** (containing thiamine 250 mg/dose) for 5 days, followed by oral thiamine and/or vitamin B compound for as long as needed (where diet is inadequate or alcohol consumption is resumed).[8] All inpatients should receive this regime as an absolute minimum.

IM thiamine preparations have a lower incidence of anaphylactic reactions than IV preparations, at 1 per 5 million pairs of ampoules of Pabrinex – far lower than many frequently used drugs that carry no special anaphylaxis warning. However this risk has resulted in fears about using parenteral preparations and the inappropriate use of oral thiamine preparations (which do not offer adequate protection). Given the risks associated with Wernicke's encephalopathy, the benefit to risk ratio grossly favours parenteral thiamine.[8,14,16] Where parenteral thiamine is used, facilities for treating anaphylaxis should be available.[17]

If Wernicke's encephalopathy is suspected the patient should be transferred to a medical unit where intravenous thiamine can be administered (see Box 4.2). If untreated, Wernicke's encephalopathy progresses to Korsakoff's syndrome (permanent memory impairment, confabulation, confusion and personality changes).

Box 4.2 Treatment for patients with suspected/established Wernicke's encephalopathy (acute medical ward)

At least 2 pairs of Pabrinex IVHP (i.e. 4 ampoules) *three times daily* for 3–5 days, followed by one pair of ampoules once daily for a further 3–5 days or longer[2,8] (until no further response is seen).

Treatment of somatic symptoms

Somatic complaints are common during assisted withdrawal. Recommended simple remedies are listed in Table 4.7.

Table 4.7 Recommended remedies for somatic symptoms in withdrawal

Symptom	Recommended treatment
Dehydration	Ensure adequate fluid intake in order to maintain hydration and electrolyte balance. Dehydration can precipitate life-threatening cardiac arrhythmia
Pain	Paracetamol (acetaminophen)
Nausea and vomiting	Metoclopramide 10 mg or prochlorperazine 5 mg 4–6 hourly
Diarrhoea	Diphenoxylate and atropine (Lomotil) or loperamide
Skin itching	Occurs commonly and not only in individuals with alcoholic liver disease: use oral antihistamines

Relapse prevention

There is no place for the continued use of benzodiazepines beyond treatment of the acute alcohol withdrawal syndrome. Acamprosate and supervised disulfiram are licensed for treatment of alcohol dependence in the UK and may be offered in combination with psychosocial treatment.[2] Treatment should be initiated by a specialist service. After 12 weeks, transfer of the prescribing to the GP may be appropriate, although specialist care may continue (shared care). Naltrexone is also recommended as an adjunct in the treatment of moderate and severe alcohol dependence.[2] As it does not have marketing authorisation for the treatment of alcohol dependence in the UK, informed consent should be sought and documented prior to commencing treatment.

Acamprosate

Acamprosate is a synthetic taurine analogue which acts as a functional glutamatergic NMDA antagonist and also increases GABA-ergic function. The number needed to treat (NNT) for the maintenance of abstinence has been calculated as 9–11.[8] The treatment effect is most pronounced at 6 months with the risk ratio (compared with placebo) of returning to drinking behaviour dropping to 0.83, though the effect has been shown to be significant for up to 12 months.[2,18] Acamprosate should be initiated as soon as possible after abstinence has been achieved (the BAP consensus guidelines[8] recommend that acamprosate should be started 'during detoxification' because of its potential neuroprotective effect). NICE recommends that acamprosate should be continued for up to 6 months, with regular (monthly) supervision. The summary of product characteristics (SPC) recommends that it is given for 1 year.

Acamprosate is relatively well tolerated; adverse effects include diarrhoea, abdominal pain, nausea, vomiting and pruritus.[2] It is contraindicated in severe renal or hepatic impairment, thus baseline liver and kidney function tests should be performed before commencing treatment. Acamprosate should be avoided in individuals who are pregnant or breastfeeding (see Box 4.3).

Box 4.3 Acamprosate: NICE Clinical Guideline 115, 2011[2]

Acamprosate should be offered for relapse prevention in moderately to severely dependent drinkers, in combination with psychosocial treatment. It should be prescribed for up to 6 months, or longer for those who perceive benefit and wish to continue taking it. The dose is 1998 mg daily (666 mg three times per day) for individuals over 60 kg. For those under 60 kg, the dose is 1332 mg daily. Treatment should be stopped in those who continue to drink for 4–6 weeks after starting the drug.

Naltrexone

Opioid blockade prevents increased dopaminergic activity after the consumption of alcohol, thus reducing its rewarding effects. Naltrexone, a non-selective opioid receptor antagonist, significantly reduces relapse to heavy drinking.[18] Although early trials used a dose of 50 mg/day, more recent US studies have used 100 mg/day. In the UK the usual dose is 50 mg/day with a trial dose of 25 mg for 2 days to check for adverse effects (see Box 4.4).

> **Box 4.4** Naltrexone: NICE Clinical Guideline 115, 2011[2]
>
> Naltrexone (50 mg/day) should be offered for relapse prevention in moderately to severely dependent drinkers, in combination with psychosocial treatment. It should be prescribed for up to 6 months, or longer for those who perceive benefit and wish to continue taking it. Treatment should be stopped in those who continue to drink for 4–6 weeks after starting the drug or in those who feel unwell while taking it.

Naltrexone is well tolerated but adverse effects include nausea (especially in the early stages of treatment), headache, abdominal pain, reduced appetite and tiredness. A comprehensive medical assessment should be carried out prior to commencing naltrexone, together with baseline renal and liver function tests. Naltrexone can be started when patients are still drinking or during medically assisted withdrawal. There is no clear evidence as to the optimal duration of treatment but 6 months appears to be an appropriate period with follow-up, including monitoring liver function.[8]

Patients on naltrexone should not be given opioid agonist drugs for analgesia; non-opioid analgesics should be used instead. In the event that opioid analgesia is necessary, it can be instituted 48–72 hours after cessation of naltrexone. Hepatotoxicity has been described with high doses of naltrexone, so use should be avoided in acute liver failure.[19]

Long-acting injectable naltrexone has been developed to improve compliance. Adverse effects are similar to those seen with the oral preparation.[20] NICE concluded that the initial evidence was encouraging but not enough to support routine use.

Nalmefene

Nalmefene is also an opioid antagonist, recommended by NICE as an option for reducing alcohol consumption for people with alcohol dependence.[2] It has been shown in one indirect meta-analysis to be superior to naltrexone in reducing heavy drinking.[21] However use of nalmefene remains controversial, with another meta-analysis suggesting that nalmefene had only limited efficacy in reducing alcohol consumption and that its value in treating alcohol addiction and relapse prevention was not fully established.[22]

Disulfiram (Antabuse)

Disulfiram inhibits the enzyme aldehyde dehydrogenase, thus preventing complete metabolism of alcohol in the liver. This results in an accumulation of the toxic intermediate product, acetaldehyde, which causes the alcohol–disulfiram reaction (see Box 4.5).

The therapeutic effect of disulfiram is thus mediated by its incompatibility with alcohol, resulting in alcohol aversion. Supervised medication optimises compliance and contributes to effectiveness.

The intensity of the intolerance reaction is dose-dependent, both with regards to the amount of alcohol consumed and the dose of disulfiram. However it is thought that much of the therapeutic effect is mediated by the mental anticipation of the aversive reaction, rather than the pharmacological action itself. Sudden death is more prevalent at doses above 1000 mg.[23] With this in mind, the value of prescribing higher doses of disulfiram must be carefully considered.

Box 4.5 Disulfiram reactions with alcohol and contraindications to use

Mild alcohol–disulfiram reaction:
- Facial flushing
- Sweating
- Nausea
- Hyperventilation
- Dyspnoea
- Tachycardia
- Hypotension

Severe alcohol–disulfiram reaction:
- Acute heart failure
- Myocardial infarction
- Arrhythmias
- Bradycardia
- Respiratory depression
- Severe hypotension

Contraindications:
- Ingestion of alcohol within the previous 24 hours
- Cardiac failure
- Coronary artery disease
- Hypertension
- Cerebrovascular disease
- Pregnancy
- Breastfeeding
- Liver disease
- Peripheral neuropathy
- Severe mental illness

Box 4.6 Disulfiram: NICE Clinical Guideline 115, 2011[2]

Disulfiram should be considered in combination with a psychological intervention for patients who wish to achieve abstinence, but for whom acamprosate or naltrexone are not suitable. Treatment should be started at least 24 hours after the last drink and should be overseen by a family member or carer. Monitoring is recommended every 2 weeks for the first 2 months, then monthly for the following 4 months. Medical monitoring should be continued at 6-monthly intervals after the first 6 months. Patients must not consume any alcohol while taking disulfiram.

Doses are 800 mg for the first dose, reducing to 100–200 mg daily for maintenance. In co-morbid alcohol and cocaine dependence doses of 500 mg daily have been given. Halitosis is a common adverse effect. If there is a sudden onset of jaundice (the rare complication of hepatotoxicity), the patient should stop the drug and seek urgent medical attention.

The evidence for disulfiram is weaker than for acamprosate and naltrexone.[2] In the UK, NICE recommends its use 'as a second-line option for moderate to severe alcohol dependence for patients who are not suitable for acamprosate or naltrexone or have a specified preference for disulfiram and who aim to stay abstinent from alcohol' (Box 4.6).[2]

Baclofen

Baclofen is a $GABA_\beta$ agonist that does not have a licence for use in alcohol dependence but is nevertheless used by some clinicians. It may have a role in reducing anxiety in severely dependent patients. It is well tolerated and can be given to alcohol-dependent patients with liver cirrhosis. Studies have used a 10 mg tds dose, but a 20 mg tds dose may have superior outcomes.[24]

Anticonvulsants

Topiramate is not licensed for use in alcohol dependence, but has been shown to reduce both the percentage of drinking days and amount of alcohol consumed on drinking days. The dose is 25 mg daily, increasing to 300 mg daily. However, its use is likely to be limited by its adverse-effect profile (paraesthesiae, dizziness, taste perversion, anorexia and weight loss, difficulties with memory and concentration). Zonisamide or levetiracetam may offer a more tolerable alternative.[25]

Gabapentin[26] and pregabalin[27] have been shown to have some efficacy in alcohol withdrawal and in reducing drinking but the evidence is limited.

Pregnancy and alcohol use

Evidence indicates that alcohol consumption during pregnancy may cause harm to the foetus. NICE advises that women should not drink any alcohol at all during pregnancy.[28] If abstinence is not tolerable, NICE advises that alcohol should be avoided in the first 3 months of pregnancy, and consumption limited to '1–2 units once or twice a week' for the rest of the pregnancy.

For alcohol-dependent pregnant women who have withdrawal symptoms, pharmacological cover for detoxification should be offered, ideally in an in-patient setting. The timing of detoxification in relation to the trimester of pregnancy should be risk-assessed against continued alcohol consumption and risks to the foetus.[8] Chlordiazepoxide has been suggested as being unlikely to pose a substantial risk, however dose-dependent malformations have been observed.[8] The Regional Drugs and Therapeutics Centre Teratology Service[29] provides national advice for health-care professionals and likes to follow up on pregnancies that require alcohol detoxification. Please refer to the references at the end of this section. Specialist advice should always be sought. (See also section on 'Drug choice in pregnancy' in Chapter 7.) No relapse prevention medication has been evaluated in pregnancy.[8]

Children and adolescents

Children and young people (10–17 years) should be assessed as outlined in NICE Clinical Guideline 115, 2011.[2]

The number of young people who are dependent and needing pharmacotherapy is likely to be small, but for those who are dependent there should be a lower threshold for admission to hospital. Doses of chlordiazepoxide for medically assisted withdrawal may need to be adjusted, but the general principles of withdrawal management are the same as for adults. All young people should have a full health screen carried out routinely to allow identification of physical and mental health problems. The evidence base for acamprosate, naltrexone and disulfiram in 16- to 19-year-olds is evolving,[8] but naltrexone is best supported in this age group.[30,31]

Older adults

There should be a lower threshold for in-patient medically assisted alcohol withdrawal for older adults.[2] While benzodiazepines remain the treatment of choice, they may need to be prescribed in lower doses and in some situations shorter-acting drugs may be preferred.[8] Older adults with alcohol use disorders should all have full routine health screens to identify physical and mental health problems. The evidence base for pharmacotherapy of alcohol use disorders in older people is limited.

Concurrent alcohol and drug use disorders

Where alcohol and drug use disorders are co-morbid, treat both conditions actively.[2]

Co-existing alcohol and benzodiazepine dependence

This is best managed with one benzodiazepine, either chlordiazepoxide or diazepam. The starting dose should take into account the requirements for medically assisted alcohol withdrawal and the typical daily equivalent dose of the relevant benzodiazepine(s).[1] In-patient treatment should be carried out over a 2- to 3-week period, possibly longer.[1]

Co-existing alcohol dependence and cocaine use

In co-morbid cocaine/alcohol dependence, naltrexone 150 mg/day resulted in reduced cocaine and alcohol use in men but not in women.[32]

Co-existing alcohol and opioid dependence

Both conditions should be treated, and attention paid to the increased mortality of individuals withdrawing from both drugs.

Co-morbid alcohol and nicotine dependence

Encourage individuals to stop smoking. Refer for smoking cessation in primary care and other settings. In in-patient settings, offer nicotine patches/inhalator during assisted alcohol withdrawal. Always promote vaping as a safer alternative to tobacco smoking.

Co-morbid mental health disorders

People with alcohol use disorders often present with other mental health disorders, particularly anxiety and depression. Public Health England has described it as 'the norm rather than the exception' and encourages a collaborative, effective and flexible approach between front-line services, stating that it is 'everyone's job' and that there is 'no wrong door'.[33]

Substance misuse disorders, including alcohol misuse, should never be a reason to exclude a patient from:

- crisis psychiatric services
- mood/anxiety/personality services once detoxed.

Depression

Depressive and anxiety symptoms occur commonly during alcohol withdrawal, but usually diminish by the third or fourth week of abstinence. Meta-analyses suggest that antidepressants with mixed pharmacology (the tricyclics imipramine or trimipramine) perform better than selective serotonin reuptake inhibitors (SSRIs – fluoxetine or sertraline) in reducing depressive symptoms in individuals with an alcohol use disorder, but the antidepressant effect is modest.[2,8] A greater antidepressant effect was seen if the diagnosis of depression was made after at least 1 week of abstinence, thus excluding those with affective symptoms caused by alcohol withdrawal. However tricyclics are not recommended in clinical practice because of their potential for cardiotoxicity and toxicity in overdose. Preliminary research on newer drugs such as mirtazapine[34] or escitalopram[35] was encouraging but a meta-analysis showed only a modest effect.[36] One trial suggested that citalopram worsened drinking outcomes.[37]

Relapse prevention medication should be considered in combination with antidepressants. Pettinati et al.[38] showed that the combination of sertraline (200 mg/day) with naltrexone (100 mg/day) had superior outcomes – improved drinking outcomes and better mood – compared with placebo and compared with each drug alone. In contrast, citalopram showed no benefit when added to naltrexone.[39]

Secondary analyses of acamprosate and naltrexone trials suggest that:

- acamprosate has an indirect modest beneficial effect on depression via increasing abstinence; and
- in depressed alcohol-dependent patients, the combination of naltrexone and an antidepressant may be better than either drug alone,[8] but findings are not consistent.[39]

Bipolar affective disorder

Bipolar patients tend to use alcohol to reduce symptoms of anxiety. Where there is co-morbidity it is important to treat the different phases as recommended in guidelines for bipolar disorder. It may be worth adding sodium valproate to lithium as two trials have shown that the combination was associated with better drinking outcomes than lithium alone. However the combination did not confer any extra benefit than lithium alone in improving mood (see BAP consensus 2012).[8] Note that, in those who continue to drink, electrolyte imbalance may precipitate lithium toxicity. Lithium is best avoided completely in binge drinkers.

Naltrexone should be offered, in the first instance, to help bipolar patients reduce their alcohol consumption.[8] If naltrexone is not effective then acamprosate should be offered. In the event that both naltrexone and acamprosate fail to promote abstinence, then disulfiram should be considered, and the risks made known to the patient.

Anxiety

Anxiety is commonly observed in alcohol-dependent individuals during intoxication, withdrawal and in the early days of abstinence. Alcohol is typically used to self-medicate anxiety disorders, particularly social anxiety. In alcohol-dependent individuals who experience anxiety it is often difficult to determine the extent to which the anxiety is a symptom of the alcohol use disorder or whether it is an independent disorder. Medically assisted withdrawal and supported abstinence for up to 8 weeks are required before a full assessment can be made. If a medically assisted withdrawal is not possible then treatment of the anxiety disorder should still be attempted, following guidelines for the respective anxiety disorder.

The use of benzodiazepines is controversial[8] because of the increased risk of benzodiazepine misuse and dependence. Benzodiazepines should only be considered following assessment in a specialist addiction service.

One meta-analysis suggests that buspirone is effective in reducing symptoms of anxiety, but not alcohol consumption.[8,40] Studies have also shown that paroxetine (up to 60 mg/day) was superior to placebo in reducing social anxiety in co-morbid patients: alcohol consumption was not affected.[8,40]

Either naltrexone or disulfiram, alone or combined, improved drinking outcomes compared with placebo in patients with PTSD and alcohol dependence. Both acamprosate and baclofen have shown benefit in reducing anxiety in *post hoc* analyses of alcohol dependence trials (see BAP consensus for references[8]). It is therefore important to ensure that these patients are enabled to become abstinent and are prescribed relapse prevention medication. Anxiety should then be treated according to the appropriate NICE guidelines.

Schizophrenia

Patients with schizophrenia who also have an alcohol use disorder should be assessed and alcohol-specific relapse prevention treatment considered, either naltrexone or acamprosate. Antipsychotic medication should be optimised[8] and clozapine may be considered. However there is insufficient evidence to recommend the use of any one antipsychotic medication over another.

References

1. Department of Health. UK Chief Medical Officers' Low Risk Drinking Guidelines. 2016. https://www.gov.uk/government/publications/alcohol-consumption-advice-on-low-risk-drinking.
2. National Institute for Health and Care Excellence. Alcohol use disorders: diagnosis, assessment and management of harmful drinking and alcohol dependence. Clinical Guidance **115**, 2011. https://www.nice.org.uk/guidance/cg115
3. National Institute for Health and Care Excellence. Alcohol-use disorders: prevention. Public Health Guideline **24**, 2010. https://www.nice.org.uk/guidance/ph24.
4. Babor T, Higgins-Biddle JC, Saunders JB, et al. *AUDIT. The Alcohol Use Disorders Identification Test: Guidelines for Use in Primary Care*, 2nd edn. Geneva: World Health Organization; 2001. http://whqlibdoc.who.int/hq/2001/WHO_MSD_MSB 01.6a.pdf?ua=1.
5. Stockwell T et al. The severity of alcohol dependence questionnaire: its use, reliability and validity. Br J Addict 1983; **78**:145–155.
6. Minozzi S et al. Anticonvulsants for alcohol withdrawal. Cochrane Database Syst Rev 2010:CD005064.

7. Brathen G et al. EFNS guideline on the diagnosis and management of alcohol-related seizures: report of an EFNS task force. Eur J Neurol 2005; **12**:575–581.

8. Lingford-Hughes AR et al. Evidence-based guidelines for the pharmacological management of substance abuse, harmful use, addiction and comorbidity: recommendations from BAP. J Psychopharmacol 2012; **26**:899–952.

9. Sullivan JT et al. Assessment of alcohol withdrawal: the revised clinical institute withdrawal assessment for alcohol scale (CIWA-Ar). Br J Addict 1989; **84**:1353–1357.

10. Gossop M et al. A Short Alcohol Withdrawal Scale (SAWS): development and psychometric properties. Addict Biol 2002; **7**:37–43.

11. National Institute for Health and Clinical Excellence. Alcohol-use disorders: physical complications. Clinical Guidance 100, 2010; last updated April 2017. https://www.nice.org.uk/guidance/cg100.

12. Amato L et al. Benzodiazepines for alcohol withdrawal. Cochrane Database Syst Rev 2010:CD005063.

13. Thomson AD et al. Time to act on the inadequate management of Wernicke's encephalopathy in the UK. Alcohol Alcohol 2013; **48**:4–8.

14. Thomson AD et al. The Royal College of Physicians report on alcohol: guidelines for managing Wernicke's encephalopathy in the accident and Emergency Department. Alcohol Alcohol 2002; **37**:513–521.

15. Day E et al. Thiamine for prevention and treatment of Wernicke-Korsakoff Syndrome in people who abuse alcohol. Cochrane Database Syst Rev 2013; **7**:CD004033.

16. Thomson AD et al. The treatment of patients at risk of developing Wernicke's encephalopathy in the community. Alcohol Alcohol 2006; **41**:159–167.

17. BNF Online. British National Formulary. 2017. https://www.medicinescomplete.com/mc/bnf/current/.

18. Donoghue K et al. The efficacy of acamprosate and naltrexone in the treatment of alcohol dependence, Europe versus the rest of the world: a meta-analysis. Addiction 2015; **110**:920–930.

19. Accord Healthcare Limited. Summary of Product Characteristics. Naltrexone Hydrochloride 50 mg Film-coated Tablets. 2014. https://www.medicines.org.uk/emc/medicine/25878.

20. Krupitsky E et al. Injectable extended-release naltrexone (XR-NTX) for opioid dependence: long-term safety and effectiveness. Addiction 2013; **108**:1628–1637.

21. Soyka M et al. Comparing nalmefene and naltrexone in alcohol dependence: are there any differences? Results from an indirect meta-analysis. Pharmacopsychiatry 2016; **49**:66–75.

22. Palpacuer C et al. Risks and benefits of nalmefene in the treatment of adult alcohol dependence: a systematic literature review and meta-analysis of published and unpublished double-blind randomized controlled trials. PLoS Med 2015; **12**:e1001924.

23. Mutschler J et al. Current findings and mechanisms of action of disulfiram in the treatment of alcohol dependence. Pharmacopsychiatry 2016; **49**:137–141.

24. Liu J et al. Baclofen for alcohol withdrawal. Cochrane Database Syst Rev 2017; **8**:Cd008502.

25. Knapp CM et al. Zonisamide, topiramate, and levetiracetam: efficacy and neuropsychological effects in alcohol use disorders. J Clin Psychopharmacol 2015; **35**:34–42.

26. Mason BJ et al. Gabapentin treatment for alcohol dependence: a randomized clinical trial. JAMA Intern Med 2014; **174**:70–77.

27. Guglielmo R et al. Pregabalin for alcohol dependence: a critical review of the literature. Adv Ther 2012; **29**:947–957.

28. National Institute for Health and Clinical Excellence. Antenatal care for uncomplicated pregnancies. Clinical Guideline 62, 2008; last updated January 2017. https://www.nice.org.uk/guidance/cg62.

29. Regional Drug and Therapeutics Centre. Regional Medicines Information Service. 2017. http://rdtc.nhs.uk/services/regional-medicines-information-service.

30. O'Malley SS et al. Reduction of alcohol drinking in young adults by naltrexone: a double-blind, placebo-controlled, randomized clinical trial of efficacy and safety. J Clin Psychiatry 2015; **76**:e207–e213.

31. Miranda R et al. Effects of naltrexone on adolescent alcohol cue reactivity and sensitivity: an initial randomized trial. Addict Biol 2014; **19**:941–954.

32. Pettinati HM et al. Gender differences with high-dose naltrexone in patients with co-occurring cocaine and alcohol dependence. J Subst Abuse Treat 2008; **34**:378–390.

33. Public Health England. Better care for people with co-occurring mental health and alcohol/drug use conditions: a guide for commissioners and service providers. 2017. https://www.gov.uk/government/uploads/system/uploads/attachment_data/file/625809/Co-occurring_mental_health_and_alcohol_drug_use_conditions.pdf.

34. Cornelius JR et al. Mirtazapine in comorbid major depression and alcohol dependence: an open-label trial. J Dual Diagn 2012; **8**:200–204.

35. Han DH et al. Adjunctive aripiprazole therapy with escitalopram in patients with co-morbid major depressive disorder and alcohol dependence: clinical and neuroimaging evidence. J Psychopharmacol 2013; **27**:282–291.

36. Foulds JA et al. Depression in patients with alcohol use disorders: systematic review and meta-analysis of outcomes for independent and substance-induced disorders. J Affect Disord 2015; **185**:47–59.

37. Charney DA et al. Poorer drinking outcomes with citalopram treatment for alcohol dependence: a randomized, double-blind, placebo-controlled trial. Alcohol Clin Exp Res 2015; **39**:1756–1765.

38. Pettinati HM et al. A double-blind, placebo-controlled trial combining sertraline and naltrexone for treating co-occurring depression and alcohol dependence. Am J Psychiatry 2010; **167**:668–675.

39. Adamson SJ et al. A randomized trial of combined citalopram and naltrexone for nonabstinent outpatients with co-occurring alcohol dependence and major depression. J Clin Psychopharmacol 2015; **35**:143–149.

40. Ipser JC et al. Pharmacotherapy for anxiety and comorbid alcohol use disorders. Cochrane Database Syst Rev 2015; **1**:Cd007505.

Opioid dependence

Prescribing for opioid dependence

Treatment of opioid dependence usually requires specialist intervention – generalists who do not have specialist experience should always contact substance misuse services before attempting to treat opioid dependence. It is strongly recommended that general adult psychiatrists *do not* initiate opioid substitute treatment unless directly advised by specialist services. It cannot be over-emphasised that the use of opioids including methadone and buprenorphine can be fatal; opioid withdrawal is not.

That having been said, self-discharge against medical advice from hospital because of intolerable opiate withdrawal also carries risks, and non-opiate medications should be used to treat opioid withdrawal until appropriate advice can be sought (see section pertaining to in-patient admission).

The pharmacological interventions used for opioid-dependent people in the UK range from harm minimisation measures such as provision of take-home naloxone, maintenance treatment with opioid substitution treatment such as methadone or buprenorphine, to naltrexone for relapse prevention. Pharmacological treatments form an integral part of recovery-orientated care alongside psychosocial treatment. The latter is not considered in this chapter and readers are referred to *Routes to Recovery* and chapter 3 of *Drug misuse and dependence: UK guidelines for clinical management* or, as it is more frequently called, the 'Orange Guidelines', to understand more about these aspects of addiction treatment.[1,2]

Opioid overdose

Opioid overdose is a preventable cause of death in the opioid-using population. This includes overdose on illicit opioids such as heroin and more recently fentanyl, and overdose on prescribed opioids such as methadone or buprenorphine. Opioid overdose is characterised clinically by the triad of **unconsciousness, a low respiratory rate** (RR <12) and **pin-point pupils**. The patient often looks cyanosed and feels cold and clammy. **Naloxone** is an opioid receptor antagonist that can reverse opioid overdose. It is available in pre-loaded syringes and should be administered intramuscularly after calling an ambulance and an initial round of chest compressions. An initial dose of 400 µg is recommended which can be repeated following three cycles of 30 chest compressions until the ambulance arrives or breathing resumes (see Figure 4.2).[3] High doses of naloxone may be necessary to displace opioids of high affinity such as buprenorphine or fentanyl.[4]

Naloxone should be written on the prn side of the drug chart for any in-patient with suspected harmful opioid use or dependence and should be kept in the resuscitation bag on the ward. Anyone can give naloxone to prevent an overdose death. Patients discharged from in-patient wards should be warned about loss of tolerance and they and their family members provided with naloxone training and take-home naloxone.[1]

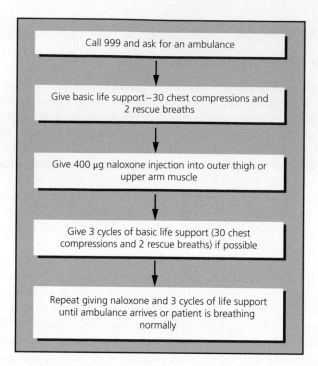

Figure 4.2 Flowchart for naloxone administration (adapted from WHO[3]).

Opioid dependence

The mainstay of pharmacological management of opioid dependence is opioid substitution treatment (OST). OST can be prescribed for detoxification, that is, at a dose to control withdrawal symptoms followed by progressive reduction and discontinuation. Alternatively, OST can be prescribed as 'maintenance', which refers to a longer period of months to years on a stable dose of OST.

The goals of OST are:

- to reduce or prevent withdrawal symptoms
- to reduce or eliminate non-prescribed drug use
- to stabilise drug intake and lifestyle
- to reduce drug-related harm (particularly injecting behaviour)
- to engage and provide an opportunity to work with the patient.

Treatment

This will depend upon:

- what pharmacotherapies and/or other interventions are available
- patient's previous history of drug use and treatment
- patient's current drug use and circumstances
- location/service where treatment is initiated.

Specialist addiction services should initiate most OST prescribing for people with mental health problems, though these patients should continue to receive appropriate psychiatric care from mental health services.[5] Some people with co-morbid opioid dependence and mental health problems will be admitted to psychiatric in-patient wards and general psychiatrists will need to take over, or initiate prescribing in the immediate term[1] (see next section).

Principles of prescribing OST

Clinicians should take care to ensure that patients meet ICD-10 criteria for opioid dependence before prescribing OST. Assessment should involve the following:

- details of what substances the person is taking, duration of use, quantity, frequency, route of administration, duration at current level and date and time of last use
- at least one positive urine or oral fluid drug screen for specific opioids
- objective signs of opioid withdrawal (see Table 4.8)
- recent sites of injection – if the patient injects drugs
- details of alcohol and other illicit drug use, including assessment for alcohol and other drug withdrawal
- details of prescribed medication, which can interact with OST (including sedating psychiatric medications and those which affect QTc)
- previous contact with treatment services
- risks related to drug use or route of administration
- collateral information from addiction services and pharmacy regarding usual dose of OST and most recently dispensed dose.

Untreated heroin withdrawal symptoms typically begin after 4–6 hours and reach their peak 32–72 hours after the last dose. Symptoms will have subsided substantially after

Table 4.8 Objective Opioid Withdrawal Scale (adapted from Handelsman et al, 1987[6])

Symptoms	Absent/normal	Mild–moderate	Severe
Lacrimation	Absent	Eyes watery	Eyes streaming/wiping eyes
Rhinorrhoea	Absent	Sniffing	Profuse secretion (wiping nose)
Agitation	Absent	Fidgeting	Can't remain seated
Perspiration	Absent	Clammy skin	Beads of sweat
Piloerection	Absent	Barely palpable hairs standing up	Readily palpable, visible
Pulse rate (BPM)	<80	>80 but <100	>100
Vomiting	Absent	Absent	Present
Shivering	Absent	Absent	Present
Yawning /10 min	<3	3–5	6 or more
Dilated pupils	Normal <4 mm	Dilated 4–6 mm	Widely dilated >6 mm

BPM, beats per minute.

CHAPTER 4

5 days. Untreated methadone withdrawal typically reaches its peak between 4 and 6 days after last dose and symptoms do not subside for 10–12 days. Untreated buprenorphine withdrawal typically lasts for up to 10 days. Specific opioid withdrawal scales are available, such as the Objective Opiate Withdrawal Scale (OOWS),[6] which can be used to help assess levels of dependence.

To prescribe OST safely:

- Use licensed medications for heroin dependence treatment (methadone and buprenorphine).
- Ensure that the patient is dependent on opioids.
- Give a safe initial dose and titrate cautiously.
- Use daily supervised consumption for the first few months of treatment or until stability is achieved (stability = abstinence from illicit opioids).
- Minimise take-away doses for first few months of treatment or until stability is achieved.

Induction and stabilisation of OST maintenance medication

Methadone and buprenorphine are the OST medications recommended by NICE for maintenance substitute prescribing. Both methadone and buprenorphine maintenance are effective in treating withdrawal symptoms and decreasing use of illicit opioids.[7] Recent guidelines and systematic reviews find that there is no evidence to support one over the other.[1] The pharmacology of methadone and buprenorphine differs. Methadone is a full agonist at μ opioid receptors while buprenorphine is a partial agonist. This difference in pharmacology affords advantages and disadvantages of each drug, tabulated in Table 4.9. The decision which to use is an individualised one based on: the client's preference; their past experience of either; polysubstance use (especially co-morbid benzodiazepine or alcohol dependence); risk of diversion; their long-term plans (including a preference for one or other as a detoxification regime); and, in the case of buprenorphine, their ability to refrain from heroin use for long enough to avoid precipitated opioid withdrawal symptoms.

In rare cases, patients may be allergic to methadone or buprenorphine or to some of the constituents within the formulations.

Methadone

Clinical effectiveness

Methadone is a long-acting opioid agonist. It has been shown to be an effective maintenance treatment of heroin dependence by retaining patients in treatment and decreasing heroin use more than non-opioid based replacement therapy.[7] Higher doses of methadone (60–100 mg/day) are recommended as they have been shown to be more effective than lower dosages in retaining patients and in reducing illicit heroin and cocaine use during treatment. According to emerging small-scale open-label

Table 4.9 Choosing between buprenorphine and methadone

	Methadone	Buprenorphine
Withdrawal syndrome	Appears to be more marked and prolonged – best for maintenance programmes	Appears to have a milder withdrawal syndrome than methadone and therefore may be preferred for detoxification programs[8,9]
Differences in initiation	Associated with increased mortality during the titration phase Need for gradual titration over a few weeks to reach therapeutic range (60–100 mg od)	Not associated with increased mortality during titration Able to reach therapeutic dose (12–16 mg od) over a few days Risk of precipitated withdrawal if patients are not already in withdrawal
Differences in retention	Methadone associated with greater retention in treatment than low dose buprenorphine (<7 mg)	Buprenorphine associated with greater drop-out from treatment only if prescribed at low and flexible doses (<7 mg)[7]
Differences in adverse effects	Methadone may be associated with QTc prolongation and torsades de pointes, which is a particular concern in patients prescribed QT-lengthening antipsychotics or those with co-morbid cocaine use	Buprenorphine is often perceived as less sedating than methadone, which can be seen as undesirable by patients[1]
Chronic pain	Patients with chronic pain conditions that frequently require additional opioid analgesia may have difficulties being treated with buprenorphine because of the 'blockade' effect although in practice this does not appear to be a major problem	Buprenorphine appears to provide greater 'blockade' effects than doses of methadone <60 mg.[10–12] If a patient on buprenorphine requires treatment for acute pain, an additional opioid may be added, titrated against response[13]
Combining with other medications	Methadone plasma levels may alter with drugs that inhibit/induce CYP3A4 such as erythromycin, several SSRIs, ribavirin and some anticonvulsants and HIV medications. This may make dose assessment difficult if a person is not consistent in their use of these CYP3A4-inhibiting drugs	Buprenorphine is less affected by drug interactions, and may be preferable for some patients
Pregnancy		Buprenorphine is associated with less severe neonatal withdrawal symptoms.[14] However, buprenorphine should not be initiated in pregnancy or switched to from methadone because of the risk of inducing withdrawal in the foetus
Diversion	Patients at greater risk of diversion of medication (e.g. past history of this; treatment in a prison setting) may be better served with methadone treatment	Sublingual buprenorphine tablets can be more easily diverted with the risk of tablets being injected Available in combination with naloxone (Suboxone) which may prevent diversion for injection
Logistics		If daily supervised consumption is not feasible, buprenorphine may be preferable[1]

HIV, human immunodeficiency virus; od, *omni die* (once a day); SSRI, selective serotonin reuptake inhibitor.

CHAPTER 4

research, methadone is of equal efficacy to buprenorphine in reducing prescription opioid abuse in prescription opioid dependence and retaining people in treatment.[15] Methadone is also associated with a reduction in drug-taking behaviours related to HIV transmission.

Prescribing information

Methadone is a Controlled Drug with a high dependency potential and a low lethal dose. For these reasons, there are special documentation requirements, including specifying the patient's name, date of birth and address on prescriptions and writing the daily dose amount and total amount prescribed in both numbers and words. Instructions such as the requirement for consumption to be supervised should also be specified, for example 'daily supervised consumption'.

Supervised daily consumption is recommended for new prescriptions, for a minimum of several months.[1] If this is not possible, instalment prescriptions for daily dispensing and collection should be used. No more than 1 week's supply should be dispensed at one time, except in exceptional circumstances.[1]

Methadone should normally be prescribed as a 1mg in 1mL oral solution.[1] The patient's address and date of birth should be included on the form, as well as the amount prescribed per day and total prescribed written in figures and words. Directions for supervision should be written clearly. Tablets can be crushed and injected and therefore should not usually be prescribed.[1,16]

Important: All patients starting a methadone treatment programme must be informed of the risks of toxicity and overdose, and the necessity for safe storage of any take-home medication.[1,17–19] Safe storage is vital, particularly if there are children in the household, as tragic deaths have occurred when children have ingested methadone. Prescribers should consider risks to children in all assessments and treatment plans of drug-using patients.

In determining the **starting dose** for patients using heroin or other opioids not already on a prescription for methadone, consideration must be given to the potential for opioid toxicity, taking into account the following:

- Tolerance to opioids can be affected by a number of factors and significantly influences an individual's risk of toxicity.[20] Of particular importance in assessing this are the client's reported current quantity, frequency and route of administration, whilst being wary of possible over-reporting. A person's tolerance to methadone can be significantly reduced within 3–4 days of not using opioids, so caution must be exercised after this time, with careful re-titration from a starting dose.
- Use of other depressant drugs, for example alcohol, benzodiazepines and psychiatric medications such as pregabalin increase risks of toxicity.
- Age. The risk of drug-related death is increased ×2.9 in patients over 45.[21]
- Co-morbid physical health problems (e.g. chronic obstructive pulmonary disease resulting in low baseline oxygen saturation).
- Long half-life of methadone, as cumulative toxicity may develop over the course of 3–10 days.[22,23] For this reason a patient should be reviewed regularly for signs of

intoxication and the dose must be omitted if there is any sign of drowsiness or other evidence of toxicity.

- Inappropriate dosing can result in fatal overdose, particularly in the first few days.[17,18,24,25] Deaths have occurred following the commencement of a daily dose of less than 30 mg methadone.[1]

It is safer to start with a low dose that can subsequently be increased at intervals if this dose later proves to be insufficient. Direct conversion tables for opioids and methadone should be viewed cautiously, as there are a number of factors influencing the values at any given time (e.g. changes in quality of street heroin). It is much safer to titrate the dose against presenting withdrawal symptoms.

The **initial total daily dose** for most cases will be in the range of **10–30 mg** methadone depending on the level of tolerance.[1,26] If this is uncertain, 10–20 mg is recommended. In an acute medical or psychiatric ward, starting doses of up to 20 mg daily are usually recommended, as patients in these settings are likely to be physically unwell in the former, or being treated with various other psychoactive drugs in the latter case.

Note: onset of action should be evident within half an hour, with peak plasma levels being achieved after approximately 2–4 hours of dosing.

Methadone induction and stabilisation in the community

This applies to patients who have not been on a prescription in the previous 3 days (including those who have been on OST and not picked up their prescription for 3 days). The initial 2 weeks of treatment with methadone are associated with a substantially increased risk of overdose mortality.[1,16,27–29] It is important that appropriate assessment, titration of doses and monitoring is performed during this period. Induction is usually undertaken in specialist services by those with appropriate competencies and after a full assessment with urine toxicology and clear evidence of opioid use and withdrawal.

- **First week.** Out-patients should attend up to three times per week to enable assessment by the prescriber and any dose titration against withdrawal symptoms. Dose increases should not exceed 5–10 mg on each occasion and not usually more than 30 mg in the first week above the initial starting dose.[26] Note that steady state plasma levels are only achieved approximately 5 days after the last dose increase. Once the patient has been stabilised on an adequate dose, methadone should be prescribed as a single regular daily dose. It should not be prescribed on a prn basis or at variable dosage. It is good practice to supervise consumption for the first few months.
- **Subsequent period.** Subsequent increases of 5–10 mg methadone can continue after the first week, but there should be at least a week between each successive increase.[1] It may take several weeks to reach the therapeutic daily dose of 60–120 mg.[1] Stabilisation is usually achieved within 6 weeks but may take longer. However it is important to consider that some patients may require more rapid stabilisation. This would need to be balanced by a high level of supervision and observation thereby allowing the ability to increase doses more rapidly. A therapeutic dose is one that eliminates opioid withdrawal symptoms and is effective in stopping on-top-of use of

heroin, without excess sedation.[30] Prescribers should take into account factors that may influence choice of methadone dose such as co-morbid cocaine use, as cocaine decreases methadone levels, and increased age as lower methadone doses appear to be associated with overdose risk in the population >45 years.[21]

Methadone cautions

- **Intoxication.** Methadone should not be given to any patient showing signs of intoxication, especially due to alcohol or other depressant drugs (e.g. benzodiazepines).[20,31] Risk of fatal overdose is greatly enhanced when methadone is taken concomitantly with alcohol and other respiratory depressant drugs, including benzodiazepines and pregabalin, which can increase the risk of overdose.[32,33] Concurrent alcohol and both prescribed and illicit drug consumption must be borne in mind when considering subsequent prescribing of methadone due to the increased risk of overdose associated with polysubstance misuse.[18,24,31,34]
- **Severe hepatic/renal dysfunction.** Metabolism and elimination of methadone may be affected, in which case the dose or dosing interval should be adjusted accordingly against clinical presentation. Because of extended plasma half-life, the interval between assessments during initial dosing may need to be extended.

Methadone overdose

In the event of methadone overdose, **naloxone** should be administered as described in the section on 'Opioid overdose'.

Methadone and risk of torsades de pointes/QT interval prolongation

It is possible that methadone, either alone or combined with other QT-prolonging agents, may increase the likelihood of QT interval prolongation on the electrocardiogram, which is associated with torsades de pointes and can be fatal.[35–37]

Recommended ECG monitoring

In 2006, the Medicines and Healthcare Product and Regulatory Authority (MHRA) recommended that patients with the following risk factors for QT interval prolongation are carefully monitored whilst taking methadone: heart or liver disease, electrolyte abnormalities, concomitant treatment with CYP3A4 inhibitors or medicines with the potential to cause QT interval prolongation (e.g. some antipsychotics and erythromycin, amongst others). Cocaine is also a QT-lengthening drug that can be associated with prolonged QT in patients taking methadone, so patients who also take cocaine should be monitored.[38] In addition, any patient requiring more than 100 mg of methadone per day should be closely monitored[39] as the risk of QTc prolongation is dose related.[35] Other patient factors increasing the risk of QT prolongation include co-morbid eating disorder, history of heart disease or stroke, liver disease, metabolic derangements such as hypokalaemia or hypocalcaemia, and HIV-positive status (irrespective of medications).[40]

Thus, individuals with the risk factors listed above should have a baseline ECG and subsequent ECG monitoring. The timeframe for the latter is not yet subject to a rigorous evidence base; annual checks in the absence of cardiac symptomatology would be a reasonable minimum frequency. It is also important to check the actions of any medications being prescribed with methadone for CYP3A4 inhibitory activity, to inform the risk–benefit analysis when commencing methadone.[41] Buprenorphine appears to be associated with less QTc prolongation and therefore may be a safer alternative in this respect,[42] although there are few studies in this area at present and there are many other factors to take into account when choosing an appropriate opioid substitute.

Remember that QT should be corrected for heart rate to produce a corrected QT (QTc) in milliseconds (ms). This is normally documented on the ECG recording. The ECG should be read by a professional with experience in reading ECGs. Brief guidelines as to actions to take are documented in Table 4.10. Always seek specialist advice where there is prolongation of the QT interval. A review of ECG monitoring suggests that there is insufficient evidence for the efficacy of QTc screening strategies for preventing cardiac morbidity and mortality in methadone-maintained patients and there is concern that in some settings the procedures involved may be 'too demanding and too stressful' and may 'interfere with the availability of patients to undergo methadone maintenance and may expose patients to health consequences of untreated opioid addiction including increased mortality risk'.[43]

Patients on or about to start methadone in in-patient settings, both medical and psychiatric wards, should always have an ECG, and patients on high doses or with other risk factors should if possible have ECGs when treated in the community, although consideration should be taken of the risks and benefits if a community patient refuses to attend for ECG monitoring.

Table 4.10 Recommended ECG monitoring for methadone-maintained patients

	Borderline prolonged QTc	Action	Prolonged QTc	Action	Very prolonged QTc	Action
Females	≥470 ms	▪ Repeat ECG ▪ Electrolytes ▪ Try to modify QT risk factors, e.g. cocaine use, methadone dose, psychotropic medications ▪ Regular ECG until normal	≥500 ms	▪ Repeat ECG ▪ Electrolytes ▪ Try to modify QT risk factors ▪ Seek Cardiology and Addictions specialist advice ▪ Reduce methadone dose ▪ If persistent QTc despite reduction, plan switch to buprenorphine ▪ Regular ECGs until normal	≥550 ms	▪ Urgent Cardiology and Addictions specialist advice ▪ Repeat ECG ▪ Electrolytes ▪ Try to modify QT risk factors ▪ Reduce methadone and re-evaluate within the week. Plan switch to buprenorphine in in-patient setting
Males	≥440 ms					

ECG, electrocardiogram.

CHAPTER 4

Buprenorphine

Clinical effectiveness

Buprenorphine (Subutex) is a synthetic partial opioid agonist with low intrinsic activity and high affinity at μ opioid receptors. This means that it produces less euphoria even at saturating doses and simultaneously blocks the action of other opioids. It is an effective treatment for use in maintenance treatment for heroin addiction if prescribed at fixed doses, although not more effective than methadone at adequate dosages.[7] It has also been found to be effective in reducing prescription opioid use and improving treatment adherence in prescription opioid dependent patients.[15] There is no significant difference between buprenorphine and methadone in terms of completion of detoxification treatment, but withdrawal symptoms may resolve more quickly with buprenorphine.[44]

Prescribing information

Buprenorphine is absorbed via the sublingual route. Each tablet takes approximately 5–10 minutes to disintegrate and be absorbed. It is effective in treating opioid dependence because:

- It alleviates/prevents opioid withdrawal and craving.
- It reduces the effects of additional opioid use because of its high receptor affinity – what patients refer to as a 'blocking' effect.[10–12]
- It is long-acting, allowing daily (or less frequent) dosing. The duration of action is related to the buprenorphine dose administered: low doses (e.g. 2 mg) exert effects for up to 12 hours; higher doses (e.g. 16–32 mg) exert effects for as long as 48–72 hours.

Prescribing buprenorphine requires the same details as when prescribing methadone. The patient's address and date of birth should be included on the form, as well as the amount prescribed per day and total prescribed written in figures and words. Directions for supervision should be written clearly.

Buprenorphine starting dose

The same principles as for methadone apply when starting treatment with buprenorphine. Doctors operating outside drug services should be aware that buprenorphine does not show up in standard multiple urine drug testing kits in the way that methadone, codeine or heroin do. It is commonly tested for using a separate urine drug screening kit which is not usually available outside addiction services. Thus, to confirm use in a timely fashion, confirmation with pharmacy regarding observed consumption and potentially specific laboratory testing of a urine sample should be considered. However, of particular interest with buprenorphine is the phenomenon of **precipitated withdrawal**. Precipitated withdrawal occurs because buprenorphine is a partial agonist with a high affinity. If it enters the brain when a full agonist (e.g. methadone or heroin) is still present, it competes for binding at the opioid receptors and replaces the full agonist. Therefore some receptors previously fully stimulated become partially stimulated. The patient experiences this change as opioid withdrawal. If the patient is already in withdrawal, they will experience the addition of a partial agonist that stimulates the receptors to a limited extent as relief of that withdrawal. Patient education is an important factor in reducing the problems during induction.

Starting buprenorphine

The first dose of buprenorphine should be administered when the patient is experiencing opioid withdrawal symptoms to reduce the risk of precipitated withdrawal. As with methadone, clear evidence of daily opioid use (including drug testing) and withdrawal symptoms are mandatory before commencing a prescription for buprenorphine.

The initial dose recommendations are shown in Table 4.11.

Table 4.11 Recommended starting doses of buprenorphine

Patient status	Dose of buprenorphine
Patient in withdrawal and no risk factors	8 mg
Patient not experiencing withdrawal and no risk factors	4 mg
Patient has concomitant risk factors (e.g. medical condition, polydrug misuse, low or uncertain severity of dependence, on other psychiatric medications)	2–4 mg

No more than 8 mg buprenorphine should be given on the first day in a non-specialist setting. In some cases 8 mg may be sufficient, but this may be increased to 12–16 mg the following day if there is continuing evidence of withdrawal and no evidence of intoxication. The dose can be given in divided doses so that it can be reviewed promptly in the event of any intoxication, though in practice this is difficult in the absence of on-site dispensing. For maintenance, the 'Orange Guidelines'[1] recommend a dose between 12 and 24 mg a day. If there is concern that doses higher than 16 mg may be required, specialist advice should be sought and the dose only increased under advice from addiction specialists.

If patients are on other respiratory sedatives such as benzodiazepines, the lower doses should be used and the patient monitored for intoxication and respiratory depression.

Transferring from methadone to buprenorphine

This should usually be under the supervision of a suitably experienced specialist prescriber. Patients transferring from methadone are at risk of experiencing precipitated withdrawal symptoms that may continue at a milder level for 1–2 weeks. Factors affecting precipitated withdrawal are listed in Table 4.12.

Transferring from methadone dose <40 mg (ideally ≤30 mg) to buprenorphine

Methadone should be ceased abruptly, and the first dose of buprenorphine given at least 24 hours after the last methadone dose. The conversion rates shown in Table 4.13 at the start of treatment are recommended but higher doses may be subsequently needed depending on clinical presentation.

Transferring from methadone 40–60 mg dose to buprenorphine

- The methadone dose should be reduced as far as possible without the patient becoming unstable or chaotic, and then abruptly stopped.
- The first buprenorphine dose should be delayed until the patient displays clear signs of withdrawal, generally 48–96 hours after the last dose of methadone. Symptomatic medication (lofexidine) may be useful to provide transitory relief.

CHAPTER 4

Table 4.12 Factors affecting risk of precipitated withdrawal with methadone to buprenorphine switch

Factor	Discussion	Recommended strategy
Dose of methadone	More likely with doses of methadone above 30 mg. Generally – the higher the dose the more severe the precipitated withdrawal[45]	Attempt transfer from doses of methadone <40 mg (preferably ≤30 mg). Transfer from >60 mg should not be attempted
Time between last methadone dose and first buprenorphine dose	Interval should be at least 24 hours. Increasing the interval reduces the incidence and severity of withdrawal[46,47]	Cease methadone and delay first dose until patient experiencing withdrawal from methadone
Dose of buprenorphine	Very low doses of buprenorphine (e.g. 2 mg) are generally inadequate to substitute for methadone. High first doses of buprenorphine (e.g. 8 mg) are more likely to precipitate withdrawal	First dose should generally be 4 mg; review patient 2–3 hours later
Patient expectancy	Patients not prepared for precipitated withdrawal are more likely to become distressed and confused by the effect	Inform patients in advance. Have contingency plan for severe symptoms
Use of other medications	Symptomatic medication (e.g. lofexidine) can be useful to relieve symptoms	Prescribe in accordance to management plan

Table 4.13 Recommended doses of buprenorphine for patients transferring from methadone (<40 mg [ideally ≤30 mg])

Last methadone dose	Day 1 initial buprenorphine dose	Day 2 buprenorphine dose
20–40 mg	4 mg	6–8 mg
10–20 mg	4 mg	4–8 mg
1–10 mg	2 mg	2–4 mg

- An initial dose of 2–4 mg should be given. The patient should then be reviewed 2–3 hours later.
- If withdrawal has been precipitated further symptomatic medication can be prescribed.
- If there has been no precipitation or worsening of withdrawal, an additional 2–4 mg of buprenorphine can be dispensed on the same day.
- The patient should be reviewed the following day, at which point the dose should be increased to between 8 and 12 mg.

Transferring from methadone doses >60 mg to buprenorphine

Such transfers should not be attempted in an out-patient setting except in exceptional circumstances by an experienced practitioner. Usually patients would be partially detoxified from methadone and transferred to buprenorphine when the methadone was at or below 30 mg daily. However, if transfer from higher dose methadone to buprenorphine is required, a referral to an in-patient unit should be considered, though the skill level of in-patient staff and extent of medical cover will also need to be considered.

Transferring from other prescribed opioids to buprenorphine

Evidence is accruing in the treatment of prescribed opioid dependence with buprenorphine and it has been found to improve adherence to drug treatment and reduce prescription opioid abuse.[15] In the UK, the Orange Guidelines recommend small divided doses be given to establish the dose required for stabilisation.[1]

Stabilisation dose of buprenorphine

Out-patients should attend regularly for the first few days to enable assessment by the prescriber and any dose titration. Dose increases should be made in increments of 2–4 mg at a time, daily if necessary, up to a maximum daily dose of 32 mg. The recommended effective maintenance doses are in the range of 12–16 mg daily[1] and patients should generally be able to achieve maintenance levels within 1–2 weeks of starting buprenorphine – usually more quickly than with methadone.

Buprenorphine less than daily dosing

Buprenorphine is licensed in the UK as a medication to be taken daily. International evidence and experience indicates that many clients can be comfortably maintained on one dose every 2–3 days.[48–51] This may be pertinent for patients in buprenorphine treatment who are considered unsuitable for take-away medication because of the risk of diversion.

The following conversion rate is recommended:

2-day buprenorphine dose = 2 × daily dose of buprenorphine (to a max 32 mg)
3-day buprenorphine dose = 3 × daily dose of buprenorphine (to a max 32 mg).

Note: In the event of patients being unable to stabilise comfortably on buprenorphine (often those transferring from methadone), the option of transferring to methadone should be available. Methadone can be commenced 24 hours after the last buprenorphine dose. Doses should be titrated cautiously according to clinical response, being mindful of the residual 'blockade' effect of buprenorphine which may last for several days, meaning that methadone toxicity can occur in a delayed manner.

Buprenorphine cautions

- **Liver function.** There is some evidence suggesting that high dose buprenorphine can cause changes in liver function in individuals with a history of liver disease.[52] Such patients should have their liver function tested before commencing, with follow-up investigations conducted 6–12 weeks after commencing buprenorphine. More frequent testing should be considered in patients of particular concern (e.g. those with severe liver disease). Elevated liver enzymes in the absence of clinically significant liver disease, however, does not necessarily contraindicate treatment with buprenorphine.

- **Intoxication.** Buprenorphine should not be given to any patient showing signs of intoxication, especially due to alcohol or other depressant drugs (e.g. benzodiazepines, sedating antipsychotics, pregabalin[32]). Buprenorphine in combination with other sedative drugs can result in respiratory depression, sedation, coma and death. Concurrent alcohol and illicit drug consumption must be borne in mind when considering subsequent prescribing of buprenorphine due to the increased risk of overdose associated with polysubstance misuse.

Overdose with buprenorphine

Buprenorphine (as a single drug in overdose) is generally regarded as safer than methadone and heroin because it causes less respiratory depression and is less likely to be associated with overdose death.[53] However, in combination with other respiratory depressant drugs the effects may be harder to manage. Very high doses of naloxone (e.g. 10–15 mg) may be needed to reverse buprenorphine effects (although lower doses such as 0.8–2 mg may be sufficient).[4] As a consequence, ventilator support is often required in cases where buprenorphine is contributing to respiratory depression (e.g. in polydrug overdose). In the event of buprenorphine overdose **always call emergency services.**

Buprenorphine with naloxone (Suboxone)

With regards to the risk of diversion and subsequent injecting of buprenorphine, consideration maybe given by the prescriber to a buprenorphine/naloxone preparation which may reduce the risk of diversion. The different sublingual and parenteral potency profiles of buprenorphine and naloxone are key: if used sublingually, the naloxone will have negligible effects. However, if the combined preparation is injected, the naloxone will have a substantial effect and can attenuate the effects of the buprenorphine in the short term and is also likely to precipitate withdrawal in opioid-dependent individuals on full opioid agonists.[54]

Alternative oral preparations

Oral methadone and buprenorphine should continue to be the mainstay of treatment;[1] other oral options such as slow release oral morphine (SROM) preparations and dihydrocodeine are not licensed in the UK for the treatment of opiate dependence.[1]

However, a specialised clinician may in very exceptional circumstances prescribe oral dihydrocodeine as maintenance therapy, where clients are unable to tolerate methadone or buprenorphine, or in other exceptional circumstances, taking into account the difficulties associated with its short half-life, supervision requirements and diversion potential.[1]

SROM preparations have been shown elsewhere in Europe to be useful as maintenance therapy in those failing to tolerate methadone, again only for prescribing by specialised clinicians.[1] A 2013 review of studies on SROM suggested that there was insufficient evidence to assess the effectiveness of this treatment.[55]

Injectable opioid maintenance prescribing

There is now compelling evidence supporting the use of injectable diamorphine maintenance prescribing for treatment of patients who fail to benefit from first-line OST.[56] Contemporary injectable prescribing differs from the previous practice of prescribing unsupervised injectable opioids in that the patient must:

- Attend in person for their prescribed injectable opioid maintenance treatment – daily or more frequently, according to the treatment plan.
- Inject their dose under the direct supervision of a competent member of staff.
- Be given no take-away injectable medication.

Oral OST is prescribed for days when supervised injectable treatment is not available if the injectable clinic is not available daily. This treatment differs from 'injecting rooms', that is, safe places with sterile equipment for people who use intravenous drugs (usually not in treatment), in that it is part of a holistic package of care with adjunctive psychosocial interventions. A Home Office licence is required to prescribe diamorphine for addictions treatment, and specialist levels of competence are required to prescribe injectable substitute opioids. Although its cost-effectiveness has been demonstrated,[57] its implementation has been limited by high set-up costs.

At present, clients should only be considered for injectable opioid prescribing in combination with psychosocial interventions, as part of a wider package of care, as an option in cases where the individual has not responded adequately to oral opioid substitution treatment, and in an area where it can be supported by locally commissioned and provided mechanisms for supervised consumption.[1,58] Patients are generally seen for supervised injecting in a specialist facility twice a day.

Treatment of opiate dependence on the psychiatric ward

Opiate overdose can occur in hospital settings. All in-patients with a history of opiate dependence should have naloxone prescribed on the prn side of the chart.

In the in-patient setting, it is imperative to manage opiate withdrawal in order to allow the patient to remain on the ward and engage in interventions tailored to the reason for their psychiatric admission. The most effective prevention of opiate withdrawal during an acute psychiatric admission is continuation of the patient's existing OST. In order to continue prescribing the same dose of OST, the following need to be confirmed independently:

- By addiction services: the prescribed dose.
- By the pharmacy where OST is dispensed: most recent supervised dose and whether any take-away doses had been given. If the most recent supervised dose is more than 3 days ago, the patient will need to have their OST re-initiated to avoid overdose (see section on 'Methadone initiation on an acute ward'). Patients admitted at weekends may have take-away doses and may not necessarily disclose these if they are not directly asked. If more than 3 days have passed since the patient's last dose of OST, they will have lost tolerance and will need to be re-initiated according to the advice of an addiction clinician.

CHAPTER 4

Continuation at the reported dose of OST should only be prescribed if the above information is confirmed and:

- The patient appears alert and comfortable on this dose.
- The patient does not appear to be intoxicated with other substances.

Note: If there is any doubt or concern regarding any factor listed previously, OST should not be prescribed.

Junior doctors may find themselves looking after a patient in opioid withdrawal in circumstances where it is not immediately possible to establish all the above information and safely prescribe OST. Opioid withdrawal, while not fatal, is highly aversive, and carries risks if it is associated with a patient in need of in-patient care self-discharging. Other medications can be helpful in managing opioid withdrawal until such help can be sought, though there is little place for them once OST is prescribed and their use during OST induction is discouraged because of the risks associated with polypharmacy and polysubstance use. The current UK clinical guidelines for the treatment of drug dependence recommend the therapies listed in Table 4.14 to target specific symptoms.[1]

Patients admitted for emergency psychiatric treatment should not be detoxified from their OST and consideration should be given to the initiation of OST in opiate-dependent patients who are not yet in treatment, with the advice of local addiction specialists. Lower doses of methadone are recommended for initiation in the in-patient setting. Although the most current national guidelines recommend splitting the dose of methadone in order to give multiple smaller doses with a lower risk of toxicity, this should be weighed against the staffing levels and skills mix present at different medication times.

Table 4.14 Treatment of symptoms of opioid withdrawal (adapted from *Drug misuse and dependence: UK guidelines for clinical management* 2017[1])

Symptom	Treatment
Diarrhoea	Loperamide 4 mg then 2 mg after each loose stool; maximum 16 mg daily for up to 5 days
Nausea, vomiting, stomach cramps	Metoclopramide 10 mg tds for a maximum of 5 days or prochlorperazine 5 mg tds or 12.5 mg IM bd
Stomach cramps	Mebeverine 135 mg tds
Agitation, anxiety and insomnia	Diazepam up to 5–10 mg tds when required or zopiclone 7.5 mg nocte for patients with a history of benzodiazepine dependence
Muscular pains and headaches	Paracetamol, aspirin or non-steroidal anti-inflammatories. Topical rubefacients can be helpful in relieving muscle aches from methadone withdrawal

bd, *bis die* (twice a day); IM, intramuscularly; nocte, at night; tds, *ter die sumendum* (three times a day).

Methadone initiation on an acute ward (or by a non-specialist in a non-addictions setting)

Induction – day 1
- The person must be exhibiting objective opioid withdrawal symptoms, as assessed on an opioid withdrawal scale such as the Objective Opiate Withdrawal Scale (Table 4.8), before any dose is prescribed.
- Give a dose of 10 mg of methadone mixture 1 mg/1 mL based on the severity of withdrawal. This should be given as a once-only dose. Methadone will start to have an effect after 20–30 minutes with peak levels being reached at 4 hours.
- Continue to monitor for signs of withdrawal 4-hourly and give a further dose of 5–10 mg as required – also observe for signs of intoxication.
- The initial daily dose (over 24 hours) will not usually be more than 30 mg.
- Prescribe naloxone as required in case of overdose.

Day 2
- Prescribe the same dose as the patient required on day 1 as a single dose, or in divided doses.
- Continue to monitor withdrawal symptoms and sedation.

Ongoing prescribing
- Consider increasing the dose further in 5–10 mg increments every 3–4 days until full relief of withdrawal symptoms is achieved, in consultation with addictions specialists.
- Once stability has been achieved, continue to prescribe the required dose.

In the acute in-patient setting it is usually advisable for the person to be maintained on a stable dose rather than commence detoxification.

Swapping from twice-daily dosing to single dosing
Patients are often transferred from acute hospitals to psychiatric care with a split dose of methadone. Split dosing in the community carries with it the risk of diversion so is discouraged apart from in pregnancy. Should the medical team wish to swap the patient from a split dose to a full dose over the course of their psychiatric admission or in preparation for discharge, this can be done incrementally by increasing the morning dose by 10 mg every 5 days or so, and monitoring for sedation.

Note: All patients leaving the ward should be trained in the use of take-home naloxone, issued with take-home naloxone[1] and have an appointment made in addiction services to continue prescribing prior to discharge.

Prescribing psychotropic medications in patients with opiate dependence

General psychiatrists often see patients with addictions with a view to treating psychiatric co-morbidity. General guidelines regarding pharmacological treatment of co-morbid psychiatric conditions are found in the British Association of Psychopharmacology guidelines for the pharmacological management of substance abuse.[59] In general, prescribers should be cautious about prescribing medication licensed for co-morbid psychiatric disorders that is sedating, because of the increased risk of respiratory depression (e.g. pregabalin, which is associated with overdose death).[32] Pregabalin and olanzapine also appear to have an abuse liability in the opioid-dependent population.[60,61] More information specific to opioid dependence is provided for depression where several RCTs concerning opioid-dependent patients specifically, rather than patients with mixed substance misuse co-morbid with depression, have been done.

Patients with opiate dependence suffer disproportionately from depression: about half of those entering treatment will meet criteria for depression. They may require 20–50% higher doses of methadone than non-depressed patients to stabilise[62] but stabilisation may precipitate remission in a majority of cases.[63] There is limited clinical trial evidence of low to moderate quality regarding antidepressant use in opioid dependence which suggests that it is of limited benefit in benefiting either mood or drug use.[59,63] Positive studies have largely been those using medication with mixed pharmacology such as tricyclic antidepressants.[64] The recommended approach to treatment of depression based on the evidence includes stabilising the patient on OST first, then if depression persists trying an SSRI first because of its relative safety, but considering mixed pharmacology antidepressants as a second line should the patient fail to respond.[64] Sertraline is the drug of choice in methadone-treated patients.

Opioid detoxification and reduction regimes

Opioid maintenance can be continued from the short term to almost indefinitely, depending on clinical need. Some patients are keen to detoxify after short periods of stability and other patients may decide to detoxify after medium- to long-term periods of stability on maintenance prescriptions. All detoxification programmes should be part of a care programme. Given the risk of serious fatal overdose post detoxification, services providing such treatment should educate the patient about these risks and supply and train them with naloxone and overdose training for emergency use.

Regarding the length of detoxification, the NICE guidelines state 'dose reduction can take place over anything from a few days to several months, with a higher initial stabilisation dose taking longer to taper', and indicate that 'up to 3 months is typical for methadone reduction, while buprenorphine reductions are typically carried out over 14 days to a few weeks'.[65] In practice, a detoxification in the community may extend over a longer period, if this facilitates the client's comfort during the process, compliance with the care plan, continued abstinence from illicit use during detoxification, and subsequent abstinence following detoxification.

Detoxification in an in-patient setting, the NICE guidelines indicate, may take place over a shorter time than in the community (suggesting 14–21 days for methadone and 7–14 days for buprenorphine) 'as the supportive environment helps a service user to tolerate emerging withdrawal symptoms'.[66] As in the community, a stabilisation on the dose of a substitute opioid is first achieved, followed by gradual dose reduction, with additive medications judiciously prescribed for withdrawal symptoms if and as needed.

Detoxification carries a recognised risk of relapse and indeed fatal overdose. Therefore if a patient is being detoxified there needs to be adequate aftercare in place, such as a rehabilitation programme and community support. For patients having emergency psychiatric or medical admissions, detoxification is not usually indicated unless it is with the support of specialist services and aftercare arrangements are in place.

Opioid withdrawal in a community setting

Methadone

Following a period of stabilisation with methadone or a longer period of maintenance, the patient and prescriber may agree a reduction programme as part of a care plan to reduce the daily methadone dose. The usual reduction would be by 5–10 mg weekly or every 2 weeks although there can be much variation in the reduction and speed of reduction. In the community setting, patient preference is the most important variable in terms of dose reduction and rate of reduction. The detoxification programme should be reviewed regularly and remain flexible to adjustments and changes, such as relapse to illicit drug use or patient anxieties about speed of reduction. Factors such as an increase in heroin or other drug use or worsening of the patient's physical, psychological or social well-being, may warrant a temporary increase, or stabilisation of the dose or a slowing-down of the reduction rate. Towards the end of the detoxification the dose reduction may be slower: 1–2 mg per week. Recent studies show that length of stability on maintenance treatment and prolonged reduction schedules (up to a year) substantially improve the chances of achieving abstinence.[67]

Buprenorphine

The same principles as for methadone apply when planning a buprenorphine detoxification regime. Dose reduction should be gradual to minimise withdrawal discomfort. A suggested reduction regime is shown in Table 4.15.

Table 4.15 Recommended dose reduction schedule for buprenorphine

Daily buprenorphine dose	Reduction rate
Above 16 mg	4 mg every 1–2 weeks
8–16 mg	2–4 mg every 1–2 weeks
2–8 mg	2 mg per week or fortnight
Below 2 mg	Reduce by 0.4–0.8 mg per week

Opioid withdrawal in a specialist addiction in-patient setting

Methadone

Patients should have a starting dose assessment of methadone, over 48 hours, by a specialist inpatient team. The dose may then be reduced following a linear regime over up to 4 weeks.[65]

Buprenorphine

Buprenorphine can be used effectively for short-term in-patient detoxifications following the same principles as for methadone.

Lofexidine

Lofexidine, an α_2-adrenergic agonist, can counteract the adrenergic hyperactivity associated with opioid withdrawal[68] (demonstrated by characteristic signs and symptoms, such as tachycardia, sweating, runny nose, hair standing on end, shivering and goose pimples). It is licensed for the management of symptoms of opioid withdrawal,[65] although additional short-term adjunctive medications may be needed, such as loperamide for diarrhoea.[1] Detoxification using lofexidine is much faster than with methadone or buprenorphine, typically lasting 5–7 days, and up to a maximum of 10 days. The usual regime commences at 800 µg daily, rising to 2.4 mg in split doses, which is then reduced over subsequent days.[1] Adverse effects may include a dry mouth, drowsiness and clinically significant hypotension and bradycardia;[2] the last two in particular must be monitored during lofexidine prescribing. Lofexidine should be used with caution in patients with cardiovascular disease or being treated with medications associated with QT prolongation.

Although lofexidine is not useful for detoxification of those with substantial opioid dependence,[1] there are certain circumstances in which this regime may have a role: where the client has made an informed and clinically appropriate decision not to use methadone or buprenorphine for detoxification; where they have made a similarly informed and clinically appropriate decision to detoxify within a short time period; and where there is only mild or uncertain opioid dependence (including young people).[65] Treatment also enables early initiation of naltrexone.

Naltrexone in relapse prevention

Evidence for the effectiveness of naltrexone as a treatment for relapse prevention in opioid misusers has been inconclusive.[69] However, for those who prefer an abstinence programme, are fully informed of the potential adverse effects and benefits of treatment, are highly motivated to remain on treatment, and have a partner supporting concordance, naltrexone treatment has been found by NICE to be a cost-effective treatment strategy in aiding abstinence from opioid misuse.[70] The naltrexone implant, not currently licensed in the UK, may also have a role to play in reducing opioid use in a motivated population of patients[71] following further research.

Close monitoring is particularly important when naltrexone treatment is initiated because of the higher risk of fatal overdose at this time. Discontinuation of naltrexone may also be associated with an increase in inadvertent overdose from illicit opioids. Thus, supervision of naltrexone administration, and careful choice of who is prescribed it (those who are abstinence-focused and motivated) are very important. Moreover, people taking naltrexone often experience adverse effects of unease (dysphoria), depression and insomnia, which can lead to relapse to illicit opioid use while on naltrexone treatment, or failure to continue on treatment. The dysphoria may be caused by either withdrawal from illicit drugs or the naltrexone treatment itself, emphasising the importance of prescribing naltrexone as part of a care programme that includes psychosocial therapy and general support.[70]

Initiating naltrexone treatment

Naltrexone has the propensity to cause a severe withdrawal reaction in patients who are either currently taking opioid drugs or who were previously taking opioid drugs and there has not been a sufficient 'wash-out' period before administering naltrexone.

The minimum recommended interval between stopping the opioid and starting naltrexone depends on the opioid used, duration of use and amount taken as a last dose. Opioid agonists with long half-lives such as methadone will require a wash-out period of up to 10 days, whereas shorter-acting opioids such as heroin may only require up to 7 days. Experience with buprenorphine indicates that a wash-out period of up to 7 days is sufficient (final buprenorphine dose >2 mg; duration of use >2 weeks) and in some cases naltrexone may be started within 2–3 days of a patient stopping (final buprenorphine dose <2 mg; duration of use <2 weeks).

A test dose of naloxone (0.2–0.8 mg), which has a much shorter half-life than naltrexone, may be given to the patient as an IM dose prior to starting naltrexone treatment. Any withdrawal symptoms precipitated will be of shorter duration than if precipitated by naltrexone.

Patients *must* be advised of the risk of withdrawal before giving the dose. It is worth thoroughly questioning the patient as to whether they have taken any opioid-containing preparation unknowingly (e.g. over-the-counter analgesic). See Box 4.7.

Box 4.7 Important points regarding prescribing naltrexone

- Ensure the client is fully informed of the increased risk of fatal opioid overdose.
- Following detoxification and any period of abstinence, an individual's tolerance to opioids will decrease markedly. At such a time, using opioids puts the individual at greatly increased risk of overdose.
- Discontinuation of naltrexone may also be associated with an increase in inadvertent overdose from illicit opioids, emphasising the need for close monitoring and support of the client at this time.

Dose of naltrexone

An initial dose of 25 mg naltrexone should be administered after a suitable opioid-free interval (and naloxone challenge if appropriate). The patient should be monitored for 4 hours after the first dose, for symptoms of opioid withdrawal. Symptomatic medication for withdrawal (lofexidine) should be available for use, if necessary, on the first day of naltrexone dosing (withdrawal symptoms may last up to 4–8 hours). Once the patient has tolerated this low naltrexone dose, subsequent doses can be increased to 50 mg daily as a maintenance dose.

Naltrexone is contraindicated in patients with hepatic dysfunction, and liver function tests should be monitored during treatment.

Pain control in patients on OST

Analgesia for methadone-prescribed patients

Non-opioid analgesics should be used in preference (e.g. paracetamol, non-steroidal anti-inflammatory drugs) initially where appropriate. If opioid analgesia (e.g. codeine, dihydrocodeine, morphine) is indicated due to the type and severity of the pain then this should be titrated accordingly for pain relief in line with usual analgesic protocols. There are specific considerations for patients receiving methadone, buprenorphine or naltrexone. In the case of patients prescribed methadone, if an opioid analgesic is appropriate, a non-methadone opioid may be co-prescribed, i.e. it is not necessary to 'rationalise' the patient's entire opioid requirements to one drug.[72] Titrating the methadone dose to provide analgesia may be appropriate in certain circumstances but this should only be carried out by experienced specialists.

As outlined elsewhere in this chapter, patients taking buprenorphine or naltrexone may be relatively refractory to opioids prescribed for analgesia, although in practice if a patient on buprenorphine requires treatment for acute pain, an additional opioid may be added titrated against response.[13]

If naltrexone is stopped to allow for the prescribing of opioid analgesia, careful monitoring will be required because of the increased risk of both relapse and overdose.[28,72]

Patients with a history of substance misuse may also need acute pain management in hospital following surgery, trauma or other illness. The primary objectives during the period of acute pain are to manage the pain and avoid the consequences of withdrawal, so it is important to maintain sufficient background medication to achieve both. Liaison with both the in-patient pain team and the local addictions services, as well as collaborative discussion with the patient, is important. The patient may be known to the addictions services, who will be able to inform the treatment plan, assist in a reliable conversion from street drugs (if these are also being taken) to prescribed analgesics and help plan a smooth transition from acute pain intervention to ongoing management of the patient's substance misuse.[28] Further details can be found in a consensus document by the British Pain Society, Royal College of Psychiatrists, Royal College of General Practitioners and The Advisory Council on the Misuse of Drugs.[72]

As advised in the consensus document, in palliative care, the principles of providing analgesia 'in substance misusers are fundamentally no different from those for other adult patients needing palliative care', although increased liaison with substance misuse services is essential. Those who are opioid dependent may receive maintenance therapy from a substance misuse service 'and this should be regarded as a separate prescription from that for analgesia when attending as a [pain clinic] outpatient', as also described in the context of chronic non-cancer pain. During admission all medication would usually be received from the in-patient unit, but with 'a clear plan for separate follow-ups for substance misuse and symptom palliation … in place on discharge except during the terminal phase of an illness'.[72] Again, further details can be found in the consensus advice document.[72] Subsequent to the publication of this document, there have been concerns regarding the abuse potential of pregabalin, a non-opioid medication used for chronic pain,[60] and the potential for prescription of pregabalin and opioids to increase the potential for overdose.[32] Therefore caution is suggested when prescribing pregabalin for chronic pain.

Pregnancy and opioid use

Substitute prescribing can occur at any time in pregnancy and carries a lower risk than continuing illicit use. Treatment should strike a balance between stabilising drug use and minimising the dose of OST in order to prevent neonatal abstinence syndrome (NAS).[1]

Women can present with opioid dependency at any stage in pregnancy, and stabilisation on substitute methadone is the treatment of choice. In the first trimester detoxification is contraindicated due to the risk of spontaneous abortion and in the third trimester it is associated with preterm delivery, foetal distress and stillbirth. If detoxification is requested, this is most safely achieved in the second trimester but should only be supervised by specialists with the appropriate competencies and with careful monitoring for any evidence of instability. Detoxification should be prescribed in small frequent decrements (e.g. 2–3 mg of methadone every 3–5 days[1]). Enforcing detoxification is contraindicated as it is likely to deter some clients from seeking help, and the majority will then return to opioid use at some point during their pregnancy;[73] fluctuating opioid concentrations in the maternal blood from intermittent use of illicit opioids may then lead to foetal withdrawal or overdose.[74,75]

Substitute prescribing during pregnancy

This should take place within a multidisciplinary team (including obstetric team, anaesthetists, neonatologists and addiction specialists) delivering a holistic package of care. The body of evidence informing treatment is small.[76] Currently, methadone and buprenorphine do not seem to differ in terms of safety. Methadone is associated with superior treatment retention and buprenorphine with less severe NAS.[76] The most recent guidelines therefore suggest allowing the patient to choose either, or to remain on whichever they are taking when they become pregnant.[1] Suboxone should be avoided in pregnancy. Changing from methadone to buprenorphine is not recommended, however, because of the risk of withdrawal for the foetus. Metabolism of methadone may increase during the third trimester, requiring split dosing.

Neonatal abstinence syndrome

The majority of neonates born to methadone-maintained mothers will require treatment for NAS.[73] NAS is characterised by a variety of signs and symptoms relating to the autonomic nervous system, gastrointestinal tract and respiratory system.[74] Infants may have a high-pitched cry, feed hungrily but ineffectively and be excessively wakeful. Severe NAS is associated with hypertonicity and seizures, but is uncommon. The NAS following methadone treatment usually commences after 48 hours[77] but can be delayed for 7–10 days.[1] In the case of any mother using drugs or OST, it is important to have access to skilled neonatal paediatric care to monitor the neonate and treat as required. Breastfeeding may reduce the severity of NAS.

It is useful to anticipate potential problems for women prescribed opioids during pregnancy with regard to opioid pain relief: such women should be managed in specialist antenatal clinics due to the increased associated risks. Antenatal assessment by anaesthetists may be recommended with regard to anticipating any anaesthetic risks, any analgesic requirements and problems with venous access.

Breastfeeding

Women prescribed methadone or buprenorphine should be encouraged to breastfeed even if they continue to use illicit opioids[1] for the following reasons:

- general health benefits to mother and infant
- specific benefits in reducing admission length and need for intervention in NAS[78]
- low concentrations of methadone and buprenorphine transferred to infant.[78]

Patients should be warned to discontinue breastfeeding gradually as abrupt cessation can cause a delayed NAS.[78] Patients who take crack cocaine or high doses of benzodiazepines should not breastfeed.[1]

References

1. Department of Health. Drug misuse and dependence: UK guidelines on clinical management. 2017. https://www.gov.uk/government/publications/drug-misuse-and-dependence-uk-guidelines-on-clinical-management.

2. Ellis K, Smith S. Routes to Recovery. 2007. http://americanradioworks.publicradio.org/features/nola/transcript.html.

3. World Health Organization. Community management of opioid overdose. 2014. http://www.who.int/substance_abuse/publications/management_opioid_overdose/en/.

4. Food and Drug Administration. FDA Advisory Committee on the Most Appropriate Dose or Doses of Naloxone to Reverse the Effects of Life-threatening Opioid Overdose in the Community Settings. 2016. https://www.fda.gov/downloads/AdvisoryCommittees/CommitteesMeetingMaterials/Drugs/AnestheticAndAnalgesicDrugProductsAdvisoryCommittee/UCM522688.pdf.

5. National Institute for Health and Care Excellence. Coexisting severe mental illness and substance misuse: community health and social care services. NICE Guideline NG58, 2016. https://www.nice.org.uk/guidance/ng58.

6. Handelsman L et al. Two new rating scales for opiate withdrawal. Am J Drug Alcohol Abuse 1987; 13:293–308.

7. Mattick RP et al. Buprenorphine maintenance versus placebo or methadone maintenance for opioid dependence. Cochrane Database Syst Rev 2014; 2:CD002207.

8. Seifert J et al. Detoxification of opiate addicts with multiple drug abuse: a comparison of buprenorphine vs. methadone. Pharmacopsychiatry 2002; 35:159–164.

9. Jasinski DR et al. Human pharmacology and abuse potential of the analgesic buprenorphine: a potential agent for treating narcotic addiction. Arch Gen Psychiatry 1978; 35:501–516.

10. Bickel WK et al. Buprenorphine: dose-related blockade of opioid challenge effects in opioid dependent humans. J Pharmacol Exp Ther 1988; 247:47–53.

11. Walsh SL et al. Acute administration of buprenorphine in humans: partial agonist and blockade effects. J Pharmacol Exp Ther 1995; 274:361–372.

12. Comer SD et al. Buprenorphine sublingual tablets: effects on IV heroin self-administration by humans. Psychopharmacology (Berl) 2001; 154:28–37.

13. Alford DP et al. Acute pain management for patients receiving maintenance methadone or buprenorphine therapy. Ann Intern Med 2006; 144:127–134.

14. Jones HE et al. Neonatal abstinence syndrome after methadone or buprenorphine exposure. N Engl J Med 2010; 363:2320–2331.

15. Nielsen S et al. Opioid agonist treatment for pharmaceutical opioid dependent people. Cochrane Database Syst Rev 2016:Cd011117.

16. Department of Health Task Force to Review Services for Drug Misusers. Report of an independent review of drug treatment services in England. HMSO.

17. Caplehorn JR. Deaths in the first two weeks of maintenance treatment in NSW in 1994: identifying cases of iatrogenic methadone toxicity. Drug Alcohol Rev 1998; 17:9–17.

18. Zador D et al. Deaths in methadone maintenance treatment in New South Wales, Australia 1990-1995. Addiction 2000; 95:77–84.

19. Hall W. Reducing the toll of opioid overdose deaths in Australia. Drug Alcohol Rev 1999; 18:213–220.

20. White JM et al. Mechanisms of fatal opioid overdose. Addiction 1999; 94:961–972.

21. Gao L et al. Risk-factors for methadone-specific deaths in Scotland's methadone-prescription clients between 2009 and 2013. Drug Alcohol Depend 2016; 167:214–223.

22. Wolff K et al. The pharmacokinetics of methadone in healthy subjects and opiate users. Br J Clin Pharmacol 1997; 44:325–334.

23. Rostami-Hodjegan A et al. Population pharmacokinetics of methadone in opiate users: characterization of time-dependent changes. Br J Clin Pharmacol 1999; 48:43–52.

24. Harding-Pink D. Methadone: one person's maintenance dose is another's poison. Lancet 1993; **341**:665–666.

25. Drummer OH et al. Methadone toxicity causing death in ten subjects starting on a methadone maintenance program. Am J Forensic Med Pathol 1992; **13**:346–350.

26. National Institute for Clinical Excellence. Methadone and buprenorphine for the management of opioid dependence. Technology Appraisal Guidance **114**, 2007. https://www.nice.org.uk/guidance/ta114.

27. Amato et al. Methadone at tapered doses for the management of opioid withdrawal. Cochrane Database Syst Rev 2013; **2**:CD003409.

28. Cornish R et al. Risk of death during and after opiate substitution treatment in primary care: prospective observational study in UK General Practice Research Database. BMJ 2010; **341**:c5475.

29. Strang J et al. Loss of tolerance and overdose mortality after inpatient opiate detoxification: follow up study. BMJ 2003; **326**:959–960.

30. Bell J. Pharmacological maintenance treatments of opiate addiction. Br J Clin Pharmacol 2014; **77**:253–263.

31. Farrell M et al. Suicide and overdose among opiate addicts. Addiction 1996; **91**:321–323.

32. Abrahamsson T et al. Benzodiazepine, z-drug and pregabalin prescriptions and mortality among patients in opioid maintenance treatment: a nation-wide register-based open cohort study. Drug Alcohol Depend 2017; **174**:58–64.

33. Pierce M et al. Impact of treatment for opioid dependence on fatal drug-related poisoning: a national cohort study in England. Addiction 2016; **111**:298–308.

34. Neale J. Methadone, methadone treatment and non-fatal overdose. Drug Alcohol Depend 2000; **58**:117–124.

35. Krantz MJ et al. Torsade de pointes associated with very-high-dose methadone. Ann Intern Med 2002; **137**:501–504.

36. Kornick CA et al. QTc interval prolongation associated with intravenous methadone. Pain 2003; **105**:499–506.

37. Martell BA et al. The impact of methadone induction on cardiac conduction in opiate users. Ann Intern Med 2003; **139**:154–155.

38. Mayet S et al. Methadone maintenance, QTc and torsade de pointes: who needs an electrocardiogram and what is the prevalence of QTc prolongation? Drug Alcohol Rev 2011; **30**:388–396.

39. Medicines and Healthcare Products Regulatory Agency. Risk of QT interval prolongation with methadone. Current Problems in Pharmacovigilance 2006; **31**:6.

40. Isbister GK et al. Drug induced QT prolongation: the measurement and assessment of the QT interval in clinical practice. Br J Clin Pharmacol 2013; **76**:48–57.

41. Cruciani RA. Methadone: to ECG or not to ECG…That is still the question. J Pain Symptom Manage 2008; **36**:545–552.

42. Wedam EF et al. QT-interval effects of methadone, levomethadyl, and buprenorphine in a randomized trial. Arch Intern Med 2007; **167**:2469–2475.

43. Pani PP et al. QTc interval screening for cardiac risk in methadone treatment of opioid dependence. Cochrane Database Syst Rev 2013; **6**:CD008939.

44. Gowing L et al. Buprenorphine for managing opioid withdrawal. Cochrane Database Syst Rev 2017; **2**:Cd002025.

45. Walsh SL, et al. Effects of buprenorphine and methadone in methadone-maintained subjects. Psychopharmacology (Berl) 1995; **119**:268–276.

46. Strain EC et al. Acute effects of buprenorphine, hydromorphone and naloxone in methadone-maintained volunteers. J Pharmacol Exp Ther 1992; **261**:985–993.

47. Strain EC et al. Buprenorphine effects in methadone-maintained volunteers: effects at two hours after methadone. J Pharmacol Exp Ther 1995; **272**:628–638.

48. Amass L et al. Alternate-day buprenorphine dosing is preferred to daily dosing by opioid-dependent humans. Psychopharmacology (Berl) 1998; **136**:217–225.

49. Amass L et al. Alternate-day dosing during buprenorphine treatment of opioid dependence. Life Sci 1994; **54**:1215–1228.

50. Johnson RE et al. Buprenorphine treatment of opioid dependence: clinical trial of daily versus alternate-day dosing. Drug Alcohol Depend 1995; **40**:27–35.

51. Eissenberg T et al. Controlled opioid withdrawal evaluation during 72 h dose omission in buprenorphine-maintained patients. Drug Alcohol Depend 1997; **45**:81–91.

52. Berson A et al. Hepatitis after intravenous buprenorphine misuse in heroin addicts. J Hepatol 2001; **34**:346–350.

53. Paone D et al. Buprenorphine infrequently found in fatal overdose in New York City. Drug Alcohol Depend 2015; **155**:298–301.

54. Stoller KB et al. Effects of buprenorphine/naloxone in opioid-dependent humans. Psychopharmacology (Berl) 2001; **154**:230–242.

55. Ferri M et al. Slow-release oral morphine as maintenance therapy for opioid dependence. Cochrane Database Syst Rev 2013; **6**:CD009879.

56. Strang J et al. Heroin on trial: systematic review and meta-analysis of randomised trials of diamorphine-prescribing as treatment for refractory heroin addiction. Br J Psychiatry 2015; **207**:5–14.

57. Byford S et al. Cost-effectiveness of injectable opioid treatment v. oral methadone for chronic heroin addiction. Br J Psychiatry 2013; **203**:341–349.

58. Strang J et al. Supervised injectable heroin or injectable methadone versus optimised oral methadone as treatment for chronic heroin addicts in England after persistent failure in orthodox treatment (RIOTT): a randomised trial. Lancet 2010; **375**:1885–1895.

59. Lingford-Hughes AR et al. Evidence-based guidelines for the pharmacological management of substance abuse, harmful use, addiction and comorbidity: recommendations from BAP. J Psychopharmacol 2012; **26**:899–952.

60. Baird CR et al. Gabapentinoid abuse in order to potentiate the effect of methadone: a survey among substance misusers. Eur Addict Res 2014; **20**:115–118.

61. James PD et al. Non-medical use of olanzapine by people on methadone treatment. BJPsych Bull 2016; **40**:314–317.

62. Tenore PL. Psychotherapeutic benefits of opioid agonist therapy. J Addict Dis 2008; **27**:49–65.

63. Nunes EV et al. Treatment of depression in patients with alcohol or other drug dependence: a meta-analysis. JAMA 2004; **291**:1887–1896.

64. Nunes EV et al. Treatment of co-occurring depression and substance dependence: using meta-analysis to guide clinical recommendations. Psychiatr Ann 2008; **38**:nihpa128505.

65. National Institute for Clinical Excellence. Drug misuse in over 16s: opioid detoxification. Clinical Guideline **52**, 2007. https://www.nice.org.uk/guidance/cg52.

66. National Institute for Clinical Excellence. Drug misuse in over 16s: psychosocial interventions. Clinical Guideline **51**, 2007. https://www.nice.org.uk/guidance/cg51.

67. Nosyk B et al. Defining dosing pattern characteristics of successful tapers following methadone maintenance treatment: results from a population-based retrospective cohort study. Addiction 2012; **107**:1621–1629.

68. Yu E et al. A Phase 3 placebo-controlled, double-blind, multi-site trial of the alpha-2-adrenergic agonist, lofexidine, for opioid withdrawal. Drug Alcohol Depend 2008; **97**:158–168.

69. Minozzi S et al. Oral naltrexone maintenance treatment for opioid dependence. Cochrane Database Syst Rev 2011; **4**:CD001333.

70. National Institute for Clinical Excellence. Naltrexone for the management of opioid dependence. Technology Appraisal **115**, 2007. https://www.nice.org.uk/guidance/ta115.

71. Kunoe N et al. Naltrexone implants after in-patient treatment for opioid dependence: randomised controlled trial. Br J Psychiatry 2009; **194**:541–546.

72. The British Pain Society et al. Pain and substance misuse: improving the patient experience. A consensus statement prepared by The British Pain Society in collaboration with The Royal College of Psychiatrists, The Royal College of General Practitioners and The Advisory Council on the Misuse of Drugs. https://www.britishpainsociety.org/static/uploads/resources/misuse_0307_v13_FINAL.pdf.

73. Winklbaur B et al. Treating pregnant women dependent on opioids is not the same as treating pregnancy and opioid dependence: a knowledge synthesis for better treatment for women and neonates. Addiction 2008; **103**:1429–1440.

74. Finnegan LP. Neonatal abstinence syndrome. In: Hoekelman RA, Friedman SB, Nelson N, et al., eds. *Primary Pediatric Care*. St Louis: Mosby; 1992, pp. 1367–1378.

75. Winklbaur B et al. Opioid dependence and pregnancy. Curr Opin Psychiatry 2008; **21**:255–259.

76. Minozzi S et al. Maintenance agonist treatments for opiate-dependent pregnant women. Cochrane Database Syst Rev 2013; **12**:CD006318.

77. Fischer G et al. Methadone versus buprenorphine in pregnant addicts: a double-blind, double-dummy comparison study. Addiction 2006; **101**:275–281.

78. Holmes AP et al. Breastfeeding considerations for mothers of infants with neonatal abstinence syndrome. Pharmacotherapy 2017; **37**:861–869.

CHAPTER 4

Nicotine and smoking cessation

Tobacco smoking is the leading preventable cause of illness and premature death worldwide. Smoking cessation interventions are clinically and cost effective for people with and without a mental illness.

In the UK, NICE recommends that every person who smokes, including those receiving community and in-patient mental health care, should be offered support to stop smoking; those people who feel unable or who are unwilling to give up should be provided with treatment to temporarily abstain whilst they are in a hospital setting.[1]

In those people wishing to make an attempt to give up there are three first-line stop-smoking medications that are recommended by NICE: nicotine replacement therapy (NRT), varenicline and bupropion, all of which at least double the chance of successfully stopping. Quit rates can be increased further if the smoker is also provided with behavioural support from a trained tobacco dependence treatment advisor.[2]

Those people who are unwilling or feel unable to give up should be encouraged to minimise harm and substitute nicotine from tobacco cigarettes with either NRT or an electronic cigarette.[3,4]

The effectiveness of smoking cessation treatments appears not to be reduced in patients with a variety of mental health problems.[5]

Nicotine replacement therapy (NRT)

NRT is licensed for smokers over the age of 12 to help those who want to stop smoking, or reduce before quitting or during a temporary period of enforced abstinence when a person is unable to smoke. It is also indicated for pregnant and breastfeeding women attempting to stop smoking.

The aim of NRT in those stopping smoking is to assist the transition from cigarette smoking to complete abstinence. This is achieved by temporarily replacing some of the nicotine obtained from tobacco cigarettes with NRT products and minimising nicotine withdrawal symptoms and the motivation to smoke. People who smoke can safely use NRT if they wish to continue using nicotine recreationally or to prevent relapse back to smoking.

NRT is a versatile stop-smoking medicine. There are currently eight licensed NRT products in the UK: transdermal patches, lozenges, gum, sublingual tablets, inhalator, nasal spray, mouth spray and oral strips (see Table 4.16).

All products are General Sales List medicines and can be bought over the counter (in the UK). NRT is formulated for systemic absorption either through the skin in the case of patches or the oral or nasal mucosa in the case of all the other products. This means that absorption of nicotine from NRT is much slower than nicotine from inhaling a tobacco cigarette and the risk of becoming addicted to NRT is minimal.[6]

Clinical effectiveness

NRT is the most studied medication for smoking cessation. There have been over 150 trials, including over 50,000 smokers. The odds ratio (OR) of abstinence for any form of NRT compared with placebo is 1.84. **Combination NRT** (i.e. combining two

Table 4.16 Nicotine replacement therapy preparations and dose

	Smoking less than 20 cigarettes/day	Smoking more than 20 cigarettes/day or people who smoke within 30 minutes of waking up
Topical patch 24-hour formulation (21 mg, 14 mg and 7 mg) 16-hour formulation (25 mg, 15 mg, 10 mg)	If smoking >20 cigarettes/day use 21 mg (24-hour) or 25 mg (16-hour) patch There is no difference in efficacy between 16-hour and 24-hour formulations The 16-hour patch should be removed at bedtime	
Nasal spray (0.5 mg/T)	One spray in each nostril when craving; no more than twice per hour; maximum 64 sprays/day	
Oral spray (1 mg/T)	1–2 sprays when craving; no more than 2 sprays per episode; no more than 4 sprays/hour; maximum 64 sprays/day	
Lozenge (1 mg, 2 mg and 4 mg)	One 1 mg hourly to prevent craving	One 2 or 4 mg hourly to prevent craving; no more than 15 2 mg/day
Gum (2 mg, 4 mg and 6 mg)	One piece of 2 mg hourly to prevent craving	One piece of 4 or 6 mg hourly to prevent craving; no more than 15 pieces 4 mg/day
Inhalator (15 mg)	No more than 6 cartridges of 15 mg/day	
Sublingual tablet (2 mg)	1–2 tablets hourly to prevent craving	2 tablets hourly to prevent craving; no more than 40 tablets/day
Mouth strips (2.5 mg)	One strip of 2.5 mg hourly to prevent craving	One strip hourly to prevent craving; no more than 15 strips/day

formulations such as a patch and an oral/nasal product) is more effective than using a single NRT product. The OR of abstinence for combination NRT compared to single NRT products is 1.43. Combination NRT has a similar efficacy to varenicline, and a greater efficacy than bupropion.[7]

Studies with smokers from the general population suggest that each cigarette provides a smoker with approximately 1–2.9 mg of nicotine.[8] Findings from studies in people with schizophrenia who smoke suggest they take more frequent puffs over a shorter period of time and, as a result, extract more nicotine from cigarettes compared with those without a mental health condition.[9] It is therefore plausible that these smokers may require higher doses of nicotine replacement.

The nicotine from oral products has to be absorbed through the cheeks, gums and back of the lips. The correct technique is to chew the gum/suck the lozenge until the taste becomes strong and then rest it between the cheek and gum; when the taste starts to fade, it is advised to repeat this process for about 20–30 minutes. Drinking coffee and carbonated drinks may block the absorption of nicotine from oral nicotine products.[10]

Adverse effects

Adverse effects from using NRT are related to the type of product, and include skin irritation from patches and irritation to the inside of the mouth from oral products. Nausea may occur if the patient is still smoking. Some sleep disturbance can be expected in the early days of treatment, though this is also a symptom of nicotine withdrawal. NRT has no known interactions with psychotropic medication.

Varenicline

Varenicline is a selective nicotinic acetylcholinergic receptor partial agonist; it mimics the action of nicotine and causes a sustained release of dopamine in the mesolimbic pathway. It also blocks dopamine release resulting from subsequent nicotine intake. This means that if it is taken as prescribed, any attempt to smoke a cigarette will be less pharmacologically rewarding and feel less satisfying to a smoker. It is indicated for smokers over the age of 18 who are motivated to stop smoking.

Clinical effectiveness

In the most recent Cochrane review the OR of continuous abstinence for varenicline compared to placebo was 2.24; varenicline was more effective when compared with bupropion (OR 1.39) and single-product NRT (OR 1.25), and was similarly effective compared with combination NRT.[11] In smokers with serious mental illness varenicline improved the odds of stopping smoking by five times compared with placebo[12] in one study and fourfold in all studies combined.[13] In a 2017 study, varenicline was more effective than nicotine patch in depressed smokers.[14]

Prescribing

People who smoke should set a target stopping date between 1 and 2 weeks after starting varenicline treatment. Those who are not willing or able to set a target date within 1–2 weeks can start treatment and then choose their own stopping date within 5 weeks. Daily doses of varenicline are shown in Table 4.17.

For people who have successfully stopped smoking at the end of 12 weeks, an additional course of 12 weeks treatment at 1 mg twice daily may be considered for the maintenance of abstinence.[15]

Table 4.17 Daily doses of varenicline

Day	Dose
1–3	0.5 mg po varenicline once daily
4–7	0.5 mg po varenicline twice daily
8–84	1 mg po varenicline twice daily

po, *per os* (by mouth).

Adverse effects

Common adverse effects include nausea, strange dreams and sleep disturbance, and headache; all occur in more than one in ten people. Varenicline has no known pharmacokinetic interaction with psychotropic medication.

Until 2016, varenicline carried a black triangle symbol, indicating that additional safety monitoring was required for people with a mental health condition. However this was removed by the European Medicines Agency following the publication of the Evaluating Adverse Events in a Global Smoking Cessation Study (EAGLES) study; this found that both varenicline and bupropion did not significantly increase the risk of neuropsychiatric adverse events (including anxiety, depression, aggression, psychosis and suicidal behaviour) when compared with placebo or nicotine patch in patients with or without a history of psychiatric disorders.[16]

Bupropion

Bupropion is an antidepressant with dopaminergic and adrenergic actions, and is additionally an antagonist at the nicotinic acetylcholinergic receptor. It is indicated for smokers over the age of 18 who are motivated to stop smoking.

Clinical effectiveness

In the most recent Cochrane review, the OR of abstinence for bupropion compared with placebo was 1.82. Bupropion was of similar efficacy to single-product NRT (risk ratio [RR] 0.99), and less effective for quitting compared with varenicline (although a trial reporting in 2017 suggests broad equality in outcome[17]) and combination NRT.[7] In smokers with serious mental illness, bupropion improved the odds of quitting by four times compared with placebo.[12]

Prescribing

People who smoke should set a target 'quit date' in the first 2 weeks of starting bupropion treatment. Daily doses are shown in Table 4.18.

Table 4.18 Daily doses of bupropion

Day	Dose
1–6	150 mg po bupropion od
7–49	150 mg po bupropion twice daily (with an interval of at least 8 hours between doses)
50–63	150 mg po bupropion twice daily (if the person has stopped smoking; discontinue if person has not quit)

od, *omni die* (once a day); po, *per os* (by mouth).

Adverse effects

Bupropion is contraindicated in those with seizure disorders, eating disorders and alcohol dependence. Clinicians should be cautious of the potential for manic switch in patients with bipolar affective disorder (very low risk but can occur[18]). Common adverse effects include dizziness, taste changes, gastrointestinal disturbance and insomnia, which can be reduced by avoiding a dose close to bedtime. Unlike NRT and varenicline, bupropion is known to interact with psychotropic medicines. It is metabolised by the cytochrome CYP2B6. Caution is advised when bupropion is co-administered with medicines known to induce (e.g. carbamazepine, phenytoin) or inhibit (e.g. valproate) cytochrome metabolism as clinical efficacy may be affected. Bupropion also inhibits the CYP2B6 pathway and therefore co-administration with medicines metabolised by this enzyme (e.g. risperidone, haloperidol) should be avoided.

Electronic cigarettes

Electronic cigarettes (e-cigarettes) are nicotine delivery devices which do not contain tobacco and do not produce smoke. They are regulated under the European Union Tobacco Products Directive (i.e. there are controls on ingredients, packaging and advertising). E-cigarette manufacturers can apply to the MHRA for a medicinal licence. To date the MHRA has licensed one e-cigarette but the manufacturers have not made this available; this means that at the time of writing no e-cigarette can be prescribed in the EU. Public Health England and The Care Quality Commission (CQC) support the use of e-cigarettes in mental health in-patient settings.[19,20]

Clinical effectiveness

A Cochrane review examining clinical trials of e-cigarettes reported that combined results from two studies showed that using an e-cigarette containing nicotine increased the chances of stopping smoking in the long term compared with using one without nicotine.[21] Other studies have found they can reduce cigarette consumption[22] and reduce withdrawal symptoms.[23] In recent years, they have become the most popular quitting aid in England; it is estimated that they contributed to an additional 18,000 long-term ex-smokers in 2015.[24] With regards to patients with mental illness, two observational studies of community and in-patients with schizophrenia or bipolar disorder who were not motivated to stop smoking found that the use of e-cigarettes was helpful in reducing or stopping smoking.[25,26] Additionally a secondary analysis of RCT data found that the use of an e-cigarette was similarly effective to NRT in motivated smokers with mental illness.[27]

Preparations and dose

In Europe, disposable prefilled cartridges and e-liquids are labelled with how many milligrams (mg) of nicotine there are per millilitre (mL), or as the percentage weight per volume (0% w/v); nicotine content ranges from zero (0%) to a maximum of 20mg/mL (or 2%).

There are several hundred e-cigarette models available; they are broadly categorised into three groups or 'generations':

1. First generation, also known as 'cigalikes', have either a non-reusable battery that can be thrown away once used or a rechargeable battery with replaceable, prefilled cartridges, which can contain nicotine.
2. Second generation, also known as personal vaporisers or tank models, come with sealed prefilled cartridges or a tank that can be filled with the vaper's choice of e-liquid.

CHAPTER 4

3. Third generation, also known as modular, 'mods' and variable voltage devices, are designed to allow modifications to individual components, including adjustable airflow, puff counters, etc.

The dose of nicotine a vaper extracts from an e-cigarette varies depending on the device, the volume of e-liquid, other ingredients in the liquid, and the frequency, size and depth of inhalation.

Adverse effects

Public Health England and the Royal College of Physicians advise that e-cigarettes offer a much less harmful alternative to tobacco for dependent smokers and bystanders.[4,19] They suggest that the hazard to health arising from long-term vapour inhalation from e-cigarettes is unlikely to exceed 5% of the harm from smoking tobacco. Mouth and throat irritation are the most commonly reported symptoms and these subside over time.

Treatment algorithms for people making an attempt to stop smoking or temporarily abstaining are supplied in Tables 4.19 and 4.20, respectively.

Table 4.19 Treatment algorithm for those people making an attempt to stop smoking

First-line quit attempt pharmacological treatment is **combination NRT** or **varenicline.** All quit attempts should be supported at least weekly by a trained tobacco dependence treatment advisor

Combination NRT quit attempt	Varenicline quit attempt
For people who smoke more than 20 cigarettes/day or who smoke within 30 minutes of waking up:	
Start 21 mg (24-hour) or 25 mg (16-hour) patch and an oral/nasal NRT product of the person's choice	
Continue patch use for up to 12 weeks, aiming to reduce patch dosage every 4 weeks	Set target 'stopping date' between 1 and 2 weeks of varenicline treatment
Continue oral/nasal product use whilst experiencing craving	Start 0.5 mg po varenicline once daily on days 1–3
	Increase to 0.5 mg po varenicline twice daily on days 4–7
For people who smoke less than 20 cigarettes/day and do not smoke within 30 minutes of waking up:	Increase to 1 mg po varenicline twice daily on days 8–84
Start 14 mg (24-hour) or 15 mg (16-hour) patch and/or an oral/nasal NRT product of the person's choice	Consider 1 mg varenicline po twice daily for an additional 12 weeks for the maintenance of abstinence in people who have successfully stopped smoking at the end of the initial 12-week course of varenicline
Continue patch use for up to 12 weeks, aiming to reduce patch dosage every 4 weeks	
Continue oral/nasal product use whilst experiencing craving	

Bupropion could be considered second line or where people who smoke express a preference for bupropion therapy

Table 4.19 (*Continued*)

Bupropion quit attempt

Set target 'stopping date' between 1 and 2 weeks of bupropion treatment
Start 150 mg po bupropion daily on day 1–6
Increase to 150 mg po bupropion twice daily on days 7–49 (with an interval of at least 8 hours between doses)
Maintain dose at 150 mg po bupropion on days 50–63 (otherwise discontinue if person has not quit)

In patients with **serious mental illness** both varenicline and bupropion have been shown to increase the odds of stopping smoking by greater than four times compared to placebo. In patients with stable psychiatric co-morbidity an NRT patch was also found to double the abstinence rates compared to placebo. Both varenicline and bupropion did not significantly increase the risk of neuropsychiatric adverse events (including anxiety, depression, aggression, psychosis and suicidal behaviour) when compared to placebo or NRT in patients with or without a history of psychiatric disorders. It is always advisable to monitor a patient's mental health when undergoing a quit attempt

People who smoke wishing to use an **e-cigarette** to quit should generally set a quit date and use the e-cigarette to stop in one go by replacing all their tobacco cigarettes with an e-cigarette as soon as possible. Alternatively, they can gradually reduce the amount they smoke over several weeks and increase the use of the e-cigarette until they have completely switched. Similar to the use of NRT, advise the service user to start with a higher strength of nicotine

NRT, nicotine replacement therapy; po, *per os* (by mouth).

Table 4.20 Treatment algorithm for those people not making an attempt to stop, i.e. those people temporarily abstaining or aiming to reduce their cigarette consumption

Those who are unwilling or feel unable to quit should be encouraged to minimise harm and substitute nicotine from tobacco cigarettes with either **combination NRT** or an **electronic cigarette**

Combination NRT	E-Cigarettes
For people who smoke more than 20 cigarettes/day or who smoke within 30 minutes of waking up:	
Start 21 mg (24-hour) or 25 mg (16-hour) patch and an oral/nasal NRT product of the person's choice	The dose of nicotine a vaper extracts from an e-cigarette varies depending on the device, the volume of e-liquid, other ingredients in the liquid, the frequency, size and depth of inhalation. The more dependent a smoker is, the higher strength of nicotine is recommended
Continue to offer NRT products even if met with initial refusal	
Smokers should have fingertip control over NRT products at times of craving	A rough guide is that smokers of:
For people who smoke less than 20 cigarettes/day and do not smoke within 30 minutes of waking up:	20 tobacco cigarettes/day require 20 mg or more of nicotine/day 40 tobacco cigarettes/day require 40 mg or more of nicotine/day 60 tobacco cigarettes/day require 60 mg or more of nicotine/day
Start 14 mg (24-hour) or 15 mg (16-hour) patch and/or an oral/nasal NRT product of the person's choice	Smokers should have fingertip control over their e-cigarette at times of craving. Similar to NRT, people who smoke should be encouraged to regularly use an e-cigarette between smoking episodes to promote smoke-free intervals
Continue to offer NRT products even if met with initial refusal	
Smokers should have fingertip control over NRT products at times of craving	

It is not currently possible to prescribe e-cigarettes in the NHS. Practitioners should consult local smoke-free polices to establish which type of e-cigarette is permitted in individual mental health in-patient settings

NRT, nicotine replacement therapy.

References

1. National Institute for Health and Care Excellence. Smoking cessation – acute, maternity and mental health services. Public Health Guideline 48, 2013. http://guidance.nice.org.uk/PH48.
2. National Institute for Health and Care Excellence. Stop smoking services. Public Health Guideline 10, 2008; last updated November 2013. https://www.nice.org.uk/guidance/ph10.
3. National Institute for Health and Care Excellence. Smoking: harm reduction. Public Health Guideline 45, 2013. https://www.nice.org.uk/guidance/ph45.
4. Royal College of Physicians. Nicotine without smoke: tobacco harm reduction. A report by the Tobacco Advisory Group of the Royal College of Physicians. 2016. https://www.rcplondon.ac.uk/projects/outputs/nicotine-without-smoke-tobacco-harm-reduction-0.
5. Tidey JW et al. Smoking cessation and reduction in people with chronic mental illness. BMJ 2015; 351:h4065.
6. Hajek P et al. Dependence potential of nicotine replacement treatments: effects of product type, patient characteristics, and cost to user. Prev Med 2007; 44:230–234.
7. Cahill K et al. Pharmacological interventions for smoking cessation: an overview and network meta-analysis. Cochrane Database Syst Rev 2013:Cd009329.
8. Henningfield JE et al. Pharmacotherapy for nicotine dependence. CA Cancer J Clin 2005; 55:281–299; quiz 322–283, 325.
9. Williams JM et al. Increased nicotine and cotinine levels in smokers with schizophrenia and schizoaffective disorder is not a metabolic effect. Schizophr Res 2005; 79:323–335.
10. Henningfield JE et al. Drinking coffee and carbonated beverages blocks absorption of nicotine from nicotine polacrilex gum. JAMA 1990; 264:1560–1564.
11. Cahill K et al. Nicotine receptor partial agonists for smoking cessation. Cochrane Database Syst Rev 2016:Cd006103.
12. Roberts E et al. Efficacy and tolerability of pharmacotherapy for smoking cessation in adults with serious mental illness: a systematic review and network meta-analysis. Addiction 2016; 111:599–612.
13. Wu Q et al. Varenicline for smoking cessation and reduction in people with severe mental illnesses: systematic review and meta-analysis. Addiction 2016; 111:1554–1567.
14. Rohsenow DJ et al. Varenicline versus nicotine patch with brief advice for smokers with substance use disorders with or without depression: effects on smoking, substance use and depressive symptoms. Addiction 2017; 112:1808–1820.
15. Hajek P et al. Varenicline in prevention of relapse to smoking: effect of quit pattern on response to extended treatment. Addiction 2009; 104:1597–1602.
16. Anthenelli RM et al. Neuropsychiatric safety and efficacy of varenicline, bupropion, and nicotine patch in smokers with and without psychiatric disorders (EAGLES): a double-blind, randomised, placebo-controlled clinical trial. Lancet 2016; 387:2507–2520.
17. Benli AR et al. A comparison of the efficacy of varenicline and bupropion and an evaluation of the effect of the medications in the context of the smoking cessation programme. Tob Induc Dis 2017; 15:10.
18. Giasson-Gariepy K et al. A case of hypomania during nicotine cessation treatment with bupropion. Addict Sci Clin Pract 2013; 8:22.
19. McNeill A et al. E-cigarettes: an evidence update. A report commissioned by Public Health England. 2015. https://www.gov.uk/government/uploads/system/uploads/attachment_data/file/457102/Ecigarettes_an_evidence_update_A_report_commissioned_by_Public_Health_England_FINAL.pdf.
20. Care Quality Commission. Brief guide: the use of 'blanket restrictions' in mental health wards. 2017. https://www.cqc.org.uk/sites/default/files/20170322_briefguide-use_of_blanket_restrictions_in_mental_health_wards.pdf.
21. Hartmann-Boyce J et al. Electronic cigarettes for smoking cessation. Cochrane Database Syst Rev 2016; 9:Cd010216.
22. Brose LS et al. Is the use of electronic cigarettes while smoking associated with smoking cessation attempts, cessation and reduced cigarette consumption? A survey with a 1-year follow-up. Addiction 2015; 110:1160–1168.
23. Dawkins L et al. First- versus second-generation electronic cigarettes: predictors of choice and effects on urge to smoke and withdrawal symptoms. Addiction 2015; 110:669–677.
24. Beard E et al. Association between electronic cigarette use and changes in quit attempts, success of quit attempts, use of smoking cessation pharmacotherapy, and use of stop smoking services in England: time series analysis of population trends. BMJ 2016; 354:i4645.
25. Caponnetto P et al. Impact of an electronic cigarette on smoking reduction and cessation in schizophrenic smokers: a prospective 12-month pilot study. Int J Environ Res Public Health 2013; 10:446–461.
26. Pratt SI et al. Appeal of electronic cigarettes in smokers with serious mental illness. Addict Behav 2016; 59:30–34.
27. O'Brien B et al. E-cigarettes versus NRT for smoking reduction or cessation in people with mental illness: secondary analysis of data from the ASCEND trial. Tob Induc Dis 2015; 13:5.

Pharmacological treatment of dependence on stimulants

The most commonly misused stimulants are cocaine (as hydrochloride or free base), amphetamine sulfate and methamphetamine hydrochloride. These drugs are usually insufflated (snorted) (e.g. cocaine HCl; amphetamine SO_4), smoked (cocaine base) or injected.

There are no effective pharmacotherapies for the treatment of stimulant dependence. A wide variety of pharmacological agents have been assessed and found lacking.[1] Effective medications are available only for some psychiatric complications of stimulant use. For example, antidepressants have a role in treating major depressive disorder associated with stimulant use[2] as do antipsychotics for amphetamine psychosis.[3] However neither class of drug is efficacious in treating stimulant dependence itself.[4–6]

Psychosocial interventions remain the recommended treatment for dependence, with the most benefits seen from approaches incorporating contingency.[2]

Cocaine

Detoxification

Symptoms of withdrawal include depressed mood, agitation and insomnia.[7] These are usually self-limiting. It should be noted that given cocaine's short half-life and the binge nature of cocaine use, many patients essentially detoxify themselves regularly, with no pharmacological therapy. Symptomatic relief such as the short-term use of hypnotics may be helpful in some but these agents may be diverted for illicit use or become agents of dependence themselves.[2]

Substitution treatment

There is little evidence for any benefit of substitution therapy for the treatment of cocaine misuse and it should not be prescribed.[2] There is inconclusive evidence that some agents may increase rates of abstinence. These include drugs that increase extracellular dopamine by stimulating dopamine release (dexamphetamine),[8,9] inhibiting dopamine reuptake (bupropion and modafinil),[8–11] or inhibiting dopamine metabolism (disulfiram).[12] A recent review[9] was conducted of several agents including bupropion, dexamfetamine, lisdexamfetamine, methylphenidate, modafinil, mazindol, methamphetamine, mixed amphetamine salts and selegiline. There was some evidence that psychostimulants improved sustained cocaine abstinence and one trial supporting the use of 300 mg/day modafinil.[13] However, the quality of evidence is low with high attrition bias. Another Cochrane review[14] found no evidence for the benefit of dopamine agonists. One recent small study suggested that topiramate may have efficacy[15] but a meta-analysis found no effect.[16]

Amphetamines

A wide variety of amphetamines are misused, including 'street' amphetamine, methamphetamine and pharmaceutical dexamfetamine. Any drug in this class is likely to have misuse potential. As with cocaine there is no evidence base for pharmacological

CHAPTER 4

treatment of withdrawal,[2,3,5] although the number of agents that have been investigated is relatively limited.[3,5] A systematic review of dexamfetamine, bupropion, methylphenidate and modafinil as replacement therapies found no reduction in amphetamine use or craving and no increase in sustained abstinence.[17] Future research may change this outcome in view of the small sample sizes and paucity of studies available for review. Naltrexone has shown promise in initial trials by attenuating the subjective effects of dexamfetamine[18] and reducing amphetamine use in dependent individuals,[19] but it appears inactive in methamphetamine dependence.[20]

Detoxification

A withdrawal syndrome is common in those who are dependent. Treatment should focus on symptomatic relief, although many symptoms of amphetamine withdrawal (low mood, listlessness, fatigue, etc.) are short-lived and self-limiting and may not be amenable to pharmacological treatment. Insomnia can be treated with short courses of hypnotics.

Maintenance

Dexamfetamine maintenance should not be initiated as there is no good evidence for this practice.[2] There are, however, patients that have been prescribed dexamfetamine as a maintenance treatment for drug dependence for many years. Ideally such patients should be gradually detoxified over several months. For some, though, the consequences of enforced detoxification may be worse than continuing to prescribe dexamfetamine. In these cases the best decision may be to continue to prescribe. A decision to continue prescribing dexamfetamine should only be made by an addiction specialist.[2]

Psychosis

A minority of individuals using amphetamines will develop marked psychosis (paranoid delusions, hallucinations and extreme agitation) requiring emergency medical and psychiatric care. More commonly users report sub-clinical psychotic symptoms that do not require high-intensity intervention. Development of psychotic symptoms is thought to be related to the cumulative quantity and the frequency of exposure to amphetamines. In one of the only RCTs of antipsychotic medications for treating amphetamine psychosis, olanzapine and haloperidol delivered at clinically relevant doses showed similar efficacy in resolving psychotic symptoms.[21] While antipsychotic medications demonstrate efficacy in providing short-term relief, there is no evidence to guide decisions regarding long-term clinical care.

Polysubstance abuse

In those that are dependent on opioids and cocaine, the provision of effective substitution therapy for treatment of the opioid dependence with either methadone or buprenorphine can lead to a reduction in cocaine use.[2]

References

1. de Lima MS et al. Pharmacological treatment of cocaine dependence: a systematic review. Addiction 2002; **97**:931–949.
2. Department of Health. Drug misuse and dependence: UK guidelines on clinical management. 2017. https://www.gov.uk/government/publications/drug-misuse-and-dependence-uk-guidelines-on-clinical-management.
3. Shoptaw SJ et al. Treatment for amphetamine psychosis. Cochrane Database Syst Rev 2009:CD003026.
4. Pani PP et al. Antidepressants for cocaine dependence and problematic cocaine use. Cochrane Database Syst Rev 2011:CD002950.
5. Srisurapanont M et al. Treatment for amphetamine dependence and abuse. Cochrane Database Syst Rev 2001:CD003022.
6. Indave BI et al. Antipsychotic medications for cocaine dependence. Cochrane Database Syst Rev 2016; **3**:CD006306.
7. Rounsaville BJ. Treatment of cocaine dependence and depression. Biol Psychiatry 2004; **56**:803–809.
8. Perez-Mana C et al. Efficacy of indirect dopamine agonists for psychostimulant dependence: a systematic review and meta-analysis of randomized controlled trials. J Subst Abuse Treat 2011; **40**:109–122.
9. Castells X et al. Psychostimulant drugs for cocaine dependence. Cochrane Database Syst Rev 2016; **9**:CD007380.
10. Anderson AL et al. Modafinil for the treatment of cocaine dependence. Drug Alcohol Depend 2009; **104**:133–139.
11. Martinez-Raga J et al. Modafinil: a useful medication for cocaine addiction? Review of the evidence from neuropharmacological, experimental and clinical studies. Curr Drug Abuse Rev 2008; **1**:213–221.
12. Pani PP et al. Disulfiram for the treatment of cocaine dependence. Cochrane Database Syst Rev 2010:CD007024.
13. Kampman KM et al. A double blind, placebo controlled trial of modafinil for the treatment of cocaine dependence without co-morbid alcohol dependence. Drug Alcohol Depend 2015; **155**:105–110.
14. Minozzi S et al. Dopamine agonists for the treatment of cocaine dependence. Cochrane Database Syst Rev 2015:CD003352.
15. Baldacara L et al. Efficacy of topiramate in the treatment of crack cocaine dependence: a double-blind, randomized, placebo-controlled trial. J Clin Psychiatry 2016; **77**:398–406.
16. Singh M et al. Topiramate for cocaine dependence: a systematic review and meta-analysis of randomized controlled trials. Addiction 2016; **111**:1337–1346.
17. Perez-Mana C et al. Efficacy of psychostimulant drugs for amphetamine abuse or dependence. Cochrane Database Syst Rev 2013; **9**:CD009695.
18. Jayaram-Lindstrom N et al. Naltrexone attenuates the subjective effects of amphetamine in patients with amphetamine dependence. Neuropsychopharmacology 2008; **33**:1856–1863.
19. Jayaram-Lindstrom N et al. Naltrexone for the treatment of amphetamine dependence: a randomized, placebo-controlled trial. Am J Psychiatry 2008; **165**:1442–1448.
20. Coffin PO et al. Extended-release naltrexone for methamphetamine dependence among men who have sex with men: a randomized placebo-controlled trial. Addiction 2017; [Epub ahead of print].
21. Leelahanaj T et al. A 4-week, double-blind comparison of olanzapine with haloperidol in the treatment of amphetamine psychosis. J Med Assoc Thai 2005; **88 Suppl** 3:S43–52.

GHB and GBL dependence

GHB (γ-hydroxybutyrate) and GBL (γ-butaryl-lactone, a pro-drug of GHB) use is uncommon but medically important because, in dependent users, withdrawal can proceed rapidly to life-threatening agitated delirium. Complications include seizures, bradycardia, cardiac arrest and renal failure. Doctors in emergency departments and psychiatric hospitals need to be able to recognise and manage acute withdrawal.

GHB and GBL are colloquially often referred to as 'G'. They reduce anxiety and produce disinhibition and sedation, primarily through actions at the GABA$_\beta$ receptor. These drugs are used recreationally for socialising and occasionally to aid sleep. Among men who have sex with men (MSM) they can be used to facilitate sex in the context of potential high-risk sexual behaviour such as 'chemsex'. Both drugs have a narrow therapeutic index, and overdose is not uncommon. Dependence is rare, but in dependent users withdrawal has a rapid onset and can produce severe delirium with paranoid delusions and life-threatening complications.[1]

The withdrawal syndrome[1,2]

Dependent users take GBL 'round the clock' (consuming doses day and night, every 1–3 hours or more frequently). Onset of withdrawal symptoms is typically a few hours following the last dose of GBL. The withdrawal syndrome is similar to alcohol withdrawal and may include symptoms such as tachycardia, insomnia, anxiety, sweating and fine tremors.[1] Untreated, this can progress to agitated delirium, often with psychotic features (including paranoid delusions and hallucinations) later followed by severe tremors, muscle rigidity and seizures.[1] Muscle rigidity may be so severe as to produce fever, rhabdomyolysis and acute renal failure. The requirement for medication to manage symptoms eases over 4–6 days, although there are case reports of more prolonged withdrawal.

Withdrawal management

The evidence base for detoxification from GBL is limited. The core principle of managing withdrawal is to treat early and so prevent the development of delirium and other complications. Once established, delirium can be difficult to control.[3] Early treatment with benzodiazepines is required. Diazepam is often used. Baclofen (a GABA$_\beta$ agonist) and phenobarbital have also been used effectively as adjunctive medications.[1,4] GHB itself has been successfully used to aid withdrawal.[5] Reducing doses are given every 3 hours over 2 weeks.

Existing alcohol withdrawal scales are unlikely to be helpful in evaluating withdrawal severity. For up-to-date guidance on the management of GHB/GBL withdrawal, it is recommended (in the UK) that information be sought from the National Poisons Information Service (NPIS), specifically the NPIS 24-hour telephone service and the poisons information database TOXBASE®.

The two scenarios with which clinicans should be conversant are unplanned acute withdrawal (Table 4.21) and planned elective withdrawal (Table 4.22) in dependent users.

Table 4.21 Management of acute unplanned withdrawal

Setting	■ Acute unplanned withdrawal is a medical emergency and should be managed in the in-patient setting ■ Severe withdrawal may require admission to an ICU
Initial pharmacotherapy	■ Initiate diazepam 20 mg po when early withdrawal symptoms are observed ■ Diazepam can be repeated at 30-minute to 4-hourly intervals until symptoms are controlled ■ Most cases of GBL withdrawal require 60–80 mg diazepam in the first 24 hours ■ High daily dosages of up to 300 mg po diazepam may be necessary ■ If the patient becomes drowsy, withhold diazepam and review diagnosis ■ One-to-one nursing care may assist in managing severe cases ■ Have flumazenil to hand should reversal of effects be required
Adjunctive pharmacotherapy	■ Initiate baclofen 10 mg po tds in combination with benzodiazepine withdrawal regimen where benzodiazepines prove inadequate ■ This can be titrated to 20 mg po tds in cases of continued anxiety and agitation although extreme caution is required ■ In cases of severe withdrawal consider addition of phenobarbital in doses of 150–450 mg/day IV* (ICU only) ■ In cases where severe withdrawal remains uncontrolled, IV anaesthetic such as propofol* may be required (ICU only)

*The respiratory-depressant effects of phenobarbital and propofol cannot be reversed; facilities for mechanical ventilation should be available.
ICU, intensive care unit; IV, intravenous; po, *per os* (by mouth); tds, *ter die sumendum* (three times a day).

Table 4.22 Management of planned elective withdrawal

Setting	■ All patients undergoing planned withdrawal should be medically supervised ■ Ambulatory community detoxification should only be attempted where there is no history of delirium or psychosis. A third party should be at home who is able to monitor and support the withdrawal process. There should be the option of transferring the patient to an in-patient unit if symptoms are not well controlled
Pre-withdrawal	■ Discuss the treatment plan with the patient and person who will be supporting them ■ Encourage the patient to keep a week-long diary of GBL use including dose frequency and quantity ■ Encourage the patient to cease 'on-top' drug use such as mephedrone, prior to elective withdrawal ■ Start baclofen 10 mg po tds 3–7 days before target withdrawal date ■ Encourage patients to reduce GBL dose as much as tolerable by reducing each dose by 0.1 mL every 1–2 days or by increasing the time between doses
Withdrawal	■ On day 1 of planned ambulatory withdrawal, ask the patient to attend having used no GBL for 2 hours, and advise them to dispose of their remaining supplies of GBL ■ Advise patients they will need to stay at the clinic for up to 4 hours on day 1, that they cannot drive motor vehicles during withdrawal and should not drink alcohol or take other sedatives during withdrawal ■ Increase baclofen to 20 mg po tds ■ Initiate benzodiazepine treatment once signs and symptoms of withdrawal develop – tachycardia, sweaty palms, fine tremor, anxiety. Start diazepam 20 mg, review after 2 hours and monitor hourly for anxiety/sedation/respiratory depression. Repeat up to 20 mg po diazepam if indicated ■ Once 6 hours have passed since last GBL usage the patient may be given up to a further 40 mg diazepam to take home, and then be seen on the following 2 days ■ At each daily visit, review diazepam dosage and titrate to symptoms. Diazepam is seldom needed beyond 7 days. Typical initial daily doses of diazepam are around 40–60 mg/day
Post-withdrawal	■ Continue baclofen 20 mg po tds following benzodiazepine withdrawal reducing over 4–6 weeks ■ After withdrawal, persisting anxiety and insomnia are common, and there is a high risk of relapse. Before initiating elective withdrawal management, a plan should be in place to monitor and support patients for 4 weeks to minimise risk of relapse

po, *per os* (by mouth); tds, *ter die sumendum* (three times a day).

References

1. Kamal RM et al. Pharmacological treatment in gamma-hydroxybutyrate (ghb) and gamma-butyrolactone (gbl) dependence: detoxification and relapse prevention. CNS Drugs 2017; **31**:51–64.
2. Bell J et al. Gamma-butyrolactone (GBL) dependence and withdrawal. Addiction 2011; **106**:442–447.
3. Novel Psychoactive Treatment UK Network (NEPTUNE). Guidance on the Clinical Management of Acute and Chronic Harms of Club Drugs and Novel Psychoactive Substances. 2015. http://neptune-clinical-guidance.co.uk/wp-content/uploads/2015/03/NEPTUNE-Guidance-March-2015.pdf.
4. LeTourneau JL et al. Baclofen and gamma-hydroxybutyrate withdrawal. Neurocrit Care 2008; **8**:430–433.
5. Dijkstra BA et al. Detoxification with titration and tapering in gamma-hydroxybutyrate (GHB) dependent patients: the Dutch GHB monitor project. Drug Alcohol Depend 2017; **170**:164–173.

Benzodiazepine misuse

Benzodiazepine prescribing increased during the 1960s and 1970s, mainly because of the improved safety profile of these drugs relative to barbiturates. However, it was soon noted that benzodiazepines have a high potential for causing dependence. Prescriptions originally started for other disorders were often continued long-term and led to the development of dependence. This was and is particularly common in elderly patients and those with anxiety spectrum disorders or depression.

Benzodiazepine dependence can be thought of as either iatrogenic (low daily doses prescribed over many years) or non-iatrogenic (high doses, illicitly obtained, consumed intermittently).

Discontinuation

A Cochrane review evaluated the evidence for pharmacological interventions for benzodiazepine mono-dependence and concluded that a gradual reduction of benzodiazepine dose by about an eighth (10–20%) of the dose per fortnight was preferable to an abrupt discontinuation.[1] A more recent review confirmed that withdrawal over a period of less than 6 months is appropriate for most patients.[2] A meta-analysis supports the effectiveness of multifaceted prescribing interventions (usually including psychological interventions/support) in reducing benzodiazepine use in older patients[3] and a recent RCT has demonstrated that a simple educational approach based on self-efficacy theory resulted in almost a quarter of long-term elderly benzodiazepine users engaging voluntarily in reducing and discontinuing use.[4]

A large number of patients presenting to addictions services may be using illicit benzodiazepines in addition to their primary substance of abuse. People with non-iatrogenic benzodiazepine dependence often consume doses greater than 100 mg diazepam a day. Although some services provide prescriptions for benzodiazepines, there is no evidence that substitute prescribing of benzodiazepines ultimately reduces benzodiazepine misuse. If benzodiazepines are prescribed, this should ideally be for a short-term, time-limited (2–3 weeks) prescription and with a view to detoxification.

If patients have been prescribed benzodiazepines for a substantial period of time, it may be preferable to convert to equivalents of diazepam as this is longer acting and so less likely to be associated with withdrawal symptoms. Benzodiazepine dependence as part of polysubstance dependence should also be treated by a gradual withdrawal of the medication. Benzodiazepines prescribed at greater than 30 mg diazepam equivalent per day may cause harm[5] and so this should be avoided if at all possible (such doses are rare in iatrogenic dependence[6]). Psychosocial interventions including contingency management have had some success at reducing benzodiazepine use.

A summary of benzodiazepine withdrawal and a withdrawal schedule are provided in Box 4.8.

Pregnancy and benzodiazepine misuse

Benzodiazepines are not major human teratogens but should ideally be gradually discontinued before a planned pregnancy. If a woman is prescribed benzodiazepines and

---

Box 4.8   Summary of benzodiazepine withdrawal

- Benzodiazepines should be withdrawn at a rate of around 1/8 of the dose every 2 weeks.
- Discontinuation should usually be completed within 6 months.
- Switching to an equivalent dose of (long-acting) diazepam before beginning withdrawal is commonplace.
- Benzodiazepine misuse is frequently seen in multisubstance misuse where opiates may be the primary drug of dependence.

Typical diazepam withdrawal schedule

Baseline	30 mg/day
Week 2	25 mg/day
Week 4	20 mg/day
Week 6	18 mg/day
Week 8	16 mg/day
Week 10	14 mg/day
Week 12	12 mg/day
Week 14	10 mg/day

Then reduce by 2 mg/day every 2 weeks if tolerated.

---

found to be pregnant, the prescription should be gradually withdrawn over as short a time as possible, being mindful of the risk of withdrawal seizures and the potential consequences for the pregnant woman and foetus. A risk–benefit analysis should be undertaken and specialist advice sought (see section on 'Drug choice in pregnancy' in Chapter 7).

References

1. Denis C et al. Pharmacological interventions for benzodiazepine mono-dependence management in outpatient settings. Cochrane Database Syst Rev 2006:CD005194.
2. Lader M et al. Withdrawing benzodiazepines in primary care. CNS Drugs 2009; 23:19–34.
3. Gould RL et al. Interventions for reducing benzodiazepine use in older people: meta-analysis of randomised controlled trials. Br J Psychiatry 2014; 204:98–107.
4. Tannenbaum C et al. Reduction of inappropriate benzodiazepine prescriptions among older adults through direct patient education: the EMPOWER cluster randomized trial. JAMA Intern Med 2014; 174:890–898.
5. Department of Health. Drug misuse and dependence: UK guidelines on clinical management. 2017. https://www.gov.uk/government/publications/drug-misuse-and-dependence-uk-guidelines-on-clinical-management.
6. Vicens C et al. Comparative efficacy of two interventions to discontinue long-term benzodiazepine use: cluster randomised controlled trial in primary care. Br J Psychiatry 2014; 204:471–479.

Synthetic cannabinoid receptor agonists (SCRAs)

The clinical importance of SCRAs relates to their acute toxicity (which is potentially life-threatening), their relationship to psychosis and their propensity to induce dependence. Doctors working in emergency departments, psychiatric settings and addiction services should be able to recognise and manage acute intoxication with synthetic cannabinoids.

Synthetic cannabinoids, or synthetic cannabinoid receptor agonists (SCRAs), are a structurally diverse group of chemicals that act as an agonist at the CB1 receptor. In the UK, they are used predominantly by vulnerable groups such as the homeless and prisoners. Most commonly, they are dissolved in alcohol and sprayed on plant material, then smoked. More than one SCRA compound may be present in a single herbal pack[1] and at the time of writing there are more than 700 street names for SCRAs,[1] the most common of which are 'Spice' and 'K2'. Many patients may not admit to SCRA use despite their recent use.[2] SCRAs are more potent in their action at the CB1 receptor and can be longer lasting than tetrahydracannabinol (THC), the active ingredient in cannabis. They also have diverse non-CB1 actions, which can influence their clinical effects.

Acute intoxication is distinct from and more severe than THC intoxication and is associated with physical harms which can be life-threatening.[3] It is estimated that the risk of requiring emergency treatment is 30 times higher than that associated with the use of cannabis.[4] SCRAs can precipitate psychosis which persists after intoxication. Around 12% of users report symptoms of dependence and a withdrawal syndrome similar to cannabis withdrawal.

Acute SCRA intoxication

Acute SCRA intoxication needs to be recognised clinically as urine drug testing for SCRAs is not possible in the acute setting because of their structural diversity.[5] Features of SCRA intoxication are detailed in Table 4.23 and are based on case series of presentations to emergency units.[2,3,6,7] Presentations and incidence of particular symptoms vary widely, which may reflect the chemical diversity of SCRAs. The most common features appear to be agitation, nausea and tachycardia.[3] Intoxication is usually short-lived, with 78% resolving within 8 hours.[7] A psychotic episode is commonly precipitated: 41% of presentations of acutely intoxicated patients to accident and emergency departments were associated with psychotic symptoms.[6]

Management of acute SCRA intoxication

Patients should be cared for in an appropriate setting so may require transfer from a psychiatric setting, such as a Place of Safety suite, to the emergency department. ECG and cardiac monitoring to detect possible arrhythmias and blood tests to detect possible complications such as renal failure, acidosis, metabolite derangements, rhabdomyolysis and hepatotoxicity[8] are useful. Treatment is supportive and commonly involves sedation using benzodiazepines or rarely anaesthesia, antipsychotics, intravenous

CHAPTER 4

Table 4.23 Features of acute SCRA intoxication

System affected	Feature
Cardiovascular system	Tachycardia Hypertension Bradycardia Hypotension Chest pain – can precipitate myocardial ischaemia Cardiac arrest
Gastrointestinal system and abdominal organs	Nausea Vomiting – often profuse Abdominal pain Hepatotoxicity Acute renal injury – acute tubular necrosis and acute interstitial nephritis
Nervous system	Agitation Anxiety Aggression Confusion Psychotic symptoms – can persist after intoxication Seizures Coma Catatonia with posturing
Other	Conjunctival injection Rhabdomyolysis

fluids, supplemental oxygen and anti-emetics.[3,5–7] Reassuringly, neither antipsychotic nor benzodiazepine use in SCRA intoxication has been associated with adverse cardiovascular effects and antipsychotics have not been associated with increased incidence of seizures.[6]

Management of SCRA-related psychosis

Psychotic symptoms are a common aspect of SCRA intoxication and can outlast the acute intoxication phase in 30%. SCRA-associated psychosis is more florid than cannabis-related psychosis and less likely to have manic features.[9] This psychosis is very commonly associated with aggression;[9] catatonia[10] and severe self-mutilation[11] are described. Thus psychiatric admission may be necessary to manage the degree of behavioural disturbance. The length of admission reported is variable, from shorter than a week to over a month.[9,12] Relative to cannabis users, SCRA psychosis seems to be more resistant to antipsychotic treatment, requiring higher doses (according to one study, mean dose of antipsychotic was equivalent to 11 mg haloperidol, whereas in cannabis users mean dose was 6 mg/day, and in those without either co-morbidity it was 3 mg/day)[13] and longer treatment.[9]

Management of SCRA dependence and withdrawal

SCRA dependence is reported in case studies and surveys and may be expected to occur at higher rates than dependence on cannabis given the higher potency of SCRA. Generic psychosocial addiction treatment approaches to SCRA dependence using motivational interviewing techniques, and drug diaries with the aim to cut down slowly are recommended. Advising patients to switch to cannabis as a lower potency (and hence less harmful) alternative should be undertaken with caution given reports that cannabis does not alleviate SCRA withdrawal[14] and with the patient having a full understanding of the legal implications – possession of cannabis is an offence whereas possession of most SCRAs is, in the UK, covered by the Psychoactive Substances Act 2016.

Patients with months of daily use experience a physiological withdrawal syndrome lasting several days with some similarities to cannabis withdrawal (potentially reflecting to some extent co-morbid cannabis dependence and complex withdrawal): disturbed sleep, strange dreams, restlessness, anxiety, craving, shivering and muscle twitching.[5,15] Increased blood pressure and heart rate are also reported.[5] Treatment with benzodiazepines has been reported to be both effective and ineffective.[14] Low dose quetiapine (50 mg) was effective[14] in the case of benzodiazepine failure.

References

1. Spice Addiction Support. 700 Street Names for Synthetic Marijuana (Spice, K2, etc.). 2017. https://spiceaddictionsupport.org/street-names-for-synthetic-marijuana/.
2. Abouchedid R et al. Analytical confirmation of synthetic cannabinoids in a cohort of 179 presentations with acute recreational drug toxicity to an Emergency Department in London, UK in the first half of 2015. Clin Toxicol (Phila) 2017; 55:338–345.
3. Tait RJ et al. A systematic review of adverse events arising from the use of synthetic cannabinoids and their associated treatment. Clin Toxicol (Phila) 2016; 54:1–13.
4. Winstock A et al. Risk of emergency medical treatment following consumption of cannabis or synthetic cannabinoids in a large global sample. J Psychopharmacol 2015; 29:698–703.
5. Novel Psychoactive Treatment UK Network (NEPTUNE). Guidance on the Clinical Management of Acute and Chronic Harms of Club Drugs and Novel Psychoactive Substances. 2015. http://neptune-clinical-guidance.co.uk/wp-content/uploads/2015/03/NEPTUNE-Guidance-March-2015.pdf.
6. Monte AA et al. Characteristics and treatment of patients with clinical illness due to synthetic cannabinoid inhalation reported by medical toxicologists: a ToxIC database study. J Med Toxicol 2017; 13:146–152.
7. Hoyte CO et al. A characterization of synthetic cannabinoid exposures reported to the National Poison Data System in 2010. Ann Emerg Med 2012; 60:435–438.
8. Gurney SM et al. Pharmacology, toxicology, and adverse effects of synthetic cannabinoid drugs. Forensic Sci Rev 2014; 26:53–78.
9. Shalit N et al. Characteristics of synthetic cannabinoid and cannabis users admitted to a psychiatric hospital: a comparative study. J Clin Psychiatry 2016; 77:e989–995.
10. Khan M et al. Catatonia secondary to synthetic cannabinoid use in two patients with no previous psychosis. Am J Addict 2016; 25:25–27.
11. Meijer KA et al. Smoking synthetic marijuana leads to self-mutilation requiring bilateral amputations. Orthopedics 2014; 37:e391–394.
12. Hurst D et al. Psychosis associated with synthetic cannabinoid agonists: a case series. Am J Psychiatry 2011; 168:1119.
13. Bassir Nia A et al. Psychiatric comorbidity associated with synthetic cannabinoid use compared to cannabis. J Psychopharmacol 2016; 30:1321–1330.
14. Nacca N et al. The synthetic cannabinoid withdrawal syndrome. J Addict Med 2013; 7:296–298.
15. Castaneto MS et al. Synthetic cannabinoids: epidemiology, pharmacodynamics, and clinical implications. Drug Alcohol Depend 2014; 144:12–41.

CHAPTER 4

Interactions between 'street drugs' and prescribed psychotropic drugs

There are some significant interactions between 'street drugs' and drugs that are prescribed for the treatment of mental illness. Information comes from case reports or theoretical assumptions, rarely from systematic investigation. A summary can be found in Table 4.24, but remember that the evidence base is poor. Always be cautious.

In all patients who misuse street drugs:

- Infection with hepatitis B and C is common. The associated liver damage may lead to a reduced ability to metabolise other drugs and increased sensitivity to adverse effects.
- Infection with HIV is common.[28,29] Antiretroviral drugs are involved in pharmacokinetic interactions with a number of prescribed and non-prescribed drugs.[30] For example, ritonavir can decrease the metabolism of ecstasy and precipitate toxicity, and a number of antiretrovirals can increase or decrease methadone metabolism.[31]
- Prescribed drugs may be used in the same way as illicit drugs (i.e. erratically and not as intended). Large quantities of prescribed drugs should not be given to out-patients.
- Additive or synergistic effects of respiratory depressants may play a contributory role in deaths from overdose with methadone or other opioid agonists.[1] Caution is needed in prescribing sedative medicines such as benzodiazepines.

Acute behavioural disturbance

Acute intoxication with street drugs may result in behavioural disturbance especially when synthetic cannabinoid agonists or cathinones are taken.[32,33] Non-drug management is preferable. If at all possible a urine drug screen should be done to determine the drugs that have been taken before prescribing any psychotropic. Note, however, that urine screening tests may not detect newer psychoactive agents. A physical examination should be done if possible (blood pressure, temperature, pulse, respiration and ECG).

If intervention with a psychotropic is unavoidable, promethazine 50 mg *or* olanzapine 10 mg po/IM are probably the safest options. Temperature, pulse, respiration and blood pressure *must* be monitored afterwards. Benzodiazepines are commonly misused with other street drugs and so standard doses may be ineffective in tolerant users. Interactions are also possible (see Table 4.24).

Table 4.24 Interactions between 'street drugs' and psychotropic drugs

	Cannabis	Heroin/methadone[1]	Cocaine, amphetamines, ecstasy, MDA, 6-APB	Alcohol	Ketamine[2]
General considerations	■ Usually smoked in cigarettes (induces CYP1A2) ■ Can be sedative ■ Dose-related tachycardia ■ THC/CBD inhibit CYP3A4 and CYP1A2[3]	■ Can produce sedation/respiratory depression ■ QTc prolongation also reported with methadone (see section on methadone)	■ Stimulants (cocaine can be sedative in higher doses) ■ Arrhythmia possible ■ Cerebral/cardiac ischaemia with cocaine – may be fatal ■ Hyperthermia/dehydration with ecstasy[4]	■ Sedative ■ Liver damage possible	■ Sedative – readily causes unconciousness ■ Onset of effects may be rapid if snorted or injected
Older antipsychotics	■ Antipsychotics reduce the psychotropic effects of almost all drugs of abuse by blocking dopamine receptors (dopamine is the neurotransmitter responsible for 'reward') ■ Patients prescribed antipsychotics may increase their consumption of illicit substances to compensate ■ Patients who have taken ecstasy may be more prone to EPS ■ Cardiotoxic or very sedative antipsychotics are best avoided, at least initially. Sulpiride is a reasonably safe first choice				
Second-generation antipsychotics	■ Risk of additive sedation ■ Cannabis smoking in tobacco can reduce plasma levels of olanzapine and clozapine via induction of CYP1A2[5] ■ Clozapine might reduce cannabis and alcohol consumption[6] ■ Outcome of THC/CBD inhibition of CYP1A2 unknown	■ Risk of additive sedation ■ Case report of methadone withdrawal being precipitated by risperidone[7] ■ Isolated report of quetiapine increasing methadone levels, especially in those with slowed CYP2D6 hepatic metabolism[8]	■ Antipsychotics may reduce craving and cocaine-induced euphoria[9-13] ■ Olanzapine may worsen cocaine dependency[14] ■ Clozapine may increase cocaine levels but diminish subjective response[15]	■ Increased risk of hypotension with olanzapine (and possibly other beta blockers)	■ Increased sedation
Antidepressants	■ Tachycardia has been reported (monitor pulse and take care with TCAs[16]) ■ Complex, unpredictable effects of CYP induction (tobacco) and CYP inhibition (THC/CBD)	■ Avoid very sedative antidepressants ■ Some SSRIs can increase methadone plasma levels[17] (citalopram is SSRI of choice but note the small risk of additive QTc prolongation) ■ Case report of serotonin syndrome occurring when sertraline prescribed with methadone for a palliative care patient[18]	■ Avoid TCAs (arrhythmia risk) ■ MAOIs contraindicated (hypertension) ■ SSRI antidepressants are generally ineffective at attenuating withdrawal effects from cocaine[19] ■ SSRIs may greatly increase plama concentrations of MDMA[20] ■ Risk of SSRIs increasing cocaine levels, especially fluoxetine[21] ■ Concomitant use of SSRIs or aripiprazole and lamotrigine with cocaine or other stimulants (especially MDA and 6-APD) could precipitate a serotonin syndrome[22,23] ■ SSRIs may enhance subjective reaction to cocaine[24]	■ Avoid very sedative antidepressants ■ Avoid antidepressants that are toxic in OD ■ Impaired psychomotor skills (not SSRIs)	■ Inhibitors of CYP3A4 (e.g. fluoxetine/paroxetine) will lengthen ketamine half-life ■ Beware hypertension with SNRIs and reboxetine

(Continued)

Table 4.24 (Continued)

	Cannabis	Heroin/methadone[1]	Cocaine, amphetamines, ecstasy, MDA, 6-APB	Alcohol	Ketamine[2]
Anticholinergics	■ Misuse is likely. Try to avoid if at all possible (by using a second-generation drug if an antipsychotic is required) ■ Can cause hallucinations, elation and cognitive impairment				
Lithium	■ Very toxic if taken erratically ■ Always consider the effects of dehydration (particularly problematic with alcohol or ecstasy)				
Carbamazepine/valproate	■ Carbamazepine (CBZ) may decrease THC concentrations via induction of CYP3A4[25]	■ Carbamazepine (CBZ) decreases methadone levels[26] (danger if CBZ stopped suddenly) ■ Valproate seems less likely to interact	■ Carbamazepine induces CYP3A4, which leads to more rapid formation of norcocaine (hepatotoxic and more cardiotoxic than cocaine)[27]	■ Monitor LFTs	■ Carbamazepine decreases ketamine plasma concentrations via CYP3A4 induction
Benzodiazepines (Always remember that benzodiazepines are liable to misuse)	■ Monitor level of sedation	■ Oversedation (and respiratory depression possible) ■ Concomitant use can lead to accidental overdose ■ Possible pharmacokinetic interaction (increased methadone levels)	■ Oversedation (if high doses of cocaine have been taken) ■ Widely used after cocaine intoxication ■ Future misuse possible detoxification	■ Oversedation (and respiratory depression) possible ■ Widely used in alcohol detoxification	■ Oversedation and respiratory depression

6-APB, 6-(2-aminopropyl)benzofuran; EPS, extrapyramidal symptoms; LFTs, liver function tests; MAOI, monoamine oxidase inhibitor; MDA, 3,4-methylenedioxyamphetamine; MDMA, 3,4-methylenedioxymethamphetamine; OD, overdose; SNRI, serotonin–noradrenaline reuptake inhibitor; SSRI, selective serotonin reuptake inhibitor; TCA, tricyclic antidepressant; THC/CBD, tetrahydrocannabinol/cannabidiol.

References

1. Department of Health. Drug misuse and dependence: UK guidelines on clinical management. 2017. https://www.gov.uk/government/publications/drug-misuse-and-dependence-uk-guidelines-on-clinical-management.
2. Pfizer Limited. Summary of Product Characteristics. Ketalar 10 mg/ml Injection. 2017. https://www.medicines.org.uk/emc/medicine/12939.
3. Arellano AL et al. Neuropsychiatric and general interactions of natural and synthetic cannabinoids with drugs of abuse and medicines. CNS Neurol Disord Drug Targets 2017; 16:554–566.
4. Gowing LR et al. The health effects of ecstasy: a literature review. Drug Alcohol Rev 2002; 21:53–63.
5. Zullino DF et al. Tobacco and cannabis smoking cessation can lead to intoxication with clozapine or olanzapine. Int Clin Psychopharmacol 2002; 17:141–143.
6. Green AI et al. Alcohol and cannabis use in schizophrenia: effects of clozapine vs. risperidone. Schizophr Res 2003; 60:81–85.
7. Wines JD Jr et al. Opioid withdrawal during risperidone treatment. J Clin Psychopharmacol 1999; 19:265–267.
8. Uehlinger C et al. Increased (R)-methadone plasma concentrations by quetiapine in cytochrome P450s and ABCB1 genotyped patients. J Clin Psychopharmacol 2007; 27:273–278.
9. Poling J et al. Risperidone for substance dependent psychotic patients. Addict Disord Treat 2005; 4:1–3.
10. Albanese MJ et al. Risperidone in cocaine-dependent patients with comorbid psychiatric disorders. J Psychiatr Pract 2006; 12:306–311.
11. Sattar SP et al. Potential benefits of quetiapine in the treatment of substance dependence disorders. J Psychiatry Neurosci 2004; 29:452–457.
12. Grabowski J et al. Risperidone for the treatment of cocaine dependence: randomized, double-blind trial. J Clin Psychopharmacol 2000; 20:305–310.
13. Kishi T et al. Antipsychotics for cocaine or psychostimulant dependence: systematic review and meta-analysis of randomized, placebo-controlled trials. J Clin Psychiatry 2013; 74:e1169–e1180.
14. Kampman KM et al. A pilot trial of olanzapine for the treatment of cocaine dependence. Drug Alcohol Depend 2003; 70:265–273.
15. Farren CK et al. Significant interaction between clozapine and cocaine in cocaine addicts. Drug Alcohol Depend 2000; 59:153–163.
16. Benowitz NL et al. Effects of delta-9-tetrahydrocannabinol on drug distribution and metabolism. Antipyrine, pentobarbital, and ethanol. Clin Pharmacol Ther 1977; 22:259–268.
17. Hemeryck A et al. Selective serotonin reuptake inhibitors and cytochrome P-450 mediated drug-drug interactions: an update. Curr Drug Metab 2002; 3:13–37.
18. Bush E et al. A case of serotonin syndrome and mutism associated with methadone. J Palliat Med 2006; 9:1257–1259.
19. Pani PP et al. Antidepressants for cocaine dependence and problematic cocaine use. Cochrane Database Syst Rev 2011:CD002950.
20. Rietjens SJ et al. Pharmacokinetics and pharmacodynamics of 3,4-methylenedioxymethamphetamine (MDMA): interindividual differences due to polymorphisms and drug-drug interactions. Crit Rev Toxicol 2012; 42:854–876.
21. Fletcher PJ et al. Fluoxetine, but not sertraline or citalopram, potentiates the locomotor stimulant effect of cocaine: possible pharmacokinetic effects. Psychopharmacology (Berl) 2004; 174:406–413.
22. Silins E et al. Qualitative review of serotonin syndrome, ecstasy (MDMA) and the use of other serotonergic substances: hierarchy of risk. Aust N Z J Psychiatry 2007; 41:649–655.
23. Kotwal A et al. Serotonin syndrome in the setting of lamotrigine, aripiprazole, and cocaine use. Case Rep Med 2015; 2015:769531.
24. Soto PL et al. Citalopram enhances cocaine's subjective effects in rats. Behav Pharmacol 2009; 20:759–762.
25. GW Pharma Ltd. Summary of Product Characteristics. Sativex Oromucosal Spray. 2015. https://www.medicines.org.uk/emc/medicine/23262.
26. Miller BL, Mena I, Giombetti R, et al. Neuropsychiatric effects of cocaine: SPECT measurements. In: Paredes A, Gorelick DA, eds. Cocaine: Physiological and Physiopathological Effects, 1st edn. New York: Haworth Press; 1993, pp. 47–58.
27. Roldan CJ, Habal R. Toxicity, cocaine. 2004. http://www.emedicine.com/med/topic400.htm.
28. Vocci FJ et al. Medication development for addictive disorders: the state of the science. Am J Psychiatry 2005; 162:1432–1440.
29. Tsuang J et al. Pharmacological treatment of patients with schizophrenia and substance abuse disorders. Addictive Disorders and Their Treatment 2005; 4:127–137.
30. Bracchi M et al. Increasing use of 'party drugs' in people living with HIV on antiretrovirals: a concern for patient safety. AIDS 2015; 29:1585–1592.
31. Gruber VA et al. Methadone, buprenorphine, and street drug interactions with antiretroviral medications. Curr HIV/AIDS Rep 2010; 7:152–160.
32. Smith CD et al. Novel psychoactive substances: a novel clinical challenge. BMJ Case Rep 2013; 2013.
33. Anderson C et al. A novel psychoactive substance poses a new challenge in the management of paranoid schizophrenia. BMJ Case Rep 2015; 2015.

CHAPTER 4

Drugs of misuse – a summary

In the UK, one in 12 adults uses illicit drugs in any one year,[1] and at least a third of those with mental illness can be classified as having a 'dual diagnosis'.[2,3] There is now compelling evidence that cannabis use increases the risk of psychosis.[4-7] Substance misuse in fully compliant patients with schizophrenia increases the relapse rate to the levels seen in those who are non-compliant[8] (i.e. substance misuse negates the benefits of antipsychotic treatment). Urine testing for illicit drugs is routine on many psychiatric wards. It is important to be aware of the duration of detection of drugs in urine and of other commonly used substances and drugs that can give a false positive result. Some false positives are unpredictable (i.e. not related to chemical similarity), for example amisulpride can give a false positive for buprenorphine.[9] False positive results are most likely with point of care immunoassay kits. If a positive result has implications for a patient's liberty, and the patient denies use of substances, a second sample should be sent to the laboratory for definitive testing.

Table 4.25 provides a basic summary of drugs of misuse.

Table 4.25 Basic summary of drugs of misuse

Drug	Physical signs/ symptoms of intoxication	Most common mental state changes[10]	Withdrawal symptoms	Duration of withdrawal	Duration of detection in the urine[11,12]	Other substances which give a positive result[13-15]
Amfetamine-type stimulants[16]	Tachycardia; increased BP; anorexia; tremor; restlessness	Visual/tactile/olfactory auditory hallucinations; paranoia; elation	Fatigue; hunger; depression; irritability, craving, social withdrawal	Peaks 7–34 hours; lasts maximum of 5 days	Depends on half-life, mostly 48–72 hours	Cough and decongestant preparations, bupropion, chloroquine, chlorpromazine, labetalol, promethazine, ranitidine, selegiline, large quantities of tyramine, tranylcypromine, trazodone, and many others
GHB/GBL	Drowsiness, coma, disinhibition	Sociability, confidence	Tremor; tachycardia; paranoia; delirium; psychosis; visual/tactile/ olfactory/auditory hallucinations	3–4 days	Difficult to detect, not routinely screened for	Not known
Benzodiazepines	Sedation; disinhibition	Relaxation; visual hallucinations; disorientation; sleep disturbance	Anxiety, insomnia, delirium, seizures; visual/ tactile/olfactory auditory hallucinations; psychosis	Usually short-lived but may last weeks to months	Up to 28 days: depending on half-life of drug taken	Nefopam, sertraline, zopiclone, efavirenz
Cannabis[6,7,17-21]	Tachycardia; lack of co-ordination; red eyes; postural hypotension	Elation; psychosis; perceptual distortions; disturbance of memory/ judgement; twofold increase in risk of developing schizophrenia	Restlessness; irritability; insomnia; anxiety	Uncertain Probably less than 1 month (longer in heavy users)	Single use: 3 days; chronic heavy use: up to 30 days	Passive 'smoking' of cannabis Efavirenz, ibuprofen, naproxen
Synthetic cannabinoid receptor agonists (SCRAs)	Tachycardia, hypertension, red eyes, agitation	Anxiety, agitation, aggression, psychotic symptoms, clouded consciousness	Anxiety, sleep disturbance, headache	Uncertain	Difficult to detect using conventional screening methods because of chemical heterogeneity	Not known

(Continued)

Table 4.25 (Continued)

Drug	Physical signs/ symptoms of intoxication	Most common mental state changes[10]	Withdrawal symptoms	Duration of withdrawal	Duration of detection in the urine[11,12]	Other substances which give a positive result[13-15]
Cocaine	Tachycardia/tachypnoea; increased BP/headache; respiratory depression; chest pain	Euphoria; paranoid psychosis; panic attacks/ anxiety; insomnia/ excitement	Fatigue; hunger; depression; irritability; craving; social withdrawal	12–18 hours	Up to 96 hours	Food/tea containing coca leaves Codeine Ephedrine/pseudoephedrine
Heroin	Pinpoint pupils; clammy skin; respiratory depression	Drowsiness; euphoria; hallucinations	Dilated pupils; nausea; diarrhoea; generalised pains; gooseflesh; runny nose/eyes	Peaks after 36–72 hours	Up to 72 hours	Diphenoxylate, naltrexone, naloxone, opiate analgesics, food/tea containing poppy seed, amisulpride, diphenhydramine, 4-quinolones, tramadol
Methadone	Pinpoint pupils; respiratory depression; pulmonary oedema	As above	As above but milder and longer lasting	Peaks after 4–6 days; can last 6 weeks	Up to 7 days with chronic use	Quetiapine
Ketamine[22-25]	Increased heart rate, increased BP, palpitations, dizziness, abdominal discomfort, lower urinary tract symptoms, ataxia	Impaired consciousness, dissociation, hallucinations, ego diffusion	Fatigue, poor appetite, drowsiness, craving, anxiety, dysphoria, restlessness, palpitations, tremor, sweating	48 hours	Ketamine – up to 2 days Norketamine – up to 14 days	Quetiapine
LSD[26]	Variable Dilated pupils Moderate increase in HR and BP, flushing, sweating, hypersalivation, increased tendon reflexes	Euphoria, introspection, illusions, pseudohallucinations, altered sense of time, altered thought processes, altered perception of body, vivid recollections of significant memories	None	N/A	Up to 4 days	Ambroxol, amitriptyline, brompheniramine, bupropion, buspirone, cephradine, chlorpromazine, desipramine, diltiazem, doxepin, ergonovine, fentanyl, fluoxetine, haloperidol, imipramine, labetalol, lysergol, methylphenidate, metoclopramide, prochlorperazine, risperidone, sertraline, thioridazine, trazodone, verapamil

For more detail, see Moeller et al, 2017.[27]

BP, blood pressure; GHB/GBL, γ-hydroxybutyrate/γ-butaryl-lactone; HR, heart rate; LSD, lysergic acid diethylamide; N/A, not applicable.

References

1. NHS Digital. Statistics on Drugs Misuse: England, 2017. 2017. http://www.content.digital.nhs.uk/catalogue/PUB23442.

2. Menezes PR et al. Drug and alcohol problems among individuals with severe mental illness in south London. Br J Psychiatry 1996; **168**:612–619.

3. Phillips P et al. Drug and alcohol misuse among in-patients with psychotic illnesses in three inner-London psychiatric units. Psychiatric Bulletin 2003; **27**:217–220.

4. Sara GE et al. The impact of cannabis and stimulant disorders on diagnostic stability in psychosis. J Clin Psychiatry 2014; **75**:349–356.

5. Di Forti M et al. High-potency cannabis and the risk of psychosis. Br J Psychiatry 2009; **195**:488–491.

6. Murray RM et al. Traditional marijuana, high-potency cannabis and synthetic cannabinoids: increasing risk for psychosis. World Psychiatry 2016; **15**:195–204.

7. Marconi A et al. Meta-analysis of the association between the level of cannabis use and risk of psychosis. Schizophr Bull 2016; **42**:1262–1269.

8. Hunt GE et al. Medication compliance and comorbid substance abuse in schizophrenia: impact on community survival 4 years after a relapse. Schizophr Res 2002; **54**:253–264.

9. Couchman L et al. Amisulpride and sulpiride interfere in the CEDIA DAU buprenorphine test. Ann Clin Psychiatry 2008; **45 Suppl** 1.

10. Truven Health Analytics. Micromedex 2.0. 2017. https://www.micromedexsolutions.com/home/dispatch.

11. Substance Abuse and Mental Health Services Administration (US). Substance abuse: clinical issues in intensive outpatient treatment. Treatment Improvement Protocol (TIP) Series, No. 47. Rockville, MD: SAMHSA; 2006.

12. Mayo Medical Laboratories. Approximate Detection Times. 2016. http://www.mayomedicallaboratories.com/test-info/drug-book.

13. Brahm NC et al. Commonly prescribed medications and potential false-positive urine drug screens. Am J Health Syst Pharm 2010; **67**:1344–1350.

14. Saitman A et al. False-positive interferences of common urine drug screen immunoassays: a review. J Anal Toxicol 2014; **38**:387–396.

15. Liu CH et al. False positive ketamine urine immunoassay screen result induced by quetiapine: a case report. J Formos Med Assoc 2017; **116**:720–722.

16. Shoptaw SJ et al. Treatment for amphetamine psychosis. Cochrane Database Syst Rev 2009:CD003026.

17. Johns A. Psychiatric effects of cannabis. Br J Psychiatry 2001; **178**:116–122.

18. Hall W et al. Long-term cannabis use and mental health. Br J Psychiatry 1997; **171**:107–108.

19. Arseneault L et al. Causal association between cannabis and psychosis: examination of the evidence. Br J Psychiatry 2004; **184**:110–117.

20. Budney AJ et al. Review of the validity and significance of cannabis withdrawal syndrome. Am J Psychiatry 2004; **161**:1967–1977.

21. Bonnet U et al. The cannabis withdrawal syndrome: current insights. Subst Abuse Rehabil 2017; **8**:9–37.

22. Novel Psychoactive Treatment UK Network (NEPTUNE). Guidance on the Clinical Management of Acute and Chronic Harms of Club Drugs and Novel Psychoactive Substances. 2015. http://neptune-clinical-guidance.co.uk/wp-content/uploads/2015/03/NEPTUNE-Guidance-March-2015.pdf.

23. Chen WY et al. Gender differences in subjective discontinuation symptoms associated with ketamine use. Subst Abuse Treat Prev Policy 2014; **9**:39.

24. Critchlow DG. A case of ketamine dependence with discontinuation symptoms. Addiction 2006; **101**:1212–1213.

25. Adamowicz P et al. Urinary excretion rates of ketamine and norketamine following therapeutic ketamine administration: method and detection window considerations. J Anal Toxicol 2005; **29**:376–382.

26. Passie T et al. The pharmacology of lysergic acid diethylamide: a review. CNS Neurosci Ther 2008; **14**:295–314.

27. Moeller KE et al. Clinical interpretation of urine drug tests: what clinicians need to know about urine drug screens. Mayo Clin Proc 2017; **92**:774–796.

CHAPTER 4

Drug treatment of special patient groups

Part 2

Drug treatment of special
patient groups

Chapter 5

Children and adolescents

Principles of prescribing practice in childhood and adolescence[1]

- **Target symptoms, not diagnoses.** Diagnosis can be difficult in children and co-morbidity is very common. Treatment should target key symptoms. While a working diagnosis is beneficial to frame expectations and help communication with patients and parents, it should be kept in mind that it could take some time for the illness to evolve.
- **Technical aspects of paediatric prescribing.** The Medicines Act 1968 and European legislation make provision for doctors to use medicines in an off-label or out-of-licence capacity or to use unlicensed medicines. However, individual prescribers are always responsible for ensuring that there is adequate information to support the quality, efficacy, safety and intended use of a drug before prescribing it. It is recognised that the informed use of unlicensed medicines, or of licensed medicines for unlicensed applications (off-label use), is often necessary in paediatric practice.
  - Prescription writing in the UK: Inclusion of age is a legal requirement in the case of prescription-only medicines for children under 12 years of age, but it is preferable to state the age for all prescriptions for children.
- **Begin with less, go slow and monitor efficacy and adverse reactions.** In out-patient care, dosage will usually commence lower in mg/kg per day terms than adults. Gradually increase the dose as needed, and finish at a dose that produces adequate symptom control with minimum adverse reactions (adverse reactions are more common in children and adolescents). In routine clinical care, regular monitoring of efficacy and adverse reactions is essential, in order to ensure that treatment is necessary and that it should continue.[2]
- **Multiple medications are often required in the severely ill.** Monotherapy is ideal. However, childhood-onset illness can be severe and may require treatment with psychosocial approaches in combination with more than one medication.[3] Co-pharmacy is using different medications for different disorders or symptoms, while poly-pharmacy is the use of multiple medications to manage the same problem. As children often have multiple co-occurring conditions, co-pharmacy is common.

The Maudsley Prescribing Guidelines in Psychiatry, Thirteenth Edition. David M. Taylor, Thomas R. E. Barnes and Allan H. Young.
© 2018 David M. Taylor. Published 2018 by John Wiley & Sons Ltd.

- **Allow time for an adequate trial of treatment.** Children are generally more ill than their adult counterparts and will often require longer periods of treatment before responding. An adequate trial of treatment for those who have required in-patient care may well be 8 weeks for depression or schizophrenia.
- **Where possible, change one drug at a time.** Make changes to one drug at a time and attempt to remove a drug when adding a new drug, if possible.
- **Monitor outcome in more than one setting.** For symptomatic treatments (such as stimulants for attention deficit hyperactivity disorder [ADHD]), bear in mind that the expression of problems may be different across settings (e.g. home and school); a dose titrated against parent reports may be too high for the daytime at school.
- **Patient and family medication education is essential.** For some child and adolescent psychiatric patients the need for medication will be life-long. The first experiences with medications are therefore crucial to long-term outcomes and adherence. Education regarding the problems, medication, adverse reactions and medication adherence should be addressed. Patients and their guardians should be encouraged to ask for changes to their treatment regimen.

References

1. Nunn K, Dey C. *The Clinician's Guide to Psychotropic Prescribing in Children and Adolescents*, 1st edn. Sydney: Glade Publishing; 2003.
2. Santosh PJ et al. Pediatric Antipsychotic Use and Outcomes Monitoring. J Child Adolesc Psychopharmacol 2017; 27:546–554.
3. Luk E, Reed E. Polypharmacy or pharmacologically rich? In: Nunn KP, Dey C, eds. *The Clinician's Guide to Psychotropic Prescribing in Children and Adolescents*, 2nd edn. Sydney: Glade Publishing; 2003, pp. 8–11.

Further reading

For detailed adverse effects of CNS Drugs in children and adolescents, see:

British Medical Association et al. *British National Formulary for Children* (July 2017). London: Pharmaceutical Press; 2017.

Elbe D, Bezchlibnyk-Butler K, Virani A et al. *Clinical Handbook of Psychotropic Drugs for Children and Adolescents*, 3rd revised edn. Oxford, UK: Hogrefe Publishing; 2015.

Gerlach M, Warnke A, Greenhill L. *Psychiatric Drugs in Children and Adolescents. Basic Pharmacology and Practical Applications*. Vienna: Springer-Verlag Wien; 2014.

Riddle MA et al. Introduction: Issues and viewpoints in pediatric psychopharmacology. Int Rev Psychiatry 2008; 20:119–120.

Martin A, Scahill L, Charney D et al. *Pediatric Psychopharmacology: Principles and Practice*, 2nd edn. New York: Oxford University Press; 2011.

Depression in children and adolescents

Psychological intervention

The UK National Institute for Health and Care Excellence (NICE) guidelines[1] and American Academy of Child and Adolescent Psychiatry (AACAP) practice parameters[2] recommend that psychological intervention be considered as first-line treatment for depression in children and adolescents and specifically so in cases of mild to moderate depression.

For moderate to severe depression in young people, both the original[1] and updated NICE guidelines[3] recommend combined therapy of medication and psychological treatment. The updated NICE guidelines[3] also recommend the use of medication at an earlier stage of treatment in moderate to severe depression.

Pharmacotherapy

NICE Clinical guideline 28[1] supports the use of selective serotonin reuptake inhibitors (SSRIs) but only in combination with psychological therapy.[1,4-7] Two US studies, Treatment of Adolescents with Depression Study (TADS)[8] and Treatment of Resistant Depression in Adolescence (TORDIA),[9] found that cognitive behavioural therapy (CBT) confers benefit when used in combination with medication. A large UK study did not establish the additional benefit of combined therapy (fluoxetine plus CBT) and a review demonstrated that the use of fluoxetine on its own in addition to routine clinical care is effective in treating moderate to severe depression.[10-12] A Cochrane review in 2014[13] found limited evidence that combination therapy is more effective than antidepressant medication alone and no evidence that combination therapy is more effective than psychological therapy alone. The NICE Surveillance Group also suggested that the additional benefit of combining CBT and antidepressant treatment compared with the administration of antidepressants alone may not be as significant as previously thought.[14] Whether CBT provides added value to treatment and outcomes remains a controversial area but guidelines do now support the administration of fluoxetine for moderate to severe depression at a much earlier stage of treatment.[3] The more severe the depressive episode the more likely it is that medication, in combination with psychological treatment or on its own, will be efficacious in the early stages of treatment.[15,16] Good initial response is a sign of improved rates of recovery and outcomes.[8,9]

The placebo response rate in randomised controlled trials (RCTs) is high in young people suffering with depression[15,17,18] although this is most prevalent in large multicentre and industry-sponsored trials.[19] On average, drug and placebo response rates in children and adolescents differ by only 10%[6] and the benefits of active treatment appear to be modest. In a meta-analysis, the rate of response to antidepressants was 61% compared to 50% to placebo.[20] The number needed to treat (NNT) is 9–10 overall and lower in adolescents.[6,20] Note that this NNT refers to the number needed for one additional person to respond to active treatment. Overall response rates are much higher than NNTs suggest. There is some evidence to suggest that dose increases can improve response.[21]

CHAPTER 5

Fluoxetine is the recommended first-line pharmacological treatment and is superior to placebo in children and adolescents.[3,4,22,23] In the UK, it is licensed for use in children and young people from 8 to 18 years to treat moderate to severe major depression which is unresponsive to psychological therapy.[4] Cochrane agree that fluoxetine is the drug of choice in this patient group.[15] Recent network meta-analyses have confirmed fluoxetine's superiority over CBT[24] and other drugs.[23,24]

Fluoxetine and **escitalopram** are the only antidepressants approved by the US Food and Drug Administration (FDA) for adolescents and fluoxetine is the only FDA-approved medication for pre-pubertal children (from age 8 years). The European Medicines Agency recommends that the use of SSRIs in children and adolescents should be restricted to their approved indications.[25]

Studies in adults have shown that the elimination half-life of fluoxetine is 1–4 days and 7–15 days for its primary metabolite, norfluoxetine, making it a preferable SSRI for adolescents who are then less likely to experience withdrawal effects when omitting a dose or stopping the medication abruptly.[26,27] Body weight influences fluoxetine concentrations and starting doses of medication have to be lowered in children. However during treatment the half-lives of most antidepressants are much lower in children than in adolescents and higher doses may have to be administered in order to achieve adequate blood concentration and therapeutic effects.[27,28]

Fluoxetine should be started at a low dose of 10 mg daily which can be increased after 1 week to achieve a minimum effective dosage of 20 mg daily.[1] Patients and their parents/carers should be informed about the potential adverse effects associated with SSRI treatment and know how to seek help in an emergency. Any pre-existing symptoms that might be interpreted as side-effects (e.g. agitation, anxiety, suicidality) should be noted.[20]

Alternative SSRIs and other antidepressants

If there is no response to fluoxetine and pharmacotherapy is still considered to be the most favourable option, an alternative SSRI such as **sertraline** or **citalopram**[1] may be used cautiously by specialists. Evidence suggests some efficacy for sertraline[1,29,30] but one RCT showed it to be inferior to CBT.[31] There is limited evidence for antidepressant efficacy of citalopram.[4,15,32,33] It should not be used in children and adolescents with congenital long QT syndrome and caution is advised in those with congenital heart disease or hepatic impairment.[34] Citalopram is more toxic in overdose.[35]

Escitalopram is the therapeutically active isomer of racemic citalopram.[36] It was shown to be efficacious in two RCTs[37,38] and is approved by the FDA for use in depression in those aged 12 years and upwards.

Sertraline, citalopram and escitalopram are quickly metabolised by children and twice daily dosing should be considered.[39,40] Sertraline, citalopram and escitalopram should also be started at low doses and titrated weekly up to minimum effective doses: sertraline 50–100 mg, citalopram 20 mg and escitalopram 10 mg.

Paroxetine is considered to be an unsuitable option.[1,4]

Tricyclic antidepressants (TCAs) are not effective in pre-pubertal children but may have marginal efficacy in adolescents.[6,41] In practice, tricyclics are not recommended in children and adolescents.[1]. Amitriptyline (up to 200 mg/day), imipramine (up to 300 mg/day) and nortriptyline have all been studied in RCTs. Because of more extensive metabolism, young people require higher mg/kg doses than adults. The side-effect burden associated with TCAs is considerable. Vertigo, orthostatic hypotension, tremor and dry mouth limit tolerability.[41] Tricyclics are also more cardiotoxic in young people than in adults. Baseline and on-treatment electrocardiograms (ECGs) should be performed. Co-prescribing with other drugs known to prolong the QTc interval should be avoided. There is no evidence that adolescents who fail to respond to SSRIs respond to tricyclics.

There is little evidence for the use of **mirtazapine**[42] but it is sometimes used in clinical practice where sleep is a problem.

Omega-3 fatty acids may be effective in childhood depression but evidence is minimal.[43]

Vitamin D supplementation may be effective in improving depressive symptoms in young people with vitamin D deficiency but evidence is minimal.[44]

St John's wort should be avoided because of the risk of interaction.

Severe depression that is life-threatening or unresponsive to other treatments may respond to electroconvulsive therapy (ECT).[45–47] ECT should not be used in children under 12.[1] The effects of ECT on the developing brain are unknown.

Safety of antidepressants

When prescribing SSRIs it is important that the dose is increased slowly to minimise the risk of treatment-emergent agitation and that patients are monitored closely for the development of treatment-emergent suicidal thoughts and acts. Patients should be seen at least weekly in the early stages of treatment. Adverse effects linked to SSRIs include sedation, insomnia and gastrointestinal symptoms; rarely SSRIs can induce bleeding, serotonin syndrome, activation and mania (more detailed reviews of these problems in adults can be found in Chapter 3).

There is evidence from meta-analyses of pooled trials that antidepressants increase the risk of suicidal behaviour[8,20,48–55] and aggression[55] in the short term although no completed suicides were reported in any of the trials in young people. The risk of spontaneously reported suicidal ideation and suicidal behaviour in adolescents treated with antidepressant medication is 1–3 out of every 100 children.[53] Conversely, some studies point to the risk of suicide associated with untreated depression.[56] Reduced prescribing of SSRIs in the USA[57] and the Netherlands[58] has been linked to an increase in the rate of suicide.

The TADS study, which compared CBT with fluoxetine, placebo and combined CBT and fluoxetine, showed that all treatment arms were effective in reducing suicidal ideation but that the combined treatment of fluoxetine and CBT reduced the risk of suicidal events to the greatest extent.[8] A review concluded that on balance there is a role for SSRIs in depression in children and adolescents.[5] Overall, the potential benefits of treatment with antidepressants outweigh the risks in relation to suicidal behaviours.

Starting and titrating the dose of SSRIs and alternative medication

The administration of all SSRIs should be monitored against the emergence of adverse effects and the dose should be reduced if adverse effects persist beyond one week. In this case the dose of the medication should be lowered to the highest tolerable dose. SSRI

CHAPTER 5

medication should be administered for a minimum of 4–6 weeks and if the child or young person fails to respond and remains symptomatic a dose increase should be considered. A recent meta-analysis reports that much of the overall improvement with SSRI medication compared to placebo occurs by week 2 and that treatment gains are greatest early in treatment in depression in young people.[59] A switch to another medication should be made if there is insufficient improvement after approximately 10–12 weeks (switch much earlier if there are *no* signs of improvement). Medication effectiveness should be initially monitored at weekly intervals and re-evaluated every 4–6 weeks.

Duration of treatment

There is little evidence regarding optimum duration of treatment.[60] Adding relapse prevention CBT to fluoxetine during continuation treatment has shown sustained remission and lower rates of relapse in comparison to medication on its own.[61,62] To consolidate the response to the acute treatment and avoid relapse, treatment with fluoxetine should continue for at least 6 and up to 12 months.[63,64] There is a significant reduction of the risk of relapse with a continuation of treatment for 6 months.[40,63]

Maintenance

Following an asymptomatic period of approximately 6–12 months, it may be appropriate to consider maintenance treatment, particularly if there is a history of recurrent, prolonged or severe depressive episodes, co-morbidity, suicidality or environmental factors.[2]

Discontinuation

At the end of treatment, the antidepressant dose should be tapered slowly to minimise discontinuation symptoms. Ideally this should be done over 6–12 weeks.[1,40] Because of fluoxetine's long duration of action it can probably be safely tapered over 2 weeks. The duration of tapering is difficult to judge in an individual because of the long period between dose reduction and emergence of discontinuation reactions (often a week or more).

Refractory depression

There are no clear clinical guidelines for the management of treatment-resistant depression in adolescents[1,2] but there is evidence from the TORDIA published studies[9] that adolescents who failed to respond to treatment with one SSRI may improve when switched to another SSRI or venlafaxine and even more so when the pharmacotherapy was combined with concurrent CBT. A switch to an SSRI was just as efficacious as a switch to venlafaxine with less severe adverse effects. TORDIA results demonstrate that with continued treatment of depression among treatment-resistant adolescents approximately one-third remit.[65] However the venlafaxine group had more adverse effects and there was an association with higher rates of suicidal events in those who entered the study with high suicidal ideation.[66] A recent meta-analysis found a significantly increased risk of suicidality for young people given venlafaxine[23] although a large cohort study suggested no increased risk of suicidality for venlafaxine.[67] NICE recommends that venlafaxine should not be used for the treatment of depression in children and adolescents.[3]

Predictors of poor response to treatment may include greater depression severity, longer duration of depressive episode, greater impairment, sub-syndromal manic symptoms, self-harm, drug and alcohol abuse, hopelessness, higher baseline suicidal ideation and family conflict.[68-70] Moderators of treatment response may include co-morbidity and a history of abuse.[68,69]

Augmentation

Augmentation with a second medication has not been studied in RCTs in depressed children and adolescents who have either not responded to treatment or have only shown a partial improvement. Case studies and post hoc TORDIA studies have demonstrated some benefits from the addition of atypical antipsychotics or lithium.[65,71]

Risk of bipolar disorder

Some young people, and especially children, will develop behavioural activation in response to the administration of SSRIs. It is estimated that 3–8% of young people prescribed SSRIs present with heightened mood, restlessness and silliness which is transitory in nature. This disinhibitory response to starting SSRI medication or being prescribed increasing doses of medication needs to be differentiated from hypomania or mania.[72] Early bipolar illness should be suspected when the presentation is one of severe depression, associated with psychosis or rapid mood shifts, and the condition worsens on treatment with antidepressants. Early studies suggested that between 20% and 40% of children and young people presenting with depression will develop bipolar affective disorder[73] when treated with antidepressants (the antidepressants presumably acting so as to reveal the disorder, not cause it). In some studies in bipolar patients treatment with antidepressants is associated with new or worsening rapid cycling in as many as 23% of bipolar patients.[74] It seems that the younger the child, the greater the risk.[75] In the case of emergent mania early treatment with atypical antipsychotics and mood stabilisers should be considered.[76] Further details regarding the treatment of bipolar depression can be found in the section on 'Bipolar illness in children and adolescents' in this chapter.

Box 5.1 summarises the treatment of depression in children and adolescents.

CHAPTER 5

Box 5.1 Summary of pharmacotherapy for depression in children and adolescents[1,3,14,25,37,38,42,65,71]

First line	Fluoxetine (FDA approved for 8 years and over in the USA)
Second line	Sertraline or citalopram*
Third line	Escitalopram (FDA approved for 12 years and over in the USA)
Fourth line	Consider augmentation of antidepressant with second-generation antipsychotic or lithium**
	Consider mirtazapine** (where sedation required)

* Caution advised in cardiac or hepatic disease (please refer to text).
** No RCTs available.

References

1. National Institute for Clinical Excellence. Depression in children and young people: identification and management in primary, community and secondary care. Clinical Guidance 28, 2005.
2. Birmaher B et al. Practice parameter for the assessment and treatment of children and adolescents with depressive disorders. J Am Acad Child Adolesc Psychiatry 2007; 46:1503–1526.
3. National Institute for Health and Care Excellence. Depression in children and young people: identification and management. Clinical Guidance 28 (updated September 2017). https://www.nice.org.uk/guidance/CG28.
4. Medicines and Healthcare Products Regulatory Agency. Selective serotonin reuptake inhibitor (SSRI) antidepressants – findings of the Committee on Safety of Medicines (CSM). 2004. http://webarchive.nationalarchives.gov.uk/20141205212747/http://www.mhra.gov.uk/Safetyinformation/Safetywarningsalertsandrecalls/Safetywarningsandmessagesformedicines/CON1004259.
5. Kratochvil CJ et al. Selective serotonin reuptake inhibitors in pediatric depression: is the balance between benefits and risks favorable? J Child Adolesc Psychopharmacol 2006; 16:11–24.
6. Tsapakis EM et al. Efficacy of antidepressants in juvenile depression: meta-analysis. Br J Psychiatry 2008; 193:10–17.
7. Whittington CJ et al. Selective serotonin reuptake inhibitors in childhood depression: systematic review of published versus unpublished data. Lancet 2004; 363:1341–1345.
8. March JS et al. The Treatment for Adolescents With Depression Study (TADS): long-term effectiveness and safety outcomes. Arch Gen Psychiatry 2007; 64:1132–1143.
9. Brent D et al. Switching to another SSRI or to venlafaxine with or without cognitive behavioral therapy for adolescents with SSRI-resistant depression: the TORDIA Randomized Controlled Trial. JAMA 2008; 299:901–913.
10. Goodyer I et al. Selective serotonin reuptake inhibitors (SSRIs) and routine specialist care with and without cognitive behaviour therapy in adolescents with major depression: randomised controlled trial. BMJ 2007; 335:142.
11. Dubicka B et al. The treatment of adolescent major depression: a comparison of the ADAPT and TADS trials. In: Yule W, ed. *Depression in Childhood and Adolescence: The Way Forward*. London: Association for Child and Adolescent Mental Health; 2009.
12. Dubicka B et al. Combined treatment with cognitive-behavioural therapy in adolescent depression: meta-analysis. Br J Psychiatry 2010; 197:433–440.
13. Cox GR et al. Psychological therapies versus antidepressant medication, alone and in combination for depression in children and adolescents. Cochrane Database Syst Rev 2014:Cd008324.
14. National Institute for Health and Care Excellence. Addendum to clinical guideline 28, depression in children and young people. 2015. https://www.nice.org.uk/guidance/cg28/evidence/addendum-pdf-193488882.
15. Hetrick SE et al. Newer generation antidepressants for depressive disorders in children and adolescents. Cochrane Database Syst Rev 2012; 11:CD004851.
16. March J et al. Fluoxetine, cognitive-behavioral therapy, and their combination for adolescents with depression: Treatment for Adolescents With Depression Study (TADS) randomized controlled trial. JAMA 2004; 292:807–820.
17. Jureidini JN et al. Efficacy and safety of antidepressants for children and adolescents. BMJ 2004; 328:879–883.
18. Vitiello B et al. Pharmacological treatment of children and adolescents with depression. Expert Opin Pharmacother 2016; 17:2273–2279.
19. Walkup JT. Antidepressant Efficacy for Depression in Children and Adolescents: industry- and NIMH-Funded Studies. Am J Psychiatry 2017; 174:430–437.
20. Bridge JA et al. Clinical response and risk for reported suicidal ideation and suicide attempts in pediatric antidepressant treatment: a meta-analysis of randomized controlled trials. JAMA 2007; 297:1683–1696.
21. Heiligenstein JH et al. Fluoxetine 40-60 mg versus fluoxetine 20 mg in the treatment of children and adolescents with a less-than-complete response to nine-week treatment with fluoxetine 10-20 mg: a pilot study. J Child Adolesc Psychopharmacol 2006; 16:207–217.
22. MacQueen GM et al. Canadian Network for Mood and Anxiety Treatments (CANMAT) 2016 Clinical Guidelines for the Management of Adults with Major Depressive Disorder: Section 6. Special Populations: Youth, Women, and the Elderly. Can J Psychiatry 2016; 61:588–603.
23. Cipriani A et al. Comparative efficacy and tolerability of antidepressants for major depressive disorder in children and adolescents: a network meta-analysis. Lancet 2016; 388:881–890.
24. Ma D et al. Comparative efficacy, acceptability, and safety of medicinal, cognitive-behavioral therapy, and placebo treatments for acute major depressive disorder in children and adolescents: a multiple-treatments meta-analysis. Curr Med Res Opin 2014; 30:971–995.
25. European Medicines Agency. European Medicines Agency finalises review of antidepressants in children and adolescents. http://www.ema.europa.eu/ema/index.jsp?curl=pages/news_and_events/news/2009/12/news_detail_000882.jsp&mid=WC0b01ac058004d5c1.
26. Wilens TE et al. Fluoxetine pharmacokinetics in pediatric patients. J Clin Psychopharmacol 2002; 22:568–575.
27. Findling RL et al. The relevance of pharmacokinetic studies in designing efficacy trials in juvenile major depression. J Child Adolesc Psychopharmacol 2006; 16:131–145.
28. Sakolsky DJ et al. Antidepressant exposure as a predictor of clinical outcomes in the Treatment of Resistant Depression in Adolescents (TORDIA) study. J Clin Psychopharmacol 2011; 31:92–97.
29. Donnelly CL et al. Sertraline in children and adolescents with major depressive disorder. J Am Acad Child Adolesc Psychiatry 2006; 45:1162–1170.
30. Rynn M et al. Long-term sertraline treatment of children and adolescents with major depressive disorder. J Child Adolesc Psychopharmacol 2006; 16:103–116.
31. Melvin GA et al. A comparison of cognitive-behavioral therapy, sertraline, and their combination for adolescent depression. J Am Acad Child Adolesc Psychiatry 2006; 45:1151–1161.

32. Wagner KD et al. A randomized, placebo-controlled trial of citalopram for the treatment of major depression in children and adolescents. Am J Psychiatry 2004; **161**:1079–1083.

33. von Knorring AL et al. A randomized, double-blind, placebo-controlled study of citalopram in adolescents with major depressive disorder. J Clin Psychopharmacol 2006; **26**:311–315.

34. Leonard HL et al. Pharmacology of the selective serotonin reuptake inhibitors in children and adolescents. J Am Acad Child Adolesc Psychiatry 1997; **36**:725–736.

35. Klein-Schwartz W et al. Comparison of citalopram and other selective serotonin reuptake inhibitor ingestions in children. Clin Toxicol (Phila) 2012; **50**:418–423.

36. Hyttel J et al. The pharmacological effect of citalopram residues in the (S)-(+)-enantiomer. J Neural Transm Gen Sect 1992; **88**:157–160.

37. Wagner KD et al. A double-blind, randomized, placebo-controlled trial of escitalopram in the treatment of pediatric depression. J Am Acad Child Adolesc Psychiatry 2006; **45**:280–288.

38. Emslie GJ et al. Escitalopram in the treatment of adolescent depression: a randomized placebo-controlled multisite trial. J Am Acad Child Adolesc Psychiatry 2009; **48**:721–729.

39. Axelson DA et al. Sertraline pharmacokinetics and dynamics in adolescents. J Am Acad Child Adolesc Psychiatry 2002; **41**:1037–1044.

40. Sakolsky D et al. Developmentally informed pharmacotherapy for child and adolescent depressive disorders. Child Adolesc Psychiatr Clin N Am 2012; **21**:313–325, viii.

41. Hazell P et al. Tricyclic drugs for depression in children and adolescents. Cochrane Database Syst Rev 2013; **6**:CD002317.

42. Haapasalo-Pesu KM et al. Mirtazapine in the treatment of adolescents with major depression: an open-label, multicenter pilot study. J Child Adolesc Psychopharmacol 2004; **14**:175–184.

43. Nemets H et al. Omega-3 treatment of childhood depression: a controlled, double-blind pilot study. Am J Psychiatry 2006; **163**:1098–1100.

44. Hogberg G et al. Depressed adolescents in a case-series were low in vitamin D and depression was ameliorated by vitamin D supplementation. Acta Paediatr 2012; **101**:779–783.

45. McKeough G. Electroconvulsive therapy. In: Nunn KP, Dey C, eds. *The Clinician's Guide to Psychotropic Prescribing in Children and Adolescents*, 1st edn. Sydney: Glade Publishing; 2003, pp. 358–365.

46. Ghaziuddin N et al. Practice parameter for use of electroconvulsive therapy with adolescents. J Am Acad Child Adolesc Psychiatry 2004; **43**:1521–1539.

47. Zhand N et al. Use of electroconvulsive therapy in adolescents with treatment-resistant depressive disorders: a case series. J ECT 2015; **31**:238–245.

48. Martinez C et al. Antidepressant treatment and the risk of fatal and non-fatal self harm in first episode depression: nested case-control study. BMJ 2005; **330**:389.

49. Kaizar EE et al. Do antidepressants cause suicidality in children? A Bayesian meta-analysis. Clin Trials 2006; **3**:73–90.

50. Mosholder AD et al. Suicidal adverse events in pediatric randomized, controlled clinical trials of antidepressant drugs are associated with active drug treatment: a meta-analysis. J Child Adolesc Psychopharmacol 2006; **16**:25–32.

51. Simon GE et al. Suicide risk during antidepressant treatment. Am J Psychiatry 2006; **163**:41–47.

52. Olfson M et al. Antidepressant drug therapy and suicide in severely depressed children and adults: a case-control study. Arch Gen Psychiatry 2006; **63**:865–872.

53. Hammad TA et al. Suicidality in pediatric patients treated with antidepressant drugs. Arch Gen Psychiatry 2006; **63**:332–339.

54. Dubicka B et al. Suicidal behaviour in youths with depression treated with new-generation antidepressants: meta-analysis. Br J Psychiatry 2006; **189**:393–398.

55. Sharma T et al. Suicidality and aggression during antidepressant treatment: systematic review and meta-analyses based on clinical study reports. BMJ 2016; **352**:i65.

56. Gibbons RD et al. Relationship between antidepressants and suicide attempts: an analysis of the Veterans Health Administration data sets. Am J Psychiatry 2007; **164**:1044–1049.

57. Libby AM et al. Decline in treatment of pediatric depression after FDA advisory on risk of suicidality with SSRIs. Am J Psychiatry 2007; **164**:884–891.

58. Gibbons RD et al. Early evidence on the effects of regulators' suicidality warnings on SSRI prescriptions and suicide in children and adolescents. Am J Psychiatry 2007; **164**:1356–1363.

59. Varigonda AL et al. Systematic review and meta-analysis: early treatment responses of selective serotonin reuptake inhibitors in pediatric major depressive disorder. J Am Acad Child Adolesc Psychiatry 2015; **54**:557–564.

60. Kennard BD et al. Relapse and recurrence in pediatric depression. Child Adolesc Psychiatr Clin N Am 2006; **15**:1057–1079, xi.

61. Kennard BD et al. Cognitive-behavioral therapy to prevent relapse in pediatric responders to pharmacotherapy for major depressive disorder. J Am Acad Child Adolesc Psychiatry 2008; **47**:1395–1404.

62. Emslie GJ et al. Continued effectiveness of relapse prevention cognitive-behavioral therapy following fluoxetine treatment in youth with major depressive disorder. J Am Acad Child Adolesc Psychiatry 2015; **54**:991–998.

63. Emslie GJ et al. Fluoxetine treatment for prevention of relapse of depression in children and adolescents: a double-blind, placebo-controlled study. J Am Acad Child Adolesc Psychiatry 2004; **43**:1397–1405.

64. Emslie GJ et al. Fluoxetine versus placebo in preventing relapse of major depression in children and adolescents. Am J Psychiatry 2008; **165**:459–467.

65. Emslie GJ et al. Treatment of Resistant Depression in Adolescents (TORDIA): week 24 outcomes. Am J Psychiatry 2010; **167**:782–791.

66. Brent DA et al. Predictors of spontaneous and systematically assessed suicidal adverse events in the treatment of SSRI-resistant depression in adolescents (TORDIA) study. Am J Psychiatry 2009; **166**:418–426.

67. Cooper WO et al. Antidepressants and suicide attempts in children. Pediatrics 2014; **133**:204–210.
68. Vitiello B et al. Long-term outcome of adolescent depression initially resistant to selective serotonin reuptake inhibitor treatment: a follow-up study of the TORDIA sample. J Clin Psychiatry 2011; **72**:388–396.
69. Asarnow JR et al. Treatment of selective serotonin reuptake inhibitor-resistant depression in adolescents: predictors and moderators of treatment response. J Am Acad Child Adolesc Psychiatry 2009; **48**:330–339.
70. Maalouf FT et al. Do sub-syndromal manic symptoms influence outcome in treatment resistant depression in adolescents? A latent class analysis from the TORDIA study. J Affect Disord 2012; **138**:86–95.
71. Pathak S et al. Adjunctive quetiapine for treatment-resistant adolescent major depressive disorder: a case series. J Child Adolesc Psychopharmacol 2005; **15**:696–702.
72. Wilens TE et al. Disentangling disinhibition. J Am Acad Child Adolesc Psychiatry 1998; **37**:1225–1227.
73. Geller B et al. Rate and predictors of prepubertal bipolarity during follow-up of 6- to 12-year-old depressed children. J Am Acad Child Adolesc Psychiatry 1994; **33**:461–468.
74. Ghaemi SN et al. Diagnosing bipolar disorder and the effect of antidepressants: a naturalistic study. J Clin Psychiatry 2000; **61**:804–808.
75. Martin A et al. Age effects on antidepressant-induced manic conversion. Arch Pediatr Adolesc Med 2004; **158**:773–780.
76. Dubicka B et al. Pharmacological treatment of depression and bipolar disorder in children and adolescents. Advances in Psychiatric Treatment 2010; **16**:402–412.

CHAPTER 5

Bipolar illness in children and adolescents

Diagnostic issues

Bipolar disorder in children has become an area of intense research interest and controversy in recent years.[1,2] While classical manic presentations fulfilling DSM-V or ICD-10 criteria are well known to clinicians treating adolescents, they are rare in younger children.[3,4] Claims that mania in pre-puberty may present as chronic (non-episodic) irritability or with extremely short (a few hours duration) episodes should be treated with great caution.[2] Short-lived episodes of exuberance are normative in children, while temper outbursts and mood lability can be seen in children presenting with a wide range of other primary diagnoses (such as conduct, anxiety, depressive, and autism spectrum disorders).[5] A detailed developmental assessment should therefore form the basis of any treatment decisions.

Clinical guidance

Before prescribing

- Establish a clinical diagnosis informed by structured instrument assessment if possible. Try to monitor symptom patterns prospectively with mood or sleep diaries. If in doubt, seek specialist advice early on.
- Explain the diagnosis to the patient and family and invest time and effort in psycho-education. This is likely to improve adherence and there is evidence that it reduces relapse rates, at least in adults.[6]
- Measure baseline symptoms of mania (e.g. Young Mania Rating Scale[7] [YMRS]), depression (e.g. Children's Depression Rating Scale[8] [CDRS]), and impairment (e.g. Clinical Global Impression – BP version[9]). Use these to set clear and realistic treatment goals.
- Measure baseline height, weight, waist circumference, pulse, ECG and blood pressure and obtain baseline bloods as appropriate (fasting blood glucose, haemoglobin A1c, fasting lipid profile, full blood count, urea and electrolytes, creatine kinase, liver function tests and prolactin).

What to prescribe?

- For the treatment of mania and hypomania in youth, NICE guidelines suggest the following similar recommendations as in adults: second-generation antipsychotics (SGA) may be used as first-line treatment, and mood stabilisers (MS) can be added after failure of two trials of SGA.[10]
- SGAs seem to show greater short-term efficacy (effect size [ES] = 0.65 compared with placebo) than MS (ES = 0.20 compared with placebo) in youth, according to a meta-analysis.[11]
- SGAs seem to produce significantly greater weight gain and somnolence in youth compared with adults.[11]
- Teratogenicity and polycystic ovary syndrome with associated infertility are particular concerns when valproate is used for adolescent girls and NICE recommends avoiding its use in women of child-bearing age.[10]

CHAPTER 5

- Adherence to lithium and blood level testing may be difficult in adolescents.
- Overall, we recommend the use of SGA as first line for the acute treatment of mania in children and adolescents (see Table 5.3), similar to recommendations in adults.

After prescribing

- Assess and measure symptoms on a regular basis to establish effectiveness.
- Monitor weight and height at each visit and repeat all fasting bloods at 3 months (then every 6 months). Offer advice on healthy lifestyle and exercise.
- The duration of most medication trials is between 3 and 5 weeks. This should guide decisions about how long to try a single drug in a patient. A complete absence of response at 1–2 weeks should prompt a switch to another SGA.
- If non-response, check compliance, measure levels (where possible), and consider increasing dose. Consider concurrent use of SGA and MS.
- Judicious extrapolation of the evidence from adults[12] is required because of the very limited evidence base in youth with bipolar disorder. This includes treatment duration and prophylaxis.[10,11,13]
- Maintenance treatment should follow adult guidelines. Consider the use of lithium early in the course of treatment, either by switching to lithium monotherapy prophylaxis or as an adjunct to a successful acute medication.

Specific issues

- Bipolar depression is a common clinical challenge and its treatment has been studied much less in youth compared to in adults (see Table 5.2). Antidepressants should be used with care and only in the presence of an antimanic agent.[10] There is limited evidence for the benefit of antidepressants in bipolar depression in adults.[14] Because of the dearth of trials in youth, we are compelled to extrapolate from adult studies[10] and recommend use of the olanzapine/fluoxetine combination or quetiapine as first-line treatment (see Table 5.4).
- The exact relationship between ADHD and bipolar disorder is still debated. Some evidence suggests that stimulants in children with ADHD and manic symptoms may be well tolerated[15] and that they may be safe and effective to use after mood stabilisation.[15] Caution and experience with prescribing these drugs are required.
- The DSM-V has introduced the new category of disruptive mood dysregulation disorder (DMDD) to capture severely irritable children (who were commonly misdiagnosed as having bipolar disorder in the USA). There is as yet no established treatment for DMDD. Lithium is ineffective,[16] but SSRIs and psychological treatment options, such as parenting interventions, may be considered.[17]

Other treatments

- There is evidence for adults and children that adjunct treatments including psycho-education, CBT and especially family-focused interventions can enhance treatment and reduce depression relapse rates in bipolar disorder.[18]
- The use of high-frequency repetitive transcranial magnetic stimulation (rTMS) in adolescents with treatment-resistant unipolar depression is only supported by

open-label studies[19] and no RCT has been done in youth with either unipolar or bipolar depression. Therefore its use is still considered experimental. In one randomised sham-controlled study, rTMS in the right prefrontal cortex was ineffective in treating acute mania in youth, as an add-on to standard pharmacotherapy (n = 26).[20]

RCT evidence and recommended first-line medication in youth in bipolar mania and depression are summarised in Tables 5.1, 5.2, 5.3 and 5.4.

Table 5.1 Summary of RCT evidence on medication used in youth with bipolar mania

Medication	Comment
Lithium	One double-blind placebo-controlled randomised trial[21] showed *significant* reductions in substance use and clinical ratings after 6 weeks, in 25 adolescents with bipolar disorder and co-morbid substance misuse. In a double-blind placebo-controlled discontinuation trial (n = 40) over 2 weeks, *no significant difference* in relapse rates was found between lithium and placebo[22]
	A more recent double-blind placebo-controlled study (n = 81), over 8 weeks, demonstrated a *significantly larger* change in YMRS score in lithium-treated youth, but with a differentiation from the placebo group only appearing after 6 weeks of treatment. There was a significant increase in thyrotropin with lithium, but no difference in weight gain[23]
	Lithium and divalproex *did not differ* in an 18-month maintenance trial in youths (n = 60) who initially stabilised on combination pharmacotherapy of lithium and divalproex.[24] However, given the compelling evidence for lithium maintenance and prophylaxis in adults, we recommend that clinicians consider its use in adolescents in preference to valproate
Valproate	In an RCT (n = 150)[25] divalproex ER (titrated to clinical response or 80–125 mg/L) *did not lead to significant differences* in mean YMRS compared with placebo at 4 weeks. (Also see risperidone and quetiapine sections below)
Oxcarbazepine	A double-blind placebo-controlled study (n = 116) *did not show significant differences* between placebo and oxcarbazepine (mean dose 1515 mg/day) in reducing mania rating at 7 weeks[26]
Olanzapine	A double-blind placebo-controlled study (n = 161)[27] showed olanzapine (5–20 mg/day) to be *significantly more effective* than placebo in YMRS mean score reduction over a period of 3 weeks. Note the higher weight gain in the treatment group (weight gain was 3.7 kg for olanzapine versus 0.3 kg for placebo) and the associated significantly increased fasting glucose, total cholesterol, AST, ALT and uric acid
Risperidone	A double-blind placebo-controlled study (n = 169) showed risperidone (at doses 0.5–2.5 or 3–6 mg) to be *significantly more effective* than placebo in YMRS mean score reduction in a 3-week follow-up.[28] The lower dose seems to lead to the same benefits at a lower risk of adverse effects. Sleepiness and fatigue were common in the treatment arms. Note, mean weight increase in treatment groups (0.7 kg versus 1.7 kg for the low and 1.4 kg for the high dose arm)
	In the Treatment of Early Age Mania (TEAM) study, *higher response rates* (and metabolic adverse effects) occurred with risperidone (mean dose of 2.57 mg) versus lithium (mean level of 1.09 mmol/L) and divalproex sodium (mean level of 113.6 mg/L).[29] A randomised follow-up of this study showed again the superiority of risperidone as an alternative treatment for non-responders to lithium and divalproex sodium, and as an add-on treatment to partial responders to the two MS.[30] However, these results need to be interpreted with caution as the definition of mania was broad and different to how bipolar disorder is defined by most UK clinicians. Similar reasons provoke caution when considering another placebo-controlled double-blind trial showing significantly better results for risperidone (mean dose 0.5 mg) versus valproic acid (mean level 81 mg/L) in 3- to 7-year-old children supposedly diagnosed with mania[31]

(Continued)

Table 5.1 (*Continued*)

Medication	Comment
Quetiapine	A double-blind placebo-controlled study (n=277)[32] showed quetiapine (at doses of 400 mg/day or 600 mg/day) to be *significantly better* than placebo in reducing mean YMRS scores at 3 weeks. The most common adverse effects included somnolence and sedation. Weight gain was 1.7 kg in the quetiapine group versus 0.4 kg for placebo
	Quetiapine is *effective* as an adjunct to valproate compared with valproate alone (n=30, 6 weeks)[33] and was *as effective* as valproate in a double-blind trial (n=50, 4 weeks)[34]
Aripiprazole	A double-blind placebo-controlled study[35,36] showed aripiprazole (at doses 10 mg/day or 30 mg/day) to be *significantly better* than placebo in reducing mean YMRS scores at both 4 weeks (n=296)[35] and 30 weeks (n=210).[36] Note the significantly higher incidence of extrapyramidal symptoms in the treatment groups (especially the higher dose). Weight gain was *significantly higher* in the treatment groups compared to placebo (3.0 kg versus 6.5 kg for the low and 6.6 kg for the high dose arm) at week 30 but not at week 4
Ziprasidone	A double-blind placebo-controlled trial (n=237)[37] showed ziprasidone (at flexible doses 40–160 mg) to be *significantly more effective* than placebo in reducing mean YMRS scores at 4 weeks. Sedation and somnolence were the most common adverse effects, while it demonstrated a neutral metabolic profile and no QTc prolongation
	Ziprasidone is not marketed in the UK and some other countries
Asenapine	A 3-week double-blind placebo-controlled study (n=350) demonstrated statistical superiority of asenapine over placebo for each of the doses used (2.5, 5 or 10 mg bd), with significant difference as early as day 4. However, many adverse effects were reported, including weight gain of more than 7% from baseline (8–12% incidence in asenapine group versus 1.1% in placebo group), metabolic changes (increase in fasting insulin, lipids, glucose), as well as somnolence, sedation, oral hypoaesthesia and paraesthesia[38]

ALT, alanine transaminase; AST, aspartate aminotransferase; ER, extended release; MS, mood stabilisers; RCT, randomised controlled trial; YMRS, Young Mania Rating Scale.

Table 5.2 Summary of RCT evidence on medication used in youth with bipolar depression

Medication	Comment
Quetiapine	In adults, there is considerably better evidence for efficacious treatments (see Chapter 2), such as quetiapine.[39,40] Surprisingly, however, a small study in 32 adolescents,[41] followed by a larger RCT (n=193),[42] failed to show effectiveness. This latest study had a high placebo response, which is not present in adult quetiapine studies[43] and which may reflect issues that have been noted before about phenotyping of mood disorders and multi-site studies[44]
Olanzapine/fluoxetine combination	The only double-blind randomised placebo-controlled trial with positive results for the treatment of bipolar depression in youth is a large study (n=255) of the olanzapine/fluoxetine combination (either 6/25 or 12/50 mg daily) for 8 weeks.[45] Between-group differences were significant at week 1 and all subsequent visits. Most frequent adverse effects were weight gain (4.4 kg for the olanzapine/fluoxetine combination versus 0.5 kg for placebo), somnolence and hyperlipidaemia. The olanzapine/fluoxetine combination is recommended by NICE guidelines,[10] along with quetiapine, as first-line treatment for bipolar depression in youth, as in adults. Although the olanzapine/fluoxetine combination is not currently available as a single preparation in the UK, its effects can be achieved by combining olanzapine and fluoxetine (e.g. 5/20 mg or 10/40 mg)
Lurasidone	Lurasidone has been shown to be effective in bipolar depression in adults[46–48] and it does not seem to cause weight gain and other metabolic disturbances. It is safe and effective in treating schizophrenia in adolescents[49] and is currently undergoing clinical trials in youth with bipolar depression
Lamotrigine	Lamotrigine has only modest, if any, effects in adult bipolar depression;[50] it has not been studied in RCTs for the treatment of acute bipolar depression in children and adolescents and is, therefore, not recommended as a first line. Moreover, a placebo-controlled randomised withdrawal study of adjunctive lamotrigine for bipolar disorder in youth, lasting over 36 weeks, failed to show any benefit in preventing time to occurrence of a bipolar event[51]

RCT, randomised controlled trial.

Table 5.3 Recommended first-line treatments for acute mania*

Drug	Dose
Aripiprazole	10 mg daily
Olanzapine	5–20 mg daily
Quetiapine	Up to 400 mg daily
Risperidone	0.5–2.5 mg daily
Asenapine	2.5–10 mg bd

* Continue acutely effective dosing regimen as prophylaxis, and consider need for lithium.

Table 5.4 Recommended first-line treatments for bipolar depression*

Drug	Dose
Olanzapine/fluoxetine	6/25–12/50 mg daily
Quetiapine	Up to 300 mg daily
Lurasidone	20(17) to 80(74) mg daily

* Continue acutely effective dosing regimen as prophylaxis, and consider need for lithium.

References

1. Carlson GA et al. Phenomenology and diagnosis of bipolar disorder in children, adolescents, and adults: complexities and developmental issues. Dev Psychopathol 2006; 18:939–969.
2. Leibenluft E. Severe mood dysregulation, irritability, and the diagnostic boundaries of bipolar disorder in youths. Am J Psychiatry 2011; 168:129–142.
3. Costello EJ et al. The Great Smoky Mountains Study of Youth. Goals, design, methods, and the prevalence of DSM-III-R disorders. Arch Gen Psychiatry 1996; 53:1129–1136.
4. Stringaris A et al. Youth meeting symptom and impairment criteria for mania-like episodes lasting less than four days: an epidemiological enquiry. J Child Psychol Psychiatry 2010; 51:31–38.
5. Krieger FV et al. Bipolar disorder and disruptive mood dysregulation in children and adolescents: assessment, diagnosis and treatment. Evid Based Ment Health 2013; 16:93–94.
6. Colom F et al. A randomized trial on the efficacy of group psychoeducation in the prophylaxis of recurrences in bipolar patients whose disease is in remission. Arch Gen Psychiatry 2003; 60:402–407.
7. Young RC et al. A rating scale for mania: reliability, validity and sensitivity. Br J Psychiatry 1978; 133:429–435.
8. Poznanski EO et al. Preliminary studies of the reliability and validity of the children's depression rating scale. J Am Acad Child Psychiatry 1984; 23:191–197.
9. Spearing MK et al. Modification of the Clinical Global Impressions (CGI) Scale for use in bipolar illness (BP): the CGI-BP. Psychiatry Res 1997; 73:159–171.
10. National Institute for Health and Care Excellence. Bipolar disorder: assessment and management: Clinical Guidance 185 (February 2016 update). 2016. https://www.nice.org.uk/guidance/cg185.
11. Correll CU et al. Antipsychotic and mood stabilizer efficacy and tolerability in pediatric and adult patients with bipolar I mania: a comparative analysis of acute, randomized, placebo-controlled trials. Bipolar Disord 2010; 12:116–141.
12. Geddes JR et al. Treatment of bipolar disorder. Lancet 2013; 381:1672–1682.
13. Diaz-Caneja CM et al. Practitioner review: long-term pharmacological treatment of pediatric bipolar disorder. J Child Psychol Psychiatry 2014; 55:959–980.

CHAPTER 5

14. Pacchiarotti I et al. The International Society for Bipolar Disorders (ISBD) task force report on antidepressant use in bipolar disorders. Am J Psychiatry 2013; 170:1249–1262.

15. Goldsmith M et al. Antidepressants and psychostimulants in pediatric populations: is there an association with mania? Paediatr Drugs 2011; 13:225–243.

16. Dickstein DP et al. Randomized double-blind placebo-controlled trial of lithium in youths with severe mood dysregulation. J Child Adolesc Psychopharmacol 2009; 19:61–73.

17. Vidal-Ribas P et al. The status of irritability in psychiatry: a conceptual and quantitative review. J Am Acad Child Adolesc Psychiatry 2016; 55:556–570.

18. Miklowitz DJ. Evidence-based family interventions for adolescents and young adults with bipolar disorder. J Clin Psychiatry 2016; 77 Suppl E1:e5.

19. Wall CA et al. Magnetic Resonance imaging-guided, open-label, high-frequency repetitive transcranial magnetic stimulation for adolescents with major depressive disorder. J Child Adolesc Psychopharmacol 2016; 26:582–589.

20. Pathak V et al. Efficacy of adjunctive high frequency repetitive transcranial magnetic stimulation of right prefrontal cortex in adolescent mania: a randomized sham-controlled study. Clin Psychopharmacol Neurosci 2015; 13:245–249.

21. Geller B et al. Double-blind and placebo-controlled study of lithium for adolescent bipolar disorders with secondary substance dependency. J Am Acad Child Adolesc Psychiatry 1998; 37:171–178.

22. Kafantaris V et al. Lithium treatment of acute mania in adolescents: a placebo-controlled discontinuation study. J Am Acad Child Adolesc Psychiatry 2004; 43:984–993.

23. Findling RL et al. Lithium in the acute treatment of bipolar i disorder: a double-blind, placebo-controlled study. Pediatrics 2015; 136:885–894.

24. Findling RL et al. Double-blind 18-month trial of lithium versus divalproex maintenance treatment in pediatric bipolar disorder. J Am Acad Child Adolesc Psychiatry 2005; 44:409–417.

25. Wagner KD et al. A double-blind, randomized, placebo-controlled trial of divalproex extended-release in the treatment of bipolar disorder in children and adolescents. J Am Acad Child Adolesc Psychiatry 2009; 48:519–532.

26. Wagner KD et al. A double-blind, randomized, placebo-controlled trial of oxcarbazepine in the treatment of bipolar disorder in children and adolescents. Am J Psychiatry 2006; 163:1179–1186.

27. Tohen M et al. Olanzapine versus placebo in the treatment of adolescents with bipolar mania. Am J Psychiatry 2007; 164:1547–1556.

28. Haas M et al. Risperidone for the treatment of acute mania in children and adolescents with bipolar disorder: a randomized, double-blind, placebo-controlled study. Bipolar Disord 2009; 11:687–700.

29. Geller B et al. A randomized controlled trial of risperidone, lithium, or divalproex sodium for initial treatment of bipolar I disorder, manic or mixed phase, in children and adolescents. Arch Gen Psychiatry 2012; 69:515–528.

30. Walkup JT et al. Treatment of Early-Age Mania: Outcomes for Partial and Nonresponders to Initial Treatment. J Am Acad Child Adolesc Psychiatry 2015; 54:1008–1019.

31. Kowatch RA et al. Placebo-controlled trial of valproic acid versus risperidone in children 3-7 years of age with bipolar I disorder. J Child Adolesc Psychopharmacol 2015; 25:306–313.

32. Pathak S et al. Efficacy and safety of quetiapine in children and adolescents with mania associated with bipolar I disorder: a 3-week, double-blind, placebo-controlled trial. J Clin Psychiatry 2013; 74:e100–e109.

33. Delbello MP et al. A double-blind, randomized, placebo-controlled study of quetiapine as adjunctive treatment for adolescent mania. J Am Acad Child Adolesc Psychiatry 2002; 41:1216–1223.

34. Delbello MP et al. A double-blind randomized pilot study comparing quetiapine and divalproex for adolescent mania. J Am Acad Child Adolesc Psychiatry 2006; 45:305–313.

35. Findling RL et al. Acute treatment of pediatric bipolar I disorder, manic or mixed episode, with aripiprazole: a randomized, double-blind, placebo-controlled study. J Clin Psychiatry 2009; 70:1441–1451.

36. Findling RL et al. Aripiprazole for the treatment of pediatric bipolar I disorder: a 30-week, randomized, placebo-controlled study. Bipolar Disord 2013; 15:138–149.

37. Findling RL et al. Ziprasidone in adolescents with schizophrenia: results from a placebo-controlled efficacy and long-term open-extension study. J Child Adolesc Psychopharmacol 2013; 23:531–544.

38. Findling RL et al. Asenapine for the acute treatment of pediatric manic or mixed episode of bipolar I disorder. J Am Acad Child Adolesc Psychiatry 2015; 54:1032–1041.

39. Calabrese JR et al. A randomized, double-blind, placebo-controlled trial of quetiapine in the treatment of bipolar I or II depression. Am J Psychiatry 2005; 162:1351–1360.

40. Thase ME et al. Efficacy of quetiapine monotherapy in bipolar I and II depression: a double-blind, placebo-controlled study (the BOLDER II study). J Clin Psychopharmacol 2006; 26:600–609.

41. Delbello MP et al. A double-blind, placebo-controlled pilot study of quetiapine for depressed adolescents with bipolar disorder. Bipolar Disord 2009; 11:483–493.

42. Findling RL et al. Efficacy and safety of extended-release quetiapine fumarate in youth with bipolar depression: an 8 week, double-blind, placebo-controlled trial. J Child Adolesc Psychopharmacol 2014; 24:325–335.

43. Suttajit S et al. Quetiapine for acute bipolar depression: a systematic review and meta-analysis. Drug Des Devel Ther 2014; 8:827–838.

44. Bridge JA et al. Clinical response and risk for reported suicidal ideation and suicide attempts in pediatric antidepressant treatment: a meta-analysis of randomized controlled trials. JAMA 2007; 297:1683–1696.

45. Detke HC et al. Olanzapine/fluoxetine combination in children and adolescents with bipolar I depression: a randomized, double-blind, placebo-controlled trial. J Am Acad Child Adolesc Psychiatry 2015; 54:217–224.

46. Loebel A et al. Lurasidone monotherapy in the treatment of bipolar I depression: a randomized, double-blind, placebo-controlled study. Am J Psychiatry 2014; 171:160–168.

47. Suppes T et al. Lurasidone adjunctive with lithium or valproate for bipolar depression: a placebo-controlled trial utilizing prospective and retrospective enrolment cohorts. J Psychiatr Res 2016; 78:86–93.

48. Suppes T et al. Lurasidone for the treatment of major depressive disorder with mixed features: a randomized, double-blind, placebo-controlled study. Am J Psychiatry 2016; 173:400–407.

49. Goldman R et al. Efficacy and safety of lurasidone in adolescents with schizophrenia: a 6-week, randomized placebo-controlled study. J Child Adolesc Psychopharmacol 2017; 27:516–525.

50. Calabrese JR et al. Lamotrigine in the acute treatment of bipolar depression: results of five double-blind, placebo-controlled clinical trials. Bipolar Disord 2008; 10:323–333.

51. Findling RL et al. Adjunctive maintenance lamotrigine for pediatric bipolar I disorder: a placebo-controlled, randomized withdrawal study. J Am Acad Child Adolesc Psychiatry 2015; 54:1020–1031.e1023.

Psychosis in children and adolescents

Schizophrenia is rare in children but the incidence increases rapidly in adolescence. A detailed developmental and physical assessment is often needed before the diagnosis is made.[1] Early-onset schizophrenia-spectrum (EOSS) disorder is often chronic and in the majority of cases requires long-term treatment with antipsychotic medication.[2]

There have been three major RCTs of first-generation antipsychotics, all of them showing high rates of extrapyramidal symptoms (EPS) and significant sedation.[2] Treatment-emergent dyskinesias can also be problematic.[3] First-generation antipsychotics (FGAs) should generally be avoided in children.

There have been a number of RCTs of second-generation antipsychotics in EOSS disorder. Olanzapine,[4–6] risperidone,[4,5,7,8] aripiprazole,[9,10] quetiapine,[10,11] paliperidone,[12] asenapine[13] and ziprasidone[14] have all been shown to be effective in the treatment of psychosis. There is evidence from a systematic review to suggest comparable efficacy for most second-generation antipsychotics with the exception of ziprasidone (inferior efficacy) and asenapine (unclear efficacy).[15] Concerns have been raised about the cardiac safety of ziprasidone.[16,17]

Children and adolescents are at greater risk than adults for adverse effects such as extrapyramidal symptoms, raised prolactin, sedation (even with aripiprazole[10]), weight gain and metabolic effects.[18]

There is evidence that clozapine is effective in treatment-resistant psychosis in adolescents, although this population may be more prone to neutropenia and seizures than adults.[19–22] Based on data obtained from the treatment of younger adults, olanzapine should probably be tried before moving to clozapine.[23]

Overall, algorithms for treating psychosis in children and adolescents are the same as those for adult patients (see Chapter 1). NICE[24] recommends oral antipsychotics in conjunction with family interventions and individual CBT. Starting doses should be at the lower end of, or below the adult range.

When prescribing antipsychotics in children and adolescents always measure baseline parameters and monitor as per the guidance in Chapter 1. For children and adolescents also include waist and hip circumference, assessment of any movement disorders and assessment of nutritional status, diet and level of physical activity.[24]

References

1. Pina-Camacho L et al. Autism spectrum disorder and schizophrenia: boundaries and uncertainties. BJPsych Advances 2016; **22**:316–324.
2. Kumra S et al. Efficacy and tolerability of second-generation antipsychotics in children and adolescents with schizophrenia. Schizophr Bull 2008; **34**:60–71.
3. Connor DF et al. Neuroleptic-related dyskinesias in children and adolescents. J Clin Psychiatry 2001; **62**:967–974.
4. Sikich L et al. A pilot study of risperidone, olanzapine, and haloperidol in psychotic youth: a double-blind, randomized, 8-week trial. Neuropsychopharmacology 2004; **29**:133–145.
5. Sikich L et al. Double-blind comparison of first- and second-generation antipsychotics in early-onset schizophrenia and schizo-affective disorder: findings from the treatment of early-onset schizophrenia spectrum disorders (TEOSS) study. Am J Psychiatry 2008; **165**:1420–1431.
6. Kryzhanovskaya L et al. Olanzapine versus placebo in adolescents with schizophrenia: a 6-week, randomized, double-blind, placebo-controlled trial. J Am Acad Child Adolesc Psychiatry 2009; **48**:60–70.
7. Haas M et al. A 6-week, randomized, double-blind, placebo-controlled study of the efficacy and safety of risperidone in adolescents with schizophrenia. J Child Adolesc Psychopharmacol 2009; **19**:611–621.
8. Haas M et al. Efficacy, safety and tolerability of two dosing regimens in adolescent schizophrenia: double-blind study. Br J Psychiatry 2009; **194**:158–164.
9. Findling RL et al. A multiple-center, randomized, double-blind, placebo-controlled study of oral aripiprazole for treatment of adolescents with schizophrenia. Am J Psychiatry 2008; **165**:1432–1441.

10. Pagsberg AK et al. Quetiapine extended release versus aripiprazole in children and adolescents with first-episode psychosis: the multicentre, double-blind, randomised tolerability and efficacy of antipsychotics (TEA) trial. Lancet Psychiatry 2017; 4:605–618.

11. Findling RL et al. Efficacy and safety of quetiapine in adolescents with schizophrenia investigated in a 6-week, double-blind, placebo-controlled trial. J Child Adolesc Psychopharmacol 2012; 22:327–342.

12. Singh J et al. A randomized, double-blind study of paliperidone extended-release in treatment of acute schizophrenia in adolescents. Biol Psychiatry 2011; 70:1179–1187.

13. Findling RL et al. Safety and efficacy from an 8 week double-blind trial and a 26 week open-label extension of asenapine in adolescents with schizophrenia. J Child Adolesc Psychopharmacol 2015; 25:384–396.

14. Findling RL et al. Ziprasidone in adolescents with schizophrenia: results from a placebo-controlled efficacy and long-term open-extension study. J Child Adolesc Psychopharmacol 2013; 23:531–544.

15. Pagsberg AK et al. Acute antipsychotic treatment of children and adolescents with schizophrenia-spectrum disorders: a systematic review and network meta-analysis. J Am Acad Child Adolesc Psychiatry 2017; 56:191–202.

16. Scahill L et al. Sudden death in a patient with Tourette syndrome during a clinical trial of ziprasidone. J Psychopharmacol 2005; 19:205–206.

17. Blair J et al. Electrocardiographic changes in children and adolescents treated with ziprasidone: a prospective study. J Am Acad Child Adolesc Psychiatry 2005; 44:73–79.

18. Correll CU. Addressing adverse effects of antipsychotic treatment in young patients with schizophrenia. J Clin Psychiatry 2011; 72:e01.

19. Kumra S et al. Childhood-onset schizophrenia. A double-blind clozapine-haloperidol comparison. Arch Gen Psychiatry 1996; 53:1090–1097.

20. Shaw P et al. Childhood-onset schizophrenia: A double-blind, randomized clozapine-olanzapine comparison. Arch Gen Psychiatry 2006; 63:721–730.

21. Kumra S et al. Clozapine and "high-dose" olanzapine in refractory early-onset schizophrenia: a 12-week randomized and double-blind comparison. Biol Psychiatry 2008; 63:524–529.

22. Schneider C et al. Systematic review of the efficacy and tolerability of clozapine in the treatment of youth with early onset schizophrenia. Eur Psychiatry 2014; 29:1–10.

23. Agid O et al. An algorithm-based approach to first-episode schizophrenia: response rates over 3 prospective antipsychotic trials with a retrospective data analysis. J Clin Psychiatry 2011; 72:1439–1444.

24. National Institute for Health and Care Excellence. Psychosis and schizophrenia in children and young people: recognition and management. Clinical Guidance 155, 2013 (last updated October 2016). https://www.nice.org.uk/guidance/cg155.

Further reading

Masi G et al. Management of schizophrenia in children and adolescents: focus on pharmacotherapy. Drugs 2011; 71:179–208.

CHAPTER 5

Anxiety disorders in children and adolescents

Diagnostic issues

Fear and worry are common in children and they are part of normal development. At the same time, anxiety disorders often begin in childhood and adolescence[1] and they are the most common psychiatric disorders in this age group, with overall prevalence between 8% and 30% depending on the impairment cut-offs used.[2] Anxiety disorders may be even more common in children with neurodevelopment disorders.[3]

In children, the more obvious clinical presentation with distress and avoidance may be masked by prominent behavioural symptoms (e.g. irritability and angry outbursts linked to avoidance). Therefore, the assessment and treatment of anxiety disorders in children needs to be undertaken by clinicians who can discriminate normal, developmentally appropriate worries, fears and shyness from anxiety disorders that significantly impair a child's functioning, and who can appreciate developmental variations in the presentation of symptoms.

Clinical guidance

Anxiety symptoms in children and adolescents often improve with age, presumably in parallel to the development of the prefrontal cortex and, in particular, executive functions. However, anxiety disorders are distressing and impairing conditions that need to be treated promptly. Chronic stress mediators may have significant impact on brain development[4] and functional impairment linked to anxiety symptoms may prevent young people from accessing normative experiences that are critical for social, emotional, and cognitive development. Finally, early and effective treatment may prevent continuity of psychopathology into adulthood: for example, young people with anxiety disorders are three times more likely to have anxiety and depression in adult life compared to non-anxious youths.[5]

Guidelines for treatment of anxiety disorders in children and adolescents have been made available in the UK and the USA. NICE guidelines focus on the treatment of social anxiety disorder in children and adolescents, suggesting the use of CBT and cautioning against the routine use of pharmacological treatment for social anxiety in this age group.[6] Guidelines from AACAP cover the treatment of all non-obsessive compulsive disorder (OCD), non-post-traumatic stress disorder (PTSD) anxiety disorders.[7] AACAP guidelines suggest multimodal treatment including psycho-education, psychotherapy (e.g. a 12-session course of exposure-based CBT), and pharmacotherapy. Drug treatment is endorsed for moderate-to-severe anxiety symptoms, when impairment makes participation in psychotherapy difficult, or when psychotherapy leads to only partial response.

Prescribing for anxiety disorders in children and adolescents

Before prescribing

- **Exclude other diagnoses.** Anxiety symptoms can be mimicked by a range of psychiatric disorders including depression (inattention, sleep problems), bipolar disorder (irritability, sleep problems, restlessness), oppositional-defiant disorder (irritability,

CHAPTER 5

oppositional behaviour), psychotic disorders (social withdrawal, restlessness), ADHD (inattention, restlessness), Asperger's syndrome (social withdrawal, poor social skills, repetitive behaviours and routines), and learning disabilities. They may also be mimicked by a range of endocrine (hyperthyroidism, hypoglycaemia, pheochromocytoma), neurological (migraine, seizures, delirium, brain tumours), cardiovascular (cardiac arrhythmias) and respiratory (asthma) conditions and lead intoxication. Anxiety-like symptoms can be observed in response to several drugs and substances including anti-asthma medications, sympathomimetics, steroids, SSRIs, antipsychotics (akathisia), diet pills, cold medicines, caffeine and energy drinks.

- **Beware contraindications to SSRIs and potential interactions.**
- **Measure baseline severity.** Structured interviews include the Anxiety Disorders Interview Schedule (ADIS) and the Kiddie-Schedule for Affective Disorders and Schizophrenia (Kiddie-SADS). Questionnaires include the Revised Children's Anxiety and Depression Scale (RCADS), Screen for Child Anxiety and Related Emotional Disorders (SCARED), or the Multidimensional Anxiety Scale for Children (MASC). Measures of functional impairment include the Children's Global Assessment Scale (CGAS) and the Clinical Global Impression scales (CGI).
- **Obtain consent.** Discuss treatment with the young person and the family (e.g. name of medication, starting/estimated ending dose, titration timeline, possible adverse effects and strategies to monitor/minimise them, strategies to monitor progress, interventions for treatment-resistant cases). Document consent in writing.

What to prescribe

- **SSRIs** are the medications of choice for the treatment of anxiety disorders in children and adolescents. A Cochrane systematic review[8] showed that there are seven short-term RCTs (<16 weeks; n treatment = 453, n control = 389) testing the efficacy of SSRIs (fluoxetine, fluvoxamine, paroxetine, sertraline) on changes in impairment for anxiety disorders in young people (CGI-I), with an overall relative risk of response of 2.38 [95% CI = 2.01–2.83] over placebo, NNT of 2–3, and no significant difference among SSRIs. The Childhood Anxiety Multimodal Study (CAMS) showed that monotherapy with sertraline (55% response) is as effective as CBT for anxiety (60% response) compared with placebo (24% response), and that combined therapy with sertraline and CBT is most likely to be successful (81% response).[9] Sertraline, fluoxetine and fluvoxamine have been approved by the FDA for treatment of paediatric OCD, and fluoxetine and escitalopram have been approved for treatment of paediatric depression. The FDA issued in 2004 a Black Box warning for concerns related to worsening of depression, agitation and suicidal ideation linked to SSRIs. These concerns were based on a review of studies of adolescents with depression rather than young people with anxiety.
- **Serotonin–norepinephrine reuptake inhibitors (SNRIs).** Venlafaxine was tested in two short-term RCTs (n treatment = 295, n control = 311) with a relative risk of response of 1.46 [95% CI = 1.25–1.71] over placebo. Duloxetine was tested in a short-term RCT (n treatment = 135, n control = 137) with relative risk of response of 1.98 [95% CI = 1.19–3.30] over placebo[10] and have been approved by the FDA for treatment of paediatric generalised anxiety disorder. Although there are no head-to-head trials

testing comparative efficacy of SSRIs and SNRIs, the adverse effects of SNRIs are generally less well tolerated than those of SSRIs.[11] Nevertheless, because of the different pharmacodynamic actions, SNRIs could be considered a third-line treatment for anxiety disorders when two trials with different SSRIs prove ineffective.

- The efficacy and safety of **buspirone** and **mirtazapine** in young people with anxiety disorders are not known, although open-label studies[12,13] suggest that they might be effective in relieving anxiety symptoms.
- Benzodiazepine use is not supported by controlled trials in children,[14] and may lead to paradoxical disinhibition in some children. Nevertheless, benzodiazepine use is at times considered in clinical practice to 'potentiate' therapeutic effect during initial titration of SSRIs (or to mitigate adverse effects) and for rapid tranquillisation.

Table 5.5 summarises the medications and doses used in the treatment of anxiety disorders in children and adolescents.

Table 5.5 Typical dosage of medications for treatment of anxiety disorders in children and adolescents

Medication	Starting dose (mg)	Dose range (mg)
SSRI		
Sertraline	12.5–25	25–200 od
Fluoxetine	5–10	10–60 od
Fluvoxamine	12.5–25	50–200 (bd if >50)
Paroxetine	5–10	10–40 od
Citalopram*	5–10	10–40 od
SNRI		
Venlafaxine XR	37.5	37.5–225 od
Duloxetine	30	30–120 od
5-HT1A partial agonist		
Buspirone*	5 tds	15–60 od
Tetracyclic		
Mirtazapine*	7.5–15	7.5–30 at night
Benzodiazepine (prn)		
Clonazepam*	0.25–0.5	–
Lorazepam*	0.5–1	–

Note – always check dose with latest formal guidance, e.g. British National Formulary for Children.

* Treatments not supported by RCT evidence.

bd, *bis die* (twice a day); od, *omni die* (once a day); prn, *pro re nata* (as required); SNRI, serotonin–noradrenaline reuptake inhibitor; SSRI, selective serotonin reuptake inhibitor; tds, *ter die sumendus* (three times a day).

After prescribing

- Acute phase
  - Start at the lowest available dose.
  - Monitor adverse effects. SSRIs are generally well tolerated during treatment for anxiety disorders in young people. Psychological adverse effects include worsening of anxiety symptoms, agitation and disinhibition. Physical adverse effects including gastrointestinal symptoms (e.g. nausea, vomiting, dyspepsia, abdominal pain, diarrhoea, constipation), headache, increased motor activity and insomnia may occur, often in mild and transient form.
  - After 1 week of treatment with SSRIs (2 weeks for SNRIs) when the child is compliant with medications and does not manifest more than minimal side effects, titrate incrementally with weekly intervals to the minimal therapeutic dose.
  - Monitor adverse effects (as listed previously) and response (e.g. RCADS, SCARED, MASC, CGAS, CGI-I) frequently and systematically.
  - Dosage for treatment with SSRIs is often similar to dosage in adults because of faster metabolism in children.
  - Therapeutic effect should appear by 6–8 weeks of treatment. It is important to communicate this to families.
  - If partial or non-response, consider accuracy of diagnosis, adequacy of medication trial and compliance of patient.
  - To improve response, consider: adding CBT, changing medication (e.g. switch SSRIs, other classes), or combining medications (e.g. for co-morbidities, to treat adverse effects, to potentiate action). Augmentation strategies with buspirone, benzodiazepines, atypical antipsychotics, and stimulant medications have been proposed but lack empirical support.[7]
- Maintenance phase
  - Continue maintenance treatment for at least 1 year of stable improvement.
  - Monitor response and adverse effects regularly.
- Discontinuation phase
  - Because of lack of information on long-term safety and possible improvement in symptoms with age and learning, consider discontinuing treatment after a period of stable improvement. A trial off medication should be started at a period of low stress/demands. Discontinuation should also be considered if the medication is no longer working or the adverse effects are too severe. Taper SSRIs slowly (e.g. 25–50% weekly) to minimise risk of discontinuation symptoms. Monitor closely for recurrence of symptoms/relapse and, if deterioration is noted, promptly restart medications.

Specific issues

Treatment of anxiety disorders in pre-school children must routinely focus on psychotherapy. In rare cases when a very young child has extreme ongoing symptoms and impairment, clinicians should reconsider diagnosis and case formulation, and reassess the adequacy of the psychotherapy trial. There are no RCTs of pharmacological interventions for anxiety in pre-school children but case reports suggest potential benefit of fluoxetine and buspirone.[15] Therefore, any prescription in pre-school children is off-label.[16]

CHAPTER 5

There has also been an interest in the role of pharmacological intervention to augment the effect of exposure therapy in PTSD.[17] An RCT showed that administration of D-cycloserine, a partial agonist of the NMDA receptor involved in fear learning and extinction, potentiates the therapeutic effect of psychotherapy in adults with social anxiety.[18] No study has tested this effect in young people.

References

1. Kessler RC et al. Lifetime prevalence and age-of-onset distributions of DSM-IV disorders in the National Comorbidity Survey Replication. Arch Gen Psychiatry 2005; 62:593–602.
2. Merikangas KR et al. Lifetime prevalence of mental disorders in U.S. adolescents: results from the National Comorbidity Survey Replication – Adolescent Supplement (NCS-A). J Am Acad Child Adolesc Psychiatry 2010; 49:980–989.
3. Simonoff E et al. Psychiatric disorders in children with autism spectrum disorders: prevalence, comorbidity, and associated factors in a population-derived sample. J Am Acad Child Adolesc Psychiatry 2008; 47:921–929.
4. Danese A et al. Adverse childhood experiences, allostasis, allostatic load, and age-related disease. Physiol Behav 2012; 106:29–39.
5. Pine DS et al. The risk for early-adulthood anxiety and depressive disorders in adolescents with anxiety and depressive disorders. Arch Gen Psychiatry 1998; 55:56–64.
6. National Institute for Health and Care Excellence. Social anxiety disorder: recognition, assessment and treatment. Clinical Guidance 159. http://www.nice.org.uk/guidance/cg159.
7. Connolly SD et al. Practice parameter for the assessment and treatment of children and adolescents with anxiety disorders. J Am Acad Child Adolesc Psychiatry 2007; 46:267–283.
8. Ipser JC et al. Pharmacotherapy for anxiety disorders in children and adolescents. Cochrane Database Syst Rev 2009:CD005170.
9. Walkup JT et al. Cognitive behavioral therapy, sertraline, or a combination in childhood anxiety. N Engl J Med 2008; 359:2753–2766.
10. Strawn JR et al. A randomized, placebo-controlled study of duloxetine for the treatment of children and adolescents with generalized anxiety disorder. J Am Acad Child Adolesc Psychiatry 2015; 54:283–293.
11. Uthman OA et al. Comparative efficacy and acceptability of pharmacotherapeutic agents for anxiety disorders in children and adolescents: a mixed treatment comparison meta-analysis. Curr Med Res Opin 2010; 26:53–59.
12. Buitelaar JK et al. Buspirone in the management of anxiety and irritability in children with pervasive developmental disorders: results of an open-label study. J Clin Psychiatry 1998; 59:56–59.
13. Mrakotsky C et al. Prospective open-label pilot trial of mirtazapine in children and adolescents with social phobia. J Anxiety Disord 2008; 22:88–97.
14. Simeon JG et al. Clinical, cognitive, and neurophysiological effects of alprazolam in children and adolescents with overanxious and avoidant disorders. J Am Acad Child Adolesc Psychiatry 1992; 31:29–33.
15. Gleason MM et al. Psychopharmacological treatment for very young children: contexts and guidelines. J Am Acad Child Adolesc Psychiatry 2007; 46:1532–1572.
16. Mohatt J et al. Treatment of separation, generalized, and social anxiety disorders in youths. Am J Psychiatry 2014; 171:741–748.
17. Parsons RG et al. Implications of memory modulation for post-traumatic stress and fear disorders. Nat Neurosci 2013; 16:146–153.
18. Hofmann SG et al. Augmentation of exposure therapy with D-cycloserine for social anxiety disorder. Arch Gen Psychiatry 2006; 63:298–304.

CHAPTER 5

Obsessive compulsive disorder (OCD) in children and adolescents

The treatment of OCD in children follows the same principles as in adults (see Chapter 3). CBT is effective in this patient group and is the treatment of first choice[1,2] although it may be combined with medication.[3]

Drug treatment

Sertraline[4-6] (from age 6 years) and **fluvoxamine** (from age 8 years) are the SSRIs licensed in the UK for the treatment of OCD in young people. Studies spanning 20 years have established the efficacy of SSRIs in the paediatric population in placebo-controlled trials. Fluoxetine, fluvoxamine, paroxetine, citalopram, escitalopram and sertraline have all been shown to be efficacious and safe in young people with OCD. Paroxetine is not recommended for use in children and young people. Dosage limitations now recommended when using both citalopram and escitalopram have restricted the medications' utility in a disorder that tends to favour an approach of using the 'maximum tolerated dosing schedule'.

Clomipramine is a tricyclic with strong serotonin reuptake inhibition activity. Clomipramine remains a useful drug for some individuals, although its adverse-effect profile (sedation, dry mouth, potential for cardiac adverse effects) tends to limit its use in this age group. There is on-going debate as to whether clomipramine is indeed more efficacious than the SSRIs in treating OCD in children and young people. As a consequence, SSRIs generally remain the recommended first choice medication for children and young people with OCD. All SSRIs appear to be equally effective, although they have different pharmacokinetics and side-effects.[5] A meta-analysis of 12 RCTs of pharmacotherapy against control, in young people (under 19 years of age), showed that medication is consistently significantly more effective than placebo, and that there is no evidence that there are any clinically relevant differences between SSRIs.[5] The SSRIs have a medium to large effect size in the treatment of OCD in children and young people.[7]

Initiation of treatment with medication

Clomipramine and SSRIs show a similar slow and incremental effect on obsessions and compulsions from as early as 1–2 weeks after initiation and placebo-referenced improvements continue for at least 24 weeks. In some cases, positive impact on mood may be noted before the initial incremental changes in OCD symptoms.[8] The effects on core OCD schema may take some weeks to months to become noticeable. In the UK, NICE therefore recommends treatment trials of SSRIs for OCD of 3 months and increasing towards the maximum tolerated effective dosage. Carefully explaining these temporal effects to patients can be important in sustaining compliance. In addition, the earliest signs of improvement may be apparent to an informant before the patient. Use of an observer-rated quantitative measure such as the Children's Yale-Brown Obsessive Compulsive Scale (CY-BOCS)[9] may therefore be helpful to monitor progress in clinical settings. The British Association for Psychopharmacology suggests starting at the lowest dose known to be effective and waiting for up to 12 weeks before evaluating effectiveness.[10] Upward dosage titration is recommended if there is insufficient clinical response. In clinical practice, a balance must be struck between tolerability and the rate of dosage increase in busy clinical services.

Prescribing SSRIs in children

In 2004, the British Medicines and Healthcare products Regulatory Agency (MHRA) cautioned against the use of SSRIs in children and young people, owing to a possible increased risk of suicidal ideation.[11] Subsequent reanalysis of SSRI use in depressed adolescents showed a modest two-fold rise in suicidal ideation or behaviours. There were no completed suicides in over 4400 children and adolescents. Careful reanalysis of treatment data highlights that SSRIs are clearly more efficacious in the OCD group of patients than they are in the treatment of moderate depressive episodes in children and young people.[7] Investigators concluded that in the paediatric OCD group, the pooled risk for suicidal ideation and attempts was less than 1% across all studies. This of course is an important risk and should be explained and carefully monitored. Nonetheless, the naturalistic course of untreated OCD is that it tends not to spontaneously remit and has tremendous morbidity. It is also now known that untreated OCD is associated with very significant morbidity including a ten-fold increased risk of completed suicide compared to the general population.[12] These factors need to be carefully considered and discussed with the patient and their carers or family in making informed choices about treatment.

On occasion, medications (SSRIs) other than sertraline, fluvoxamine and clomipramine may be used as 'off-label' preparations with the appropriate and suitable caution. Indeed, NICE guidance[13] for the treatment of OCD recommends the use of SSRIs before use of clomipramine, due to the latter drug's greater propensity for side-effects and need for cardiac monitoring. Factors guiding the choice of other medications may include issues such as the presence of other disorders (fluoxetine for OCD with co-morbid depression); a good treatment response to a certain drug in other family members; as well as cost and availability. Compliance with medication can be an issue with some young people which can guide the choice of preparation in some instances. For instance, young people with patchy compliance may be better suited to treatment with fluoxetine considering its long half-life when compared with other SSRIs. Some children find tablets or capsules hard to swallow and the availability of licensed liquid formulations is limited in most countries.

Some young people are very reluctant to engage in CBT as part of the treatment. Whilst CBT is the backbone of treatment packages for OCD it is important to remember that a medication alone may be the only viable therapeutic option. Some children have very poor insight or find accessing CBT particularly difficult. This very often includes patients with learning problems or autism spectrum disorders and co-morbid OCD. In these scenarios, where medication is being used as the only evidence-based treatment, it is essential that this remains under review so that motivation and ability to engage with CBT is regularly revisited, as part of clinical reviews. As the young person develops, their motivation for change likewise often changes.

NICE guidelines for the assessment and treatment of OCD

NICE published guidelines in 2005 on the evidence-based treatment options for OCD (and body dysmorphic disorder) for young people and adults. NICE recommends a 'stepped care' model, with increasing intensity of treatment according to clinical severity and complexity.[13] The assessment of the severity and impact of OCD can be aided by the use of the CY-BOCS questionnaire or other quantitative measures, both at baseline and as a helpful monitoring tool.[9]

The summary treatment algorithm from the NICE guideline is shown in Figure 5.1.

CBT and medication in the treatment of childhood OCD

Medication has occasionally been used as initial treatment where there is no CBT available, or if the child is unable or unwilling to engage in CBT. Studies now show convincingly that CBT is superior to placebo and that efforts should be made to try and ensure access to a suitably experienced CBT practitioner. On other occasions medication may be commenced before starting CBT, for instance in the context of significant co-morbid anxiety or depressed mood.

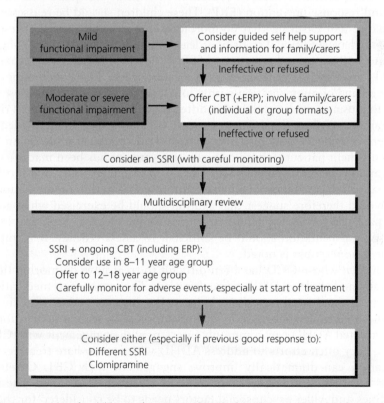

Figure 5.1 Treatment options for children and young people with obsessive-compulsive disorder. CBT, cognitive behavioural therapy; ERP, exposure and response prevention; SSRI, selective serotonin reuptake inhibitor. Adapted from NICE guidance[13] and reproduced from Heyman et al.[14] with permission from BMJ Publishing Group Ltd.

The principal study that directly compared the efficacy of CBT, sertraline, and their combination, in children and adolescents, concluded that children with OCD should begin treatment with CBT alone or CBT plus an SSRI.[2] The addition of an SSRI to a CBT treatment package has been shown to significantly address the differential response to CBT treatment alone, seen between experienced and less experienced therapists.[4]

Some children, particularly those with developmental disabilities, can find CBT extremely challenging. Efforts to tailor treatment protocols can be efficacious in many instances. For some children, however, the experience of anxiety during exposure tasks can be overwhelming. On occasions the use of a beta blocker such as propranolol can moderate the physical concomitants of anxiety to a degree such that CBT can continue.

Treatment-refractory OCD in children

Evidence from randomised trials suggests that up to three-quarters of medicated patients make an adequate response to treatment. Roughly one-quarter of children with OCD will therefore fail to respond to an initial SSRI, administered for at least 12 weeks at the maximum tolerated dose, in combination with an adequate trial of CBT and exposure and response prevention (ERP). These children should be reassessed, clarifying compliance and ensuring that co-morbidity is not being missed. These children should usually have additional trials of at least one other SSRI. Research suggests that approximately 40% respond to a second SSRI.[15] Following this, if the response is limited, a child should usually be referred to a specialist centre. Trials of clomipramine may be considered and/or augmentation with a low dose of risperidone.[14,16] Research hints at the fact that using a medication with a different method of action such as risperidone or clomipramine may benefit patients who have failed to respond to two adequate SSRI trials.[8] There is evidence that low dose antipsychotic augmentation, as an 'off-label' therapy, can benefit patients whose response to treatment has been inadequate despite at least 3 months of maximal tolerated SSRI. Unfortunately, only one-third of treatment-resistant adult cases showed a meaningful response to this augmentation strategy. The data would therefore suggest that caution should be exercised when augmenting treatment packages for OCD in children and young people. A 6-week trial of low dose antipsychotic augmentation should be sufficient to assess efficacy. It is important to discontinue if no response is noted.

Often children whose OCD has been difficult to treat have co-morbidities such as autism spectrum disorder, ADHD, or tic disorders. The response to medication can be differentially affected by these co-morbidities. For instance, cases with tic disorders may be benefitted somewhat more by augmentation with second-generation antipsychotics. Untreated ADHD can commonly interfere with engagement with CBT due to poor focus. Very often efforts to address ADHD with appropriate treatments including medication can dramatically improve engagement with CBT. Careful clinical review and reformulation is important in OCD treatment resistance. The impact of co-morbidities and wider psychosocial factors needs to be considered for their impact on the treatment response overall. The evidence base around systemic factors and their application in OCD is poor. Very often clinical experience shows that it can be vital to extensively support families and carers during treatment. This goes across all areas of the care plan but often requires helping families drop well-established patterns of accommodation around OCD.

Neither ketamine,[17] D-cycloserine nor riluzole[18] is effective in refractory childhood OCD.

Duration of treatment and long-term follow-up

Untreated OCD runs a chronic course. A series of adult studies have shown that discontinuation of medication tends to result in symptomatic relapse. Some authors have suggested that those with co-morbidities are at the greatest risk of relapse. Given that studies frequently exclude cases with additional co-morbidities, it is likely that the relapse rates have been underestimated. In the UK, NICE guidelines recommend that if a young person has responded to medication, treatment should continue for at least 6 months after remission. This recommendation was based on clinical consensus rather than as the product of carefully conducted research trials. Clinical experience would suggest that when discontinuation of treatment is attempted it should be done slowly, cautiously and in a transparent manner with the patient and their family. Once again, the careful use of clinical outcome measures should be considered when stopping medication. The role of maintenance CBT and medication is under increasing scrutiny. Individuals with developmental disabilities often struggle to generalise the lessons taken from successful CBT. Therefore, this population benefits from concerted and close review in follow-up after treatment. Both appear to offer promise in maintaining gains made after initial treatment. It is important that throughout childhood, adolescence and into adult life, the individual with OCD should have access to health-care professionals, treatment opportunities and other support as needed, and NICE recommends that if relapse occurs, people with OCD should be seen as soon as possible rather than placed on a routine waiting list.

References

1. O'Kearney RT et al. Behavioural and cognitive behavioural therapy for obsessive compulsive disorder in children and adolescents. Cochrane Database Syst Rev 2006:CD004856.
2. Freeman JB et al. Cognitive behavioral treatment for young children with obsessive-compulsive disorder. Biol Psychiatry 2007; **61**:337–343.
3. Mancuso E et al. Treatment of pediatric obsessive-compulsive disorder: a review. J Child Adolesc Psychopharmacol 2010; **20**:299–308.
4. Pediatric OCD Treatment Study (POTS) Team. Cognitive-behavior therapy, sertraline, and their combination for children and adolescents with obsessive-compulsive disorder: the Pediatric OCD Treatment Study (POTS) randomized controlled trial. JAMA 2004; **292**:1969–1976.
5. Geller DA et al. Which SSRI? A meta-analysis of pharmacotherapy trials in pediatric obsessive-compulsive disorder. Am J Psychiatry 2003; **160**:1919–1928.
6. March JS et al. Treatment benefit and the risk of suicidality in multicenter, randomized, controlled trials of sertraline in children and adolescents. J Child Adolesc Psychopharmacol 2006; **16**:91–102.
7. Garland J et al. Update on the use of SSRIs and SNRIs with children and adolescents in clinical practice. J Can Acad Child Adolesc Psychiatry 2016; **25**:4–10.
8. Bloch MH et al. Assessment and management of treatment-refractory obsessive-compulsive disorder in children. J Am Acad Child Adolesc Psychiatry 2015; **54**:251–262.
9. Scahill L et al. Children's Yale-Brown Obsessive Compulsive Scale: reliability and validity. J Am Acad Child Adolesc Psychiatry 1997; **36**:844–852.
10. Baldwin DS et al. Evidence-based pharmacological treatment of anxiety disorders, post-traumatic stress disorder and obsessive-compulsive disorder: a revision of the 2005 guidelines from the British Association for Psychopharmacology. J Psychopharmacol 2014; **28**:403–439.

CHAPTER 5

11. Medicines and Healthcare Products Regulatory Agency. Report of the CSM expert working group on the safety of selective serotonin reuptake inhibitor antidepressants. London, MRHA; 2004.

12. Fernandez de la Cruz L et al. Suicide in obsessive-compulsive disorder: a population-based study of 36 788 Swedish patients. Mol Psychiatry 2017; 22:1626–1632.

13. National Institute for Clinical Excellence. Obsessive-compulsive disorder: Core interventions in the treatment of obsessive-compulsive disorder and body dysmorphic disorder. Clinical Guidance 31, 2005. https://www.nice.org.uk/guidance/cg31.

14. Heyman I et al. Obsessive-compulsive disorder. BMJ 2006; 333:424–429.

15. Grados M et al. Pharmacotherapy in children and adolescents with obsessive-compulsive disorder. Child Adolesc Psychiatr Clin N Am 1999; 8:617–634, x.

16. Bloch MH et al. A systematic review: antipsychotic augmentation with treatment refractory obsessive-compulsive disorder. Mol Psychiatry 2006; 11:622–632.

17. Bloch MH et al. Effects of ketamine in treatment-refractory obsessive-compulsive disorder. Biol Psychiatry 2012; 72:964–970.

18. Grant PJ et al. 12-week, placebo-controlled trial of add-on riluzole in the treatment of childhood-onset obsessive-compulsive disorder. Neuropsychopharmacology 2014; 39:1453–1459.

| Post-traumatic stress disorder in children and adolescents |

Diagnostic issues

Traumatic events and PTSD are common in young people. One in four children experiences traumatic events[1] and nearly 1 in 10 children develops PTSD[2] before age 18. The prevalence of PTSD in adolescents is 4% in males and 6% in females from the general population,[3] and could be as high as 30% in young people attending emergency departments. Furthermore, young people with significant PTSD symptoms but sub-threshold criteria for diagnosis may show similar impairment and distress to children and adolescents with a diagnosis of PTSD and thus require treatment.[4] Response to trauma may also involve other anxiety disorders, depression, self-harm, aggression and substance abuse.

A diagnosis of PTSD is based on the triad of intrusive re-experiencing, avoidance of stimuli associated with the trauma, and hyper-arousal after trauma exposure. However, in children re-experiencing may not be reported in the form of distressing visual flashbacks but rather could be noted as compulsive repetition of aspects of trauma in play, drawings or verbalisation, or as nightmares. Furthermore, certain types of avoidance (sense of a foreshortened future, inability to recall important aspects of the event) may not be detectable because of insufficient abilities with abstract cognition or verbal expression. In adolescents, PTSD symptoms are often associated with and may be masked by impulsive and aggressive behaviours.[5,6] Because of the varied clinical manifestations, the assessment and treatment of PTSD in children and adolescents needs to be undertaken by clinicians who can appreciate developmental variations in the presentation of symptoms.

Clinical guidance

Guidelines for treatment of PTSD in children and adolescents are available in the UK and the USA. NICE guidelines advise that treatment should be 12 sessions of trauma-focused CBT for PTSD resulting from a single event (longer for chronic or recurrent events) and discourage routine prescription of medications.[7] Guidelines by AACAP recommend trauma-focused CBT as first-line treatment for young people with PTSD and use of pharmacotherapy if the child's symptom severity, lack of response or co-morbidity suggests a need for additional interventions.[8] The AACAP guidelines discuss treatment with SSRIs, but also treatment with anti-adrenergic and second-generation antipsychotic medications. Psychological therapies have a robust evidence base in PTSD in younger people.[9]

Prescribing for anxiety disorders in young people

Before prescribing

- Exclude other diagnoses (see section on 'Anxiety disorders in children and adolescents').
- Beware contraindication to SSRIs and potential interactions.
- Measure baseline severity. Structured interviews include the Anxiety Disorders Interview Schedule (ADIS) and the Kiddie-Schedule for Affective Disorders and Schizophrenia (Kiddie-SADS). Questionnaires include the Child PTSD Symptom

CHAPTER 5

Scale (CPSS) and the UCLA Posttraumatic Stress Disorder Reaction Index. Measures of functional impairment include the Children's Global Assessment Scale (CGAS) and the Clinical Global Impression scales (CGI).

- **Obtain consent** (see section on 'Anxiety disorders in children and adolescents').

What to prescribe

- SSRIs have shown only minimal evidence of clinical efficacy for the treatment of PTSD in children and adolescents, despite their efficacy in adults.[10] A small 12-week RCT of add-on **sertraline** (n = 11) to routine trauma-focused CBT (TF-CBT) treatment showed only marginal benefit of pharmacological treatment over TF-CBT and placebo (n = 11), which was not statistically significant.[11] A larger 10-week RCT with flexibly dosed sertraline (n treated = 67; n placebo = 64) failed to detect a benefit over placebo.[12] A small (n = 8) open-label study suggests potential efficacy of **citalopram**.[13] It is possible that SSRIs may be more effective for the treatment of PTSD in young people in the presence of co-morbid major depressive episode, anxiety disorders and OCD, although the evidence base for this is minimal. Finally, the tricyclic antidepressant **imipramine** has also been shown to be effective in adults in a small (n = 10) trial[14] but given its poor tolerability and cardiotoxicity it is rarely used in children. There is a single study in 'acute stress disorder' in children with severe burns.[15]

- Anti-adrenergic medications have been studied for the treatment of PTSD in young people because of the evidence of noradrenergic hyperactivity in PTSD[16,17] and the suggestive evidence of efficacy in adults.[18] **Clonidine** is an α_2-adrenergic agonist that reduces norepinephrine release. Clonidine is used off-label in several paediatric conditions and an open-label trial (n = 7) in children showed that clonidine can improve PTSD symptoms, in particular re-living symptoms.[19] **Guanfacine** is also an α_2-adrenergic agonist. A case study suggested that guanfacine can improve PTSD symptoms, again particularly re-living symptoms, in young people.[20] An open-label study (n = 19) reported benefits across all symptom domains.[21] The most common side-effects of α_2-adrenergic agonists are dry mouth and dizziness. Blood pressure should be monitored regularly and discontinuation should be slow to avoid rebound hypertension.

- **Prazosin** is an α_1-adrenergic antagonist that reduces the post-synaptic effect of norepinephrine. Evidence in children and adolescents is limited to case reports which showed improvement of PTSD symptoms.[22,23] Prazosin should be titrated slowly (e.g. 1 mg/week) and blood pressure (risk of orthostatic hypotension) should be carefully monitored, particularly early in treatment. **Propranolol** is a beta-antagonist that reduces the post-synaptic effect of norepinephrine. In an on-off-on study, propranolol was shown to improve PTSD in children and adolescents.[24] The most common adverse effects include hypotension, bradycardia, dizziness and bronchospasm. Blood pressure should be monitored regularly during titration.

- Second-generation antipsychotics have been studied for treatment of PTSD in children and adolescents based on the role of dopamine in various aspects of fear conditioning[25] and on the efficacy of **risperidone, olanzapine** and **aripiprazole** (either as monotherapy or adjunctive to SSRI therapy) on PTSD in adults.[18,26] Evidence in children and adolescents is limited to case series and case studies with risperidone[27] and quetiapine,[28] which showed positive results.

Table 5.6 Typical dosage of medications for treatment of PTSD in children and adolescents. These clinical guidelines are based on less than robust research evidence (e.g. case series) in children and adolescents and on extrapolation of data from adult trials

Medication	Starting dose (mg)	Dose range (mg)
SSRI		
Sertraline	12.5–25	50–200 od
Citalopram	5–10	10–40 od
Tricyclic		
Imipramine	10	25–100*
Anti-adrenergic		
Clonidine	0.05 nocte	0.1–0.2 nocte
Guanfacine	0.5 bd	1–3 nocte
Prazosin	1 nocte	2–4 nocte
Propranolol	10 tds	40–80/day
Second-generation antipsychotic		
Risperidone	0.5	0.5–1 od
Quetiapine	25–50	50–200 od (at night)

Always check dose against latest formal guidance, e.g. British National Formulary for Children.
* Approximately 1 mg/kg. ECG monitoring required.
bd, *bis die* (twice a day); nocte, at night; od, *omni die* (once a day); tds, *ter die sumendus* (three times a day).

- Mood stabilisers have been studied for the treatment of PTSD in adults, generally adjunctively in combination with SSRIs, and have been found to be effective.[18] The literature in children and adolescents is limited to one open-label study (n = 28) with **carbamazepine**[29] and one open-label study (n = 12) with **valproate semisodium**[30] that showed positive results.

A summary of the medications and doses used in the treatment of PTSD is shown in Table 5.6.

After prescribing

- **Acute phase**
  - Start at low dose and titrate at regular (e.g. weekly) intervals.
  - Monitor response (e.g. CPSS, CGAS, CGI-I) frequently and systematically.
  - Monitor adverse effects.
  - If partial or non-response, consider (1) accuracy of diagnosis, (2) adequacy of medication trial, and (3) compliance of patient.
- **Maintenance phase**
  - Monitor response and adverse effects regularly.

- Discontinuation phase
  - Consider discontinuing treatment after a period of stable improvement.
  - A trial off medication should be started at a period of low stress/demands.
  - Discontinuation should also be considered if the medication is no longer working or the adverse effects are too severe.
  - Taper medications slowly to minimise risk of withdrawal symptoms.
  - Monitor closely for recurrence of symptoms/relapse.

Specific issues

Treatment of PTSD in pre-school children must routinely focus on psychotherapy with either child–parent psychotherapy (CPP) or pre-school CBT. Pharmacological treatment of PTSD in pre-school children is not recommended.[31]

There has been an interest in preventive psychopharmacological interventions in the aftermath of trauma exposure, based on the findings that arousal and noradrenergic hyperactivity may promote consolidation of trauma memories.[32] After initial positive results with the use of **propranolol**,[33] subsequent larger studies and also studies in children and adolescents[34] failed to detect significant protective effects. **Morphine** has similar ability to inhibit noradrenergic activity, and studies in children and adolescents[35] and adults[36] suggest that morphine use after trauma might be effective in preventing development of PTSD. These findings require replication and morphine should not be used to prevent PTSD in routine clinical practice.

There has also been an interest in the role of pharmacological intervention to augment the effect of exposure therapy in PTSD.[37] An RCT showed that administration of **D-cycloserine**, a partial agonist of the NMDA receptor involved in fear learning and extinction, potentiated the therapeutic effect of psychotherapy in adults with PTSD.[38] A recent meta-analysis has shown that D-cycloserine is associated with a small augmentation effect on exposure therapy for anxiety disorders including PTSD.[39] No study has tested this effect in children and adolescents.

References

1. Costello EJ et al. The prevalence of potentially traumatic events in childhood and adolescence. J Trauma Stress 2002; 15:99–112.
2. Breslau N et al. Traumatic events and posttraumatic stress disorder in an urban population of young adults. Arch Gen Psychiatry 1991; 48:216–222.
3. Kilpatrick DG et al. Violence and risk of PTSD, major depression, substance abuse/dependence, and comorbidity: results from the National Survey of Adolescents. J Consult Clin Psychol 2003; 71:692–700.
4. Carrion VG et al. Toward an empirical definition of pediatric PTSD: the phenomenology of PTSD symptoms in youth. J Am Acad Child Adolesc Psychiatry 2002; 41:166–173.
5. Scheeringa MS et al. PTSD in children and adolescents: toward an empirically based algorithm. Depress Anxiety 2011; 28:770–782.
6. Meiser-Stedman R et al. The posttraumatic stress disorder diagnosis in preschool- and elementary school-age children exposed to motor vehicle accidents. Am J Psychiatry 2008; 165:1326–1337.
7. National Institute for Health and Care Excellence. Post-traumatic stress disorder: management. Clinical Guideline 26, 2005. http://www.nice.org.uk/guidance/CG26.
8. Cohen JA et al. Practice parameter for the assessment and treatment of children and adolescents with posttraumatic stress disorder. J Am Acad Child Adolesc Psychiatry 2010; 49:414–430.
9. Morina N et al. Interventions for children and adolescents with posttraumatic stress disorder: a meta-analysis of comparative outcome studies. Clin Psychol Rev 2016; 47:41–54.
10. Stein DJ et al. Pharmacotherapy for post traumatic stress disorder (PTSD). Cochrane Database Syst Rev 2006:CD002795.
11. Cohen JA et al. A pilot randomized controlled trial of combined trauma-focused CBT and sertraline for childhood PTSD symptoms. J Am Acad Child Adolesc Psychiatry 2007; 46:811–819.

12. Robb AS et al. Sertraline treatment of children and adolescents with posttraumatic stress disorder: a double-blind, placebo-controlled trial. J Child Adolesc Psychopharmacol 2010; 20:463–471.

13. Seedat S et al. An open trial of citalopram in adolescents with post-traumatic stress disorder. Int Clin Psychopharmacol 2001; 16:21–25.

14. Burstein A. Treatment of post-traumatic stress disorder with imipramine. Psychosomatics 1984; 25:681–687.

15. Robert R et al. Imipramine treatment in pediatric burn patients with symptoms of acute stress disorder: a pilot study. J Am Acad Child Adolesc Psychiatry 1999; 38:873—882.

16. Geracioti TD, Jr. et al. CSF norepinephrine concentrations in posttraumatic stress disorder. Am J Psychiatry 2001; 158:1227–1230.

17. De Bellis MD et al. Urinary catecholamine excretion in sexually abused girls. J Am Acad Child Adolesc Psychiatry 1994; 33:320–327.

18. Strawn JR et al. Psychopharmacologic treatment of posttraumatic stress disorder in children and adolescents: a review. J Clin Psychiatry 2010; 71:932–941.

19. Harmon RJ et al. Clonidine for posttraumatic stress disorder in preschool children. J Am Acad Child Adolesc Psychiatry 1996; 35:1247–1249.

20. Horrigan JP. Guanfacine for PTSD nightmares. J Am Acad Child Adolesc Psychiatry 1996; 35:975–976.

21. Connor DF et al. An open-label study of guanfacine extended release for traumatic stress related symptoms in children and adolescents. J Child Adolesc Psychopharmacol 2013; 23:244–251.

22. Strawn JR et al. Prazosin treatment of an adolescent with posttraumatic stress disorder. J Child Adolesc Psychopharmacol 2009; 19:599–600.

23. Akinsanya A et al. Prazosin in children and adolescents with posttraumatic stress disorder who have nightmares: a systematic review. J Clin Psychopharmacol 2017; 37:84–88.

24. Famularo R et al. Propranolol treatment for childhood posttraumatic stress disorder, acute type. A pilot study. Am J Dis Child 1988; 142:1244–1247.

25. Pezze MA et al. Mesolimbic dopaminergic pathways in fear conditioning. Prog Neurobiol 2004; 74:301–320.

26. Pae CU et al. The atypical antipsychotics olanzapine and risperidone in the treatment of posttraumatic stress disorder: a meta-analysis of randomized, double-blind, placebo-controlled clinical trials. Int Clin Psychopharmacol 2008; 23:1–8.

27. Keeshin BR et al. Risperidone treatment of an adolescent with severe posttraumatic stress disorder. Ann Pharmacother 2009; 43:1374.

28. Stathis S et al. A preliminary case series on the use of quetiapine for posttraumatic stress disorder in juveniles within a youth detention center. J Clin Psychopharmacol 2005; 25:539–544.

29. Looff D et al. Carbamazepine for PTSD. J Am Acad Child Adolesc Psychiatry 1995; 34:703–704.

30. Steiner H et al. Divalproex sodium for the treatment of PTSD and conduct disordered youth: a pilot randomized controlled clinical trial. Child Psychiatry Hum Dev 2007; 38:183–193.

31. Gleason MM et al. Psychopharmacological treatment for very young children: contexts and guidelines. J Am Acad Child Adolesc Psychiatry 2007; 46:1532–1572.

32. Cahill L et al. Beta-adrenergic activation and memory for emotional events. Nature 1994; 371:702–704.

33. Vaiva G et al. Immediate treatment with propranolol decreases posttraumatic stress disorder two months after trauma. Biol Psychiatry 2003; 54:947–949.

34. Nugent NR et al. The efficacy of early propranolol administration at reducing PTSD symptoms in pediatric injury patients: a pilot study. J Trauma Stress 2010; 23:282–287.

35. Saxe G et al. Relationship between acute morphine and the course of PTSD in children with burns. J Am Acad Child Adolesc Psychiatry 2001; 40:915–921.

36. Holbrook TL et al. Morphine use after combat injury in Iraq and post-traumatic stress disorder. N Engl J Med 2010; 362:110–117.

37. Parsons RG et al. Implications of memory modulation for post-traumatic stress and fear disorders. Nat Neurosci 2013; 16:146–153.

38. de Kleine RA et al. A randomized placebo-controlled trial of D-cycloserine to enhance exposure therapy for posttraumatic stress disorder. Biol Psychiatry 2012; 71:962–968.

39. Mataix-Cols D et al. D-Cycloserine augmentation of exposure-based cognitive behavior therapy for anxiety, obsessive-compulsive, and post-traumatic stress disorders: a systematic review and meta-analysis of individual participant data. JAMA Psychiatry 2017; 74:501–510.

CHAPTER 5

Attention deficit hyperactivity disorder

Attention Deficit Hyperactivity Disorder (ADHD) in children

- A diagnosis of attention deficit hyperactivity disorder (ADHD) should be made only after a comprehensive assessment by a specialist with expertise in ADHD.[1] Appropriate psychological, psychosocial and behavioural interventions should be put in place. Drug treatments should be only a part of the overall treatment plan.
- The indication for drug treatment is the presence of impairment resulting from ADHD; in mild to moderate cases the first treatments are usually behaviour therapy and education; medication is indicated as first line of therapy only in severe cases (e.g. those diagnosed as hyperkinetic disorder), and as second line when psychological approaches have not been successful within a reasonable time (e.g. 8 weeks) or are inappropriate.
- **Methylphenidate** is usually first line when a drug is indicated. It is a central nervous stimulant with a large evidence base from trials. Adverse effects include insomnia, anorexia, raised blood pressure and growth deceleration – which can usually be managed by symptomatic management and/or dose reduction. In the UK, there are several modified-release preparations with different release profiles available, including generic options (see Box 5.2).
- **Dexamfetamine** is an alternative central nervous system (CNS) stimulant; effects and adverse reactions are broadly similar to methylphenidate, but there is much less evidence on efficacy and safety than exists for methylphenidate, and dexamfetamine

---

Box 5.2 Summary of NICE guidance for ADHD in children[1]

- Drug treatment should only be initiated by a specialist and only after comprehensive assessment of mental and physical health and social influences.
- For cases with moderate (or lesser) degrees of severity, psychological interventions are recommended as initial therapy, with medication subsequently if still required.
- For severe cases (i.e. those with pervasive impairment from their ADHD), medication will usually be the first line of treatment.
- Methylphenidate, dexamfetamine/lisdexamfetamine, atomoxetine and guanfacine are recommended within their licensed indications.
- Methylphenidate is usually first choice of medication, but the decision should include consideration of:
  - co-morbid conditions (tics, Tourette's, epilepsy)
  - tolerability and adverse effects
  - convenience of dosing
  - potential for diversion
  - patient/parent preference.
- If using methylphenidate, consider modified-release preparations (convenience of single-day dosage, improving adherence, reducing stigma, acceptability to schools); or multiple doses of immediate-release (greater flexibility in controlling time-course of action, closer initial titration).
- Where more than one agent is considered suitable, the product with the lowest cost should be prescribed.
- Monitoring should include measurement of height and weight (with entry on growth charts) and recording of blood pressure and heart rate.

is probably more likely to be diverted and misused. Both methylphenidate and dexamfetamine are Controlled Drugs; prescriptions should be written appropriately and for a maximum supply of 28 days (in the UK).

- **Lisdexamfetamine** is a prodrug; the dexamfetamine is complexed with the amino acid lysine and in this form is inactive. It is broken down (in red blood cells) so that dexamfetamine is gradually made available. It therefore has a similar practical role to extended-release preparations of methylphenidate and, like them, is unlikely to be abused for recreational or dependency-driven purposes. Several randomised controlled trials have established it as superior to placebo in children[2,3] and adolescents.[4] Effect size from preliminary research appears to be at least as great as that of OROS-methylphenidate[3] and it seems to have a similar range of adverse effects.[5,6] A recent network meta-analysis found lisdexafetamine to be more effective than methylphenidate.[7] Long-term data suggest that it can be considered as an alternative to extended-release methylphenidate.[8]

- **Atomoxetine**[9–12] is a suitable first-line alternative. It may be particularly useful for children who do not respond to stimulants, where stimulant diversion is a problem or when 'dopaminergic' adverse effects (such as tics, anxiety and stereotypies) become problematic on stimulants. Parents should be warned of the possibilities of suicidal thinking and liver disease emerging and advised of the possible features that they might notice. It is less effective than stimulants.[7,10,13,14]

- Third-line drugs include the alpha$_2$-agonists **clonidine**[15] and **guanfacine**. A licensed modified-release preparation of guanfacine was approved in the UK in January 2016[16] for use in children with ADHD and can be considered as an alternative non-stimulant medication to atomoxetine. Very few children should receive these drugs alone for ADHD although guanfacine may be at least as effective as atomoxetine.[7]

- There is some evidence supporting the efficacy of **tricyclic antidepressants**[17,18] and **bupropion**.[19,20] **Modafinil** appears to be effective[21,22] but has not been compared with standard treatments and its safety is not established.

- There is no evidence to support the use of **second-generation antipsychotics**[23,24] for ADHD symptoms, but risperidone may be helpful in reducing severe coexistent levels of aggression and agitation, especially in those with moderate learning disability.[25]

- Co-morbid psychiatric illness is common in children with ADHD. Stimulants are often helpful overall[17] but are unlikely to be appropriate for children who have a psychotic illness, and problems with substance misuse should be managed in their own right alongside ADHD treatment.[26]

- Combinations of stimulants and atomoxetine have been used, but there are few trials and no clear evidence for efficacy.[27]

- Once stimulant treatment has been established, it is appropriate for repeat prescriptions to be supplied through general practitioners.[1]

ADHD in adults

Adult ADHD is recognised by both ICD-10 and DSM-V. NICE guidance regards the first line of treatment as medication (Box 5.3), following the same principles as for drug treatment in children.

CHAPTER 5

Box 5.3 Summary of NICE guidance for ADHD in adults[1]

- Drug treatment should only be initiated by a specialist and only after comprehensive assessment of mental and physical health and social influences.
- Drug treatment should be:
  - the first-line treatment unless the person prefers a psychological approach
  - part of a comprehensive treatment program addressing psychological behavioural, educational and/or occupational needs.
- Methylphenidate, dexamfetamine/lisdexamfetamine and atomoxetine are recommended for use in adults.
- Methylphenidate is usually first choice of medication, but the decision should include consideration of:
  - co-morbid conditions (tics, Tourette's, epilepsy, anxiety, substance abuse)
  - tolerability and adverse effects
  - convenience of dosing
  - potential for diversion
  - patient preference.
- Consider atomoxetine as first-line treatment if there are concerns about drug misuse and diversion.
- If using methylphenidate, consider modified-release preparations (convenience of single-day dosage, improving adherence, reducing stigma, acceptability within educational/occupational settings), or multiple doses of immediate-release (greater flexibility in controlling time-course of action, closer initial titration).
- For adults with ADHD and drug or alcohol addiction disorders, there should be close liaison between the professional treating the ADHD and an addiction specialist.
- Where more than one agent is considered suitable, the product with the lowest cost should be prescribed.
- Monitoring should include measurement of weight, blood pressure and heart rate.
- Consider group or individual CBT for adults who:
  - are stabilised on medication but have persisting functional impairment associated with ADHD
  - have partial or no response to drug treatment or who are intolerant to it
  - have made an informed choice not to have drug treatment
  - have difficulty accepting the diagnosis of ADHD and accepting and adhering to drug treatment
  - have remitting symptoms and psychological treatment is considered sufficient to treat mild to moderate residual functional impairment.

- At least 25% of children with ADHD will still have symptoms at the age of 30. It is appropriate to **continue treatment started in childhood** in adults whose symptoms remain disabling.
- A first-time diagnosis of ADHD in an adult should only be made after a comprehensive assessment. Whenever possible this should include information from other informants and from adults who knew the patient as a child. It is recommended to establish the symptoms and impairments of ADHD using a validated diagnostic interview assessment such as the Diagnostic Interview for DSM-IV ADHD (DIVA).[28]
- The prevalence of substance misuse and antisocial personality disorder are high in adults whose ADHD was not recognised in childhood.[29] Methylphenidate can be effective in this population,[30] but caution is appropriate in prescribing and monitoring.
- **Methylphenidate** is usually the first choice of medication. **Dexamfetamine, lisdexamfetamine** and **atomoxetine** are considered second-line choices of medication.

- For **atomoxetine,** monitoring for symptoms of liver dysfunction and suicidal thinking is advised.
- **Atomoxetine** and lisdexamfetamine are the only medications licensed for first-time use in adults with ADHD. Other drugs such as extended formulations of methylphenidate are licensed for continued treatment when this was initiated before the age of 18 years. Despite this, current NICE guidance is to use methylphenidate as the first-line treatment when treating ADHD in adults.

Prescribing in ADHD

Prescribing in ADHD is summarised in Table 5.7.

Table 5.7 Prescribing in attention deficit hyperactivity disorder

Medication	Onset and duration of action	Dose	Notes	Recommended monitoring/general notes
Methylphenidate immediate release Branded products (Ritalin, Medikinet) and various generic preparations available[31-33]	Onset: 20–60 min Duration: 2–4 hours	Initially 5–10 mg daily titrated up in weekly increments of 5–10 mg to a maximum of 2.1 mg/kg/day in divided doses. Licensed maximum dose 60 mg daily (or after specialist review up to 90 mg daily, NB unlicensed)[1]	Methylphenidate usually first-line treatment in ADHD Generally well tolerated[34]	For methylphenidate, dexamfetamine and lisdexamfetamine: ■ blood pressure[35] ■ pulse ■ height ■ weight Monitor for insomnia, mood and appetite change and the development of tics,[36] although some evidence suggests tics are not associated with psychostimulants[37] Discontinue if no benefits seen in 1 month Controlled Drug
Methylphenidate sustained release*			An afternoon dose of immediate-release methylphenidate may be necessary in some children to optimise treatment	
Concerta XL[31,32,38-40] Bioequivalent versions of Concerta XL: Matoride XL, Xenidate XL, Delmosart modified release	Onset: 30 min–2 hours Duration: 12 hours	Initially 18 mg in the morning, titrated up to a licensed maximum dose of 54 mg daily (or after specialist review up to 108 mg daily, NB unlicensed) 18 mg = 15 mg methylphenidate immediate release	Consists of an immediate-release component (22% of the dose) and a modified-release component (78% of the dose)	
Equasym XL[41,42]	Onset: 20–60 min Duration: 8 hours	Initially 10 mg in the morning, titrated up to a licensed maximum dose of 60 mg daily	Consists of an immediate-release component (30% of the dose) and a modified-release component (70% of the dose)	
Medikinet XL	Onset: 20–60 min Duration: up to 8 hours	Dose as for Equasym XL	Consists of an immediate-release component (50% of the dose) and a modified-release component (50% of the dose) Capsules can be opened and sprinkled[43]	
Dexamfetamine immediate release[34,44]	Onset: 20–60 min Duration: 3–6 hours	Initially 2.5–10 mg daily, titrated up in weekly increments of 2.5–5 mg, to a maximum of 20 mg daily in divided doses (occasionally up to 40 mg daily necessary)	Considered to be less well tolerated than methylphenidate[34]	
Lisdexamfetamine (Elvanse)[2-4]	Onset: 20–60 min Duration: 13+ hours	Initially 30 mg in the morning, titrated up to a licensed maximum dose of 70 mg daily	Prodrug, gradually hydrolysed to dexamfetamine Capsules can be opened and sprinkled[45]	

References

| **Atomoxetine**[46,47] | Approximately 4–6 weeks (atomoxetine is a noradrenaline reuptake inhibitor) | When switching from a stimulant, continue stimulant for first 4 weeks of therapy
For children <70 kg: initially 0.5 mg/kg/day for 7 days, then increase according to response. Recommended maintenance dose 1.2 mg/kg/day (in single or divided doses) and up to 1.8 mg/kg/day, to a maximum of 120 mg daily if necessary[1]
For children >70 kg: initially 40 mg daily for 7 days, then increase according to response. Recommended maintenance dose 80 mg daily | Less effective than stimulants (see main ADHD text)[10,14]
May be useful where stimulant diversion is a problem[48] | Blood pressure[49]
Pulse
Height
Weight
Monitor for insomnia, mood and appetite change and the development of tics
Not a Controlled Drug
Licensed in adults |

* For details of other preparations available elsewhere, see Cortese et al., 2017.[50]

References

1. National Institute for Health and Care Excellence. Attention Deficit Hyperactivity Disorder: diagnosis and management of ADHD in children, young people and adults. Clinical Guidance CG72, 2008. Last updated February 2016. https://www.nice.org.uk/guidance/cg72.

2. Biederman J et al. Lisdexamfetamine dimesylate and mixed amphetamine salts extended-release in children with ADHD: a double-blind, placebo-controlled, crossover analog classroom study. Biol Psychiatry 2007; 62:970–976.

3. Coghill D et al. European, randomized, phase 3 study of lisdexamfetamine dimesylate in children and adolescents with attention-deficit/hyperactivity disorder. Eur Neuropsychopharmacol 2013; 23:1208–1218.

4. Findling RL et al. Efficacy and safety of lisdexamfetamine dimesylate in adolescents with attention-deficit/hyperactivity disorder. J Am Acad Child Adolesc Psychiatry 2011; 50:395–405.

5. Heal DJ et al. Amphetamine, past and present – a pharmacological and clinical perspective. J Psychopharmacol 2013; 27:479–496.

6. Coghill DR et al. Long-term safety and efficacy of lisdexamfetamine dimesylate in children and adolescents with ADHD: a phase IV, 2-year, open-label study in Europe. CNS Drugs 2017; 31:625–638.

7. Joseph A et al. Comparative efficacy and safety of attention-deficit/hyperactivity disorder pharmacotherapies, including guanfacine extended release: a mixed treatment comparison. Eur Child Adolesc Psychiatry 2017; 26:875–897.

8. Findling RL et al. Long-term effectiveness and safety of lisdexamfetamine dimesylate in school-aged children with attention-deficit/hyperactivity disorder. CNS Spectr 2008; 13:614–620.

9. Michelson D et al. Once-daily atomoxetine treatment for children and adolescents with attention deficit hyperactivity disorder: a randomized, placebo-controlled study. Am J Psychiatry 2002; 159:1896–1901.

10. Kratochvil CJ et al. Atomoxetine and methylphenidate treatment in children with ADHD: a prospective, randomized, open-label trial. J Am Acad Child Adolesc Psychiatry 2002; 41:776–784.

11. Weiss M et al. A randomized, placebo-controlled study of once-daily atomoxetine in the school setting in children with ADHD. J Am Acad Child Adolesc Psychiatry 2005; 44:647–655.

12. Kratochvil CJ et al. A double-blind, placebo-controlled study of atomoxetine in young children with ADHD. Pediatrics 2011; 127:e862–e868.

13. Catala-Lopez F et al. The pharmacological and non-pharmacological treatment of attention deficit hyperactivity disorder in children and adolescents: a systematic review with network meta-analyses of randomised trials. PLoS One 2017; 12:e0180355.

14. Liu Q et al. Comparative efficacy and safety of methylphenidate and atomoxetine for attention-deficit hyperactivity disorder in children and adolescents: meta-analysis based on head-to-head trials. J Clin Exp Neuropsychol 2017:1–12.

15. Connor DF et al. A meta-analysis of clonidine for symptoms of attention-deficit hyperactivity disorder. J Am Acad Child Adolesc Psychiatry 1999; 38:1551–1559.

16. National Institute for Health and Care Excellence. Attention deficit hyperactivity disorder in children and young people: guanfacine prolonged-release. Evidence summary ESNM70, 2016. https://www.nice.org.uk/advice/esnm70/chapter/Key-points-from-the-evidence.

17. Hazell P. Tricyclic antidepressants in children: is there a rationale for use? CNS Drugs 1996; 5:233–239.

18. Otasowie J et al. Tricyclic antidepressants for attention deficit hyperactivity disorder (ADHD) in children and adolescents. Cochrane Database Syst Rev 2014:CD006997.

19. Gorman DA et al. Canadian guidelines on pharmacotherapy for disruptive and aggressive behaviour in children and adolescents with attention-deficit hyperactivity disorder, oppositional defiant disorder, or conduct disorder. Can J Psychiatry 2015; 60:62–76.

20. Ng QX. A systematic review of the use of bupropion for attention-deficit/hyperactivity disorder in children and adolescents. J Child Adolesc Psychopharmacol 2017; 27:112–116.

21. Biederman J et al. A comparison of once-daily and divided doses of modafinil in children with attention-deficit/hyperactivity disorder: a randomized, double-blind, and placebo-controlled study. J Clin Psychiatry 2006; 67:727–735.

22. Wang SM et al. Modafinil for the treatment of attention-deficit/hyperactivity disorder: a meta-analysis. J Psychiatr Res 2017; 84:292–300.

23. Einarson TR et al. Novel antipsychotics for patients with attention-deficit hyperactivity disorder: a systematic review. Ottawa: Canadian Coordinating Office for Health Technology Assessment (CCOHTA) 2001:Technology Report No 17.

24. Pringsheim T et al. The pharmacological management of oppositional behaviour, conduct problems, and aggression in children and adolescents with attention-deficit hyperactivity disorder, oppositional defiant disorder, and conduct disorder: a systematic review and meta-analysis. Part 2: antipsychotics and traditional mood stabilizers. Can J Psychiatry 2015; 60:52–61.

25. Correia Filho AG et al. Comparison of risperidone and methylphenidate for reducing ADHD symptoms in children and adolescents with moderate mental retardation. J Am Acad Child Adolesc Psychiatry 2005; 44:748–755.

26. Humphreys KL et al. Stimulant medication and substance use outcomes: a meta-analysis. JAMA Psychiatry 2013; 70:740–749.

27. Treuer T et al. A systematic review of combination therapy with stimulants and atomoxetine for attention-deficit/hyperactivity disorder, including patient characteristics, treatment strategies, effectiveness, and tolerability. J Child Adolesc Psychopharmacol 2013; 23:179–193.

28. DIVA Foundation. DIVA 2.0: Diagnostic Interview for ADHD in adults (DIVA), 2010. http://www.divacenter.eu/Content/VertalingPDFs/DIVA_2_EN_FORM%20-%20invulbaar.pdf.

29. Cosgrove PVF. Attention deficit hyperactivity disorder. Primary Care Psychiatry 1997; 3:101–114.

30. Spencer T et al. A double-blind, crossover comparison of methylphenidate and placebo in adults with childhood-onset attention-deficit hyperactivity disorder. Arch Gen Psychiatry 1995; 52:434–443.

31. Wolraich ML, Doffing MA. Pharmacokinetic considerations in the treatment of attention-deficit hyperactivity disorder with methylphenidate. CNS Drugs 2004; 18:243–250.

32. BNF Online. British National Formulary, 2017. https://www.medicinescomplete.com/mc/bnf/current/.

33. Electronic Medicines Compendium. Summary of Product Characteristics, 2017. Methylphenidate hydrochloride. https://www.medicines.org. uk/emc/.

34. Efron D et al. Side effects of methylphenidate and dexamphetamine in children with attention deficit hyperactivity disorder: a double-blind, crossover trial. Pediatrics 1997; 100:662–666.

35. Hennissen L et al. Cardiovascular effects of stimulant and non-stimulant medication for children and adolescents with ADHD: a systematic review and meta-analysis of trials of methylphenidate, amphetamines and atomoxetine. CNS Drugs 2017; 31:199–215.

36. Gadow KD et al. Efficacy of methylphenidate for attention-deficit hyperactivity disorder in children with tic disorder. Arch Gen Psychiatry 1995; 52:444–455.

37. Cohen SC et al. Meta-analysis: risk of tics associated with psychostimulant use in randomized, placebo-controlled trials. J Am Acad Child Adolesc Psychiatry 2015; 54:728–736.

38. Hoare P et al. 12-month efficacy and safety of OROS MPH in children and adolescents with attention-deficit/hyperactivity disorder switched from MPH I. Eur Child Adolesc Psychiatry 2005; 14:305–309.

39. Remschmidt H et al. Symptom control in children and adolescents with attention-deficit/hyperactivity disorder on switching from immediate-release MPH to OROS MPH. Results of a 3-week open-label study. Eur Child Adolesc Psychiatry 2005; 14:297–304.

40. Wolraich ML et al. Randomized, controlled trial of OROS methylphenidate once a day in children with attention-deficit/hyperactivity disorder. Pediatrics 2001; 108:883–892.

41. Findling RL et al. Comparison of the clinical efficacy of twice-daily Ritalin and once-daily Equasym XL with placebo in children with Attention Deficit/Hyperactivity Disorder. Eur Child Adolesc Psychiatry 2006; 15:450–459.

42. Anderson VR et al. Spotlight on Methylphenidate Controlled-Delivery Capsules (Equasym XL™) in the treatment of children and adolescents with Attention-Deficit Hyperactivity Disorder. CNS Drugs 2007; 21:173–175.

43. Flynn Pharma Ltd. Summary of Product Characteristics. Medikinet XL, 2017. https://www.medicines.org.uk/emc/medicine/19510.

44. Cyr M et al. Current drug therapy recommendations for the treatment of attention deficit hyperactivity disorder. Drugs 1998; 56:215–223.

45. Shire Pharmaceuticals Limited. Summary of Product Characteristics. Elvanse 20 mg, 30 mg, 40 mg, 50 mg, 60 mg & 70 mg Capsules, hard (lisdexafetamine), 2016. https://www.medicines.org.uk/emc/medicine/27442.

46. Kelsey DK et al. Once-daily atomoxetine treatment for children with attention-deficit/hyperactivity disorder, including an assessment of evening and morning behavior: a double-blind, placebo-controlled trial. Pediatrics 2004; 114:e1–e8.

47. Wernicke JF et al. Cardiovascular effects of atomoxetine in children, adolescents, and adults. Drug Saf 2003; 26:729–740.

48. Heil SH et al. Comparison of the subjective, physiological, and psychomotor effects of atomoxetine and methylphenidate in light drug users. Drug Alcohol Depend 2002; 67:149–156.

49. Reed VA et al. The safety of atomoxetine for the treatment of children and adolescents with attention-deficit/hyperactivity disorder: a comprehensive review of over a decade of research. CNS Drugs 2016; 30:603–628.

50. Cortese S et al. New formulations of methylphenidate for the treatment of attention-deficit/hyperactivity disorder: pharmacokinetics, efficacy, and tolerability. CNS Drugs 2017; 31:149–160.

CHAPTER 5

Autism spectrum disorder

Autism spectrum disorder (ASD) is a complex condition characterised by core deficits in three areas of development: language, social interaction and behaviour (stereotypies and/or restricted and unusual patterns of interests). The autism spectrum comprises autism, Asperger's syndrome and pervasive developmental disorders not otherwise specified (PDD-NOS) and is categorised under pervasive developmental disorders (PDD) in ICD 10. DSM-V no longer includes these sub-groups but defines ASD in one single category. Rett's syndrome and childhood disintegrative disorder are also categorised under PDD in the ICD, though they are aetiologically distinct, with different characteristics and outcomes from ASD.

The heterogeneity of ASD in presentation poses assessment and treatment challenges. Evidence suggests a high prevalence of psychiatric co-morbid conditions in ASD (70% have at least one and 41% more than one).[1] These include attention deficit hyperactivity disorder (ADHD), disruptive behavioural disorders, anxiety, obsessive compulsive and mood disorders. Other associated problems include intellectual disability, epilepsy, sleep disturbance, self-harm, irritability and aggression towards others. The presence of co-morbid neurodevelopmental, medical and psychiatric disorders may complicate the symptom profile and affect outcome and overall prognosis. Evaluating and optimally treating co-morbid conditions and/or associated problem behaviours is, therefore, essential.

Currently there are no validated pharmacological treatments that alleviate core ASD symptoms.[2,3] Targeting problem behaviours and co-morbid psychiatric conditions with pharmacological interventions is, however, common practice.

Pharmacotherapies are commonly used in individuals with ASD as adjuncts to psychological interventions. The bulk of the high-level evidence to date is for the efficacy of risperidone, aripiprazole, methylphenidate and some selective serotonin reuptake inhibitors (SSRIs) in the treatment of problem behaviours or co-existing disorders in ASD. Despite being widely used, the evidence for sodium valproate, atomoxetine and other psychotropic medication is relatively poor. There is a potential role for alpha$_2$-agonists, cholinergic agonists, glutamatergic agents and oxytocin but these require further investigation.[3–5]

Individuals with ASD are likely to experience more severe adverse effects than typically developing counterparts.[2,3] Therefore, achieving an effective dose with minimum adverse effects can be a challenging task. Treatment should be initiated in small doses and increased about every five half-lives of the drug, and it may take 4–6 weeks of titration to determine the therapeutic dose for every individual case.[6] Excluding any medical conditions, the presence of pain or any other physical discomfort such as gastro-oesophageal reflux must be a priority before managing problem behaviour with psychotropic drugs. A comprehensive physical examination should be part of standard practice.

The efficacy and adverse effects associated with pharmacotherapy in individuals with ASD should be systematically monitored, in view of their impaired communication and the increased propensity for more adverse effects. Standardised behaviour ratings scales and adverse effect checklists are an essential tool in monitoring progress.[7]

Pharmacological treatment of core symptoms of ASD

Restricted repetitive behaviours and interests

Restricted repetitive behaviours and interests (RRBIs) are distressing and disruptive to functioning and therefore an important treatment target to improve overall outcomes in ASD.[8] Behavioural therapies should be used as first line. When RRBIs are severe with significant impact on functioning and/or pose risks to others or self, then pharmacotherapy can be considered.

SSRIs were thought to be effective and have therefore become perhaps the most widely prescribed medications to treat RRBIs in paediatric ASD populations. The SSRIs that have been studied include fluoxetine, fluvoxamine, sertraline, citalopram and escitalopram. While adverse effects have generally been considered to be mild, increased behavioural activation and agitation occurred in some subjects. However, the evidence supporting the effectiveness of SSRIs in this respect mainly comes from single case studies and open-label trials with only a few RCTs published to date.[9-11] The available literature reports inconsistent benefit from SSRIs and there remains uncertainty about the optimal dose regime, which may be lower than those used for treatment of depression in typically developing individuals.[12,13] The mean dose of fluoxetine is around 10 mg per day, starting with 2.5 mg (see Box 5.5). A Cochrane review published in 2013 found 'no evidence of effect of SSRIs in children and emerging evidence of harm'.[14]

Other potential pharmacological treatments include second-generation antipsychotics,[15] anticonvulsants[16] and the neuropeptide, oxytocin.[17] Research with respect to risperidone indicates that it is effective in reducing repetitive behaviours in children who have high levels of irritability or aggression.[18] Reductions in stereotypical behaviours have also been reported.[3,15,19-21]

Social and communication impairment

Currently, no drug has been consistently shown to improve the core social and communication impairments in ASD.[6] **Risperidone** may have a secondary effect through improvement in irritability.[22] Analysis of data from two multicentre trials suggested that risperidone was effective for the treatment of social disability in children with ASD.[23] Glutamatergic drugs and oxytocin are currently the most promising.[24] However, a recent meta-analysis of 12 RCTs suggested that **oxytocin** has no significant effect on these two domains even though individual RCTs (7 out of the 11 studies that examined social cognition and one out of the 4 studies on RRBIs) had reported improvements from oxytocin.[25] Given the limited number of RCTs, the findings on the effectiveness of oxytocin in ASD should still be considered as unproven. Larger studies with better methodology are needed.[26] **Sulforaphane**,[27] and **insulin growth factor 1** (IGF-1)[28] await further work to prove their efficacy in modifying ASD core symptoms, as do **glutamatergic agents**.[29] **Acetylcysteine**[30] is probably not effective.

Pharmacological treatment of co-morbid problem behaviours in ASD

Inattention, overactivity and impulsiveness in ASD (symptoms of ADHD)

Children with ASD have high rates of inattention, overactivity and impulsiveness and in an around one-third these symptoms merit the diagnosis of ADHD.[1,31] Adequate numbers of controlled trials of pharmacotherapy to treat these symptoms in children with ASD are lacking.[32]

The largest controlled trial to date has been with **methylphenidate** and was conducted by the Research Units on Paediatric Psychopharmacology (RUPP) Autism Network.[33,34] In a previous retrospective and prospective study of children with ASD, Santosh and colleagues[35] reported positive benefits of treatment with methylphenidate. In general, methylphenidate produces highly variable responses in children with ASD and ADHD symptoms. These responses range from a marked improvement with few adverse effects through to poor response with or without problematic adverse effects. A large double-blind placebo-controlled trial of methylphenidate in children with intellectual disability and ADHD showed that optimal dosing with methylphenidate was effective in some.[36] Adverse effects are more commonly reported than in children with ADHD alone.[37–39] However, where ADHD symptoms are severe and/or disabling, it is reasonable to proceed with a treatment trial of methylphenidate. It is advisable to warn parents of the lower likelihood of response and the potential adverse effects and to proceed with a low initial dose (~0.125 mg/kg three times daily, depending on the preparation) increasing with small increments. Treatment should be stopped immediately if behaviour deteriorates or there are unacceptable adverse effects.

There are no published data on the efficacy of **amphetamines** in children with ASD even though they have been used to treat ADHD in these patients as well as typically developed children. **Lisdexamfetamine** (a prodrug containing D-amphetamine bound to the amino acid lysine) has been found to have efficacy and tolerability in treating ADHD in children and young people[40] but there are no specific data about those with ASD.

Atomoxetine is a noradrenergic reuptake inhibitor licensed to treat ADHD. There is preliminary evidence from small open-label trials and a handful of randomised double-blind trials[41,42] that it may be useful in children with ASD but large-scale RCTs are awaited.[43] A recent review has suggested that atomoxetine is more effective in individuals with milder ASD symptoms.[44] Whilst the number of open-label and RCTs is increasing, the evidence of benefit across the severity of ASD spectrum remains conflicting.

There is some evidence from controlled studies supporting the use of **risperidone** and **alpha$_2$-agonists** (clonidine and guanfacine). A recent multisite RCT of extended-release guanfacine compared with placebo in children with ASD (mean age 8.5 years) over a period of 8 weeks showed that it is safe and effective in managing hyperactivity in this group.[45]

There is little or no evidence to support the use of **SSRIs, venlafaxine, benzodiazepines** or anti-epileptic **mood stabilisers**.[46]

Irritability (aggression, self-injurious behaviour, severe disruptive behaviours)

Aggression towards others and the self are common problems in ASD. Although behavioural and environment approaches should be first-line treatments, more severe and dangerous behaviours usually necessitate pharmacotherapy.[47] Duration of recommended treatment is difficult to derive from published evidence but treatment appears to be beneficial for up to 6–12 months.[48] Efforts to reduce and possibly discontinue such treatment at the end of this period should be strongly considered.[47,48]

Second-generation antipsychotics (SGAs) are the first-line pharmacological treatment for children and adolescents with ASD and associated irritability.[48–50] **Risperidone**[51,52] and **aripiprazole**[53] have been (relatively) reliably shown to help irritability, disruptive behaviours, aggression and hyperactivity.[2] Both have been approved by the FDA to treat irritability associated with ASD. A recent systematic review[54] carried out a meta-analysis of data from 46 RCTs comparing efficacy of risperidone, aripiprazole and other compounds with placebo. Risperidone and aripiprazole were the most effective, with large effect sizes. Although other compounds showed some efficacy with perhaps better tolerability, these results were yielded from single studies. A recent review and meta-analysis of short-term (8 weeks) aripiprazole in the treatment of irritability in ASD children aged 6–17 years[55] found there to be a significant reduction in irritability with a moderate effect size, when compared with placebo. The most recent Cochrane review,[56] which is an update of the previous one,[57] concluded that aripiprazole may be beneficial in managing irritability, hyperactivity and stereotypies in children with ASD. The usual recommended clinical dose of aripiprazole for maintenance is between 5 and 15 mg daily.[48] The starting dose of aripiprazole is 2 mg/day. The dosing of risperidone is rather more complicated; FDA-recommended dosages for risperidone are outlined in Box 5.4.

Despite risperidone and aripiprazole offering promise, adverse effects such as weight gain and metabolic changes, increased appetite and somnolence (even with aripiprazole) can be problematic.[21,58–61] One long-term, placebo discontinuation study found that relapse rates did not differ between those who stayed on aripiprazole versus those randomised to switch to only placebo, suggesting that re-evaluation of aripiprazole use after a period of stabilisation in irritability symptoms is warranted.[56] There is only one study that makes a direct head-to-head comparison[62] showing similar tolerability and efficacy profiles for risperidone and aripiprazole. Of course, risperidone usually causes hyperprolactinaemia which may not be symptomatic but which may have longer-term effects. Close monitoring is advised.

Box 5.4 FDA guidance for risperidone dosing in children and adolescents[78]

Doses of risperidone in paediatric patients with autism spectrum disorders (by total mg/day)

Weight categories	Days 1–3	Days 4–18	Increments if dose increases are needed	Dose range
<20 kg*	0.25 mg	0.5 mg	+0.25 mg at ≥2 week intervals	0.5–3 mg**
≥20 kg	0.5 mg	1.0 mg	+0.5 mg at ≥2 week intervals	1.0–3 mg***

* Caution should be exercised for children <15 kg – no dosing data available.
** Therapeutic effect plateaus at 1 mg/day.
*** Those weighing >45 kg may require higher doses – therapeutic effect plateaus at 3 mg.

General considerations

- Risperidone can be administered once daily or twice daily.
- Patients experiencing somnolence may benefit from taking the whole daily dose at bedtime.
- Once sufficient clinical response has been achieved and maintained, consideration may be given to gradually lowering the dose to achieve the optimal balance of efficacy and safety.
- There is insufficient evidence from controlled trials to indicate how long treatment should continue.

Adverse effects

Weight gain, somnolence and hyperglycaemia require monitoring, and the long-term safety of risperidone in children and adolescents with ASD remains to be fully determined.

The effectiveness of other SGAs such as **olanzapine**,[16] **quetiapine, ziprasidone** and **clozapine** has not been tested in adequately powered RCTs. Whilst controlled studies support the use of mood stabilisers such as **lithium**[63,64] and **sodium valproate**[65] as being effective in the treatment of persistent aggression in the paediatric population, available data suggest that mood stabilisers and anticonvulsants may not be as effective as SGAs for the treatment of irritability in ASD.[66] Limited data support the combination of risperidone and **topiramate** being better than risperidone alone.[67] Further RCTs are warranted of brain-derived neurotrophic factor stimulators such as loxapine and amitriptyline.[68]

Using **benzodiazepines** to manage irritability and aggression in ASD is not recommended. However, it may be necessary to manage acute aggression with a benzodiazepine. The possibility of behavioural disinhibition which may worsen aggression must be borne in mind.

Sleep disturbance

Children with ASD have significant sleep problems[69] with sleep-onset insomnia, sleep-maintenance insomnia, and irregularities of the sleep–wake cycle being the typical problems encountered. It is essential to understand the aetiology of the sleep problem before embarking on a course of treatment. Abnormalities in the melatonin system have received some attention.[70]

Melatonin has been shown in 17 studies to be beneficial in children with ASD.[71] More recent RCTs continue to show promising results although larger RCTs are needed.[48] Doses ranged from 1 mg to 10 mg. Melatonin is usually very well tolerated.[72,73] An RCT published in 2013 showed that whilst melatonin improved sleep onset, the child's behaviour during the day did not improve.[74]

Risperidone may benefit sleep difficulties in those with extreme irritability. In the anxious or depressed child, antidepressants may be beneficial. Insomnia due to hyperarousal may benefit from clonidine or clonazepam.[75]

Anxiety and depression

SSRIs (sertraline, fluvoxamine, citalopram), despite being widely used to treat anxiety and depression in typically developing young people and those with ASD, have yet to show specific efficacy in ASD. There are some data on **buspirone** effectively targeting anxiety in ASD[76] and propranolol showing positive cognitive effects in ASD.[77] However, further evaluation is needed.

Use of risperidone in children and adolescents (Box 5.4)

Risperidone is indicated for the treatment of irritability associated with autistic disorder in children (aged 5 and over) and adolescents in the UK/EU and USA.

The dosage of risperidone should be individualised according to the response of the patient.

> ### Box 5.5   Use of fluoxetine in children and adolescents
>
> **Liquid fluoxetine:** (as hydrochloride) 20 mg/5 mL
>
> 2.5 mg/day a day for 1 week; note that 2.5 mg = 0.625 mL, which is difficult to measure accurately.
>
> Follow with flexible titration schedule based on weight, tolerability and adverse effects up to a maximum dose of 0.8 mg/kg/day (0.3 mg/kg for week 2, 0.5 mg/kg/day for week 3, and 0.8 mg/kg/day subsequently). Reduction may be indicated if adverse effects are problematic.
>
> **Adverse effects**
>
> - Monitor for treatment-emergent **suicidal** behaviour, self-harm and hostility, particularly at the beginning of treatment.
> - Hyponatraemia is also possible – see section in Chapter 3.

Use of fluoxetine in children and adolescents

When using fluoxetine to treat repetitive behaviours in ASD patients, doses much lower than those used to treat depression are normally required. It is advisable to use a liquid preparation and begin at the lowest possible dose, monitoring for adverse effects. A suitable regime is outlined in Box 5.5.

References

1. Simonoff E et al. Psychiatric disorders in children with autism spectrum disorders: prevalence, comorbidity, and associated factors in a population-derived sample. J Am Acad Child Adolesc Psychiatry 2008; **47**:921–929.
2. Accordino RE et al. Psychopharmacological interventions in autism spectrum disorder. Expert Opin Pharmacother 2016; **17**:937–952.
3. Ji N et al. An update on pharmacotherapy for autism spectrum disorder in children and adolescents. Curr Opin Psychiatry 2015; **28**:91–101.
4. Canitano R. New experimental treatments for core social domain in autism spectrum disorders. Front Pediatr 2014; **2**:61.
5. Politte LC et al. Psychopharmacological interventions in autism spectrum disorder. Harv Rev Psychiatry 2014; **22**:76–92.
6. Santosh P. Medication in autism spectrum disorder. Cut Edge Psychiatry Pract 2014; **1**:143–155.
7. Greenhill LL. Assessment of safety in pediatric psychopharmacology. J Am Acad Child Adolesc Psychiatry 2003; **42**:625–626.
8. Leekam SR et al. Restricted and repetitive behaviors in autism spectrum disorders: a review of research in the last decade. Psychol Bull 2011; **137**:562–593.
9. McDougle CJ et al. A double-blind, placebo-controlled study of fluvoxamine in adults with autistic disorder. Arch Gen Psychiatry 1996; **53**:1001–1008.
10. Buchsbaum MS et al. Effect of fluoxetine on regional cerebral metabolism in autistic spectrum disorders: a pilot study. Int J Neuropsychopharmacol 2001; **4**:119–125.
11. Hollander E et al. A placebo controlled crossover trial of liquid fluoxetine on repetitive behaviors in childhood and adolescent autism. Neuropsychopharmacology 2005; **30**:582–589.
12. Aman MG et al. Medication patterns in patients with autism: temporal, regional, and demographic influences. J Child Adolesc Psychopharmacol 2005; **15**:116–126.
13. Soorya L et al. Psychopharmacologic interventions for repetitive behaviors in autism spectrum disorders. Child Adolesc Psychiatr Clin N Am 2008; **17**:753–771.
14. Williams K et al. Selective serotonin reuptake inhibitors (SSRIs) for autism spectrum disorders (ASD). Cochrane Database Syst Rev 2013; **8**:CD004677.
15. McDougle CJ et al. Risperidone for the core symptom domains of autism: results from the study by the autism network of the research units on pediatric psychopharmacology. Am J Psychiatry 2005; **162**:1142–1148.
16. Hollander E et al. A double-blind placebo-controlled pilot study of olanzapine in childhood/adolescent pervasive developmental disorder. J Child Adolesc Psychopharmacol 2006; **16**:541–548.
17. Hollander E et al. Oxytocin infusion reduces repetitive behaviors in adults with autistic and Asperger's disorders. Neuropsychopharmacology 2003; **28**:193–198.
18. McDougle CJ et al. A double-blind, placebo-controlled study of risperidone addition in serotonin reuptake inhibitor-refractory obsessive-compulsive disorder. Arch Gen Psychiatry 2000; **57**:794–801.

CHAPTER 5

19. McCracken JT et al. Risperidone in children with autism and serious behavioral problems. N Engl J Med 2002; 347:314–321.
20. Arnold LE et al. Parent-defined target symptoms respond to risperidone in RUPP autism study: customer approach to clinical trials. J Am Acad Child Adolesc Psychiatry 2003; 42:1443–1450.
21. Dinnissen M et al. Clinical and pharmacokinetic evaluation of risperidone for the management of autism spectrum disorder. Expert Opin Drug Metab Toxicol 2015; 11:111–124.
22. Canitano R et al. Risperidone in the treatment of behavioral disorders associated with autism in children and adolescents. Neuropsychiatr Dis Treat 2008; 4:723–730.
23. Scahill L et al. Brief Report: social disability in autism spectrum disorder: results from Research Units on Pediatric Psychopharmacology (RUPP) Autism Network trials. J Autism Dev Disord 2013; 43:739–746.
24. Posey DJ et al. Developing drugs for core social and communication impairment in autism. Child Adolesc Psychiatr Clin N Am 2008; 17:787–801.
25. Ooi YP et al. Oxytocin and autism spectrum disorders: a systematic review and meta-analysis of randomized controlled trials. Pharmacopsychiatry 2017; 50:5–13.
26. Alvares GA et al. Beyond the hype and hope: critical considerations for intranasal oxytocin research in autism spectrum disorder. Autism Res 2017; 10:25–41.
27. Singh K et al. Sulforaphane treatment of autism spectrum disorder (ASD). Proc Natl Acad Sci U S A 2014; 111:15550–15555.
28. Riikonen R. Treatment of autistic spectrum disorder with insulin-like growth factors. Eur J Paediatr Neurol 2016; 20:816–823.
29. Fung LK et al. Developing medications targeting glutamatergic dysfunction in autism: progress to date. CNS Drugs 2015; 29:453–463.
30. Dean OM et al. A randomised, double blind, placebo-controlled trial of a fixed dose of N-acetyl cysteine in children with autistic disorder. Aust N Z J Psychiatry 2017; 51:241–249.
31. Lee YJ et al. Advanced pharmacotherapy evidenced by pathogenesis of autism spectrum disorder. Clin Psychopharmacol Neurosci 2014; 12:19–30.
32. Mahajan R et al. Clinical practice pathways for evaluation and medication choice for attention-deficit/hyperactivity disorder symptoms in autism spectrum disorders. Pediatrics 2012; 130 Suppl 2:S125–S138.
33. Research Units on Pediatric Psychopharmacology (RUPP) Autism Network. Randomized, controlled, crossover trial of methylphenidate in pervasive developmental disorders with hyperactivity. Arch Gen Psychiatry 2005; 62:1266–1274.
34. Posey DJ et al. Positive effects of methylphenidate on inattention and hyperactivity in pervasive developmental disorders: an analysis of secondary measures. Biol Psychiatry 2007; 61:538–544.
35. Santosh PJ et al. Impact of comorbid autism spectrum disorders on stimulant response in children with attention deficit hyperactivity disorder: a retrospective and prospective effectiveness study. Child Care Health Dev 2006; 32:575–583.
36. Simonoff E et al. Randomized controlled double-blind trial of optimal dose methylphenidate in children and adolescents with severe attention deficit hyperactivity disorder and intellectual disability. J Child Psychol Psychiatry 2013; 54:527–535.
37. Sung M et al. What's in the pipeline? Drugs in development for autism spectrum disorder. Neuropsychiatr Dis Treat 2014; 10:371–381.
38. Siegel M et al. Psychotropic medications in children with autism spectrum disorders: a systematic review and synthesis for evidence-based practice. J Autism Dev Disord 2012; 42:1592–1605.
39. Williamson ED et al. Psychotropic medications in autism: practical considerations for parents. J Autism Dev Disord 2012; 42:1249–1255.
40. Coghill D et al. European, randomized, phase 3 study of lisdexamfetamine dimesylate in children and adolescents with attention-deficit/hyperactivity disorder. Eur Neuropsychopharmacol 2013; 23:1208–1218.
41. Arnold LE et al. Atomoxetine for hyperactivity in autism spectrum disorders: placebo-controlled crossover pilot trial. J Am Acad Child Adolesc Psychiatry 2006; 45:1196–1205.
42. Harfterkamp M et al. A randomized double-blind study of atomoxetine versus placebo for attention-deficit/hyperactivity disorder symptoms in children with autism spectrum disorder. J Am Acad Child Adolesc Psychiatry 2012; 51:733–741.
43. Aman MG et al. A review of atomoxetine effects in young people with developmental disabilities. Res Dev Disabil 2014; 35:1412–1424.
44. Ghanizadeh A. Atomoxetine for treating ADHD symptoms in autism: a systematic review. J Atten Disord 2013; 17:635–640.
45. Scahill L et al. Extended-release guanfacine for hyperactivity in children with autism spectrum disorder. Am J Psychiatry 2015; 172:1197–1206.
46. Aman MG et al. Treatment of inattention, overactivity, and impulsiveness in autism spectrum disorders. Child Adolesc Psychiatr Clin N Am 2008; 17:713–738, vii.
47. National Institute for Health and Care Excellence. Autism spectrum disorder in under 19s: support and management. Clinical Guidance 170, 2013. https://www.nice.org.uk/cg170.
48. Kaplan G et al. Psychopharmacology of autism spectrum disorders. Pediatr Clin North Am 2012; 59:175–187, xii.
49. McDougle CJ et al. Atypical antipsychotics in children and adolescents with autistic and other pervasive developmental disorders. J Clin Psychiatry 2008; 69 Suppl 4:15–20.
50. Parikh MS et al. Psychopharmacology of aggression in children and adolescents with autism: a critical review of efficacy and tolerability. J Child Adolesc Psychopharmacol 2008; 18:157–178.
51. Jesner OS et al. Risperidone for autism spectrum disorder. Cochrane Database Syst Rev 2007:CD005040.
52. Scahill L et al. Risperidone approved for the treatment of serious behavioral problems in children with autism. J Child Adolesc Psychiatr Nurs 2007; 20:188–190.
53. Curran MP. Aripiprazole: in the treatment of irritability associated with autistic disorder in pediatric patients. Paediatr Drugs 2011; 13:197–204.

CHAPTER 5

54. Fung LK et al. Pharmacologic treatment of severe irritability and problem behaviors in autism: a systematic review and meta-analysis. Pediatrics 2016; **137 Suppl** 2:S124–135.

55. Douglas-Hall P et al. Aripiprazole: a review of its use in the treatment of irritability associated with autistic disorder patients aged 6–17. J Cent Nerv Syst Dis 2011; **3**:1–11.

56. Hirsch LE et al. Aripiprazole for autism spectrum disorders (ASD). Cochrane Database Syst Rev 2016:CD009043.

57. Ching H et al. Aripiprazole for autism spectrum disorders (ASD). Cochrane Database Syst Rev 2012; **5**:CD009043.

58. Caccia S. Safety and pharmacokinetics of atypical antipsychotics in children and adolescents. Paediatr Drugs 2013; **15**:217–233.

59. Sharma A et al. Efficacy of risperidone in managing maladaptive behaviors for children with autistic spectrum disorder: a meta-analysis. J Pediatr Health Care 2012; **26**:291–299.

60. Kent JM et al. Risperidone dosing in children and adolescents with autistic disorder: a double-blind, placebo-controlled study. J Autism Dev Disord 2013; **43**:1773–1783.

61. Maayan L et al. Weight gain and metabolic risks associated with antipsychotic medications in children and adolescents. J Child Adolesc Psychopharmacol 2011; **21**:517–535.

62. Ghanizadeh A et al. A head-to-head comparison of aripiprazole and risperidone for safety and treating autistic disorders, a randomized double blind clinical trial. Child Psychiatry Hum Dev 2014; **45**:185–192.

63. Campbell M et al. Lithium in hospitalized aggressive children with conduct disorder: a double-blind and placebo-controlled study. J Am Acad Child Adolesc Psychiatry 1995; **34**:445–453.

64. Malone RP et al. A double-blind placebo-controlled study of lithium in hospitalized aggressive children and adolescents with conduct disorder. Arch Gen Psychiatry 2000; **57**:649–654.

65. Donovan SJ et al. Divalproex treatment for youth with explosive temper and mood lability: a double-blind, placebo-controlled crossover design. Am J Psychiatry 2000; **157**:818–820.

66. Stigler KA et al. Pharmacotherapy of irritability in pervasive developmental disorders. Child Adolesc Psychiatr Clin N Am 2008; **17**:739–752.

67. Rezaei V et al. Double-blind, placebo-controlled trial of risperidone plus topiramate in children with autistic disorder. Prog Neuropsychopharmacol Biol Psychiatry 2010; **34**:1269–1272.

68. Hellings JA et al. Dopamine antagonists for treatment resistance in autism spectrum disorders: review and focus on BDNF stimulators loxapine and amitriptyline. Expert Opin Pharmacother 2017; **18**:581–588.

69. Krakowiak P et al. Sleep problems in children with autism spectrum disorders, developmental delays, and typical development: a population-based study. J Sleep Res 2008; **17**:197–206.

70. Sanchez-Barcelo EJ et al. Clinical uses of melatonin in pediatrics. Int J Pediatr 2011; **2011**:892624.

71. Doyen C et al. Melatonin in children with autistic spectrum disorders: recent and practical data. Eur Child Adolesc Psychiatry 2011; **20**:231–239.

72. Andersen IM et al. Melatonin for insomnia in children with autism spectrum disorders. J Child Neurol 2008; **23**:482–485.

73. Rossignol DA et al. Melatonin in autism spectrum disorders: a systematic review and meta-analysis. Dev Med Child Neurol 2011; **53**:783–792.

74. Gringras P et al. Melatonin for sleep problems in children with neurodevelopmental disorders: randomised double masked placebo controlled trial. BMJ 2012; **345**:e6664.

75. Johnson KP et al. Sleep in children with autism spectrum disorders. Curr Treat Options Neurol 2008; **10**:350–359.

76. Buitelaar JK et al. Buspirone in the management of anxiety and irritability in children with pervasive developmental disorders: results of an open-label study. J Clin Psychiatry 1998; **59**:56–59.

77. Narayanan A et al. Effect of propranolol on functional connectivity in autism spectrum disorder – a pilot study. Brain Imaging Behav 2010; **4**:189–197.

78. FDA. Highlights of Prescribing Information: RISPERDAL® (risperidone) tablets, RISPERDAL® (risperidone) oral solution, RISPERDAL® M-TAB® (risperidone) orally disintegrating tablets. 2009. https://www.accessdata.fda.gov/drugsatfda_docs/label/2009/020272s056,020588 s044,021346s033,021444s03lbl.pdf.

CHAPTER 5

Tics and Tourette's syndrome

Transient tics occur in 5–20% of children. Tourette's syndrome (TS) occurs in about 1% of children and is defined by persistent motor and vocal tics. As many as 65% of individuals with TS will have no or only very mild tics by adult life. Tics wax and wane over time and are variably exacerbated by external factors such as stress, inactivity and fatigue, depending on the individual. Tics are about 2–3 times more common in boys than girls.[1]

Detection and treatment of co-morbidity

Co-morbid OCD, ADHD, depression, anxiety and behavioural problems are more prevalent than would be expected by chance, and often cause the major impairment in people with tic disorders.[2] These co-morbid conditions are usually treated first before assessing the level of disability caused by the tics.[3]

Education and behavioural treatments

Most people with tics do not require pharmacological treatment; education for the individual with tics, their family and the people they interact with, especially schools, is crucial. Treatment aimed primarily at reducing tics is warranted if they cause distress to the patient or are functionally disabling. There has been a resurgence of interest in behavioural programs, and a recent RCT of a comprehensive behavioural intervention achieved an effect size of 0.68 which is comparable to the effect sizes achieved with medication for tics.[4] Habit reversal and exposure and response prevention are the behavioural treatments of choice.[5]

Pharmacological treatments

Studies of pharmacological interventions in TS are difficult to interpret for several reasons:

- There is a large inter-individual variation in tic frequency and severity. Small, randomised studies may include patients who are very different at baseline.
- The severity of tics in a given individual varies markedly over time, making it difficult to separate drug effect from natural variation.
- The bulk of the literature consists of case reports, case series, open studies and under-powered, randomised studies. Publication bias is also likely to be an issue.
- A high proportion of patients have co-morbid psychiatric illness. It can be difficult to disentangle any direct effect on tics from an effect on the co-morbid illness. This makes it difficult to interpret studies that report improvements in global functioning rather than specific reductions in tics.
- Large numbers of individuals attending clinics with TS appear to use complementary or alternative therapies and around 50% report benefit from these.[6]
- The placebo effect in clinical trials of tic disorders is not as large as previously thought.[7]
- Most of the published literature concerns children and adolescents.

Adrenergic α_2 agonists

Clonidine has been shown in open studies to reduce the severity and frequency of tics but in one study this effect did not seem to be convincingly larger than placebo.[8] Other studies have shown more substantial reductions in tics.[9-12] Therapeutic doses of clonidine are in the order of 3-5 µg/kg, and the dose should be built up gradually. A transdermal patch has also shown effectiveness.[13] Main adverse effects are sedation, postural hypotension and depression. Patients and their families should be informed not to stop clonidine suddenly because of the risk of rebound hypertension. Guanfacine has also been shown to be effective in the treatment of tics[14,15] and may merit a therapeutic trial in specific individuals (e.g. those with ADHD).

Antipsychotics

Adverse effects of antipsychotics may outweigh beneficial effects in the treatment of tics and so it is recommended that clonidine or guanfacine are always tried first. Antipsychotics may however be more effective than α_2-adrenergic agonists in alleviating tics in some individuals.

A number of first-generation antipsychotics have been used in TS.[16] In a Cochrane review, pimozide demonstrated robust efficacy in a meta-analysis of six trials.[17] In these trials, pimozide was compared with haloperidol (one trial), placebo (one trial), haloperidol and placebo (two trials) and risperidone (two trials) and was found to be more effective than placebo, as effective as risperidone and slightly less effective than haloperidol in reducing tics. It was associated with fewer adverse reactions compared with haloperidol but did not differ from risperidone in that respect. ECG monitoring is essential for pimozide and haloperidol. Haloperidol is often poorly tolerated. Given their adverse-effect profile, most authors recommend the use of second-generation rather than first-generation antipsychotics in the treatment of TS.[16]

More recent studies are suggestive that aripiprazole is an effective and well-tolerated treatment of children with TS (and also tics[18]). A 10-week multicentre double-blind randomised placebo-controlled trial (n=61) demonstrated the efficacy of aripiprazole in tic reduction in TS. Aripiprazole treatment was associated with significantly decreased serum prolactin concentration and increased mean body weight (by 1.6 kg), body mass index and waist circumference.[19] Several case series also support the use of aripiprazole.[20-23] A study evaluating the metabolic adverse effects of aripiprazole (n=25) and pimozide (n=25) in TS over a 24-month period demonstrated that treatment was not associated with significant increase in body mass index. However, pimozide treatment was associated with increases in blood glucose which did not plateau from 12 to 24 months, aripiprazole treatment was associated with increased cholesterol, and both medications were associated with increased triglycerides.[24] Two meta-analyses support the efficacy of aripiprazole.[25,26] A recent study[27] suggests twice weekly administration may be better tolerated than daily dosing.

Risperidone has, in addition to the studies previously mentioned, also been shown to be more effective than placebo in a small (n=34), randomised study.[28] Fatigue and increased appetite were problematic in the risperidone arm and a mean weight gain of 2.8 kg over 8 weeks was reported. One small RCT found risperidone and clonidine to

CHAPTER 5

be equally effective.[29] A small double-blind crossover study suggested that **olanzapine**[30] may be more effective than pimozide. **Sulpiride** has been shown to be effective and relatively well tolerated,[31] as has **ziprasidone**.[32] Open studies support the efficacy of **quetiapine**[33] and **olanzapine**.[34,35] One very small crossover study (n = 7) found no effect for **clozapine**.[36]

Overall, metabolic adverse effects and weight gain are common with second-generation antipsychotics so benefit/risk ratios need careful discussion.[16]

Other drugs

A small, double-blind, placebo-controlled, crossover trial of **baclofen** was suggestive of beneficial effects in overall impairment rather than a specific effect on tics.[37] The numerical benefits shown in this study did not reach statistical significance. Similarly, a double-blind, placebo-controlled trial of **nicotine** augmentation of haloperidol found beneficial effects in overall impairment rather than a specific effect on tics.[38] These benefits persisted for several weeks after nicotine (in the form of patches) was withdrawn. Nicotine patches were associated with a high prevalence of nausea and vomiting (71% and 40% respectively). The authors suggest that *pro re nata* (prn) use may be appropriate. **Pergolide** (a D_1-D_2-D_3 agonist) given in low dose significantly reduced tics in a double-blind, placebo-controlled, crossover study in children and adolescents.[39] Adverse effects included sedation, dizziness, nausea and irritability. Pergolide was also evaluated in a randomised trial in children and adolescents with chronic tics and TS, and showed significant tic reduction compared with placebo.[40] **Flutamide**, an anti-androgen, has been the subject of a small RCT in adults with TS. Modest, short-lived effects were seen in motor but not phonic tics.[41] A small RCT has shown significant advantages for **metoclopramide** over placebo[42] and for **topiramate** over placebo.[43] A meta-analysis identified 14 RCTs (all from China) comparing topiramate with haloperidol or **tiapride**. It concluded that owing to the overall low quality of the study designs, there is not enough evidence to support the routine use of topiramate in clinical practice.[44] Most recently the use of the monoamine depleting agent **deutetrabenazine** has been shown to be effective.[45] **Tetrabenazine** may also be useful as an add-on treatment.[46]

Case reports or case series describing positive effects for **ondansetron**,[47] **clomiphene**,[48] **tramadol**,[49] **ketanserin**,[50] **cyproterone**,[51] **levetiracetam**,[52] **pregabalin**[53] and **cannabis**[54] have been published. A Cochrane review of cannabinoids concluded that there was little if any current evidence for efficacy.[55] Many other drugs have been reported to be effective in single case reports. Patients in these reports all had co-morbid psychiatric illness, making it difficult to determine the effect of these drugs on TS alone.

Botulinum toxin has been used to treat bothersome or painful focal motor tics, particularly those affecting neck muscles.[16]

There may be a sub-group of children who develop tics and/or OCD in association with streptococcal or other infections/triggers. This group has been given, in the case of streptococcus, the acronym PANDAS (Paediatric Autoimmune Neuropsychiatric Disorder Associated with Streptococcus)[56] or more broadly the acronym PANS (Paediatric Acute-onset Neuropsychiatric Syndrome).[57] This is thought to be an

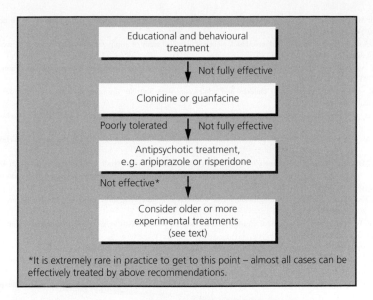

Figure 5.2 Summary of recommendations for treatment of tic/Tourette's syndrome.

autoimmune-mediated effect, and there have been trials of immune-modulatory therapy in these children as well as treatment with antibiotics for active infections and preventatively. More research in this area is warranted.

Recommended treatments for tic/Tourette's syndrome are summarised in Figure 5.2.

References

1. Murphy TK et al. Practice parameter for the assessment and treatment of children and adolescents with tic disorders. J Am Acad Child Adolesc Psychiatry 2013; 52:1341–1359.
2. Cath DC et al. European clinical guidelines for Tourette syndrome and other tic disorders. Part I: assessment. Eur Child Adolesc Psychiatry 2011; 20:155–171.
3. Singer HS. Treatment of tics and Tourette syndrome. Curr Treat Options Neurol 2010; 12:539–561.
4. Piacentini J et al. Behavior therapy for children with Tourette disorder: a randomized controlled trial. JAMA 2010; 303:1929–1937.
5. Verdellen C et al. European clinical guidelines for Tourette syndrome and other tic disorders. Part III: behavioural and psychosocial interventions. Eur Child Adolesc Psychiatry 2011; 20:197–207.
6. Kompoliti K et al. Complementary and alternative medicine use in Gilles de la Tourette syndrome. Mov Disord 2009; 24:2015–2019.
7. Cubo E et al. Impact of placebo assignment in clinical trials of tic disorders. Mov Disord 2013; 28:1288–1292.
8. Goetz CG et al. Clonidine and Gilles de la Tourette's syndrome: double-blind study using objective rating methods. Ann Neurol 1987; 21:307–310.
9. Leckman JF et al. Clonidine treatment of Gilles de la Tourette's syndrome. Arch Gen Psychiatry 1991; 48:324–328.
10. Tourette's Syndrome Study Group. Treatment of ADHD in children with tics: a randomized controlled trial. Neurology 2002; 58:527–536.
11. Du YS et al. Randomized double-blind multicentre placebo-controlled clinical trial of the clonidine adhesive patch for the treatment of tic disorders. Aust N Z J Psychiatry 2008; 42:807–813.
12. Hedderick EF et al. Double-blind, crossover study of clonidine and levetiracetam in Tourette syndrome. Pediatr Neurol 2009; 40:420–425.
13. Song PP et al. The efficacy and tolerability of the clonidine transdermal patch in the treatment for children with tic disorders: a prospective, open, single-group, Self-Controlled Study. Front Neurol 2017; 8:32.
14. Scahill L et al. A placebo-controlled study of guanfacine in the treatment of children with tic disorders and attention deficit hyperactivity disorder. Am J Psychiatry 2001; 158:1067–1074.
15. Cummings DD et al. Neuropsychiatric effects of guanfacine in children with mild Tourette syndrome: a pilot study. Clin Neuropharmacol 2002; 25:325–332.
16. Roessner V et al. Pharmacological treatment of tic disorders and Tourette Syndrome. Neuropharmacology 2013; 68:143–149.
17. Pringsheim T et al. Pimozide for tics in Tourette's syndrome. Cochrane Database Syst Rev 2009:CD006996.

CHAPTER 5

18. Yoo HK et al. An open-label study of the efficacy and tolerability of aripiprazole for children and adolescents with tic disorders. J Clin Psychiatry 2007; **68**:1088–1093.

19. Yoo HK et al. A multicenter, randomized, double-blind, placebo-controlled study of aripiprazole in children and adolescents with Tourette's disorder. J Clin Psychiatry 2013; **74**:e772–e780.

20. Davies L et al. A case series of patients with Tourette's syndrome in the United Kingdom treated with aripiprazole. Hum Psychopharmacol 2006; **21**:447–453.

21. Seo WS et al. Aripiprazole treatment of children and adolescents with Tourette disorder or chronic tic disorder. J Child Adolesc Psychopharmacol 2008; **18**:197–205.

22. Murphy TK et al. Open label aripiprazole in the treatment of youth with tic disorders. J Child Adolesc Psychopharmacol 2009; **19**:441–447.

23. Wenzel C et al. Aripiprazole for the treatment of Tourette syndrome: a case series of 100 patients. J Clin Psychopharmacol 2012; **32**:548–550.

24. Rizzo R et al. Metabolic effects of aripiprazole and pimozide in children with Tourette syndrome. Pediatr Neurol 2012; **47**:419–422.

25. Liu Y et al. Effectiveness and tolerability of aripiprazole in children and adolescents with Tourette's disorder: a meta-analysis. J Child Adolesc Psychopharmacol 2016; **26**:436–441.

26. Wang S et al. The efficacy and safety of aripiprazole for tic disorders in children and adolescents: a systematic review and meta-analysis. Psychiatry Res 2017; **254**:24–32.

27. Ghanizadeh A. Twice-weekly aripiprazole for treating children and adolescents with tic disorder, a randomized controlled clinical trial. Ann Gen Psychiatry 2016; **15**:21.

28. Scahill L et al. A placebo-controlled trial of risperidone in Tourette syndrome. Neurology 2003; **60**:1130–1135.

29. Gaffney GR et al. Risperidone versus clonidine in the treatment of children and adolescents with Tourette's syndrome. J Am Acad Child Adolesc Psychiatry 2002; **41**:330–336.

30. Onofrj M et al. Olanzapine in severe Gilles de la Tourette syndrome: a 52-week double-blind cross-over study vs. low-dose pimozide. J Neurol 2000; **247**:443–446.

31. Robertson MM et al. Management of Gilles de la Tourette syndrome using sulpiride. Clin Neuropharmacol 1990; **13**:229–235.

32. Sallee FR et al. Ziprasidone treatment of children and adolescents with Tourette's syndrome: a pilot study. J Am Acad Child Adolesc Psychiatry 2000; **39**:292–299.

33. Mukaddes NM et al. Quetiapine treatment of children and adolescents with Tourette's disorder. J Child Adolesc Psychopharmacol 2003; **13**:295–299.

34. Budman CL et al. An open-label study of the treatment efficacy of olanzapine for Tourette's disorder. J Clin Psychiatry 2001; **62**:290–294.

35. McCracken JT et al. Effectiveness and tolerability of open label olanzapine in children and adolescents with Tourette syndrome. J Child Adolesc Psychopharmacol 2008; **18**:501–508.

36. Caine ED et al. The trial use of clozapine for abnormal involuntary movement disorders. Am J Psychiatry 1979; **136**:317–320.

37. Singer HS et al. Baclofen treatment in Tourette syndrome: a double-blind, placebo-controlled, crossover trial. Neurology 2001; **56**:599–604.

38. Silver AA et al. Transdermal nicotine and haloperidol in Tourette's disorder: a double-blind placebo-controlled study. J Clin Psychiatry 2001; **62**:707–714.

39. Gilbert DL et al. Tourette's syndrome improvement with pergolide in a randomized, double-blind, crossover trial. Neurology 2000; **54**:1310–1315.

40. Gilbert DL et al. Tic reduction with pergolide in a randomized controlled trial in children. Neurology 2003; **60**:606–611.

41. Peterson BS et al. A double-blind, placebo-controlled, crossover trial of an antiandrogen in the treatment of Tourette's syndrome. J Clin Psychopharmacol 1998; **18**:324–331.

42. Nicolson R et al. A randomized, double-blind, placebo-controlled trial of metoclopramide for the treatment of Tourette's disorder. J Am Acad Child Adolesc Psychiatry 2005; **44**:640–646.

43. Jankovic J et al. A randomised, double-blind, placebo-controlled study of topiramate in the treatment of Tourette syndrome. J Neurol Neurosurg Psychiatry 2010; **81**:70–73.

44. Yang CS et al. Topiramate for Tourette's syndrome in children: a meta-analysis. Pediatr Neurol 2013; **49**:344–350.

45. Jankovic J et al. Deutetrabenazine in tics associated with Tourette syndrome. Tremor Other Hyperkinet Mov (N Y) 2016; **6**:422.

46. Porta M et al. Tourette's syndrome and role of tetrabenazine: review and personal experience. Clin Drug Invest 2008; **28**:443–459.

47. Toren P et al. Ondansetron treatment in patients with Tourette's syndrome. Int Clin Psychopharmacol 1999; **14**:373–376.

48. Sandyk R. Clomiphene citrate in Tourette's syndrome. Int J Neurosci 1988; **43**:103–106.

49. Shapira NA et al. Novel use of tramadol hydrochloride in the treatment of Tourette's syndrome. J Clin Psychiatry 1997; **58**:174–175.

50. Bonnier C et al. Ketanserin treatment of Tourette's syndrome in children. Am J Psychiatry 1999; **156**:1122–1123.

51. Izmir M et al. Cyproterone acetate treatment of Tourette's syndrome. Can J Psychiatry 1999; **44**:710–711.

52. Awaad Y et al. Use of levetiracetam to treat tics in children and adolescents with Tourette syndrome. Mov Disord 2005; **20**:714–718.

53. Hienert M et al. Pregabalin in Tourette's syndrome: a case series. Am J Psychiatry 2016; **173**:1242–1243.

54. Sandyk R et al. Marijuana and Tourette's syndrome. J Clin Psychopharmacol 1988; **8**:444–445.

55. Curtis A et al. Cannabinoids for Tourette's Syndrome. Cochrane Database Syst Rev 2009:CD006565.

56. Martino D et al. The PANDAS subgroup of tic disorders and childhood-onset obsessive-compulsive disorder. J Psychosom Res 2009; **67**:547–557.

57. Chang K et al. Clinical evaluation of youth with pediatric acute-onset neuropsychiatric syndrome (PANS): recommendations from the 2013 PANS Consensus Conference. J Child Adolesc Psychopharmacol 2015; **25**:3–13.

Melatonin in the treatment of insomnia in children and adolescents

Insomnia is a common symptom in childhood. Underlying causes may be behavioural (inappropriate sleep associations or bedtime resistance), physiological (delayed sleep phase syndrome) or related to underlying mood disorders (anxiety, depression and bipolar disorder). All forms of insomnia are more common in children with learning difficulties, autism, ADHD and sensory impairments (particularly visual). Although behavioural interventions should be the primary intervention and have a robust evidence base, exogenous melatonin is now the 'first-line' medication prescribed for childhood insomnia.[1]

Melatonin is a hormone that is produced by the pineal gland in a circadian manner. The evening rise in melatonin, enabled by darkness, precedes the onset of natural sleep by about 2 hours.[2] Melatonin is involved in the induction of sleep and in synchronisation of the circadian system.

There are a wide variety of unlicensed fast-release, slow-release and liquid preparations of melatonin. Many products rely on food-grade rather than pharmaceutical-grade melatonin and some are expensive. A prolonged-release formulation of melatonin (Circadin) was licensed in the UK in April 2008 as a short-term treatment of insomnia in patients over 55 years of age. Many children are unable to swallow these tablets, and although they can be crushed (and become immediate-release) the Product Licence has limited children's access to a pharmaceutical-grade prolonged-release preparation. A prolonged-release melatonin (PedPRM) minitablet mimicking the endogenous release profile of the hormone at night, was recently developed and evaluated in a phase III multicentre randomized, placebo-controlled study of children with autism. The study began with a 13-week double-blind treatment period followed by an extended open-label period with continued efficacy and safety monitoring. Data available to date show clinically significant improvement in caregivers' diary-reported sleep initiation and maintenance (sleep latency, total sleep time, longest sleep period).[3] Effects were maintained in the long-term period. The medication was well tolerated and no unexpected safety issues were reported. Secondary outcomes showed improvements in child's social functioning and behaviour, and caregivers' well-being. Results from the study will form part of a Marketing Authorisation submission and in time a licensed paediatric melatonin product. Until then, use of melatonin in this population will be off-label but with clinicians following MHRA guidance to prescribe a licensed formulation where possible (i.e. Circadin).[4]

Lack of any 'head to head' studies means that there are still no good data on whether, or when, immediate- or slow-release melatonin preparations should be used but data suggest they have similar effects on sleep latency and duration. There are additionally a number of melatonin analogues already produced, or in development,[5] although they are virtually never used in the paediatric population. There is no evidence from equivalence studies of any superiority over melatonin itself.

Efficacy

Two meta-analyses on the use of melatonin in sleep disorders have been published.[6,7] Both pooled data from studies in children and adults. The first considered melatonin in primary sleep disorders (not accompanied by any medical or psychiatric disorder likely to account for the sleep problem) and showed improvements in the time taken to fall asleep of just over 10 minutes across the group, but this improved to nearly 40 minutes if delayed sleep phase syndrome was the underlying cause. The study considering melatonin in secondary sleep disorders found no significant effect on sleep latency in this rather heterogeneous group.

Since these meta-analyses, many smaller RCTs comparing melatonin with placebo in children have been published.[8-14] Studies have considered diverse groups including children with sleep phase delay, ADHD, ASD, intellectual disability and epilepsy. Results are surprisingly consistent considering the different underlying disorders. Children in these studies fall asleep about 30 minutes quicker and their total time asleep increases by a similar amount of time (roughly 20–50 minutes). The effect size for sleep latency is much greater than that for total sleep time, confirming that melatonin is of most use for sleep initiation, rather than sleep maintenance. Importantly, over time, a number of children who fall asleep earlier on melatonin will also start to wake up earlier on melatonin.

The two largest RCTs to date considered the use of melatonin for children with ASD and neurodevelopmental delay.[15,16] Both employed a behavioural intervention, although with different designs. Together they demonstrated the value of a sleep behavioural intervention before melatonin treatment, and the value of continuing the behavioural intervention during melatonin administration. Both studies showed similar effectiveness of melatonin for sleep latency, but total sleep time was increased more in the study that used a combined slow-/fast-release preparation of melatonin.

Adverse effects

Many of the children who have received melatonin in RCTs and published case series had developmental problems and/or sensory deficits. The scope for detecting subtle adverse effects in this population is limited. Screening for adverse effects was not routine in all studies. Early reports included a very small case series where melatonin was reported to worsen seizures[17] and exacerbate asthma[18,19] in the short term. Other reported adverse effects include headache, depression, restlessness, confusion, nausea, tachycardia and pruritus.[20,21] In the more recent largest placebo-controlled studies to date involving children with learning difficulty, autism and epilepsy,[12,14,15] and the most recent (PedPRM) minitablet study, there were no excess adverse effects in the treatment group over that recorded for placebo, and in particular seizures were not worsened. A recent Cochrane review found no worsening of seizure frequency in patients with epilepsy given melatonin.[22]

Dose

The cut-off point between physiological and pharmacological doses in children is less than 500 µg. Physiological doses of melatonin may result in very high receptor occupancy. The doses used in RCTs and published case series vary hugely with between 500 µg and 5 mg being the most common doses although much lower and higher doses have been used. The optimal dose is unknown and there is no evidence to support a direct relationship between dose and response.[23] In one large RCT, 18% of children

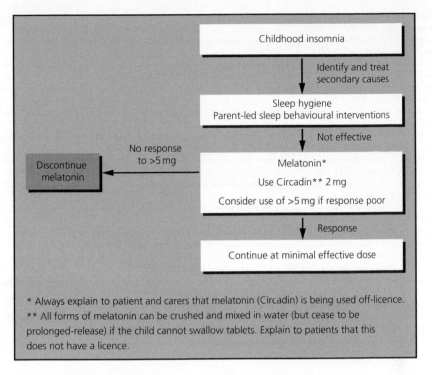

Figure 5.3 Summary of recommendations for the use of melatonin.

seemed to respond to a 500 µg dose but others seemed to require much higher doses (12 mg).[15] Increasing doses above 5 mg is likely to provoke the direct sedative effects of melatonin, rather than its sleep phase shifting properties. This might be necessary and helpful for some children with severe and bilateral brain injury.

The use of salivary melatonin measurements is an expensive but effective way to identify those children with the most delayed sleep phase (likely to have the best response to exogenous melatonin) and those children who are slow metabolisers of melatonin in whom serum levels accumulate during the daytime (particularly on higher doses) and in whom efficacy will eventually be lost.

See Figure 5.3 for a summary of recommendations for the use of melatonin.

References

1. Gringras P. When to use drugs to help sleep. Arch Dis Child 2008; 93:976–981.
2. Macchi MM et al. Human pineal physiology and functional significance of melatonin. Front Neuroendocrinol 2004; 25:177–195.
3. Gringras P et al. Efficacy and safety of pediatric prolonged-release melatonin for insomnia in children with autism spectrum disorder. J Am Acad Child Adolesc Psychiatry 2017; 56:948–957.
4. Medicines and Healthcare Products Regulatory Agency. Restrictions on the import of unlicensed Melatonin products following the grant of a marketing authorisation for Circadin ® 2mg tablets. 2008. http://www.mhra.gov.uk.
5. Arendt J et al. Melatonin and its agonists: an update. Br J Psychiatry 2008; 193:267–269.
6. Buscemi N et al. The efficacy and safety of exogenous melatonin for primary sleep disorders. A meta analysis. J Gen Intern Med 2005; 20:1151–1158.

CHAPTER 5

7. Buscemi N et al. Efficacy and safety of exogenous melatonin for secondary sleep disorders and sleep disorders accompanying sleep restriction: meta-analysis. BMJ 2006; 332:385–393.

8. Van der Heijden KB et al. Effect of melatonin on sleep, behavior, and cognition in ADHD and chronic sleep-onset insomnia. J Am Acad Child Adolesc Psychiatry 2007; 46:233–241.

9. Wasdell MB et al. A randomized, placebo-controlled trial of controlled release melatonin treatment of delayed sleep phase syndrome and impaired sleep maintenance in children with neurodevelopmental disabilities. J Pineal Res 2008; 44:57–64.

10. Braam W et al. Melatonin treatment in individuals with intellectual disability and chronic insomnia: a randomized placebo-controlled study. J Intellect Disabil Res 2008; 52:256–264.

11. Gupta M et al. Add-on melatonin improves sleep behavior in children with epilepsy: randomized, double-blind, placebo-controlled trial. J Child Neurol 2005; 20:112–115.

12. Coppola G et al. Melatonin in wake-sleep disorders in children, adolescents and young adults with mental retardation with or without epilepsy: a double-blind, cross-over, placebo-controlled trial. Brain Dev 2004; 26:373–376.

13. Weiss MD et al. Sleep hygiene and melatonin treatment for children and adolescents with ADHD and initial insomnia. J Am Acad Child Adolesc Psychiatry 2006; 45:512–519.

14. Garstang J et al. Randomized controlled trial of melatonin for children with autistic spectrum disorders and sleep problems. Child Care Health Dev 2006; 32:585–589.

15. Gringras P et al. Melatonin for sleep problems in children with neurodevelopmental disorders: randomised double masked placebo controlled trial. BMJ 2012; 345:e6664.

16. Cortesi F et al. Controlled-release melatonin, singly and combined with cognitive behavioural therapy, for persistent insomnia in children with autism spectrum disorders: a randomized placebo-controlled trial. JSleep Res 2012; 21:700–709.

17. Sheldon SH. Pro-convulsant effects of oral melatonin in neurologically disabled children. Lancet 1998; 351:1254.

18. Maestroni GJ. The immunoneuroendocrine role of melatonin. J Pineal Res 1993; 14:1–10.

19. Sutherland ER et al. Elevated serum melatonin is associated with the nocturnal worsening of asthma. J Allergy Clin Immunol 2003; 112:513–517.

20. Chase JE et al. Melatonin: therapeutic use in sleep disorders. Ann Pharmacother 1997; 31:1218–1226.

21. Jan JE et al. Melatonin treatment of sleep-wake cycle disorders in children and adolescents. Dev Med Child Neurol 1999; 41:491–500.

22. Brigo F et al. Melatonin as add-on treatment for epilepsy. Cochrane Database Syst Rev 2016:CD006967.

23. Sack RL et al. Sleep-promoting effects of melatonin: at what dose, in whom, under what conditions, and by what mechanisms? Sleep 1997; 20:908–915.

Rapid tranquillisation (RT) in children and adolescents

As in adults, a comprehensive mental state assessment and appropriately implemented treatment plan along with staff skilled in the use of de-escalation techniques and appropriate placement of the patient are key to minimising the need for enforced parenteral medication.

Health-care professionals undertaking RT and/or restraint in children and adolescents should be trained and competent in undertaking these procedures in this population, and should be clear about the legal context for any restrictive practices they employ. Be particularly cautious when considering high-potency antipsychotic medication (such as haloperidol), especially in those who have not taken antipsychotic medication before, because of the increased risk of acute dystonic reactions in this age group.[1] NICE recommends using intramuscular lorazepam (and no other drug).[2]

A wide dose range is given in Table 5.8 for medication used in RT. Caution is required, especially for younger children, but in older adolescents consider the use of adult doses, especially in those who are not drug naïve and where doses in the lower end of the quoted dose range have proved ineffective.

Table 5.8 Recommended drugs for rapid tranquillisation if the oral route is refused or has proven ineffective

Medication	Dose	Onset of action	Comment
Olanzapine IM[3,4]	2.5–10 mg	15–30 min	Possibly increased risk of respiratory depression when administered with benzodiazepines, particularly if alcohol has been consumed. Separate administration by at least 1 hour
Haloperidol IM[5]	0.025–0.075 mg/kg/dose (max 2.5 mg) IM Adolescents >12 years can receive the adult dose (2.5–5 mg)	20–30 min	Must have parenteral anticholinergics present in case of laryngeal spasm or other dystonia (young people more vulnerable to severe dystonia) Adult data suggest co-administration of promethazine may reduce EPS risk[6] **ECG essential**
Lorazepam* IM[7,8]	<12 years: 0.5–1 mg; >12 years: 0.5–2 mg	20–40 min	Slower onset of action than midazolam Only treatment recommended by NICE Flumazenil is the reversing agent for all benzodiazepines
Midazolam* IM, IV or buccal[8,9]	0.1–0.15 mg/kg (IM) Buccal midazolam 300–500 µg/kg or 6–10 years = 7.5 mg >10 years = 10 mg	10–20 min IM (1–3 min IV)	Quicker onset and shorter duration of action than lorazepam or diazepam IV administration should only be used (usually as a last resort) with extreme caution and where resuscitation facilities are available. Shorter onset and duration of action than haloperidol When given as buccal liquid, onset of action is 15–30 minutes.[10] Some published data in mental health but only in adults.[11] Buccal liquid is unlicensed for this use.

(Continued)

Table 5.8 (*Continued*)

Medication	Dose	Onset of action	Comment
Diazepam* IV (not for IM administration)[12]	0.1 mg/kg/dose by slow IV injection. Max 40 mg total daily dose <12 years and 60 mg >12 years	1–3 min	Long half-life that does not correlate with length of sedation. Possibility of accumulation **Never give as IM injection**
Ziprasidone IM[13–16] (not UK)	10–20 mg	15–30 min IM	Apparently effective. QT prolongation is of concern in this patient group **ECG essential**
Aripiprazole IM[17,18]	9.75 mg	15–30 min	Evidence of effectiveness in adults but no data for children and adolescents
Promethazine IM	<12 years: 5–25 mg (max 50 mg/day) >12 years: 25–50 mg (max 100 mg/day)	Up to 60 min	An effective sedative, although has a slow onset of action. Useful if the cause of behavioural disturbance is unknown and there is concern about the use of antipsychotic medication in a child or young person

* Note that young people are particularly vulnerable to disinhibitory reactions with benzodiazepines.
ECG, electrocardiogram; EPS, extrapyramidal symptoms; IM, intramuscular; IV, intravenous.

Oral medication should always be offered (and repeated if necessary if the young person is willing to take it), before resorting to parenteral treatment. Buccal midazolam[11] and inhaled loxapine[19] have not been widely investigated in children in RT at the time of writing. Buccal midazolam is commonly used for seizures in children. Monitoring after RT is the same as in adults (see section on RT, Chapter 3).

References

1. National Institute for Health and Care Excellence. Psychosis and schizophrenia in children and young people: recognition and management. Clinical Guideline 155, 2013 (last updated October 2016). https://www.nice.org.uk/guidance/cg155.
2. National Institute for Health and Care Excellence. Violence and aggression: short-term management in mental health, health and community settings. NICE Guideline 10, 2015. https://www.nice.org.uk/guidance/ng10.
3. Breier A et al. A double-blind, placebo-controlled dose-response comparison of intramuscular olanzapine and haloperidol in the treatment of acute agitation in schizophrenia. Arch Gen Psychiatry 2002; 59:441–448.
4. Lindborg SR et al. Effects of intramuscular olanzapine vs. haloperidol and placebo on QTc intervals in acutely agitated patients. Psychiatry Res 2003; 119:113–123.
5. Powney MJ et al. Haloperidol for psychosis-induced aggression or agitation (rapid tranquillisation). Cochrane Database Syst Rev 2012; 11:CD009377.
6. TREC Collaborative Group. Rapid tranquillisation for agitated patients in emergency psychiatric rooms: a randomised trial of midazolam versus haloperidol plus promethazine. BMJ 2003; 327:708–713.
7. Sorrentino A. Chemical restraints for the agitated, violent, or psychotic pediatric patient in the emergency department: controversies and recommendations. Curr Opin Pediatr 2004; 16:201–205.
8. Nobay F et al. A prospective, double-blind, randomized trial of midazolam versus haloperidol versus lorazepam in the chemical restraint of violent and severely agitated patients. Acad Emerg Med 2004; 11:744–749.
9. Kennedy RM et al. The "ouchless emergency department". Getting closer: advances in decreasing distress during painful procedures in the emergency department. Pediatr Clin North Am 1999; 46:1215–1247.
10. Schwagmeier R et al. Midazolam pharmacokinetics following intravenous and buccal administration. Br J Clin Pharmacol 1998; 46:203–206.
11. Taylor D et al. Buccal midazolam for agitation on psychiatric intensive care wards. Int J Psychiatry Clin Pract 2008; 12:309–311.

12. Nunn K, Dey C. Medication Table In: Nunn K, Dey C, eds. *The Clinician's Guide to Psychotropic Prescribing in Children and Adolescents*, 1st edn. Sydney: Glade Publishing.; 2003, pp. 383–452.

13. Khan SS et al. A naturalistic evaluation of intramuscular ziprasidone versus intramuscular olanzapine for the management of acute agitation and aggression in children and adolescents. J Child Adolesc Psychopharmacol 2006; 16:671–677.

14. Staller JA. Intramuscular ziprasidone in youth: a retrospective chart review. J Child Adolesc Psychopharmacol 2004; 14:590–592.

15. Hazaray E et al. Intramuscular ziprasidone for acute agitation in adolescents. J Child Adolesc Psychopharmacol 2004; 14:464–470.

16. Barzman DH et al. A retrospective chart review of intramuscular ziprasidone for agitation in children and adolescents on psychiatric units: prospective studies are needed. J Child Adolesc Psychopharmacol 2007; 17:503–509.

17. Sanford M, Scott LJ. Intramuscular aripiprazole: a review of its use in the management of agitation in schizophrenia and bipolar I disorder. CNS Drugs 2008; 22:335–352.

18. National Institute for Health and Care Excellence. Aripiprazole for schizophrenia in people aged 15 to 17 years – Technology Appraisal 13, 2011. https://www.nice.org.uk/guidance/ta213.

19. Lesem MD et al. Rapid acute treatment of agitation in individuals with schizophrenia: multicentre, randomised, placebo-controlled study of inhaled loxapine. Br J Psychiatry 2011; 198:51–58.

Doses of commonly used psychotropic drugs in children and adolescents

See Table 5.9 for doses of commonly used psychotropic drugs in children and adolescents.

Table 5.9 Starting doses of commonly used psychotropic drugs in children and adolescents[1,2]*

Drug	Starting dose**	Comment
Antipsychotics		
Aripiprazole	2 mg	Increase to 5–15 mg daily according to response
Clozapine	6.25–12.5 mg	Use plasma levels to determine maintenance dose
Olanzapine	2.5–5 mg	Use plasma levels to determine maintenance dose
Quetiapine	25 mg	Effective dose usually in the range 150–200 mg daily
Risperidone	0.25–2 mg	Adjust dose according to response and adverse effects
Antidepressants		
Fluoxetine	5–10 mg/day	Adjust dose according to response and adverse effects
Sertraline	25–50 mg daily	Effective dose 50–100 mg, sometimes higher
Citalopram	10 mg daily	Effective dose 10–40 mg (note QT effects)
Escitalopram	5 mg daily	Effective dose 10–20 mg (note QT effects)
Other drugs		
Lithium	100–200 mg/day lithium carbonate	Use plasma levels to determine maintenance dose
Valproate	10–20 mg/kg/day in divided doses	Use plasma levels to determine maintenance dose. Avoid use in females of child-bearing age
Melatonin	2 mg at night	The optimal dose of melatonin is unknown: 500 µg exceeds physiological production, 2 mg is effective, doses above 5 mg may be more effective because of a direct sedative effect

*We have removed haloperidol, amitriptyline and carbamazepine from this table as none of these is recommended in children.

**Suggested approximate oral starting doses (see primary literature for doses in individual indications). Lower dose in suggested range is for children weighing less than 25 kg.

References

1. BNF Online. British National Formulary, 2017. https://www.medicinescomplete.com/mc/bnf/current/.
2. BNFC Online. British National Formulary for Children, 2017. https://www.medicinescomplete.com/mc/bnfc/current/.

Chapter 6

Prescribing in older people

General principles

The pharmacokinetics and pharmacodynamics of most drugs are altered to an important extent in older people. These changes in drug handling and action must be taken into account if treatment is to be effective and adverse effects minimised. Older people often have a number of concurrent illnesses and may require treatment with several drugs. This leads to a greater chance of problems arising because of drug interactions and to a higher rate of drug-induced problems in general.[1] It is reasonable to assume that all drugs are more likely to cause adverse effects in older patients than in younger patients.

How drugs affect the ageing body (altered pharmacodynamics)

As we age, control over reflex actions such as blood pressure and temperature regulation is reduced. Receptors may become more sensitive. This results in an increased incidence and severity of adverse effects. For example, drugs that decrease gut motility are more likely to cause constipation (e.g. anticholinergics and opioids) and drugs that affect blood pressure are more likely to cause falls (e.g. tricyclic antidepressants [TCAs] and diuretics). Older people demonstrate an exaggerated response to central nervous system (CNS)-active drugs such as benzodiazepines and opioids. This is partly due to an age-related decline in CNS function and partly due to increased pharmacodynamic sensitivity to these drugs.[2] Therapeutic response to medication can also be delayed; for example, older adults may take longer to respond to antidepressants than younger adults.[3]

Older people may be more prone to develop serious adverse effects such as agranulocytosis[4] and neutropenia[5] with clozapine, stroke with antipsychotic drugs[6] and bleeding with selective serotonin reuptake inhibitors (SSRIs).

The Maudsley Prescribing Guidelines in Psychiatry, Thirteenth Edition. David M. Taylor, Thomas R. E. Barnes and Allan H. Young.
© 2018 David M. Taylor. Published 2018 by John Wiley & Sons Ltd.

How ageing affects drug therapy (altered pharmacokinetics)[7]

Absorption

Gut motility decreases with age, as does secretion of gastric acid. This leads to drugs being absorbed more slowly, resulting in a slower onset of action. The same *amount* of drug is absorbed as in a younger adult, but rate of absorption is slower.

Distribution

Older adults have more body fat, less body water and less albumin than younger adults. This leads to an increased volume of distribution and a longer duration of action for some fat-soluble drugs (e.g. diazepam), higher concentrations of some drugs at the site of action (e.g. digoxin) and a reduction in the amount of drug bound to albumin (increased amounts of active 'free drug'; e.g. warfarin, phenytoin).

Metabolism

The majority of drugs are hepatically metabolised. Liver size is reduced in the elderly, but in the absence of hepatic disease or significantly reduced hepatic blood flow, there is no significant reduction in metabolic capacity. The magnitude of pharmacokinetic interactions is unlikely to be altered but the pharmacodynamic consequences of these interactions may be amplified.

Excretion

Renal function declines with age: 35% of function is lost by the age of 65 years and 50% by the age of 80.

More function is lost if there are concurrent medical problems such as heart disease, diabetes or hypertension. Measurement of serum creatinine or urea can be misleading in the elderly because muscle mass is reduced, so less creatinine is produced. It is particularly important that estimated glomerular filtration rate (eGFR)[8] is used as a measure of renal function in this age group. It is best to assume that all elderly patients have at most two-thirds of normal renal function.

Most drugs are eventually (after metabolism) excreted by the kidney. A few do not undergo biotransformation first. Lithium and sulpiride are important examples. Drugs primarily excreted via the kidney will accumulate in the elderly, leading to toxicity and adverse effects. Dosage reduction is likely to be required (see section on renal failure and psychotropics).

Drug interactions

Some drugs have a narrow therapeutic index (a small increase in dose can cause toxicity and a small reduction in dose can cause a loss of therapeutic action). The most commonly prescribed ones are digoxin, warfarin, theophylline, phenytoin and lithium. Changes in the way these drugs are handled in older people and the greater chance of interaction with other drugs mean that toxicity and therapeutic failure are more likely.

> **Box 6.1**　Reducing drug-related risk in older people
>
> Adherence to the following principles will reduce drug-related morbidity and mortality.
> - Use drugs only when absolutely necessary.
> - Avoid, if possible, drugs that block α_1 adrenoceptors, have anticholinergic adverse effects, are very sedative, have a long half-life or are potent inhibitors of hepatic metabolising enzymes.
> - Start with a low dose and increase slowly but do not undertreat. Some drugs still require the full adult dose.
> - Try not to treat the adverse effects of one drug with another drug. Find a better-tolerated alternative.
> - Keep therapy simple; that is, once daily administration whenever possible.

These drugs can be used safely but extra care must be taken and blood concentrations should be measured where possible. See Box 6.1.

Some drugs inhibit or induce hepatic metabolising enzymes. Important examples include some SSRIs, erythromycin and carbamazepine. This may lead to the metabolism of another drug being altered. Many drug interactions occur through this mechanism. Details of individual interactions and their consequences can be found in Appendix 1 of the *BNF*.[9] Most can be predicted by a sound knowledge of pharmacology.

Administering medicines in foodstuffs[10–12]

Sometimes patients may refuse treatment with medicines, even when such treatment is thought to be in their best interests. In the UK, where the patient has a mental illness or has capacity, the Mental Health Act should be used, but if the patient lacks capacity, this option may not be desirable. Medicines should never be administered covertly to elderly patients with dementia without a full discussion with the multidisciplinary team and the patient's relatives. The outcome of this discussion should be clearly documented in the patient's clinical notes. Medicines should be administered covertly only if the clear and express purpose is to reduce suffering for the patient. (For further information, see section on 'Covert administration of medicines within food and drink' in this chapter.)

For advice on dosing of psychotropic drugs in the elderly, see the section on 'A guide to medication doses of commonly used psychotropic drugs in older adults' in this chapter.

References

1. Royal College of Physicians. Medication for older people. Summary and recommendations of a report of a working party of The Royal College of Physicians. J R Coll Physicians Lond 1997; 31:254–257.
2. Bowie MW et al. Pharmacodynamics in older adults: a review. Am J Geriatr Pharmacother 2007; 5:263–303.
3. Baldwin R et al. Management of depression in later life. Adv Psychiatr Treat 2004; 10:131–139.
4. Munro J et al. Active monitoring of 12,760 clozapine recipients in the UK and Ireland. Beyond pharmacovigilance. Br J Psychiatry 1999; 175:576–580.
5. O'Connor DW et al. The safety and tolerability of clozapine in aged patients: a retrospective clinical file review. World J Biol Psychiatry 2010; 11:788–791.
6. Douglas IJ et al. Exposure to antipsychotics and risk of stroke: self controlled case series study. BMJ 2008; 337:a1227.

7. Mayersohn M. Special pharmacokinetic considerations in the elderly. In: Evans W, Schentage J, Jusko J, eds. *Applied Pharmacokinetics: Principles of Therapeutic Drug Monitoring*. Vancouver, WA: Applied Therapeutics Inc; 1992.

8. Morriss R et al. Lithium and eGFR: a new routinely available tool for the prevention of chronic kidney disease. Br J Psychiatry 2008; **193**:93–95.

9. BMJ Group and Pharmaceutical Press, BMJ. *British National Formulary*, 72nd edn. https://www.medicinescomplete.com/mc/2017.

10. Royal College of Psychiatrists. College Statement on Covert Administration of Medicines. Psychiatr Bull 2004; **28**:385–386.

11. Haw C et al. Administration of medicines in food and drink: a study of older inpatients with severe mental illness. Int Psychogeriatr 2010; **22**:409–416.

12. Haw C et al. Covert administration of medication to older adults: a review of the literature and published studies. J Psychiatr Ment Health Nurs 2010; **17**:761–768.

Dementia

Dementia is a progressive degenerative neurological syndrome affecting around 5% of those aged over 65 years, rising to 20% in the over-80s. This age-related disorder is characterised by cognitive decline, impaired memory and thinking, and a gradual loss of skills needed to carry out activities of daily living. Often, other mental functions may also be affected, including changes in mood, personality and social behaviour.[1]

The various types of dementia are classified according to the different disease processes affecting the brain. The most common cause of dementia is Alzheimer's disease (AD), accounting for around 60% of all cases. Vascular dementia and dementia with Lewy bodies (DLB) are responsible for most other cases. Alzheimer's disease and vascular dementia may co-exist and are often difficult to separate clinically. Dementia is also encountered in about 30–70% of patients with Parkinson's disease.[1]

Alzheimer's disease

Cognitive enhancers used in Alzheimer's disease

Acetylcholinesterase (AChE) inhibitors

The cholinergic hypothesis of AD is predicated on the observation that the cognitive deterioration associated with the disease results from progressive loss of cholinergic neurons and decreasing levels of acetylcholine (ACh) in the brain.[2] More recent studies however have called this theory into question and it is no longer widely believed that cholinergic depletion alone is responsible for the symptoms of AD.[3]

Three inhibitors of AChE (AChE-Is) are currently licensed in the UK and elsewhere for the treatment of mild to moderate dementia in AD: donepezil, rivastigmine and galantamine. In addition, rivastigmine is licensed in the treatment of mild to moderate dementia associated with Parkinson's disease. Both acetylcholinesterase (AChE) and butyrylcholinesterase (BuChE) have been found to play an important role in the degradation of ACh.[4] Cholinesterase inhibitors differ in pharmacological action: donepezil selectively inhibits AChE, rivastigmine affects both AChE and BuChE, and galantamine selectively inhibits AChE and also has nicotinic receptor agonist properties.[5] To date, these differences have not been shown to result in important differences in efficacy or tolerability. See Table 6.1 for comparison of AChE inhibitors.

Memantine

Memantine is licensed in the UK for the treatment of moderate to severe dementia in AD. It is believed to exert its therapeutic effect by acting as a low-to-moderate affinity, non-competitive N-methyl-D-aspartate (NMDA) receptor antagonist that binds preferentially to open NMDA receptor-operated calcium channels. This activity-dependent binding blocks NMDA-mediated ion flux and is thought to mitigate the effects of sustained and pathologically elevated levels of glutamate (excitotoxicity) that may lead to neuronal dysfunction.[6] See Table 6.1.

CHAPTER 6

Table 6.1 Characteristics of cognitive enhancers[7–15]

Characteristic	Donepezil	Rivastigmine	Galantamine	Memantine
Primary mechanism	AChE-I (selective + reversible)	AChE-I (reversible, non-competitive inhibitor)	AChE-I (competitive + reversible)	Glutamate receptor antagonist
Other mechanism	None	BuChE-I	Nicotine receptor agonist	5-HT$_3$ receptor antagonist
Starting dose	5 mg daily	1.5 mg bd (oral) (or 4.6 mg/24 hours patch)	4 mg bd (or 8 mg XL daily)	5 mg daily
Usual treatment dose (and max dose)	10 mg daily	3–6 mg bd (oral) or 9.5 mg/24 hours patch	8–12 mg bd (or 16–24 mg XL daily)	20 mg daily or (10 mg bd)
Recommended minimum interval between dose increases	4 weeks (increase by 5 mg daily)	2 weeks for oral (increase by 1.5 mg twice a day) 4 weeks for patch (increase to 9.5 mg/24 hours) (can consider increase to 13.3 mg/24 hours after 6 months if tolerated and meaningful cognitive/functional decline occurs on 9.5 mg/24 hours)	4 weeks (increase by 4 mg twice a day or 8 mg XL daily)	1 week (increase by 5 mg weekly)
Adverse effects[7–14]	Diarrhoea*, nausea*, headache*, common cold, anorexia, hallucinations, agitation, aggressive behaviour, abnormal dreams and nightmares, syncope, dizziness, insomnia, vomiting, abdominal disturbance, rash, pruritus, muscle cramps, urinary incontinence, fatigue, pain	Anorexia*, dizziness*, nausea*, vomiting*, diarrhoea*, decreased appetite, nightmares, agitation, confusion, anxiety, headache, somnolence, tremor, abdominal pain and dyspepsia, sweating fatigue and asthenia malaise, weight loss (frequency of adverse effects with the patch may differ from capsules)	Nausea*, vomiting*, decreased appetite, hallucination, depression, syncope, dizziness, tremor, headache, somnolence, lethargy, bradycardia, hypertension, abdominal pain and discomfort, diarrhoea, dyspepsia, muscle spasms, fatigue, asthenia, malaise, weight loss, fall	Drug hypersensitivity, somnolence, dizziness, balance disorders, hypertension, dyspnoea, constipation, elevated liver function test, headache
Half-life (hours)	~70	~1 (oral) 3.4 (patch)	7–8 (tablets/oral solution) 8–10 (XL capsules)	60–100

Metabolism	CYP3A4 CYP2D6 (minor)	Minimal involvement of CYP isoenzymes	CYP3A4 CYP2D6	Primarily non-hepatic
Drug–drug interactions	Yes (see Table 6.2)	Interactions unlikely	Yes (see Table 6.2)	Yes (see Table 6.2)
Effect of food on absorption	None	Delays rate and extent of absorption	Delays rate but not extent of absorption	None
Cost of preparations[7,15] (for 1-month treatment at usual, i.e. max dose in UK)	Tablets: £1.10 Orodispersible tablets: £7.92 Oral solution (1 mg/mL): £89.60	Capsules: £42.46 Oral solution (2 mg/mL): £135.55 Patches 9.5 mg: £30.00 4.6 mg and 13.3 mg: £77.97	Tablets: £74.10 Capsules MR: £79.80 Oral solution (Reminyl®) (4 mg/mL): £201.60	Tablets: £1.39 Oral solution (10 mg/mL): £61.25 NB: Bottles supplied with a dosing pump dispensing 5 mg in 0.5 mL per actuation
Relative cost	$	$$	$$$	$
Patent status	Generic available	Generic available	Generic available (branded oral solution cheaper than generic)	Generic available

* Very common: ≥1/10 and common: ≥1/100.

AChE-I, acetylcholinesterase inhibitor; bd, *bis die* (twice a day); BuChE-I, butyrylcholinesterase inhibitor; CYP, cytochrome P450; ER, extended release; MR, modified release; NMDA, N-methyl-D-aspartate; XL, extended release.

Efficacy of drugs used in dementia

Currently there is no cure for dementia, and no treatment exists to modify or reverse its progression. Therapeutic interventions are therefore targeted to treat symptoms or improve cognitive function. Acetylcholinesterase inhibitors may provide some modest cognitive, functional and global benefits in mild to moderate AD.[16]

All three AChE-Is seem to have broadly similar clinical effects, as measured with the Mini Mental State Examination (MMSE), a 30-point basic evaluation of cognitive function, and the Alzheimer's Disease Assessment Scale – cognitive subscale (ADAS-cog), a 70-point evaluation largely of cognitive dysfunction. Estimates of the number needed to treat (NNT) (for an improvement of >4 points ADAS-cog) range from 4 to 12.[17]

Cochrane reviews for all three AChE-Is have been carried out, both collectively as a group and for each drug separately. In the review for all AChE-Is, which included 10 randomised controlled trials (RCTs), results demonstrated that treatment over 6 months produced improvements in cognitive function of on average –2.7 points on the ADAS-cog scale. Benefits were also noted on measures of activities of daily living (ADL) and behaviour, although none of these treatment effects was large. Despite the slight variations in the mode of action of the three drugs, there is no evidence of any differences between them with respect to efficacy.[18]

A recent systematic review and meta-analysis of RCTs (including 16,106 patients) comparing AChE-Is and placebo found that AChE-Is improved cognitive function (effect size = 0.38), global symptomatology (effect size = 0.28) and functional capacity (effect size = 0.16) but not neuropsychiatric symptoms. (See section on 'Management of behavioural and psychological symptoms of dementia'.) All-cause discontinuation was higher with AChE-Is (odds ratio [OR] = 1.66), as was discontinuation due to adverse effects (OR = 1.75). Rivastigmine was associated with a worse rate of all-cause discontinuation than other drugs and donepezil with a relatively higher efficacy on global change. The proportion of patients with serious adverse effects decreased with age. Mortality was lower with AChE-Is than with placebo (OR = 0.65),[19] a finding confirmed by a more recent trial.[20]

A review of the NICE Technology Appraisal for AChE-Is and memantine concluded that the additional clinical effectiveness evidence identified continues to suggest clinical benefit from AChE-Is in alleviating AD symptoms although there is considerable debate about the magnitude of effect. There is also some evidence that AChE-Is have an impact on controlling disease progression.[21] Although there is also new evidence for the effectiveness of memantine, overall it remains less robust than the evidence supporting AChE-Is.[22]

Donepezil

Pivotal trials of donepezil[23–25] suggest an advantage over placebo of 2.5–3.1 points on the ADAS-cog scale. Results from the donepezil Cochrane review suggested statistically significant improvements for both 5 and 10 mg/day at 24 weeks compared with placebo on the ADAS-cog scale with a 2.01 point and a 2.80 point reduction, respectively.[26] A long-term placebo-controlled trial of donepezil in 565 patients with mild to moderate

AD found a small but significant benefit on cognition compared with placebo. This was reflected in a 0.8 point difference in the MMSE score.[27] The size of the effect is similar to other trials.

Rivastigmine

Studies for rivastigmine[28,29] suggest an advantage of 2.6–4.9 points on the ADAS-cog scale over placebo. In the rivastigmine Cochrane review, patients on rivastigmine (6–12 mg/day by mouth, or 9.5 mg/day by skin patch) were better on three outcomes than those on placebo, after 6 months of treatment. The differences were quite small for cognitive function (2 points, using the ADAS-cog, which has a range of 70 points) and activities of daily living (effect size of 0.20). Patients on rivastigmine were more likely to show overall improvement compared with those on placebo (OR 1.47), however there was no difference for behavioural changes or impact on caregivers. Patients on rivastigmine were also about twice as likely to experience adverse events, although this risk might have been slightly less for patients using patches compared with capsules.[30] Rivastigmine transdermal patch (9.5 mg/24 hours) has been shown to be as effective as the highest doses of capsules but with a superior tolerability profile in a 6-month double-blind, placebo-controlled RCT[31] and more recently confirmed in a Chinese study.[32] A nasal spray has also been developed.[33]

Galantamine

Studies with galantamine[34–36] suggest an advantage over placebo of 2.9–3.9 points on the ADAS-cog scale. The Cochrane review of galantamine reported that treatment with the drug led to a significantly greater proportion of subjects with improved or unchanged global rating scale rating at all doses except for 8 mg/day. Point estimate of effect was lower for 8 mg/day but similar for 16–36 mg/day. Treatment effect for 24 mg/day over 6 months was a 3.1 point reduction in ADAS-cog.[37] Data from two trials of galantamine in mild cognitive impairment suggest marginal clinical benefit but a yet unexplained excess in death rate.[37] Galantamine has been shown to be effective (albeit marginally so) in severe AD in people with MMSE scores of 5–12 points.[38]

Memantine

An NNT analysis of memantine found it to have an NNT of 3–8[39] for improved cognitive function. The efficacy of memantine was evaluated using the ADAS-cog subscale to assess cognitive abilities in mild to moderate AD and the severe impairment battery (SIB) to evaluate cognitive functions in moderate to severe AD. The SIB is a 40-item test with scores ranging from 0 to 100, higher scores reflecting higher levels of cognitive ability.[40] Trials in moderate to severe dementia found that memantine showed significant benefits on both scales.[41] A Cochrane review of memantine concluded that it had a small beneficial effect at 6 months in moderate to severe AD. In patients with mild to moderate dementia, the small beneficial effect on cognition was not clinically detectable in those with vascular dementia and barely detectable in those with AD.[42] A recent systematic review and meta-analysis including nine studies and 2433 patients found that memantine monotherapy significantly improved cognitive function (effect size = –0.27), behavioural disturbances (effect size = –0.12), activities of daily living

CHAPTER 6

(effect size = −0.09), global function assessment (effect size = −0.18) and stage of dementia (effect size = −0.23) scores. It was superior to placebo in terms of discontinuation because of inefficacy (risk ratio [RR] = 0.36). Moreover, memantine was associated with less agitation compared with placebo (RR = 0.68). There were no significant differences in the rate of discontinuation because of all causes, all adverse events and individual adverse effects other than agitation between the memantine monotherapy and placebo groups.[6]

Quantifying the effects of drugs in dementia

All the above results need to be interpreted with caution because of differences in the populations included in the different studies, and especially as so few head-to-head studies[43] have been published. Alzheimer's disease is characterised by inexorable cognitive decline, which is generally well quantified by tests such as ADAS-cog and MMSE. The average annual rate of decline in untreated patients ranges between 6 and 12 points on the ADAS-cog (and the annual increase in ADAS-cog in patients with untreated moderate AD has been estimated to be as much as 9–11 points per year). A 4-point change in the ADAS-cog score is considered clinically meaningful.[44] It is difficult to predict treatment effect in individual patients.

Switching between drugs used in dementia

The benefits of treatment with AChE-Is are rapidly lost when drug administration is interrupted[45] and may not be fully regained when drug treatment is reinitiated.[46] Poor tolerability with one agent does not rule out good tolerability with another.[47] The recently revised British Association for Psychopharmacology (BAP) Guidelines for Dementia confirm that previous comparative trials have failed to consistently demonstrate any significant differences in efficacy between the three AChE-Is, the main differences found being in frequency and type of adverse events. As a result, their recommendation that a significant proportion of patients (up to 50%) appear to both tolerate and benefit from switching between AChE-Is if they cannot tolerate one, remains valid.[48]

Several cases of discontinuation syndrome upon stopping donepezil have been published[49,50] suggesting that a gradual withdrawal should be carried out where possible. However, a study comparing abrupt versus stepwise switching from donepezil to memantine found no clinically relevant differences in adverse effects despite patients in the abrupt group experiencing more frequent adverse effects than the stepwise discontinuation group (46% vs 32% respectively).[51] (For switching to rivastigmine patch see section on 'Tolerability'.)

Following a systematic review of the literature,[52] a practical approach to switching between AChE-Is has been proposed: in the case of intolerance, switching to another agent should be done only after complete resolution of adverse effects following discontinuation of the initial agent. In the case of lack of efficacy, switching can be done overnight, with a quicker titration scheme thereafter. Switching to another AChE-I is not recommended in individuals who show loss of benefit several years after initiation of therapy.

Other effects

AChE inhibitors may also affect non-cognitive aspects of AD and other dementias. Several studies have investigated their safety and efficacy in managing the non-cognitive symptoms of dementia. For more information about the management of these symptoms, see section on 'Management of behavioural and psychological symptoms of dementia (BPSD)'.

Dosing

Different titration schedules do, to some extent, differentiate AChE-Is (see Table 6.1 for dosing information). Donepezil has been perhaps the easiest to use as it is given once daily whereas both rivastigmine and galantamine at least initially needed to be given twice daily and have prolonged titration schedules. These factors may be important to prescribers, patients and caregivers. This was demonstrated in an early retrospective analysis of the patterns of use of AChE-Is, where it was shown that donepezil was significantly more likely to be prescribed at an effective dose than either rivastigmine or galantamine.[53] Galantamine however is now usually given once daily as the controlled release formulation and rivastigmine is now available as a patch. Memantine once daily dosing has been found to be similar in safety and tolerability to twice daily dosing and may be more practical.[54]

Recently, the US Food and Drug Administration (FDA) approved a higher daily dose of **donepezil sustained release (23 mg)** for moderate to severe AD on the basis of positive phase III trial results. Donepezil, 23 mg/day, is currently marketed in the US and parts of Asia. In a global phase III study in patients with moderate to severe AD, donepezil 23 mg/day demonstrated significantly greater cognitive benefits than donepezil 10 mg/day, with a between-treatment difference in mean change in the SIB score of 2.2 points in the overall study population and 3.1 points in patients with advanced AD. Dose escalation was somewhat challenging given the increased incidence of adverse gastrointestinal (GI) effects observed when increasing the dose of donepezil from 10 to 23 mg daily. These adverse effects seldom persist beyond a 1-month period. Using stepwise titration strategies may address these adverse GI effects and could potentially involve increasing the dose of donepezil from 10 to 23 mg over a 1- to 2-month period by taking one 10 mg tablet plus one 5 mg tablet once daily for 1 month followed by a 23 mg tablet once daily or a 10 mg tablet and 23 mg tablet on alternate days. A study in South Korea has been designed to determine the optimal dose escalation strategy for successful up-titration to 23 mg/day.[55] Clinical recommendations emphasise the importance of patient selection (AD severity, tolerability of lower doses of donepezil and absence of contraindications), a stepwise titration strategy for dose escalation, and appropriate monitoring and counselling of patients and caregivers in the management of patients with AD.[55]

Memantine extended release (ER) 28 mg once daily capsule formulation was approved in the US in 2010 and became available more recently. Its efficacy was demonstrated in a large, multinational, phase III trial which showed that the addition of memantine ER to ongoing cholinesterase inhibitors improved key outcomes compared with cholinesterase inhibitor monotherapy, including measures of cognition and global status. The most common adverse events were headache, diarrhoea and dizziness.[56]

Combination treatment

The benefits of adding memantine to AChE-Is are not clear but the combination appears to be well tolerated[57,58] and may even result in a decreased incidence of GI adverse effects compared with monotherapy with an AChE-I.[59] Studies investigating the benefits of combining AChE-Is with memantine have found conflicting results. A large multicentre study[60] concluded that the efficacy of donepezil and of memantine did not differ significantly in the presence or absence of the other and that there were no significant benefits for the combination over donepezil alone. A retrospective study on the benefits of combined memantine and AChE-I treatment in older patients affected with AD (MEMAGE study), which included 240 patients, found that combined treatment was effective in slowing cognitive impairment and preventing onset of agitation and aggression.[61] A systematic review and meta-analysis including 7 studies and 2182 patients found that combination therapy was superior to monotherapy with AChE-I in terms of behavioural disturbances, activities of daily living and global assessment. In addition, cognitive function scores exhibited favourable trends with combination therapy. The effects of combination therapy were more significant in the moderate to severe AD subgroup in terms of all efficacy outcome scores. The discontinuation rate was similar in both groups, and there were no significant differences in individual adverse effects.[62] The European Academy of Neurology (EAN) Guidelines now recommend the use of a combination of an AChE-I plus memantine rather than AChE-I alone in patients with moderate to severe AD, although the strength of the evidence supporting this recommendation is said to be weak.[63] Studies have confirmed that there are no pharmacokinetic or pharmacodynamic interactions between AChE-Is and memantine.[64,65]

Tolerability

Drug tolerability may differ between AChE-Is, but, again, in the absence of sufficient direct comparisons, it is difficult to draw definitive conclusions. Overall tolerability can be broadly evaluated by reference to the numbers withdrawing from clinical trials. Withdrawal rates in trials of donepezil[23,24] ranged from 4% to 16% (placebo 1–7%). With rivastigmine,[28,29] rates ranged from 7% to 29% (placebo 7%) and with galantamine[34-36] from 7% to 23% (placebo 7–9%). These figures relate to withdrawals specifically associated with adverse effects. The number needed to harm (NNH) has been reported to be 12.[17] A study of the French pharmacovigilance database identified age, the use of antipsychotic drugs, antihypertensives and drugs targeting the alimentary tract and metabolism as factors associated with serious reactions to AChE-Is.[66]

Tolerability seems to be affected by speed of titration and, perhaps less clearly, by dose. Most adverse effects occurred in trials during titration, and slower titration schedules are recommended in clinical use. This may mean that these drugs are equally well tolerated in practice.

Rivastigmine patches may offer convenience and a superior tolerability profile to rivastigmine capsules.[31,32] Data from three trials found that rivastigmine patch was better tolerated than the capsules with fewer GI adverse effects and fewer discontinuations due to these adverse effects.[67] Data support recommendations for patients on high doses of rivastigmine capsules (>6 mg/day) to switch directly to the 9.5 mg/24 hour patch, while those on lower doses (≤6 mg/day) should start on the 4.6 mg/24 hour patch for 4 weeks before increasing to the 9.5 mg/24 hour patch. This latter switch is also recommended for patients switching from other oral cholinesterase inhibitors to the rivastigmine patch (with a 1-week washout period in patients sensitive to adverse effects or those who have very low body weight or a history of bradycardia).[68] It is possible to consider increasing the dose to 13.3 mg/24 hours after 6 months on 9.5 mg/24 hours if tolerated and meaningful cognitive or functional decline occurs. A 48-week RCT found the higher strength patch (13.3 mg) to significantly reduce deterioration in instrumental activities of daily living (IADL) compared with the 9.5 mg/24 hour patch and was well tolerated.[69]

Memantine appears to be well tolerated[70,71] and the only conditions associated with warnings include hepatic impairment and epilepsy/seizures.[72]

Adverse effects

Cholinesterase inhibitors

When adverse effects occur with AChE-Is, they are largely predictable: excess cholinergic stimulation can lead to nausea, vomiting, dizziness, insomnia and diarrhoea.[73] Such effects are most likely to occur at the start of therapy or when the dose is increased. They are dose-related and tend to be transient. Urinary incontinence has also been reported.[74] There appear to be no important differences between drugs in respect to type or frequency of adverse events, although clinical trials generally suggest a relatively lower frequency of adverse events for donepezil. This may simply be a reflection of the aggressive titration schedules used in trials of other drugs. Gastrointestinal effects appeared to be more common with oral rivastigmine in clinical trials than with other cholinesterase inhibitors, however slower titration, ensuring oral rivastigmine is taken with food or using the patch reduces the risk of GI effects.

An analysis of 16 years of individual case safety reports from VigiBase found that the most common adverse effects reported with AChE-Is were neuropsychiatric symptoms (31.4%), GI disorders (15.9%) and general disorders and administration site conditions (11.9%). Cardiovascular adverse drug reactions (ADRs) accounted for 11.7% of ADRs.[75]

In view of their pharmacological action, AChE-Is can be expected to have vagotonic effects on heart rate (i.e. bradycardia). The potential for this action may be of particular importance in patients with 'sick sinus syndrome' or other supraventricular cardiac conduction disturbances, such as sinoatrial or atrioventricular block.[7–13]

Concerns over the potential cardiac adverse effects associated with AChE-Is were raised following findings from controlled trials of galantamine in mild cognitive impairment (MCI) in which increased mortality was associated with galantamine compared with placebo (1.5% vs 0.5%, respectively).[76] Although no specific cause of death was dominant, half the deaths reported were due to cardiovascular disorders. As a result, the FDA issued a warning restricting galantamine in patients with MCI. The relevance to AD remains unclear.[77] A Cochrane review of pooled data from RCTs of the AChE-Is revealed that there was a significantly higher incidence of syncope amongst the AChE-I groups compared with the placebo groups (3.43% vs 1.87%). A population-based study using a case-time-control design examined health records for 1.4 million older adults in

Ontario and found that treatment with AChE-Is was associated with a doubled risk of hospitalisation for bradycardia. (The drugs were resumed at discharge in over half the cases suggesting that cardiovascular toxicity of AChE-Is is underappreciated by clinicians.[78]) It seems that patients with Lewy body dementia are more susceptible to the bradyarrhythmic adverse effects of these drugs owing to the autonomic insufficiency associated with the disease.[79] A similar study found hospital visits for syncope were also more frequent in people receiving AChE-Is than in controls: 31.5 versus 18.6 events per 1000 person-years (adjusted hazard ratio [HR] 1.76).[80]

The manufacturers of all three agents therefore advise that the drugs should be used with caution in patients with cardiovascular disease or in those taking concurrent medicines that reduce heart rate (e.g. digoxin or beta blockers). Although a pre-treatment mandatory ECG has been suggested,[77] a review of published evidence showed that the incidence of cardiovascular adverse effects is low and that serious adverse effects are rare. In addition, the value of pre-treatment screening and routine ECGs is questionable and is not currently recommended by NICE. However, in patients with a history of cardiovascular disease or those who are prescribed concomitant negative chronotropic drugs with AChE-Is, an ECG is advised. (See Yorkshire and the Humber Clinical Networks guidelines – The Assessment of Cardiac Status Before Prescribing Acetyl Cholinesterase Inhibitors for Dementia, 2016.[81])

In a study of 204 elderly patients with AD, each had their ECG and blood pressure assessed before and after starting AChE-I therapy. It was noted that none of the AChE-Is was associated with increased negative chronotropic, arrhythmogenic or hypotensive effects and therefore a preferred drug could not be established with regards to vagotonic effects.[82] Similarly, a Danish retrospective cohort study[83] found no substantial differences in the risk of myocardial infarction (MI) or heart failure between participants on donepezil and those using the other AChE-Is. Memantine was in fact associated with greatest risk of all-cause mortality, although sicker individuals were selected for memantine therapy. A Swedish cohort study[84] found that AChE-Is were associated with a 35% reduced risk of MI or death in patients with AD. These associations were stronger with increasing doses of AChE-Is. RCTs are required in order to confirm findings from this observational study, but they fit well with other observations of reduced mortality.

A review of the cardiovascular effects of dementia drugs[85] found that although such events with AChE-Is are very uncommon, there was evidence that they are associated with small but significant increase in the risk of syncope and bradycardia. There are also a few reports that they may occasionally be associated with QT prolongation and torsades de pointes.

Guidelines for managing cardiovascular risk prior to and during treatment with AChE-Is in AD are summarised in Figure 6.1.

Memantine

Although little is known about the cardiovascular effects of memantine, there have been reports of bradycardia and reduced cardiovascular survival associated with its use.[85]

An analysis of pooled prospective data for **memantine** revealed that the most frequently reported adverse effects in placebo-controlled trials included agitation (7.5% memantine vs 12% placebo), falls (6.8% vs 7.1%), dizziness (6.3% vs 5.7%),

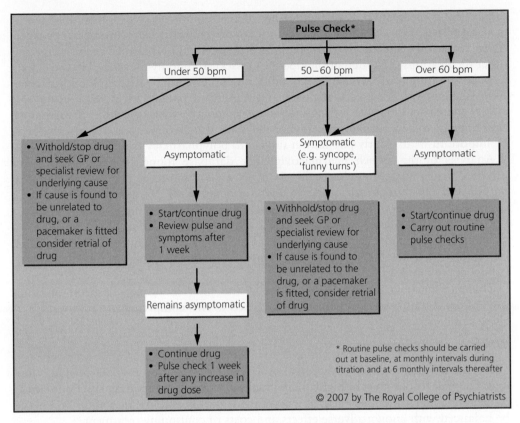

Figure 6.1 Suggested guidelines for managing cardiovascular risk prior to and during treatment with AChE-Is in AD.[81,86] Reproduced with permission from Rowland et al, 2007.[86]

accidental injury (6.0% vs 7.2%), influenza-like symptoms (6.0% vs 5.8%), headache (5.2% vs 3.7%) and diarrhoea (5.0% vs 5.6%).[87]

An analysis of the French Pharmacovigilance Database compared adverse effects reported with **donepezil** with **memantine**. The most frequent ADRs with donepezil alone and memantine alone were respectively: bradycardia (10% vs 7%), weakness (5% vs 6%) and convulsions (4% vs 3%). Although it is well known that donepezil is often associated with bradycardia and memantine associated with seizures, this analysis suggests that memantine can also induce bradycardia and donepezil seizures, thus high-lighting the care required when treating patients with dementia who have a history of bradycardia or epilepsy.[88]

Interactions

Potential for interaction may also differentiate currently available AChE-Is. Donepezil[89] and galantamine[90] are metabolised by cytochromes 2D6 and 3A4 and so drug levels may be altered by other drugs affecting the function of these enzymes. AChE-Is them-selves may also interfere with the metabolism of other drugs, although this is perhaps a theoretical consideration. Rivastigmine has almost no potential for interaction since it is metabolised at the site of action and does not affect hepatic cytochromes. A prospective pharmacodynamic analysis of potential drug interactions between rivastigmine and other medications (22 different therapeutic classes) commonly prescribed in the elderly population compared adverse effects odds ratios between rivastigmine and placebo. Rivastigmine was not associated with any significant pattern of increase in adverse effects that would indicate a drug interaction compared with placebo.[91] Rivastigmine thus appears to be least likely to cause problematic drug interactions, a factor that may be important in an elderly population subject to polypharmacy (see Table 6.2).

Analysis of the French pharmacovigilance database found that the majority of reported drug interactions concerning AChE-Is were found to be pharmacodynamic in nature and most frequently involved the combination of AChE-Is and bradycardic drugs (beta blockers, digoxin, amiodarone, calcium-channel antagonists). Almost a third of these interactions resulted in cardiovascular ADRs such as bradycardia, atrioventricular block and arterial hypotension. The second most frequent drug interaction reported was the combination of AChE-I with anticholinergic drugs leading to pharmacological antagonism.[94]

The pharmacodynamics, pharmacokinetic and pharmacogenetic aspects of drugs used in dementia have recently been summarised in two comprehensive reviews.[95,96]

When to stop treatment

The evidence base to guide withdrawal of dementia medication in older people is limited. These decisions must be highly individualised and patient-centred. Discontinuation of dementia medication may lead to worsening cognition and function and risks should be balanced with known adverse effects and costs of continuing treatment.[97]

A large multicentre study[60] of community-dwelling patients with moderate or severe AD investigated the long-term effects of donepezil over 12 months compared with stopping donepezil after 3 months, switching to memantine, or combining donepezil with memantine. Continued treatment with donepezil was associated with continued cognitive benefits, and patients with a Mini Mental State Examination (MMSE) score as low as 3 also benefitted from treatment. This suggests that patients should continue treatment with AChE-Is for as long as possible and there should not be a cut-off MMSE score where treatment is stopped automatically. Moreover, secondary and post hoc analyses of this study found that withdrawal of donepezil in patients with moderate to severe AD increased the risk of nursing home placement during 12 months of treatment, but made no difference during the following 3 years of follow-up. This highlights the point that decisions to stop or continue treatment should be informed by potential risks of withdrawal, even if the perceived benefits of continued treatment are not clear.[98]

In addition to this, a meta-analysis evaluating the efficacy of the three AChE-Is and memantine in relation to the severity of AD found that the efficacy of all drugs except memantine was independent of dementia severity in all domains. The effect of memantine on functional impairment was actually better in patients with more severe AD. Results clearly demonstrated that patients in differing stages of AD retain the ability to respond to treatment with AChE-Is and memantine. Medication effects are therefore substantially independent from disease severity, and patients with a wide range of

Table 6.2 Drug–drug interactions[8–13,92,93]

Drug	Metabolism	Plasma levels increased by	Plasma levels decreased by	Pharmacodynamic interactions
Donepezil (Aricept®)	Substrate at 3A4 and 2D6	**Ketoconazole** **Itraconazole** **Erythromycin** **Quinidine** **Fluoxetine** **Paroxetine**	**Rifampicin** **Phenytoin** **Carbamazepine** **Alcohol**	Antagonistic with **anticholinergic drugs** and **competitive neuromuscular blockers** (e.g. **tubocurarine**) Potential for synergistic activity with **cholinomimetics** such as **depolarising neuromuscular blocking agents** (e.g. **succinylcholine**), **cholinergic agonists** and **peripherally acting cholinesterase inhibitors** (e.g. **neostigmine**). **Beta blockers, amiodarone or calcium-channel blockers** may have additive effects on cardiac conduction. Caution with concomitant use of **drugs known to induce QT prolongation and/or torsades de pointes**. Movement disorders and neuroleptic malignant syndrome have occurred with concomitant use of **antipsychotics** and cholinesterase inhibitors Concurrent use with **seizure lowering agents** may result in reduced seizure threshold
Rivastigmine (Exelon®)	Non-hepatic metabolism	Metabolic interactions appear unlikely Rivastigmine may inhibit the butyryl-cholinesterase mediated metabolism of other substances, e.g. **cocaine** Smoking **tobacco** increases the clearance of rivastigmine		Antagonistic effects with **anticholinergic** and **competitive neuromuscular blockers** (e.g. **tubocurarine**). Potential for synergistic activity with **cholinomimetics** such as **depolarising neuromuscular blocking** agents (e.g. **succinylcholine**), **cholinergic agonists** (e.g. **bethanechol**) or **peripherally acting cholinesterase inhibitors** (e.g. **neostigmine**). Synergistic effects on cardiac conduction with **beta blockers, amiodarone, calcium-channel blockers**. Caution with concomitant use of **drugs known to induce QT prolongation and/or torsades de pointes**. Movement disorders and neuroleptic malignant syndrome have occurred with concomitant use of **antipsychotics** and cholinesterase inhibitors. Concurrent use with **metoclopramide** may result in increased risk of EPS
Galantamine (Reminyl®)	Substrate at 3A4 and 2D6	**Ketoconazole** **Erythromycin** **Ritonavir** **Quinidine** **Paroxetine** **Fluoxetine** **Fluvoxamine** **Amitriptyline**	None known	Antagonistic effects with **anticholinergic** and **competitive neuromuscular blockers** (e.g. **tubocurarine**). Potential for synergistic activity with **cholinomimetics** such as **depolarising neuromuscular blocking agents** (e.g. **succinylcholine**), **cholinergic agonists** and **peripherally acting cholinesterase inhibitors** (e.g. **neostigmine**). Possible interaction with agents that significantly reduce heart rate (e.g. **digoxin, beta blockers, certain calcium-channel blockers** and **amiodarone**). Caution with concomitant use of drugs known to induce QT prolongation and/or torsades de pointes (manufacturer recommends ECG in such cases). Movement disorders and neuroleptic malignant syndrome have occurred with concomitant use of **antipsychotics** and cholinesterase inhibitors

(Continued)

Table 6.2 (*Continued*)

Drug	Metabolism	Plasma levels increased by	Plasma levels decreased by	Pharmacodynamic interactions
Memantine (Exiba®)	Primarily non-hepatic metabolism Renally eliminated	**Cimetidine** **Ranitidine** **Procainamide** **Quinidine** **Quinine** **Nicotine** **Trimethoprim** Isolated cases of INR increases reported with concomitant warfarin (close monitoring of prothrombin time or INR advisable) Drugs that alkalinise urine (pH ~8) may reduce renal elimination of memantine (e.g. **carbonic anhydrase inhibitors, sodium bicarbonate**).	None known (Possibility of reduced serum level of **hydrochlorothiazide** when co-administered with memantine)	Effects of **L-dopa, dopaminergic agonists, selegiline** and **anticholinergics** may be enhanced Effects of **barbiturates** and **antipsychotics** may be reduced Avoid concomitant use with **amantadine, ketamine** and **dextromethorphan** – increased risk of CNS toxicity. One published case report on possible risk for **phenytoin** and memantine combination Dosage adjustment may be necessary for **antispasmodic agents, dantrolene** or **baclofen** when administered with memantine A single case report of myoclonus and confusion when co-administered with **co-trimoxazole** or **trimethoprim**

NB: This list is not exhaustive – caution with other drugs that are also inhibitors or enhancers of CYP3A4 and CYP2D6 enzymes.
CNS, central nervous system; EPS, extrapyramidal symptoms; INR, international normalised ratio.

> **Box 6.2** Reasons for stopping treatment
>
> ▪ When the patient/caregiver decides to stop (after being advised on the risks and benefits of stopping treatment).
> ▪ When the patient refuses to take the medication (but see section on 'Covert administration of medicines within food and drink').
> ▪ When there are problems with patient compliance which cannot be reasonably resolved.
> ▪ When the patient's cognitive, functional or behavioural decline is worsened by treatment.
> ▪ When there are intolerable adverse effects.
> ▪ When co-morbidities make treatment risky or futile (e.g. terminal illness).
> ▪ Where there is no clinically meaningful benefit to continuing therapy (clinical judgement should be used here rather than ceasing treatment when a patient reaches a certain score on a cognitive outcome or when they are institutionalised).
> ▪ When dementia has progressed to a severely impaired stage (Global Deterioration Scale stage 7: development of swallowing difficulties).

severities can benefit from drug therapy. This suggests that the severity of a patient's illness should not preclude treatment with these drugs.[99]

Guidance for discontinuation of dementia medication in clinical practice has been summarised in Box 6.2.[97]

When a decision is made to stop therapy (for reasons other than lack of tolerability), tapering of the dose and monitoring the patient for evidence of significant decline during the next 1–3 months are advised. If such decline occurs, reinstatement of therapy should be considered.

NICE recommendations

NICE Guidance on Dementia[1] was last updated in September 2016 and has been amended to incorporate the updated NICE technology appraisal of drugs for AD,[100] also updated in May 2016. See Box 6.3.

Other treatments (where the evidence remains less certain)

Gingko biloba

A Cochrane review found that although *Gingko biloba* appears to be safe with no excess adverse effects compared with placebo, there was no convincing evidence that it is efficacious for dementia and cognitive impairment. Many of the trials were too small and used unsatisfactory methods and publication bias could not be excluded. The review concluded that gingko's clinical benefit in dementia or cognitive impairment is somewhat inconsistent and unconvincing.[102] A later randomised, double-blind trial which compared *Gingko biloba*, donepezil or both combined found no statistically significant or clinically relevant differences between the three groups with respect to efficacy. In addition, it was noted that combined treatment adverse effects were less frequent than with donepezil alone.[103] Two recent meta-analyses suggest useful efficacy for gingko,[104,105] notwithstanding numerous methodological concerns. Several reports have noted that gingko may increase the risk of bleeding.[106] The drug is widely used in Germany but less so elsewhere.

CHAPTER 6

Box 6.3 Summary of NICE guidance for the treatment of Alzheimer's disease[1,100]

- The three acetylcholinesterase inhibitors donepezil, galantamine and rivastigmine are recommended for managing mild to moderate AD.
- Memantine is recommended for managing moderate AD for people who are intolerant of or have a contraindication to AChE-Is, or for managing severe AD.
- Treatment should be under the following conditions:
  Prescribers should only start treatment with donepezil, galantamine, rivastigmine or memantine on the advice of a clinician who has the necessary knowledge and skills. This could include:
  - secondary care medical specialists such as psychiatrists, geriatricians and neurologists
  - other health-care professionals such as GPs, nurse consultants and advanced nurse practitioners with specialist expertise in diagnosing and treating AD.
- Ensure that local arrangements for prescribing, supply and treatment review follow the NICE guideline on medicines optimisation.[101]
- Treatment should be continued only when it is considered to be having a worthwhile effect on cognitive, global, functional or behavioural symptoms.
- Therapy with AChE-Is should be initiated with a drug with the lowest acquisition cost (taking into account required daily dose and the price per dose once shared care has started). An alternative may be considered on the basis of adverse effects profile, expectations about adherence, medical co-morbidity, possibility of drug interactions and dosing profiles.
- When assessing the severity of AD and the need for treatment, health-care professionals should not rely solely on cognition scores in circumstances in which it would be inappropriate to do so, and should take into account any physical, sensory or learning disabilities, or communication difficulties that could affect the results. Any adjustments considered appropriate should be made.

Vitamins

A Cochrane review of **vitamin E** for AD and MCI examined three studies. The authors' conclusions were that there is no evidence of efficacy of vitamin E in prevention or treatment of AD or MCI and that further research is required in order to identify its role in this area.[107]

Interest in vitamin D has declined.

A placebo-controlled pilot RCT of 1 mg **folic acid** supplementation of AChE-Is over 6 months in 57 patients with AD showed significant benefit in combined IADL and social behaviour scores (folate + 1.50 [SD 5.32] vs placebo –2.29 [SD 6.16] [p = 0.03]) but no change in MMSE scores.[108] Another RCT examining the efficacy of **multivitamins and folic acid** as an adjunct to AChE-Is over 26 weeks in 89 patients with AD found no statistically significant benefits between the two groups on cognition or ADL function.[109] A Cochrane review found no evidence that **folic acid** with or without **vitamin B_{12}** improves cognitive function of unselected elderly people with or without dementia.[110]

Whilst elevated homocysteine, decreased folate and low vitamin B_{12} serum levels have previously been associated with poor cognitive function, cognitive decline and dementia, prospective studies have not found a relationship between dementia and high homocysteine.[111] A systematic and critical review of the literature did not provide any clear evidence that supplementation with vitamin B_{12} and/or folate improves cognition or dementia even though these supplements might normalise homocysteine levels.[112]

Omega-3 fatty acids

A Cochrane review of omega-3 fatty acids for the treatment of dementia included three trials that investigated 632 people with mild to moderate AD. The review found that taking omega-3 polyunsaturated fatty acid supplements for 6 months had no effect on cognition (learning and understanding), everyday functioning, quality of life or mental health. It also had no effect on ratings of the overall severity of the illness. The trials did not report adverse effects very well, but none of the studies described significant harmful effects on health.[113]

Ginseng

A prospective open-label study of ginseng in AD measured cognitive performance in 97 patients randomly assigned ginseng or placebo for 12 weeks and then 12 weeks after the ginseng had been discontinued. After ginseng treatment, the cognitive subscales of ADAS and MMSE score began to show improvement continued up to 12 weeks but scores declined to levels of the control group following discontinuation of ginseng.[114] A recent systematic review and meta-analysis[115] including four RCTs involving 259 participants showed that the effects of ginseng on AD remain unproven. The main limitations of the available studies were small sample sizes, poor methodological qualities and no placebo controls. Larger, well-designed studies are needed to test the effect of ginseng on AD in the future.

Dimebon

Dimebon (also known as latrepirdine), a non-selective antihistamine previously approved in Russia but later discontinued for commercial reasons, has been assessed for safety, tolerability and efficacy in the treatment of patients with mild to moderate AD. It acts as a weak inhibitor of butyrylcholinesterase and acetylcholinesterase, weakly blocks the NMDA-receptor signalling pathway and inhibits the mitochondrial permeability transition pore opening.[116] A recent Cochrane review concluded that there was no beneficial effect of dimebon on cognition and function in mild to moderate AD, though there appeared to be modest benefit for behaviour.[117]

Hirudin

Natural hirudin, isolated from salivary gland of medicinal leeches, is a direct thrombin inhibitor and has been used for many years in China. A small 20-week open-label RCT of 84 patients receiving donepezil or donepezil plus hirudin (3 g/day) found that patients on the combination showed significant decrease in ADAS-cog scores and significant increase in ADL scores compared with donepezil alone. However haemorrhage and hypersensitivity reactions were more common in the combination group compared with the donepezil group (11.9% and 7.1% vs 2.4% and 2.4%, respectively).[118] The potential haemorrhagic effects of hirudin need further exploration before it can be considered for clinical use.

Huperzine A

Huperzine A, an alkaloid isolated from the Chinese herb *Huperzia serrata*, is a potent, highly selective, reversible AChE-I used for treating AD since 1994 in China and available as a nutraceutical in the USA. A meta-analysis found that huperzine A 300–500 μg daily

CHAPTER 6

for 8–24 weeks in AD led to significant improvements in MMSE (mean change 3.5) and ADL with effect size shown to increase over treatment time. Most adverse effects were cholinergic in nature and no serious adverse effects occurred.[119] A later meta-analysis produced similarly positive, if uncertain, results.[120] A Cochrane review of huperzine A in vascular dementia, however, found no convincing evidence for its value in vascular dementia.[121] Similarly, a Cochrane review of huperzine A for MCI concluded that the current evidence is insufficient for this indication as no eligible trials were identified.[122]

Saffron

There is increasing evidence to suggest possible efficacy of *Crocus sativus* (saffron) in the management of AD. In a 16-week placebo-controlled RCT, saffron produced a significantly better outcome on cognitive function in mild to moderate AD than placebo and there were no significant differences between the two groups in terms of observed adverse events.[123] A 22-week double-blind study included 55 patients randomly assigned to saffron capsules 15 mg bd or donepezil 5 mg bd. Results found no significant differences between the two groups in terms of efficacy or adverse effects, although vomiting occurred significantly more frequently in the donepezil group.[124] In a randomised double-blind parallel-group study, 68 patients with moderate to severe AD received memantine (20 mg/day) or saffron extract (30 mg/day) capsules for 12 months. Participants were evaluated every month by the Severe Cognitive Impairment Rating Scale (SCIRS) and functional assessment staging (FAST) in addition to recording the probable adverse events. There was no significant difference between the two groups in the scores changes from baseline to the endpoint on SCIRS and FAST. The frequency of adverse events was not significantly different between the two groups either.[125]

Cerebrolysin

Cerebrolysin is a parenterally administered, porcine brain-derived peptide preparation that has pharmacodynamic properties similar to those of endogenous neurotrophic factors. A meta-analysis included six RCTs comparing cerebrolysin 30 mg/day with placebo in mild to moderate AD. Cerebrolysin was significantly more effective than placebo at 4 weeks regarding cognitive function and at 4 weeks and 6 months regarding global clinical change and 'global benefit'. The safety of cerebrolysin was comparable to placebo.[126] In addition, a large RCT comparing cerebrolysin, donepezil or combination therapy showed beneficial effects on global measures and cognition for all three treatment groups compared with baseline.[127] A Cochrane review assessed the efficacy and safety of cerebrolysin in vascular dementia. It concluded that cerebrolysin may have positive effects on cognitive function and global function in patients with vascular dementia of mild to moderate severity, but there was still insufficient evidence to recommend it as a routine treatment for vascular dementia due to the limited number of included trials, wide variety of treatment durations and short-term follow-up in most of the trials.[128] Cerebrolysin was generally well tolerated in trials with dizziness being the most frequently reported adverse event.[127]

Statins

In AD, amyloid protein is deposited in the form of extracellular plaques, and studies have determined that amyloid protein generation is cholesterol-dependent.

Hypercholesterolaemia has also been implicated in the pathogenesis of vascular dementia. Because of the role of statins in cholesterol reduction, they have been explored as a
means to treat dementia. A Cochrane review however found that there is still insufficient evidence to recommend statins for the treatment of dementia. Analysis from the
studies available indicate that statins have no benefit on the outcome measures ADAS-
cog or MMSE.[129] A further Cochrane review examined whether statins could prevent
dementia. Initial evidence from observational studies was very promising. However,
indication bias may have been a factor in these studies and the evidence from subsequent RCTs has been negative.[130]

Cocoa

Sixty older people were studied in a clinical trial of neurovascular coupling and
cognition in response to 30 days of cocoa consumption. Two cups of cocoa daily for
30 days resulted in higher neurovascular coupling (NVC) and individuals with higher
NVC had better cognitive function and greater cerebral white matter structural
integrity.[131]

Souvenaid

Souvenaid is a medical food for the dietary management of early AD. The mix of nutri-
ents in this drink is suggested to have a beneficial effect on cognitive function; however
health claims for medical foods are not checked by government agencies. Souvenaid has
been investigated in three clinical trials. The first trial showed that Souvenaid produced
a significant improvement in delayed verbal recall, but not in other psychological
tests.[132] The second and largest trial showed no effect on any outcome.[133] A third trial
showed no significant effect at 12 or 24 weeks, but a significant difference in the
24-week time course of the composite memory score.[134] However none of these outcomes was clearly specified as a primary outcome at trial registration. There is currently
therefore no convincing proof that Souvenaid benefits cognitive function. Further regulated and robust efficacy data are required.

Idalopirdine

Idalopirdine is a 5-HT$_6$ receptor antagonist. Given that the 5-HT$_6$ receptor is expressed
in areas of the CNS involved with memory and that there is evidence suggesting that
blocking of these receptors induces acetylcholine release, it has become a promising
approach that 5-HT$_6$ antagonism could restore ACh levels in a deteriorated cholinergic
system.[135] A double-blind, placebo-controlled RCT (LADDER) including 278 patients
found that idalopirdine improved cognitive function in donepezil-treated patients with
moderate AD. At week 24, the change from baseline in ADAS-cog total score was
+1.38 in the placebo group and –0.77 in the idalopirdine group (treatment difference
of –2.16 points). The most common adverse events (occurring in >3% of patients)
were increased γ-glutamyltransferase (14 [10%] in the idalopirdine group vs 2 [2%] in
the placebo group), diarrhoea (6 [4%] vs 9 [7%]), urinary tract infections (3 [2%] vs
9 [7%]), fall (3 [2%] vs 8 [6%]), increased alanine aminotransferase (9 [6%] vs none),
and benign prostatic hyperplasia (2 [5%] vs none). Serious adverse events were
reported by 14 (10%) patients in the idalopirdine group and 13 (10%) patients in the
placebo group.[136]

CHAPTER 6

Anti-inflammatory drugs

A large number of RCTs of anti-inflammatory agents in AD have failed to reach primary outcomes. Large-scale studies of non-steroidal anti-inflammatory drugs (NSAIDs) including indometacin, naproxen and rofecoxib in AD have been unsuccessful. RCTs with a range of other anti-inflammatory drugs including prednisolone, hydroxychloroquine, simvastatin, atorvastatin, aspirin and rosiglitazone have also shown no clinically significant changes in primary cognitive outcomes in patients with AD.[48]

Trazodone and dibenzoylmethane

Two existing compounds have recently been found to be markedly neuroprotective in mouse models of neurodegeneration, using clinically relevant doses over a prolonged period of time, without systemic toxicity. Trazodone, an antidepressant in the serotonin antagonist and reuptake inhibitor class which has additional anxiolytic and hypnotic effects, has been shown to reduce behavioural and psychological symptoms of dementia in AD but no study had previously looked at the progression of neurodegeneration with trazodone treatment. Dibenzoylmethane (DBM) is a minor constituent of liquorice that has been found to have antineoplastic effects, with efficacy against prostate and mammary tumours. In prion-diseased mice, both trazodone and DBM treatment restored memory deficits, abrogated development of neurological signs, prevented neurodegeneration and significantly prolonged survival. In tauopathy-frontotemporal dementia mice, both drugs were neuroprotective, rescued memory deficits and reduced hippocampal atrophy. Further, trazodone reduced p-tau burden. These compounds therefore represent potential new disease-modifying treatments for dementia.[137] Trazodone in particular should now be tested in prospective trials in patients, however at the time of writing there is insufficient evidence to recommend routine prescription of trazodone to reduce rate of cognitive decline. There are no available observational data suggesting that trazodone reduces risk of dementia but some data that suggest important adverse outcomes in older people.[138]

Novel treatments

Three new drugs have failed to improve clinical outcomes in phase III trials for Alzheimer's disease. These include:

- **Semagacestat,** a γ-secretase inhibitor;[139] the trials including 3000 patients were discontinued in 2010 because of the absence of improvement in cognition in the study group and worsening cognition at higher doses compared to controls. Incidence of skin cancer was also higher in the study group.[140]
- **Solanezumab** is a humanised monoclonal antibody that binds soluble forms of amyloid and promotes its clearance from the brain.[141] Despite failing to reach predefined endpoints in phase III trials in patients with mild to moderate AD, subsequent pooled analysis showed that cognitive scores in a subgroup of patients with milder symptoms showed small benefits.[140] However, an eagerly awaited third trial investigating solanezumab (EXPEDITION3) in older patients with a clinical diagnosis of early AD and amyloid deposits that was seen as a 'major test' of the

amyloid cascade hypothesis also found negative results which were announced in November 2016 – solanezumab did not slow cognitive decline in adults with mild AD.[142]

- **Bapineuzumab**; a humanised anti-amyloid-β monoclonal antibody.[143] A recent meta-analysis of RCTs with bapineuzumab confirmed its lack of clinical efficacy and, owing to its associations with serious adverse effects (vasogenic oedema), its use is not recommended in patients with mild to moderate AD.[144]

Vascular dementia

Vascular dementia (VaD) has been reported to comprise 10–50% of dementia cases and is the second most common type of dementia after AD. It is caused by ischaemic damage to the brain and is associated with cognitive impairment and behavioural disturbances. The management options are currently very limited and focus on controlling the underlying risk factors for cerebrovascular disease.[145]

None of the currently available drugs is formally licensed in the UK for VaD. The management of VaD has been summarised.[146,147] Unlike the situation with stroke, there is no conclusive evidence that treatment of hyperlipidaemia with statins or treatment of blood clotting abnormalities with acetylsalicylic acid have an effect on VaD incidence or disease progression.[148] Similarly a Cochrane review found that there were no studies supporting the role of statins in the treatment of VaD.[130] There is however growing evidence for donepezil,[149,150] rivastigmine,[151,152] galantamine[153–155] and memantine.[156,157] The largest clinical trial of donepezil in VaD found small but significant improvement on the vascular ADAS-cog subscale but no difference was seen on the Clinician's Interview-Based Impression of Change (CIBIC-Plus).[158] These results are consistent with prior trials suggesting that donepezil may have a greater impact on cognitive rather than global outcomes in VaD. The Cochrane review for donepezil in vascular cognitive impairment however found evidence to support its benefit in improving cognition function, clinical global impression and ADL after 6 months treatment.[150] In a Cochrane review for galantamine for vascular cognitive impairment,[18,159] there were limited data suggesting some advantage over placebo in areas of cognition and global clinical state. However the authors thought more studies were needed to confirm these results. Trials of galantamine reported high rates of GI adverse effects. The Cochrane review for rivastigmine in vascular cognitive impairment found some evidence of benefit, however the conclusion was based on one large study and adverse effects with rivastigmine led to withdrawal in a significant proportion of patients.[130,160] Furthermore a meta-analysis of RCTs found that cholinesterase inhibitors and memantine produce small benefits in cognition of uncertain clinical significance and concluded that data were insufficient to support widespread use of these agents in VaD.[145]

Note that it is impossible to diagnose with certainty vascular or Alzheimer's dementia, and much dementia has mixed causation. This might explain why certain AChE-Is do not always provide consistent results in probable VaD, and the data indicating efficacy in cognitive outcomes were derived from older patients, who were therefore likely to have concomitant AD pathology.[161]

CHAPTER 6

Dementia with Lewy bodies

It has been suggested that dementia with Lewy bodies (DLB) may account for 15–25% of cases of dementia (although autopsy suggests much lower rates). Characteristic symptoms are dementia with fluctuation of cognitive ability, early and persistent visual hallucinations and spontaneous motor features of parkinsonism. Falls, syncope, transient disturbances of consciousness, neuroleptic sensitivity and hallucinations in other modalities are also common.[162]

A Cochrane review for AChE-Is in DLB and Parkinson's disease (PD) dementia and cognitive impairment found evidence supporting their use in PD, but no statistically significant improvement was observed in patients with DLB and the review concluded that further trials were necessary to clarify their effects in this patient group.[163] A comparative analysis of cholinesterase inhibitors in DLB, which included open-label trials as well as the placebo-controlled randomised trial of rivastigmine, found that there was no compelling evidence that one AChE-I is better than the other in DLB.[164] Comprehensive reviews[165] of the treatment of DLB and meta-analysis of trials[166,167] are available, however no substantial new data regarding the use of antipsychotic drugs or AChE-Is have been published recently and so recommendations made in these areas remain unchanged.[48] Despite certain reports of patients with DLB worsening or responding adversely when exposed to memantine,[168] an RCT of memantine (funded by the manufacturer) found it to be mildly beneficial in terms of global clinical status and behavioural symptoms in patients with DLB.[169] A systematic review and meta-analysis, however, found memantine to have no significant effects on motor function, cognition, neuropsychiatric symptoms or ADL scores, but it was superior to placebo for the overall impression of the disorders.[170] These results do not show a consistent pattern of treatment response which highlights the considerable variation in sensitivity to treatment effects in this population.[48]

Mild cognitive impairment

Mild cognitive impairment (MCI) is hypothesised to represent a pre-clinical stage of dementia but forms a heterogeneous group with variable prognosis. A Cochrane review assessing the safety and efficacy of AChE-Is in MCI found there was very little evidence that they affect progression to dementia or cognitive test scores. This weak evidence was countered by the increased risk of adverse effects, particularly GI effects, meaning that AChE-Is could not be recommended in MCI.[171] A systematic review[172] found that there was no replicated evidence that any intervention was effective for MCI including AChE-Is and the NSAID rofecoxib. A recent review summarises the management of MCI in older people.[173]

Other dementias

A systematic review of RCTs for **frontotemporal dementias** showed that certain drugs may be effective in reducing behavioural symptoms (e.g. SSRIs, trazodone) but none of these had an effect on cognition.[174]

A Cochrane review assessed the efficacy and safety of AChE-Is for **rare dementias associated with neurological conditions**. The sample sizes of most trials were very small

Table 6.3 Summary of BAP recommendations

	First choice	Second choice
Alzheimer's disease	AChE-Is	Memantine
Vascular dementia	None	None
Mixed dementia	AChE-Is	Memantine
Dementia with Lewy bodies	AChE-Is	Memantine
Mild cognitive impairment	None	None
Dementia with Parkinson's disease	AChE-Is	None
Frontotemporal dementia	None	None

AChE-I, acetylcholinesterase inhibitor.

and efficacy on cognitive function and ADL was found to be unclear, although AChE-Is were associated with more GI adverse effects compared with placebo.[175]

Summary of clinical practice guidance with anti-dementia drugs from BAP[48]

AChE-Is and memantine are effective in AD with a broad range of severity. Other drugs including statins, anti-inflammatory drugs, vitamin E, nutritional supplements and gingko cannot be recommended, either for the treatment or prevention of AD. Neither AChE-Is nor memantine are effective in MCI. AChE-Is are not effective in frontotemporal dementia and may cause agitation. AChE-Is may be used for people with LBDs (both PD dementia and DLB), and memantine may be helpful. No drug is clearly effective in VaD, though AChE-Is are beneficial in mixed dementia. Early evidence suggests that multifactorial interventions may have potential to prevent or delay the onset of dementia. Many novel pharmacological approaches involving strategies to reduce amyloid and/or tau deposition in those with or at high risk of AD are in progress. Although results of pivotal studies in early (prodromal/mild) AD are awaited, results to date in more established (mild to moderate) AD have been equivocal and no disease-modifying agent is either licensed or can be currently recommended for clinical use. See Table 6.3.

References

1. National Institute for Health and Care Excellence. Dementia: supporting people with dementia and their carers in health and social care. Clinical Guideline 42, 2011; updated September 2016. https://www.nice.org.uk/guidance/cg42.
2. Francis PT et al. The cholinergic hypothesis of Alzheimer's disease: a review of progress. J Neurol Neurosurg Psychiatry 1999; 66:137–147.
3. Craig LA et al. Revisiting the cholinergic hypothesis in the development of Alzheimer's disease. Neurosci Biobehav Rev 2011; 35:1397–1409.
4. Mesulam M et al. Widely spread butyrylcholinesterase can hydrolyze acetylcholine in the normal and Alzheimer brain. Neurobiol Dis 2002; 9:88–93.
5. Weinstock M. Selectivity of cholinesterase inhibition: clinical implications for the treatment of Alzheimer's disease. CNS Drugs 1999; 12:307–323.
6. Matsunaga S et al. Memantine monotherapy for Alzheimer's disease: a systematic review and meta-analysis. PLoS One 2015; 10:e0123289.
7. BNF Online. British National Formulary. 2017. https://www.medicinescomplete.com/mc/bnf/current/.

CHAPTER 6

8. Eisai Ltd. Summary of Product Characteristics. Aricept tablets (donepezil hydrochloride). 2016. https://www.medicines.org.uk/emc/medicine/577.

9. Novartis Pharmaceuticals UK Limited. Summary Of Product Characteristics. Exelon 4.6 mg/24h, 9.5 mg/24h, 13.3 mg/24h transdermal patch. 2015. https://www.medicines.org.uk/emc/medicine/20232.

10. Sandoz Limited. Summary of Product Characteristics. Rivastigmine Sandoz 1.5 mg, 3 mg, 4.5 mg, 6 mg hard capsules. 2016. https://www.medicines.org.uk/emc/medicine/25164.

11. Shire Pharmaceuticals Limited. Summary of Product Characteristics. Reminyl XL 8mg, 16mg and 24mg prolonged release capsules.2017. https://www.medicines.org.uk/emc/medicine/16219.

12. Shire Pharmaceuticals Limited. Summary of Product Characteristics. Reminyl Oral Solution. 2017. https://www.medicines.org.uk/emc/medicine/10337.

13. Shire Pharmaceuticals Limited. Summary of Product Characteristics. Reminyl Tablets. 2017. https://www.medicines.org.uk/emc/medicine/10335.

14. Lundbeck Limited. Summary of Product Characteristics. Ebixa 5mg/pump actuation oral solution, 20mg and 10 mg Tablets and Treatment Initiation Pack. 2014. https://www.medicines.org.uk/emc/medicine/10175.

15. NHS Prescription Services. Drug Tariff. 2017. https://www.nhsbsa.nhs.uk/pharmacies-gp-practices-and-appliance-contractors/drug-tariff.

16. Buckley JS et al. A risk-benefit assessment of dementia medications: systematic review of the evidence. Drugs Aging 2015; 32:453–467.

17. Lanctot KL et al. Efficacy and safety of cholinesterase inhibitors in Alzheimer's disease: a meta-analysis. CMAJ 2003; 169:557–564.

18. Birks J. Cholinesterase inhibitors for Alzheimer's disease. Cochrane Database Syst Rev 2006:CD005593.

19. Blanco-Silvente L et al. Discontinuation, efficacy, and safety of cholinesterase inhibitors for alzheimer's disease: a meta-analysis and meta-regression of 43 randomized clinical trials enrolling 16 106 patients. Int J Neuropsychopharmacol 2017; 20:519–528.

20. Mueller C et al. Associations of acetylcholinesterase inhibitor treatment with reduced mortality in Alzheimer's disease: a retrospective survival analysis. Age Ageing 2017:1–7.

21. Farlow MR. Do cholinesterase inhibitors slow progression of Alzheimer's disease? Int J Clin Pract Suppl 2002:37–44.

22. Bond M et al. The effectiveness and cost-effectiveness of donepezil, galantamine, rivastigmine and memantine for the treatment of Alzheimer's disease (review of Technology Appraisal No. 111): a systematic review and economic model. Health Technol Assess 2012; 16:1–470.

23. Rogers SL et al. Donepezil improves cognition and global function in Alzheimer disease: a 15-week, double-blind, placebo-controlled study. Donepezil Study Group. Arch Intern Med 1998; 158:1021–1031.

24. Rogers SL et al. A 24-week, double-blind, placebo-controlled trial of donepezil in patients with Alzheimer's disease. Donepezil Study Group. Neurology 1998; 50:136–145.

25. Rogers SL et al. Long-term efficacy and safety of donepezil in the treatment of Alzheimer's disease: final analysis of a US multicentre open-label study. Eur Neuropsychopharmacol 2000; 10:195–203.

26. Birks J et al. Donepezil for dementia due to Alzheimer's disease. Cochrane Database Syst Rev 2006:CD001190.

27. AD2000 Collaborative Group. Long-term donepezil treatment in 565 patients with Alzheimer's disease (AD2000): randomised double-blind trial. Lancet 2004; 363:2105–2115.

28. Corey-Bloom J et al. A randomized trial evaluating the efficacy and safety of ENA 713 (rivastigmine tartrate), a new acetylcholinesterase inhibitor, in patients with mild to moderately severe Alzheimer's disease. Int J Geriatr Psychopharmacol 1998; 1:55–64.

29. Rosler M et al. Efficacy and safety of rivastigmine in patients with Alzheimer's disease: international randomised controlled trial. BMJ 1999; 318:633–638.

30. Birks JS et al. Rivastigmine for Alzheimer's disease. Cochrane Database Syst Rev 2015; 9:CD001191.

31. Winblad B et al. A six-month double-blind, randomized, placebo-controlled study of a transdermal patch in Alzheimer's disease – rivastigmine patch versus capsule. Int J Geriatr Psychiatry 2007; 22:456–467.

32. Zhang ZX et al. Rivastigmine patch in Chinese patients with probable Alzheimer's disease: a 24-week, randomized, double-blind parallel-group study comparing rivastigmine patch (9.5 mg/24 h) with capsule (6 mg twice daily). CNS Neurosci Ther 2016; 22:488–496.

33. Morgan TM et al. Absolute bioavailability and safety of a novel rivastigmine nasal spray in healthy elderly individuals. Br J Clin Pharmacol 2017; 83:510–516.

34. Tariot PN et al. A 5-month, randomized, placebo-controlled trial of galantamine in AD. The Galantamine USA-10 Study Group. Neurology 2000; 54:2269–2276.

35. Raskind MA et al. Galantamine in AD: A 6-month randomized, placebo-controlled trial with a 6-month extension. The Galantamine USA-1 Study Group. Neurology 2000; 54:2261–2268.

36. Wilcock GK et al. Efficacy and safety of galantamine in patients with mild to moderate Alzheimer's disease: multicentre randomised controlled trial. Galantamine International-1 Study Group. BMJ 2000; 321:1445–1449.

37. Loy C et al. Galantamine for Alzheimer's disease and mild cognitive impairment. Cochrane Database Syst Rev 2006:CD001747.

38. Burns A et al. Safety and efficacy of galantamine (Reminyl) in severe Alzheimer's disease (the SERAD study): a randomised, placebo-controlled, double-blind trial. Lancet Neurol 2009; 8:39–47.

39. Livingston G et al. The place of memantine in the treatment of Alzheimer's disease: a number needed to treat analysis. Int J Geriatr Psychiatry 2004; 19:919–925.

40. Schmitt FA et al. The severe impairment battery: concurrent validity and the assessment of longitudinal change in Alzheimer's disease. The Alzheimer's Disease Cooperative Study. Alzheimer Dis Assoc Disord 1997; 11 Suppl 2:S51–S56.

41. Mecocci P et al. Effects of memantine on cognition in patients with moderate to severe Alzheimer's disease: post-hoc analyses of ADAS-cog and SIB total and single-item scores from six randomized, double-blind, placebo-controlled studies. Int J Geriatr Psychiatry 2009; 24:532–538.

42. McShane R et al. Memantine for dementia. Cochrane Database Syst Rev 2006:CD003154.

43. Kobayashi H et al. The comparative efficacy and safety of cholinesterase inhibitors in patients with mild-to-moderate Alzheimer's disease: a Bayesian network meta-analysis. Int J Geriatr Psychiatry 2016; 31:892–904.

44. Stern RG et al. A longitudinal study of Alzheimer's disease: measurement, rate, and predictors of cognitive deterioration. Am J Psychiatry 1994; 151:390–396.

45. Burns A et al. Efficacy and safety of donepezil over 3 years: an open-label, multicentre study in patients with Alzheimer's disease. Int J Geriatr Psychiatry 2007; 22:806–812.

46. Doody RS et al. Open-label, multicenter, phase 3 extension study of the safety and efficacy of donepezil in patients with Alzheimer disease. Arch Neurol 2001; 58:427–433.

47. Farlow MR et al. Effective pharmacologic management of Alzheimer's disease. Am J Med 2007; 120:388–397.

48. O'Brien JT et al. Clinical practice with anti-dementia drugs: a revised (third) consensus statement from the British Association for Psychopharmacology. J Psychopharmacol 2017; 31:147–168.

49. Singh S et al. Discontinuation syndrome following donepezil cessation. Int J Geriatr Psychiatry 2003; 18:282–284.

50. Bidzan L et al. Withdrawal syndrome after donepezil cessation in a patient with dementia. Neurol Sci 2012; 33:1459–1461.

51. Waldemar G et al. Tolerability of switching from donepezil to memantine treatment in patients with moderate to severe Alzheimer's disease. Int J Geriatr Psychiatry 2008; 23:979–981.

52. Massoud F et al. Switching cholinesterase inhibitors in older adults with dementia. Int Psychogeriatr 2011; 23:372–378.

53. Dybicz SB et al. Patterns of cholinesterase-inhibitor use in the nursing home setting: a retrospective analysis. Am J Geriatr Pharmacother 2006; 4:154–160.

54. Jones RW et al. Safety and tolerability of once-daily versus twice-daily memantine: a randomised, double-blind study in moderate to severe Alzheimer's disease. Int J Geriatr Psychiatry 2007; 22:258–262.

55. Sabbagh M et al. Clinical recommendations for the use of donepezil 23 mg in moderate-to-severe Alzheimer's disease in the Asia-Pacific region. Dement Geriatr Cogn Dis Extra 2016; 6:382–395.

56. Plosker GL. Memantine extended release (28 mg once daily): a review of its use in Alzheimer's disease. Drugs 2015; 75:887–897.

57. Tariot PN et al. Memantine treatment in patients with moderate to severe Alzheimer disease already receiving donepezil: a randomized controlled trial. JAMA 2004; 291:317–324.

58. Hartmann S et al. Tolerability of memantine in combination with cholinesterase inhibitors in dementia therapy. Int Clin Psychopharmacol 2003; 18:81–85.

59. Olin JT et al. Safety and tolerability of rivastigmine capsule with memantine in patients with probable Alzheimer's disease: a 26-week, open-label, prospective trial (Study ENA713B US32). Int J Geriatr Psychiatry 2010; 25:419–426.

60. Howard R et al. Donepezil and memantine for moderate-to-severe Alzheimer's disease. N Engl J Med 2012; 366:893–903.

61. Gareri P et al. Retrospective study on the benefits of combined Memantine and cholinEsterase inhibitor treatMent in AGEd Patients affected with Alzheimer's Disease: the MEMAGE study. J Alzheimers Dis 2014; 41:633–640.

62. Matsunaga S et al. Combination therapy with cholinesterase inhibitors and memantine for Alzheimer's disease: a systematic review and meta-analysis. Int J Neuropsychopharmacol 2014; 18.

63. Schmidt R et al. EFNS-ENS/EAN Guideline on concomitant use of cholinesterase inhibitors and memantine in moderate to severe Alzheimer's disease. Eur J Neurol 2015; 22:889–898.

64. Periclou AP et al. Lack of pharmacokinetic or pharmacodynamic interaction between memantine and donepezil. Ann Pharmacother 2004; 38:1389–1394.

65. Grossberg GT et al. Rationale for combination therapy with galantamine and memantine in Alzheimer's disease. J Clin Pharmacol 2006; 46:17S–26S.

66. Pariente A et al. Factors associated with serious adverse reactions to cholinesterase inhibitors: a study of spontaneous reporting. CNS Drugs 2010; 24:55–63.

67. Sadowsky CH et al. Safety and tolerability of rivastigmine transdermal patch compared with rivastigmine capsules in patients switched from donepezil: data from three clinical trials. Int J Clin Pract 2010; 64:188–193.

68. Sadowsky C et al. Switching from oral cholinesterase inhibitors to the rivastigmine transdermal patch. CNS Neurosci Ther 2010; 16:51–60.

69. Cummings J et al. Randomized, double-blind, parallel-group, 48-week study for efficacy and safety of a higher-dose rivastigmine patch (15 vs. 10 cm(2)) in Alzheimer's disease. Dement Geriatr Cogn Disord 2012; 33:341–353.

70. Parsons CG et al. Memantine is a clinically well tolerated N-methyl-D-aspartate (NMDA) receptor antagonist – a review of preclinical data. Neuropharmacology 1999; 38:735–767.

71. Reisberg B et al. Memantine in moderate-to-severe Alzheimer's disease. N Engl J Med 2003; 348:1333–1341.

72. Jones RW. A review comparing the safety and tolerability of memantine with the acetylcholinesterase inhibitors. Int J Geriatr Psychiatry 2010; 25:547–553.

73. Dunn NR et al. Adverse effects associated with the use of donepezil in general practice in England. J Psychopharmacol 2000; 14:406–408.

74. Hashimoto M et al. Urinary incontinence: an unrecognised adverse effect with donepezil. Lancet 2000; 356:568.

75. Kroger E et al. Adverse drug reactions reported with cholinesterase inhibitors: an analysis of 16 years of individual case safety reports from vigibase. Ann Pharmacother 2015; 49:1197–1206.

76. FDA Alert for Healthcare Professionals. Galantamine hydrobromide (marketed as Razadyne, formerly Reminyl). 2005. https://www.fda.gov/Drugs/DrugSafety/ucm109350.htm.

77. Malone DM et al. Cholinesterase inhibitors and cardiovascular disease: a survey of old age psychiatrists' practice. Age Ageing 2007; 36:331–333.

78. Park-Wyllie LY et al. Cholinesterase inhibitors and hospitalization for bradycardia: a population-based study. PLoS Med 2009; 6:e1000157.
79. Rosenbloom MH et al. Donepezil-associated bradyarrhythmia in a patient with dementia with Lewy bodies (DLB). Alzheimer Dis Assoc Disord 2010; 24:209–211.
80. Gill SS et al. Syncope and its consequences in patients with dementia receiving cholinesterase inhibitors: a population-based cohort study. Arch Intern Med 2009; 169:867–873.
81. NHS Yorkshire and Humber Clinical Networks. The Assessment of Cardiac Status Before Prescribing Acetyl Cholinesterase Inhibitors for Dementia. Version 1. 2016. http://www.yhscn.nhs.uk/media/PDFs/mhdn/Dementia/ECG%20Documents/ACHEIGuidance%20V1_Final.pdf.
82. Isik AT et al. Which cholinesterase inhibitor is the safest for the heart in elderly patients with Alzheimer's disease? Am J Alzheimers Dis Other Demen 2012; 27:171–174.
83. Fosbol EL et al. Comparative cardiovascular safety of dementia medications: a cross-national study. J Am Geriatr Soc 2012; 60:2283–2289.
84. Nordstrom P et al. The use of cholinesterase inhibitors and the risk of myocardial infarction and death: a nationwide cohort study in subjects with Alzheimer's disease. Eur Heart J 2013; 34:2585–2591.
85. Howes LG. Cardiovascular effects of drugs used to treat Alzheimer's disease. Drug Saf 2014; 37:391–395.
86. Rowland JP et al. Cardiovascular monitoring with acetylcholinesterase inhibitors: a clinical protocol. Adv Psychiatr Treat 2007; 13:178–184.
87. Farlow MR et al. Memantine for the treatment of Alzheimer's disease: tolerability and safety data from clinical trials. Drug Saf 2008; 31:577–585.
88. Babai S et al. Comparison of adverse drug reactions with donepezil versus memantine: analysis of the French Pharmacovigilance Database. Therapie 2010; 65:255–259.
89. Dooley M et al. Donepezil: a review of its use in Alzheimer's disease. Drugs Aging 2000; 16:199–226.
90. Scott LJ et al. Galantamine: a review of its use in Alzheimer's disease. Drugs 2000; 60:1095–1122.
91. Grossberg GT et al. Lack of adverse pharmacodynamic drug interactions with rivastigmine and twenty-two classes of medications. Int J Geriatr Psychiatry 2000; 15:242–247.
92. Medicines Complete. Stockley's Drug Interactions. 2017. https://www.medicinescomplete.com/about/.
93. Truven Health Analytics. Micromedex 2.0. 2017. https://www.micromedexsolutions.com/home/dispatch/ssl/true.
94. Tavassoli N et al. Drug interactions with cholinesterase inhibitors: an analysis of the French pharmacovigilance database and a comparison of two national drug formularies (Vidal, British National Formulary). Drug Saf 2007; 30:1063–1071.
95. Noetzli M et al. Pharmacodynamic, pharmacokinetic and pharmacogenetic aspects of drugs used in the treatment of Alzheimer's disease. Clin Pharmacokinet 2013; 52:225–241.
96. Pasqualetti G et al. Potential drug-drug interactions in Alzheimer patients with behavioral symptoms. Clin Interv Aging 2015; 10:1457–1466.
97. Parsons C. Withdrawal of antidementia drugs in older people: who, when and how? Drugs Aging 2016; 33:545–556.
98. Howard R et al. Nursing home placement in the Donepezil and Memantine in Moderate to Severe Alzheimer's Disease (DOMINO-AD) trial: secondary and post-hoc analyses. Lancet Neurol 2015; 14:1171–1181.
99. Di Santo SG et al. A meta-analysis of the efficacy of donepezil, rivastigmine, galantamine, and memantine in relation to severity of Alzheimer's disease. J Alzheimers Dis 2013; 35:349–361.
100. National Institute for Health and Care Excellence. Donepezil, galantamine, rivastigmine and memantine for the treatment of Alzheimer's disease. Technology Appraisal Guidance TA217 (last updated May 2016). http://www.nice.org.uk/guidance/index.jsp?action=byID&o=134192011.
101. National Institute for Health and Care Excellence. Medicines optimisation: the safe and effective use of medicines to enable the best possible outcomes. NICE Guideline 5, 2015. https://www.nice.org.uk/guidance/ng5.
102. Birks J et al. Ginkgo biloba for cognitive impairment and dementia. Cochrane Database Syst Rev 2009:CD003120.
103. Yancheva S et al. Ginkgo biloba extract EGb 761(R), donepezil or both combined in the treatment of Alzheimer's disease with neuropsychiatric features: a randomised, double-blind, exploratory trial. Aging Ment Health 2009; 13:183–190.
104. Tan MS et al. Efficacy and adverse effects of ginkgo biloba for cognitive impairment and dementia: a systematic review and meta-analysis. J Alzheimers Dis 2015; 43:589–603.
105. Yang G et al. Ginkgo biloba for mild cognitive impairment and Alzheimer's disease: a systematic review and meta-analysis of randomized controlled trials. Curr Top Med Chem 2016; 16:520–528.
106. Bent S et al. Spontaneous bleeding associated with ginkgo biloba: a case report and systematic review of the literature: a case report and systematic review of the literature. J Gen Intern Med 2005; 20:657–661.
107. Farina N et al. Vitamin E for Alzheimer's dementia and mild cognitive impairment. Cochrane Database Syst Rev 2017; 1:CD002854.
108. Connelly PJ et al. A randomised double-blind placebo-controlled trial of folic acid supplementation of cholinesterase inhibitors in Alzheimer's disease. Int J Geriatr Psychiatry 2008; 23:155–160.
109. Sun Y et al. Efficacy of multivitamin supplementation containing vitamins B6 and B12 and folic acid as adjunctive treatment with a cholinesterase inhibitor in Alzheimer's disease: a 26-week, randomized, double-blind, placebo-controlled study in Taiwanese patients. Clin Ther 2007; 29:2204–2214.
110. Malouf R et al. Folic acid with or without vitamin B12 for the prevention and treatment of healthy elderly and demented people. Cochrane Database Syst Rev 2008:CD004514.
111. Ho RC et al. Is high homocysteine level a risk factor for cognitive decline in elderly? A systematic review, meta-analysis, and meta-regression. Am J Geriatr Psychiatry 2011; 19:607–617.

112. Vogel T et al. Homocysteine, vitamin B12, folate and cognitive functions: a systematic and critical review of the literature. Int J Clin Pract 2009; 63:1061–1067.

113. Burckhardt M, et al. Omega-3 fatty acids for the treatment of dementia. Cochrane Database Syst Rev 2016; 4:CD009002.

114. Lee ST et al. Panax ginseng enhances cognitive performance in Alzheimer disease. Alzheimer Dis Assoc Disord 2008; 22:222–226.

115. Wang Y et al. Ginseng for Alzheimer's disease: a systematic review and meta-analysis of randomized controlled trials. Curr Top Med Chem 2016; 16:529–536.

116. Doody RS et al. Effect of dimebon on cognition, activities of daily living, behaviour, and global function in patients with mild-to-moderate Alzheimer's disease: a randomised, double-blind, placebo-controlled study. Lancet 2008; 372:207–215.

117. Chau S et al. Latrepirdine for Alzheimer's disease (Dimebon). Cochrane Database Syst Rev 2015:CD009524.

118. Li DQ et al. Donepezil combined with natural hirudin improves the clinical symptoms of patients with mild-to-moderate Alzheimer's disease: a 20-week open-label pilot study. Int J Med Sci 2012; 9:248–255.

119. Wang BS et al. Efficacy and safety of natural acetylcholinesterase inhibitor huperzine A in the treatment of Alzheimer's disease: an updated meta-analysis. J Neural Transm 2009; 116:457–465.

120. Yang G et al. Huperzine A for Alzheimer's disease: a systematic review and meta-analysis of randomized clinical trials. PLoS One 2013; 8:e74916.

121. Hao Z et al. Huperzine A for vascular dementia. Cochrane Database Syst Rev 2009:CD007365.

122. Yue J et al. Huperzine A for mild cognitive impairment. Cochrane Database Syst Rev 2012; 12:CD008827.

123. Akhondzadeh S et al. Saffron in the treatment of patients with mild to moderate Alzheimer's disease: a 16-week, randomized and placebo-controlled trial. J Clin Pharm Ther 2010; 35:581–588.

124. Akhondzadeh S et al. A 22-week, multicenter, randomized, double-blind controlled trial of Crocus sativus in the treatment of mild-to-moderate Alzheimer's disease. Psychopharmacology (Berl) 2010; 207:637–643.

125. Farokhnia M et al. Comparing the efficacy and safety of Crocus sativus L. with memantine in patients with moderate to severe Alzheimer's disease: a double-blind randomized clinical trial. Hum Psychopharmacol 2014; 29:351–359.

126. Gauthier S et al. Cerebrolysin in mild-to-moderate Alzheimer's disease: a meta-analysis of randomized controlled clinical trials. Dement Geriatr Cogn Disord 2015; 39:332–347.

127. Plosker GL et al. Spotlight on cerebrolysin in dementia. CNS Drugs 2010; 24:263–266.

128. Chen N et al. Cerebrolysin for vascular dementia. Cochrane Database Syst Rev 2013:CD008900.

129. McGuinness B et al. Cochrane review on 'Statins for the treatment of dementia'. Int J Geriatr Psychiatry 2013; 28:119–126.

130. McGuinness B et al. Statins for the prevention of dementia. Cochrane Database Syst Rev 2016:CD003160.

131. Sorond FA et al. Neurovascular coupling, cerebral white matter integrity, and response to cocoa in older people. Neurology 2013; 81:904–909.

132. Scheltens P et al. Efficacy of a medical food in mild Alzheimer's disease: a randomized, controlled trial. Alzheimer's Dement 2010; 6:1–10.

133. Shah RC et al. The S-Connect study: results from a randomized, controlled trial of Souvenaid in mild-to-moderate Alzheimer's disease. Alzheimers Res Ther 2013; 5:59.

134. Scheltens P et al. Efficacy of Souvenaid in mild Alzheimer's disease: results from a randomized, controlled trial. J Alzheimers Dis 2012; 31:225–236.

135. Galimberti D et al. Idalopirdine as a treatment for Alzheimer's disease. Expert Opin Investig Drugs 2015; 24:981–987.

136. Wilkinson D et al. Safety and efficacy of idalopirdine, a 5-HT6 receptor antagonist, in patients with moderate Alzheimer's disease (LADDER): a randomised, double-blind, placebo-controlled phase 2 trial. Lancet Neurol 2014; 13:1092–1099.

137. Halliday M et al. Repurposed drugs targeting eIF2alpha-P-mediated translational repression prevent neurodegeneration in mice. Brain 2017; 140:1768–1783.

138. Coupland C et al. Antidepressant use and risk of adverse outcomes in older people: population based cohort study. BMJ 2011; 343:d4551.

139. Doody RS et al. A phase 3 trial of semagacestat for treatment of Alzheimer's disease. N Engl J Med 2013; 369:341–350.

140. Briggs R et al. Drug treatments in Alzheimer's disease. Clin Med (Lond) 2016; 16:247–253.

141. Doody RS et al. Phase 3 trials of solanezumab for mild-to-moderate Alzheimer's disease. N Engl J Med 2014; 370:311–321.

142. Le Couteur DG et al. Solanezumab and the amyloid hypothesis for Alzheimer's disease. BMJ 2016; 355:i6771.

143. Salloway S et al. Two phase 3 trials of bapineuzumab in mild-to-moderate Alzheimer's disease. N Engl J Med 2014; 370:322–333.

144. Abushouk AI et al. Bapineuzumab for mild to moderate Alzheimer's disease: a meta-analysis of randomized controlled trials. BMC Neurol 2017; 17:66.

145. Kavirajan H et al. Efficacy and adverse effects of cholinesterase inhibitors and memantine in vascular dementia: a meta-analysis of randomised controlled trials. Lancet Neurol 2007; 6:782–792.

146. Bocti C et al. Management of dementia with a cerebrovascular component. Alzheimers Dement 2007; 3:398–403.

147. Demaerschalk BM et al. Treatment of vascular dementia and vascular cognitive impairment. Neurologist 2007; 13:37–41.

148. Baskys A et al. Pharmacological prevention and treatment of vascular dementia: approaches and perspectives. Exp Gerontol 2012; 47:887–891.

149. Roman GC et al. Donepezil in vascular dementia: combined analysis of two large-scale clinical trials. Dement Geriatr Cogn Disord 2005; 20:338–344.

150. Malouf R et al. Donepezil for vascular cognitive impairment. Cochrane Database Syst Rev 2004:CD004395.

151. Moretti R et al. Rivastigmine superior to aspirin plus nimodipine in subcortical vascular dementia: an open, 16-month, comparative study. Int J Clin Pract 2004; 58:346–353.

CHAPTER 6

152. Moretti R et al. Rivastigmine in subcortical vascular dementia: a randomized, controlled, open 12-month study in 208 patients. Am J Alzheimers Dis Other Demen 2003; 18:265–272.

153. Small G et al. Galantamine in the treatment of cognitive decline in patients with vascular dementia or Alzheimer's disease with cerebrovascular disease. CNS Drugs 2003; 17:905–914.

154. Kurz AF et al. Long-term safety and cognitive effects of galantamine in the treatment of probable vascular dementia or Alzheimer's disease with cerebrovascular disease. Eur J Neurol 2003; 10:633–640.

155. Erkinjuntti T et al. Efficacy of galantamine in probable vascular dementia and Alzheimer's disease combined with cerebrovascular disease: a randomised trial. Lancet 2002; 359:1283–1290.

156. Wilcock G et al. A double-blind, placebo-controlled multicentre study of memantine in mild to moderate vascular dementia (MMM500). Int Clin Psychopharmacol 2002; 17:297–305.

157. Orgogozo JM et al. Efficacy and safety of memantine in patients with mild to moderate vascular dementia: a randomized, placebo-controlled trial (MMM 300). Stroke 2002; 33:1834–1839.

158. Roman GC et al. Randomized, placebo-controlled, clinical trial of donepezil in vascular dementia: differential effects by hippocampal size. Stroke 2010; 41:1213–1221.

159. Craig D et al. Galantamine for vascular cognitive impairment. Cochrane Database Syst Rev 2006:CD004746.

160. Birks J et al. Rivastigmine for vascular cognitive impairment. Cochrane Database Syst Rev 2013; 5:CD004744.

161. Wang J et al. Cholinergic deficiency involved in vascular dementia: possible mechanism and strategy of treatment. Acta Pharmacol Sin 2009; 30:879–888.

162. Wild R et al. Cholinesterase inhibitors for dementia with Lewy bodies. Cochrane Database Syst Rev 2003:CD003672.

163. Rolinski M et al. Cholinesterase inhibitors for dementia with Lewy bodies, Parkinson's disease dementia and cognitive impairment in Parkinson's disease. Cochrane Database Syst Rev 2012; 3:CD006504.

164. Bhasin M et al. Cholinesterase inhibitors in dementia with Lewy bodies: a comparative analysis. Int J Geriatr Psychiatry 2007; 22:890–895.

165. Boot BP. Comprehensive treatment of dementia with Lewy bodies. Alzheimers Res Ther 2015; 7:45.

166. Stinton C et al. Pharmacological management of Lewy body dementia: a systematic review and meta-analysis. Am J Psychiatry 2015; 172:731–742.

167. Wang HF et al. Efficacy and safety of cholinesterase inhibitors and memantine in cognitive impairment in Parkinson's disease, Parkinson's disease dementia, and dementia with Lewy bodies: systematic review with meta-analysis and trial sequential analysis. J Neurol Neurosurg Psychiatry 2015; 86:135–143.

168. Sabbagh MN et al. The use of memantine in dementia with Lewy bodies. J Alzheimers Dis 2005; 7:285–289.

169. Emre M et al. Memantine for patients with Parkinson's disease dementia or dementia with Lewy bodies: a randomised, double-blind, placebo-controlled trial. Lancet Neurol 2010; 9:969–977.

170. Matsunaga S et al. Memantine for Lewy body disorders: systematic review and meta-analysis. Am J Geriatr Psychiatry 2015; 23:373–383.

171. Russ TC et al. Cholinesterase inhibitors for mild cognitive impairment. Cochrane Database Syst Rev 2012; 9:CD009132.

172. Cooper C et al. Treatment for mild cognitive impairment: systematic review. Br J Psychiatry 2013; 203:255–264.

173. Eshkoor SA et al. Mild cognitive impairment and its management in older people. Clin Interv Aging 2015; 10:687–693.

174. Nardell M et al. Pharmacological treatments for frontotemporal dementias: a systematic review of randomized controlled trials. Am J Alzheimers Dis Other Demen 2014; 29:123–132.

175. Li Y et al. Cholinesterase inhibitors for rarer dementias associated with neurological conditions. Cochrane Database Syst Rev 2015:CD009444.

> ### Safer prescribing for physical conditions in dementia

People with dementia are more susceptible to cognitive adverse effects of drugs. Drugs may affect cognition through their action on cholinergic, histaminergic or opioid neurotransmitter pathways or through more complex actions. Medications prescribed for physical disorders may also interact with cognitive-enhancing medication.

Anticholinergic drugs

Anticholinergic drugs reduce the efficacy of acetylcholinesterase inhibitors[1,2] and also cause sedation, cognitive impairment, delirium[3] and falls.[4] These effects may be more severe in older patients with dementia.[5] Table 6.4 summarises the anticholinergic effect on cognition (AEC) of drugs commonly used in older adults in the UK.[6] Combining several drugs with anticholinergic activity increases the anticholinergic burden for an individual. One study showed that a high anticholinergic burden total score was associated with a greater decline in MMSE score and a higher mortality.[7]

It is good practice to keep the anticholinergic burden to a minimum (preferably zero) in older people, especially if they have cognitive impairment. See Box 6.4.

Where possible, drugs with an equivalent therapeutic effect but a mode of action which does not affect the cholinergic system should be used. If this is not possible, the prescription of a drug with low anticholinergic activity or high specificity to the site of action (and thus minimal central activity) should be encouraged. Anticholinergic drugs that do not cross the blood–brain barrier (BBB) have less profound effects on cognitive function.[8] The AEC scale takes all of these factors into account.

Safety of physical health medication prescribed in dementia

Anticholinergic drugs used in urinary incontinence

Oxybutynin easily penetrates the CNS and has consistently been associated with deterioration in cognitive function. Although studies of **tolterodine** found no adverse CNS effects,[9] case reports have described adverse effects including memory loss, hallucinations and delirium.[10–12] In contrast, **darifenacin**, an M_3 selective receptor antagonist, has been investigated in healthy elderly subjects for its effects on cognitive function and was noted to have no significant effects on cognitive tests compared with placebo,[13,14] although studies in dementia are lacking. **Solifenacin** has been shown to cause impairment of working memory[15] although it was investigated in stroke patients and was found not to affect their short-term cognitive performance.[16] A study looking at the use of **trospium** with galantamine in patients with Alzheimer's disease found no significant change in cognitive function.[17] There are no *in vivo* studies investigating whether or not **fesoterodine** causes cognitive impairment but *in vitro* evaluation found that its active metabolite 5-hydroxy-methyl-tolterodine (5-HMT) had one of the highest detectable serum anticholinergic activities and therefore it has potential to induce central anticholinergic adverse effects. However anticholinergic activity measured in serum does not necessarily reflect brain concentrations[18] and theoretically fesoterodine has a very low ability to cross the BBB.[15]

Table 6.4 Anticholinergic effect on cognition (AEC) scores[6] (updated September 2017)

Adcal – 0	Clarithromycin – NK	Gabapentin – 0	Naproxen – 0	Sitagliptin – 0
Alendronic acid (alendronate) – 0	Clemastine – 3	Galantamine – 0	Nifedipine – 0	Solifenacin – 1
Alfuzosin – 0	Clomipramine – 3	Gaviscon – 0	Nimodipine – 0	Sotalol – 0
Alimemazine (trimeprazine) – 3	Clonazepam – NK	Gliclazide – 0	Nitrofurantoin – NK	Spironolactone – NK
Allopurinol – NK	Clonidine – NK	Granisetron – 0	Nortriptyline – 3	Sulfasalazine – 0
Alprazolam – 0	Clopidogrel – 0	Haloperidol – 0	Olanzapine – 2	Sulpiride – 0
Alverine – 0	Clozapine – 3	Heparin – 0	Omeprazole – 0	Tamoxifen – NK
Amantadine – 2	Co-beneldopa – 0	Hydrochlorothiazide – 0	Ondansetron – 0	Tamsulosin – 0
Amiloride – 0	Co-careldopa – 0	Hydrocodone – NK	Orlistat – 0	Temazepam – 1
Aminophylline – 0	Codeine – NK	Hydrocortisone – NK	Orphenadrine – 3	Tetracycline – 0
Amiodarone – 1	Colchicine – NK	Hydroxyzine – 1	Oxcarbazepine – NK	Theophylline – NK
Amisulpride – 0	Co-tenidone – 0	Hyoscine hydrobromide – 3	Oxybutynin – 3	Thiamine – 0
Amitriptyline – 3	Cyclizine – 1	Hyoscine butylbromide (Buscopan) – 1	Oxycodone – NK	Tiotropium bromide (inhalation) – 0
Amlodipine – 0	Cyproheptadine – 3	Ibuprofen – 0	Paliperidone – 1	Tizanidine – NK
Amoxicillin – 0	Dabigatran – NK	Iloperidone – 1	Pantoprazole – 0	Tolcapone – 0
Anastrozole – NK	Darifenacin – 0	Imipramine – 3	Paracetamol – 0	Tolterodine – 2
Apixaban – NK	Desipramine – 2	Indapamide – 0	Paroxetine – 2	Topiramate – NK
Apomorphine – 0	Dexamethasone – NK	Insulin – 0	Penicillin – 0	Tramadol – 0
Aripiprazole – 1	Dexamfetamine (dexamphetamine) – 0	Ipratropium bromide – 0	Peppermint oil – 0	Trazodone – 0
Aspirin – 0	Dextropropoxyphene – NK	Irbesartan – NK	Pergolide – 0	Trifluoperazine – 2
Atenolol – 0	Diazepam – 1	Isocarboxazid – 1	Perindopril – 0	Trihexyphenidyl (benzhexol) – 3
Atomoxetine – 0	Diclofenac – 0	Isosorbide dinitrate – 0	Perphenazine – 1	Trimethoprim – 0

Atorvastatin – 0	Dicycloverine (dicyclomine) – 2	Isosorbide mononitrate – 0	Pethidine – 2	Trimipramine – 3
Atropine – 3	Digoxin – NK	Ketorolac – 0	Phenelzine – 1	Trospium – 0
Atropine eye drops – 1	Dihydrocodeine – NK	Labetalol – 0	Phenytoin – NK	Valproate – 0
Azathioprine – 0	Diltiazem – 0	Lactulose – 0	Pimozide – 2	Venlafaxine – 0
Baclofen – NK	Dimenhydrinate – 2	Lamotrigine – 0	Pirenzepine – 1	Verapamil – NK
Beclometasone dipropionate (inhaler) – 0	Diphenhydramine – 2	Lansoprazole – NK	Pravastatin – 0	Vitamin B_{12} – 0
Bendroflumethiazide – 0	Dipyridamole – 0	Lercanidipine – 0	Prazosin – 0	Vitamins – 0
Benztropine – 3	Disopyramide – 2	Levetiracetam – NK	Prednisolone – 1	Vortioxetine – 0
Betahistine – 0	Docusate sodium – 0	Levodopa – 0	Pregabalin – NK	Warfarin – 0
Bezafibrate – 0	Domperidone – 1	Levomepromazine (methotrimeprazine) – 2	Prochlorperazine – 2	Ziprasidone – 0
Bisacodyl – 0	Donepezil – 0	Levothyroxine (thyroxine) – 0	Procyclidine – 3	Zolpidem – 0
Bisoprolol – NK	Dothiepin (dosulepin) – 3	Liraglutide – 0	Promazine – 2	Zopiclone – NK
Bromocriptine – 1	Doxazosin – 0	Lisinopril – 0	Promethazine – 3	Zotepine – 2
Budesonide (inhaler) – 0	Doxepin – 3	Lithium – 1	Propantheline – 2	Zuclopentixol (zuclopenthixol) – 1
Bumetanide – NK	Doxycycline – 0	Lofepramine – 3	Propranolol – 0	
Buprenorphine – 0	Dulaglutide – 0	Loperamide – 0	Quetiapine – 2	
Bupropion – 0	Duloxetine – 0	Loratadine – 0	Quinidine – 1	
Buspirone – 1	Enalapril – 0	Lorazepam – 0	Quinine – 1	
Cabergoline – 0	Enoxaparin – 0	Losartan – 0	Rabeprazole – 0	
Calcium – 0	Entacapone – 0	Lovastatin – 0	Ramipril – NK	
Calcium and vitamin D – 0	Erythromycin – NK	Lurasidone – 0	Ranitidine – 0	
Candesartan – 0	Exanatide – 0	Macrogol – 0	Rasagiline – 0	

(Continued)

Table 6.4 (*Continued*)

Captopril – NK	Ezetimibe – 0	Magnesium – 0	Reboxetine – 0
Carbachol – 0	Felodipine – 0	Mebeverine – 0	Risedronate – 0
Carbamazepine – 1	Fentanyl – 1	Melatonin – 0	Risperidone – 0
Carbimazole – NK	Ferrous sulphate – 0	Meloxicam – 0	Rivaroxaban – NK
Carbocisteine – 0	Fesoterodine – 0	Memantine – 0	Rivastigmine – 0
Carvedilol – NK	Fexofenadine – 0	Mesalazine – 0	Ropinirole – 0
Cefalexin (cephalexin) – 0	Finasteride – 0	Metformin – NK	Rosiglitazone – 0
Cetirizine – 0	Flavoxate* – NK	Methocarbamol – NK	Rosuvastatin – NK
Chloral hydrate – NK	Flecainide – 0	Methotrexate – NK	Salbutamol – 0
Chlordiazepoxide – 0	Flucloxacillin – 0	Metoclopramide – 0	
Chlorphenamine – 2	Fludrocortisone – NK	Metoprolol – 0	Salmeterol (inhaler) – 0
Chlorpromazine – 3	Fluoxetine – 1	Midazolam – 1	Selegiline – 0
Chlortalidone – NK	Flupentixol (flupenthixol) – 1	Minocycline – 0	Senna – 0
Cimetidine – 0	Fluphenazine – 1	Mirabegron – 0	Sertindole – 1
Cinnarizine – 1	Fluvoxamine – 0	Mirtazapine – 1	Sertraline – 1
Ciprofloxacin – 0	Folic acid – 0	Moclobemide – 0	Sildenafil – 0
Citalopram – 1	Furosemide – 0	Morphine – 0	Simvastatin – 0

The AEC scale is available as a regularly updated web-based app. Please go to www.medichec.com.
NK, not known.

All tertiary amine drugs (i.e. oxybutynin, tolterodine, fesoterodine and darifenacin) are metabolised by cytochrome P450 (CYP450) enzymes. Increasing age or co-administration of drugs that inhibit these enzymes (e.g. erythromycin, fluoxetine) can lead to higher serum levels and therefore increased adverse effects. The metabolism of **trospium** is unknown, although metabolism via the CYP450 system does not occur, meaning that pharmacokinetic drug interactions are unlikely with this drug.[9] See Table 6.5 for a summary of the physiochemical properties of anticholinergic drugs used in urinary incontinence.

Alpha blockers for urinary retention

Alpha blockers such as **tamsulosin, alfuzosin** and **prazosin** are reported to cause drowsiness, dizziness and depression.[21] There is no published literature reporting their effects on cognition, and alpha blockers do not feature on any anticholinergic cognitive burden list.

Drugs used in gastrointestinal disorders

Loperamide
Although loperamide may have some anticholinergic activity, there are no data to suggest that it can worsen cognitive function in patients with dementia. It may add to the anticholinergic cognitive burden if used in conjunction with other anticholinergic drugs however.

Laxatives
There is no evidence to suggest that laxatives have any negative impact on cognitive function. In fact, since constipation can lead to behavioural and psychological symptoms of dementia (BPSD), treating it can improve these symptoms in many cases.

Anti-emetics
Cyclizine is a first-generation histamine antagonist and can impair cognitive and psychomotor performance (see 'Antihistamines' section).[22]

Metoclopramide has little anticholinergic action, but the D_2 receptor antagonism of both metoclopramide and prochlorperazine can produce movement disorders and so these drugs must be used with great caution in people with dementia.

CHAPTER 6

Table 6.5 Physiochemical properties of anticholinergic drugs in urinary incontinence[15,19] (adapted with permission[20])

Drug	Muscarinic receptor (M$_3$:M$_1$ affinity ratio)	Polarity	Lipophilicity	Molecular weight (kDa)	P-gp substrate	Theoretical ability to cross BBB	Effect on cognition
Darifenacin	Mainly M$_3$ (9.3:1)	Neutral	High	507.5 (relatively large)	Yes	High (but bladder-selective and P-gp substrate)	–
Fesoterodine	Non-selective	Neutral	Very low	411.6	Yes	Very low	No data yet
Oxybutynin	Non-selective	Neutral	Moderate	357 (relatively small)	No	Moderate/high	+++
Solifenacin	Mainly M$_3$ (2.5:1)	Neutral	Moderate	480.6	No	Moderate	–/+
Tolterodine	Non-selective	Neutral	Low	475.6	No	Low	+
Trospium chloride	Non-selective	Positively charged	Not lipophilic	428	Yes	Almost none	–

– No reports of adverse effects on cognition.
+ Some adverse effects on cognition reported.
+++ Consistent reports of adverse effects on cognition.

Domperidone is a dopamine D_2 receptor antagonist that does not usually cross the BBB. However, since BBB alterations can occur in dementia, CNS penetration of domperidone and resulting adverse effects can occur.[23] Recent reports have highlighted a small increased risk of serious cardiac adverse effects with domperidone, especially in older people. The maximum dose has been reduced to 30mg/day and the maximum treatment duration should not exceed 1 week. Domperidone is now contraindicated in those with underlying cardiac conditions or severe hepatic impairment and in patients receiving other medications known to prolong the QT interval or potent CYP3A4 inhibitors.[24]

Serotonin 5-HT$_3$ receptor antagonists, used for treating chemotherapy-induced nausea and vomiting, do not have adverse effects on cognition and may have some cognitive-enhancing action.[25] These drugs carry cardiovascular warnings and should be used cautiously in patients with cardiac co-morbidities or taking concomitant arrhythmogenic drugs or drugs known to prolong the QT interval. **Granisetron** allows for once daily administration, which is preferable in elderly patients with memory problems or swallowing difficulties. Granisetron is metabolised exclusively via a single CYP family (CYP3A4) and thus has lower propensity for drug interactions.[26] All 5-HT$_3$ antagonists cause constipation.

Antispasmodics

Hyoscine hydrobromide (scopolamine) is a centrally acting anticholinergic which is lipophilic and penetrates the BBB easily. It impairs memory, speed of processing and attention. Older patients suffer these symptoms at lower doses and are more vulnerable to confusion and hallucinations.[27] People with Alzheimer's disease have experienced clinically significant cognitive impairment at lower doses compared with healthy, age-matched controls.[5] The effect that hyoscine has on cognition is so significant that it is used in trials to produce memory deficits similar to those seen in dementia (the scopolamine challenge test).[28]

Hyoscine butylbromide (Buscopan) exerts topical spasmolytic action on smooth muscle of the GI tract. Hyoscine butylbromide is not thought to enter the CNS, and so anticholinergic adverse effects at the CNS are extremely rare.[29]

Alverine, **mebeverine** and **peppermint oil** are relaxants of intestinal smooth muscle and do not appear to have an effect on cognition.

Bronchodilators

Beta agonists

In patients with co-existing Parkinson's disease or essential tremor, tremor induced by beta agonists may result in misdiagnosis and over-treatment of Parkinson's disease.[30] Tremor is a common adverse effect of cholinesterase inhibitors so caution should be exercised when these drugs are used with beta agonists.

Anticholinergic bronchodilators

Inhaled anticholinergic drugs have few systemic adverse effects compared with oral medication.[30] A randomised, double-blind, placebo-controlled comparison of ipratropium and theophylline treatment was unable to detect a negative effect with either drug on the psychometric test performance of elderly patients. This suggests that treatment with inhaled ipratropium is not associated with significant cognitive impairment in older people.[31]

Theophylline

As with cholinesterase inhibitors, nausea and vomiting are common adverse effects of theophylline. Neurological effects such as headaches, anxiety, behavioural disturbances, depression and seizures can occur in 50% of patients on theophylline. Although seizures are rare, they are significantly more likely in older people than younger people. Theophylline does not cause significant cognitive impairment.[31]

Hypersalivation

Oral anticholinergic agents used for hypersalivation (e.g. hyoscine hydrobromide) should be avoided in the elderly because of the risk of cognitive impairment, delirium and constipation. Pirenzepine is a relatively selective M_1 and M_4 muscarinic receptor antagonist which is not thought to cross the BBB and therefore has little CNS penetration.[32]

   Atropine solution, given sublingually or used as a mouthwash, is sometimes used to manage hypersalivation. There are no data available for the extent of penetration through the BBB when atropine is administered by this route.

Myasthenia gravis (MG)

Unlike acetylcholinesterase inhibitors used in Alzheimer's disease (donepezil, rivastigmine and galantamine), those used in MG (**pyridostigmine, neostigmine**) act peripherally and do not cross the BBB (so as to minimise unwanted central effects).[33] It is possible that combining peripheral and central acetylcholinesterase inhibitors may add to the cholinomimetic adverse effect burden (e.g. nausea, vomiting, diarrhoea, abdominal cramps and increased salivation). Memantine may be an alternative to cholinesterase inhibitors in cases where the combined cholinomimetic effects of drugs used for MG and AD are not tolerated.

Analgesics

Non-steroidal anti-inflammatory drugs and paracetamol

Paracetamol (acetaminophen) is a safe drug and there is no evidence that it causes cognitive impairment other than in overdose when it may cause delirium.[34] There is some evidence that chronic use of aspirin can cause confusional states.[35] Case reports implicate NSAIDs in causing delirium and psychosis[36] although clinical trials have not demonstrated significant adverse effects on cognition with naproxen[37] or indometacin.[38] NSAIDs are difficult to use in older people due to their cardiovascular risk and risk of gastrointestinal bleeding.[39] It is good practice to prescribe gastroprotection with these drugs. Although there is little evidence for their efficacy and safety in dementia, consideration should be given to the use of topical NSAIDs (if clinically appropriate), to reduce GI risk.

Opiates

Sedation is a potential problem with all opiates.[40] Delirium induced by opioids may be associated with agitation, hallucinations or delusions.[40] **Pethidine** is associated with a high risk of cognitive impairment as its metabolites have anticholinergic properties and accumulate rapidly if renal function is impaired.[41] **Codeine** may increase the risk of falls, and both tramadol and codeine have a high risk of drug–drug interactions as well as considerable variation in response and adverse effects.[42] **Fentanyl patches**, useful as they can be in chronic pain and palliative care, should not be used to initiate opioid analgesia in frail older people[43] because of their long duration of action even after the patch is removed, making the treatment of adverse effects more difficult.[42] **Morphine** is a very effective analgesic but is likely to cause cognitive problems and other adverse effects in elderly patients.[44] **Oxycodone** has a short half-life, few drug–drug interactions and more predictable dose–response relationships than other opiates. It is therefore, theoretically at least, a good candidate for oral analgesia in dementia.[42] **Buprenorphine** transdermal patches probably have fewer adverse effects than many other opiates.

Antihistamines

First-generation H_1 antihistamines include **chlorphenamine, hydroxyzine, cyclizine** and **promethazine**. They are non-selective, have anticholinergic activity and readily penetrate the BBB, which can lead to unwanted cognitive adverse effects. They can impair cognitive and psychomotor performance and can trigger seizures, dyskinesia, dystonia and hallucinations. The second-generation H_1 antihistamines (e.g. **loratadine, cetirizine** and **fexofenadine**) penetrate poorly into the CNS and are considerably less likely to cause these adverse effects. Moreover, they lack any anticholinergic effects.[22]

Statins

A Cochrane review assessed the clinical efficacy and tolerability of statins in the treatment of dementia[45] and showed that there was no significant benefit from statins in terms of cognitive function, but equally no evidence that statins were detrimental to cognition. Earlier case reports had highlighted subjective complaints of memory loss associated with the use of statins.[46] This tended to occur in the first 2 months after starting the drug, and was most commonly associated with simvastatin. In the event of a patient experiencing cognitive problems on simvastatin it may be worth first stopping the drug, and if the complaint resolves, trying atorvastatin or pravastatin instead, as these drugs are less likely to cross the BBB. A more recent Cochrane review[47] assessed the efficacy of statins in the prevention of dementia and concluded that there was no evidence that statins given in late life to people at risk of vascular disease prevented cognitive decline or dementia.

Antihypertensives

Mid-life hypertension has negative effects on cognition and increases the risk of a person developing dementia.[48] A systematic review found that treatment reduced the risk of all-cause dementia by 9% in comparison with the control group.[49] Antihypertensive treatment, regardless of drug class, had a positive effect on global cognition and on all cognitive functions except language. Angiotensin II receptor blockers (ARBs) were more effective than beta blockers, diuretics and angiotensin-converting enzyme inhibitors in improving scores of cognition. A Cochrane review[50] looked at the effects of withdrawing antihypertensive medications on cognition or prevention of dementia but results were uncertain. Withdrawing antihypertensive drugs was however associated with increased blood pressure. It is unlikely to increase mortality at 3–4 months' follow-up, although there was a signal from one large study looking at withdrawal after stroke that withdrawal was associated with an increase in cardiovascular events.

Other cardiac drugs

Digoxin has been associated with acute confusional states at therapeutic drug concentrations.[51] It has also been reported to cause nightmares.[52] However one study showed that treatment of cardiac failure with digoxin improved cognitive performance in 25% of patients treated (and in 23% of the patients treated who did not have cardiac failure).[53] There are some case reports of amiodarone being associated with delirium.[54,55]

H₂ antagonists and proton pump inhibitors

Although H_2 receptor antagonists (e.g. cimetidine, ranitidine) are not used widely now, it is not uncommon to see patients with dementia who have been prescribed these drugs for several years. CNS reactions to these drugs have been reviewed.[56] Neurotoxicity in the form of delirium, sometimes with agitation and hallucinations, generally occurred in the first 2 weeks of therapy and resolved within 3 days of stopping the drug. The estimated incidence of these reactions was 0.2% or less in out-patients, but much higher in hospitalised patients, particularly in patients with hepatic and liver failure.[57] If someone with dementia is stable on an H_2 antagonist, there is no reason to stop it. Proton pump inhibitors appear less likely to cause cognitive problems.

Antibiotics

Many antibiotics have been associated rarely with delirium but there is no consistent pattern of them causing cognitive impairment. Given the importance of treating infection in dementia, the most appropriate antibiotic for the infection being treated should be used. The evidence might suggest that if there is a choice between either a quinolone or macrolide antibiotic with another class of antibiotic, the other class might be preferred for someone with dementia given the possible risk of these two classes of drugs triggering cognitive disorders. Antituberculous therapy, particularly isoniazid, has attracted some case reports of adverse psychiatric reactions.[58]

Table 6.6 summarises those drugs that are recommended for use in dementia and the drugs to avoid.

Table 6.6 Recommended drugs and drugs to avoid in dementia (adapted with permission[20])

Condition	Drug class or drug name	Drugs to avoid in dementia	Recommended drugs in dementia
Allergic conditions	Antihistamines	Chlorphenamine Promethazine Hydroxyzine Cyproheptadine Cyclizine (and other first-generation antihistamines)	Cetirizine Loratadine Fexofenadine (and other second-generation antihistamines)
Asthma/COPD	Bronchodilators		Beta agonists Inhaled anticholinergics (have not been reported to affect cognition) Theophylline
Constipation	Laxatives	No evidence to suggest that laxatives have any negative impact on cognitive function. Constipation itself may worsen cognition	
Diarrhoea	Loperamide	Low-potency anticholinergic. Not known to have effects on cognitive function, however may add to the anticholinergic cognitive burden if used in combination with other anticholinergics	
Hyperlipidaemia	Statins		All are safe but atorvastatin and pravastatin less likely to cross BBB
Hypersalivation	Anticholinergics	Hyoscine hydrobromide	Pirenzepine Atropine (sublingually)
Hypertension	Antihypertensives	Beta blockers (avoidance may not always be possible)	Calcium-channel blockers, angiotensin-converting enzyme inhibitors, and angiotensin receptor blockers may all improve cognitive function
Infections	Antibiotics	Delirium reported mostly with quinolone and macrolide antibiotics. But given the importance of treating infections, the most appropriate antibiotic for the infections should be used	
Myasthenia gravis	Peripheral acetylcholinesterase inhibitors, e.g. neostigmine and pyridostigmine	May add to the cholinergic adverse effects of central acetylcholinesterase inhibitors (e.g. donepezil, etc.) in patients with dementia, i.e. increased risk of nausea/vomiting, etc.	
Nausea/vomiting	Anti-emetics	Cyclizine Metoclopramide Prochlorperazine	Domperidone (see main text for restrictions) Serotonin 5-HT$_3$ receptor antagonists
Other gastrointestinal conditions	Antispasmodics	Atropine sulphate Dicycloverine hydrochloride	Alverine, mebeverine, peppermint oil Hyoscine-n-butylbromide Propantheline bromide

CHAPTER 6

(Continued)

Table 6.6 (Continued)

Condition	Drug class or drug name	Drugs to avoid in dementia	Recommended drugs in dementia
Pain	Analgesics	Pethidine Pentazocine Dextropropoxyphene Codeine Tramadol Methadone	Paracetamol Oxycodone Buprenorphine Topical NSAIDs (where appropriate)
		Fentanyl patches (caution in opioid naïve patients) Morphine (may be indicated in treatment-resistant pain or palliative care – use cautiously due to associated cognitive and other adverse effects)	
Urinary frequency	Anticholinergic drugs used in overactive bladder	Oxybutynin Tolterodine	Darifenacin Trospium Solifenacin (use if others not available – some reports of cognitive adverse effects)
		Data for fesoterodine are still lacking – it is non-selective and has high central anticholinergic activity but theoretically has very low ability to cross the BBB	
Urinary retention	Alpha blockers	Not known to have effects on cognitive function	

BBB, blood–brain barrier; COPD, chronic obstructive pulmonary disease; NSAIDs, non-steroidal anti-inflammatory drugs.

References

1. Sink KM et al. Dual use of bladder anticholinergics and cholinesterase inhibitors: long-term functional and cognitive outcomes. J Am Geriatr Soc 2008; **56**:847–853.
2. Lu CJ et al. Chronic exposure to anticholinergic medications adversely affects the course of Alzheimer disease. Am J Geriatr Psychiatry 2003; **11**:458–461.
3. Modi A et al. Concomitant use of anticholinergics with acetylcholinesterase inhibitors in Medicaid recipients with dementia and residing in nursing homes. J Am Geriatr Soc 2009; **57**:1238–1244.
4. Aizenberg D et al. Anticholinergic burden and the risk of falls among elderly psychiatric inpatients: a 4-year case-control study. Int Psychogeriatr 2002; **14**:307–310.
5. Sunderland T et al. Anticholinergic sensitivity in patients with dementia of the Alzheimer type and age-matched controls. A dose-response study. Arch Gen Psychiatry 1987; **44**:418–426.
6. Bishara D et al. Anticholinergic effect on cognition (AEC) of drugs commonly used in older people. Int J Geriatr Psychiatry 2017; **32**:650–656.
7. Fox C et al. Anticholinergic medication use and cognitive impairment in the older population: the medical research council cognitive function and ageing study. J Am Geriatr Soc 2011; **59**:1477–1483.
8. Wagg A. The cognitive burden of anticholinergics in the elderly – implications for the treatment of overactive bladder. European Urological Review 2012; **7**:42–49.
9. Pagoria D et al. Antimuscarinic drugs: review of the cognitive impact when used to treat overactive bladder in elderly patients. Curr Urol Rep 2011; **12**:351–357.
10. Womack KB et al. Tolterodine and memory: dry but forgetful. Arch Neurol 2003; **60**:771–773.
11. Tsao JW et al. Transient memory impairment and hallucinations associated with tolterodine use. N Engl J Med 2003; **349**:2274–2275.
12. Edwards KR et al. Risk of delirium with concomitant use of tolterodine and acetylcholinesterase inhibitors. J Am Geriatr Soc 2002; **50**:1165–1166.
13. Kay G et al. Differential effects of the antimuscarinic agents darifenacin and oxybutynin ER on memory in older subjects. Eur Urol 2006; **50**:317–326.
14. Lipton RB et al. Assessment of cognitive function of the elderly population: effects of darifenacin. J Urol 2005; **173**:493–498.

15. Chancellor MB et al. Blood-brain barrier permeation and efflux exclusion of anticholinergics used in the treatment of overactive bladder. Drugs Aging 2012; **29**:259–273.

16. Park JW. The effect of solifenacin on cognitive function following stroke. Dement Geriatr Cogn Dis Extra 2013; **3**:143–147.

17. Isik AT et al. Trospium and cognition in patients with late onset Alzheimer disease. J Nutr Health Aging 2009; **13**:672–676.

18. Jakobsen SM et al. Evaluation of brain anticholinergic activities of urinary spasmolytic drugs using a high-throughput radio receptor bioassay. J Am Geriatr Soc 2011; **59**:501–505.

19. Kay GG et al. Preserving cognitive function for patients with overactive bladder: evidence for a differential effect with darifenacin. Int J Clin Pract 2008; **62**:1792–1800.

20. Bishara D et al. Safe prescribing of physical health medication in patients with dementia. Int J Geriatr Psychiatry 2014; **29**:1230–1241.

21. BNF Online. British National Formulary. 2017. https://www.medicinescomplete.com/mc/bnf/current/.

22. Mahdy AM et al. Histamine and antihistamines. Anaesth Intensive Care Med 2011; **12**:324–329.

23. Roy-Desruisseaux J et al. Domperidone-induced tardive dyskinesia and withdrawal psychosis in an elderly woman with dementia. Ann Pharmacother 2011; **45**:e51.

24. Medicines and Healthcare Products Regulatory Agency. Domperidone: risks of cardiac side effects – indication restricted to nausea and vomiting, new contraindications, and reduced dose and duration of use. 2014. https://www.gov.uk/drug-safety-update/domperidone-risks-of-cardiac-side-effects.

25. Bentley KR et al. Therapeutic potential of serotonin 5-HT3 antagonists in neuropsychiatric disorders. CNS Drugs 1995; **3**:363–392.

26. Gridelli C. Same old story? Do we need to modify our supportive care treatment of elderly cancer patients? Focus on antiemetics. Drugs Aging 2004; **21**:825–832.

27. Flicker C et al. Hypersensitivity to scopolamine in the elderly. Psychopharmacology (Berl) 1992; **107**:437–441.

28. Ebert U et al. Scopolamine model of dementia: electroencephalogram findings and cognitive performance. Eur J Clin Invest 1998; **28**:944–949.

29. Sanofi. Summary of Product Characteristics. Buscopan 10 mg Tablets. 2017. https://www.medicines.org.uk/emc/medicine/30089.

30. Gupta P et al. Potential adverse effects of bronchodilators in the treatment of airways obstruction in older people: recommendations for prescribing. Drugs Aging 2008; **25**:415–443.

31. Ramsdell JW et al. Effects of theophylline and ipratropium on cognition in elderly patients with chronic obstructive pulmonary disease. Ann Allergy Asthma Immunol 1996; **76**:335–340.

32. Fritze J et al. Pirenzepine for clozapine-induced hypersalivation. Lancet 1995; **346**:1034.

33. Pohanka M. Acetylcholinesterase inhibitors: a patent review (2008–present). Expert Opin Ther Pat 2012; **22**:871–886.

34. Gray SL et al. Drug-induced cognition disorders in the elderly: incidence, prevention and management. Drug Saf 1999; **21**:101–122.

35. Bailey RB et al. Chronic salicylate intoxication. A common cause of morbidity in the elderly. J Am Geriatr Soc 1989; **37**:556–561.

36. Hoppmann RA et al. Central nervous system side effects of nonsteroidal anti-inflammatory drugs. Aseptic meningitis, psychosis, and cognitive dysfunction. Arch Intern Med 1991; **151**:1309–1313.

37. Wysenbeek AJ et al. Assessment of cognitive function in elderly patients treated with naproxen. A prospective study. Clin Exp Rheumatol 1988; **6**:399–400.

38. Bruce-Jones PN et al. Indomethacin and cognitive function in healthy elderly volunteers. Br J Clin Pharmacol 1994; **38**:45–51.

39. Barber JB et al. Treatment of chronic non-malignant pain in the elderly: safety considerations. Drug Saf 2009; **32**:457–474.

40. Ripamonti C et al. CNS adverse effects of opioids in cancer patients. CNS Drugs 1997; **8**:21–37.

41. Alagiakrishnan K et al. An approach to drug induced delirium in the elderly. Postgrad Med J 2004; **80**:388–393.

42. McLachlan AJ et al. Clinical pharmacology of analgesic medicines in older people: impact of frailty and cognitive impairment. Br J Clin Pharmacol 2011; **71**:351–364.

43. Dosa DM et al. Frequency of long-acting opioid analgesic initiation in opioid-naive nursing home residents. J Pain Symptom Manage 2009; **38**:515–521.

44. Tannenbaum C et al. A systematic review of amnestic and non-amnestic mild cognitive impairment induced by anticholinergic, antihistamine, GABAergic and opioid drugs. Drugs Aging 2012; **29**:639–658.

45. McGuinness B et al. Statins for the treatment of dementia. Cochrane Database Syst Rev 2014:CD007514.

46. Wagstaff LR et al. Statin-associated memory loss: analysis of 60 case reports and review of the literature. Pharmacotherapy 2003; **23**:871–880.

47. McGuinness B et al. Statins for the prevention of dementia. Cochrane Database Syst Rev 2016:CD003160.

48. Qiu C et al. The age-dependent relation of blood pressure to cognitive function and dementia. Lancet Neurol 2005; **4**:487–499.

49. Levi MN et al. Antihypertensive classes, cognitive decline and incidence of dementia: a network meta-analysis. J Hypertens 2013; **31**:1073–1082.

50. Jongstra S et al. Antihypertensive withdrawal for the prevention of cognitive decline. Cochrane Database Syst Rev 2016; **11**:CD011971.

51. Eisendrath SJ et al. Toxic neuropsychiatric effects of digoxin at therapeutic serum concentrations. Am J Psychiatry 1987; **144**:506–507.

52. Brezis M et al. Nightmares from digoxin. Ann Intern Med 1980; **93**:639–640.

53. Laudisio A et al. Digoxin and cognitive performance in patients with heart failure: a cohort, pharmacoepidemiological survey. Drugs Aging 2009; **26**:103–112.

54. Athwal H et al. Amiodarone-induced delirium. Am J Geriatr Psychiatry 2003; **11**:696–697.

55. Foley KT et al. Separate episodes of delirium associated with levetiracetam and amiodarone treatment in an elderly woman. Am J Geriatr Pharmacother 2010; **8**:170–174.

56. Cantu TG et al. Central nervous system reactions to histamine-2 receptor blockers. Ann Intern Med 1991; **114**:1027–1034.

57. Vial T et al. Side effects of ranitidine. Drug Saf 1991; **6**:94–117.

58. Kass JS et al. Nervous system effects of antituberculosis therapy. CNS Drugs 2010; **24**:655–667.

Management of behavioural and psychological symptoms of dementia

Behavioural and psychological symptoms of dementia (BPSD) can include a wide range of difficulties including: aggression, agitation, wandering, hoarding, sexual disinhibition, hallucinations, delusions, apathy and shouting,[1] as well as less externally challenging symptoms such as low mood and anxiety. These symptoms affect more than 90% of patients to varying degrees.[2] The number, type and severity of these symptoms vary amongst patients and the fact that several types occur simultaneously in individuals makes it difficult to target specific ones therapeutically. The safe and effective management of these symptoms is the subject of a long-standing debate because treatment is not well informed by properly conducted studies[3] and many available agents have been linked to serious adverse effects.

Non-drug measures

Since the publication in the UK of the influential report *The use of antipsychotic medication for people with dementia: time for action*, which detailed the risks associated with antipsychotic use in dementia,[4] there has been a drive to review evidence for antipsychotics and to formulate non-pharmacological treatment pathways for BPSD. Systematic reviews have been completed,[5] new models of care developed[6,7] and guidance documents written.[8] The key themes include:

1. The move towards an individualised approach to treatment.
2. The importance of ensuring that treatable physical causes or exacerbating factors are addressed as a first step. These include pain (see section on 'Analgesics'), delirium and physical illness, constipation and medication adverse effects (see section on 'Safer prescribing for physical conditions in dementia'). All these factors can cause distress and lead to BPSD.
3. The importance of understanding 'problem behaviours' as expressions of distress and unmet need.[6,7]
4. The gathering of an extensive life history, direct observation of care being given, collecting structured information (e.g. through the use of sleep, pain or Antecedent-Behaviour-Consequence [ABC] charts), all to support the understanding of what that unmet need might be.[8]
5. Formulation meetings to pull the information into a model to understand factors leading to and perpetuating the behaviour.
6. Clear and pragmatic care plans developed with carers to address the unmet needs identified through steps 1–5.
7. Care plans are reviewed and adjusted accordingly.

A variety of non-pharmacological methods for the management of BPSD[9] have been developed and some are reasonably well supported by cogent research.[10] These interventions can be useful to consider as part of an individualised care plan but are better if implemented by working closely with caregivers and supported by more personalised interventions and developing the skills of the caregiver(s). Behavioural management techniques and caregiver psycho-education centred on the individual patient's behaviour have been found to be generally successful and the effects can last for months.[11]

Snoezelen (specially designed rooms with a soothing and stimulating environment) have shown some short-term benefits in the past,[12] however a 2009 Cochrane Summary found that two new trials did not show any significant effects on behaviour, interactions and mood of people with dementia.[13] A number of different complementary therapies[14] have been used in dementia including massage, reflexology, administration of herbal medicines and aromatherapy. **Aromatherapy**[15,16] is the fastest growing of these therapies, with extracts from lavender and *Melissa* balm most commonly used.[9] While some positive results from controlled trials have shown significant reduction in agitation,[17] when assessed using a rigorous blinded RCT, there was no evidence that *Melissa* aromatherapy was superior to placebo or donepezil.[18] Overall, the evidence base remains sparse and the adverse-effect profile relatively unexplored.[19] A systematic review of aromatherapy use in non-cognitive symptoms of dementia identified adverse effects including vomiting, dizziness, abdominal pain and wheezing when essential oils were taken orally, and diarrhoea, allergic skin reactions, drowsiness and serious unspecified adverse events when administered topically or by inhalation.[16] Two recent systematic reviews[20,21] suggest that **music therapy** is very effective for the management of agitation in institutionalised patients with AD, particularly when the intervention includes individualised and interactive music. Bright light therapy has little and possibly no clinically significant effect. **Therapeutic touch** is effective for reducing physical non-aggressive behaviours but is not superior to simulated therapeutic touch or usual care for reducing physically aggressive and verbally agitated behaviours. Behavioural management techniques are generally not superior to placebo or pharmacological therapies for managing agitation in AD. However, given concerns over almost all drug therapies, non-pharmacological measures should always be considered first.

Recommendation: evidence-based, non-drug measures (e.g. music therapy) are first-line treatments for BPSD.

Pharmacological measures

Analgesics

It has been suggested that pain in patients with impaired language and abstract thinking may manifest as agitation and therefore treatment of undiagnosed pain may contribute to the overall prevention and management of agitation.[22] An RCT investigating the effects of a stepwise protocol of treatment with analgesics in patients with moderate to severe dementia and agitation noted significant improvement in agitation, overall neuropsychiatric symptoms and pain. The majority of patients in the study received only paracetamol (acetaminophen).

A Cochrane review investigated the clinical efficacy and safety of opioids for agitation in people with dementia.[23] RCTs of opioids compared with placebo were assessed, however there was insufficient evidence to establish the clinical efficacy or safety of opioids in this patient group. Lack of data meant authors were unable to determine if opioids either relieve or exacerbate agitation.

Recommendation: the assessment and effective treatment of pain is important. Even in people without overt pain, a trial of analgesics (usually paracetamol) is worthwhile.

CHAPTER 6

Antipsychotic drugs in behavioural and psychological symptoms of dementia

First-generation antipsychotic drugs (FGAs) have been widely used for decades for BPSD. They are probably effective[24] but, because of extrapyramidal and other adverse effects, are less well tolerated[25,26] than second-generation antipsychotic drugs (SGAs). SGAs have been shown to be comparable in efficacy to FGAs for behavioural symptoms of dementia,[27-29] with one study finding risperidone to be superior to haloperidol.[30] SGAs were once widely recommended in dementia-related behaviour disturbance[31] but their use is now highly controversial.[32,33] There are three reasons for this: effect size is small,[34-37] tolerability is poor[37-39] and there is an association with increased mortality.[40]

Various reviews and trials support the modest efficacy of olanzapine,[27,41] risperidone,[42-46] quetiapine,[29,47-49] aripiprazole[50-52] and amisulpride.[53,54] One study comparing olanzapine with risperidone[36] and one comparing quetiapine with risperidone[55] found no significant differences between treatment groups. However data outlined in the next paragraph have led to risperidone (licensed) followed by olanzapine (unlicensed) being the treatments of choice in managing psychosis or aggression in dementia. One study found clozapine to be beneficial in treatment-resistant agitation associated with dementia.[56]

The most compelling data come from the CATIE-AD trial. This study[57] showed very minor effectiveness advantages for olanzapine and risperidone (but not for quetiapine) over placebo in terms of time to discontinuation, but all drugs were poorly tolerated because of sedation, confusion and extrapyramidal symptoms (EPS), the last of these not being a problem with quetiapine. Similarly, in a second report,[48] greater improvement was noted with olanzapine or risperidone on certain neuropsychiatric rating scales compared with placebo (but not with quetiapine). A Cochrane review[58] of atypical antipsychotics for aggression and psychosis in AD found that evidence suggests that risperidone and olanzapine are useful in reducing aggression and risperidone reduces psychosis. **However, the authors concluded that because of modest efficacy and significant increase in adverse effects, neither risperidone nor olanzapine should be routinely used to treat dementia patients unless there is severe distress or a serious risk of physical harm to those living or working with the patient.**

Increased mortality with antipsychotic drugs in dementia

Following analysis of published and unpublished data in 2004, initial warnings were issued in the UK and USA regarding increased mortality in patients with dementia with certain SGAs (mainly risperidone and olanzapine).[59-61] These warnings have been extended to include all SGAs as well as conventional antipsychotic drugs[61,62] in view of more recent data. A warning about a possible risk of cerebrovascular events has now been added to product labelling for all FGAs and SGAs.

Several published analyses support these warnings,[40,63] confirming an association between SGAs and stroke.[64,65] The magnitude of increased mortality with FGAs has been shown to be similar[66-68] to that with SGAs and possibly even greater.[69-73] Some studies suggested that the risk of cerebrovascular accidents (CVAs) in elderly users of antipsychotic drugs may not be cumulative.[74,75] The risk was found to be elevated especially during the first weeks of treatment but then to decrease over time, returning to base level after 3 months. In contrast, a long-term study (24–54 months) deduced that mortality was progressively increased over time for antipsychotic-treated (risperidone and FGAs) patients compared with those receiving placebo.[76] At present this is not a widely held view.

Whether the risk of mortality differs from one antipsychotic drug to another has been investigated in several studies. The first study[77] found that among nursing home residents prescribed antipsychotic drugs, when compared with risperidone, haloperidol users had an increased risk of mortality whereas quetiapine users had a decreased risk. No clinically meaningful differences were observed for the other drugs investigated: olanzapine, aripiprazole and ziprasidone. The effects were strongest shortly after the start of treatment and remained after adjustment for dose. There was a dose–response relation for all drugs except quetiapine.[77] The second study[78] confirmed these findings. This study included elderly patients with dementia and also assessed risk of mortality with valproic acid. Haloperidol was associated with the highest rates of mortality, followed by risperidone, olanzapine, valproic acid and then quetiapine. Another study[79] investigated adjusted hazard ratios of death of 14 individual antipsychotic drugs compared with risperidone in new users of antipsychotic drugs. A higher risk of death was found for haloperidol, levomepromazine and zuclopenthixol and to a lesser extent for melperone compared with risperidone. Lower risks were observed for quetiapine, olanzapine, clozapine and flupenthixol, amongst other antipsychotic drugs. No statistically significant difference was found for amisulpride. A further study[80] determined the absolute mortality risk increase and numbers needed to harm (NNH) of antipsychotic drugs and valproic acid relative to either no treatment or antidepressant treatment. Compared with matched non-users, patients receiving haloperidol had an increased mortality risk (3.8% and NNH of 26), followed by risperidone (3.7% and NNH of 27), olanzapine (2.5% and NNH of 40) and quetiapine (2.0% and NNH of 50). The antidepressant group had only slightly increased risk of death relative to matched non-users; the risk difference for valproic acid was not significantly different from 0, providing no clear evidence for increased mortality. This increased risk of mortality is higher than previously reported for antipsychotic drugs. In addition, analyses suggested a dose–response relationship between atypical antipsychotic drugs and risk of mortality.

Several mechanisms have been postulated for the underlying causes of CVAs with antipsychotic drugs.[81] Orthostatic hypotension may aggravate the deficit in cerebral perfusion in an individual with cerebrovascular insufficiency or atherosclerosis thus causing a CVA. Tachycardia may similarly decrease cerebral perfusion or dislodge a thrombus in a patient with atrial fibrillation (see Chapter 10 on psychotropics in AF). Following an episode of orthostatic hypotension, there could be a rebound excess of catecholamines with vasoconstriction thus aggravating cerebral insufficiency. In addition, hyperprolactinaemia could in theory accelerate atherosclerosis, and sedation might cause dehydration and haemoconcentration, each of which is a possible mechanism for increased risk of CVA.[81] One study[74] suggests that affinity for M_1 and α_2 receptors predicts effects on stroke.

A review of the literature comparing the safety of FGAs and SGAs in elderly patients with dementia found conflicting results. One study found that, overall, both were associated with similar increased risk for all-cause mortality and CVAs. Patients being

CHAPTER 6

treated with FGAs had an increased risk of cardiac arrhythmias and extrapyramidal symptoms relative to SGA users who were exposed to an increased risk of venous thromboembolism and aspiration pneumonia. Also, despite metabolic effects having consistently been documented in studies with atypical antipsychotic drugs, this effect tended to be attenuated with advancing age and in elderly patients with dementia.[82] Conversely, a recent observational study[83] found a 1.14-fold increase in 180-day mortality for FGA initiators compared to SGA initiators. Analyses suggested that stroke, ventricular arrhythmia, myocardial infarction and pneumonia might explain 15–45% of this mortality difference.

Risperidone clinical trial data were recently examined to look for individual patient characteristics associated with CVAs and death and for any treatment-emergent risk factors.[84] Baseline complications of depression and delusions were found to be associated with a lower relative risk of CVAs in risperidone-treated patients. For mortality, the only significant baseline predictor in patients treated with risperidone was depression, which was associated with a lower relative risk. The relative risk of death was higher in risperidone patients treated with anti-inflammatory medications.

Both typical[85] and atypical antipsychotic drugs[86] may also hasten cognitive decline in dementia, although there is some evidence to refute this.[55,87,88]

Recommendation: use of risperidone (licensed for persistent aggression in AD) and olanzapine may be justified in some cases. Effect is modest at best. When prescribed, regular review is recommended.

Clinical information for antipsychotic use in dementia

Antipsychotic drugs should not be used routinely to treat agitation and aggression in people with dementia.[89]

Risperidone is the only drug licensed in the UK for the management of non-cognitive symptoms associated with dementia and is therefore the agent of choice. It is specifically indicated for short-term treatment (up to 6 weeks) of persistent aggression in patients with moderate to severe AD unresponsive to non-pharmacological approaches and when there is a risk of harm to self or others.[90] Risperidone is licensed up to 1 mg twice a day,[91] although the optimal dose in dementia has been found to be 500 µg twice a day (1 mg daily).[92]

Alternative antipsychotic drugs may be used (off-licence) if risperidone is contraindicated or not tolerated. Olanzapine has some positive efficacy data for reducing aggression in dementia,[58] work is underway investigating the efficacy and tolerability of amisulpride in dementia,[93,94] and quetiapine (although not as effective as risperidone and olanzapine) may be considered in patients with Parkinson's disease or Lewy body dementia (at very small doses) because of its low propensity for causing movement disorders.

Only prescribe antipsychotics after:

- careful risk assessment, balancing the cerebrovascular risk (taking into account hypertension, diabetes, smoking, atrial fibrillation and previous stroke)

- discussion of possible risks and benefits with the carer (and patient if she/he has capacity)
- clear documentation of the above.[89]

It is recommended that all patients prescribed antipsychotic drugs should have the following tests at **baseline,** at **3 months** and **annually:**

1. blood pressure and pulse
2. weight (ideally also monitor monthly for the first 3 months)
3. blood tests
   a. fasting glucose or HbA1c
   b. urea and electrolytes (U&Es) including estimated glomerular filtration rate (eGFR)
   c. full blood count (FBC)
   d. lipids (if possible fasting)
   e. liver function tests (LFTs)
   f. prolactin levels
4. ECG (repeat at between 4 weeks and 3 months or when clinically indicated).

- In-patients, very ill or physically frail patients may need more frequent physical health monitoring than this.
- Review of the antipsychotic drug needs to be done at 4–6 weeks (maybe earlier for in-patients), then at 3 months and then every 6 months if physically stable and there are no adverse effects. Consider trying to stop the antipsychotic drug at each review, where appropriate. See Table 6.7.

Table 6.7 Reduction or discontinuation regimen for antipsychotic drugs in BPSD – a guide[95]

Antipsychotic	Usual dose range in dementia	Suggested regimen for reduction/discontinuation (generally reduce over 2–4 weeks, ideally over 4 weeks if possible)
Amisulpride	25–50 mg/day	Reduce by 12.5–25 mg every 1–2 weeks (depending on dose) then stop
Aripiprazole	5–15 mg/day	Reduce by 5 mg every 1–2 weeks (depending on dose) then stop (if patient is on 5 mg daily, reduce to 2.5 mg for 2 weeks, however note that tablets are not scored and liquid is expensive – contact local pharmacist for advice)
Haloperidol	Not recommended in older people with dementia (except in delirium) Reduce by 0.25–0.5 mg every 1–2 weeks (depending on dose) then stop	
Olanzapine	2.5–10 mg/day	Reduce by 2.5 mg every 1–2 weeks (depending on dose) then stop
Quetiapine	12.5–300 mg/day	For doses 12.5–100 mg/day, reduce by 12.5–25 mg every 1–2 weeks (depending on dose) then stop
		For doses >100–300 mg/day, reduce by 25–50 mg every 1–2 weeks (depending on dose) then stop
		If dose is 300 mg/day, reduce to 150–200 mg/day for 1 week then by 50–mg per week
Risperidone	0.25–2 mg/day	Reduce by 0.25–0.5 mg every 1–2 weeks (depending on dose) then stop

For higher doses, reduce gradually over 4 weeks.
NB: If serious adverse effects occur, stop antipsychotic drug immediately.

CHAPTER 6

Other pharmacological agents in BPSD

Cognitive enhancers

Donepezil,[96,97] rivastigmine[98–101] and galantamine[102–104] may afford some benefit in reducing behavioural disturbance in dementia. Their effect seems apparent only after several weeks of treatment.[105] However, the evidence is somewhat inconsistent and a study of donepezil in agitation associated with dementia found no apparent benefit compared with placebo.[106] Rivastigmine has shown positive results for neuropsychiatric symptoms associated with vascular[98] and Lewy body dementia.[98,107] A meta-analysis investigating the impact of cholinesterase inhibitors on non-cognitive symptoms of dementia found a statistically significant reduction in symptoms among patients with AD, however the clinical relevance of this effect remained unclear.[108] A systematic review of RCTs concluded that AChE-Is have, at best, a modest impact on non-cognitive symptoms of dementia. However, in the absence of alternative safe and effective pharmacological options, a trial of an AChE-I is an appropriate pharmacological strategy for the management of behavioural disturbances in AD.[109]

NICE guidance suggests considering a cholinesterase inhibitor only for:[1,110]

- people with Lewy body dementia who have BPSD causing significant distress or leading to behaviour that challenges
- people with mild to moderate AD who have non-cognitive symptoms and/or behaviour that challenges, causing significant distress or potential harm to the individual if:
  - a non-pharmacological approach is inappropriate or has been ineffective, and
  - antipsychotic drugs are inappropriate or have been ineffective.

Growing evidence for memantine also suggests benefits for neuropsychiatric symptoms associated with AD.[111–113] A Cochrane review of memantine found that slightly fewer patients with moderate to severe AD taking memantine developed agitation, but one study[114] found no effect for memantine in established agitation. The review also suggested that memantine may have a small beneficial effect on behaviour in mild to moderate VaD but this was not supported by clinical global measures.[115] A double-blind, placebo-controlled RCT[116] compared memantine and antipsychotic drugs for the long-term treatment of neuropsychiatric symptoms in people with AD (MAIN-AD). The study indicated no benefits for memantine. Despite apparently positive findings in studies (often manufacturer-sponsored), the use of cognitive-enhancing agents for behavioural disturbance remains controversial.

NICE guidance[1] suggests considering memantine only for:

- people with moderate AD who have non-cognitive symptoms and/or behaviour that challenges and are intolerant of or have a contraindication to AChE-Is, as well as people with severe AD provided:
  - a non-pharmacological approach is inappropriate or has been ineffective, and
  - antipsychotic drugs are inappropriate or have been ineffective.

Recommendation: use of AChE-Is or memantine can be justified in the situations described here. Effect is modest at best.

Benzodiazepines

Benzodiazepines[117,118] are widely used but their use is poorly supported. Benzodiazepines have been associated with cognitive decline,[117] risk of dementia,[119] risk of pneumonia,[120] and an increase in all-cause mortality[121] and may contribute to increased frequency of falls and hip fractures[118,122] in the elderly population.

Recommendation: avoid benzodiazepines.

Antidepressants

Substantial evidence suggests that depression can be considered both a cause and consequence of AD. Depression is considered causative because it is a risk factor for AD. In fact, the prevalence rate of depression and AD co-morbidity is estimated to be 30–50%.[123] Two potential mechanisms by which antidepressants affect cognition in depression have been postulated: a direct effect caused by the pharmacological action of the drugs on specific neurotransmitters and a secondary effect caused by improvement of depression.[124]

Despite reports of a possible modest advantage over placebo, **SSRIs** have ultimately shown doubtful efficacy in non-cognitive symptoms of dementia in the past.[125,126] One review, however, contradicted previous findings and indicated that antidepressants (mainly SSRIs) not only showed efficacy in treating non-cognitive symptoms but were also well tolerated.[127] The authors noted that the most common antidepressants used in dementia were sertraline followed by citalopram and trazodone. Some of the clinical evidence demonstrating the beneficial effects of SSRIs in AD patients, either alone or in combination with AChE-Is, has been summarised in recent papers.[123,128] The Citalopram for Agitation in AD Study (CitAD)[129] found that the addition of citalopram titrated up to 30 mg/day significantly reduced agitation and caregivers' distress compared with placebo in 186 patients who were receiving psychosocial intervention. A secondary analysis[130] evaluated the effect of citalopram on 12 neuropsychiatric symptom domains assessed by the neuropsychiatric inventory (NPI). Citalopram showed efficacy for agitation/aggression, including reductions in the frequency of irritability, anxiety, delusions and hallucinations, but an increase in the severity of sleep/night-time behaviour disorders. Considering several covariates together[131] allowed the identification of responders. Those with moderate agitation and with lower levels of cognitive impairment were more likely to benefit from citalopram, and those with more severe agitation and greater cognitive impairment were at greater risk for adverse responses. This is perhaps of academic interest only, as the maximum dose of citalopram in this group of patients is 20 mg a day because of the drug's effect on cardiac QT interval.

Findings suggest that in AD patients treated with AChE-Is, SSRIs may exert some degree of protection against the negative effects of depression on cognition. To date, literature analysis does not clarify if the combined effect of SSRIs and AChE-Is is synergistic, additive or independent.[124] In addition, it is still unclear whether SSRIs have beneficial effects on cognition in AD patients who are not actively manifesting mood or behavioural problems.[128]

Trazodone[132,133] is sometimes used for non-cognitive symptoms although evidence is limited. It has been found to reduce irritability and cause a slight reduction in agitation, most probably by means of its sedative effects.[132,133] A Cochrane review of trazodone for agitation in dementia[132] however found insufficient evidence from RCTs to support its use in dementia.

A second, more recent, Cochrane review investigating the efficacy and safety of anti-depressants for agitation and psychosis in dementia has also been published.[134] The authors concluded that there are currently relatively few studies available but there is some evidence to support the use of certain antidepressants for agitation and psychosis in dementia. The SSRIs sertraline and citalopram were associated with a reduction in symptoms of agitation when compared with placebo in two studies. Both SSRIs and trazodone appear to be tolerated reasonably well when compared with placebo, typical antipsychotics and atypical antipsychotics. Future studies involving more subjects are required however to determine the effectiveness and safety of SSRIs, trazodone or other antidepressants in managing these symptoms.

A Cochrane review investigating whether antidepressants are clinically effective and acceptable for the treatment of patients with depression in the context of dementia concluded that antidepressants are not necessarily ineffective in dementia but rather there is not much evidence to support their efficacy and therefore they should be used with caution.[135] Furthermore, a large, independent, parallel group RCT found no difference in depression scores when comparing placebo, sertraline or mirtazapine in patients with dementia, suggesting that first-line treatment for depression in AD should be reconsidered.[136]

Whilst some emerging studies have found that antidepressant use in older people may be associated with an increased risk of dementia, it is important to keep in mind that previous studies have shown that late-life depression is associated with an increased risk for dementia. Hence any comparisons of antidepressant users to non-depressed non-users are subject to indication bias as the increased dementia risk could be due to depression, not the medication. A retrospective cohort study[137] was conducted including 3688 patients aged 60 years or older without dementia enrolled in a depression screening study in primary care clinics. Information on antidepressant use and incident dementia during follow-up was retrieved from electronic medical records. SSRI users had significantly higher dementia risk than non-users with severe depression (HR = 2.26, p = 0.0005). Future research is needed to confirm these results in other populations and to explore the potential mechanism underlying the observed association, if one indeed exists.

The association between mortality risk and use of antidepressants in people with dementia is not known. A Swedish study[138] included 20,050 memory clinic patients diagnosed with incident dementia and collected data on antidepressant use at the time of dementia diagnosis and over the 3-year period before a dementia diagnosis. Use of antidepressant treatment for 3 consecutive years before a dementia diagnosis was associated with a lower mortality risk for all dementia disorders and in AD.

Tricyclic antidepressants are best avoided in patients with dementia. They can cause falls, possibly via orthostatic hypotension, and increase confusion because of their potent anticholinergic adverse effects.[139]

Recommendation: although evidence is weak, use of SSRIs is justified in people with dementia who have clear symptoms of moderate or severe depression, especially if non-pharmacological approaches have been ineffective.

Mood stabilisers/anticonvulsants

RCTs of mood stabilisers in non-cognitive symptoms of dementia have been completed for **oxcarbazepine**,[140] **carbamazepine**[141] and **valproate**.[142] **Gabapentin**, lamotrigine and topiramate have also been used.[143] Of the mood stabilisers, carbamazepine has the most robust evidence of efficacy in non-cognitive symptoms.[144] However its serious adverse effects (especially Stevens–Johnson syndrome) and its potential for drug interactions somewhat limit its use. One RCT of valproate that included an open-label extension found valproate to be ineffective in controlling symptoms. Seven of the 39 patients enrolled died during the 12-week extension phase study period, although the deaths could not be attributed to the drug.[145] A study investigating the optimal dose of valproic acid in dementia found that whilst serum levels between 40 and 60 µg/L and relatively low doses (7–12 mg/kg per day) are associated with improvements in agitation in some patients, similar levels produced no significant improvements in others and led to substantial adverse effects.[146] A Cochrane review of valproate for the treatment of agitation in dementia found no evidence of efficacy but advocated the need for further research into its use in dementia.[147] Valproate does not delay emergence of agitation in dementia.[148] Literature reviews of anticonvulsants in non-cognitive symptoms of dementia found that valproate, oxcarbazepine and lithium showed low or no evidence of efficacy and that more RCTs are needed to strengthen the evidence for gabapentin, topiramate and lamotrigine.[144] Although clearly beneficial in some patients, anticonvulsant mood stabilisers cannot be recommended for routine use in the treatment of neuropsychiatric symptoms in dementia at present.[143]

Recommendation: limited evidence to support use – use may be justified where other treatments are contraindicated or ineffective. Valproate is best avoided.

Melatonin and sleep disturbances in AD

Evidence regarding the effectiveness of melatonin supplementation on sleep in patients with AD is limited. Six double-blind, randomised, placebo-controlled trials, mostly of limited sample size, have been published. Although it is clear that melatonin has no significant adverse effects, even at high doses, the results of studies have been equivocal. Some studies showed beneficial effects, mainly improvement of day/night-time sleep ratio, and decrease of nocturnal activity whilst other studies failed to demonstrate objective effectiveness.[149] Non-pharmacological management of sleep disturbances should be considered.[150]

Recommendation: limited evidence to support use, but safe to use and may be justified in some cases where benefits are seen. Non-pharmacological management of sleep disturbances should be considered.

A Cochrane review[151] of pharmacotherapies for sleep disturbances in dementia found no RCTs of many drugs that are widely prescribed for sleep problems in dementia, including the benzodiazepine and non-benzodiazepine hypnotics, although there is considerable uncertainty about the balance of benefits and risks associated with these common treatments. From the studies identified, there was no evidence that melatonin (up to 10 mg) helped sleep problems in patients with moderate to severe dementia due to AD. There was some evidence to support the use of a low dose (50 mg) of trazodone, although a larger trial is needed to allow a more definitive conclusion to be reached on the balance of risks and benefits. There was no evidence of any effect of ramelteon on sleep in patients with mild to moderate dementia due to AD. This is an area with a high need for pragmatic trials, particularly of those drugs that are in common clinical use for sleep problems in dementia.

Sedating antihistamines (e.g. promethazine)

Promethazine is frequently used in BPSD for its sedative effects. It has strong anticholinergic effects and readily penetrates the BBB therefore potentially causing significant cognitive impairment.[152]

Recommendation: may be used for short-term use only but evidence is minimal.

Miscellaneous agents

There is some evidence for the effects of *Gingko biloba* on neuropsychiatric symptoms of dementia, especially for apathy, anxiety, depression and irritability.[153] A once daily dose of 240 mg was safe and effective in patients with mild to moderate dementia.[154]

Recommendation: limited evidence to support use, but safe to use in mild to moderate dementia.

Electroconvulsive therapy (ECT)

A small study[155] examined the clinical records of 25 patients with dementia and a pre-existing psychiatric disorder treated with ECT. Twenty-nine acute ECT courses and 15 maintenance courses were reviewed. Treatment effectiveness and cognitive adverse effects were assessed as well as factors associated with response to treatment including pre-existing psychiatric disorders, concomitant pharmacological treatment and types of dementia. The study showed meaningful clinical effectiveness and good tolerability of ECT in patients with severe neuropsychiatric symptoms of dementia. Clinically meaningful response was seen in 72% of acute treatment courses and maintenance ECT was effective in maintaining response in 87% of treatment courses although there were two cases of significant cognitive adverse effects. Use of antipsychotic or antidepressant medications, pre-existing psychiatric disorder or gender were not associated with response.

Recommendation: insufficient evidence to recommend ECT use in BPSD. Caution: can cause significant cognitive adverse effects.

Summary

The evidence base available to guide treatment in this area is insufficient to allow specific recommendations on appropriate management and drug choice. The basic approach is to try non-drug measures and analgesia before resorting to the use of psychotropic drugs. Whichever drug is chosen, the approach outlined in Box 6.5 should be noted.

Box 6.5 Approach to the patient with BPSD

- Exclude physical illness potentially precipitating non-cognitive symptoms of dementia, e.g. constipation, infection, pain.
- Target the symptoms requiring treatment.
- Consider non-pharmacological methods.
- Carry out a risk–benefit analysis tailored to individual patient needs when selecting a drug.
- Make evidence-based decisions when choosing a drug.
- Discuss treatment options and explain the risks to patient (if they have capacity) and family/ caregivers.
- Titrate the drug from a low starting dose and maintain the lowest dose possible for the shortest period necessary.
- Review appropriateness of treatment regularly so that an ineffective drug is not continued unnecessarily.
- Monitor for adverse effects.
- Document clearly treatment choices and discussions with patient, family or caregivers.

References

1 National Institute for Health and Care Excellence. Dementia. Supporting people with dementia and their carers in health and social care. Clinical Guideline 42, 2011; updated September 2016. https://www.nice.org.uk/guidance/cg42.

2 Steinberg M et al. Point and 5-year period prevalence of neuropsychiatric symptoms in dementia: the Cache County Study. Int J Geriatr Psychiatry 2008; 23:170–177.

3 Salzman C et al. Elderly patients with dementia-related symptoms of severe agitation and aggression: consensus statement on treatment options, clinical trials methodology, and policy. J Clin Psychiatry 2008; 69:889–898.

4 Department of Health. The use of antipsychotic medication for people with dementia: Time for action. A report for the Minister of State for Care Services by Professor Sube Banerjee. 2009. https://www.rcpsych.ac.uk/pdf/Antipsychotic%20Bannerjee%20Report.pdf.

5. Livingston G et al. A systematic review of the clinical effectiveness and cost-effectiveness of sensory, psychological and behavioural interventions for managing agitation in older adults with dementia. Health Technol Assess 2014; 18:1–226, v–vi.

6. Kales HC et al. Assessment and management of behavioral and psychological symptoms of dementia. BMJ 2015; 350:h369.

7. James IA. *Understanding Behaviour in Dementia That Challenges: A Guide to Assessment and Treatment.* London: Jessica Kingsley Publishers; 2011.

8. Brechin D et al. British Psychological Society. Briefing paper. Alternatives to antipsychotic medication: Psychological approaches in managing psychological and behavioural distress in people with dementia. 2013. http://www.bps.org.uk/system/files/Public%20files/antipsychotic.pdf.

9. Douglas S et al. Non-pharmacological interventions in dementia. Adv Psychiatr Treat 2004; 10:171–177.

10. Ayalon L et al. Effectiveness of nonpharmacological interventions for the management of neuropsychiatric symptoms in patients with dementia: a systematic review. Arch Intern Med 2006; 166:2182–2188.

11. Livingston G et al. Systematic review of psychological approaches to the management of neuropsychiatric symptoms of dementia. Am J Psychiatry 2005; 162:1996–2021.

12. Chung JC et al. Snoezelen for dementia. Cochrane Database Syst Rev 2002:CD003152.

13. Chung JCC et al. Cochrane Summary – No evidence of the efficacy of snoezelen or multi-sensory stimulation programmes for people with dementia. 2009. http://www.cochrane.org/CD003152/DEMENTIA_no-evidence-of-the-efficacy-of-snoezelen-or-multi-sensory-stimulation-programmes-for-people-with-dementia.

14. McCarney R et al. Homeopathy for dementia. Cochrane Database Syst Rev 2003:CD003803.

15. Forrester LT et al. Aromatherapy for dementia. Cochrane Database Syst Rev 2014:CD003150.

16. Fung JK et al. A systematic review of the use of aromatherapy in treatment of behavioral problems in dementia. Geriatr Gerontol Int 2012; 12:372–382.

17. Ballard CG et al. Aromatherapy as a safe and effective treatment for the management of agitation in severe dementia: the results of a double-blind, placebo-controlled trial with Melissa. J Clin Psychiatry 2002; 63:553–558.

18. Burns A et al. A double-blind placebo-controlled randomized trial of Melissa officinalis oil and donepezil for the treatment of agitation in Alzheimer's disease. Dement Geriatr Cogn Disord 2011; 31:158–164.

19. Nguyen QA et al. The use of aromatherapy to treat behavioural problems in dementia. Int J Geriatr Psychiatry 2008; 23:337–346.

20. Millan-Calenti JC et al. Optimal nonpharmacological management of agitation in Alzheimer's disease: challenges and solutions. Clin Interv Aging 2016; 11:175–184.

21. Livingston G et al. Non-pharmacological interventions for agitation in dementia: systematic review of randomised controlled trials. Br J Psychiatry 2014; 205:436–442.

22. Husebo BS et al. Efficacy of treating pain to reduce behavioural disturbances in residents of nursing homes with dementia: cluster randomised clinical trial. BMJ 2011; 343:d4065.

CHAPTER 6

23. Brown R et al. Opioids for agitation in dementia. Cochrane Database Syst Rev 2015:CD009705.
24. Devanand DP et al. A randomized, placebo-controlled dose-comparison trial of haloperidol for psychosis and disruptive behaviors in Alzheimer's disease. Am J Psychiatry 1998; 155:1512–1520.
25. Chan WC et al. A double-blind randomised comparison of risperidone and haloperidol in the treatment of behavioural and psychological symptoms in Chinese dementia patients. Int J Geriatr Psychiatry 2001; 16:1156–1162.
26. Tariot PN et al. Quetiapine treatment of psychosis associated with dementia: a double-blind, randomized, placebo-controlled clinical trial. Am J Geriatr Psychiatry 2006; 14:767–776.
27. Verhey FR et al. Olanzapine versus haloperidol in the treatment of agitation in elderly patients with dementia: results of a randomized controlled double-blind trial. Dement Geriatr Cogn Disord 2006; 21:1–8.
28. De Deyn PP et al. A randomized trial of risperidone, placebo, and haloperidol for behavioral symptoms of dementia. Neurology 1999; 53:946–955.
29. Savaskan E et al. Treatment of behavioural, cognitive and circadian rest-activity cycle disturbances in Alzheimer's disease: haloperidol vs. quetiapine. Int J Neuropsychopharmacol 2006; 9:507–516.
30. Suh GH et al. Comparative efficacy of risperidone versus haloperidol on behavioural and psychological symptoms of dementia. Int J Geriatr Psychiatry 2006; 21:654–660.
31. Lee PE et al. Atypical antipsychotic drugs in the treatment of behavioural and psychological symptoms of dementia: systematic review. BMJ 2004; 329:75.
32. Jeste DV et al. Atypical antipsychotics in elderly patients with dementia or schizophrenia: review of recent literature. Harv Rev Psychiatry 2005; 13:340–351.
33. Jeste DV et al. ACNP White Paper: update on use of antipsychotic drugs in elderly persons with dementia. Neuropsychopharmacology 2008; 33:957–970.
34. Aupperle P. Management of aggression, agitation, and psychosis in dementia: focus on atypical antipsychotics. Am J Alzheimers Dis Other Demen 2006; 21:101–108.
35. Yury CA et al. Meta-analysis of the effectiveness of atypical antipsychotics for the treatment of behavioural problems in persons with dementia. Psychother Psychosom 2007; 76:213–218.
36. Deberdt WG et al. Comparison of olanzapine and risperidone in the treatment of psychosis and associated behavioral disturbances in patients with dementia. Am J Geriatr Psychiatry 2005; 13:722–730.
37. Schneider LS et al. Efficacy and adverse effects of atypical antipsychotics for dementia: meta-analysis of randomized, placebo-controlled trials. Am J Geriatr Psychiatry 2006; 14:191–210.
38. Anon. How safe are antipsychotics in dementia? Drug Ther Bull 2007; 45:81–86.
39. Rosack J. Side-effect risk often tempers antipsychotic use for dementia. Psychiatr News 2006; 41:1–38.
40. Schneider LS et al. Risk of death with atypical antipsychotic drug treatment for dementia: meta-analysis of randomized placebo-controlled trials. JAMA 2005; 294:1934–1943.
41. Street JS et al. Olanzapine treatment of psychotic and behavioural symptoms in patients with Alzheimer disease in nursing care facilities: a double-blind, randomized, placebo-controlled trial. The HGEU Study Group. Arch Gen Psychiatry 2000; 57:968–976.
42. Bhana N et al. Risperidone: a review of its use in the management of the behavioural and psychological symptoms of dementia. Drugs Aging 2000; 16:451–471.
43. Katz I et al. The efficacy and safety of risperidone in the treatment of psychosis of Alzheimer's disease and mixed dementia: a meta-analysis of 4 placebo-controlled clinical trials. Int J Geriatr Psychiatry 2007; 22:475–484.
44. Onor ML et al. Clinical experience with risperidone in the treatment of behavioral and psychological symptoms of dementia. Prog Neuropsychopharmacol Biol Psychiatry 2007; 31:205–209.
45. Rabinowitz J et al. Treating behavioral and psychological symptoms in patients with psychosis of Alzheimer's disease using risperidone. Int Psychogeriatr 2007; 19:227–240.
46. Kurz A et al. Effects of risperidone on behavioral and psychological symptoms associated with dementia in clinical practice. Int Psychogeriatr 2005; 17:605–616.
47. McManus DQ et al. Quetiapine, a novel antipsychotic: experience in elderly patients with psychotic disorders. Seroquel Trial 48 Study Group. J Clin Psychiatry 1999; 60:292–298.
48. Onor ML et al. Efficacy and tolerability of quetiapine in the treatment of behavioral and psychological symptoms of dementia. Am J Alzheimers Dis Other Demen 2006; 21:448–453.
49. Zhong KX et al. Quetiapine to treat agitation in dementia: a randomized, double-blind, placebo-controlled study. Curr Alzheimer Res 2007; 4:81–93.
50. Laks J et al. Use of aripiprazole for psychosis and agitation in dementia. Int Psychogeriatr 2006; 18:335–340.
51. De Deyn P et al. Aripiprazole for the treatment of psychosis in patients with Alzheimer's disease: a randomized, placebo-controlled study. J Clin Psychopharmacol 2005; 25:463–467.
52. Mintzer JE et al. Aripiprazole for the treatment of psychoses in institutionalized patients with Alzheimer dementia: a multicenter, randomized, double-blind, placebo-controlled assessment of three fixed doses. Am J Geriatr Psychiatry 2007; 15:918–931.
53. Mauri M et al. Amisulpride in the treatment of behavioural disturbances among patients with moderate to severe Alzheimer's disease. Acta Neurol Scand 2006; 114:97–101.
54. Lim HK et al. Amisulpride versus risperidone treatment for behavioral and psychological symptoms in patients with dementia of the Alzheimer type: a randomized, open, prospective study. Neuropsychobiology 2006; 54:247–251.

55. Rainer M et al. Quetiapine versus risperidone in elderly patients with behavioural and psychological symptoms of dementia: efficacy, safety and cognitive function. Eur Psychiatry 2007; **22**:395–403.

56. Lee HB et al. Clozapine for treatment-resistant agitation in dementia. J Geriatr Psychiatry Neurol 2007; **20**:178–182.

57. Schneider LS et al. Effectiveness of atypical antipsychotic drugs in patients with Alzheimer's disease. N Engl J Med 2006; **355**:1525–1538.

58. Ballard C et al. Atypical antipsychotics for aggression and psychosis in Alzheimer's disease (review). Cochrane Database Syst Rev 2006:DOI: 10.1002/14651858.CD14003476.

59. Pharmacovigilance Working Party. Antipsychotics and cerebrovascular accident. SPC wording for antipsychotics. 2005.

60. Duff G. Atypical antipsychotic drugs and stroke – Committee on Safety of Medicines. 2004. http://www.mhra.gov.uk/home/groups/pl-p/documents/websiteresources/con019488.pdf.

61. FDA. Information on Conventional Antipsychotics – FDA Alert 6/16/2008. http://www.fda.gov.

62. European Medicines Agency. CHMP Assessment Report on conventional antipsychotics. 2008. http://www.emea.europa.eu.

63. Kryzhanovskaya LA et al. A review of treatment-emergent adverse events during olanzapine clinical trials in elderly patients with dementia. J Clin Psychiatry 2006; **67**:933–945.

64. Herrmann N et al. Do atypical antipsychotics cause stroke? CNS Drugs 2005; **19**:91–103.

65. Douglas IJ et al Exposure to antipsychotics and risk of stroke: self controlled case series study. BMJ 2008; **337**:a1227.

66. Kales HC et al. Mortality risk in patients with dementia treated with antipsychotics versus other psychiatric medications. Am J Psychiatry 2007; **164**:1568–1576.

67. Herrmann N et al. Atypical antipsychotics and risk of cerebrovascular accidents. Am J Psychiatry 2004; **161**:1113–1115.

68. Trifiro G et al. All-cause mortality associated with atypical and typical antipsychotics in demented outpatients. Pharmacoepidemiol Drug Saf 2007; **16**:538–544.

69. Nasrallah HA et al. Lower mortality in geriatric patients receiving risperidone and olanzapine versus haloperidol: preliminary analysis of retrospective data. Am J Geriatr Psychiatry 2004; **12**:437–439.

70. Gill SS et al. Antipsychotic drug use and mortality in older adults with dementia. Ann Intern Med 2007; **146**:775–786.

71. Sacchetti E et al. Risk of stroke with typical and atypical anti-psychotics: a retrospective cohort study including unexposed subjects. J Psychopharmacol 2008; **22**:39–46.

72. Wang PS et al. Risk of death in elderly users of conventional vs. atypical antipsychotic medications. N Engl J Med 2005; **353**:2335–2341.

73. Hollis J et al. Antipsychotic medication dispensing and risk of death in veterans and war widows 65 years and older. Am J Geriatr Psychiatry 2007; **15**:932–941.

74. Wu CS et al. Association of stroke with the receptor-binding profiles of antipsychotics – a case-crossover study. Biol Psychiatry 2013; **73**:414–421.

75. Kleijer BC et al. Risk of cerebrovascular events in elderly users of antipsychotics. J Psychopharmacol 2009; **23**:909–14.

76. Ballard C et al. The dementia antipsychotic withdrawal trial (DART-AD): long-term follow-up of a randomised placebo-controlled trial. Lancet Neurol 2009; **8**:151–157.

77. Huybrechts KF et al. Differential risk of death in older residents in nursing homes prescribed specific antipsychotic drugs: population based cohort study. BMJ 2012; **344**:e977.

78. Kales HC et al. Risk of mortality among individual antipsychotics in patients with dementia. Am J Psychiatry 2012; **169**:71–79.

79. Schmedt N et al. Comparative risk of death in older adults treated with antipsychotics: a population-based cohort study. Eur Neuropsychopharmacol 2016; **26**:1390–1400.

80. Maust DT et al. Antipsychotics, other psychotropics, and the risk of death in patients with dementia: number needed to harm. JAMA Psychiatry 2015; **72**:438–445.

81. Smith DA et al. Association between risperidone treatment and cerebrovascular adverse events: examining the evidence and postulating hypotheses for an underlying mechanism. J Am Med Dir Assoc 2004; **5**:129–132.

82. Trifiro G et al. Use of antipsychotics in elderly patients with dementia: do atypical and conventional agents have a similar safety profile? Pharmacol Res 2009; **59**:1–12.

83. Jackson JW et al. Mediators of first- versus second-generation antipsychotic-related mortality in older adults. Epidemiology 2015; **26**:700–709.

84. Howard R et al. Baseline characteristics and treatment-emergent risk factors associated with cerebrovascular event and death with risperidone in dementia patients. Br J Psychiatry 2016; **209**:378–384.

85. McShane R et al. Do neuroleptic drugs hasten cognitive decline in dementia? Prospective study with necropsy follow up. BMJ 1997; **314**:266–270.

86. Ballard C et al. Quetiapine and rivastigmine and cognitive decline in Alzheimer's disease: randomised double blind placebo controlled trial. BMJ 2005; **330**:874.

87. Livingston G et al. Antipsychotics and cognitive decline in Alzheimer's disease: the LASER-Alzheimer's disease longitudinal study. J Neurol Neurosurg Psychiatry 2007; **78**:25–29.

88. Paleacu D et al. Quetiapine treatment for behavioural and psychological symptoms of dementia in Alzheimer's disease patients: a 6-week, double-blind, placebo-controlled study. Int J Geriatr Psychiatry 2008; **23**:393–400.

89. Corbett A et al. Don't use antipsychotics routinely to treat agitation and aggression in people with dementia. BMJ 2014; **349**:g6420.

90. Janssen-Cilag Ltd. Summary of Product Characteristics. Risperdal Tablets, Liquid & Quicklet. 2015. https://www.medicines.org.uk/.

91. BNF Online. British National Formulary. 2017. https://www.medicinescomplete.com/mc/bnf/current/.

CHAPTER 6

92. Katz IR et al. Comparison of risperidone and placebo for psychosis and behavioral disturbances associated with dementia: a randomized, double-blind trial. Risperidone Study Group. J Clin Psychiatry 1999; 60:107–115.

93. NHS Health Research Authority. Optimisation of amisulpride prescribing in older people. 2012. https://www.hra.nhs.uk/planning-and-improving-research/application-summaries/research-summaries/optimisation-of-amisulpride-prescribing-in-older-people/.

94. Reeves S et al. A population approach to characterise amisulpride pharmacokinetics in older people and Alzheimer's disease. Psychopharmacology (Berl) 2016; 233:3371–3381.

95. NHS PrescQIPP. Reducing Antipsychotic Prescribing in Dementia Toolkit. 2014. https://www.prescqipp.info/resources/send/109-reducing-antipsychotic-prescribing-in-dementia-toolkit/1353-reducing-antipsychotic-prescribing-in-dementia-toolkit.

96. Terao T et al. Can donepezil be considered a mild antipsychotic in dementia treatment? A report of donepezil use in 6 patients. J Clin Psychiatry 2003; 64:1392–1393.

97. Weiner MF et al. Effects of donepezil on emotional/behavioral symptoms in Alzheimer's disease patients. J Clin Psychiatry 2000; 61:487–492.

98. Figiel G et al. A systematic review of the effectiveness of rivastigmine for the treatment of behavioral disturbances in dementia and other neurological disorders. Curr Med Res Opin 2008; 24:157–166.

99. Finkel SI. Effects of rivastigmine on behavioral and psychological symptoms of dementia in Alzheimer's disease. Clin Ther 2004; 26:980–990.

100. Rosler M et al. Effects of two-year treatment with the cholinesterase inhibitor rivastigmine on behavioural symptoms in Alzheimer's disease. Behav Neurol 1998; 11:211–216.

101. Cummings JL et al. Effects of rivastigmine treatment on the neuropsychiatric and behavioral disturbances of nursing home residents with moderate to severe probable Alzheimer's disease: a 26-week, multicenter, open-label study. Am J Geriatr Pharmacother 2005; 3:137–148.

102. Cummings JL et al. Reduction of behavioral disturbances and caregiver distress by galantamine in patients with Alzheimer's disease. Am J Psychiatry 2004; 161:532–538.

103. Herrmann N et al. Galantamine treatment of problematic behavior in Alzheimer disease: post-hoc analysis of pooled data from three large trials. Am J Geriatr Psychiatry 2005; 13:527–534.

104. Tangwongchai S et al. Galantamine for the treatment of BPSD in Thai patients with possible Alzheimer's disease with or without cerebro-vascular disease. Am J Alzheimers Dis Other Demen 2008; 23:593–601.

105. Barak Y et al. Donepezil for the treatment of behavioral disturbances in Alzheimer's disease: a 6-month open trial. Arch Gerontol Geriatr 2001; 33:237–241.

106. Howard RJ et al. Donepezil for the treatment of agitation in Alzheimer's disease. N Engl J Med 2007; 357:1382–1392.

107. McKeith I et al. Efficacy of rivastigmine in dementia with Lewy bodies: a randomised, double-blind, placebo-controlled international study. Lancet 2000; 356:2031–2036.

108. Campbell N et al. Impact of cholinesterase inhibitors on behavioral and psychological symptoms of Alzheimer's disease: a meta-analysis. Clin Interv Aging 2008; 3:719–728.

109. Rodda J et al. Are cholinesterase inhibitors effective in the management of the behavioral and psychological symptoms of dementia in Alzheimer's disease? A systematic review of randomized, placebo-controlled trials of donepezil, rivastigmine and galantamine. Int Psychogeriatr 2009; 21:813–824.

110. National Institute for Health and Care Excellence. Donepezil, galantamine, rivastigmine and memantine for the treatment of Alzheimer's disease. Technology Appraisal Guidance TA217, 2011; last updated May 2016. https://www.nice.org.uk/guidance/ta217.

111. Cummings JL et al. Behavioral effects of memantine in Alzheimer disease patients receiving donepezil treatment. Neurology 2006; 67:57–63.

112. Wilcock GK et al. Memantine for agitation/aggression and psychosis in moderately severe to severe Alzheimer's disease: a pooled analysis of 3 studies. J Clin Psychiatry 2008; 69:341–348.

113. Gauthier S et al. Improvement in behavioural symptoms in patients with moderate to severe Alzheimer's disease by memantine: a pooled data analysis. Int J Geriatr Psychiatry 2007; 23:537–545.

114. Fox C et al. Efficacy of memantine for agitation in Alzheimer's dementia: a randomised double-blind placebo controlled trial. PLoS One 2012; 7:e35185.

115. McShane R et al. Memantine for dementia. Cochrane Database Syst Rev 2006:CD003154.

116. Ballard C et al. A double-blind randomized placebo-controlled withdrawal trial comparing memantine and antipsychotics for the long-term treatment of function and neuropsychiatric symptoms in people with Alzheimer's disease (MAIN-AD). J Am Med Dir Assoc 2015; 16:316–322.

117. Verdoux H et al. Is benzodiazepine use a risk factor for cognitive decline and dementia? A literature review of epidemiological studies. Psychol Med 2005; 35:307–315.

118. Lagnaoui R et al. Benzodiazepine utilization patterns in Alzheimer's disease patients. Pharmacoepidemiol Drug Saf 2003; 12:511–515.

119. Billioti de Gage S et al. Benzodiazepine use and risk of dementia: prospective population based study. BMJ 2012; 345:e6231.

120. Taipale H et al. Risk of pneumonia associated with incident benzodiazepine use among community-dwelling adults with Alzheimer disease. CMAJ 2017; 189:e519–e529.

121. Palmaro A et al. Benzodiazepines and risk of death: results from two large cohort studies in France and UK. Eur Neuropsychopharmacol 2015; 25:1566–1577.

122. Chang CM et al. Benzodiazepine and risk of hip fractures in older people: a nested case-control study in Taiwan. Am J Geriatr Psychiatry 2008; 16:686–692.

CHAPTER 6

123. Aboukhatwa M et al. Antidepressants are a rational complementary therapy for the treatment of Alzheimer's disease. Mol Neurodegener 2010; **5**:10.

124. Rozzini L et al. Efficacy of SSRIs on cognition of Alzheimer's disease patients treated with cholinesterase inhibitors. Int Psychogeriatr 2010; **22**:114–119.

125. Deakin JB et al. Paroxetine does not improve symptoms and impairs cognition in frontotemporal dementia: a double-blind randomized controlled trial. Psychopharmacology (Berl) 2004; **172**:400–408.

126. Finkel SI et al. A randomized, placebo-controlled study of the efficacy and safety of sertraline in the treatment of the behavioral manifestations of Alzheimer's disease in outpatients treated with donepezil. Int J Geriatr Psychiatry 2004; **19**:9–18.

127. Henry G et al. Efficacy and tolerability of antidepressants in the treatment of behavioral and psychological symptoms of dementia, a literature review of evidence. Am J Alzheimers Dis Other Demen 2011; **26**:169–183.

128. Chow TW et al. Potential cognitive enhancing and disease modification effects of SSRIs for Alzheimer's disease. Neuropsychiatr Dis Treat 2007; **3**:627–636.

129. Porsteinsson AP et al. Effect of citalopram on agitation in Alzheimer disease: the CitAD randomized clinical trial. JAMA 2014; **311**:682–691.

130. Leonpacher AK et al. Effects of citalopram on neuropsychiatric symptoms in Alzheimer's dementia: evidence from the CitAD study. Am J Psychiatry 2016; **173**:473–480.

131. Schneider LS et al. Heterogeneity of treatment response to citalopram for patients with Alzheimer's disease with aggression or agitation: the CitAD Randomized Clinical Trial. Am J Psychiatry 2016; **173**:465–472.

132. Martinon-Torres G et al. Trazodone for agitation in dementia. Cochrane Database Syst Rev 2004:CD004990.

133. Lopez-Pousa S et al. Trazodone for Alzheimer's disease: a naturalistic follow-up study. Arch Gerontol Geriatr 2008; **47**:207–215.

134. Seitz DP et al. Antidepressants for agitation and psychosis in dementia. Cochrane Database Syst Rev 2011; **2**:CD008191.

135. Bains J et al. The efficacy of antidepressants in the treatment of depression in dementia. Cochrane Database Syst Rev 2002:CD003944.

136. Banerjee S et al. Sertraline or mirtazapine for depression in dementia (HTA-SADD): a randomised, multicentre, double-blind, placebo-controlled trial. Lancet 2011; **378**:403–411.

137. Wang C et al. Antidepressant use in the elderly is associated with an increased risk of dementia. Alzheimer Dis Assoc Disord 2016; **30**:99–104.

138. Enache D et al. Antidepressants and mortality risk in a dementia cohort: data from SveDem, the Swedish Dementia Registry. Acta Psychiatr Scand 2016; **134**:430–440.

139. Ballard C et al. Management of neuropsychiatric symptoms in people with dementia. CNS Drugs 2010; **24**:729–739.

140. Sommer OH et al. Effect of oxcarbazepine in the treatment of agitation and aggression in severe dementia. Dement Geriatr Cogn Disord 2009; **27**:155–163.

141. Tariot PN et al. Efficacy and tolerability of carbamazepine for agitation and aggression in dementia. Am J Psychiatry 1998; **155**:54–61.

142. Lonergan E et al. Valproate preparations for agitation in dementia. Cochrane Database Syst Rev 2009:CD003945.

143. Konovalov S et al. Anticonvulsants for the treatment of behavioral and psychological symptoms of dementia: a literature review. Int Psychogeriatr 2008; **20**:293–308.

144. Yeh YC et al. Mood stabilizers for the treatment of behavioral and psychological symptoms of dementia: an update review. Kaohsiung J Med Sci 2012; **28**:185–193.

145. Sival RC et al. Sodium valproate in aggressive behaviour in dementia: a twelve-week open label follow-up study. Int J Geriatr Psychiatry 2004; **19**:305–312.

146. Dolder CR et al. Valproic acid in dementia: does an optimal dose exist? J Pharm Pract 2012; **25**:142–150.

147. Lonergan E et al. Valproate preparations for agitation in dementia. Cochrane Database Syst Rev 2009:CD003945.

148. Tariot PN et al. Chronic divalproex sodium to attenuate agitation and clinical progression of Alzheimer disease. Arch Gen Psychiatry 2011; **68**:853–861.

149. Peter-Derex L et al. Sleep and Alzheimer's disease. Sleep Med Rev 2015; **19**:29–38.

150. David R et al. Non-pharmacologic management of sleep disturbance in Alzheimer's disease. J Nutr Health Aging 2010; **14**:203–206.

151. McCleery J et al. Pharmacotherapies for sleep disturbances in dementia. Cochrane Database Syst Rev 2016; **11**:CD009178.

152. Bishara D et al. Anticholinergic effect on cognition (AEC) of drugs commonly used in older people. Int J Geriatr Psychiatry 2017; **32**:650–656.

153. Scripnikov A et al. Effects of Ginkgo biloba extract EGb 761 on neuropsychiatric symptoms of dementia: findings from a randomised controlled trial. Wien Med Wochenschr 2007; **157**:295–300.

154. Bachinskaya N et al. Alleviating neuropsychiatric symptoms in dementia: the effects of Ginkgo biloba extract EGb 761. Findings from a randomized controlled trial. Neuropsychiatr Dis Treat 2011; **7**:209–215.

155. Isserles M et al. Clinical effectiveness and tolerability of electroconvulsive therapy in patients with neuropsychiatric symptoms of dementia. J Alzheimers Dis 2017; **57**:45–51.

A guide to medication doses of commonly used psychotropic drugs in older adults

See Table 6.8.

References

1. Generics UK T/A Mylan. Summary of Product Characteristics. Clomipramine 25 mg Capsules, Hard. 2017. https://www.medicines.org.uk/emc/medicine/33260.
2. Prescribers' Digital Reference. Desvenlafaxine – Drug Summary. 2017.
3. Eli Lilly and Company Limited. Summary of Product Characteristics. Cymbalta 30mg hard gastro-resistant capsules, Cymbalta 60mg hard gastro-resistant capsules. 2017. https://www.medicines.org.uk/emc/medicine/15694.
4. Zentiva. Summary of Product Characteristics. Molipaxin 100mg/ Trazodone 100mg Capsules. 2015. https://www.medicines.org.uk/emc/medicine/26734.
5. Prescribers' Digital Reference. Trintellix (vortioxetine) – drug information. 2017. http://www.pdr.net/drug-information/trintellix?druglabelid=3348.
6. Muller MJ et al. Amisulpride doses and plasma levels in different age groups of patients with schizophrenia or schizoaffective disorder. J Psychopharmacol 2009; 23:278–286.
7. Psarros C et al. Amisulpride for the treatment of very-late-onset schizophrenia-like psychosis. Int J Geriatr Psychiatry 2009; 24:518–522.
8. Clark-Papasavas C et al. Towards a therapeutic window of D2/3 occupancy for treatment of psychosis in Alzheimer's disease, with [F]fallypride positron emission tomography. Int J Geriatr Psychiatry 2014; 29:1001–1009.
9. Prescribers' Digital Reference. Brexpiprazole – Drug Summary. 2017. http://www.pdr.net/drug-summary/Rexulti-brexpiprazole-3759.
10. Prescribers' Digital Reference. Vraylar (cariprazine) – drug information. 2017. http://www.pdr.net/drug-information/vraylar?druglabelid=3792.
11. Jeste DV et al. Conventional vs. newer antipsychotics in elderly patients. Am J Geriatr Psychiatry 1999; 7:70–76.
12. Karim S et al. Treatment of psychosis in elderly people. Advances in Psychiatric Treatment 2005; 11:286–296.
13. The Parkinson Study Group. Low-dose clozapine for the treatment of drug-induced psychosis in Parkinson's disease. N Engl J Med 1999; 340:757–763.
14. Sunovion Pharmaceuticals Europe Ltd. Summary of Product Characteristics. Latuda 18.5mg, 37mg and 74mg film-coated tablets. 2016. https://www.medicines.org.uk/emc/medicine/29125.
15. Otsuka Pharmaceutical (UK) Ltd. Summary of Product Characteristics. Abilify Maintena 300mg & 400mg powder and solvent for prolonged-release suspension for injection and suspension for injection in pre filled syringe. 2016. https://www.medicines.org.uk/emc/medicine/31386.
16. Janssen-Cilag Limited. Summary of Product Characteristics. TREVICTA 175mg, 263mg, 350mg, 525mg prolonged release suspension for injection. 2016. https://www.medicines.org.uk/emc/medicine/32050.
17. Janssen-Cilag Limited. Summary of Product Characteristics. RISPERDAL CONSTA 25 mg powder and solvent for prolonged-release suspension for intramuscular injection. 2016. https://www.medicines.org.uk/emc/medicine/9939.
18. Sanofi. Summary of Product Characteristics. Priadel 200mg prolonged release tablets. 2015. https://www.medicines.org.uk/emc/medicine/25501.
19. Pfizer Limited. Summary of Product Characteristics. Lyrica Capsules. 2017. https://www.medicines.org.uk/emc/medicine/14651.

Table 6.8 Guide to medication doses of commonly used psychotropic drugs in older adults

Drug	Specific indication/additional notes	Starting dose	Usual maintenance dose	Maximum dose in elderly
Antidepressants				
Agomelatine	Depression Monitor LFTs Data suggest agomelatine is not effective in patients >75 years	25 mg nocte	25–50 mg daily	50 mg nocte
Citalopram	Depression/anxiety disorder	10 mg mane	10–20 mg mane	20 mg mane
Clomipramine	Depression/phobic and obsessional states	10 mg nocte (dose increases should be cautious)	30–75 mg daily[1] should be reached after about 10 days	75 mg daily[1]
Desvenlafaxine	No formal recommendations are available for dosing in older adults.[2] For older adults, possible reduced renal clearance of desvenlafaxine should be considered when determining an appropriate dose Dosage in renal impairment: CrCl 50–80 mL/minute: no dosage adjustment needed CrCl 30–50 mL/minute: 50 mg daily is the recommended daily and maximum dose CrCl <30 mL/minute or end-stage renal disease (ESRD): 50 mg every other day is the recommended daily and maximum dose Older adults are also at greater risk for developing clinically significant hyponatraemia[2]			400 mg daily[2]
Duloxetine	Depression/anxiety disorder	30 mg daily*	60 mg daily	120 mg daily[3] (caution as limited data in elderly for this dose)
Escitalopram	Depression/anxiety disorder	5 mg mane	5–10 mg mane	10 mg mane
Fluoxetine	Depression/anxiety disorder Caution as long half-life and inhibitor of several CYP enzymes	20 mg mane	20 mg mane	40 mg mane usually (but 60 mg can be used)
Lofepramine	Depression	35 mg nocte*	70 mg nocte*	140 mg nocte or in divided doses* (occasionally 210 mg nocte required)
Mirtazapine	Depression	7.5 mg nocte or usually 15 mg nocte*	15–30 mg nocte	45 mg nocte

(Continued)

Table 6.8 (*Continued*)

Drug	Specific indication/additional notes	Starting dose	Usual maintenance dose	Maximum dose in elderly
Sertraline	Depression/anxiety disorder	25–50 mg mane (25 mg can be increased to 50 mg mane after 1 week)	50–100 mg mane*	100 mg (occasionally up to 150 mg mane)*
Trazodone	Depression	100 mg daily in divided doses or as a single night-time dose[4]	100–200 mg daily*	300 mg daily[4]
	Agitation in dementia Avoid single doses >100 mg	25 mg bd*	25–100 mg daily*	200 mg daily* (in divided doses)
Venlafaxine	Depression/anxiety disorder Monitor BP on initiation	37.5 mg mane (increased to 75 mg XL mane after 1 week) *	75–150 mg (XL) mane*	150 mg daily (occasionally 225 mg daily necessary)*
Vortioxetine	Major depressive disorder	5–10 mg daily[5]	5–20 mg daily[5]	20 mg daily[5]
Antipsychotics				
Amisulpride	Chronic schizophrenia	50 mg daily*	100–200 mg daily*	400 mg daily[6] (caution >200 mg daily)*
	Late-life psychosis	25–50 mg daily*	50–100 mg daily* (increase in 25 mg steps)	200 mg daily[7] (caution >100 mg daily)*
	Agitation/psychosis in dementia Caution QTc prolongation	25 mg nocte[8]	25–50 mg daily[8]	50 mg daily[8]
Aripiprazole	Schizophrenia, mania (oral)	5 mg mane*	5–15 mg daily*	20 mg mane*
	Control of agitation (IM injection)	5.25 mg*	5.25–9.75 mg*	15 mg daily* (combined oral + IM)
Brexpiprazole	Dosage not established in older adults[9]			
Cariprazine	Dosage not established in older adults[10]			
Clozapine	Schizophrenia	6.25–12.5 mg daily[11,12] increased by no more than 6.25–12.5 mg once or twice a week[11]	50–100 mg daily[11,12]	100 mg daily[11,12]
	Parkinson's related psychosis	6.25 mg daily[13]	25–37.5 mg daily[13]	50 mg daily[13]

	IM injection	The oral bioavailability of clozapine is about half that of the IM injection, e.g. 50mg daily of the IM injection is roughly equivalent to 100mg daily of the tablets/oral solution. After each injection has been given the patient must be observed every 15 minutes for the first 2 hours to check for excess sedation. NB: If IM lorazepam is required leave at least ONE HOUR between administration of IM clozapine and IM lorazepam		
Iloperidone		No formal recommendations are available for dosing in older adults		
Lurasidone		Dosing recommendations for elderly patients with normal renal function (CrCl ≥80 mL/minute) are the same as for adults with normal renal function. However, because elderly patients may have diminished renal function, dose adjustments may be required according to their renal function status[14]		Limited data on higher doses used in older adults. No data are available in elderly people treated with 148mg. Caution should be exercised when treating patients ≥65 years of age with higher doses[14]
Olanzapine	Schizophrenia	2.5mg nocte*	5–10mg daily*	15mg nocte[12]
	Agitation/psychosis in dementia	2.5mg nocte*	2.5–10mg daily*	10mg nocte* (optimal dose is 5mg daily)[12]
Quetiapine	Schizophrenia	12.5–25mg daily[12]	75–125mg daily[11]	200–300mg daily[12]
	Agitation/psychosis in dementia	12.5–25mg daily*	50–100mg daily*	100–300mg daily[12]
Risperidone	Psychosis	0.5mg bd (0.25–0.5mg daily in some cases)[12]	1–2.5mg daily[11]	4mg daily
	Late-onset psychosis	0.5mg daily*	1mg daily*	2mg daily* (optimal dose is 1mg daily)
	Agitation/psychosis in dementia	0.25mg daily* or bd	0.5mg bd	2mg daily (optimal dose is 1mg daily)[12]
Haloperidol	Psychosis	0.25–0.5mg daily[11]	1–3.5mg daily[11]	Caution >3.5mg – assess tolerability and ECG Max 10mg/day (oral) Max 5mg/day (IM)
	Agitation Avoid in older adults (except in delirium) owing to risk of QTc prolongation	0.25–0.5mg daily*	0.5–1.5mg daily or bd	

(Continued)

Table 6.8 (*Continued*)

Drug	Specific indication/additional notes	Starting dose	Usual maintenance dose	Maximum dose in elderly
Long-acting conventional antipsychotic drugs				
Flupentixol decanoate (Depixol)		Test dose: 5–10 mg	After at least 7 days of test dose: 10–20 mg every 2–4 weeks* Dose increased gradually according to response and tolerability in steps of 5–10 mg every 2 weeks*	40 mg every 2 weeks* (extend frequency to every 3–4 weeks if EPS develop) (Occasionally up to 50 or 60 mg every 2 weeks* may be used if tolerated)
Fluphenazine decanoate	Caution – high risk of EPS	Test dose 6.25 mg	After 4–7 days of test dose: 12.5–25 mg every 2–4 weeks Dose increased gradually according to response and tolerability in steps of 12.5 mg every 2–4 weeks*	50 mg every 4 weeks*
Haloperidol decanoate	Risk of EPS and QTc prolongation	(No test dose) 12.5–25 mg every 4 weeks	12.5–25 mg every 4 weeks	50 mg every 4 weeks*
Zuclopenthixol decanoate (Clopixol)		Test dose: 25–50 mg	After at least 7 days of test dose: 50–200 mg every 2–4 weeks*	200 mg every 2 weeks*
Long-acting atypical antipsychotic drugs				
Aripiprazole long-acting injection	No formal recommendations are available for dosing in older adults. However no detectable effect of age on pharmacokinetics[15]			
Paliperidone palmitate	Dose based on renal function Because elderly patients may have diminished renal function, they are dosed as in mild renal impairment even if tests show normal renal function*	Loading doses: Day 1: 100 mg Day 8: 75 mg (lower loading doses may be appropriate in some)*	25–100 mg monthly*	100 mg monthly*

Drug	Notes			
Paliperidone palmitate 3-monthly injection	Dose based on renal function. Because elderly patients may have diminished renal function, they are dosed as in mild renal impairment even if tests show normal renal function*	If the last dose of 1-monthly paliperidone palmitate injectable is: 50 mg 75 mg 100 mg	Initiate the 3-monthly injection at the following doses: 175 mg 263 mg 350 mg (There is no equivalent dose for the 25 mg dose of 1-monthly paliperidone palmitate injection)[16]	350 mg 3-monthly*
Risperidone long-acting injection	Monitor renal function	25 mg every 2 weeks	25 mg every 2 weeks	25 mg every 2 weeks Consider 37.5 mg every 2 weeks in patients treated with oral risperidone doses >4 mg/day[17]
Mood stabilisers				
Carbamazepine	Bipolar disorder Caution – drug interactions Check LFTs, FBC and U&Es Consider checking plasma levels	50 mg bd or 100 mg bd*	200–400 mg/day*	600–800 mg/day*
Lamotrigine	Bipolar disorder (titration as in young adults) Check for interactions and make appropriate dose alterations (see BNF)	25 mg daily (monotherapy) 25 mg on alternate days (if with valproate) 50 mg daily (if with carbamazepine)	Increase by 25 mg steps every 14 days Increase by 25 mg steps every 14 days Increase by 50 mg steps every 14 days	200 mg/day* 100 mg/day* 100 mg bd*
Lithium carbonate MR	Bipolar disorder Mania/depression Caution – drug interactions Check renal and thyroid function and regularly monitor plasma levels	100*–200 mg nocte	200–600 mg daily*	600–1200 mg daily (aim for plasma levels 0.4–0.8 mmol/L in elderly)[18]

(Continued)

Table 6.8 (Continued)

Drug	Specific indication/additional notes	Starting dose	Usual maintenance dose	Maximum dose in elderly
Sodium valproate	Bipolar disorder Check LFTs and consider checking plasma levels	Sodium valproate: 100–200 mg bd* Semi-sodium valproate: 250 mg daily or bd*	Sodium valproate: 200–400 mg bd* Semi-sodium valproate: 500 mg–1 g daily*	Sodium valproate: 400 mg bd* Semi-sodium valproate: 1 g daily*
	Agitation in dementia (not licensed and not recommended) Check response, tolerability and plasma levels for guide	Sodium valproate: 50 mg bd (liquid) or 100 mg bd*	Sodium valproate: 100–200 mg bd*	Sodium valproate: 200 mg bd*
Anxiolytics/hypnotics				
Clonazepam	Agitation	0.5 mg daily	1–2 mg/day*	4 mg/day*
Diazepam	Agitation	1 mg tds		6 mg/day*
Lorazepam	Prn only – avoid regular use due to short half-life and risk of dependence	0.5 mg daily	0.5–2 mg daily*	2 mg/day
Melatonin	Insomnia – short-term use (up to 13 weeks)	2 mg (modified release) once daily (1–2 hours before bedtime)		
Pregabalin	Generalised anxiety disorder Dose adjustment based on renal function (see product information)[19]	Usually 25 mg bd (increase by 25 mg bd weekly) Up to 75 mg bd (if healthy and normal renal function)	Usually 150 mg daily* Up to 150 mg bd (if healthy and normal renal function)	150–300 mg/day*
Zolpidem	Insomnia (short-term use – up to 4 weeks)	5 mg nocte	5 mg nocte	5 mg nocte
Zopiclone	Insomnia (short-term use – up to 4 weeks)	3.75 mg nocte	3.75–7.5 mg nocte	7.5 mg nocte

* There is no information available in the literature for these drug doses in elderly patients – the doses stated are a guide only. Where there are no data, the maximum doses are conservative and may be exceeded if the drug is well tolerated and following clinician's assessment.

All doses are from the *British National Formulary* (73rd edition 2017) unless otherwise indicated.

bd, *bis die* (twice a day); BP, blood pressure; CrCl, creatinine clearance; CYP, cytochrome P450; ECG, electrocardiogram; EPS, extrapyramidal symptoms; FBC, full blood count; IM, intramuscular; LFTs, liver function tests; mane, morning; nocte, at night; prn, *pro re nata* (as required); tds, *ter die sumendum* (three times a day); U&Es, urea and electrolytes; XL, prolonged release.

Covert administration of medicines within food and drink

This section deals with covert medication provision within UK law only.

In mental health settings it is common for patients to refuse medication. Some patients with cognitive disorders may lack capacity to make an informed choice about whether medication will be beneficial to them or not. In these cases, the clinical team may consider whether it would be in the patient's best interests to conceal medication in food or drink. This practice is known as covert administration. Guidance from the UK Nursing and Midwifery Council[1] and the Royal College of Psychiatrists[2] has been published in order to protect patients from the unlawful and inappropriate administration of medication in this way. In the UK, the legal framework for such interventions is either the Mental Capacity Act (MCA)[3] or, more rarely, the Mental Health Act (MHA).[4]

Assessment of mental capacity[3,5,6]

When it applies to the covert administration of medicines, the assessment of capacity regarding treatment is primarily a matter for doctors treating the patient.[3,5] Nurses will also have to be mindful of their own codes of professional practice and should be satisfied that the doctor's assessment is reasonable. In assessing capacity it is important to make the assessment in relation to the particular treatment proposed. Capacity can vary over time and the assessment should be made at the time of the proposed treatment. The assessment should be documented in the patient's notes and recorded in the care plan.

A patient is presumed to have the capacity to make treatment decisions unless he/she is unable to:

- understand the information relevant to the decision
- retain that information
- use or weigh that information as part of the process of making the decision, or
- communicate his/her decision (whether by talking, using sign language or any other means).

Guidance on covert administration

If a patient has the capacity to give a valid refusal to medication and is not detainable under the Mental Health Act, their refusal should be respected.

If a patient has the capacity to give a valid refusal and is either being treated under the Mental Health Act or is legally detainable under the Act, the provisions of the Mental Health Act with regard to treatment will apply (which are outside the scope of this chapter). In general the Mental Health Act will only be used if the person is actively resisting admission and treatment. Someone who passively assents to admission and treatment can be admitted and treated without the Mental Health Act being used. If such a patient lacks capacity the legal framework under which the patient is being treated is the Mental Capacity Act.

The administration of medicines to patients who lack the capacity to consent and who are unable to appreciate that they are taking medication (e.g. unconscious patients)

CHAPTER 6

should not need to be carried out covertly. However some patients who lack the capacity to consent would be aware of receiving medication, if they were not deceived into thinking otherwise,[7] for example a patient with moderate dementia who has no insight and does not believe he needs to take medication, but will take liquid medication if this is mixed with his tea without him being aware of this. It is this group to whom the rest of this guidance applies.

Treatment may be given to people who lack capacity if it has been concluded that that treatment is in the patient's best interests (Section 5 MCA[3]) and is proportionate to the harm to be avoided (Chapter 6.41, MCA Code of Practice[6]). So, there should be a clear expectation that the patient will benefit from covert administration and that this will avoid significant harm (either mental or physical) to the patient or others. The treatment must be necessary to save the patient's life, to prevent deterioration in health or to ensure an improvement in physical or mental health.[3,6]

The decision to administer medication covertly should not be made by a single individual but should involve discussion with the multidisciplinary team caring for the patient and the patient's relatives or informal carers. It is good practice to hold a 'Best Interests Meeting'. If it were determined at the Best Interests Meeting that the provision of covert medication would amount to a deprivation of liberty (where previously there was none), then an application for Deprivation of Liberty Safeguards (DoLS) authorisation should be made. Decisions regarding covert administration of medication should be carefully documented in the patient's medical records with a clear management plan, including details of how the covert medication plan will be reviewed. This documentation must be easily accessible on viewing the person's records and the decision should be subject to regular review.

It is not necessary to have a new Best Interests Meeting each time there is a change in medication. However, when covert medication is first considered, health-care professionals should consider what types of changes in medication may be anticipated in future and should agree on the thresholds of what changes may require a new Best Interests Meeting. This management plan should be recorded in the patient's notes. If significant changes that could cause adverse effects are envisaged, then a new Best Interests Meeting should be held before these changes are made.

In deciding how often capacity assessments should be repeated, clinicians should follow the guidance within the Practical Guide to the Mental Capacity Act.[5] If there is any evidence that the patient has re-gained capacity, an immediate capacity assessment must be done. Decisions in the patient's best interests can no longer be made, their DoLS authorisation will no longer be valid and covert administration of medication must cease immediately.

Recent case law[8] has dealt with the relationship between the use of covert medication and the need for a DoLS authorisation. A person is deprived of their liberty when they are under continuous supervision and control and are not free to leave. The administration of covert medication will only in itself lead to a deprivation of liberty where that covert medication affects the person's behaviour or mental health or it acts as a sedative to such an extent that it will deprive the person of their liberty. The use of covert medication within a care plan must be clearly identified within the DoLS assessment and authorisation.

When considering covert use of psychiatric medication the following must be taken into account:[9]

1. If the patient meets the criteria for the MHA, this must be used in preference to the MCA.
2. The MCA can be used as authority for covert use of psychiatric medication in patients not under the MHA if the medication is necessary to prevent deterioration or ensure an improvement in the patient's mental health and it is in the person's best interest to receive the drug. The usual procedures for covert medication including documentation of capacity assessment, Best Interests Meeting and pharmacist's review should be followed.
3. Caution is needed in the use of medication which may sedate or reduce a patient's physical mobility (see paragraph above), as use of such drugs may constitute a Deprivation of Liberty and require the patient to be under the DoLs framework. Documentation of whether the proposed use of a covert psychiatric drug constitutes a Deprivation of Liberty is important.

Summary of process

The process for covert administration of medicines should include the following safeguards.

- The assurance that all efforts have been made to give medication openly in its normal form before considering covert administration.
- Assessment of capacity of the patient to make a decision regarding their treatment with medication. If the patient has capacity their wishes should be respected and covert medication not administered.
- A record of the examination of the patient's capacity must be made in the clinical notes, and evidence for incapacity documented.
- If the patient lacks capacity there should be a Best Interests Meeting which should be attended by relevant health professionals and a person who can communicate the views and interests of the patient (family member, friend or independent mental capacity advocate [IMCA]). If the patient has an attorney appointed under the MCA for health and welfare decisions then this person should be present at the meeting.
- Those attending the meeting should ascertain whether the patient has made an Advanced Decision refusing a particular medication or treatment which can be used to guide decision-making.
- The Best Interests Meeting should consider whether a formal legal procedure such as the MHA DoLs is appropriate. Discussion of the indications and use of this legislation in the context of covert medication is outside the scope of this guidance but specialist psychiatric and/or legal opinion should be sought in individual circumstances if necessary.
- Medication should not be administered covertly until a Best Interests Meeting has been held. If the situation is urgent it is acceptable for a less formal discussion to occur between caregiver/nursing staff, prescriber and family/advocate in order to make an urgent decision but a formal meeting should be arranged as soon as possible.

- After the meeting there should be clear documentation of the outcome of the meeting. If the decision is to use covert administration of medication, a check should be made with the pharmacy to determine whether the properties of the medications are likely to be affected by crushing and/or being mixed with food or drink. The prescription card should be amended to describe how the medication is to be administered.
- When the medication is administered in foodstuff, it is the responsibility of the dispensing nurse to ensure that the medication is taken. This can be facilitated by direct observation or by nominating another member of the clinical team to observe the patient taking the medication.
- A plan to review on a regular basis the need for continued covert administration of medicines should be made.

Additional information:

- For patients in care homes, the NICE Guidelines – Managing medicines in care homes (March 2014) – should be referred to.[10,11] The basic principles of this NICE guidance are the same as this policy. Mental health practitioners have a duty to inform the care home manager if they suspect the correct procedures are not being followed as regards covert medication, and to discuss with their team leader possible safeguarding referral if the home manager does not act on their advice.
- There are no specific restrictions to state that relatives or other informal caregivers cannot give medication covertly and in certain cases it may be acceptable as long as they have been advised to do so by a health professional (e.g. GP) and all standards of the policy have been met.

The procedure for assessing the need for and establishing covert administration of medication is outlined in Figure 6.2.

References

1. Nursing and Midwifery Council. Standards for medicines management (minor updates to references and the Code 2015). https://www.nmc.org.uk/globalassets/sitedocuments/standards/nmc-standards-for-medicines-management.pdf.
2. Royal College of Psychiatrists. College Statement on Covert Administration of Medicines. Psychiatric Bulletin 2004; 28:385–386.
3. Office of Public Sector Information. Mental Capacity Act 2005 – Chapter 9. 2005. http://www.legislation.gov.uk/ukpga/2005/9/pdfs/ukpga_20050009_en.pdf.
4. The National Archives. Mental Health Act 2007. http://www.legislation.gov.uk/ukpga/2007/12/contents.
5. British Medical Association and the Law Society. *Assessment of Mental Capacity. A Practical Guide for Doctors and Lawyers*, 4th edn. London: Law Society Publishing; 2015.
6. Office of the Public Guardian. Mental Capacity Act Code of Practice (updated 2016). https://www.gov.uk/government/publications/mental-capacity-act-code-of-practice.
7. Department for Constitutional Affairs. Mental Capacity Act 2005 – Code of Practice. http://www.justice.gov.uk/.
8. Hempsons. Newsflash: Covert medication and DOLS – new court guidance. 2016. http://www.hempsons.co.uk/news/newsflash-covert-medication-dols-new-court-guidance/.
9. Care Quality Commission. Brief guide: covert medication in mental health services. 2016. https://www.cqc.org.uk/sites/default/files/20161122_briefguide-covert_medication.pdf.
10. National Institute for Health and Care Excellence. Managing medicines in care homes. Social Care Guideline SC1, 2014. https://www.nice.org.uk/guidance/sc1.
11. PrescQIPP. Bulletin 101 – Best practice guidance in covert administration of medication. 2015. https://www.prescqipp.info/resources/send/216-care-homes-covert-administration/2147-b101-covert-administration.

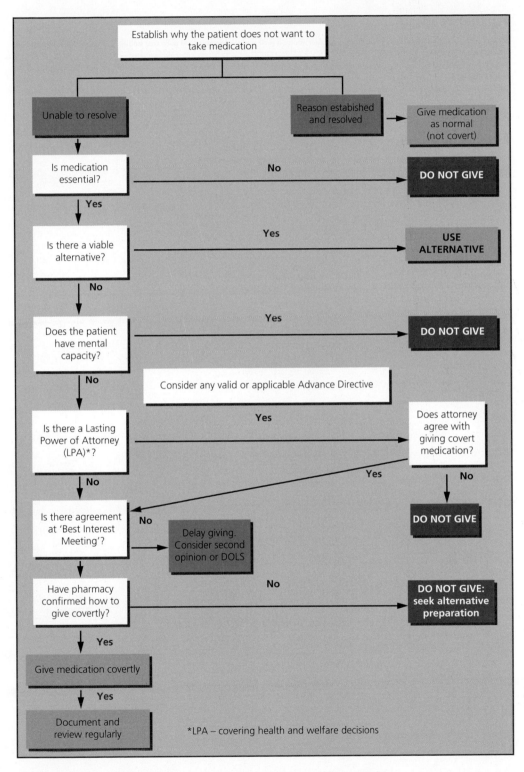

Figure 6.2 Algorithm for determining whether or not to administer medicine covertly.

CHAPTER 6

Further reading

Haw C et al. Covert administration of medication to older adults: a review of the literature and published studies. J Psychiatr Ment Health Nurs 2010; 17:761–768.

Haw C et al. Administration of medicines in food and drink: a study of older inpatients with severe mental illness. Int Psychogeriatr 2010; 22:409–416.

Joyce T. Best interests: guidance on determining the best interests of adults who lack the capacity to make a decision (or decisions) for themselves. England and Wales. A report published by the Professional Practice Board of the British Psychological Society. 2007. http://www.bps.org.uk/.

For Scotland

Mental Welfare Commission for Scotland. Good Practice Guide: Covert Medication. 2013.
http://www.mwcscot.org.uk/media/140485/covert_medication_finalnov_13.pdf.

Chapter 7

Pregnancy and breastfeeding

Drug choice in pregnancy

A 'normal' outcome to pregnancy can never be guaranteed. The spontaneous abortion rate in confirmed early pregnancy is 10–20% and the risk of spontaneous major malformation is 2–3% (approximately 1 in 40 pregnancies).[1]

Lifestyle factors have an important influence on pregnancy outcome. It is well established that smoking cigarettes, eating a poor diet and drinking alcohol during pregnancy can have adverse consequences for the foetus. Moderate maternal caffeine consumption has been associated with low birth weight,[2] and pre-pregnancy obesity increases the risk of neural tube defects (obese women seem to require higher doses of folate supplementation than women who have a body mass index [BMI] in the healthy range[3]).

In addition, psychiatric illness during pregnancy is an independent risk factor for congenital malformations, stillbirths and neonatal deaths.[4] Perinatal mental disorders are associated with risks for a broad range of negative child outcomes, many of which can persist into late adolescence.[5] Affective illness, anxiety disorders, eating disorders and other mental disorders increase the risk of pre-term delivery.[6,7] Note that pre-term delivery is also associated with an increased risk of depression, bipolar disorder and schizophrenia spectrum disorders in subsequent adult life.[8]

The potential risks of psychotropic drug use in pregnancy include major malformation (first-trimester exposure), neonatal toxicity (third-trimester exposure), longer-term neurobehavioural effects and increased risk of physical health problems in adult life.

The safety of psychotropic drugs in pregnancy cannot be clearly established because robust, prospective trials are obviously unethical. Individual decisions on psychotropic use in pregnancy are therefore based on database studies that have many limitations (e.g. failure to control for the effects of illness, smoking, obesity, other medications and other confounders, multiple statistical tests increasing the risk of Type 2 error and exposure status based on pharmacy data), limited prospective data from teratology information centres, and published case reports which are known to be biased towards

The Maudsley Prescribing Guidelines in Psychiatry, Thirteenth Edition. David M. Taylor,
Thomas R. E. Barnes and Allan H. Young.
© 2018 David M. Taylor. Published 2018 by John Wiley & Sons Ltd.

selective reporting of adverse outcomes. At worst there may be no human data at all, but only animal data from early preclinical studies. With new drugs, early reports of adverse outcomes may or may not be replicated and a 'best guess' assessment must be made of the risks and benefits associated with withdrawal or continuation of drug treatment. Even with established drugs, data related to long-term outcomes are rare.

It is also important to note that pregnancy does not protect against mental illness and may even elevate overall risk if medication is stopped. In late pregnancy and early post partum there is an increased risk of relapse, irrespective of medication use.

The patient's view of risks and benefits will have paramount importance. Clinicians should be aware of the importance of prescribing medication to women with a severe mental illness. Perinatal suicides are notable for being associated with lack of active treatment, specifically treatment with psychotropic medication.[9]

This section provides a brief summary of the relevant issues and evidence to date. Box 7.1 outlines the general principles of prescribing in pregnancy.

What to include in discussions with pregnant women[15]

Discussions should include:

- The woman's ability to be treated with non-pharmacological interventions. This should include previous response to non-pharmacological interventions.
- The potential impact of an untreated mental disorder on the foetus or infant.
- The risks from stopping medication abruptly.
- Severity of previous episodes, response to treatment and the woman's preference.
- The background risk of foetal malformations for pregnant women without a mental disorder.
- The increased risk of harm associated with drug treatments during pregnancy and the post-natal period, including the risk in overdose (and acknowledge uncertainty surrounding risks).
- The possibility that stopping a drug with known teratogenic risk after pregnancy is confirmed may not remove the risk of malformations.
- Breastfeeding.

Where possible, written material should be provided to explain the risks (preferably individualised). Absolute and relative risks should be discussed. Risks should be described using natural frequencies rather than percentages (for example, 1 in 10 rather than 10%) and common denominators (for example, 1 in 100 and 25 in 100, rather than 1 in 100 and 1 in 4).

Psychosis during pregnancy and post partum

- Pregnancy does not protect against relapse.
- Psychosis during pregnancy predicts post-partum psychosis.[16]
- The incidence of post-partum psychosis is 0.1–0.25% in the general population (around 1–2 psychiatric hospitalisations per 1000 births).
- Women with bipolar disorder have an increased risk of post-partum psychosis with around one in five experiencing a psychotic relapse post partum.[17]

Box 7.1 General principles of prescribing in pregnancy

In all women of child-bearing potential

- Always discuss the possibility of pregnancy – half of all pregnancies are unplanned.[10]
- Avoid using drugs that are contraindicated during pregnancy in women of reproductive age (especially valproate and carbamazepine). If these drugs are prescribed, women should be made fully aware of their teratogenic properties even if not planning pregnancy. Consider prescribing folate. Valproate should be reserved for post-menopausal women only. Its use in younger women should be treatment of last resort.

If mental illness is newly diagnosed in a pregnant woman

- Try to avoid all drugs in the first trimester (when major organs are being formed) unless benefits outweigh risks.
- If non-drug treatments are not effective/appropriate, use an established drug at the lowest effective dose.

If a woman taking psychotopic drugs is planning a pregnancy

- Consideration should be given to discontinuing treatment if the woman is well and at low risk of relapse.
- Discontinuation of treatment for women with severe mental illness and at a high risk of relapse is unwise, but consideration should be given to switching to a low risk drug. Be aware that switching drugs may increase the risk of relapse.

If a woman taking psychotropic medication discovers that she is pregnant

- Abrupt discontinuation of treatment post conception for women with severe mental illness and at a high risk of relapse is unwise; relapse may ultimately be more harmful to the mother and child than continued, effective drug therapy.
- Consider remaining with current (effective) medication rather than switching, to minimise the risk of relapse and hence the number of drugs to which the foetus is exposed.

If the patient smokes (smoking is more common in pregnant women with psychiatric illness)[11]

- Always encourage switching to nicotine replacement therapy – smoking has numerous adverse outcomes, nicotine replacement therapy does not.[12] Referral to smoking cessation services is mandated by the National Institute for Health and Care Excellence (NICE) and engagement should therefore be encouraged and supported where possible.

In all pregnant women

- Ensure that the parents are as involved as possible in all decisions.
- Use the lowest effective dose.
- Use the drug with the lowest known risk to mother and foetus.
- Prescribe as few drugs as possible, both simultaneously and in sequence.
- Be prepared to adjust doses as pregnancy progresses and drug handling is altered. Dose increases are frequently required in the third trimester[13] when blood volume expands by around 30%. Plasma level monitoring may be helpful, where available. Note that hepatic enzyme activity changes markedly during pregnancy; CYP2D6 activity is increased by almost 50% by the end of pregnancy while the activity of CYP1A2 is reduced by up to 70%.[14]
- Consider referral to specialist perinatal services.
- Ensure adequate foetal screening.
- Be aware of potential problems with individual drugs around the time of delivery.
- Inform the obstetric team of psychotropic use and possible complications.
- Monitor the neonate for withdrawal effects after birth.
- Document all decisions.

- There is a high risk of relapse in women with a family history of post-partum psychosis or a personal history of post-partum psychosis.[18]
- The mental health of the mother in the perinatal period influences fetal well-being, obstetric outcome and child development.

The risks of not treating psychosis include:

- harm to the mother through poor self-care or judgement, lack of obstetric care or impulsive acts including suicide
- harm to the foetus or neonate (ranging from neglect to infanticide).

It has long been established that people with schizophrenia are more likely to have minor physical anomalies than the general population. Some of these anomalies may be apparent at birth, while others are more subtle and may not be obvious until later in life. This background risk complicates assessment of the effects of antipsychotic drugs. (Psychiatric illness itself during pregnancy is an independent risk factor for congenital malformations and perinatal mortality.)

Treatment with antipsychotics

First-generation antipsychotics

- First-generation antipsychotics (FGAs) are generally considered to have minimal risk of teratogenicity,[19,20] although data are not conclusive, as might be expected.
- Most initial data originated from studies that included primarily women with hyperemesis gravidarum (a condition associated with an increased risk of congenital malformations) treated with low doses of phenothiazines. The modest increase in risk identified in some of these studies, along with no clear clustering of congenital abnormalities, suggests that the condition being treated may be responsible rather than drug treatment.
- A prospective study that included 284 women who took an FGA (mostly haloperidol, promethazine or flupentixol) during pregnancy concluded that pre-term birth and low birth weight were more common with FGAs than second-generation antipsychotics (SGAs) or no antipsychotic exposure.[21] In total, 20% of neonates exposed to an FGA in the last week of gestation experienced early somnolence and jitteriness. The rate of major malformations, at 5%, was double that of controls (no antipsychotic exposure) but there was no clustering of abnormalities.
- However, in a recent large American study including over a million women, no meaningful increase in the risk of major malformations or cardiac malformations was seen in 733 women prescribed an FGA.[22]
- There may be an association between haloperidol and limb defects (based on a small number of cases), but if real, the risk is likely to be extremely low.
- Neonatal dyskinesia has been reported with FGAs.[23]
- Neonatal jaundice has been reported with phenothiazines.[19]

It remains uncertain whether FGAs are entirely without risk to the foetus or to later development.[19,20] However, this continued uncertainty and the wide use of these drugs over several decades suggest that any risk is small – an assumption borne out by most studies.[24]

Second-generation antipsychotics

- SGAs are unlikely to be major teratogens.
- In a large American study including over a million women no meaningful increase in the risk of major malformations or cardiac malformations was seen in 9258 women prescribed an SGA. A small increase in absolute risk was seen with risperidone. The authors suggest that this particular finding should be interpreted with caution and be seen as an initial safety signal which requires further investigation.[22] In a separate study of 214 women taking an SGA the absolute risk of major malformation was estimated to be 1.4% compared with 1.1% in the control group.[25]
- A prospective study that included 561 women who took an SGA (mostly olanzapine, quetiapine, clozapine, risperidone or aripiprazole) during pregnancy concluded that SGA exposure was associated with increased birth weight, a modestly increased risk of cardiac septal defects (possibly due to screening bias or co-exposure to selective serotonin reuptake inhibitors [SSRIs]), and, as with FGAs, withdrawal effects in 15% of neonates.[20]
- There are most data for olanzapine, which has been associated with both lower birth weight and increased risk of intensive care admission,[26] a large head circumference[27] and with microsomia;[28] the last of these is consistent with the reported increase in the risk of gestational diabetes.[19,27,29,30] Olanzapine seems to be relatively safe with respect to congenital malformations; the prevalence being consistent with population norms in a study that reported on 610 prospectively followed pregnancies.[31] Olanzapine has however been associated with a range of problems including hip dysplasia,[32] meningocele, ankyloblepharon[33] and neural tube defects[19] (an effect that could be related to pre-pregnancy obesity rather than drug exposure[2]). Importantly there is no clustering of congenital malformations.
- The use of clozapine appears to present no increased risk of malformation, although gestational diabetes and neonatal seizures may be more likely to occur.[29] There is a single case report of maternal overdose resulting in foetal death[19] and there are theoretical concerns about the risk of agranulocytosis in the foetus/neonate.[19] NICE has in the past recommended that pregnant women should be switched from clozapine to another antipsychotic,[15] but this recommendation has since been removed and clozapine is now included in medications that may be prescribed in pregnancy. Lower mean adaptive behaviour scores have been reported in infants exposed to clozapine *in utero* compared with risperidone, quetiapine or olanzapine. Higher rates of disturbed sleep and lability were reported in clozapine-exposed infants in the same study.[34] On the balance of evidence available, clozapine should usually be continued.
- The risk of gestational diabetes may be increased with all SGAs.[27]
- The effect of SGAs on long-term neurodevelopment remains unclear.[35] A small prospective case control study reported that babies who were exposed to antipsychotics *in utero* had delayed cognitive, motor and social–emotional development at 2 and 6 months old but not at 12 months.[36] The clinical significance of this finding, if any, is unclear.

Overall, these data do not allow an assessment of relative risks associated with different agents and certainly do not confirm absolutely the safety of any particular drug. At least two studies have suggested a small increased risk of malformation,[21,26] however a

CHAPTER 7

> **Box 7.2** Recommendations – psychosis in pregnancy
>
> - Patients with a history of psychosis who are maintained on antipsychotic medication should be advised to discuss a planned pregnancy as early as possible.
> - Be aware that drug-induced hyperprolactinaemia may prevent pregnancy. Consider switching to an alternative drug if hyperprolactinaemia occurs and a pregnancy is planned.
> - If a pregnant woman is stable on an antipsychotic and likely to relapse without medication, advise her to continue the antipsychotic.[15] Switching medication is generally not advised owing to the risk of relapse. Consider using the antipsychotic that has worked best for the woman after discussion of benefits and risks.[38] This may minimise foetal exposure by avoiding the need for higher doses if the woman relapses, and/or multiple drugs should relapse occur.
> - The most reproductive safety data are available for quetiapine, olanzapine, risperidone and haloperidol, with more limited data for clozapine, aripiprazole and ziprasidone. Quetiapine has a relatively low rate of placental passage.[38]
> - Advise pregnant women taking antipsychotic medication about diet and monitor for excessive weight gain.
> - Women taking an antipsychotic during pregnancy should be monitored for gestational diabetes. NICE recommends that women be offered an oral glucose tolerance test.
> - NICE recommends avoiding depot preparations and anticholinergic drugs in pregnancy unless a depot is needed to keep a woman well through the perinatal period.
> - Antipsychotic discontinuation symptoms can occur in the neonate (e.g. crying, agitation, increased suckling). This is thought to be a class effect.[39] When antipsychotics are taken in pregnancy it is recommended that the woman gives birth in a unit that has access to paediatric intensive care facilities.[21] Some centres used mixed (breast/bottle) feeding to minimise withdrawal symptoms.

more recent study including over a million women found no meaningful increase in the risk of malformations with FGAs or SGAs after correcting for key confounders.[22] Antipsychotic use during pregnancy may be associated with an increased risk of caesarean section[26] and stillbirth,[37] though this may be due to confounding. As with other drugs, decisions must be based on the latest available information and an individualised assessment of probable risks and benefits. If possible, specialist advice should be sought, and primary reference sources consulted. Recommendations for the treatment of psychosis in pregnancy are summarised in Box 7.2.

Depression during pregnancy and post partum[40–42]

- Approximately 10% of pregnant women develop a depressive illness. Around a third of cases of post-partum depression begin before birth.
- Risk may be at least partially genetically determined.
- There is a significant increase in new psychiatric episodes in the first 3 months after delivery. At least 80% are mood disorders, primarily depression.
- Women who have had a previous episode of depressive illness (post-partum or not) are at higher risk of further episodes during pregnancy and post partum. The risk is highest in women with bipolar illness.
- There is some evidence that depression increases the risk of spontaneous abortion, having a low birth weight or small for gestational age baby, or of pre-term delivery, though effects are small.[5,43,44] The mental health of the mother influences foetal well-being, obstetric outcome and child development.

The risks of not treating depression include:

- harm to the mother through poor self-care, lack of obstetric care or self-harm
- harm to the foetus or neonate (ranging from neglect to infanticide).

Treatment with antidepressants

The use of antidepressants during pregnancy is common; in the Netherlands, up to 2% of women are prescribed antidepressants during the first trimester,[45] and in the USA around 10% of women are prescribed antidepressants at some point during their pregnancy,[43,46] and this rate is increasing.[47] The majority of prescriptions are for SSRIs. In the UK, the large majority of women who are prescribed antidepressants stop taking them in very early pregnancy (<6 weeks gestation),[48] most likely because of concerns about teratogenicity. A large Danish study has also noted that pregnant women are considerably less likely to be prescribed antidepressants than women who are not pregnant.[49]

Relapse rates are higher in those with a history of depression who discontinue medication compared to those who continue. One study found that 68% of women who were well on antidepressant treatment and stopped during pregnancy relapsed, compared with 26% who continued antidepressants.[40]

Some data suggest that antidepressants may increase the risk of spontaneous abortion (but note that confounding factors were not controlled for), pre-term delivery, low birth weight, respiratory distress in the neonate, a low APGAR score at birth and admission to a special care baby unit.[43,50–58] Most studies are observational and do not control for maternal depression. In a large cohort study the presence of depressive symptoms but not antidepressant use[59] was associated with pre-term birth and babies small for gestational age. Interestingly, a large Finnish study found SSRI use to be associated with a lower risk of pre-term birth and caesarean delivery compared with unexposed women diagnosed with a psychiatric illness,[60] and untreated maternal depression itself is associated with an increased risk of both low birth weight and pre-term birth.[61] SSRIs do not appear to increase the risk of stillbirth or neonatal mortality.[62,63]

While it is reasonably certain that commonly used antidepressants are not major teratogens,[64] some antidepressants have been associated with specific congenital malformations,[65] many of which are rare. Most of these potential associations remain unreplicated.[43] There are conflicting data on the issue of the influence of duration of antidepressant use.[66,67]

The effects on early growth and neurodevelopment are poorly studied; the limited data that do exist are reassuring.[54,68,69] One small study reported abnormal general movements in neonates exposed to SSRIs *in utero*.[70] A small increase in the risk of childhood autism has also been suggested[71,72] but not confirmed by several large studies[73–75] and a meta-analysis which found that pre-conception exposure was more consistently associated with autism spectrum disorders than any trimester exposure, suggesting confounding by indication.[76] SSRIs may be associated with a higher risk of poor neonatal adaptation syndrome than serotonin–noradrenaline reuptake inhibitors (SNRIs).[77] Increased levels of anxiety symptoms have been reported in exposed children.[78]

CHAPTER 7

Women who take antidepressants during pregnancy may be at increased risk of developing hypertension,[79] pre-eclampsia[80] and post-partum haemorrhage.[81–83] It has been suggested that SSRIs may cause the last of these by reducing serotonin-mediated uterine contraction as well as interfering with haemostasis.[84] A subsequent smaller study did not confirm this association, possibly because it was underpowered to do so.[85] Depression itself may increase the risk of pre-eclampsia.[86]

There is also some evidence that successful antidepressant use can be beneficial for child behavioural outcomes, for example a Danish study on antidepressant exposure found that adverse outcomes were more likely in depressed women not taking antidepressants.[83]

Tricyclic antidepressants

- Foetal exposure to tricyclic antidepressants (TCAs) via umbilicus and amniotic fluid is high.[87,88]
- TCAs have been widely used throughout pregnancy without apparent detriment to the foetus.[64,89,90]
- A weak association between clomipramine use and cardiovascular defects cannot be excluded[91] and the European summary of product characteristics (SPC) for Anafranil states: 'Neonates whose mothers had taken tricyclic antidepressants until delivery have developed dyspnoea, lethargy, colic, irritability, hypotension or hypertension, tremor or spasms, during the first few hours or days. Studies in animals have shown reproductive toxicity. Anafranil is not recommended during pregnancy and in women of childbearing potential not using contraception.' One case of neonatal QT prolongation and torsades de pointes has been reported following maternal clomipramine use,[92] and one case of Timothy syndrome 1, a disorder characterised by severe QT prolongation, in a newborn whose mother took amitriptyline in early pregnancy.[93]
- Some authorities recommend the use of nortriptyline and desipramine (not available in the UK) if using TCAs because these drugs are less anticholinergic and hypotensive than amitriptyline and imipramine (respectively, their tertiary amine parent molecules).
- TCA use during pregnancy increases the risk of pre-term delivery.[89,90,94]
- Use of TCAs in the third trimester is well known to produce neonatal withdrawal effects: agitation, irritability, seizures, respiratory distress and endocrine and metabolic disturbances.[89] These are usually mild and self-limiting.
- Little is known of the developmental effects of pre-natal exposure to TCAs, although one small study detected no adverse consequences.[95] Limited data suggest *in utero* exposure to TCAs has no effects on later development.[95,96]

Selective serotonin reuptake inhibitors

- Sertraline appears to result in the least placental exposure.[97]
- SSRIs appear not to be major teratogens,[64,67,89,98] with most data supporting the safety of fluoxetine.[95,99–102] Note, though, that one study revealed a slight overall increase in rate of malformation with SSRIs.[103,104] Database and case-control studies have reported an association between SSRIs and anencephaly, craniosynostosis, omphalocele, persistent pulmonary hypertension, clubfoot and increased umbilical cord length[105] in the newborn.[106–108] Paroxetine has been specifically associated with cardiac malformations,[109–111] particularly after high dose (>25 mg/day) first-trimester

exposure.[112] However some studies have failed to replicate this finding for paroxetine,[89,113] and have implicated other SSRIs.[114-116] A higher risk of some cardiac birth defects has been reported to be associated with paroxetine and fluoxetine compared with other SSRIs.[117] Other studies have found no association between any SSRI and an increased risk of cardiac septal defects[107,118,119] and other heart defects.[120-122] Note that one database study reported that foetal alcohol disorders were 10 times more common in those exposed to SSRIs *in utero* than controls,[123] and that alcohol use during pregnancy (which may be used as self-medication for depression) is associated with an increased risk of cardiac defects in the foetus.[91]

- SSRIs have also been associated with decreased gestational age[124] (usually a few days, which is of questionable clinical significance[125]), spontaneous abortion[126] and decreased birth weight (mean 175 g).[99,100,127] It is possible that these effects are primarily associated with maternal depression rather than specifically with antidepressant treatment.[125] The longer the duration of *in utero* exposure, the greater the chance of low birth weight and respiratory distress.[66] Three groups of symptoms are seen in neonates exposed to antidepressants in late pregnancy: those associated with serotonergic toxicity, those associated with antidepressant discontinuation symptoms and those related to early birth.[128] Neonatal discontinuation syndrome may be associated with prematurity.[129] Third-trimester exposure to sertraline has been associated with reduced early APGAR scores.[99] Third-trimester use of paroxetine may give rise to neonatal complications, presumably related to abrupt withdrawal.[130,131] Other SSRIs have similar, possibly less severe effects.[131,132] Body temperature instability, poor feeding, respiratory distress, cardiac rhythm disturbance, lethargy, muscle tone anomalies, jitteriness, jerky movements and seizures have been reported.[91]
- Data relating to neurodevelopmental outcome of foetal exposure to SSRIs are less than conclusive.[95,96,133-136] Depression itself may have more obvious adverse effects on development.[95] Maternal SSRI use has been associated with autism spectrum disorders.[137-139] However, large studies have either failed to show this association after accounting for maternal illness[73-75] or have found it to be no longer significant.[140,141]
- Problems with speech and language,[142-144] behaviour[145,146] and fine motor control have been reported[147] but it is not clear whether or not this is due to confounding.
- When taken in late pregnancy, SSRIs may increase the risk of persistent pulmonary hypertension of the newborn. The absolute risk appears to be small and more modest than previously estimated[148] and may exist only in late pregnancy exposure.[149] Note this increased risk is compared with population norms, not women with depression in whom the risk is unquantified.[150]
- An association between SSRIs and an increased risk of post-partum haemorrhage has been reported.[82] However, SSRIs have also been shown not to significantly increase the risk of blood loss at delivery.[151]

Other antidepressants

- No specific risks were identified with duloxetine in a study that prospectively followed 233 women through pregnancy and delivery.[152] However, a case of suspected withdrawal syndrome requiring hospitalisation has been reported.[153]
- Rather more scarce data suggest the absence of teratogenic potential with moclobemide[154] and reboxetine.[155] Venlafaxine has been associated with cardiac defects,

CHAPTER 7

> **Box 7.3** Recommendations – depression in pregnancy
>
> - Patients who are already receiving antidepressants and are at high risk of relapse are best maintained on the same antidepressant during and after pregnancy.
> - Those who develop a moderate-severe or severe depressive illness during pregnancy should be treated with antidepressant drugs.
> - If initiating an antidepressant during pregnancy or for a woman considering pregnancy, previous response to treatment must be taken into account. The antidepressant that has previously proved to be effective should be considered. For previously untreated patients, sertraline may be considered.
> - Screen for alcohol use and be vigilant for the development of hypertension and pre-eclampsia. Women who take SSRIs may be at increased risk of post-partum haemorrhage.
> - When taken in late pregnancy, SSRIs may increase the risk of persistent pulmonary hypertension of the newborn. The absolute risk is very low.
> - The neonate may experience discontinuation symptoms, which are usually mild, such as agitation and irritability, or rarely respiratory distress and convulsions (with SSRIs). The risk is assumed to be particularly high with short half-life drugs such as paroxetine and venlafaxine. Continuing to breastfeed and then 'weaning' by switching to mixed (breast/bottle) feeding may help reduce the severity of reactions.

anencephaly and cleft palate,[156] neonatal withdrawal and poor neonatal adaptation syndrome.[100] However, newer data suggest that first-trimester use appears not to be associated with an increased risk of major congenital malformations.[157] Second-trimester exposure to venlafaxine has been associated with babies being born small for gestational age.[52] Similarly, trazodone, bupropion (amfebutamone) and mirtazapine have few data supporting their safety.[100,158,159] Data suggest that both bupropion and mirtazapine are not associated with malformations but, like SSRIs, may be linked to an increased rate of spontaneous abortion.[160–162] First-trimester exposure to bupropion may be associated with a slightly elevated risk of ventricular septal defects.[163] Bupropion exposure *in utero* has been associated with an increased risk of attention deficit hyperactivity disorder (ADHD) in young children.[164,165]

- **Monoamine oxidase inhibitors** (MAOIs) should be avoided in pregnancy because of a suspected increased risk of congenital malformations and because of the risk of hypertensive crisis.[166]
- There is no evidence to suggest that **electroconvulsive therapy** (ECT) causes harm to either the mother or foetus during pregnancy[167] although general anaesthesia is of course not without risks. In resistant depression, NICE recommends that ECT is used before/instead of drug combinations.

Box 7.3 summarises recommendations for the treatment of depression in pregnancy.

Bipolar illness during pregnancy and post partum

- The risk of relapse during pregnancy if mood-stabilising medication is discontinued is high; one study found that bipolar women who were euthymic at conception and discontinued mood stabilisers were twice as likely to relapse and spent five times as long in relapse than women who continued mood stabilisers.[168]
- The risk of relapse after delivery is hugely increased.

- The mental health of the mother influences foetal well-being, obstetric outcome and child development.
- Women with bipolar illness are 50% more likely than controls to have their labour induced or a caesarean delivery, a pre-term delivery and a neonate that is small for gestational age; the neonate is also more likely to have hypoglycaemia and micro-cephaly.[7] These associations hold true in both treated and untreated women.
- Bipolar illness itself does not seem to significantly increase the malformation rate; any such association is with mood-stabilising drugs.[7]

The risks of not stabilising mood include:

- harm to the mother through poor self-care, lack of obstetric care or self-harm
- harm to the foetus or neonate (ranging from neglect to infanticide).

Treatment with mood stabilisers

- **Lithium** completely equilibrates across the placenta.[169]
- Although the overall risk of major malformations in infants exposed *in utero* has prob-ably been overestimated, lithium should be avoided in pregnancy if possible. However, if lithium is the best drug for the woman, and the drug most likely to keep her well, the woman should be advised of the increased risk but supported to stay on lithium.
- If discontinuation is planned, slow discontinuation before conception is the preferred course of action[29,170] because abrupt discontinuation is suspected of worsening the risk of relapse. The relapse rate post partum may be as high as 70% in women who discontinued lithium before conception.[171] If discontinuation is unsuccessful during pregnancy, restart and continue.
- Lithium use during pregnancy has a well-known association with the cardiac malfor-mation Ebstein's anomaly. However, more recent data suggest that the magnitude of the effect is much smaller than previously estimated.[172,173] Furthermore, a large sur-veillance study of 5.6 million births found an association with maternal mental health problems generally rather than specifically with lithium.[174]
- The period of maximum risk to the foetus is 2–6 weeks after conception,[175] before many women know that they are pregnant. The risk of atrial and ventricular septal defects may also be increased.[26] A 2012 review suggests the exact nature and inci-dence of congenital malformation is 'uncertain'.[173]
- If lithium is continued during pregnancy, high-resolution ultrasound and echocardi-ography should be performed in liaison with foetal medicine obstetric services.
- In the third trimester, the use of lithium may be problematic because of changing pharmacokinetics: an increasing dose of lithium is required to maintain the lithium level during pregnancy as total body water increases, but the requirements return abruptly to pre-pregnancy levels immediately after delivery.[176] NICE recommends lithium plasma levels are monitored every 4 weeks until 36 weeks and weekly there-after. The dose should be adjusted to maintain the plasma level within the woman's therapeutic range. Lithium should be stopped during labour and the plasma level checked 12 hours after her last dose.[15] Women taking lithium should deliver in hos-pital where fluid balance can be monitored and maintained.
- Neonatal goitre, hypotonia, lethargy and cardiac arrhythmia can occur.

CHAPTER 7

Most data relating to **carbamazepine, valproate** and lamotrigine come from studies in epilepsy, a condition associated with increased neonatal malformation. These data may not be precisely relevant to use in mental illness.

- Both carbamazepine and valproate have a clear causal link with increased risk of a variety of foetal abnormalities, particularly neural tube defects including spina bifida.[177] Both drugs should be avoided, if possible, and an antipsychotic prescribed instead. Valproate confers a higher risk (around 10%) than carbamazepine[178–180] and should not be used in women of child-bearing age except where all other treatment has failed. Although 1 in 20 women of child-bearing age who are in long-term contact with mental health services are prescribed mood-stabilising drugs, awareness of the teratogenic potential of these drugs amongst psychiatrists is low.[177]
- There is no evidence that folate protects against anticonvulsant-induced neural tube defects if given during pregnancy,[181] but it may do so if given prior to conception (the neural tube is essentially formed by 8 weeks of pregnancy[182] before many women realise they are pregnant). However, folate supplementation may be beneficial with regard to early neurodevelopment and so should always be offered.[181]
- Valproate monotherapy has also been associated with an increased relative risk of atrial septal defects, cleft palate, hypospadias, polydactyly and craniosynostosis, although absolute risks are low.[183] Valproate is also associated with a reduced head circumference in the neonate.[184] The risk of major malformations with valproate may be increased by using doses above 1g/day.[185,186]
- There appears to be a clear causal association between valproate use in pregnancy and motor and neurodevelopmental problems in exposed children. A review of studies by the European Medicines Agency showed that up to 40% of pre-school children exposed to valproate *in utero* experienced some form of developmental delay, including delayed walking and talking, memory problems, difficulty with speech and language and a lower intellectual ability. Poorer outcomes have been shown in language functioning, attention, memory, executive functioning and adaptive behaviour compared with carbamazepine and lamotrigine exposure. Lower IQs and an increased diagnosis rate of autistic spectrum disorder are also reported.[187,188]
- Where continued use of carbamazepine is deemed essential, low-dose (but effective) monotherapy is strongly recommended, as the teratogenic effect is probably dose-related.[189,190] Use of carbamazepine in the third trimester may necessitate maternal vitamin K.
- There is growing evidence that **lamotrigine** is safer in pregnancy than carbamazepine or valproate across a range of outcomes.[181,187,191,192] Clearance of lamotrigine seems to increase radically during pregnancy[193] and then reduces post partum[194] so frequent lamotrigine levels are necessary.
- Lower APGAR scores at birth have been reported with carbamazepine, valproate and topiramate. If an association exists, the absolute risk is low.[195]
- Major malformations, specifically orofacial clefts, have been reported with topiramate.[196]

Box 7.4 summarises the recommendations for the treatment of bipolar disorder in pregnancy.

> **Box 7.4** Recommendations – bipolar disorder in pregnancy
>
> - For women who have had a long period without relapse, the possibility of switching to a safer drug (antipsychotic) or withdrawing treatment completely before conception and for at least the first trimester should be considered.
> - The risk of relapse both pre and post partum is very high if medication is discontinued abruptly.
> - No mood stabiliser is clearly safe. NICE recommends the use of mood-stabilising antipsychotics as a preferable alternative to continuation with a mood stabiliser.
> - Women with severe illness or who are known to relapse quickly after discontinuation of a mood stabiliser should be advised to continue their medication following discussion of the risks.
> - NICE recommends that if lithium is considered essential in a woman planning pregnancy, the woman be informed of the risk of foetal malformations and the risk of toxicity in the baby if lithium is continued during breastfeeding. Lithium plasma levels should be monitored more frequently throughout pregnancy and the post-natal period, and lithium should be stopped during labour. Women prescribed lithium should undergo appropriate monitoring of the foetus in liaison with foetal medicine obstetric services to screen for Ebstein's anomaly.
> - NICE advises against the use of valproate in pregnancy. Valproate should be discontinued before a woman becomes pregnant. Women taking valproate who are planning a pregnancy should be advised to gradually stop the drug because of the high risk of foetal malformations and adverse neurodevelopment outcomes after any exposure in pregnancy. If valproate is the only drug that works for a particular woman, and this is seen as the only option for her during pregnancy, then she needs to be given a clear briefing of the risks and to sign a consent form confirming that she understands the risk of malformations and developmental delays.
> - NICE advises discussing the possibility of stopping carbamazepine if a woman is planning a pregnancy or becomes pregnant. If carbamazepine is used, prophylactic vitamin K should be administered to the mother and neonate after delivery.
> - In acute mania in pregnancy use an antipsychotic and if this is ineffective consider ECT.
> - In bipolar depression during pregnancy use cognitive behavioural therapy (CBT) for moderate depression and an SSRI for more severe depression. Lamotrigine is also an option.

Sedatives

Anxiety disorders and insomnia are commonly seen in pregnancy.[197] Preferred treatments are CBT and sleep-hygiene measures respectively.

- First-trimester exposure to **benzodiazepines** has been associated with an increased risk of oral clefts in newborns,[198] although two subsequent studies have failed to confirm this association.[199,200]
- Benzodiazepines have been associated with pyloric stenosis and alimentary tract atresia.[199] A large Swedish cohort study (n = 1406 women who took a benzodiazepine during pregnancy) did not confirm these associations or suggest others.[200] Note that data on elective terminations were not available.
- Benzodiazepine use in pregnancy has been associated with caesarean delivery, neonatal ventilatory support, low birth weight, pre-term delivery and small for gestational age babies.[50,199,201,202]
- Third-trimester use is commonly associated with neonatal difficulties (floppy baby syndrome).[203]
- **Promethazine** has been used in hyperemesis gravidarum and appears not to be teratogenic, although data are limited.

CHAPTER 7

- Data on Z drugs are limited. However, available data suggest that Z drugs are not associated with an increased risk of congenital malformations.[204]
- Zolpidem may be associated with an increased risk of pre-term delivery and low birth weight, and increased likelihood of caesarean section.[205]

Rapid tranquillisation

There is almost no published information on the use of rapid tranquillisation in pregnant women. The acute use of short-acting benzodiazepines such as lorazepam and of the sedative antihistamine promethazine is unlikely to be harmful. Presumably, the use of either drug will be problematic immediately before birth. NICE also recommends the use of an antipsychotic but does not specify a particular drug.[15] Where sedative drugs have been given during labour, an anaesthetist and neonatologist should be present for resuscitation of the baby in cases of respiratory depression.

Table 7.1 Recommendations* – psychotropic drugs in pregnancy. *Minimise the number of drugs the foetus is exposed to*

Psychotropic group	Recommendations
Antidepressants	Women who are at a high risk of relapse are best maintained on the same antidepressant during and after pregnancy
	When initiating an antidepressant in a woman planning pregnancy, previous response must be taken into account. Sertraline is an option
Antipsychotics	There is no clear evidence that any antipsychotic is a major teratogen. Consider using/continuing the drug the mother has previously responded to rather than switching prior to/during pregnancy
	Screen for adverse metabolic effects. Offer the woman an oral glucose tolerance test. Arrange for the woman to give birth in a unit with access to neonatal intensive care facilities
	When initiating an antipsychotic in a woman planning pregnancy, previous response must be taken into account. Quetiapine has a relatively low rate of placental passage
Mood stabilisers	Valproate should be stopped if a woman becomes pregnant
	Avoid other anticonvulsants unless risks and consequences of relapse outweigh the known risk of teratogenesis
	Consider using a mood-stabilising antipsychotic
	Lamotrigine is also an option (bipolar depression only)
Sedatives	Non-drug measures are preferred
	Benzodiazepines, zopiclone and zolpidem are probably not teratogenic but are best avoided in late pregnancy. Promethazine is widely used but supporting safety data are scarce

*It cannot be overstated that treatment needs to be individualised for each patient. This summary table is not intended to suggest that all patients should be switched to a recommended drug. For each patient, take into account their current prescription, response to treatment, history of response to other treatments and the risks known to apply in pregnancy (both for current treatment and for switching).

Attention deficit hyperactivity disorder

Limited data suggest that methylphenidate is not a major teratogen.[206]

Table 7.1 summarises the recommendations for the use of psychotropic drugs in pregnancy.

References

1. McElhatton PR. Pregnancy: (2) General principles of drug use in pregnancy. Pharm J 2003; **270**:232–234.
2. Care Study Group. Maternal caffeine intake during pregnancy and risk of fetal growth restriction: a large prospective observational study. BMJ 2008; **337**:a2332.
3. Rasmussen SA et al. Maternal obesity and risk of neural tube defects: a metaanalysis. Am J Obstet Gynecol 2008; **198**:611–619.
4. Schneid-Kofman N et al. Psychiatric illness and adverse pregnancy outcome. Int J Gynaecol Obstet 2008; **101**:53–56.
5. Stein A et al. Effects of perinatal mental disorders on the fetus and child. Lancet 2014; **384**:1800–1819.
6. MacCabe JH et al. Adverse pregnancy outcomes in mothers with affective psychosis. Bipolar Disorders 2007; **9**:305–309.
7. Boden R et al. Risks of adverse pregnancy and birth outcomes in women treated or not treated with mood stabilisers for bipolar disorder: population based cohort study. BMJ 2012; **345**:e7085.
8. Nosarti C et al. Preterm birth and psychiatric disorders in young adult life. Arch Gen Psychiatry 2012; **69**:E1–E8.
9. Khalifeh H et al. Suicide in perinatal and non-perinatal women in contact with psychiatric services: 15 year findings from a UK national inquiry. Lancet Psychiatry 2016; **3**:233–242.
10. de La Rochebrochard E et al. Children born after unplanned pregnancies and cognitive development at 3 years: social differentials in the United Kingdom Millennium Cohort. Am J Epidemiol 2013; **178**:910–920.
11. Goodwin RD et al. Mental disorders and nicotine dependence among pregnant women in the United States. Obstet Gynecol 2007; **109**:875–883.
12. Royal College of Physicians. Nicotine without smoke: tobacco harm reduction. A report by the Tobacco Advisory Group of the Royal College of Physicians. 2016. https://www.rcplondon.ac.uk/projects/outputs/nicotine-without-smoke-tobacco-harm-reduction-0.
13. Sit DK et al. Changes in antidepressant metabolism and dosing across pregnancy and early postpartum. J Clin Psychiatry 2008; **69**:652–658.
14. Ter Horst PG et al. Pharmacological aspects of neonatal antidepressant withdrawal. Obstet Gynecol Surv 2008; **63**:267–279.
15. National Institute for Health and Care Excellence. Antenatal and postnatal mental health: clinical management and service guidance. Clinical Guideline 192, 2014; last updated August 2017. https://www.nice.org.uk/guidance/cg192.
16. Harlow BL et al. Incidence of hospitalization for postpartum psychotic and bipolar episodes in women with and without prior prepregnancy or prenatal psychiatric hospitalizations. Arch Gen Psychiatry 2007; **64**:42–48.
17. Wesseloo R et al. Risk of postpartum relapse in bipolar disorder and postpartum psychosis: a systematic review and meta-analysis. Am J Psychiatry 2016; **173**:117–127.
18. Jones I et al. Bipolar disorder, affective psychosis, and schizophrenia in pregnancy and the post-partum period. Lancet 2014; **384**:1789–1799.
19. Gentile S. Antipsychotic therapy during early and late pregnancy. A systematic review. Schizophr Bull 2010; **36**:518–544.
20. Diav-Citrin O et al. Safety of haloperidol and penfluridol in pregnancy: a multicenter, prospective, controlled study. J Clin Psychiatry 2005; **66**:317–322.
21. Habermann F et al. Atypical antipsychotic drugs and pregnancy outcome: a prospective, cohort study. J Clin Psychopharmacol 2013; **33**:453–462.
22. Huybrechts KF et al. Antipsychotic use in pregnancy and the risk for congenital malformations. JAMA Psychiatry 2016; **73**:938–946.
23. Collins KO et al. Maternal haloperidol therapy associated with dyskinesia in a newborn. Am J Health Syst Pharm 2003; **60**:2253–2255.
24. Trixler M et al. Use of antipsychotics in the management of schizophrenia during pregnancy. Drugs 2005; **65**:1193–1206.
25. Cohen LS et al. Reproductive safety of second-generation antipsychotics: current data from the Massachusetts General Hospital National Pregnancy Registry for Atypical Antipsychotics. Am J Psychiatry 2016; **173**:263–270.
26. Reis M et al. Maternal use of antipsychotics in early pregnancy and delivery outcome. J Clin Psychopharmacol 2008; **28**:279–288.
27. Boden R et al. Antipsychotics during pregnancy: relation to fetal and maternal metabolic effects. Arch Gen Psychiatry 2012; **69**:715–721.
28. Newham JJ et al. Birth weight of infants after maternal exposure to typical and atypical antipsychotics: prospective comparison study. Br J Psychiatry 2008; **192**:333–337.
29. Ernst CL et al. The reproductive safety profile of mood stabilizers, atypical antipsychotics, and broad-spectrum psychotropics. J Clin Psychiatry 2002; 63 Suppl 4:42–55.
30. McKenna K et al. Pregnancy outcome of women using atypical antipsychotic drugs: a prospective comparative study. J Clin Psychiatry 2005; **66**:444–449.
31. Brunner E et al. Olanzapine in pregnancy and breastfeeding: a review of data from global safety surveillance. BMC Pharmacol Toxicol 2013; **14**:38.
32. Spyropoulou AC et al. Hip dysplasia following a case of olanzapine exposed pregnancy: a questionable association. Arch Womens Ment Health 2006; **9**:219–222.
33. Arora M et al. Meningocele and ankyloblepharon following in utero exposure to olanzapine. Eur Psychiatry 2006; **21**:345–346.

CHAPTER 7

34. Shao P et al. Effects of clozapine and other atypical antipsychotics on infants development who were exposed to as fetus: a post-hoc analysis. PLoS One 2015; **10**:e0123373.
35. Gentile S et al. Neurodevelopmental outcomes in infants exposed in utero to antipsychotics: a systematic review of published data. CNS Spectr 2017; **22**:273–281.
36. Peng M et al. Effects of prenatal exposure to atypical antipsychotics on postnatal development and growth of infants: a case-controlled, prospective study. Psychopharmacology (Berl) 2013; **228**:577–584.
37. Sorensen MJ et al. Risk of fetal death after treatment with antipsychotic medications during pregnancy. PLoS One 2015; **10**:e0132280.
38. McAllister-Williams RH et al. British Association for Psychopharmacology consensus guidance on the use of psychotropic medication pre-conception, in pregnancy and postpartum 2017. J Psychopharmacol 2017; **31**:519–552.
39. European Medicines Agency. Antipsychotics – risk of extrapyramidal effects and withdrawal symptoms in newborns after exposure during pregnancy. Pharmacovigilance Working Party, July 2011 plenary meeting. Issue 1107. 2011. http://www.ema.europa.eu/docs/en_GB/document_library/Report/2011/07/WC500109581.pdf.
40. Cohen LS et al. Relapse of major depression during pregnancy in women who maintain or discontinue antidepressant treatment. JAMA 2006; **295**:499–507.
41. Munk-Olsen T et al. New parents and mental disorders: a population-based register study. JAMA 2006; **296**:2582–2589.
42. Mahon PB et al. Genome-wide linkage and follow-up association study of postpartum mood symptoms. Am J Psychiatry 2009; **166**:1229–1237.
43. Yonkers KA et al. The management of depression during pregnancy: a report from the American Psychiatric Association and the American College of Obstetricians and Gynecologists. Gen Hosp Psychiatry 2009; **31**:403–413.
44. Engelstad HJ et al. Perinatal outcomes of pregnancies complicated by maternal depression with or without selective serotonin reuptake inhibitor therapy. Neonatology 2014; **105**:149–154.
45. Ververs T et al. Prevalence and patterns of antidepressant drug use during pregnancy. Eur J Clin Pharmacol 2006; **62**:863–870.
46. Andrade SE et al. Use of antidepressant medications during pregnancy: a multisite study. Am J Obstet Gynecol 2008; **198**:194–195.
47. Alwan S et al. Patterns of antidepressant medication use among pregnant women in a united states population. J Clin Pharmacol 2010; **51**:264–270.
48. Petersen I et al. Pregnancy as a major determinant for discontinuation of antidepressants: an analysis of data from The Health Improvement Network. J Clin Psychiatry 2011; **72**:979–985.
49. Munk-Olsen T et al. Prevalence of antidepressant use and contacts with psychiatrists and psychologists in pregnant and postpartum women. Acta Psychiatr Scand 2012; **125**:318–324.
50. Calderon-Margalit R et al. Risk of preterm delivery and other adverse perinatal outcomes in relation to maternal use of psychotropic medications during pregnancy. Am J Obstet Gynecol 2009; **201**:579.e1–8.
51. Lund N et al. Selective serotonin reuptake inhibitor exposure in utero and pregnancy outcomes. Arch Pediatr Adolesc Med 2009; **163**:949–54.
52. Ramos E et al. Association between antidepressant use during pregnancy and infants born small for gestational age. Can J Psychiatry 2010; **55**:643–652.
53. Jensen HM et al. Maternal depression, antidepressant use in pregnancy and Apgar scores in infants. Br J Psychiatry 2013; **202**:347–351.
54. Wisner KL et al. Does fetal exposure to SSRIs or maternal depression impact infant growth? Am J Psychiatry 2013; **170**:485–493.
55. Leibovitch L et al. Short-term neonatal outcome among term infants after in utero exposure to serotonin reuptake inhibitors. Neonatology 2013; **104**:65–70.
56. Cantarutti A et al. Is the Risk of preterm birth and low birth weight affected by the use of antidepressant agents during pregnancy? A population-based investigation. PLoS One 2016; **11**:e0168115.
57. Norby U et al. Neonatal morbidity after maternal use of antidepressant drugs during pregnancy. Pediatrics 2016; **138**.
58. Nakhai-Pour HR et al. Use of antidepressants during pregnancy and the risk of spontaneous abortion. CMAJ 2010; **182**:1031–1037.
59. Venkatesh KK et al. Association of antenatal depression symptoms and antidepressant treatment with preterm birth. Obstet Gynecol 2016; **127**:926–933.
60. Malm H et al. Pregnancy complications following prenatal exposure to ssris or maternal psychiatric disorders: results from population-based national register data. Am J Psychiatry 2015; **172**:1224–1232.
61. Jarde A et al. Neonatal outcomes in women with untreated antenatal depression compared with women without depression: a systematic review and meta-analysis. JAMA Psychiatry 2016; **73**:826–837.
62. Jimenez-Solem E et al. SSRI use during pregnancy and risk of stillbirth and neonatal mortality. Am J Psychiatry 2013; **170**:299–304.
63. Stephansson O et al. Selective serotonin reuptake inhibitors during pregnancy and risk of stillbirth and infant mortality. JAMA 2013; **309**:48–54.
64. Ban L et al. Maternal depression, antidepressant prescriptions, and congenital anomaly risk in offspring: a population-based cohort study. BJOG 2014; **121**:1471–1481.
65. Berard A et al. Antidepressant use during pregnancy and the risk of major congenital malformations in a cohort of depressed pregnant women: an updated analysis of the Quebec Pregnancy Cohort. BMJ open 2017; **7**:e013372.
66. Oberlander TF et al. Effects of timing and duration of gestational exposure to serotonin reuptake inhibitor antidepressants: population-based study. Br J Psychiatry 2008; **192**:338–343.
67. Ramos E et al. Duration of antidepressant use during pregnancy and risk of major congenital malformations. Br J Psychiatry 2008; **192**:344–350.
68. Nulman I et al. Neurodevelopment of children following prenatal exposure to venlafaxine, selective serotonin reuptake inhibitors, or untreated maternal depression. Am J Psychiatry 2012; **169**:1165–1174.

69. Suri R et al. A prospective, naturalistic, blinded study of early neurobehavioral outcomes for infants following prenatal antidepressant exposure. J Clin Psychiatry 2011; 72:1002–1007.
70. de Vries NK et al. Early neurological outcome of young infants exposed to selective serotonin reuptake inhibitors during pregnancy: results from the observational SMOK study. PLoSOne 2013; 8:e64654.
71. Hviid A et al. Use of selective serotonin reuptake inhibitors during pregnancy and risk of autism. N Engl J Med 2013; 369:2406–2415.
72. Rai D et al. Parental depression, maternal antidepressant use during pregnancy, and risk of autism spectrum disorders: population based case-control study. BMJ 2013; 346:f2059.
73. Brown HK et al. Association between serotonergic antidepressant use during pregnancy and autism spectrum disorder in children. JAMA 2017; 317:1544–1552.
74. Sujan AC et al. Associations of maternal antidepressant use during the first trimester of pregnancy with preterm birth, small for gestational age, autism spectrum disorder, and attention-deficit/hyperactivity disorder in offspring. JAMA 2017; 317:1553–1562.
75. Castro VM et al. Absence of evidence for increase in risk for autism or attention-deficit hyperactivity disorder following antidepressant exposure during pregnancy: a replication study. Transl Psychiatry 2016; 6:e708.
76. Mezzacappa A et al. Risk for autism spectrum disorders according to period of prenatal antidepressant exposure: a systematic review and meta-analysis. JAMA Pediatr 2017; 171:555–563.
77. Kieviet N et al. Risk factors for poor neonatal adaptation after exposure to antidepressants in utero. Acta Paediatr 2015; 104:384–391.
78. Brandlistuen RE et al. Behavioural effects of fetal antidepressant exposure in a Norwegian cohort of discordant siblings. Int J Epidemiol 2015; 44:1397–1407.
79. De Vera MA et al. Antidepressant use during pregnancy and the risk of pregnancy-induced hypertension. Br J Clin Pharmacol 2012; 74: 362–369.
80. Palmsten K et al. Antidepressant use and risk for preeclampsia. Epidemiology 2013; 24:682–691.
81. Bruning AH et al. Antidepressants during pregnancy and postpartum hemorrhage: a systematic review. Eur J Obstet Gynecol Reprod Biol 2015; 189:38–47.
82. Hanley GE et al. Postpartum hemorrhage and use of serotonin reuptake inhibitor antidepressants in pregnancy. Obstet Gynecol 2016; 127:553–561.
83. Grzeskowiak LE et al. Antidepressant use in late gestation and risk of postpartum haemorrhage: a retrospective cohort study. BJOG 2016; 123:1929–1936.
84. Palmsten K et al. Use of antidepressants near delivery and risk of postpartum hemorrhage: cohort study of low income women in the United States. BMJ 2013; 347:f4877.
85. Lupattelli A et al. Risk of vaginal bleeding and postpartum hemorrhage after use of antidepressants in pregnancy: a study from the Norwegian Mother and Child Cohort Study. J Clin Psychopharmacol 2014; 34:143–48.
86. Uguz F. Is there any association between use of antidepressants and preeclampsia or gestational hypertension?: a systematic review of current studies. J Clin Psychopharmacol 2017; 37:72–77.
87. Loughhead AM et al. Placental passage of tricyclic antidepressants. Biol Psychiatry 2006; 59:287–290.
88. Loughhead AM et al. Antidepressants in amniotic fluid: another route of fetal exposure. Am J Psychiatry 2006; 163:145–147.
89. Davis RL et al. Risks of congenital malformations and perinatal events among infants exposed to antidepressant medications during pregnancy. Pharmacoepidemiol Drug Saf 2007; 16:1086–1094.
90. Kallen B. Neonate characteristics after maternal use of antidepressants in late pregnancy. Arch Pediatr Adolesc Med 2004; 158:312–316.
91. Gentile S. Tricyclic antidepressants in pregnancy and puerperium. Expert Opin Drug Saf 2014; 13:207–225.
92. Fukushima N et al. A neonatal prolonged QT syndrome due to maternal use of oral tricyclic antidepressants. Eur J Pediatr 2016; 175: 1129–1132.
93. Corona-Rivera JR et al. Unusual retrospective prenatal findings in a male newborn with Timothy syndrome type 1. Eur J Med Genet 2015; 58:332–335.
94. Maschi S et al. Neonatal outcome following pregnancy exposure to antidepressants: a prospective controlled cohort study. BJOG 2008; 115: 283–289.
95. Nulman I et al. Child development following exposure to tricyclic antidepressants or fluoxetine throughout fetal life: a prospective, controlled study. Am J Psychiatry 2002; 159:1889–1895.
96. Nulman I et al. Neurodevelopment of children exposed in utero to antidepressant drugs. N Engl J Med 1997; 336:258–262.
97. Hendrick V et al. Placental passage of antidepressant medications. Am J Psychiatry 2003; 160:993–996.
98. Gentile S. Selective serotonin reuptake inhibitor exposure during early pregnancy and the risk of birth defects. Acta Psychiatr Scand 2011; 123:266–275.
99. Hallberg P et al. The use of selective serotonin reuptake inhibitors during pregnancy and breast-feeding: a review and clinical aspects. J Clin Psychopharmacol 2005; 25:59–73.
100. Gentile S. The safety of newer antidepressants in pregnancy and breastfeeding. Drug Saf 2005; 28:137–152.
101. Kallen BA et al. Maternal use of selective serotonin re-uptake inhibitors in early pregnancy and infant congenital malformations. Birth Defects Res A Clin Mol Teratol 2007; 79:301–308.
102. Einarson TR et al. Newer antidepressants in pregnancy and rates of major malformations: a meta-analysis of prospective comparative studies. Pharmacoepidemiol Drug Saf 2005; 14:823–827.
103. Wogelius P et al. Maternal use of selective serotonin reuptake inhibitors and risk of congenital malformations. Epidemiology 2006; 17: 701–704.
104. Jordan S et al. Selective serotonin reuptake inhibitor (SSRI) antidepressants in pregnancy and congenital anomalies: analysis of linked databases in Wales, Norway and Funen, Denmark. PLoS One 2016; 11:e0165122.

105. Kivisto J et al. Maternal use of selective serotonin reuptake inhibitors and lengthening of the umbilical cord: indirect evidence of increased foetal activity – a retrospective cohort study. PLoS One 2016; 11:e0154628.

106. Chambers CD et al. Selective serotonin-reuptake inhibitors and risk of persistent pulmonary hypertension of the newborn. N Engl J Med 2006; 354:579–587.

107. Alwan S et al. Use of selective serotonin-reuptake inhibitors in pregnancy and the risk of birth defects. N Engl J Med 2007; 356:2684–2692.

108. Yazdy MM et al. Use of selective serotonin-reuptake inhibitors during pregnancy and the risk of clubfoot. Epidemiology 2014; 25:859–865.

109. Thormahlen GM. Paroxetine use during pregnancy: is it safe? Ann Pharmacother 2006; 40:1834–1837.

110. Myles N et al. Systematic meta-analysis of individual selective serotonin reuptake inhibitor medications and congenital malformations. Aust N Z J Psychiatry 2013; 47:1002–1012.

111. Berard A et al. The risk of major cardiac malformations associated with paroxetine use during the first trimester of pregnancy: a systematic review and meta-analysis. Br J Clin Pharmacol 2016; 81:589–604.

112. Berard A et al. First trimester exposure to paroxetine and risk of cardiac malformations in infants: the importance of dosage. Birth Defects Res B Dev Reprod Toxicol 2007; 80:18–27.

113. Einarson A et al. Evaluation of the risk of congenital cardiovascular defects associated with use of paroxetine during pregnancy. Am J Psychiatry 2008; 165:749–752.

114. Diav-Citrin O et al. Paroxetine and fluoxetine in pregnancy: a prospective, multicentre, controlled, observational study. Br J Clin Pharmacol 2008; 66:695–705.

115. Louik C et al. First-trimester use of selective serotonin-reuptake inhibitors and the risk of birth defects. N Engl J Med 2007; 356: 2675–2683.

116. Berard A et al. Sertraline use during pregnancy and the risk of major malformations. Am J Obstet Gynecol 2015; 212:795.e1–e12.

117. Reefhuis J et al. Specific SSRIs and birth defects: Bayesian analysis to interpret new data in the context of previous reports. BMJ 2015; 351:h3190.

118. Margulis AV et al. Use of selective serotonin reuptake inhibitors in pregnancy and cardiac malformations: a propensity-score matched cohort in CPRD. Pharmacoepidemiol Drug Saf 2013; 22:942–951.

119. Riggin L et al. The fetal safety of fluoxetine: a systematic review and meta-analysis. J Obstet Gynaecol Can 2013; 35:362–369.

120. Furu K et al. Selective serotonin reuptake inhibitors and venlafaxine in early pregnancy and risk of birth defects: population based cohort study and sibling design. BMJ 2015; 350:h1798.

121. Petersen I et al. Selective serotonin reuptake inhibitors and congenital heart anomalies: comparative cohort studies of women treated before and during pregnancy and their children. J Clin Psychiatry 2016; 77:e36–42.

122. Wang S et al. Selective serotonin reuptake inhibitors (SSRIs) and the risk of congenital heart defects: a meta-analysis of prospective cohort studies. J Am Heart Assoc 2015; 4.

123. Malm H et al. Selective serotonin reuptake inhibitors and risk for major congenital anomalies. Obstet Gynecol 2011; 118:111–120.

124. Ross LE et al. Selected pregnancy and delivery outcomes after exposure to antidepressant medication: a systematic review and meta-analysis. JAMA Psychiatry 2013; 70:436–443.

125. Andrade C. Antenatal exposure to selective serotonin reuptake inhibitors and duration of gestation. J Clin Psychiatry 2013; 74:e633–e635.

126. Hemels ME et al. Antidepressant use during pregnancy and the rates of spontaneous abortions: a meta-analysis. Ann Pharmacother 2005; 39:803–809.

127. Oberlander TF et al. Neonatal outcomes after prenatal exposure to selective serotonin reuptake inhibitor antidepressants and maternal depression using population-based linked health data. Arch Gen Psychiatry 2006; 63:898–906.

128. Boucher N et al. A new look at the neonate's clinical presentation after in utero exposure to antidepressants in late pregnancy. J Clin Psychopharmacol 2008; 28:334–339.

129. Yang J et al. Neonatal discontinuation syndrome in serotonergic antidepressant-exposed neonates. J Clin Psychiatry 2017; 78:605–611.

130. Haddad PM et al. Neonatal symptoms following maternal paroxetine treatment: serotonin toxicity or paroxetine discontinuation syndrome? J Psychopharmacol 2005; 19:554–557.

131. Sanz EJ et al. Selective serotonin reuptake inhibitors in pregnant women and neonatal withdrawal syndrome: a database analysis. Lancet 2005; 365:482–487.

132. Koren G. Discontinuation syndrome following late pregnancy exposure to antidepressants. Arch Pediatr Adolesc Med 2004; 158:307–308.

133. Gentile S. SSRIs in pregnancy and lactation: emphasis on neurodevelopmental outcome. CNS Drugs 2005; 19:623–633.

134. Casper RC et al. Follow-up of children of depressed mothers exposed or not exposed to antidepressant drugs during pregnancy. J Pediatr 2003; 142:402–408.

135. Hermansen TK et al. Prenatal SSRI exposure: effects on later child development. Child Neuropsychol 2015; 21:543–569.

136. Kaplan YC et al. Maternal SSRI discontinuation, use, psychiatric disorder and the risk of autism in children: a meta-analysis of cohort studies. Br J Clin Pharmacol 2017; 83:2798–2806.

137. Boukhris T et al. Antidepressant use in pregnancy and the risk of attention deficit with or without hyperactivity disorder in children. Paediatr Perinat Epidemiol 2017; 31:363–373.

138. Croen LA et al. Antidepressant use during pregnancy and childhood autism spectrum disorders. Arch Gen Psychiatry 2011; 68: 1104–1112.

139. Healy D et al. Links between serotonin reuptake inhibition during pregnancy and neurodevelopmental delay/spectrum disorders: a systematic review of epidemiological and physiological evidence. Int J Risk Saf Med 2016; 28:125–141.

140. Clements CC et al. Prenatal antidepressant exposure is associated with risk for attention-deficit hyperactivity disorder but not autism spectrum disorder in a large health system. Mol Psychiatry 2015; 20:727–734.

141. Brown HK et al. The association between antenatal exposure to selective serotonin reuptake inhibitors and autism: a systematic review and meta-analysis. J Clin Psychiatry 2017; 78:e48–e58.

142. Brown AS et al. Association of selective serotonin reuptake inhibitor exposure during pregnancy with speech, scholastic, and motor disorders in offspring. JAMA Psychiatry 2016; 73:1163–1170.

143. Skurtveit S et al. Prenatal exposure to antidepressants and language competence at age three: results from a large population-based pregnancy cohort in Norway. BJOG 2014; 121:1621–1631.

144. Handal M et al. Prenatal exposure to folic acid and antidepressants and language development: a population-based cohort study. J Clin Psychopharmacol 2016; 36:333–339.

145. Hanley GE et al. Prenatal exposure to serotonin reuptake inhibitor antidepressants and childhood behavior. Pediatr Res 2015; 78:174–180.

146. Johnson KC et al. Preschool outcomes following prenatal serotonin reuptake inhibitor exposure: differences in language and behavior, but not cognitive function. J Clin Psychiatry 2016; 77:e176–182.

147. Partridge MC et al. Fine motor differences and prenatal serotonin reuptake inhibitors exposure. J Pediatr 2016; 175:144–149.e1.

148. Huybrechts KF et al. Antidepressant use late in pregnancy and risk of persistent pulmonary hypertension of the newborn. JAMA 2015; 313: 2142–2151.

149. Byatt N et al. Exposure to selective serotonin reuptake inhibitors in late pregnancy increases the risk of persistent pulmonary hypertension of the newborn, but the absolute risk is low. Evid Based Nurs 2015; 18:15–16.

150. Grigoriadis S et al. Prenatal exposure to antidepressants and persistent pulmonary hypertension of the newborn: systematic review and meta-analysis. BMJ 2014; 348:f6932.

151. Kim DR et al. Is third trimester serotonin reuptake inhibitor use associated with postpartum hemorrhage? J Psychiatr Res 2016; 73:79–85.

152. Hoog SL et al. Duloxetine and pregnancy outcomes: safety surveillance findings. Int J Med Sci 2013; 10:413–419.

153. Abdy NA et al. Duloxetine withdrawal syndrome in a newborn. Clin Pediatr (Phila) 2013; 52:976–977.

154. Rybakowski JK. Moclobemide in pregnancy. Pharmacopsychiatry 2001; 34:82–83.

155. Pharmacia Ltd. Erdronax: use on pregnancy, renally and hepatically impaired patients. Personal Communication. 2003.

156. Polen KN et al. Association between reported venlafaxine use in early pregnancy and birth defects, national birth defects prevention study, 1997–2007. Birth Defects Res A Clin Mol Teratol 2013; 97:28–35.

157. Lassen D et al. First-trimester pregnancy exposure to venlafaxine or duloxetine and risk of major congenital malformations: a systematic review. Basic Clin Pharmacol Toxicol 2016; 118:32–36.

158. Einarson A et al. A multicentre prospective controlled study to determine the safety of trazodone and nefazodone use during pregnancy. Can J Psychiatry 2003; 48:106–110.

159. Rohde A et al. Mirtazapine (Remergil) for treatment resistant hyperemesis gravidarum: rescue of a twin pregnancy. Arch Gynecol Obstet 2003; 268:219–221.

160. Djulus J et al. Exposure to mirtazapine during pregnancy: a prospective, comparative study of birth outcomes. J Clin Psychiatry 2006; 67:1280–1284.

161. Cole JA et al. Bupropion in pregnancy and the prevalence of congenital malformations. Pharmacoepidemiol Drug Saf 2007; 16:474–484.

162. Smit M et al. Mirtazapine in pregnancy and lactation – a systematic review. Eur Neuropsychopharmacol 2016; 26:126–135.

163. Louik C et al. First-trimester exposure to bupropion and risk of cardiac malformations. Pharmacoepidemiol Drug Saf 2014; 23: 1066–1075.

164. Figueroa R. Use of antidepressants during pregnancy and risk of attention-deficit/hyperactivity disorder in the offspring. J Dev Behav Pediatr 2010; 31:641–648.

165. Forsberg L et al. School performance at age 16 in children exposed to antiepileptic drugs in utero – a population-based study. Epilepsia 2010; 52:364–369.

166. Hendrick V et al. Management of major depression during pregnancy. Am J Psychiatry 2002; 159:1667–1673.

167. Miller LJ. Use of electroconvulsive therapy during pregnancy. Hosp Community Psychiatry 1994; 45:444–450.

168. Viguera AC et al. Risk of recurrence in women with bipolar disorder during pregnancy: prospective study of mood stabilizer discontinuation. Am J Psychiatry 2007; 164:1817–1824.

169. Newport DJ et al. Lithium placental passage and obstetrical outcome: implications for clinical management during late pregnancy. Am J Psychiatry 2005; 162:2162–2170.

170. Dodd S et al. The pharmacology of bipolar disorder during pregnancy and breastfeeding. Expert Opin Drug Saf 2004; 3:221–229.

171. Viguera AC et al. Risk of recurrence of bipolar disorder in pregnant and nonpregnant women after discontinuing lithium maintenance. Am J Psychiatry 2000; 157:179–184.

172. Diav-Citrin O et al. Pregnancy outcome following in utero exposure to lithium: a prospective, comparative, observational study. Am J Psychiatry 2014; 171:785–794.

173. McKnight RF et al. Lithium toxicity profile: a systematic review and meta-analysis. Lancet 2012; 379:721–728.

174. Boyle B et al. The changing epidemiology of Ebstein's anomaly and its relationship with maternal mental health conditions: a European registry-based study. Cardiol Young 2017; 27:677–685.

175. Yonkers KA et al. Lithium during pregnancy: drug effects and therapeutic implications. CNS Drugs 1998; 4:269.

176. Blake LD et al. Lithium toxicity and the parturient: case report and literature review. Int J Obstet Anesth 2008; 17:164–169.

177. James L et al. Informing patients of the teratogenic potential of mood stabilising drugs; a case notes review of the practice of psychiatrists. J Psychopharmacol 2007; 21:815–819.

178. Wide K et al. Major malformations in infants exposed to antiepileptic drugs in utero, with emphasis on carbamazepine and valproic acid: a nation-wide, population-based register study. Acta Paediatr 2004; 93:174–176.

179. Wyszynski DF et al. Increased rate of major malformations in offspring exposed to valproate during pregnancy. Neurology 2005; **64**: 961–965.

180. Weston J et al. Monotherapy treatment of epilepsy in pregnancy: congenital malformation outcomes in the child. The Cochrane Database Syst Rev 2016; **11**:CD010224.

181. Campbell E et al. Malformation risks of antiepileptic drug monotherapies in pregnancy: updated results from the UK and Ireland Epilepsy and Pregnancy Registers. J Neurol Neurosurg Psychiatry, 2014; **85**:1029–1034.

182. Bestwick JP et al. Prevention of neural tube defects: a cross-sectional study of the uptake of folic acid supplementation in nearly half a million women. PLoSOne 2014; **9**:e89354.

183. Jentink J et al. Valproic acid monotherapy in pregnancy and major congenital malformations. N Engl J Med 2010; **362**:2185–2193.

184. Tomson T et al. Teratogenic effects of antiepileptic drugs. Lancet Neurol 2012; **11**:803–813.

185. Tomson T et al. Dose-dependent teratogenicity of valproate in mono- and polytherapy: an observational study. Neurology 2015; **85**: 866–872.

186. Thomas SV et al. Malformation risk of antiepileptic drug exposure during pregnancy in women with epilepsy: results from a pregnancy registry in South India. Epilepsia 2017; **58**:274–281.

187. Bromley R et al. Treatment for epilepsy in pregnancy: neurodevelopmental outcomes in the child. Cochrane Database Syst Rev 2014: CD010236.

188. Bromley RL et al. Fetal antiepileptic drug exposure and cognitive outcomes. Seizure 2017; **44**:225–231.

189. Vajda FJ et al. Critical relationship between sodium valproate dose and human teratogenicity: results of the Australian register of anti-epileptic drugs in pregnancy. J Clin Neurosci 2004; **11**:854–858.

190. Vajda FJ et al. Maternal valproate dosage and foetal malformations. Acta Neurol Scand 2005; **112**:137–143.

191. Tomson T et al. Dose-dependent risk of malformations with antiepileptic drugs: an analysis of data from the EURAP epilepsy and pregnancy registry. Lancet Neurol 2011; **10**:609–617.

192. Molgaard-Nielsen D et al. Newer-generation antiepileptic drugs and the risk of major birth defects. JAMA 2011; **305**:1996–2002.

193. de Haan GJ et al. Gestation-induced changes in lamotrigine pharmacokinetics: a monotherapy study. Neurology 2004; **63**:571–573.

194. Clark CT et al. Lamotrigine dosing for pregnant patients with bipolar disorder. Am J Psychiatry 2013; **170**:1240–1247.

195. Christensen J et al. Apgar-score in children prenatally exposed to antiepileptic drugs: a population-based cohort study. BMJ Open 2015; **5**:e007425.

196. Bromley RL et al. Cognition in school-age children exposed to levetiracetam, topiramate, or sodium valproate. Neurology 2016; **87**: 1943–1953.

197. Ross LE et al. Anxiety disorders during pregnancy and the postpartum period: a systematic review. J Clin Psychiatry 2006; **67**:1285–1298.

198. Dolovich LR et al. Benzodiazepine use in pregnancy and major malformations or oral cleft: meta-analysis of cohort and case-control studies. BMJ 1998; **317**:839–843.

199. Wikner BN et al. Use of benzodiazepines and benzodiazepine receptor agonists during pregnancy: neonatal outcome and congenital malformations. Pharmacoepidemiol Drug Saf 2007; **16**:1203–1210.

200. Reis M et al. Combined use of selective serotonin reuptake inhibitors and sedatives/hypnotics during pregnancy: risk of relatively severe congenital malformations or cardiac defects. A register study. BMJ Open 2013; **3**:e002166.

201. Okun ML et al. A review of sleep-promoting medications used in pregnancy. Am J Obstet Gynecol 2015; **212**:428–441.

202. Yonkers KA et al. Maternal antidepressant use and pregnancy outcomes. JAMA 2017; **318**:665–666.

203. McElhatton PR. The effects of benzodiazepine use during pregnancy and lactation. Reprod Toxicol 1994; **8**:461–475.

204. Wikner BN et al. Are hypnotic benzodiazepine receptor agonists teratogenic in humans? J Clin Psychopharmacol 2011; **31**:356–359.

205. Wang LH et al. Increased risk of adverse pregnancy outcomes in women receiving zolpidem during pregnancy. Clin Pharmacol Ther 2010; **88**:369–374.

206. Pottegard A et al. First-trimester exposure to methylphenidate: a population-based cohort study. J Clin Psychiatry 2014; **75**:e88–e93.

Further reading

Howard LM et al. Non-psychotic mental disorders in the perinatal period. Lancet 2014; **384**:1775–1788.

Jones I et al. Bipolar disorder, affective psychosis, and schizophrenia in pregnancy and the post-partum period. Lancet 2014; **384**:1789–1799.

McAllister-Williams RH et al. British Association for Psychopharmacology consensus guidance on the use of psychotropic medication preconception, in pregnancy and postpartum 2017. J Psychopharmacol 2017; **31**:519–552.

Other sources of information

National Teratology Information Service. http://www.uktis.org/

Breastfeeding

The long-term benefits of breastfeeding on child physical health and cognitive development are well known. Women are generally encouraged to breastfeed for at least 6 months. One factor that may influence a mother's decision to breastfeed is the safety of a drug taken whilst breastfeeding. With some notable exceptions most psychotropic drugs should be continued in breastfeeding women because of the benefits of breastfeeding and the lack of evidence of harm for most drugs. However current evidence suggests that for a few drugs, described in the following sections, the woman should be advised not to breastfeed if such medications are the best option for her care.

Data on the safety of psychotropic medication in breastfeeding are largely derived from small studies or case reports and case series. Reported infant and neonatal outcomes in most cases are limited to short-term acute adverse effects. Long-term safety cannot therefore be guaranteed for the psychotropic drugs mentioned here. The information presented must be interpreted with caution with respect to the limits of the data from which it is derived and the need for such information to be regularly updated.

Infant exposure

All psychotropic drugs are excreted in breast milk to varying degrees. The most direct measure of infant exposure is, of course, infant plasma levels but these data are rarely available. Instead, many publications report only drug concentrations in breast milk and in maternal plasma. Breast milk drug concentrations can be used to estimate the daily infant dose (by assuming a milk intake of 150 mL/kg/day). The infant weight-adjusted dose when expressed as a proportion of the maternal weight-adjusted dose is known as the relative infant dose (RID). The RID should be used as a guide only, as values are estimates and these estimates vary widely in the literature for individual drugs.

Drugs with an RID below 10% are usually regarded as safe in breastfeeding. Where measured, infant plasma levels below 10% of average maternal plasma levels have also been proposed as safe in breastfeeding.[1]

General principles of prescribing psychotropic drugs in breastfeeding

- The safety of individual drugs in breastfeeding should be taken into account when prescribing psychotropic medication for women considering pregnancy.
- Discussions about the safety of drugs in breastfeeding should be held as early as possible, ideally before conception or early in pregnancy. Decisions about the use of drugs in pregnancy should include the discussion about breastfeeding. Switching drugs at the end of pregnancy or in the days after birth is not advisable because of the high risk of relapse.
- Where a mother has taken a particular psychotropic during pregnancy and until delivery, continuation with the drug while breastfeeding will usually be appropriate (see notable exceptions as follows), as this may minimise withdrawal symptoms in the infant.
- In each case the benefits of breastfeeding to the mother and infant must be weighed against the risk of drug exposure in the infant.

CHAPTER 7

- It is usually inappropriate to stop breastfeeding except when the currently prescribed drug is contraindicated in breastfeeding. As treatment of maternal mental illness is the priority, in such cases treatment should not be withheld but the mother should be advised to bottlefeed with formula milk.
- When **initiating** a drug post partum it is:
  - important to consider the mother's previous response to treatment
  - best to avoid a psychotropic drug with high reported infant plasma levels or a high RID
  - important to consider the half-lives of the drugs: drugs with a long half-life can accumulate in breast milk and infant serum.
- Neonates and infants do not have the same capacity for drug clearance as adults. Premature infants and infants with renal, hepatic, cardiac or neurological impairment are at a greater risk from exposure to drugs.
- Infants should be monitored for any specific adverse effects of the drugs as well as for abnormalities in feeding patterns and growth and development.
- Infant plasma levels should be monitored if toxicity is suspected.
- Women receiving sedating medication should be strongly advised not to breastfeed in bed as they may fall asleep and roll onto the baby, with a potential risk of hypoxia to the baby.
- Sedation may affect a woman's ability to interact with her children. Women receiving sedating drugs should be monitored for this effect.
- Wherever possible:
  - Use the lowest effective dose.
  - Avoid polypharmacy.
  - Continue the regimen prescribed during pregnancy.

Table 7.2 summarises the recommendations for drug use in breastfeeding. Further information is provided in Tables 7.3–7.7.

Table 7.2 Summary of recommendations. It is usually advisable to continue the drug that has been used during pregnancy

Drug group	Recommended drugs
Antidepressants	It is usually advisable to continue the drug that has been used during pregnancy. When initiating an antidepressant post partum **sertraline or mirtazapine** may be considered. Other drugs may be used. See Table 7.3
Antipsychotics	It is usually advisable to continue the drug that has been used during pregnancy. The exception is clozapine. Women taking clozapine should be advised against breastfeeding and clozapine should be continued
	When initiating an antipsychotic post partum **olanzapine or quetiapine** may be considered. Other drugs may be used. See Table 7.4
Mood stabilisers	It is usually advisable to continue the drug that has been used during pregnancy. The exception is lithium. Women taking lithium should be advised against breastfeeding and lithium should be continued
	When initiating a mood stabiliser post partum a mood-stabilising antipsychotic such as **olanzapine or quetiapine** may be considered. Other drugs may be used. See Table 7.5
Sedatives	Best avoided. Use a drug with a short half-life. **Lorazepam** may be considered

Antidepressant drugs in breastfeeding

Table 7.3 provides information on individual drugs in breastfeeding based on available published data in late 2017. Manufacturers' formal advice on drugs in breastfeeding is available in the summary of product characteristics or European Public Assessment Report for individual drugs. Table 7.3 does not include this advice (which is often uninformative), but instead uses primary reference sources.

It is usually advisable to continue the antidepressant prescribed during pregnancy. Switching drugs post partum for the purpose of breastfeeding is usually not sensible. Table 7.3 should be used as a guide when initiating treatment post partum. In each case previous response to treatment must be considered.

Antipsychotic drugs in breastfeeding

Table 7.4 provides information on individual drugs in breastfeeding based on available published data in late 2017. Manufacturers' formal advice on drugs in breastfeeding is available in the summary of product characteristics or European Public Assessment Report for individual drugs. Table 7.4 does not include this advice (which is often uninformative), but instead uses primary reference sources. It is usually advisable to continue the antipsychotic prescribed during pregnancy. Switching drugs post partum for the purpose of breastfeeding is usually not sensible. The exception to this is clozapine – clozapine should continue but breastfeeding should be avoided. Table 7.4 should be used as a guide when initiating treatment post partum. In each case the previous response (and lack of response) to treatment must be considered.

Mood stabilisers in breastfeeding

Table 7.5 provides information on individual drugs in breastfeeding based on available published data in late 2017. Manufacturers' formal advice on drugs in breastfeeding is available in the summary of product characteristics or European Public Assessment Report for individual drugs. Table 7.5 does not include this advice (which is often uninformative), but instead uses primary reference sources. It is usually advisable to continue the mood stabiliser prescribed during pregnancy. Switching drugs post partum for the purpose of breastfeeding is usually not sensible. The exception to this is lithium. Lithium should be continued but breastfeeding should not be permitted. Table 7.5 should be used as a guide when initiating treatment post partum. In each case the previous response (and lack of response) to treatment must be considered.

Hypnotic drugs in breastfeeding

Table 7.6 provides information on individual drugs in breastfeeding based on available published data in late 2017. Manufacturers' formal advice on drugs in breastfeeding is available in the summary of product characteristics or European Public Assessment Report for individual drugs. Table 7.6 does not include this advice (which is often uninformative), but instead uses primary reference sources.

CHAPTER 7

Table 7.3 Antidepressants in breastfeeding

Drug	Infant plasma concentrations	Relative infant dose (RID)	Reported acute adverse effects in infant	Reported developmental effects in infant
Agomelatine[2,3]	Not assessed	Not available	None reported but not studied	None reported but not studied
Bupropion[3-11]	Undetectable or low	0.2–2%	Two reports of seizure-like activity in 6-month-olds In one of the cases the infant experienced sleep disturbance, severe emesis and somnolence. The infant plasma levels were below the level required for quantification. The mother was also taking escitalopram	None reported but not studied
Citalopram[1,3,9,12-21]	Undetectable to up to 10% of maternal plasma levels Higher than for fluvoxamine, sertraline, paroxetine and escitalopram, but lower than for fluoxetine	3–10%	Sleep disturbance (which resolved on halving maternal dose), colic, decreased feeding, and irritability and restlessness One case of irregular breathing, sleep disorder and hypo- and hypertonia in an infant exposed to citalopram *in utero*. Symptoms attributed to withdrawal syndrome despite the mother continuing citalopram post partum	None reported In a study of 78 infants of mothers taking an SSRI or venlafaxine no difference in weight was noted at 6 months compared with the 'normative' weight In a study of 11 infants normal neurodevelopment was observed up to 1 year. One of the children was unable to walk at 1 year, however neurological status of the child was deemed normal 6 months later
Duloxetine[3,9,22-24]	<1% of maternal plasma levels	<1%	Dizziness, nausea, fatigue	None reported but not assessed
Escitalopram[3,9,11,25-30]	Undetectable or low	3–8.3%	Necrotising enterocolitis in 5-day infant (necessitating intensive care admission and intravenous antibiotic treatment). Infant was exposed to escitalopram *in utero*. Symptoms were lethargy, decreased oral intake and blood in the stools Seizure-like activity, sleep disturbance, severe emesis and somnolence in 6-month-old. Mother was also taking bupropion	None reported but not studied

Drug	Relative infant dose	Infant plasma level	Adverse effects	Other
Fluoxetine[1,3,9,12,21,31–42]	1.6–14.6%	Variable: can be >10% of maternal plasma levels. Highest reported levels of SSRIs	Colic, excessive crying, decreased sleep, diarrhoea, vomiting, somnolence, decreased feeding, hypotonia, moaning, grunting and hyperactivity. One case of seizure activity at 3 weeks, 4 months and then 5 months. Mother was also taking carbamazepine. One case of tachypnoea, jitteriness, irritability, fever and compensated metabolic acidosis. Infant plasma levels were in the adult therapeutic range. The authors diagnosed serotonin syndrome. Mother was taking fluoxetine 60 mg	Normal weight gain and neurological development has been reported for many infants. One retrospective study found lower growth curves compared with non-exposed infants. One case of a reduction in platelet serotonin
Fluvoxamine[3,9,12,43–50]	1–2%	Undetectable to up to half the maternal plasma level	Neonatal jaundice, severe diarrhoea, mild vomiting, decreased sleep and agitation	None reported. In a study of 78 infants of mothers taking an SSRI or venlafaxine no difference in weight was noted at 6 months compared with the 'normative' weight
MAOIs	No published data found			
Mianserin[3,51]	Not assessed	Not assessed	None reported	None reported but not studied
Mirtazapine[3,9,52–56]	0.5–4.4%	Undetectable or low. There is one case of higher mirtazapine plasma levels. The authors suggest there may be a large difference in mirtazapine elimination rates between individual infants	In a study of 54 infants exposed to mirtazapine in utero the incidence of poor neonatal adaptation syndrome was significantly diminished in those who were breastfed	No abnormalities reported. In a study of 8 infants weights for 3 were observed to be between the 10th and 25th percentiles. All 3 were noted to also have a low birth weight
Moclobemide[3,57,58]	3.4%	Low	None reported	None reported but not studied
Paroxetine[1,3,9,12,21,35,43,59–68]	0.5–2.8%	Undetectable or low	Vomiting and irritability, which were attributed to severe hyponatraemia. In a study of 72 infants adverse effects were noted in 9 infants. Insomnia, restlessness and constant crying were most commonly reported	None reported. In a study of 78 infants of mothers taking an SSRI or venlafaxine no difference in weight was noted at 6 months compared with the 'normative' weight. Breastfed infants of 27 women taking paroxetine reached the usual developmental milestones at 3, 6 and 12 months, similar to a control group

(Continued)

Table 7.3 (*Continued*)

Drug	Infant plasma concentrations	Relative infant dose (RID)	Reported acute adverse effects in infant	Reported developmental effects in infant
Reboxetine[3,9,69]	Undetectable or low	1–3%	None reported	In a study of 4 infants, 3 reached normal milestones. The fourth had developmental problems thought not to be related to reboxetine
Sertraline[3,9,21,35,63,70–78]	Undetectable or low. There is one report of an unusually high infant serum level (half maternal serum level). The infant was reported to be 'clinically thriving'	0.5–3%	Serotonergic overstimulation reported in pre-term infant also exposed to sertraline *in utero*. Symptoms included hyperthermia, shivering, myoclonus, tremor, and irritability, high-pitched crying, decreased suckling reflex and reactivity Withdrawal symptoms (agitation, restlessness, insomnia and an enhanced startle reaction) developed in a breastfed neonate after abrupt withdrawal of maternal sertraline. The neonate was exposed to sertraline *in utero*	None reported In a study of 78 infants of mothers taking an SSRI or venlafaxine no difference in weight was noted at 6 months compared with the 'normative' weight
Trazodone[3,79]	Not assessed	2.8%	None reported but not assessed	None reported but not assessed
Tricyclic antidepressants (TCAs)[3,12,80–88]	Undetectable or low	Nortriptyline, amitriptyline, clomipramine: 1–3%	Adverse effects have not been reported in infants exposed to nortriptyline, clomipramine, imipramine, dosulepin and desipramine through breast milk Severe sedation and poor feeding reported with amitriptyline Poor suckling, muscle hypotonia, drowsiness and respiratory depression reported with doxepin	None reported A study of 15 children did not show a negative outcome in regard to cognitive development in breastfed children 3–5 years post partum
Venlafaxine[3,9,21,35,63,89–96]	Undetectable to up to 37% of maternal plasma levels	6–9%	Lethargy, jitteriness, rapid breathing, poor suckling and dehydration in an infant also exposed *in utero*. Symptoms subsided over a week on breastfeeding. Authors suggested that breastfeeding may have helped manage infant withdrawal symptoms post partum	None reported In a study of 78 infants of mothers taking an SSRI or venlafaxine no difference in weight was noted at 6 months compared with the 'normative' weight
Vortioxetine	Published data not available			

MAOI, monoamine oxidase inhibitor; SSRI, selective serotonin reuptake inhibitor.

Table 7.4 Antipsychotic drugs in breastfeeding

Drug	Infant plasma concentration	Estimated daily infant dose as proportion of maternal dose (RID)	Acute adverse effects in infant	Developmental effects in infant
Amisulpride[3,92,97,98]	Not reported	10.7%	None reported	None reported
Aripiprazole[3,99-104]	4% of maternal plasma. A proportion of the drug detected may have been due to placental transfer following *in utero* exposure	0.9–8.3%	None reported	None reported
Asenapine	Published data not available			
Brexpiprazole	No published data available			
Butyrophenones[3,12,35,80,98,105-107]	Not reported	Haloperidol: 0.2–12%	None reported	Delayed development was noted in 3 infants exposed to a combination of haloperidol and chlorpromazine in breast milk Normal development has also been reported
Cariprazine	No published data available			
Clozapine[3,12,35,80,106,108-110] NB: Avoid	Not reported	1.4%	Sedation, agranulocytosis, decreased sucking reflex, irritability, seizures and cardiovascular instability	There is one report of delayed speech acquisition. The infant was also exposed to clozapine *in utero*
Lurasidone	No published data available			
Olanzapine[3,12,35,80,98,111-122]	Undetectable or low One case of plasma levels decreasing over 5 months. The authors proposed that the infant's capacity to metabolise olanzapine 'developed rapidly' around the age of 4 months	1.0–1.6%	Somnolence, drowsiness, irritability, tremor, insomnia, lethargy, poor suckling and shaking One case of jaundice and sedation. Infant was exposed *in utero* and had cardiomegaly	One case of lower developmental age than chronological age. Mother was taking additional psychotropic medication One case of speech delay and one of motor developmental delay Two cases of failure to gain weight Normal development has also been reported

(Continued)

Table 7.4 (*Continued*)

Drug	Infant plasma concentration	Estimated daily infant dose as proportion of maternal dose (RID)	Acute adverse effects in infant	Developmental effects in infant
Paliperidone	No specific data available. See risperidone			
Phenothiazines[3,12,80,105–107]	Variable	Chlorpromazine: 0.3%	Lethargy	Delayed development in 3 infants exposed to a combination of chlorpromazine and haloperidol
Quetiapine[3,93,120,123–132]	Undetectable	0.09–0.1%	Excessive sleep. Mother was also taking mirtazapine and a benzodiazepine	In a small study of quetiapine augmentation of maternal antidepressant there were two cases of mild developmental delays, thought not to be related to quetiapine
Risperidone[3,133–137]	Risperidone: undetectable 9-hydoxyrisperidone: low	Risperidone: 2.8–9.1% 9-hydoxyrisperidone: 3.46–4.7%	None reported	None reported
Sertindole	Published data not available			
Sulpiride[3,138–142]	Not reported	2.7–20.7%	None reported	None reported but not assessed
Thioxanthenes[3,12,107,143–145]	Not reported	Zuclopentixol: 0.4–0.9%	None reported	None reported for flupentixol Not assessed for zuclopentixol
Ziprasidone[3,20,107,146]	Not reported	0.07–1.2%	None reported	None reported
Iloperidone	Published data not available			

Table 7.5 Mood stabilisers in breastfeeding

Drug	Infant plasma concentration	Estimated daily infant dose as proportion of maternal dose (RID)	Acute adverse effects in infant	Developmental effects in infant
Carbamazepine[3,12,147–157]	Generally low although one report of an infant plasma level within adult therapeutic range	1.1–7.3%	Adverse effects have not been reported for a number of infants One case of cholestatic hepatitis, one of transient hepatic dysfunction with hyperbilirubinaemia and elevated GGT. The adverse effects in the first case resolved after discontinuation of breastfeeding and the second resolved despite continued feeding One case of seizure-like activity, drowsiness, irritability and high-pitched crying. Mother was taking multiple agents Poor suckling, poor feeding and 2 cases of hyperexcitability	None reported A prospective study of children of women with epilepsy found no adverse development at ages 6–36 months. The study assessed outcomes in children exposed to anticonvulsants in utero who were subsequently breastfed compared with those who were not A study of 199 infants exposed to anti-epileptic medications in utero and through breast milk failed to show a difference in IQ between breastfed and non-breastfed infants at the age of 3 years A study of 181 children concluded that IQ was not adversely affected by anticonvulsant exposure through breast milk
Lamotrigine[3,150,155,158–167]	Undetectable to 48% of maternal plasma levels	9.2–18.3%	No adverse effects have been reported in a number of infants 7 cases of thrombocytosis One case of a severe cyanotic episode (preceded by mild episodes of apnoea) requiring resuscitation. Neonatal serum concentration was in the upper therapeutic range. Infant exposed in utero. The mother was taking a high dose (850 mg/day) Three cases of rash. In one case the rash was attributed to eczema, and to soy allergy in another. The third case resolved spontaneously	No abnormalities reported A prospective study of children of women with epilepsy found that breastfeeding whilst taking an anticonvulsant was not associated with adverse development of infants at ages 6–36 months. The study assessed outcomes in children exposed to anticonvulsants in utero who were subsequently breastfed compared with those who were not A study of 199 infants exposed to anti-epileptic medications during breastfeeding failed to show a difference in IQ between breastfed and non-breastfed infants at the age of 3 years. The infants were exposed to anti-epileptic medications in utero A study of 181 children concluded that IQ was not adversely affected by anticonvulsant exposure through breast milk

(Continued)

Table 7.5 (*Continued*)

Drug	Infant plasma concentration	Estimated daily infant dose as proportion of maternal dose (RID)	Acute adverse effects in infant	Developmental effects in infant
Lithium[3,104,147,149,168–171] NB: Avoid	Undetectable to 57% of maternal plasma levels	12–30.1%	Early feeding problems, increased urea, raised creatinine, non-specific signs of toxicity One case of elevated TSH. *In utero* exposure One case of cyanosis, lethargy, hypothermia, hypotonia and a heart murmur. *In utero* exposure No adverse effects have been reported in others	None reported
Topiramate[172,173]	Undetectable to 20% of maternal plasma levels	3–35%	Diarrhoea	None reported but not assessed
Valproate[3,12,147–150,155,174,175]	<2% of maternal plasma levels	1.4–1.7%	Thrombocytopenia and anaemia which reversed on stopping breastfeeding. *In utero* exposure	A prospective study of children of women with epilepsy found that breastfeeding whilst taking an anticonvulsant was not associated with adverse development of infants at ages 6–36 months. The study assessed outcomes in children exposed to anticonvulsants *in utero* who were subsequently breastfed compared with those who were not A study of 199 infants exposed to anti-epileptic medications during breastfeeding failed to show a difference in IQ between breastfed and non-breastfed infants at the age of 3 years. The infants were exposed to antiepileptic medications *in utero* A study of 181 children concluded that IQ was not adversely affected by anticonvulsant exposure through breast milk

GGT, γ-glutamyl transferase; TSH, thyroid-stimulating hormone.

Table 7.6 Hypnotic drugs in breastfeeding

Drug	Infant plasma concentration	Estimated daily infant dose as proportion of maternal dose (RID)	Acute adverse effects in infant	Developmental effects in infant
Benzodiazepines[3,12,35,176-183]	Not reported	Clonazepam: 2.8% Diazepam: 7.1% Lorazepam: 2.6–2.9% Oxazepam: 0.28–1%	Sedation, lethargy, weight loss and mild jaundice One case of persistent apnoea with clonazepam Restlessness and mild drowsiness with alprazolam In a telephone survey of 124 women, 2 reported CNS depression in their breastfeeding neonates. One of the children was exposed to benzodiazepines *in utero* No adverse effects have been reported in others	None reported but not studied
Promethazine	No published data available			
Zopiclone, zolpidem and zaleplon[3,184-186]	Not reported	Zaleplon: 1.5% Zopiclone: 1.5% Zolpidem: 0.02–0.18%	None reported	None reported but not studied

CNS, central nervous system.

Table 7.7 Stimulant drugs in breastfeeding

Drug	Infant plasma concentration	Estimated daily infant dose as proportion of maternal dose (RID)	Acute adverse effects in infant	Developmental effects in infant
Atomoxetine	No published data available			
Dexamfetamine[187]	Undetectable to 14% of maternal plasma level	5.7%	None reported	None reported but not assessed
Lisdexamfetamine	No published data available			
Methylphenidate[188–190]	Undetectable	0.16–0.7%	None reported	None reported

Stimulant drugs in breastfeeding

Table 7.7 provides information on individual drugs in breastfeeding based on available published data in late 2017. Manufacturers' formal advice on drugs in breastfeeding is available in the summary of product characteristics or European Public Assessment Report for individual drugs. Table 7.7 does not include this advice (which is often uninformative), but instead uses primary reference sources. It is usually advisable to continue the drug prescribed during pregnancy. Switching drugs post partum for the purpose of breastfeeding is usually not sensible. Table 7.7 should be used as a guide when initiating treatment post partum. In each case the previous response (and lack of response) to treatment must be considered.

References

1. Weissman AM et al. Pooled analysis of antidepressant levels in lactating mothers, breast milk, and nursing infants. Am J Psychiatry 2004; 161:1066–1078.
2. Schmidt FM et al. Agomelatine in breast milk. Int J Neuropsychopharmacol 2013; 16:497–499.
3. Hale TW, Rowe HE. Medications and Mothers' Milk, 17th edn. New York: Springer Publishing Ltd; 2017.
4. Briggs GG et al. Excretion of bupropion in breast milk. Ann Pharmacother 1993; 27:431–433.
5. Chaudron LH et al. Bupropion and breastfeeding: a case of a possible infant seizure. J Clin Psychiatry 2004; 65:881–882.
6. Nonacs RM et al. Bupropion SR for the treatment of postpartum depression: a pilot study. Int J Neuropsychopharmacol 2005; 8:445–449.
7. Haas JS et al. Bupropion in breast milk: an exposure assessment for potential treatment to prevent post-partum tobacco use. Tob Control 2004; 13:52–56.
8. Baab SW et al. Serum bupropion levels in 2 breastfeeding mother-infant pairs. J Clin Psychiatry 2002; 63:910–911.
9. Berle JO, Spigset O. Antidepressant use during breastfeeding. Curr Womens Health Rev 2011; 7:28–34.
10. Davis MF et al. Bupropion levels in breast milk for 4 mother-infant pairs: more answers to lingering questions. J Clin Psychiatry 2009; 70:297–298.
11. Neuman G et al. Bupropion and escitalopram during lactation. Ann Pharmacother 2014; 48:928–931.
12. Burt VK et al. The use of psychotropic medications during breast-feeding. Am J Psychiatry 2001; 158:1001–1009.
13. Lee A et al. Frequency of infant adverse events that are associated with citalopram use during breast-feeding. Am J Obstet Gynecol 2004; 190:218–221.
14. Heikkinen T et al. Citalopram in pregnancy and lactation. Clin Pharmacol Ther 2002; 72:184–191.
15. Jensen PN et al. Citalopram and desmethylcitalopram concentrations in breast milk and in serum of mother and infant. Ther Drug Monit 1997; 19:236–239.
16. Spigset O et al. Excretion of citalopram in breast milk. Br J Clin Pharmacol 1997; 44:295–298.
17. Rampono J et al. Citalopram and demethylcitalopram in human milk; distribution, excretion and effects in breast fed infants. Br J Clin Pharmacol 2000; 50:263–268.
18. Schmidt K et al. Citalopram and breast-feeding: serum concentration and side effects in the infant. Biol Psychiatry 2000; 47:164–165.

19. Franssen EJ et al. Citalopram serum and milk levels in mother and infant during lactation. Ther Drug Monit 2006; 28:2–4.
20. Werremeyer A. Ziprasidone and citalopram use in pregnancy and lactation in a woman with psychotic depression. Am J Psychiatry 2009; 166:1298.
21. Hendrick V et al. Weight gain in breastfed infants of mothers taking antidepressant medications. J Clin Psychiatry 2003; 64:410–412.
22. Boyce PM et al. Duloxetine transfer across the placenta during pregnancy and into milk during lactation. Arch Womens Ment Health 2011; 14:169–172.
23. Briggs GG et al. Use of duloxetine in pregnancy and lactation. Ann Pharmacother 2009; 43:1898–1902.
24. Lobo ED et al. Pharmacokinetics of duloxetine in breast milk and plasma of healthy postpartum women. Clin Pharmacokinet 2008; 47:103–109.
25. Gentile S. Escitalopram late in pregnancy and while breast-feeding (Letter). Ann Pharmacother 2006; 40:1696–1697.
26. Castberg I et al. Excretion of escitalopram in breast milk. J Clin Psychopharmacol 2006; 26:536–538.
27. Rampono J et al. Transfer of escitalopram and its metabolite demethylescitalopram into breastmilk. Br J Clin Pharmacol 2006; 62:316–322.
28. Potts AL et al. Necrotizing enterocolitis associated with in utero and breast milk exposure to the selective serotonin reuptake inhibitor, escitalopram. J Perinatol 2007; 27:120–122.
29. Ilett KF et al. Estimation of infant dose and assessment of breastfeeding safety for escitalopram use in postnatal depression. Ther Drug Monit 2005; 27:248.
30. Bellantuono C et al. The safety of escitalopram during pregnancy and breastfeeding: a comprehensive review. Hum Psychopharmacol 2012; 27:534–539.
31. Yoshida K et al. Fluoxetine in breast-milk and developmental outcome of breast-fed infants. Br J Psychiatry 1998; 172:175–178.
32. Lester BM et al. Possible association between fluoxetine hydrochloride and colic in an infant. J Am Acad Child Adolesc Psychiatry 1993; 32:1253–1255.
33. Hendrick V et al. Fluoxetine and norfluoxetine concentrations in nursing infants and breast milk. Biol Psychiatry 2001; 50:775–782.
34. Hale TW et al. Fluoxetine toxicity in a breastfed infant. Clin Pediatr 2001; 40:681–684.
35. Malone K et al. Antidepressants, antipsychotics, benzodiazepines, and the breastfeeding dyad. Perspect Psychiatr Care 2004; 40:73–85.
36. Heikkinen T et al. Pharmacokinetics of fluoxetine and norfluoxetine in pregnancy and lactation. Clin Pharmacol Ther 2003; 73:330–337.
37. Epperson CN et al. Maternal fluoxetine treatment in the postpartum period: effects on platelet serotonin and plasma drug levels in breast-feeding mother-infant pairs. Pediatrics 2003; 112:e425.
38. Taddio A et al. Excretion of fluoxetine and its metabolite, norfluoxetine, in human breast milk. J Clin Pharmacol 1996; 36:42–47.
39. Brent NB et al. Fluoxetine and carbamazepine concentrations in a nursing mother/infant pair. Clin Pediatr (Phila) 1998; 37:41–44.
40. Kristensen JH et al. Distribution and excretion of fluoxetine and norfluoxetine in human milk. Br J Clin Pharmacol 1999; 48:521–527.
41. Burch KJ et al. Fluoxetine/norfluoxetine concentrations in human milk. Pediatrics 1992; 89:676–677.
42. Morris R et al. Serotonin syndrome in a breast-fed neonate. BMJ Case Rep 2015; 2015.
43. Hendrick V et al. Use of sertraline, paroxetine and fluvoxamine by nursing women. Br J Psychiatry 2001; 179:163–166.
44. Piontek CM et al. Serum fluvoxamine levels in breastfed infants. J Clin Psychiatry 2001; 62:111–113.
45. Yoshida K et al. Fluvoxamine in breast-milk and infant development. Br J Clin Pharmacol 1997; 44:210–211.
46. Hagg S et al. Excretion of fluvoxamine into breast milk. Br J Clin Pharmacol 2000; 49:286–288.
47. Arnold LM et al. Fluvoxamine concentrations in breast milk and in maternal and infant sera. J Clin Psychopharmacol 2000; 20:491–492.
48. Kristensen JH et al. The amount of fluvoxamine in milk is unlikely to be a cause of adverse effects in breastfed infants. J Hum Lact 2002; 18:139–143.
49. Wright S et al. Excretion of fluvoxamine in breast milk. Br J Clin Pharmacol 1991; 31:209.
50. Uguz F. Gastrointestinal side effects in the baby of a breastfeeding woman treated with low-dose fluvoxamine. J Hum Lact 2015; 31:371–373.
51. Buist A et al. Mianserin in breast milk (Letter). Br J Clin Pharmacol 1993; 36:133–134.
52. Aichhorn W et al. Mirtazapine and breast-feeding. Am J Psychiatry 2004; 161:2325.
53. Klier CM et al. Mirtazapine and breastfeeding: maternal and infant plasma levels. Am J Psychiatry 2007; 164:348–349.
54. Kristensen JH et al. Transfer of the antidepressant mirtazapine into breast milk. Br J Clin Pharmacol 2007; 63:322–327.
55. Tonn P et al. High mirtazapine plasma levels in infant after breast feeding: case report and review of the literature. J Clin Psychopharmacol 2009; 29:191–192.
56. Smit M et al. Mirtazapine in pregnancy and lactation: data from a case series. J Clin Psychopharmacol 2015; 35:163–167.
57. Buist A et al. Plasma and human milk concentrations of moclobemide in nursing mothers. Hum Psychopharmacol 1998; 13:579–582.
58. Pons G et al. Moclobemide excretion in human breast milk. Br J Clin Pharmacol 1990; 29:27–31.
59. Begg EJ et al. Paroxetine in human milk. Br J Clin Pharmacol 1999; 48:142–147.
60. Stowe ZN et al. Paroxetine in human breast milk and nursing infants. Am J Psychiatry 2000; 157:185–189.
61. Misri S et al. Paroxetine levels in postpartum depressed women, breast milk, and infant serum. J Clin Psychiatry 2000; 61:828–832.
62. Ohman R et al. Excretion of paroxetine into breast milk. J Clin Psychiatry 1999; 60:519–523.
63. Berle JO et al. Breastfeeding during maternal antidepressant treatment with serotonin reuptake inhibitors: infant exposure, clinical symptoms, and cytochrome p450 genotypes. J Clin Psychiatry 2004; 65:1228–1234.
64. Merlob P et al. Paroxetine during breast-feeding: infant weight gain and maternal adherence to counsel. Eur J Pediatr 2004; 163:135–139.
65. Abdul Aziz A et al. Severe paroxetine induced hyponatremia in a breast fed infant. J Bahrain Med Soc 2004; 16:195–198.
66. Hendrick V et al. Paroxetine use during breast-feeding. J Clin Psychopharmacol 2000; 20:587–589.
67. Spigset O et al. Paroxetine level in breast milk. J Clin Psychiatry 1996; 57:39.

CHAPTER 7

68. Uguz F et al. Short-term safety of paroxetine and sertraline in breastfed infants: a retrospective cohort study from a university hospital. Breastfeed Med 2016; 11:487–489.

69. Hackett LP et al. Transfer of reboxetine into breastmilk, its plasma concentrations and lack of adverse effects in the breastfed infant. Eur J Clin Pharmacol 2006; 62:633–638.

70. Llewellyn A et al. Psychotropic medications in lactation. J Clin Psychiatry 1998; 59 Suppl 2:41–52.

71. Mammen OK et al. Sertraline and norsertraline levels in three breastfed infants. J Clin Psychiatry 1997; 58:100–103.

72. Altshuler LL et al. Breastfeeding and sertraline: a 24-hour analysis. J Clin Psychiatry 1995; 56:243–245.

73. Dodd S et al. Sertraline analysis in the plasma of breast-fed infants. Aust N Z J Psychiatry 2001; 35:545–546.

74. Dodd S et al. Sertraline in paired blood plasma and breast-milk samples from nursing mothers. Hum Psychopharmacol 2000; 15:161–264.

75. Epperson N et al. Maternal sertraline treatment and serotonin transport in breast-feeding mother-infant pairs. Am J Psychiatry 2001; 158:1631–1637.

76. Stowe ZN et al. The pharmacokinetics of sertraline excretion into human breast milk: determinants of infant serum concentrations. J Clin Psychiatry 2003; 64:73–80.

77. Muller MJ et al. Serotonergic overstimulation in a preterm infant after sertraline intake via breastmilk. Breastfeed Med 2013; 8:327–329.

78. Wisner KL et al. Serum sertraline and N-desmethylsertraline levels in breast-feeding mother-infant pairs. Am J Psychiatry 1998; 155:690–692.

79. Verbeeck RK et al. Excretion of trazodone in breast milk. Br J Clin Pharmacol 1986; 22:367–370.

80. Yoshida K et al. Psychotropic drugs in mothers' milk: a comprehensive review of assay methods, pharmacokinetics and of safety of breast-feeding. J Psychopharmacol 1999; 13:64–80.

81. Misri S et al. Benefits and risks to mother and infant of drug treatment for postnatal depression. Drug Saf 2002; 25:903–911.

82. Yoshida K et al. Investigation of pharmacokinetics and of possible adverse effects in infants exposed to tricyclic antidepressants in breast-milk. J Affect Disord 1997; 43:225–237.

83. Frey OR et al. Adverse effects in a newborn infant breast-fed by a mother treated with doxepin. Ann Pharmacother 1999; 33:690–693.

84. Ilett KF et al. The excretion of dothiepin and its primary metabolites in breast milk. Br J Clin Pharmacol 1992; 33:635–639.

85. Kemp J et al. Excretion of doxepin and N-desmethyldoxepin in human milk. Br J Clin Pharmacol 1985; 20:497–499.

86. Buist A et al. Effect of exposure to dothiepin and northiaden in breast milk on child development. Br J Psychiatry 1995; 167:370–373.

87. Khachman D et al. Clomipramine in breast milk: a case study (article in French). Journal de Pharmacie Clinique 2007; 28:33–38.

88. Uguz F. Poor feeding and severe sedation in a newborn nursed by a mother on a low dose of amitriptyline. Breastfeed Med 2017; 12:67–68.

89. Koren G et al. Can venlafaxine in breast milk attenuate the norepinephrine and serotonin reuptake neonatal withdrawal syndrome. J Obstet Gynaecol Can 2006; 28:299–302.

90. Ilett KF et al. Distribution of venlafaxine and its O-desmethyl metabolite in human milk and their effects in breastfed infants. Br J Clin Pharmacol 2002; 53:17–22.

91. Newport DJ et al. Venlafaxine in human breast milk and nursing infant plasma: determination of exposure. J Clin Psychiatry 2009; 70:1304–1310.

92. Ilett KF et al. Assessment of infant dose through milk in a lactating woman taking amisulpride and desvenlafaxine for treatment-resistant depression. Ther Drug Monit 2010; 32:704–707.

93. Misri S et al. Quetiapine augmentation in lactation: a series of case reports. J Clin Psychopharmacol 2006; 26:508–511.

94. Hendrick V et al. Venlafaxine and breast-feeding. Am J Psychiatry 2001; 158:2089–2090.

95. Rampono J et al. Estimation of desvenlafaxine transfer into milk and infant exposure during its use in lactating women with postnatal depression. Arch Womens Ment Health 2011; 14:49–53.

96. Ilett KF et al. Distribution and excretion of venlafaxine and O-desmethylvenlafaxine in human milk. Br J Clin Pharmacol 1998; 45:459–462.

97. Teoh S et al. Estimation of rac-amisulpride transfer into milk and of infant dose via milk during its use in a lactating woman with bipolar disorder and schizophrenia. Breastfeed Med 2010; 6:85–88.

98. Uguz F. Breastfed infants exposed to combined antipsychotics: two case reports. Am J Ther 2016; 23:e1962–1964.

99. Schlotterbeck P et al. Aripiprazole in human milk. Int J Neuropsychopharmacol 2007; 10:433.

100. Lutz UC et al. Aripiprazole in pregnancy and lactation: a case report. J Clin Psychopharmacol 2010; 30:204–205.

101. Watanabe N et al. Perinatal use of aripiprazole: a case report. J Clin Psychopharmacol 2011; 31:377–379.

102. Mendhekar DN et al. Aripiprazole use in a pregnant schizoaffective woman. Bipolar Disord 2006; 8:299–300.

103. Nordeng H et al. Transfer of aripiprazole to breast milk: a case report. J Clin Psychopharmacol 2014; 34:272–275.

104. Frew JR. Psychopharmacology of bipolar I disorder during lactation: a case report of the use of lithium and aripiprazole in a nursing mother. Arch Womens Ment Health 2015; 18:135–136.

105. Yoshida K et al. Breast-feeding and psychotropic drugs. International Review of Psychiatry (Abingdon, England) 1996; 8:117–124.

106. Patton SW et al. Antipsychotic medication during pregnancy and lactation in women with schizophrenia: evaluating the risk. Can J Psychiatry 2002; 47:959–965.

107. Klinger G et al. Antipsychotic drugs and breastfeeding. Pediatr Endocrinol Rev 2013; 10:308–317.

108. Mendhekar DN. Possible delayed speech acquisition with clozapine therapy during pregnancy and lactation. J Neuropsychiatry Clin Neurosci 2007; 19:196–197.

109. Barnas C et al. Clozapine concentrations in maternal and fetal plasma, amniotic fluid, and breast milk. Am J Psychiatry 1994; 151:945.

110. Shao P et al. Effects of clozapine and other atypical antipsychotics on infants development who were exposed to as fetus: a post-hoc analysis. PLoS One 2015; 10:e0123373.

111. Goldstein DJ et al. Olanzapine-exposed pregnancies and lactation: early experience. J Clin Psychopharmacol 2000; **20**:399–403.

112. Croke S et al. Olanzapine excretion in human breast milk: estimation of infant exposure. Int J Neuropsychopharmacol 2002; **5**:243–247.

113. Gardiner SJ et al. Transfer of olanzapine into breast milk, calculation of infant drug dose, and effect on breast-fed infants. Am J Psychiatry 2003; **160**:1428–1431.

114. Ambresin G et al. Olanzapine excretion into breast milk: a case report. J Clin Psychopharmacol 2004; **24**:93–95.

115. Lutz UC et al. Olanzapine treatment during breast feeding: a case report. Ther Drug Monit 2008; **30**:399–401.

116. Whitworth A et al. Olanzapine and breast-feeding: changes of plasma concentrations of olanzapine in a breast-fed infant over a period of 5 months. J Psychopharmacol 2010; **24**:121–123.

117. Eli Lilly and Company Limited. Personal Correspondence – Olanzapine – Use in Pregnant or Nursing Women. 2011.

118. Gilad O et al. Outcome of infants exposed to olanzapine during breastfeeding. Breastfeed Med 2010; **6**:55–58.

119. Goldstein DJ et al. Olanzapine use during breast-feeding. Schizophr Res 2002; **53** (Suppl 1):185.

120. Aydin B et al. Olanzapine and quetiapine use during breastfeeding: excretion into breast milk and safe breastfeeding strategy. J Clin Psychopharmacol 2015; **35**:206–208.

121. Stiegler A et al. Olanzapine treatment during pregnancy and breastfeeding: a chance for women with psychotic illness? Psychopharmacology (Berl) 2014; **231**:3067–3069.

122. Var L et al. Management of postpartum manic episode without cessation of breastfeeding: a longitudinal follow up of drug excretion into breast milk. Eur Neuropsychopharmacol 2013; **23** (Suppl 1):S382.

123. Lee A et al. Excretion of quetiapine in breast milk. Am J Psychiatry 2004; **161**:1715–1716.

124. Gentile S. Quetiapine-fluvoxamine combination during pregnancy and while breastfeeding (Letter). Arch Womens Ment Health 2006; **9**:158–159.

125. Seppala J. Quetiapine (Seroquel) is effective and well tolerated in the treatment of psychotic depression during breast feeding. Eur Neuropsychopharmacol 2004:S245.

126. Kruninger U et al. Pregnancy and lactation under treatment with quetiapine. Psychiatr Prax 2007; **34** Suppl 1:S75–S76.

127. Ritz S. Quetiapine monotherapy in post-partum onset bipolar disorder with a mixed affective state. Eur Neuropsychopharmacol 2005; **15** Suppl 3:S407.

128. Rampono J et al. Quetiapine and breast feeding. Ann Pharmacother 2007; **41**:711–714.

129. Tanoshima R et al. Quetiapine in human breast milk – population PK analysis of milk levels and simulated infant exposure. J Popul Ther Clin Pharmacol 2012; **19**:e259-e98–e98.

130. Yazdani-Brojeni P et al. Quetiapine in human milk and simulation-based assessment of infant exposure. Clin Pharmacol Ther 2010; **87** Suppl 1:S3–S4.

131. Var L et al. Management of postpartum manic episode without cessation of breastfeeding: a longitudinal follow up of drug excretion into breast milk. Eur Neuropsychopharmacol 2013; **23** Suppl 2:S382.

132. Van Boekholt AA et al. Quetiapine concentrations during exclusive breastfeeding and maternal quetiapine use. Ann Pharmacother 2015; **49**:743–744.

133. Hill RC et al. Risperidone distribution and excretion into human milk: case report and estimated infant exposure during breast feeding. J Clin Psychopharmacol 2000; **20**:285–286.

134. Aichhorn W et al. Risperidone and breast-feeding. J Psychopharmacol 2005; **19**:211–213.

135. Ilett KF et al. Transfer of risperidone and 9-hydroxyrisperidone into human milk. Ann Pharmacother 2004; **38**:273–276.

136. Ratnayake T et al. No complications with risperidone treatment before and throughout pregnancy and during the nursing period. J Clin Psychiatry 2002; **63**:76–77.

137. Weggelaar NM et al. A case report of risperidone distribution and excretion into human milk: how to give good advice if you have not enough data available. J Clin Psychopharmacol 2011; **31**:129–131.

138. Ylikorkala O et al. Treatment of inadequate lactation with oral sulpiride and buccal oxytocin. Obstet Gynecol 1984; **63**:57–60.

139. Ylikorkala O et al. Sulpiride improves inadequate lactation. Br Med J 1982; **285**:249–251.

140. Aono T et al. Augmentation of puerperal lactation by oral administration of sulpiride. J Clin Endocrinol Metab 1970; **48**:478–482.

141. Polatti F. Sulpiride isomers and milk secretion in puerperium. Clin Exp Obstet Gynecol 1982; **9**:144–147.

142. Aono T et al. Effect of sulpiride on poor puerperal lactation. Am J Obstet Gynecol 1982; **143**:927–932.

143. Matheson I et al. Milk concentrations of flupenthixol, nortriptyline and zuclopenthixol and between-breast differences in two patients. Eur J Clin Pharmacol 1988; **35**:217–220.

144. Kirk L et al. Concentrations of Cis(Z)-flupentixol in maternal serum, amniotic fluid, umbilical cord serum, and milk. Psychopharmacology (Berl) 1980; **72**:107–108.

145. Aaes-Jorgensen T et al. Zuclopenthixol levels in serum and breast milk. Psychopharmacology (Berl) 1986; **90**:417–418.

146. Schlotterbeck P et al. Low concentration of ziprasidone in human milk: a case report. Int J Neuropsychopharmacol 2009; **12**:437–438.

147. Chaudron LH et al. Mood stabilizers during breastfeeding: a review. J Clin Psychiatry 2000; **61**:79–90.

148. Wisner KL et al. Serum levels of valproate and carbamazepine in breastfeeding mother-infant pairs. J Clin Psychopharmacol 1998; **18**:167–169.

149. Ernst CL et al. The reproductive safety profile of mood stabilizers, atypical antipsychotics, and broad-spectrum psychotropics. J Clin Psychiatry 2002; **63** Suppl 4:42–55.

150. Meador KJ et al. Effects of breastfeeding in children of women taking antiepileptic drugs. Neurology 2010; **75**:1954–1960.

151. Zhao M et al. [A case report of monitoring on carbamazepine in breast feeding woman]. Beijing Da Xue Xue Bao 2010; **42**:602–603.

152. Froescher W et al. Carbamazepine levels in breast milk. Ther Drug Monit 1984; **6**:266–271.

CHAPTER 7

153. Frey B et al. Transient cholestatic hepatitis in a neonate associated with carbamazepine exposure during pregnancy and breast-feeding. EurJ Pediatr 1990;**150**:136–138.

154. Merlob P et al. Transient hepatic dysfunction in an infant of an epileptic mother treated with carbamazepine during pregnancy and breast-feeding. Ann Pharmacother 1992;**26**:1563–1565.

155. Veiby G et al. Early child development and exposure to antiepileptic drugs prenatally and through breastfeeding: a prospective cohort study on children of women with epilepsy. JAMA Neurol 2013;**70**:1367–1374.

156. Pynnonen S et al. Letter: Carbamazepine and mother's milk. Lancet 1975;**2**:563.

157. Meador KJ et al. Breastfeeding in children of women taking antiepileptic drugs: cognitive outcomes at age 6 years. JAMA Pediatr 2014;**168**:729–736.

158. Ohman I et al. Lamotrigine in pregnancy: pharmacokinetics during delivery, in the neonate, and during lactation. Epilepsia 2000;**41**:709–713.

159. Liporace J et al. Concerns regarding lamotrigine and breast-feeding. Epilepsy Behav 2004;**5**:102–105.

160. Gentile S. Lamotrigine in pregnancy and lactation (Letter). Arch Womens Ment Health 2005;**8**:57–58.

161. Page-Sharp M et al. Transfer of lamotrigine into breast milk (Letter). Ann Pharmacother 2006;**40**:1470–1471.

162. Rambeck B et al. Concentrations of lamotrigine in a mother on lamotrigine treatment and her newborn child. Eur J Clin Pharmacol 1997;**51**:481–484.

163. Tomson T et al. Lamotrigine in pregnancy and lactation: a case report. Epilepsia 1997;**38**:1039–1041.

164. Newport DJ et al. Lamotrigine in breast milk and nursing infants: determination of exposure. Pediatrics 2008;**122**:e223–e231.

165. Fotopoulou C et al. Prospectively assessed changes in lamotrigine-concentration in women with epilepsy during pregnancy, lactation and the neonatal period. Epilepsy Res 2009;**85**:60–64.

166. Nordmo E et al. Severe apnea in an infant exposed to lamotrigine in breast milk. Ann Pharmacother 2009;**43**:1893–1897.

167. Wakil L et al. Neonatal outcomes with the use of lamotrigine for bipolar disorder in pregnancy and breastfeeding: a case series and review of the literature. Psychopharmacol Bull 2009;**42**:91–98.

168. Moretti ME et al. Monitoring lithium in breast milk: an individualized approach for breast-feeding mothers. Ther Drug Monit 2003;**25**:364–366.

169. Viguera AC et al. Lithium in breast milk and nursing infants: clinical implications. Am J Psychiatry 2007;**164**:342–345.

170. Bogen DL et al. Three cases of lithium exposure and exclusive breastfeeding. Arch Womens Ment Health 2012;**15**:69–72.

171. Tunnessen WW, Jr. et al. Toxic effects of lithium in newborn infants: a commentary. J Pediatr 1972;**81**:804–807.

172. Westergren T et al. Probable topiramate-induced diarrhea in a 2-month-old breast-fed child — a case report. Epilepsy Behav Case Rep 2014;**2**:22–23.

173. Gentile S. Topiramate in pregnancy and breastfeeding. Clin Drug Investig 2009;**29**:139–141.

174. Piontek CM et al. Serum valproate levels in 6 breastfeeding mother-infant pairs. J Clin Psychiatry 2000;**61**:170–172.

175. Bjornsson E. Hepatotoxicity associated with antiepileptic drugs. Acta Neurol Scand 2008;**118**:281–290.

176. Spigset O et al. Excretion of psychotropic drugs into breast milk: pharmacokinetic overview and therapeutic implications. CNS Drugs 1998;**9**:111–134.

177. Hagg S et al. Anticonvulsant use during lactation. Drug Saf 2000;**22**:425–440.

178. Iqbal MM et al. Effects of commonly used benzodiazepines on the fetus, the neonate, and the nursing infant. Psychiatr Serv 2002;**53**:39–49.

179. Buist A et al. Breastfeeding and the use of psychotropic medication: a review. J Affect Disord 1990;**19**:197–206.

180. Fisher JB et al. Neonatal apnea associated with maternal clonazepam therapy: a case report. Obstet Gynecol 1985;**66**:34S–35S.

181. Davanzo R et al. Benzodiazepine e allattamento materno. Medico e Bambino 2008;**27**:109–114.

182. Kelly LE et al. Neonatal benzodiazepines exposure during breastfeeding. J Pediatr 2012;**161**:448–451.

183. Birnbaum CS et al. Serum concentrations of antidepressants and benzodiazepines in nursing infants: a case series. Pediatrics 1999;**104**:e11.

184. Darwish M et al. Rapid disappearance of zaleplon from breast milk after oral administration to lactating women. J Clin Pharmacol 1999;**39**:670–674.

185. Pons G et al. Excretion of psychoactive drugs into breast milk. Pharmacokinetic principles and recommendations. Clin Pharmacokinet 1994;**27**:270–289.

186. Matheson I et al. The excretion of zopiclone into breast milk. Br J Clin Pharmacol 1990;**30**:267–271.

187. Ilett KF et al. Transfer of dexamphetamine into breast milk during treatment for attention deficit hyperactivity disorder. Br J Clin Pharmacol 2007;**63**:371–375.

188. Hackett LP et al. Methylphenidate and breast-feeding. Ann Pharmacother 2006;**40**:1890–1891.

189. Bolea-Alamanac BM et al. Methylphenidate use in pregnancy and lactation: a systematic review of evidence. Br J Clin Pharmacol 2014;**77**:96–101.

190. Marchese M et al. Is it safe to breastfeed while taking methylphenidate? Can Fam Physician 2015;**61**:765–766.

Hepatic and renal impairment

Hepatic impairment

Patients with hepatic impairment may have:

- **Reduced capacity to metabolise** biological waste products, dietary proteins and foreign substances such as drugs. Clinical consequences include hepatic encephalopathy and increased dose-related adverse effects from drugs.
- **Reduced ability to synthesise** plasma proteins and vitamin K-dependent clotting factors. Clinical consequences include hypoalbuminaemia, leading in extreme cases to ascites. Increased toxicity from highly protein-bound drugs should be anticipated. There is also an increased risk of bleeding from drugs that irritate the gastrointestinal tract and perhaps with selective serotonin reuptake inhibitors (SSRIs).
- **Reduced hepatic blood flow.** Clinical consequences include oesophageal varices and elevated plasma levels of drugs subject to first pass metabolism.

General principles of prescribing in hepatic impairment

Liver function tests (LFTs) are a poor marker of hepatic metabolising capacity, as the hepatic reserve is large. Note that many patients with chronic liver disease are asymptomatic or have fluctuating clinical symptoms. Always consider the clinical presentation rather than adhere to rigid rules involving LFTs.

There are few clinical studies relating to the use of psychotropic drugs in people with hepatic disease. The following principles should be adhered to:

1. Prescribe as **few drugs** as possible.
2. Use **lower starting doses**, particularly of drugs that are highly protein bound. Tricyclic antidepressants (TCAs), SSRIs (except citalopram), trazodone and antipsychotic drugs may have increased free plasma levels, at least initially. This will not be reflected in measured (total) plasma levels. Use lower doses of drugs known to be subject to extensive first pass metabolism. Examples include TCAs and haloperidol.

The Maudsley Prescribing Guidelines in Psychiatry, Thirteenth Edition. David M. Taylor,
Thomas R. E. Barnes and Allan H. Young.
© 2018 David M. Taylor. Published 2018 by John Wiley & Sons Ltd.

3. Be cautious with drugs that are extensively hepatically metabolised (most psychotropic drugs). Lower doses may be required. Exceptions are sulpiride, amisulpride, lithium and gabapentin, which all undergo no or minimal hepatic metabolism.
4. Leave longer intervals between dosage increases. Remember that the half-life of most drugs is prolonged in hepatic impairment, so it will take longer for plasma levels to reach steady state.
5. If albumin is reduced, consider the implications for drugs that are highly protein bound, and if ascites is present consider the increased volume of distribution for water-soluble drugs.
6. Avoid medicines with a long half-life or those that require to be metabolised to render them active (pro-drugs)
7. Always monitor carefully for adverse effects, which may be delayed.
8. Avoid drugs that are very sedative because of the risk of precipitating hepatic encephalopathy.
9. Avoid drugs that are very constipating because of the risk of precipitating hepatic encephalopathy.
10. Avoid drugs that are known to be hepatotoxic in their own right (e.g. monoamine oxidase inhibitors [MAOIs], chlorpromazine).
11. Choose a low-risk drug (see Table 8.5) and monitor LFTs weekly, at least initially. If LFTs deteriorate after a new drug is introduced, consider switching to another drug.

These rules should always be observed in severe liver disease (low albumin, increased clotting time, ascites, jaundice, encephalopathy, etc.). The information presented here should be interpreted in the context of the patient's clinical presentation.

Antipsychotic medications in hepatic impairment

One-third of patients who are prescribed antipsychotic medication have at least one abnormal LFT, and in 4% at least one LFT is elevated three times above the upper limit of normal. Transaminases are most often affected and this generally occurs within 1–6 weeks of treatment initiation. Only rarely does clinically significant hepatic damage result.[1] Recommendations for the use of antipsychotic medications in hepatic impairment are summarised in Table 8.1.

Table 8.1 Antipsychotic medications in hepatic impairment

Drug	Comments
Amisulpride[2,3]	Predominantly renally excreted, so dosage reduction should not be necessary as long as renal function is normal
Aripiprazole[2–5]	Extensively hepatically metabolised. Limited data that hepatic impairment has minimal effect on pharmacokinetics. SPC states no dosage reduction required in mild–moderate hepatic impairment, but caution required in severe impairment. Limited clinical experience. Caution required. Small number of reports of hepatotoxicity; increased LFTs, hepatitis and jaundice[1,6,7]
Asenapine[2,3,5]	Hepatically metabolised. SPC recommends avoid in severe hepatic disease; no dose adjustment required in mild to moderate disease.[8] Elevation in ALT and AST reported in paediatric clinical trials[3]
Brexpiprazole[9]	Little information. Use no more than 3 mg/day in moderate or severe hepatic failure. Long half-life (~90 hours)
Cariprazine[10]	Occasional increases in ALT. No dosage adjustment is required in patients with mild or moderate hepatic failure; contraindicated in severe hepatic disease. Long half-life (~2–4 days)
Clozapine[2,3,11–13]	Very sedative and constipating. Contraindicated in active liver disease associated with nausea, anorexia or jaundice, progressive liver disease or hepatic failure. In less severe disease, start with 12.5 mg and increase slowly, using plasma levels to gauge metabolising capacity and guide dosage adjustment. Transient elevations in AST, ALT and GGT to over twice the normal range occur in over 10% of physically healthy people. Clozapine-induced hepatitis, jaundice, cholestasis and liver failure have been reported. If jaundice develops, clozapine should be discontinued. See section on clozapine adverse effects (Chapter 1)
Flupentixol/ zuclopenthixol[2,3,14,15]	Both are extensively hepatically metabolised. Abnormal LFTs and (rarely) jaundice have been reported with flupentixol.[2] Small, transient elevations in transaminases, cholestatic hepatitis and jaundice[2] have been reported in some patients treated with zuclopenthixol. One report of flupentixol-induced hepatitis.[16] No other literature reports of use or harm.[17] Depot preparations are best avoided, as altered pharmacokinetics will make dosage adjustment difficult and adverse effects from dosage accumulation more likely
Haloperidol[2]	UK SPC states 'caution in liver disease'. Isolated reports of cholestasis, acute hepatic failure, hepatitis and abnormal LFTs often used in low doses (5 mg/day) for nausea and vomitting in hepatic impairment in paliative care[2,3]
Iloperidone[3,5,18]	Hepatically metabolised. Reduce dose in moderate impairment (two-fold increase in active metabolites) and avoid completely in severe hepatic impairment (no studies done). No dose reduction necessary in mild impairment. Infrequent reports of cholelithiasis
Lurasidone[2,3,5]	Hepatically metabolised. SPC recommends starting dose of 18.5 mg in hepatic impairment, maximum dose of 74 mg/day in moderate hepatic impairment, and 37 mg in severe impairment. No dose adjustment is required in mild hepatic impairment. Increases in ALT reported infrequently
Olanzapine[2,3,5,11]	Although extensively hepatically metabolised, the pharmacokinetics of olanzapine seem to change little in severe hepatic impairment. It is sedative and anticholinergic (can cause constipation) so caution is advised. Start with 5 mg/day and consider using plasma levels to guide dosage (aim for 20–40 μg/L). Dose related, transient, asymptomatic elevations in ALT and AST reported in physically healthy adults, particularly early in treatment. People with liver disease or those taking other hepatotoxic drugs may be at increased risk. Rare cases of hepatitis in the literature

(Continued)

Table 8.1 (*Continued*)

Drug	Comments
Paliperidone[2,3,5]	Mainly excreted unchanged by the kidneys so no dosage adjustment required for mild–moderate impairment. However, no data are available with respect to severe hepatic impairment and clinical experience is limited; caution required. Rises in transaminases and GGT reported, some cases of jaundice. May be a good choice for patients with pre-existing hepatic disease[19–22]
Phenothiazines[2,3]	All cause sedation and constipation. Transient abnormalities in LFTs reported. Associated with cholestasis and some reports of fulminant hepatic cirrhosis. Best avoided completely in hepatic impairment; some phenothiazines are actively contraindicated. Chlorpromazine is particularly hepatotoxic; rare cases of immune-mediated obstructive jaundice which may progress to liver disease
Quetiapine[2,3,5,23]	Extensively hepatically metabolised but short half-life. Clearance reduced by a mean of 30% in hepatic impairment so start at 25 mg/day (IR preparation) or 50 mg/day (XL preparation) and increase in 25–50 mg/day increments. Can cause sedation and constipation. Transient rises in AST, ALT and GGT reported, rarely jaundice and hepatitis. Several cases of fatal hepatic failure and of hepatocellular damage reported in the literature. A number of studies describe use in patients with alcohol dependence[24–26]
Risperidone[2,3,5,11]	Extensively hepatically metabolised and highly protein bound. Manufacturers recommend a halved starting dose and slower dose titration. Those with severe impairment should start at 0.5 mg bd, and increase by 0.5 mg bd at a maximum rate of 3 times a week. Risperidone Consta can be started at 12.5 mg fortnightly, or 25 mg every 2 weeks if 2 mg daily oral dosing has been tolerated. Transient, asymptomatic elevations in LFTs, cholestatic hepatitis, jaundice, and rare cases of hepatic failure have been reported. Steatohepatitis may arise as a result of weight gain[27]
Sulpiride[2,3]	Almost completely renally excreted with a low potential to cause sedation or constipation. Dosage reduction should not be required. Rises in hepatic enzymes are common. Isolated case reports of cholestatic jaundice and primary biliary cirrhosis

ALT, alanine aminotransferase; AST, aspartate aminotransferase; bd, *bis die* (twice a day); GGT, γ-glutamyl transferase; IR, immediate release; LFT, liver function test; SPC, summary of product characteristics; XL, extended release.

Antidepressant medications in hepatic impairment

Of those treated with antidepressants, 0.5–3% develop asymptomatic mild elevation of hepatic transaminases. Onset is normally between several days and 6 months of treatment initiation and the elderly are more vulnerable. Frank, clinically significant liver damage however is rare and mostly idiosyncratic (unpredictable and not related to dose). Cross toxicity within class has been described.[28] Recommendations for the use of antidepressant medications in hepatic impairment are summarised in Table 8.2.

Table 8.2 Antidepressant medications in hepatic impairment

Drug	Comments
Agomelatine[2,3,28–30]	Liver injury including hepatic failure, liver enzyme increases more than 10× ULN, and hepatitis reported, most commonly in first months of treatment. Contraindicated in established liver disease. Dose-related increase in transaminases reported; perform LFTs at baseline, 3, 6, 12, 24 weeks and thereafter where clinically indicated. Stop treatment if transaminases rise more than 3× ULN. Use cautiously where other risk factors for hepatic disease are present
Duloxetine[2,3,31–35]	Hepatically metabolised. Clearance markedly reduced even in mild impairment. Reports of hepatocellular injury and, less commonly, jaundice. Isolated case report of fulminant hepatic failure. Contraindicated in hepatic impairment
Fluoxetine[2,3,36–40]	Extensively hepatically metabolised with a long half-life. Kinetic studies demonstrate accumulation in compensated cirrhosis. Although dosage reduction (of at least 50%) or alternate day dosing is recommended, it would take many weeks to reach steady-state serum levels, making fluoxetine complex to use. Asymptomatic increases in LFTs found in 0.5% of healthy adults. Rare cases of hepatitis reported
MAOIs[2,3,41]	Rare cases of fatal hepatic necrosis, hepatotoxicity and jaundice with phenelzine, rarely hepatitis with tranylcypromine and one isolated case of fatal hepatotoxicity with moclobemide. Doses of moclobemide should be reduced by 30–50% in hepatic impairment, or the dosing interval increased. Non-selective MAOIs are contraindicated in patients with hepatic impairment
Mirtazapine[2,3,42]	Hepatically metabolised and sedative. 50% dose reduction recommended based on kinetic data. Mild, asymptomatic increases in LFTs seen in healthy adults (ALT >3 times the upper limit of normal in 2%). Few cases of cholestatic and hepatocellular damage reported. Used in some liver units for affect on appetite and sleep
Other SSRIs[2,3,35,40,43–52]	All are hepatically metabolised and accumulate on chronic dosing. Dosage reduction (including reduction of maximum dose by 50%[53] and/or reduced dosing frequency) may be required (see individual SPCs for details). Sertraline has been found to be both safe and effective in a placebo-controlled RCT of the management of cholestatic pruritus. Raised LFTs and rare cases of hepatitis, including chronic active hepatitis, have been reported with paroxetine. Sertraline and fluvoxamine have also been associated with hepatitis. Citalopram, escitalopram and paroxetine have minimal effects on hepatic enzymes and may be the SSRIs of choice although occasional hepatotoxicity has been reported. Paroxetine is used by some specialised liver units with few apparent problems. Be aware of increased risk of bleeding
Reboxetine[2,3,54]	50% reduction in starting dose recommended. Does not seem to be associated with hepatotoxicity
TCAs[2,3,55]	All are hepatically metabolised, highly protein bound and will accumulate. They vary in their propensity to cause sedation and constipation. All are associated with raised LFTs and rare cases of hepatitis. Sedative TCAs such as trimipramine, imipramine, dosulepin (dothiepin) and amitriptyline are best avoided
Venlafaxine/ desvenlafaxine[2,3,56,57]	Dosage reduction of 50% advised in mild and moderate hepatic impairment. Rare cases of hepatitis reported

ALT, alanine aminotransferase; LFT, liver function test; MAOI, monoamine oxidase inhibitor; RCT, randomised controlled trial; SPC, summary of product characteristics; SSRI, selective serotonin reuptake inhibitor; TCA, tricyclic antidepressant; ULN, upper limit of normal.

CHAPTER 8

Mood stabilisers in hepatic impairment[2,3,58]

Recommendations for the use of mood-stabilising medications in hepatic impairment are summarised in Table 8.3.

Table 8.3 Mood stabilisers in hepatic impairment

Drug	Comments
Carbamazepine[58]	Extensively hepatically metabolised and potent inducer of CYP450 enzymes. In chronic stable disease, caution advised. Avoid use in acute liver disease. Reduce starting dose by 50%, and titrate up slowly, using plasma levels to guide dosage. Stop if LFTs deteriorate. Associated with hepatitis, cholangitis, cholestatic and hepatocellular jaundice, and hepatic failure (rare). Adverse hepatic effects are most common in the first month of treatment. Hepatocellular damage is often associated with a poor outcome. Vulnerability to carbamazepine-induced hepatic damage may be genetically determined
Lamotrigine	Manufacturers recommend 50% reduction in initial dose, dose escalation and maintenance dose in moderate hepatic impairment and 75% in severe hepatic impairment. Discontinue if lamotrigine-induced rash (which can be serious). Extreme caution advised, particularly if co-prescribed with valproate. Elevated LFTs and hepatitis reported
Lithium	Not metabolised so dosage reduction not required as long as renal function is normal. Use serum levels to guide dosage and monitor more frequently if ascites status changes (volume of distribution will change). One case of ascites and one of hyperbilirubinaemia reported over many decades of lithium use worldwide
Valproate[59]	Highly protein bound and hepatically metabolised. Dosage reduction with close monitoring of LFTs in moderate hepatic impairment. Use plasma levels (measure free levels – total concentrations may appear to be normal) to guide dosage. Caution advised. Contraindicated in severe and/or active hepatic impairment, or family history of severe impairment; impairment of usual metabolic pathway can lead to generation of hepatotoxic metabolites via alternative pathway. Risk of liver toxicity is increased in people with hepatic insufficiency if salicylates are used concomitantly. Associated with elevated LFTs and serious hepatotoxicity including fulminant hepatic failure. Mitochondrial disease, learning disability, polypharmacy, metabolic disorders and underlying hepatic disease may be risk factors. Particularly hepatotoxic in very young children. The greatest risk is in the first 3 months of treatment

LFT, liver function test.

Stimulants in hepatic impairment[2,3,60]

Recommendations for the use of stimulant medications in hepatic impairment are summarised in Table 8.4.

Table 8.4 Stimulant medications in hepatic impairment

Drug	Comments
Atomoxetine[61]	Reduce initial and target dose by 50% in moderate impairment, and by 75% in severe impairment. Very rare reports of liver toxicity, manifested by elevated hepatic enzymes, and raised bilirubin with jaundice. SPC states 'discontinue in patients with jaundice or laboratory evidence of liver injury, and do not restart'
Methylphenidate	Rare reports of liver dysfunction and hypersensitivity reactions

SPC, summary of product characteristics.

Psychotropic medications in hepatic impairment

Table 8.5 summarises recommended psychotropic medications in hepatic impairment.

Table 8.5 Recommended psychotropic medications in hepatic impairment

Drug group	Recommended drugs
Antipsychotics	**Sulpiride/amisulpride**: no dosage reduction required if renal function is normal **Paliperidone**: if depot required
Antidepressants	**Sertraline or mirtazapine**: start at low dose. Titrate slowly (if required)
Mood stabilisers	**Lithium**: use plasma levels to guide dosage. Care needed if ascites status changes
Sedatives	**Lorazepam**, **oxazepam**, **temazepam**: as short half-life with no active metabolites. Use low doses with caution with longer dosing intervals, as sedative drugs can accumulate and precipitate hepatic encephalopathy **Zopiclone**: 3.75 mg with care in moderate hepatic impairment

Drug-induced hepatic damage

Hy's rule, defined as alanine aminotransferase (ALT) >3 times the upper limit of normal combined with serum bilirubin >2 times the upper limit of normal, is recommended by the US Food and Drug Administration (FDA) to assess the hepatotoxicity of new drugs.[58]

Drug-induced hepatic damage can be due to:

- Direct dose-related hepatotoxicity (Type 1 ADR). A small number of drugs fall into this category, e.g. paracetamol, alcohol.
- Hypersensitivity reactions (Type 2 ADR). These can present with rash, fever and eosinophilia. Almost all drugs have been associated with cases of hepatotoxicity; frequency varies.

Almost any type of liver damage can occur, ranging from mild transient asymptomatic increases in LFTs to fulminant hepatic failure. See Tables 8.1, 8.2, 8.3 and 8.4 for details of the hepatotoxic potential of individual drugs.

Risk factors for drug-induced hepatotoxicity include:[62]

- increasing age
- female gender
- alcohol consumption
- co-prescription of enzyme-inducing drugs
- genetic predisposition
- obesity
- pre-existing liver disease (small effect).

When interpreting LFTs, remember that:[63]

- 12% of the healthy adult population have one LFT outside (above or below) the normal reference range.
- Up to 10% of patients with clinically significant hepatic disease have normal LFTs.
- Individual LFTs lack specificity for the liver, but >1 abnormal test greatly increases the likelihood of liver pathology.
- The absolute values of LFTs are a poor indicator of disease severity.

When monitoring LFTs:

- Ideally LFTs should be measured before treatment starts so that 'baseline' values are available.
- LFT elevations of <2 times the upper limit of the normal reference range are rarely clinically significant.
- Most drug-related LFT elevations occur early in treatment (first month) and are transient. They may indicate adaptation of the liver to the drug rather than damage per se. Transient LFT elevations may also occur during periods of weight gain.[64]
- If LFTs are persistently elevated >3-fold, continuing to rise or accompanied by clinical symptoms, the suspected drugs should be withdrawn.
- When tracking change, >20% change in liver enzymes is required to exclude biological or analytical variation.

References

1. Marwick KF et al. Antipsychotics and abnormal liver function tests: systematic review. Clin Neuropharmacol 2012; 35:244–253.
2. Datapharm Communications Ltd. Electronic Medicines Compendium. 2017. https://www.medicines.org.uk/emc/.
3. Truven Health Analytics. Micromedix Software Product. 2018. http://truvenhealth.com/products/micromedex.
4. Mallikaarjun S et al. Effects of hepatic or renal impairment on the pharmacokinetics of aripiprazole. Clin Pharmacokinet 2008; 47: 533–542.
5. Preskorn SH. Clinically important differences in the pharmacokinetics of the ten newer "atypical" antipsychotics: Part 3. Effects of renal and hepatic impairment. J Psychiatr Pract 2012; 18:430–437.
6. Chico G et al. Clinical vignettes 482 aripiprazole causes cholelithiasis and hepatitis: a rare finding. Am J Gastroenterol 2005; 100:S164.
7. Kornischka J et al. Acute drug-induced hepatitis during aripiprazole monotherapy: a case report. J Pharmacovigil 2016; 4:201.
8. Peeters P et al. Asenapine pharmacokinetics in hepatic and renal impairment. Clin Pharmacokinet 2011; 50:471–481.
9. Parikh NB et al. Clinical role of brexpiprazole in depression and schizophrenia. Ther Clin Risk Manag 2017; 13:299–306.
10. Scarff JR. Cariprazine for schizophrenia and bipolar disorder. Innov Clin Neurosci 2016; 13:49–52.
11. Atasoy N et al. A review of liver function tests during treatment with atypical antipsychotic drugs: a chart review study. Prog Neuropsychopharmacol Biol Psychiatry 2007; 31:1255–1260.
12. Brown CA et al. Clozapine toxicity and hepatitis. J Clin Psychopharmacol 2013; 33:570–571.
13. Tucker P. Liver toxicity with clozapine. Aust N Z J Psychiatry 2013; 47:975–976.
14. Amdisen A et al. Zuclopenthixol acetate in viscoleo – a new drug formulation. An open Nordic multicentre study of zuclopenthixol acetate in Viscoleo in patients with acute psychoses including mania and exacerbation of chronic psychoses. Acta Psychiatr Scand 1987; 75:99–107.
15. Wistedt B et al. Zuclopenthixol decanoate and haloperidol decanoate in chronic schizophrenia: a double-blind multicentre study. Acta Psychiatr Scand 1991; 84:14–21.
16. Demuth N et al. [Flupentixol-induced acute hepatitis]. Gastroenterol Clin Biol 1999; 23:152–153.
17. Nolen WA et al. Disturbances of liver function of long acting neuroleptic drugs. Pharmakopsychiatr Neuropsychopharmakol 1978; 11:199–204.
18. Novartis Pharmaceuticals Corporation. Highlights of Prescribing Information. FANAPT® (iloperidone) tablets. 2017. http://www.fanapt.com/product/pi/pdf/fanapt.pdf.
19. Amatniek J et al. Safety of paliperidone extended-release in patients with schizophrenia or schizoaffective disorder and hepatic disease. Clin Schizophr Relat Psychoses 2014; 8:8–20.
20. Macaluso M et al. Pharmacokinetic drug evaluation of paliperidone in the treatment of schizoaffective disorder. Expert Opin Drug Metab Toxicol 2017; 13:871–879.
21. Chou HW et al. Using paliperidone as a monotherapeutic agent on a schizophrenic patient with cirrhosis of the liver. J Neuropsychiatry Clin Neurosci 2013; 25:E37.
22. Paulzen M et al. Remission of drug-induced hepatitis after switching from risperidone to paliperidone. Am J Psychiatry 2010; 167: 351–352.
23. Das A et al. Liver injury associated with quetiapine: an illustrative case report. J Clin Psychopharmacol 2017; 37:623–625.
24. Monnelly EP et al. Quetiapine for treatment of alcohol dependence. J Clin Psychopharmacol 2004; 24:532–535.
25. Brown ES et al. A randomized, double-blind, placebo-controlled trial of quetiapine in patients with bipolar disorder, mixed or depressed phase, and alcohol dependence. Alcohol Clin Exp Res 2014; 38:2113–2118.
26. Vatsalya V et al. Safety assessment of liver injury with quetiapine fumarate XR management in very heavy drinking alcohol-dependent patients. Clin Drug Investig 2016; 36:935–944.
27. Holtmann M et al. Risperidone-associated steatohepatitis and excessive weight-gain. Pharmacopsychiatry 2003; 36:206–207.
28. Voican CS et al. Antidepressant-induced liver injury: a review for clinicians. Am J Psychiatry 2014; 171:404–415.
29. Freiesleben SD et al. A systematic review of agomelatine-induced liver injury. J Mol Psychiatry 2015; 3:4.
30. Gahr M et al. Safety and tolerability of agomelatine: focus on hepatotoxicity. Curr Drug Metab 2014; 15:694–702.
31. Hanje AJ et al. Case report: fulminant hepatic failure involving duloxetine hydrochloride. Clin Gastroenterol Hepatol 2006; 4:912–917.
32. Vuppalanchi R et al. Duloxetine hepatotoxicity: a case-series from the drug-induced liver injury network. Aliment Pharmacol Ther 2010; 32:1174–1183.
33. Lin ND et al. Hepatic outcomes among adults taking duloxetine: a retrospective cohort study in a US health care claims database. BMC Gastroenterol 2015; 15:134.
34. McIntyre RS et al. The hepatic safety profile of duloxetine: a review. Expert Opin Drug Metab Toxicol 2008; 4:281–285.
35. Bunchorntavakul C et al. Drug hepatotoxicity: newer agents. Clin Liver Dis 2017; 21:115–134.
36. Schenker S et al. Fluoxetine disposition and elimination in cirrhosis. Clin Pharmacol Ther 1988; 44:353–359.
37. Cai Q et al. Acute hepatitis due to fluoxetine therapy. Mayo Clin Proc 1999; 74:692–694.
38. Friedenberg FK et al. Hepatitis secondary to fluoxetine treatment. Am J Psychiatry 1996; 153:580.
39. Johnston DE et al. Chronic hepatitis related to use of fluoxetine. Am J Gastroenterol 1997; 92:1225–1226.
40. Hale AS. New antidepressants: use in high-risk patients. J Clin Psychiatry 1993; 54 Suppl:61–70.
41. Stoeckel K et al. Absorption and disposition of moclobemide in patients with advanced age or reduced liver or kidney function. Acta Psychiatr Scand Suppl 1990; 360:94–97.
42. Thomas E et al. Mirtazapine-induced steatosis. Int J Clin Pharmacol Ther 2017; 55:630–632.
43. Benbow SJ et al. Paroxetine and hepatotoxicity. BMJ 1997; 314:1387.

44. Kuhs H et al. A double-blind study of the comparative antidepressant effect of paroxetine and amitriptyline. Acta Psychiatr Scand Suppl 1989; 350:145–146.

45. de Bree H et al. Fluvoxamine maleate: disposition in men. Eur J Drug Metab Pharmacokinet 1983; 8:175–179.

46. Green BH. Fluvoxamine and hepatic function. Br J Psychiatry 1988; 153:130–131.

47. Milne RJ et al. Citalopram. A review of its pharmacodynamic and pharmacokinetic properties, and therapeutic potential in depressive illness. Drugs 1991; 41:450–477.

48. Lopez-Torres E et al. Hepatotoxicity related to citalopram (Letter). Am J Psychiatry 2004; 161:923–924.

49. Colakoglu O et al. Toxic hepatitis associated with paroxetine. Int J Clin Pract 2005; 59:861–862.

50. Rao N. The clinical pharmacokinetics of escitalopram. Clin Pharmacokinet 2007; 46:281–290.

51. Suen CF et al. Acute liver injury secondary to sertraline. BMJ Case Rep 2013; 2013.

52. Mayo MJ et al. Sertraline as a first-line treatment for cholestatic pruritus. Hepatology 2007; 45:666–674.

53. Mullish BH et al. Review article: depression and the use of antidepressants in patients with chronic liver disease or liver transplantation. Aliment Pharmacol Ther 2014; 40:880–892.

54. Tran A et al. Pharmacokinetics of reboxetine in volunteers with hepatic impairment. Clin Drug Investig 2000; 19:473–477.

55. Committee on Safety in Medicines. Lofepramine (Gamanil) and abnormal blood tests of liver function. Current Problems 1988; 23:2.

56. Archer DF et al. Cardiovascular, cerebrovascular, and hepatic safety of desvenlafaxine for 1 year in women with vasomotor symptoms associated with menopause. Menopause 2013; 20:47–56.

57. Baird-Bellaire S et al. An open-label, single-dose, parallel-group study of the effects of chronic hepatic impairment on the safety and pharmacokinetics of desvenlafaxine. Clin Ther 2013; 35:782–794.

58. Bjornsson E. Hepatotoxicity associated with antiepileptic drugs. Acta Neurol Scand 2008; 118:281–290.

59. Krahenbuhl S et al. Mitochondrial diseases represent a risk factor for valproate-induced fulminant liver failure. Liver 2000; 20:346–348.

60. Panei P et al. Safety of psychotropic drug prescribed for attention-deficit/hyperactivity disorder in Italy. Adverse Drug Reaction Bulletin 2010;999–1002.

61. Reed VA et al. The safety of atomoxetine for the treatment of children and adolescents with attention-deficit/hyperactivity disorder: a comprehensive review of over a decade of research. CNS Drugs 2016; 30:603–628.

62. Grattagliano I et al. Biochemical mechanisms in drug-induced liver injury: certainties and doubts. World J Gastroenterol 2009; 15:4865–4876.

63. Rosalki SB et al. Liver function profiles and their interpretation. Br J Hosp Med 1994; 51:181–186.

64. Rettenbacher MA et al. Association between antipsychotic-induced elevation of liver enzymes and weight gain: a prospective study. J Clin Psychopharmacol 2006; 26:500–503.

Renal impairment

Using drugs in patients with renal impairment needs careful consideration. This is because some drugs are nephrotoxic and also because pharmacokinetics (absorption, distribution, metabolism, excretion) of drugs are altered in renal impairment. Essentially, **patients with renal impairment have a reduced capacity to excrete drugs** and their metabolites.

General principles of prescribing in renal impairment

- *Estimate* **the excretory capacity of the kidney** by calculating the glomerular filtration rate (GFR). GFR is assessed by measurement of:
  - an ideal filtration marker, e.g. inulin or ethylenediaminetetra-acetic acid (EDTA) – gives accurate estimate but expensive and invasive
  - serum creatinine – an easy and cheap method but inaccurate
  - cystatin C protein – a more expensive test than creatinine but more accurate.
- Check proteinuria by measuring urinary albumin and calculate the albumin:creatinine ratio.
- Or by using the equations in Boxes 8.1 and 8.2 to improve the precision of GFR determination using serum creatinine and cystatin C. Note that these estimates are still inherently inaccurate.[1,2] CKD-EPI is more accurate than MDRD and is now preferred.

When calculating **drug doses**, use estimated creatinine clearance (CrCl) from the Cockcroft–Gault equation. Do not use the CKD-EPI or MDRD formulae for dose calculation because **most** current dose recommendations are based on the CrCl estimations from the Cockcroft–Gault equation.

Box 8.1 The Cockcroft–Gault equation*

$$CrCl\,(mL/min) = \frac{F(140 - age\ (in\ years)) \times ideal\ body\ weight\ (kg))}{Serum\ creatinine\ (\mu mol/L)}$$

F = 1.23 (men) and 1.04 (women).
Ideal body weight should be used for patients at extremes of body weight or else the result of the calculation is a poor estimate:

- For men, ideal body weight (kg) = 50 kg + 2.3 kg per inch over 5 feet
- For women, ideal body weight (kg) = 45.5 kg + 2.3 kg per inch over 5 feet

An online calculator is available at https://www.nuh.nhs.uk/staff-area/antibiotics/creatinine-clearance-calculator/

*This equation is not accurate if plasma creatinine is unstable (e.g. in acute renal failure), in obesity, in pregnant women, in children or in diseases causing production of abnormal amounts of creatinine. It has only been validated in White patients. CrCl is relatively less representative of GFR in severe renal failure.

> **Box 8.2** The Chronic Kidney Disease Epidemiology Collaboration (CKD-EPI) formula
>
> This replaces the previously used Modification of Diet in Renal Disease (MDRD) equation.[1] Note that some pathology departments still use MDRD.
>
> $$GFR = 141 \times \min(S_{cr}/\kappa, 1)^{\alpha} \times \max(S_{cr}/\kappa, 1)^{-1.209} \times 0.993^{Age} \times 1.018 \,[\text{if female}] \times 1.159 \,[\text{if Black}]$$
>
> - S_{cr} is serum creatinine in mg/dL
> - κ is 0.7 for females and 0.9 for males
> - α is −0.329 for females and −0.411 for males
> - min indicates the minimum of S_{cr}/κ or 1
> - max indicates the maximum of S_{cr}/κ or 1.
>
> An online calculator is available at: https://www.kidney.org/professionals/kdoqi/gfr_calculator
>
> **Use the Cockcroft–Gault equation for drug dose calculation.**

Classify the stage of renal impairment

See Figure 8.1.[2]

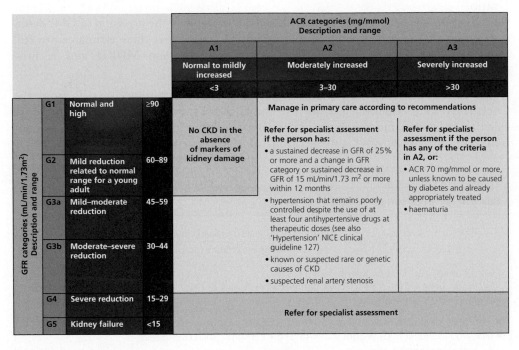

Figure 8.1 Classification of renal impairment. ACR, albumin:creatinine ratio; CKD, chronic kidney disease; GFR, glomerular filtration rate.

Notes

- **Older adults (>65 years) should be assumed to have at least mild renal impairment.** Their serum creatinine may not be raised because they have a smaller muscle mass.
- **Avoid drugs that are nephrotoxic** (e.g. lithium) where renal reserve is limited.

- Be cautious when using drugs that are extensively renally cleared (e.g. sulpiride, amisulpride, lithium).
- Start at a low dose and increase slowly because, in renal impairment, the half-life of a drug and the time for it to reach steady state are often prolonged. Plasma level monitoring may be useful for some drugs.
- Try to avoid long-acting drugs (e.g. depot preparations). Their dose and frequency cannot be easily adjusted should renal function change.
- Prescribe as few drugs as possible. Patients with renal failure take many medications requiring regular review. Interactions and adverse effects can be avoided if fewer drugs are used.
- Monitor the patient for adverse effects. Patients with renal impairment are more likely to experience adverse effects and these may take longer to develop than in healthy patients. Adverse effects such as sedation, confusion and postural hypotension can be more common.
- Be cautious when using drugs with anticholinergic effects, since they may cause urinary retention.
- There are few clinical studies of the use of psychotropic drugs in people with renal impairment. Advice about drug use in renal impairment is often based on knowledge of the drug's pharmacokinetics in healthy patients.
- The effect of renal replacement therapies (e.g. dialysis) on drugs is difficult to predict. See Tables 8.6–8.11 in this chapter. Seek specialist advice.
- Try to avoid drugs known to prolong QTc interval. Electrolyte changes are common in established renal failure so it is probably best to avoid antipsychotic drugs with the greatest risk of QTc prolongation (see Chapter 1).
- Monitor weight carefully. Weight gain predisposes to diabetes, which can contribute to rhabdomyolysis[3] and renal failure. Psychotropic medications commonly cause weight gain.
- Be vigilant for serotonin syndrome with antidepressants, and dystonias and neuroleptic malignant syndrome (NMS) with antipsychotics. The resulting rhabdomyolysis can cause renal failure and there are case reports of rhabdomyolysis occurring with antipsychotics without other symptoms of NMS.[4–6]
- Depression is common in chronic kidney disease but evidence for effectiveness of antidepressants in this condition is lacking.[7,8] In chronic kidney disease, starting some antidepressants at a higher versus a lower dose reduces mortality risk.[9]
- Both schizophrenia and bipolar disorder are associated with an increased risk of chronic kidney disease.[10,11]
- Antipsychotics (e.g. olanzapine, quetiapine) may be associated with acute kidney injury,[12] possibly via their effects on blood pressure and urinary retention but studies are conflicting.[13]
- Mood-stabilising anticonvulsants used in bipolar disorder are associated with an increased rate of chronic kidney disease.[11]

Antipsychotic medications in renal impairment

Recommendations for the use of antipsychotic medications in renal impairment are summarised in Table 8.6.

Antidepressant medications in renal impairment

Recommendations for the use of antidepressant medications in renal impairment are summarised in Table 8.7.

Mood-stabilising medications in renal impairment

Recommendations for the use of mood-stabilising medications in renal impairment are summarised in Table 8.8.

Anxiolytic and hypnotic medications in renal impairment

Recommendations for the use of anxiolytic and hypnotic medications in renal impairment are summarised in Table 8.9.

Table 8.6 Antipsychotic medications in renal impairment

Drug	Comments
Amisulpride[1,4–17]	Primarily renally excreted. 50% excreted unchanged in urine. Limited experience in renal disease. Manufacturer states no data with doses of >50 mg but recommends the following dosing: 50% of dose if GFR is 30–60 mL/min; 33% of dose if GFR is 10–30 mL/min; no recommendations for GFR <10 mL/min so **best avoided in established renal failure**
Aripiprazole[14,15,17–20]	Less than 1% of unchanged aripiprazole renally excreted. Manufacturer states no dose adjustment required in renal failure as pharmacokinetics are similar in healthy and severely renally diseased patients. There is one case report of safe use of oral aripiprazole 5 mg in an 83-year-old man having haemodialysis. Avoid depot formulation – no current experience
Asenapine[15,17,21]	Manufacturer states no dose adjustment required for patients with renal impairment but no experience with use if GFR <15 mL/min. A 5 mg single-dose study in renal impairment suggests that no dose adjustment is needed
Chlorpromazine[14,15,17,22,23]	Less than 1% excreted unchanged in urine. Manufacturer advises avoiding in renal dysfunction. Dosing: GFR 10–50 mL/min, dose as in normal renal function; GFR <10 mL/min, start with a small dose because of an increased risk of anticholinergic, sedative and hypotensive adverse effects. Monitor carefully
Clozapine[15,17,24 27]	Only trace amounts of unchanged clozapine excreted in urine; however there are rare case reports of interstitial nephritis and acute renal failure. Nocturnal enuresis and urinary retention are common adverse effects. Contraindicated by manufacturer in severe renal disease. Anticholinergic, sedative and hypotensive adverse effects occur more frequently in patients with renal disease. Dosing: GFR 10–50 mL/min as in normal renal function but with caution; GFR <10 mL/min start with a low dose and titrate slowly (based on renal expert opinion). Levels are useful to guide dosing. May cause and aggravate diabetes, a common cause of renal disease. Case reports exist of successful continuation after renal transplantation[28]
Flupentixol[14,15,17]	Negligible renal excretion of unchanged flupentixol. Dosing: GFR 10–50 mL/min, dose as in normal renal function; GFR <10 mL/min, start with ¼ to ½ of normal dose and titrate slowly. May cause hypotension and sedation in renal impairment and can accumulate. Manufacturer recommends caution in renal failure. Avoid depot preparations in renal impairment
Haloperidol[5,14,15,17,29,30]	Less than 1% excreted unchanged in urine. Manufacturer advises caution in renal failure. Dosing: GFR 10–50 mL/min, dose as in normal renal function; GFR <10 mL/min, start with a lower dose as can accumulate with repeated dosing. A case report of haloperidol use in renal failure suggests starting at a low dose and increasing slowly. Has been used to treat uraemia-associated nausea in renal failure. Avoid depot preparations in renal impairment
Lurasidone[31]	9% excreted unchanged in urine. Manufacturer recommends dose adjustment if GFR <50 mL/min (starting dose is 18.75 mg/day, maximum 74 mg/day) and avoiding if GFR <15 mL/min. Renal failure has been reported rarely
Olanzapine[4,14,15,17,30,32]	57% of olanzapine is excreted mainly as metabolites (7% excreted unchanged) in urine. Dosing: GFR <50 mL/min, initially 5 mg daily and titrate as necessary. Avoid long-acting preparations in renal impairment unless the oral dose is well tolerated and effective. Manufacturer recommends a lower long-acting injection starting dose of 150 mg 4-weekly in patients with renal impairment. May cause and aggravate diabetes, a common cause of renal disease. Hypothermia has been reported when used in renal failure

(Continued)

Table 8.6 (*Continued*)

Drug	Comments
Paliperidone[14,15,17]	Paliperidone is also a metabolite of risperidone. 59% excreted unchanged in urine. Dosing: GFR 50–80 mL/min, 3 mg daily and increase according to response to max of 6 mg daily; GFR 10–50 mL/min, 1.5 mg daily increasing to 3 mg daily according to response. Use with caution as clearance is reduced by 71% in severe kidney disease. Manufacturer contraindicates oral form if GFR <10 mL/min due to lack of experience, and both depot preparations if GFR <50 mL/min (reduced loading and maintenance doses if GFR 50 to <80 mL/min). There is a single case report of successful paliperidone monthly injection use in a patient with renal failure undergoing haemodialysis[33]
Pimozide[14,15,17]	Less than 1% of pimozide excreted unchanged in urine; dose reductions not usually needed in renal impairment. Dosing: GFR 10–50 mL/min, dose as in normal renal function; GFR <10 mL/min, start at a low dose and increase according to response. Manufacturer cautions in renal failure
Quetiapine[14,15,17,34,35]	Less than 5% of quetiapine excreted unchanged in urine. Plasma clearance reduced by an average of 25% in patients with a GFR <30 mL/min. In patients with GFR of <10 to 50 mL/min start at 25 mg/day and increase in daily increments of 25–50 mg to an effective dose. Two separate case reports (one of thrombotic thrombocytopenic purpura and another of non-NMS rhabdomyolysis), both resulting in acute renal failure with quetiapine, have been published
Risperidone[14,15,17,30,36–38]	Clearance of risperidone and the active metabolite of risperidone is reduced by 60% in patients with moderate to severe renal disease. Dosing: GFR < 50 mL/min, 0.5 mg twice daily for at least 1 week then increasing by 0.5 mg twice daily to 1–2 mg bd. The manufacturer advises caution when using risperidone in renal impairment. The long-acting injection should only be used after titration with oral risperidone as described above. If 2 mg orally is tolerated, 25 mg intramuscularly every 2 weeks can be administered. There is a case report of successful use of risperidone long-acting injection at a dose of 50 mg 2-weekly in a patient on haemodialysis. Another describes the successful use of risperidone in a child with steroid-induced psychosis and nephrotic syndrome
Sulpiride[3,14,15,17,39]	Almost totally renally excreted, with 95% excreted in urine and faeces as unchanged sulpiride. Dosing regime: GFR 30–60 mL/min, give 70% of normal dose; GFR 10–30 mL/min, give 50% of normal dose; GFR <10 mL/min, give 34% of normal dose. There is a case report of renal failure with sulpiride due to diabetic coma and rhabdomyolysis. **Probably best avoided in renal impairment**
Trifluoperazine[17]	Less than 1% excreted unchanged in urine. Dosing: GFR <10–50 mL/min, as for normal renal function – start with a low dose. Very limited data
Ziprasidone[14,30,40,41]	Less than 1% renally excreted unchanged. No dose adjustment needed for GFR >10 mL/min but care needed with using the injection as it contains a renally eliminated excipient (cyclodextrin sodium). Case report of 80 mg twice daily dose used in a patient on haemodialysis who then developed agranulocytosis[42]
Zuclopentixol[14,15,17]	10–20% of unchanged drug and metabolites excreted unchanged in urine. Manufacturer cautions use in renal disease as can accumulate. Dosing: 10–50 mL/min, dose as in normal renal function; GFR <10 mL/min, start with 50% of the dose and titrate slowly. Avoid both depot preparations (acetate and decanoate) in renal impairment

bd, *bis die* (twice a day); GFR, glomerular filtration rate; NMS, neuroleptic malignant syndrome.

Table 8.7 Antidepressant medications in renal impairment[7]

Drug	Comments
Agomelatine[15]	Negligible renal excretion of unchanged agomelatine. No data on use in renal disease. Manufacturer says pharmacokinetics unchanged in small study of 25 mg dose in severe renal impairment but cautions use in moderate or severe renal disease. Nephroprotective effects have been observed in rats[43,44]
Amitriptyline[14,15,17,23,30,45–47]	Less than 2% excreted unchanged in urine; no dose adjustment needed in renal failure. Dose as in normal renal function but start at a low dose and increase slowly. Monitor patient for urinary retention, confusion, sedation and postural hypotension. Has been used to treat pain in those with renal disease. Plasma level or ECG monitoring may be useful
Bupropion (amfebutamone)[14,15,17,23,30,48,49]	0.5% excreted unchanged in urine. Dosing: GFR <50 mL/min, 150 mg once daily. A single-dose study in haemodialysis patients (stage 5 disease) recommended a dose of 150 mg every 3 days. Metabolites may accumulate in renal impairment and clearance is reduced. Elevated levels increase risk of seizures
Citalopram[14,15,17,30,50–55]	Less than 13% of citalopram excreted unchanged in urine. Single-dose studies in mild and moderate renal impairment show no change in the pharmacokinetics of citalopram. Dosing is as for normal renal function; however, use with caution if GFR <10 mL/min due to reduced clearance. The manufacturer does not advise use if GFR <20 mL/min. Renal failure has been reported with citalopram overdose. Citalopram can treat depression in chronic renal failure and improve quality of life. A case report of hyponatraemia has been reported in a renal transplant patient on citalopram
Clomipramine[14,15,17,23,56]	2% of unchanged clomipramine excreted in urine. Dosing: GFR 20–50 mL/min, dose as for normal renal function; GFR <20 mL/min, effects unknown, start at a low dose and monitor patient for urinary retention, confusion, sedation and postural hypotension as accumulation can occur. There is a case report of clomipramine-induced interstitial nephritis and reversible acute renal failure
Desvenlafaxine[7,14,57,58]	45% of desvenlafaxine excreted unchanged in urine. Dosing advice is conflicting. Manufacturer recommends: GFR 30–50 mL/min, 50 mg per day; GFR <30 mL/min, 50 mg every other day. However other authors[7] recommend 25 mg/day in all stages of renal impairment. Half-life is prolonged and desvenlafaxine accumulates as GFR decreases. Urinary retention, delay when starting to pass urine and proteinuria have been reported as adverse effects
Dosulepin[14,17,59] (dothiepin)	56% of mainly active metabolites renally excreted. They have a long half-life and may accumulate, resulting in excessive sedation. Dosing: GFR 20–50 mL/min, dose as for normal renal function; GFR <20 mL/min, start with a small dose and titrate to response. Monitor patient for urinary retention, confusion, sedation and postural hypotension
Doxepin[14,15,17,23]	Less than 1% excreted unchanged in urine. Dosing: GFR 10–50 mL/min, as in normal renal function but monitor patient for urinary retention, confusion, sedation and postural hypotension; GFR <10 mL/min, start with a small dose and increase slowly. Manufacturer advises using with caution. Haemolytic anaemia with renal failure has been reported with doxepin
Duloxetine[14,17,60,61]	Less than 1% excreted unchanged in urine. Manufacturer states no dose adjustment is necessary for GFR >30 mL/min; however, starting at a low dose and increasing slowly is advised. Duloxetine is contraindicated in patients with a GFR <30 mL/min as it can accumulate in chronic kidney disease. Licensed to treat diabetic neuropathic pain and stress incontinence in women. Diabetes is a common cause of renal impairment. There is a case report of acute renal failure with duloxetine. Serotonin syndrome has been reported in a patient with chronic kidney disease on trazodone and duloxetine[62]

CHAPTER 8

(Continued)

Table 8.7 (*Continued*)

Drug	Comments
Escitalopram[14,17,63–65]	8% excreted unchanged in urine. The manufacturer states dosage adjustment is not necessary in patients with mild or moderate renal impairment but caution is advised if GFR <30 mL/min so start with a low dose and increase slowly. A case study of reversible renal tubular defects and another of renal failure have been reported with escitalopram. One study says effective versus placebo in end-stage renal disease
Fluoxetine[8,14,15,17,23,30,66–68]	2.5–5% of fluoxetine and 10% of the active metabolite norfluoxetine excreted unchanged in urine. Dosing: GFR 20–50 mL/min, dose as normal renal function; GFR <20 mL/min, use a low dose or on alternate days and increase according to response. Plasma levels after 2 months treatment with 20 mg (in patients on dialysis with GFR <10 mL/min) are similar to those with normal renal function. Efficacy studies of fluoxetine in depression and renal disease are conflicting. One small placebo-controlled study of fluoxetine in patients on chronic dialysis found no significant differences in depression scores between the two groups after 8 weeks of treatment. Another found fluoxetine effective
Fluvoxamine[14,17,23,30]	2% excreted unchanged in urine. Little information on its use in renal impairment. Manufacturer cautions in renal impairment. Dosing: GFR 10–50 mL/min, dose as for normal renal function; GFR <10 mL/min, as for normal renal function but start on a low dose and titrate slowly. Acute renal failure has been reported
Imipramine[14,15,17,23,45]	Less than 5% excreted unchanged in urine. No specific dose adjustment necessary in renal impairment (GFR <10–50 mL/min). Monitor patient for urinary retention, confusion, sedation and postural hypotension. Renal impairment with imipramine has been reported and manufacturer advises caution in severe renal impairment. Renal damage reported rarely
Lofepramine[14,15,17,69]	There is little information about the use of lofepramine in renal impairment. Less than 5% is excreted unchanged in the urine. Dosing: GFR 10–50 mL/min, dose as in normal renal function; GFR <10 mL/min, start with a small dose and titrate slowly. Manufacturer contraindicates in severe renal impairment
Mirtazapine[14,15,17,70]	75% excreted unchanged in urine. Clearance is reduced by 30% in patients with a GFR of 11–39 mL/min and by 50% in patients with a GFR <10 mL/min. Dosing advice: GFR 10–50 mL/min, dose as for normal renal function; GFR <10 mL/min, start at a low dose and monitor closely. Mirtazapine has been used to treat pruritus caused by renal failure and appetite loss in patients on dialysis.[71] Is associated with kidney calculus formation
Moclobemide[14,15,17,72,73]	Less than 1% of parent drug excreted unchanged in urine. However, an active metabolite was found to be raised in patients with renal impairment but was not thought to affect dosing. The manufacturer advises that dose adjustments are not required in renal impairment. Dosing: GFR <10–50 mL/min, dose as in normal renal function
Nortriptyline[14,17,23,30,45,74]	Less than 5% excreted unchanged in urine. If GFR 10–50 mL/min, dose as in normal renal function; if GFR <10 mL/min, start at a low dose. Plasma level monitoring recommended at doses of >100 mg/day, as plasma concentrations of active metabolites are raised in renal impairment. Worsening of GFR in elderly patients has also been reported. Plasma level monitoring can be useful

Table 8.7 *(Continued)*

Drug	Comments
Paroxetine[14,15,17,23,75–78]	Less than 2% of oral dose excreted unchanged in urine. Single-dose studies show increased plasma concentrations of paroxetine when GFR <30 mL/min. Dosing advice differs: GFR 30–50 mL/min, dose as normal renal function; GFR <10–30 mL/min, start at 10 mg/day (other source says start at 20 mg) and increase dose according to response. Paroxetine 10 mg daily and psychotherapy have been used sucessfully to treat depression in patients on chronic haemodialysis. Rarely associated with Fanconi syndrome and acute renal failure
Phenelzine[14,17]	Approximately 1% excreted unchanged in urine. No dose adjustment required in renal failure
Reboxetine[14,15,17,79,80]	Approximately 10% of unchanged drug excreted unchanged in urine. Dosing: GFR <20 mL/min, 2 mg twice daily, adjusting dose according to response. Half-life is prolonged as renal function decreases
Sertraline[14,15,17,23,81–84]	Less than 0.2% of unchanged sertraline excreted in urine. Pharmacokinetics in renal impairment are unchanged in single-dose studies but no published data on multiple dosing. Dosing is as for normal renal function. Sertraline has been used to treat dialysis-associated hypotension[85] and uraemic pruritus; however, acute renal failure has been reported so it should be used with caution. An RCT (CAST study) of sertraline in kidney disease is ongoing, as is a trial of sertraline versus CBT in patients on haemodialysis (ASCEND study).[86] Another small RCT (ASSertID study) in patients with depression on haemodialysis reported no difference between sertraline and placebo.[87] Has been associated with serotonin syndrome when used in patients on haemodialysis. May reduce CRP in patients on haemodialysis with depression[88]
Trazodone[14,15,17,89]	Less than 5% excreted unchanged in urine but care needed as approximately 70% of active metabolite also excreted. Dosing: GFR 20–50 mL/min, dose as normal renal function; GFR 10–20 mL/min, dose as normal renal function but start with small dose and increase gradually; GFR <10 mL/min, start with small doses and increase gradually. Serotonin syndrome reported in a patient with chronic kidney disease on trazodone and duloxetine[62]
Trimipramine[14,17,23,45,90,91]	No dose reduction required in renal impairment; however, elevated urea, acute renal failure and interstitial nephritis have been reported. As with all tricyclic antidepressants, monitor patient for urinary retention, confusion, sedation and postural hypotension as patients with renal impairment are at increased risk of having these adverse effects
Venlafaxine[14,15,23,92–94]	1–10% excreted unchanged in urine (30% as the active metabolite). Clearance is decreased and half-life prolonged in renal impairment. Dosing advice differs: GFR 30–50 mL/min, dose as in normal renal function or reduce by 50%; GFR 10–30 mL/min, reduce dose by 50% and give tablets once daily; GFR <10 mL/min, reduce dose by 50% and give once daily. Rhabdomyolysis and renal failure have been reported rarely with venlafaxine. Has been used to treat peripheral diabetic neuropathy in haemodialysis patients. High doses may cause hypertension
Vortioxetine[15,95]	Negligible amounts excreted unchanged in urine. Manufacturer advises that no dose adjustment is needed in renal impairment and end-stage disease but advises caution

CBT, cognitive behavioural therapy; CRP, C-reactive protein; ECG, electrocardiogram; GFR, glomerular filtration rate; RCT, randomised controlled trial.

CHAPTER 8

Table 8.8 Mood-stabilising medications in renal impairment

Drug	Comments
Carbamazepine[14,15,17,96–103]	2–3% of dose excreted unchanged in urine. Dose reduction not necessary in renal disease, although cases of renal failure, tubular necrosis and tubulointerstitial nephritis have been reported rarely and metabolites may accumulate. Can cause Stevens–Johnson syndrome and toxic epidermal necrolysis, which may result in acute renal failure. Maintenance therapy in bipolar disorder is associated with an increased rate of chronic kidney disease[11]
Lamotrigine[14,15,17,104–108]	Less than 10% of lamotrigine excreted unchanged in urine. Single-dose studies in renal failure show pharmacokinetics are little affected; however, inactive metabolites can accumulate (effects unknown) and half-life can be prolonged. Renal failure and interstitial nephritis have also been reported. Dosing: GFR <10–50 mL/min, use cautiously, start with a low dose, increase slowly and monitor closely. One source suggests in GFR <10 mL/min use 100 mg every other day
Lithium[14,15,17,23,109,110]	Lithium is nephrotoxic and contraindicated in severe renal impairment; 95% is excreted unchanged in the urine. Long-term treatment may result in impaired renal function ('creatinine creep'), permanent changes in kidney histology, nephrogenetic diabetes insipidus, nephrotic syndrome and both reversible and irreversible kidney damage.[111,112] However, shorter studies in younger populations do not show declining GFR[113] or the development of end-stage renal disease.[11] If lithium is used in renal impairment, toxicity is more likely. Lithium toxicity increases the risk of renal impairment. The manufacturer contraindicates lithium in renal impairment. Dosing: GFR 10–50 mL/min, avoid or reduce dose (50–75% of normal dose) and monitor levels; GFR <10 mL/min, avoid if possible; however if used it is essential to reduce dose (25–50% of normal dose). Renal damage is more likely with chronic toxicity than acute
Valproate[14,15,17,114–120]	Approximately 2% excreted unchanged. Dose adjustment usually not required in renal impairment; however, free valproate levels may be increased. Renal impairment, interstitial nephritis, Fanconi syndrome, renal tubular acidosis and renal failure have been reported. Dose as in normal renal function; however, in severe impairment (GFR <10 mL/min) it may be necessary to alter doses according to free (unbound) valproate levels. May be less likely than lithium to cause chronic kidney disease in patients with bipolar disorder[121]

GFR, glomerular filtration rate.

Table 8.9 Anxiolytic and hypnotic medications in renal impairment

Drug	Comments
Buspirone[14,15,17,23]	Less than 1% is excreted unchanged; however, active metabolite is renally excreted. Dosing advice contradictory, suggest: GFR 10–50 mL/min dose as normal; GFR <10 mL/min, avoid if possible due to accumulation of active metabolites; if essential, reduce dose by 25–50% if patient is anuric. Manufacturer contraindicates in severe renal impairment
Chlordiazepoxide[15,17,23]	1–2% excreted unchanged but chlordiazepoxide has a long-acting active metabolite that can accumulate. Dosing: GFR 10–50 mL/min, dose as normal renal function; GFR <10 mL/min, reduce dose by 50%. Monitor for excessive sedation. Manufacturer cautions in chronic renal disease
Clomethiazole[14,15,17,122] (chlormethiazole)	0.1–5% of unchanged drug excreted unchanged in urine. Dose as in normal renal function but monitor for excessive sedation. Manufacturer recommends caution in renal disease
Clonazepam[14,15,17,123]	Less than 0.5% of clonazepam excreted unchanged in urine. Dose adjustment not required in impaired renal function; however, with long-term administration active metabolites may accumulate so start at a low dose and increase according to response. Monitor for excessive sedation. Has been used for insomnia in patients on haemodialysis
Diazepam[14,17,23,124]	Less than 0.5% excreted unchanged. Dosing: GFR 20–50 mL/min, dose as in normal renal function; GFR <20 mL/min, use small doses and titrate to response. Long-acting, active metabolites accumulate in renal impairment; monitor patients for excessive sedation and encephalopathy. One case of interstitial nephritis with diazepam has been reported in a patient with chronic renal failure
Eszopiclone[125]	Less than 10% excreted unchanged in urine. No dose adjustment is needed in renal impairment
Lorazepam[14,15,17,23,126–131]	Less than 1% excreted unchanged in urine. Dose as in normal renal function but carefully according to response as some may need lower doses. Monitor for excessive sedation. Impaired elimination reported in two patients with severe renal impairment and also reports of propylene glycol in lorazepam injection causing renal impairment and acute tubular necrosis. However lorazepam injection has been successfully used to treat catatonia in two patients with renal failure
Nitrazepam[15,17]	Less than 5% excreted unchanged in urine. Dosing GFR 10–50 mL/min, as per normal renal function; GFR <10 mL/min, start with small dose and increase slowly. Manufacturer advises reducing dose in renal impairment. Monitor patient for sedation
Oxazepam[14,17,23,132]	Less than 1% excreted unchanged in urine. Dose adjustment needed in severe renal impairment. Oxazepam may take longer to reach steady state in patients with renal impairment. Dosing: GFR 10–50 mL/min, dose as in normal renal function; GFR <10 mL/min, start at a low dose and increase according to response. Monitor for excessive sedation
Promethazine[14,15,17,23,133]	Dose reduction usually not necessary; however, promethazine has a long half-life so monitor for excessive sedative effects in patients with renal impairment. Manufacturer advises caution in renal impairment. There is a case report of interstitial nephritis in a patient who was a poor metaboliser of promethazine
Temazepam[14,15,17,23]	Less than 2% excreted unchanged in urine. In renal impairment the inactive metabolite can accumulate. Monitor for excessive sedative effects. Dosing: GFR 20–50 mL/min, dose as normal renal function; GFR <20 mL/min, dose as in normal renal function but start with 5 mg
Zolpidem[14,15,17,123,134]	Clearance moderately reduced in renal impairment. No dose adjustment required in renal impairment. Zolpidem 1 mg has been used to treat insomnia in patients on haemodialysis
Zopiclone[14,15,17,135,136]	Less than 5% excreted unchanged in urine. Manufacturer states no accumulation of zopiclone in renal impairment but suggests starting at 3.75 mg. Dosing: GFR <10 mL/min, start with lower dose. Interstitial nephritis reported rarely

GFR, glomerular filtration rate.

Anti-dementia medications in renal impairment

Recommendations for the use of anti-dementia medications in renal impairment are summarised in Table 8.10.

Table 8.10 Anti-dementia medications in renal impairment

Drug	Comments
Donepezil[15,17,137–139]	17% excreted unchanged in urine. Dosing is as in normal renal function for GFR <10–50 mL/min. Manufacturer states that clearance is not affected by renal impairment. Single-dose studies find similar pharmacokinetics in moderate and severe renal impairment compared with healthy controls. Has been used at a dose of 3 mg/day in an elderly patient with Alzheimer's dementia on dialysis. Single case of rhabdomyolysis causing acute renal failure[140]
Galantamine[15,17]	18–22% excreted unchanged in urine. Dose as in normal renal function for GFR 10–50 mL/min; at GFR <10 mL/min, start at a low dose and increase slowly. Manufacturer contraindicates use in GFR <10 mL/min. Plasma levels may be increased in patients with moderate and severe renal impairment
Memantine[14,15,141]	Manufacturers recommend a 10 mg dose if GFR 5–29 mL/min; 10 mg daily for 7 days then increased to 20 mg daily if tolerated for GFR >30–49 mL/min. Renal tubular acidosis, severe urinary tract infections and alkalisation of urine (e.g. by drastic dietary changes) can increase plasma levels of memantine. Acute renal failure has been reported
Rivastigmine[15,17]	0% excreted unchanged in urine. Dosing advice for GFR <50 mL/min, start at a low dose and gradually increase. Steady state plasma concentrations are not affected by renal function[142]

GFR, glomerular filtration rate.

Summary – psychotropic medications in renal impairment

Where renal function declines while on existing drug treatment, rule out existing drugs as a cause of reduced function and continue at a dose suggested in Tables 8.6, 8.7, 8.8, 8.9 and 8.10. Where new drug treatment is required, follow the suggestions in Table 8.11.

Table 8.11 Recommended psychotropic medications in renal impairment

Drug group	Recommended drugs
Antipsychotics	No agent clearly preferred to another, however: ■ avoid sulpiride and amisulpride ■ avoid highly anticholinergic agents because they can contribute to urinary retention ■ first-generation antipsychotic – suggest **haloperidol** 2–6 mg/day ■ second-generation antipsychotic – suggest **olanzapine** 5 mg/day
Antidepressants	No agent clearly preferred to another, however: ■ **citalopram (care: QTc-prolonging effects)** and **sertraline** are suggested as reasonable choices
Mood stabilisers	No agent clearly preferred to another, however: ■ avoid lithium if possible ■ suggest start one of the following at a low dose, increase slowly and monitor for adverse effects: **valproate**, **carbamazepine** or **lamotrigine**
Anxiolytics and hypnotics	No agent clearly preferred to another, however: ■ excessive sedation is more likely to occur in patients with renal impairment, so monitor all patients carefully ■ **lorazepam** and **zopiclone** are suggested as reasonable choices
Anti-dementia drugs	No agent clearly preferred to another, however: ■ **rivastigmine** is a reasonable choice

References

1. Levey AS et al. A new equation to estimate glomerular filtration rate. Ann Intern Med 2009; **150**:604–612.
2. National Institute for Health and Care Excellence. Chronic kidney disease in adults: assessment and management. Clinical Guideline 182, 2014; last updated January 2015. https://www.nice.org.uk/guidance/cg182.
3. Toprak O et al. New-onset type II diabetes mellitus, hyperosmolar non-ketotic coma, rhabdomyolysis and acute renal failure in a patient treated with sulpiride. Nephrol Dial Transplant 2005; **20**:662–663.
4. Baumgart U et al. Olanzapine-induced acute rhabdomyolysis – a case report. Pharmacopsychiatry 2005; **38**:36–37.
5. Marsh SJ et al. Rhabdomyolysis and acute renal failure during high-dose haloperidol therapy. Ren Fail 1995; **17**:475–478.
6. Smith RP et al. Quetiapine overdose and severe rhabdomyolysis. J Clin Psychopharmacol 2004; **24**:343.
7. Nagler EV et al. Antidepressants for depression in stage 3–5 chronic kidney disease: a systematic review of pharmacokinetics, efficacy and safety with recommendations by European Renal Best Practice (ERBP). Nephrol Dial Transplant 2012; **27**:3736–3745.
8. Palmer SC et al. Antidepressants for treating depression in adults with end-stage kidney disease treated with dialysis. Cochrane Database Syst Rev 2016:Cd004541.
9. Dev V et al. Higher anti-depressant dose and major adverse outcomes in moderate chronic kidney disease: a retrospective population-based study. BMC Nephrol 2014; **15**:79.
10. Tzeng NS et al. Is schizophrenia associated with an increased risk of chronic kidney disease? A nationwide matched-cohort study. BMJ Open 2015; **5**:e006777.
11. Kessing LV et al. Use of lithium and anticonvulsants and the rate of chronic kidney disease: a nationwide population-based study. JAMA Psychiatry 2015; **72**:1182–1191.
12. Jiang Y et al. A retrospective cohort study of acute kidney injury risk associated with antipsychotics. CNS Drugs 2017; **31**:319–326.
13. Ryan PB et al. Atypical antipsychotics and the risks of acute kidney injury and related outcomes among older adults: a replication analysis and an evaluation of adapted confounding control strategies. Drugs Aging 2017; **34**:211–219.
14. Truven Health Analytics. Micromedex 2.0. 2017. https://www.micromedexsolutions.com/home/dispatch.
15. Datapharm Ltd. Electronic Medicines Compendium. 2017. https://www.medicines.org.uk/emc/.
16. Noble S et al. Amisulpride: a review of its clinical potential in dysthymia. CNS Drugs 1999; **12**:471–483.
17. Ashley C, Currie A. *The Renal Drug Handbook*, 4th edn. Oxford: Radcliffe Publishing Ltd; 2014.
18. Aragona M. Tolerability and efficacy of aripiprazole in a case of psychotic anorexia nervosa comorbid with epilepsy and chronic renal failure. Eat Weight Disord 2007; **12**:e54–e57.
19. Mallikaarjun S et al. Effects of hepatic or renal impairment on the pharmacokinetics of aripiprazole. Clin Pharmacokinet 2008; **47**:533–542.
20. Tzeng NS et al. Delusional parasitosis in a patient with brain atrophy and renal failure treated with aripiprazole: case report. Prog Neuropsychopharmacol Biol Psychiatry 2010; **34**:1148–1149.
21. Peeters P et al. Asenapine pharmacokinetics in hepatic and renal impairment. Clin Pharmacokinet 2011; **50**:471–481.
22. Fabre J et al. Influence of renal insufficiency on the excretion of chloroquine, phenobarbital, phenothiazines and methacycline. Helv Med Acta 1967; **33**:307–316.
23. Aronoff GR et al. *Drug Prescribing in Renal Failure: Dosing Guidelines for Adults and Children*, 5th edn. Philadelphia: American College of Physicians; 2007.
24. Fraser D et al. An unexpected and serious complication of treatment with the atypical antipsychotic drug clozapine. Clin Nephrol 2000; **54**:78–80.
25. Au AF et al. Clozapine-induced acute interstitial nephritis. Am J Psychiatry 2004; **161**:1501.
26. Elias TJ et al. Clozapine-induced acute interstitial nephritis. Lancet 1999; **354**:1180–1181.
27. Siddiqui BK et al. Simultaneous allergic interstitial nephritis and cardiomyopathy in a patient on clozapine. NDT Plus 2008; **1**:55–56.
28. Lim AM et al. Clozapine, immunosuppressants and renal transplantation. Asian J Psychiatr 2016; **23**:118.
29. Lobeck F et al. Haloperidol concentrations in an elderly patient with moderate chronic renal failure. J Geriatr Drug Ther 1986; **1**:91–97.
30. Cohen LM et al. Update on psychotropic medication use in renal disease. Psychosomatics 2004; **45**:34–48.
31. Sunovion Pharmaceuticals Europe Ltd. Summary of Product Characteristics. Latuda 18.5 mg, 37 mg and 74 mg film-coated tablets. 2016. https://www.medicines.org.uk/emc/medicine/29125.
32. Kansagra A et al. Prolonged hypothermia due to olanzapine in the setting of renal failure: a case report and review of the literature. Ther Adv Psychopharmacol 2013; **3**:335–339.
33. Samalin L et al. Interest of clozapine and paliperidone palmitate plasma concentrations to monitor treatment in schizophrenic patients on chronic hemodialysis. Schizophr Res 2015; **166**:351–352.
34. Thyrum PT et al. Single-dose pharmacokinetics of quetiapine in subjects with renal or hepatic impairment. Prog Neuropsychopharmacol Biol Psychiatry 2000; **24**:521–533.
35. Huynh M et al. Thrombotic thrombocytopenic purpura associated with quetiapine. Ann Pharmacother 2005; **39**:1346–1348.
36. Snoeck E et al. Influence of age, renal and liver impairment on the pharmacokinetics of risperidone in man. Psychopharmacology (Berl) 1995; **122**:223–229.
37. Herguner S et al. Steroid-induced psychosis in an adolescent: treatment and prophylaxis with risperidone. Turk J Pediatr 2006; **48**:244–247.
38. Batalla A et al. Antipsychotic treatment in a patient with schizophrenia undergoing hemodialysis. J Clin Psychopharmacol 2010; **30**:92–94.
39. Bressolle F et al. Pharmacokinetics of sulpiride after intravenous administration in patients with impaired renal function. Clin Pharmacokinet 1989; **17**:367–373.

CHAPTER 8

40. Aweeka F et al. The pharmacokinetics of ziprasidone in subjects with normal and impaired renal function. Br J Clin Pharmacol 2000; **49**: 27S–33S.

41. Roerig. Highlights of Prescribing Information: GEODON® (ziprasidone HCl) capsules; GEODON® (ziprasidone mesylate) injection for intramuscular use. 2017. http://labeling.pfizer.com/ShowLabeling.aspx?id=584.

42. Iskandar JW et al. Transient agranulocytosis associated with ziprasidone in a 45-year-old man on hemodialysis. J Clin Psychopharmacol 2015; **35**:347–348.

43. Basol N et al. Beneficial effects of agomelatine in experimental model of sepsis-related acute kidney injury. Ulus Travma Acil Cerrahi Derg 2016; **22**:121–126.

44. Karaman A et al. A novel approach to contrast-induced nephrotoxicity: the melatonergic agent agomelatine. Br J Radiol 2016; **89**:20150716.

45. Lieberman JA et al. Tricyclic antidepressant and metabolite levels in chronic renal failure. Clin Pharmacol Ther 1985; **37**:301–307.

46. Mitas JA et al. Diabetic neuropathic pain: control by amitriptyline and fluphenazine in renal insufficiency. South Med J 1983; **76**: 462–463, 467.

47. Murphy EJ. Acute pain management pharmacology for the patient with concurrent renal or hepatic disease. Anaesth Intensive Care 2005; **33**:311–322.

48. Turpeinen M et al. Effect of renal impairment on the pharmacokinetics of bupropion and its metabolites. Br J Clin Pharmacol 2007; **64**: 165–173.

49. Worrall SP et al. Pharmacokinetics of bupropion and its metabolites in haemodialysis patients who smoke. A single dose study. Nephron Clin Pract 2004; **97**:c83–c89.

50. Joffe P et al. Single-dose pharmacokinetics of citalopram in patients with moderate renal insufficiency or hepatic cirrhosis compared with healthy subjects. Eur J Clin Pharmacol 1998; **54**:237–242.

51. Kalender B et al. Antidepressant treatment increases quality of life in patients with chronic renal failure. Ren Fail 2007; **29**:817–822.

52. Kelly CA et al. Adult respiratory distress syndrome and renal failure associated with citalopram overdose. Hum Exp Toxicol 2003; **22**: 103–105.

53. Spigset O et al. Citalopram pharmacokinetics in patients with chronic renal failure and the effect of haemodialysis. Eur J Clin Pharmacol 2000; **56**:699–703.

54. Hosseini SH et al. Citalopram versus psychological training for depression and anxiety symptoms in hemodialysis patients. Iran J Kidney Dis 2012; **6**:446–451.

55. Sran H et al. Confusion after starting citalopram in a renal transplant patient. BMJ Case Rep 2013; **2013**.

56. Onishi A et al. Reversible acute renal failure associated with clomipramine-induced interstitial nephritis. Clin Exp Nephrol 2007; **11**:241–243.

57. Wyeth Pharmaceuticals Inc. Highlights of Prescribing Information. PRISTIQ® (desvenlafaxine) Extended-Release Tablets, for oral use. 2016. http://labeling.pfizer.com/showlabeling.aspx?id=497

58. Nichols AI et al. The pharmacokinetics and safety of desvenlafaxine in subjects with chronic renal impairment. Int J Clin Pharmacol Ther 2011; **49**:3–13.

59. Rees JA. Clinical interpretation of pharmacokinetic data on dothiepin hydrochloride (Dosulepin, Prothiaden). J Int Med Res 1981; **9**:98–102.

60. Lobo ED et al. Effects of varying degrees of renal impairment on the pharmacokinetics of duloxetine: analysis of a single-dose phase I study and pooled steady-state data from phase II/III trials. Clin Pharmacokinet 2010; **49**:311–321.

61. Ho NV et al. Duloxetine-Induced Multi-System Organ Failure: A Case Report. Poster presented at American Geriatrics Society Annual Meeting, May 11–15, 2011: National Harbor, Maryland; 2011.

62. Uong C et al. Poster 91 Serotonin syndrome in chronic kidney disease patient after given a dose of duloxetine while on trazodone: a case report. PM&R 2014; **6 (Suppl)**:S214–S215.

63. Miriyala K et al. Renal failure in a depressed adolescent on escitalopram. J Child Adolesc Psychopharmacol 2008; **18**:405–408.

64. Adiga GU et al. Renal tubular defects from antidepressant use in an older adult: an uncommon but reversible adverse drug effect. Clin Drug Invest 2006; **26**:607–610.

65. Yazici AE et al. Efficacy and tolerability of escitalopram in depressed patients with end stage renal disease: an open placebo-controlled study. Bull Clin Psychopharmacol 2012; **22**:23–30.

66. Bergstrom RF et al. The effects of renal and hepatic disease on the pharmacokinetics, renal tolerance, and risk-benefit profile of fluoxetine. Int Clin Psychopharmacol 1993; **8**:261–266.

67. Blumenfield M et al. Fluoxetine in depressed patients on dialysis. Int J Psychiatry Med 1997; **27**:71–80.

68. Levy NB et al. Fluoxetine in depressed patients with renal failure and in depressed patients with normal kidney function. Gen Hosp Psychiatry 1996; **18**:8–13.

69. Lancaster SG et al. Lofepramine. A review of its pharmacodynamic and pharmacokinetic properties, and therapeutic efficacy in depressive illness. Drugs 1989; **37**:123–140.

70. Davis MP et al. Mirtazapine for pruritus. J Pain Symptom Manage 2003; **25**:288–291.

71. Shibata K et al. SP704 The effect of mirtazapine in dialysis patient with appetite loss. Nephrol Dial Transplant 2015; **30 (Suppl 3)**:iii611.

72. Schoerlin MP et al. Disposition kinetics of moclobemide, a new MAO-A inhibitor, in subjects with impaired renal function. J Clin Pharmacol 1990; **30**:272–284.

73. Stoeckel K et al. Absorption and disposition of moclobemide in patients with advanced age or reduced liver or kidney function. Acta Psychiatr Scand Suppl 1990; **360**:94–97.

74. Pollock BG et al. Metabolic and physiologic consequences of nortriptyline treatment in the elderly. Psychopharmacol Bull 1994; **30**:145–150.

75. Doyle GD et al. The pharmacokinetics of paroxetine in renal impairment. Acta Psychiatr Scand Suppl 1989; 350:89–90.

76. Ishii T et al. A rare case of combined syndrome of inappropriate antidiuretic hormone secretion and Fanconi syndrome in an elderly woman. Am J Kidney Dis 2006; 48:155–158.

77. Kaye CM et al. A review of the metabolism and pharmacokinetics of paroxetine in man. Acta Psychiatr Scand Suppl 1989; 350:60–75.

78. Koo JR et al. Treatment of depression and effect of antidepression treatment on nutritional status in chronic hemodialysis patients. Am J Med Sci 2005; 329:1–5.

79. Coulomb F et al. Pharmacokinetics of single-dose reboxetine in volunteers with renal insufficiency. J Clin Pharmacol 2000; 40:482–487.

80. Dostert P et al. Review of the pharmacokinetics and metabolism of reboxetine, a selective noradrenaline reuptake inhibitor. Eur Neuropsychopharmacol 1997; 7 Suppl 1:S23–S35.

81. Brewster UC et al. Addition of sertraline to other therapies to reduce dialysis-associated hypotension. Nephrology (Carlton) 2003; 8: 296–301.

82. Chan KY et al. Use of sertraline for antihistamine-refractory uremic pruritus in renal palliative care patients. J Palliat Med 2013; 16: 966–970.

83. Chander WP et al. Serotonin syndrome in maintenance haemodialysis patients following sertraline treatment for depression. J Indian Med Assoc 2011; 109:36–37.

84. Jain N et al. Rationale and design of the Chronic Kidney Disease Antidepressant Sertraline Trial (CAST). Contemp Clin Trials 2013; 34:136–144.

85. Razeghi E et al. A randomized crossover clinical trial of sertraline for intradialytic hypotension. Iran J Kidney Dis 2015; 9:323–330.

86. Hedayati SS et al. Rationale and design of A Trial of Sertraline vs. Cognitive Behavioral Therapy for End-stage Renal Disease Patients with Depression (ASCEND). Contemp Clin Trials 2016; 47:1–11.

87. Friedli K et al. Sertraline versus placebo in patients with major depressive disorder undergoing hemodialysis: a randomized, controlled feasibility trial. Clin J Am Soc Nephrol 2017; 12:280–286.

88. Zahed NS et al. Impact of sertraline on serum concentration of CRP in hemodialysis patients with depression. J Renal Inj Prev 2017; 6:65–69.

89. Catanese B et al. A comparative study of trazodone serum concentrations in patients with normal or impaired renal function. Boll Chim Farm 1978; 117:424–427.

90. Leighton JD et al. Trimipramine-induced acute renal failure (Letter). N Z Med J 1986; 99:248.

91. Simpson GM et al. A preliminary study of trimipramine in chronic schizophrenia. Curr Ther Res Clin Exp 1966; 99:248.

92. Troy SM et al. The effect of renal disease on the disposition of venlafaxine. Clin Pharmacol Ther 1994; 56:14–21.

93. Guldiken S et al. Complete relief of pain in acute painful diabetic neuropathy of rapid glycaemic control (insulin neuritis) with venlafaxine HCL. Diabetes Nutr Metab 2004; 17:247–249.

94. Pascale P et al. Severe rhabdomyolysis following venlafaxine overdose. Ther Drug Monit 2005; 27:562–564.

95. Takeda Pharmaceuticals America Inc. Highlights of Prescribing Information. BRINTELLIX (vortioxetine) tablets. 2014. http://us.brintellix.com/.

96. Hegarty J et al. Carbamazepine-induced acute granulomatous interstitial nephritis. Clin Nephrol 2002; 57:310–313.

97. Hogg RJ et al. Carbamazepine-induced acute tubulointerstitial nephritis. J Pediatr 1981; 98:830–832.

98. Imai H et al. Carbamazepine-induced granulomatous necrotizing angiitis with acute renal failure. Nephron 1989; 51:405–408.

99. Jubert P et al. Carbamazepine-induced acute renal failure. Nephron 1994; 66:121.

100. Nicholls DP et al. Acute renal failure from carbamazepine (Letter). Br Med J 1972; 4:490.

101. Tutor-Crespo MJ et al. Relative proportions of serum carbamazepine and its pharmacologically active 10,11-epoxy derivative: effect of polytherapy and renal insufficiency. Ups J Med Sci 2008; 113:171–180.

102. Verrotti A et al. Renal tubular function in patients receiving anticonvulsant therapy: a long-term study. Epilepsia 2000; 41:1432–1435.

103. Hung CC et al. Acute renal failure and its risk factors in Stevens-Johnson syndrome and toxic epidermal necrolysis. Am J Nephrol 2009; 29:633–638.

104. Fervenza FC et al. Acute granulomatous interstitial nephritis and colitis in anticonvulsant hypersensitivity syndrome associated with lamotrigine treatment. Am J Kidney Dis 2000; 36:1034–1040.

105. Fillastre JP et al. Pharmacokinetics of lamotrigine in patients with renal impairment: influence of haemodialysis. Drugs Exp Clin Res 1993; 19:25–32.

106. Schaub JE et al. Multisystem adverse reaction to lamotrigine. Lancet 1994; 344:481.

107. Wootton R et al. Comparison of the pharmacokinetics of lamotrigine in patients with chronic renal failure and healthy volunteers. Br J Clin Pharmacol 1997; 43:23–27.

108. Bansal AD et al. Use of antiepileptic drugs in patients with chronic kidney disease and end stage renal disease. Semin Dial 2015; 28:404–412.

109. Gitlin M. Lithium and the kidney: an updated review. Drug Saf 1999; 20:231–243.

110. Lepkifker E et al. Renal insufficiency in long-term lithium treatment. J Clin Psychiatry 2004; 65:850–856.

111. McKnight RF et al. Lithium toxicity profile: a systematic review and meta-analysis. Lancet 2012; 379:721–728.

112. Shine B et al. Long-term effects of lithium on renal, thyroid, and parathyroid function: a retrospective analysis of laboratory data. Lancet 2015; 386:461–468.

113. Clos S et al. Long-term effect of lithium maintenance therapy on estimated glomerular filtration rate in patients with affective disorders: a population-based cohort study. Lancet Psychiatry 2015; 2:1075–1083.

114. Smith GC et al. Anticonvulsants as a cause of Fanconi syndrome. Nephrol Dial Transplant 1995; 10:543–545.

115. Fukuda Y et al. Immunologically mediated chronic tubulo-interstitial nephritis caused by valproate therapy. Nephron 1996; 72:328–329.

116. Watanabe T et al. Secondary renal Fanconi syndrome caused by valproate therapy. Pediatr Nephrol 2005; 20:814–817.

117. Zaki EL et al. Renal injury from valproic acid: case report and literature review. Pediatr Neurol 2002; 27:318–319.

118. Tanaka H et al. Distal type of renal tubular acidosis after anti-epileptic therapy in a girl with infantile spasms. Clin Exp Nephrol 1999; 3:311–313.
119. Knorr M et al. Fanconi syndrome caused by antiepileptic therapy with valproic acid. Epilepsia 2004; 45:868–871.
120. Rahman MH et al. Acute hemolysis with acute renal failure in a patient with valproic acid poisoning treated with charcoal hemoperfusion. Hemodial Int 2006; 10:256–259.
121. Hayes JF et al. Adverse renal, endocrine, hepatic, and metabolic events during maintenance mood stabilizer treatment for bipolar disorder: a population-based cohort study. PLoS Med 2016; 13:e1002058.
122. Pentikainen PJ et al. Pharmacokinetics of chlormethiazole in healthy volunteers and patients with cirrhosis of the liver. Eur J Clin Pharmacol 1980; 17:275–284.
123. Dashti-Khavidaki S et al. Comparing effects of clonazepam and zolpidem on sleep quality of patients on maintenance hemodialysis. Iran J Kidney Dis 2011; 5:404–409.
124. Sadjadi SA et al. Allergic interstitial nephritis due to diazepam. Arch Intern Med 1987; 147:579.
125. Sunovion Pharmaceuticals Inc. Highlights of Prescribing Information. LUNESTA® (eszopiclone) tablets, for oral use. 2014. https://www.accessdata.fda.gov/drugsatfda_docs/label/2014/021476s030lbl.pdf.
126. Huang CE et al. Intramuscular lorazepam in catatonia in patients with acute renal failure: a report of two cases. Chang Gung Med J 2010; 33:106–109.
127. Reynolds HN et al. Hyperlactatemia, increased osmolar gap, and renal dysfunction during continuous lorazepam infusion. Crit Care Med 2000; 28:1631–1634.
128. Verbeeck RK et al. Impaired elimination of lorazepam following subchronic administration in two patients with renal failure. Br J Clin Pharmacol 1981; 12:749–751.
129. Yaucher NE et al. Propylene glycol-associated renal toxicity from lorazepam infusion. Pharmacotherapy 2003; 23:1094–1099.
130. Zar T et al. Acute kidney injury, hyperosmolality and metabolic acidosis associated with lorazepam. Nat Clin Pract Nephrol 2007; 3:515–520.
131. Hayman M et al. Acute tubular necrosis associated with propylene glycol from concomitant administration of intravenous lorazepam and trimethoprim-sulfamethoxazole. Pharmacotherapy 2003; 23:1190–1194.
132. Murray TG et al. Renal disease, age, and oxazepam kinetics. Clin Pharmacol Ther 1981; 30:805–809.
133. Leung N et al. Acute kidney injury in patients with inactive cytochrome P450 polymorphisms. Ren Fail 2009; 31:749–752.
134. Drover DR. Comparative pharmacokinetics and pharmacodynamics of short-acting hypnosedatives: zaleplon, zolpidem and zopiclone. Clin Pharmacokinet 2004; 43:227–238.
135. Goa KL et al. Zopiclone. A review of its pharmacodynamic and pharmacokinetic properties and therapeutic efficacy as an hypnotic. Drugs 1986; 32:48–65.
136. Hussain N et al. Zopiclone-induced acute interstitial nephritis. Am J Kidney Dis 2003; 41:E17.
137. Suwata J et al. New acetylcholinesterase inhibitor (donepezil) treatment for Alzheimer's disease in a chronic dialysis patient. Nephron 2002; 91:330–332.
138. Nagy CF et al. Steady-state pharmacokinetics and safety of donepezil HCl in subjects with moderately impaired renal function. Br J Clin Pharmacol 2004; 58 Suppl 1:18–24.
139. Tiseo PJ et al. An evaluation of the pharmacokinetics of donepezil HCl in patients with moderately to severely impaired renal function. Br J Clin Pharmacol 1998; 46 Suppl 1:56–60.
140. Sahin OZ et al. A rare case of acute renal failure secondary to rhabdomyolysis probably induced by donepezil. Case Rep Nephrol 2014; 2014:214359.
141. Periclou A et al. Pharmacokinetic study of memantine in healthy and renally impaired subjects. Clin Pharmacol Ther 2006; 79:134–143.
142. Lefevre G et al. Effects of renal impairment on steady-state plasma concentrations of rivastigmine: a population pharmacokinetic analysis of capsule and patch formulations in patients with Alzheimer's disease. Drugs Aging 2016; 33:725–736.

Prescribing in specialist conditions

Chapter 9

Drug treatment of other psychiatric conditions

Borderline personality disorder

Borderline personality disorder (BPD) is common in psychiatric settings with a reported prevalence of up to 20%.[1] In BPD, co-morbid depression, anxiety spectrum disorders and bipolar illness occur more frequently than would be expected by chance association alone, and the lifetime risk of having at least one co-morbid mental disorder approaches 100%.[2] The suicide rate in BPD is similar to that seen in affective disorders and schizophrenia.[3,4]

Although it is classified as a personality disorder, several symptoms of BPD may intuitively be expected to respond to drug treatment. These include affective instability, transient stress-related psychotic symptoms, suicidal and self-harming behaviours, and impulsivity.[4] A high proportion of people with BPD are prescribed psychotropic drugs,[2,5,6] often in polypharmacy regimes.[7,8]. Indeed a recent survey of prescribing practice across England found that over 90% of patients with BPD had been prescribed psychotropic medication, most commonly antidepressants or antipsychotics, particularly for affective instability.[6] The prevalence of prescribing of antipsychotics, antidepressants and mood stabilisers in those with BPD as a sole psychiatric diagnosis is not notably different than in those with BPD and a co-morbid diagnosis of schizophrenia, depression or bipolar disorder, respectively.[6] No drug is specifically licensed for the treatment of BPD.

In 2009 NICE[9] recommended that:

- Drug treatment should not be used routinely for BPD or for the individual symptoms or behaviour associated with the disorder (e.g. repeated self-harm, marked emotional instability, risk-taking behaviour and transient psychotic symptoms).
- Drug treatment may be considered in the overall treatment of co-morbid conditions.
- Short-term use of sedative medication may be considered as part of the overall treatment plan for people with BPD in a crisis. The duration of treatment should be agreed with them but should be no longer than one week.

The Maudsley Prescribing Guidelines in Psychiatry, Thirteenth Edition. David M. Taylor, Thomas R. E. Barnes and Allan H. Young.
© 2018 David M. Taylor. Published 2018 by John Wiley & Sons Ltd.

NICE guidelines were last reviewed in January 2015, when no changes were recommended.[10]

Soon after the publication of the NICE guideline for BPD, two further independent systematic reviews were published.[11,12] Essentially the same studies were considered in all three reviews, and where numerical data were combined in meta-analyses the results of these analyses were similar across all three systematic reviews. In addition, all noted that the majority of studies of drug treatment in BPD last for only 6 weeks and that the large number of different outcome measures that were used made it difficult to evaluate and compare studies.

NICE considered that the data were not robust enough to be the basis for recommendations to the NHS while the other two reviews concluded that some of the analyses showed promising results and that these were sufficiently robust to inform clinical practice. The most recent systematic review[13] updated the previous analyses by including 15 studies published between 2010 and 2017. Conclusions were little different from the earlier NICE review – that the body of evidence was insufficient to make clear clinical recommendations.

Antipsychotic medications

Open studies have found benefit for a number of first- and second-generation antipsychotic medications over a wide range of symptoms. In contrast, placebo-controlled randomised controlled trials (RCTs) generally show more modest benefits for active drug over placebo. The symptoms/symptom clusters that may respond are affect dysregulation, impulsivity and cognitive–perceptual symptoms.[11,12,14,15] Olanzapine may have the most robust effect[13,16,17] but its effect is modest, at best.[13] Open studies report reductions in aggression and self-harming behaviour with clozapine,[18–21] and clozapine has been shown to have an anti-aggressive effect in people with schizophrenia.[22] Clozapine seems to reduce the risk of hospital admission in BPD.[23]

Antipsychotic medications are associated with a wide range of adverse effects and trial dropouts are common.[13]

Antidepressant medications

Several open studies have found that selective serotonin reuptake inhibitors (SSRIs) reduce impulsivity and aggression in BPD, but these findings have not been replicated in RCTs. It can be concluded with reasonable certainty that there is no robust evidence to support the use of antidepressants in treating depressed mood or impulsivity in people with BPD.[11,12]

Mood-stabilising medications

Up to a half of people with BPD may be also be diagnosed with bipolar spectrum disorder[24] (although such diagnoses are rather controversial) and mood stabilisers are commonly prescribed.[2] There is some evidence that mood stabilisers reduce impulsivity, anger and affect dysregulation in people with BPD.[11,12] Lithium is licensed for the control of aggressive behaviour or intentional self-harm.[25] A large RCT of lamotrigine is complete and awaits publication.[26,27]

Opioid antagonists

Very limited evidence supports the efficacy of naltrexone in reducing self-harm and dissociative symptoms.[13,28]

Management of crisis

Drug treatments are often used during periods of crisis when 'symptoms' can be severe, distressing and potentially life-threatening. By their very nature, these symptoms can be expected to wax and wane.[3] Consequently, drug therapy may be required intermittently and on each episode the decision to prescribe needs to be informed by a careful consideration of the relative harms versus benefits of medication. It is generally easy to see when treatment is required, but much more difficult to decide when modest gains are worthwhile and whether or not continuation is likely to be necessary.

NICE[9] recommend that, during periods of crisis, time-limited treatment with a sedative drug may be helpful. Anticipated adverse-effect profile and potential toxicity in overdose should guide choice. For example, benzodiazepines (particularly short-acting drugs) can cause disinhibition in this group of patients,[29] potentially compounding problems; sedative antipsychotics can cause extrapyramidal symptoms (EPS) and/or considerable weight gain, and tricyclic antidepressants are particularly toxic in overdose. A sedative antihistamine such as promethazine (25–50 mg) is usually well tolerated and may be a helpful short-term treatment when used as part of a co-ordinated care plan. Its adverse effects (dry mouth, constipation) and lack of clear anxiolytic effects may militate against longer-term use.

References

1. Kernberg OF et al. Borderline personality disorder. Am J Psychiatry 2009; **166**:505–508.
2. Pascual JC et al. A naturalistic study of changes in pharmacological prescription for borderline personality disorder in clinical practice: from APA to NICE guidelines. Int Clin Psychopharmacol 2010; **25**:349–355.
3. Links PS et al. Prospective follow-up study of borderline personality disorder: prognosis, prediction of outcome, and Axis II comorbidity. Can J Psychiatry 1998; **43**:265–270.
4. Oldham JM. Guideline Watch: Practice Guideline for the Treatment of Patients With Borderline Personality Disorder. Focus 2005; **3**:396–400.
5. Baker-Glenn E et al. Use of psychotropic medication among psychiatric out-patients with personality disorder. The Psychiatrist 2010; **34**:83–86.
6. Paton C. Prescribing for people with emotionally unstable personality disorder under the care of UK mental health services. J Clin Psychiatry 2015; **76**: e512–e518.
7. Paolini E et al. Pharmacological treatment of borderline personality disorder: a retrospective observational study at inpatient unit in Italy. Int J Psychiatry Clin Pract 2017; **21**:75–79.
8. Martin-Blanco A et al. Changes over the last 15 years in the psychopharmacological management of persons with borderline personality disorder. Acta Psychiatr Scand 2017; **136**:323–331.
9. National Institute for Health and Care Excellence. Borderline personality disorder: recognition and management. Clinical Guideline 78, 2009. https://www.nice.org.uk/guidance/cg78.
10. National Institute for Health and Care Excellence. Centre for Clinical Practice – Surveillance Programme: Recommendation for Guidance Executive. Clinical guideline CG78: Borderline personality disorder: Treatment and management. 2015. https://www.nice.org.uk/guidance/CG78/documents/cg78-borderline-personality-disorder-bpd-surveillance-review-decision-january-20153.
11. Lieb K et al. Pharmacotherapy for borderline personality disorder: Cochrane systematic review of randomised trials. Br J Psychiatry 2010; **196**:4–12.

12. Ingenhoven T et al. Effectiveness of pharmacotherapy for severe personality disorders: meta-analyses of randomized controlled trials. J Clin Psychiatry 2010; 71:14–25.

13. Hancock-Johnson E et al. A focused systematic review of pharmacological treatment for borderline personality disorder. CNS Drugs 2017; 31:345–356.

14. Zanarini MC et al. A dose comparison of olanzapine for the treatment of borderline personality disorder: a 12-week randomized, double-blind, placebo-controlled study. J Clin Psychiatry 2011; 72:1353–1362.

15. Canadian Agency for Drugs and Technologies in Health. Aripiprazole for Borderline Personality Disorder: A Review of the Clinical Effectiveness. 2017. https://www.ncbi.nlm.nih.gov/pubmedhealth/PMH0096409/.

16. Shafti S et al. A comparative study on olanzapine and aripiprazole for symptom management in female patients with borderline personality disorder. Bull Clin Psychopharm 2015; 25:38–43.

17. Bozzatello P et al. Efficacy and tolerability of asenapine compared with olanzapine in borderline personality disorder: an open-label randomized controlled trial. CNS Drugs 2017; 31:809–819.

18. Benedetti F et al. Low-dose clozapine in acute and continuation treatment of severe borderline personality disorder. J Clin Psychiatry 1998; 59:103–107.

19. Frogley C et al. A case series of clozapine for borderline personality disorder. Ann Clin Psychiatry 2013; 25:125–134.

20. Chengappa KN et al. Clozapine reduces severe self-mutilation and aggression in psychotic patients with borderline personality disorder. J Clin Psychiatry 1999; 60:477–484.

21. Dickens GL et al. Experiences of women in secure care who have been prescribed clozapine for borderline personality disorder. Borderline Personal Disord Emot Dysregul 2016; 3:12.

22. Volavka J et al. Heterogeneity of violence in schizophrenia and implications for long-term treatment. Int J Clin Pract 2008; 62:1237–1245.

23. Rohde C et al. Real-world effectiveness of clozapine for borderline personality disorder: results from a 2-year mirror-image study. J Pers Disord 2017:1–15.

24. Deltito J et al. Do patients with borderline personality disorder belong to the bipolar spectrum? J Affect Disord 2001; 67:221–228.

25. Sanofi. Summary of Product Characteristics. Priadel 400mg prolonged release tablets. 2015. https://www.medicines.org.uk/emc/product/2753.

26. Crawford MJ et al. Lamotrigine versus inert placebo in the treatment of borderline personality disorder: study protocol for a randomized controlled trial and economic evaluation. Trials 2015; 16:308.

27. National Institute of Health Research. The clinical and cost effectiveness of lamotrigine for people with borderline personality disorder: Randomised controlled trial. 2013. https://www.journalslibrary.nihr.ac.uk/programmes/hta/1010301#/documentation.

28. Moghaddas A et al. The potential role of naltrexone in borderline personality disorder. Iran J Psychiatry 2017; 12:142–146.

29. Gardner DL et al. Alprazolam-induced dyscontrol in borderline personality disorder. Am J Psychiatry 1985; 142:98–100.

Eating disorders

Eating disorders are increasingly common, especially in children and adolescents.[1,2] Lifetime prevalence is 1% for anorexia nervosa, 2% for bulimia and 4% for binge eating disorder (rates for women are about three to ten times higher than for men).[3] There are many similarities between the different types of eating disorders and patients often traverse diagnoses, which can complicate treatment.[4] Other psychiatric conditions (particularly anxiety, depression and obsessive compulsive disorder) often coexist with eating disorders and this may in part explain the benefit sometimes seen with medication.

Anorexia nervosa carries considerable risk of mortality or serious physical morbidity. Patients may present with multiple physical conditions including amenorrhoea, muscle wasting, electrolyte abnormalities, cardiovascular complications and osteoporosis. Patients who purge through vomiting are at high risk of loss of tooth enamel, gastro-oesophageal erosion and dehydration.[4] Other modes of purging include laxative and diuretic misuse.

Any medicine prescribed should be accompanied by close monitoring to check for possible adverse reactions.

Anorexia nervosa

General guidance

There are few controlled trials to guide treatment with medicines for anorexia nervosa. Prompt weight restoration to a safe weight, family therapy and structured psychotherapy are the main interventions.[2,5] The aim of (physical) treatment is to improve nutritional health through re-feeding; there is very limited evidence for the use of any pharmacological interventions other than those prescribed to correct metabolic deficiencies. Medicines may be used to treat co-morbid conditions[2] but have a very limited role in weight restoration.[6] Olanzapine is the only one suggested to have any effect on weight restoration in anorexia nervosa,[7–9] and is a promising, if unlicensed, treatment. Early data for quetiapine were encouraging[10] but were not replicated in a later RCT.[11] Overall, the body of evidence for pharmacotherapy (41 studies by 2016) is said to be 'unsatisfactory'[12] and a meta-analysis found no significant effect over placebo.[13] A network meta-analysis is planned.[14]

Dronabinol, a synthetic cannabinoid agonist, may induce slight weight gain[15] but remains an experimental treatment.

Psychopharmacological studies in anorexia nervosa have a number of shortcomings including small sample sizes and a focus on weight rather than changes in psychopathology. The use of medicines to restore weight in anorexia nervosa is thus controversial; behavioural interventions are preferred.

Health-care professionals should be aware of the risk of medicines that prolong the QT interval. All patients with a diagnosis of anorexia nervosa should have an alert placed in their prescribing record noting that they are at increased risk of arrhythmias secondary to electrolyte disturbances and potential cardiac complications associated with inadequate nutrition. Electrocardiogram (ECG) monitoring should be undertaken if the prescription of any medicine that may compromise cardiac functioning is essential.[2] Caution is also necessary because of low body weight and possibly reduced hepatic function. When olanzapine is used, the starting dose should be 1.25 mg.

Physical aspects

Vitamins and minerals

Treatment with a multivitamin/multimineral supplement in oral form is recommended during both in-patient and out-patient weight restoration[2] (in the UK, Forceval or Sanatogen Gold one capsule daily may be used).

Electrolytes

Electrolyte disturbances (e.g. hypokalaemia) may develop slowly over time and may be asymptomatic and resolve with re-feeding. Hypophosphataemia may also be precipitated by re-feeding. Rapid correction may be hazardous. Oral supplementation is therefore used to prevent serious sequelae rather than simply to restore normal levels. If supplements are used, urea and electrolytes, bicarbonate, calcium, phosphorus and magnesium need to be monitored and an ECG needs to be performed.[16]

Osteoporosis

Bone loss is a serious complication of anorexia with serious consequences. Hormonal treatment using oestrogen or dehydroepiandrosterone (DHEA) does not have a positive impact on bone density and oestrogen is not recommended in children and adolescents due to the risk of premature fusion of the bones.[2] Antipsychotic drugs that raise prolactin levels can further increase the risk of bone loss and osteoporosis. Bisphosphonates are not generally recommended for women with anorexia nervosa due to the lack of data about both the benefits and also safety; they are not licensed for use in pre-menopausal girls.

Psychiatric aspects

Acute illness: antidepressants

A Cochrane review found no evidence from four placebo-controlled trials that antidepressants improved weight gain, eating disorder or associated psychopathology.[17] It has been suggested that neurochemical abnormalities in starvation may partially explain this non-response.[17] Co-prescribing nutritional supplementation (including tryptophan) with fluoxetine has not been shown to increase efficacy.[18] NICE found little evidence to support the use of antidepressants.[2] Naturalistic studies suggest an important risk of switch to mania.[19]

Other psychotropic medicines

Antipsychotics (e.g. olanzapine), minor tranquillisers or antihistamines (e.g. promethazine) are often used to reduce the high levels of anxiety associated with anorexia nervosa but they are not usually recommended for the promotion of weight gain.[2] Case reports and retrospective studies have suggested that olanzapine may reduce agitation (and possibly improve weight gain).[20,21] One RCT[8] showed that 87.5% of patients given olanzapine achieved weight restoration (55.6% placebo). Quetiapine may improve psychological symptoms but there are few data.[10] Only prolactin-sparing antipsychotics should be considered. Pooled effects of antipsychotics on weight are statistically non-existent.[13]

Many other medications[6] have been investigated in small placebo-controlled trials of varying quality and success; these include zinc,[22] naltrexone[23] and cyproheptadine.[24]

Relapse prevention

There is evidence from one small trial that fluoxetine may be useful in improving outcome and preventing relapse of patients with anorexia nervosa after weight restoration.[25] Other studies have found no benefit.[17,26] SSRIs can, albeit very rarely, elevate prolactin.

Co-morbid disorders

Antidepressants are often used to treat co-morbid major depressive disorder and obsessive compulsive disorder. However, caution should be used as these conditions may resolve with weight gain alone.[2]

Bulimia nervosa and binge eating disorder

Psychological interventions should be considered first-line treatment for bulimia.[27] Adults with bulimia nervosa (BN) and binge eating disorder (BED) may be offered a trial of an antidepressant. SSRIs (specifically fluoxetine[28–30]) are the antidepressants of first choice. The effective dose of fluoxetine is 60 mg daily.[31] Patients should be informed that this can reduce the frequency of binge eating and purging but long-term effects are unknown.[2] Early response (at 3 weeks) is a strong predictor of response overall.[32]

Antidepressants may be used for the treatment of bulimia nervosa in adolescents but they are not licensed for this age group and there is little evidence for this practice. They should not be considered as a first-line treatment in adolescent bulimia nervosa.[2]

There is some reasonable evidence that topiramate reduces the frequency of binge eating[33] and limited evidence for the usefulness of bupropion,[34] duloxetine,[35] lamotrigine,[36,37] zonisamide,[38,39] acamprosate[40] and sodium oxybate.[41] Systematic reviews[42,43] confirm the efficacy of SSRIs and also suggest benefit for lisdexamfetamine (based on a high-quality RCT[44]). Lisdexamfetamine is approved for BED in the USA.[45] It is not, at the time of writing, approved elsewhere. The starting dose is usually 30 mg daily, the maintenance dose 50–70 mg daily.

Other atypical eating disorders

There have been no studies of the use of medicines to treat atypical eating disorders other than anorexia nervosa, BN and BED.[2,46] Other eating disorders officially recognised are: avoidant/restrictive food intake disorder (ARFID), pica, rumination disorder, other specified feeding or eating disorder (OSFED) and unspecified feeding or eating disorder (UFED). There are no pharmacological RCTs in these conditions. In the absence of evidence to guide the management of other atypical eating disorders, it is recommended that the clinician considers following the guidance of the eating disorder that mostly resembles the individual patient's eating disorder.[2]

NICE guidance on eating disorders is summarised in Box 9.1.

CHAPTER 9

Box 9.1 Summary of NICE guidance on eating disorders[2]

Anorexia nervosa
- Psychological interventions are the treatments of choice and should be accompanied by monitoring of the patient's physical state.
- No pharmacological intervention is recommended although olanzapine is best supported. A range of medicines may be used in the treatment of co-morbid conditions.

Bulimia nervosa
- An evidence-based self-help programme or cognitive behavioural therapy for bulimia nervosa should be the first choice of treatment.
- A trial of fluoxetine may be offered as an alternative or additional first step.

Binge eating disorder
- An evidence-based self-help programme or cognitive behavioural therapy for binge eating disorder should be the first choice of treatment.
- A trial of an SSRI can be considered as an alternative or additional first step.
- Lisdexamfetamine is also an option.

References

1. Zeiler M et al. Prevalence of eating disorder risk and associations with health-related quality of life: results from a large school-based population screening. Eur Eating Disord Rev 2016; 24:9–18.
2. National Institute for Health and Care Excellence. Eating disorders: recognition and treatment. NICE guideline 69, 2017. https://www.nice.org.uk/guidance/ng69.
3. Keski-Rahkonen A et al. Epidemiology of eating disorders in Europe: prevalence, incidence, comorbidity, course, consequences, and risk factors. Curr Opin Psychiatry 2016; 29:340–345.
4. Steffen KJ et al. Emerging drugs for eating disorder treatment. Expert Opin Emerg Drugs 2006; 11:315–336.
5. American Psychiatric Association. Treatment of patients with eating disorders, third edition. Am J Psychiatry 2006; 163:4–54.
6. Crow SJ et al. What potential role is there for medication treatment in anorexia nervosa? Int J Eat Disord 2009; 42:1–8.
7. Dunican KC et al. The role of olanzapine in the treatment of anorexia nervosa. Ann Pharmacother 2007; 41:111–115.
8. Bissada H et al. Olanzapine in the treatment of low body weight and obsessive thinking in women with anorexia nervosa: a randomized, double-blind, placebo-controlled trial. Am J Psychiatry 2008; 165:1281–1288.
9. Leggero C et al. Low-dose olanzapine monotherapy in girls with anorexia nervosa, restricting subtype: focus on hyperactivity. J Child Adolesc Psychopharmacol 2010; 20:127–133.
10. Court A et al. Investigating the effectiveness, safety and tolerability of quetiapine in the treatment of anorexia nervosa in young people: a pilot study. J Psychiatr Res 2010; 44:1027–1034.
11. Powers PS et al. Double-blind placebo-controlled trial of quetiapine in anorexia nervosa. Eur Eat Disord Rev 2012; 20:331–334.
12. Miniati M et al. Psychopharmacological options for adult patients with anorexia nervosa. CNS Spectr 2016; 21:134–142.
13. de Vos J et al. Meta analysis on the efficacy of pharmacotherapy versus placebo on anorexia nervosa. J Eat Disord 2014; 2:27.
14. Wade TD et al. Comparative efficacy of pharmacological and non-pharmacological interventions for the acute treatment of adult outpatients with anorexia nervosa: study protocol for the systematic review and network meta-analysis of individual data. J Eat Disord 2017; 5:24.
15. Andries A et al. Dronabinol in severe, enduring anorexia nervosa: a randomized controlled trial. Int J Eat Disord 2014; 47:18–23.
16. Connan F et al. Biochemical and endocrine complications. Eur Eat Disord Rev 2000; 8:144–157.
17. Claudino AM et al. Antidepressants for anorexia nervosa. Cochrane Database Syst Rev 2006:CD004365.
18. Barbarich NC et al. Use of nutritional supplements to increase the efficacy of fluoxetine in the treatment of anorexia nervosa. Int J Eat Disord 2004; 35:10–15.
19. Rossi G et al. Pharmacological treatment of anorexia nervosa: a retrospective study in preadolescents and adolescents. Clin Pediatr (Phila) 2007; 46:806–811.
20. Malina A et al. Olanzapine treatment of anorexia nervosa: a retrospective study. Int J Eat Disord 2003; 33:234–237.
21. La Via MC et al. Case reports of olanzapine treatment of anorexia nervosa. Int J Eat Disord 2000; 27:363–366.
22. Su JC et al. Zinc supplementation in the treatment of anorexia nervosa. Eat Weight Disord 2002; 7:20–22.
23. Marrazzi MA et al. Naltrexone use in the treatment of anorexia nervosa and bulimia nervosa. Int Clin Psychopharmacol 1995; 10:163–172.
24. Halmi KA et al. Anorexia nervosa. Treatment efficacy of cyproheptadine and amitriptyline. Arch Gen Psychiatry 1986; 43:177–181.
25. Kaye WH et al. Double-blind placebo-controlled administration of fluoxetine in restricting- and restricting-purging-type anorexia nervosa. Biol Psychiatry 2001; 49:644–652.
26. Walsh BT et al. Fluoxetine after weight restoration in anorexia nervosa: a randomized controlled trial. JAMA 2006; 295:2605–2612.

27. Vocks S et al. Meta-analysis of the effectiveness of psychological and pharmacological treatments for binge eating disorder. Int J Eat Disord 2010; **43**:205–217.

28. Fluoxetine in the treatment of bulimia nervosa. A multicenter, placebo-controlled, double-blind trial. Fluoxetine Bulimia Nervosa Collaborative Study Group. Arch Gen Psychiatry 1992; **49**:139–147.

29. Goldstein DJ et al. Long-term fluoxetine treatment of bulimia nervosa. Fluoxetine Bulimia Nervosa Research Group. Br J Psychiatry 1995; **166**:660–666.

30. Romano SJ et al. A placebo-controlled study of fluoxetine in continued treatment of bulimia nervosa after successful acute fluoxetine treatment. Am J Psychiatry 2002; **159**:96–102.

31. Bacaltchuk J et al. Antidepressants versus placebo for people with bulimia nervosa. Cochrane Database Syst Rev 2003:CD003391.

32. Sysko R et al. Early response to antidepressant treatment in bulimia nervosa. Psychol Med 2010; **40**:999–1005.

33. Arbaizar B et al. Efficacy of topiramate in bulimia nervosa and binge-eating disorder: a systematic review. Gen Hosp Psychiatry 2008; **30**:471–475.

34. White MA et al. Bupropion for overweight women with binge-eating disorder: a randomized, double-blind, placebo-controlled trial. J Clin Psychiatry 2013; **74**:400–406.

35. Leombruni P et al. Duloxetine in obese binge eater outpatients: preliminary results from a 12-week open trial. Hum Psychopharmacol 2009; **24**:483–488.

36. Guerdjikova AI et al. Lamotrigine in the treatment of binge-eating disorder with obesity: a randomized, placebo-controlled monotherapy trial. Int Clin Psychopharmacol 2009; **24**:150–158.

37. Trunko ME et al. A pilot open series of lamotrigine in DBT-treated eating disorders characterized by significant affective dysregulation and poor impulse control. Borderline Personal Disord Emot Dysregul 2017; **4**:21.

38. Ricca V et al. Zonisamide combined with cognitive behavioral therapy in binge eating disorder: a one-year follow-up study. Psychiatry (Edgmont) 2009; **6**:23–28.

39. Guerdjikova AI et al. Zonisamide in the treatment of bulimia nervosa: an open-label, pilot, prospective study. Int J Eat Disord 2013; **46**:747–750.

40. McElroy SL et al. Acamprosate in the treatment of binge eating disorder: a placebo-controlled trial. Int J Eat Disord 2011; **44**:81–90.

41. McElroy SL et al. Sodium oxybate in the treatment of binge eating disorder: an open-label, prospective study. Int J Eat Disord 2011; **44**:262–268.

42. Brownley KA et al. Binge-eating disorder in adults: a systematic review and meta-analysis. Ann Intern Med 2016; **165**:409–420.

43. Peat CM et al. Comparative effectiveness of treatments for binge-eating disorder: systematic review and network meta-analysis. Eur Eating Disord Rev 2017; **25**:317–328.

44. McElroy SL et al. Efficacy and safety of lisdexamfetamine for treatment of adults with moderate to severe binge-eating disorder: a randomized clinical trial. JAMA Psychiatry 2015; **72**:235–246.

45. Citrome L. Lisdexamfetamine for binge eating disorder in adults: a systematic review of the efficacy and safety profile for this newly approved indication – what is the number needed to treat, number needed to harm and likelihood to be helped or harmed? Int J Clin Pract 2015; **69**:410–421.

46. Leombruni P et al. A 12 to 24 weeks pilot study of sertraline treatment in obese women binge eaters. Hum Psychopharmacol 2006; **21**:181–188.

Further reading

Himmerich H et al. Psychopharmacological advances in eating disorders. Expert review of clinical pharmacology 2018; **11**:95–108.

Bello NT et al. Safety of pharmacotherapeutic options for bulimia nervosa and binge eating disorder. Expert Opin Drug Safety 2018; **17**:17–23.

Delirium

Delirium is a common neuropsychiatric condition that presents in medical and surgical settings and is known by various names including organic brain syndrome, intensive care psychosis and acute confusional state.[1]

Diagnostic criteria for delirium[2]

- **Disturbance of consciousness** (reduced clarity of awareness of the environment) with reduced ability to focus, sustain or shift attention.
- A **change in cognition** (such as memory deficit, disorientation, language disturbance or perceptual disturbance) not better explained by a pre-existing or evolving dementia.
- The disturbance develops over a **short period of time** (usually hours to days) and tends to fluctuate over the course of the day.
- There is often evidence from the history, physical examination or laboratory findings that the disturbance is due to concomitant medications, a medical condition, substance intoxication or substance withdrawal.

Tools for evaluation[3]

A brief cognitive assessment should be included in the examination of patients at risk of delirium. A standardised tool, the Confusion Assessment Method (CAM), is a brief, validated algorithm currently used to diagnose delirium. CAM relies on the presence of acute onset of symptoms, fluctuating course, inattention and either disorganised thinking or an altered level of consciousness.

Clinical subtypes of delirium[4-6]

- **Hyperactive delirium:** characterised by increased motor activity with agitation, hallucinations and inappropriate behaviour.
- **Hypoactive delirium:** characterised by reduced motor activity and lethargy (has a poorer prognosis).
- **Mixed delirium:** features of both increased and reduced motor activity.

Prevalence

Delirium is present in 10% of hospitalised medical patients and a further 10–30% develop delirium after admission.[4] Postoperative delirium occurs in 15–53% of patients and in 70–87% of those in intensive care.[7]

Risk factors

Delirium is almost invariably multifactorial and it is often impossible to isolate a single precipitant as the cause.[4] The most important risk factors[4,5,8,9] have consistently emerged as:

- prior cognitive impairment or dementia
- older age (>65 years)
- multiple co-morbidities
- previous history of delirium, stroke, neurological disease, falls or gait disorder

- psychoactive drug use
- polypharmacy (>4 medications)
- anticholinergic drug use.

Outcome

Patients with delirium have an increased length of hospital stay, increased mortality and increased risk of long-term institutional placement.[1,5] Hospital mortality rates of patients with delirium range from 6% to 18% and are twice that of matched controls.[5] In older people, the 1-year mortality rate associated with cases of delirium is 35–40%.[7] Up to 60% of individuals suffer persistent cognitive impairment following delirium and these patients are also three times more likely to develop dementia.[1,5]

Management

Preventing delirium is the most effective strategy for reducing its frequency and complications.[7] Delirium is a medical emergency and the identification and treatment of the underlying cause should be the first aim of management.[10]

Non-pharmacological or environmental support strategies should be instituted wherever possible. These include co-ordinating nursing care, preventing sensory deprivation and disorientation, and maintaining competence.[5,11] Pharmacological treatment should be directed first at the underlying cause (if known) and then at the relief of specific symptoms of delirium.

The common errors in the pharmacological management of delirium are to use antipsychotic medications in excessive doses, to give them too late or to over-use benzodiazepines.[4]

General principles of delirium management[4,5,12–14]

- Keep the use of sedatives and antipsychotic medications to a minimum.
- Use one drug at a time.
- Tailor doses according to age, body size and degree of agitation.
- Titrate doses to effect.
- Use small doses regularly, rather than large doses less frequently.
- Review at least every 24 hours.
- Increase scheduled doses if regular 'as needed' doses are required after the initial 24-hour period.
- Maintain at an effective dose and discontinue 7–10 days after symptoms resolve.
- Ensure that the diagnosis of delirium is documented both in the patient's hospital notes and in their primary health record (include in discharge letter or summary).

Choice of drug[15,16]

High-quality trials of pharmacological treatments for delirium are lacking, with available studies often comprising heterogeneous populations and clinical outcomes, and producing conflicting results. There is insufficient evidence to recommend any single drug treatment over others. Different patient populations may derive less benefit from antipsychotic treatment (e.g. those in palliative care[17]). Treatment choice should therefore be informed by the likelihood of interaction with coexisting medical conditions or other medications (see Table 9.1).

Table 9.1 Drugs used to treat delirium

Drug	Dose	Adverse effects	Notes
First-generation antipsychotics			
Haloperidol[1,5,7,11,18-21]	Oral 0.5–1 mg bd with additional doses every 4 hourly as needed. (peak effect: 4–6 h) IM 0.5–1 mg, observe for 30–60 minutes and repeat if necessary (peak effect: 20–40 minutes)	EPS can occur especially at doses above 3 mg Prolonged QT interval Increased risk of stroke in patients with dementia	Considered first-line agent. No trial data has demonstrated superiority of other antipsychotics over haloperidol, however care must be taken to monitor for extrapyramidal and cardiac adverse effects Baseline ECG is recommended for all patients, and especially for the elderly or those with a family or personal history of cardiac disease Regular monitoring of the ECG and potassium levels should be carried out if there are other conditions present that may prolong the QT interval Avoid in Lewy body dementia and Parkinson's disease Avoid intravenous use where possible. However in the medical ICU setting, IV is often used with close continuous ECG monitoring
Second-generation antipsychotics			
Amisulpride[11,12,22,23]	Oral 50–300 mg od, up to a maximum of 800 mg od Doses higher than 300 mg should be given in two divided doses	Prolonged QT interval Increased risk of stroke in patients with dementia	Very limited evidence in delirium As amisulpride is almost entirely excreted via the kidneys it is imperative to monitor renal function when used in medically ill or elderly patients
Aripiprazole[11,12,22-24]	Oral 5–15 mg/day, up to a maximum of 30 mg/day	EPS less likely than with haloperidol Akathisia or worsening sleep cycle may be problematic Increased risk of stroke in patients with dementia	Very limited evidence The rapid-acting intramuscular preparation has not been assessed in the treatment of delirium
Olanzapine[25-29]	Oral 2.5–5 mg od, up to a maximum of 20 mg/day	EPS less likely than with haloperidol Sedation is the most commonly reported adverse effect Increased risk of stroke in patients with dementia	A trial comparing olanzapine, risperidone, haloperidol and quetiapine showed that all were equally efficacious and safe in the treatment of delirium, but the response rate to olanzapine was poorer in the older age group (>75 years)[30] The rapid-acting IM preparation has not been assessed in the treatment of delirium

Table 9.1 (*Continued*)

Drug	Dose	Adverse effects	Notes
Risperidone[27,28,31–36]	Oral 0.5 mg bd with additional doses every 4 hourly as needed Usual maximum 4 mg/day	The most commonly reported adverse effects are hypotension and EPS Increased risk of stroke in patients with dementia	A trial comparing risperidone with olanzapine showed that both were equally effective in reducing delirium symptoms but the response to risperidone was poorer in the older age group (>70 years)[28]
Quetiapine[37–42]	Oral 12.5–50 mg bd This may be increased every 12 hours to 200 mg daily if it is well tolerated	Sedation and postural hypotension are the most common reported adverse effects Increased risk of stroke in patients with dementia	There are an increasing number of trials demonstrating safety and efficacy of low-dose quetiapine compared with haloperidol both in and outside the medical ICU. Now first choice agent in many units
Ziprasidone[43]	IM 10 mg every 2 hourly Usual maximum 40 mg/day	QT prolongation Increased risk of stroke in patients with dementia	Very limited evidence. Not available in the UK
Benzodiazepines			
Lorazepam[1,5,7]	Oral/IM 0.25–1 mg every 2 to 4 hourly as needed Usual maximum 3 mg in 24 hours IV use is usually reserved for emergencies	More likely than antipsychotics to cause respiratory depression, over-sedation and paradoxical excitement Associated with prolongation and worsening of delirium symptoms	Used in alcohol or sedative/hypnotic withdrawal, Parkinson's disease and NMS Otherwise – avoid
Diazepam[44]	Starting oral dose of 5–10 mg In the elderly a starting dose of 2 mg is recommended	Much longer half-life than lorazepam Associated with prolongation and worsening of delirium symptoms	Used in alcohol or sedative/hypnotic withdrawal, Parkinson's disease and NMS Otherwise – avoid
Cholinesterase inhibitors			
Donepezil[45,46]	Oral 5 mg od	Reasonably well tolerated compared with placebo. Nausea, vomiting and diarrhoea are the most common adverse effects reported	Very limited evidence. In the small studies where it has been used, clinical benefits have not been convincing. Not recommended
Rivastigmine[47,48]	Oral 1.5–6 mg bd	A study which added rivastigmine to usual care (haloperidol) showed that rivastigmine did not decrease the duration of delirium but in fact was associated with a more severe type of delirium, a longer stay in intensive care and higher mortality compared with placebo	Use of rivastigmine to treat delirium in critically ill patients is not recommended. May have a place in delirium prevention[40]

(*Continued*)

Table 9.1 (*Continued*)

Drug	Dose	Adverse effects	Notes
Other drugs			
Melatonin[50]	Oral 2 mg od	Sedation is the most commonly reported adverse effect	Very limited experience, used mainly to correct altered sleep–wake cycle. Not recommended
Trazodone[4,7]	25–150 mg nocte	Over-sedation is problematic	Limited experience – used only in uncontrolled studies. Not recommended
Sodium valproate[51,52]	Oral/IM/IV 250 mg bd increased to around 1500 mg/day, or 20 mg/kg/day Target plasma levels have not been validated for this indication. Note that physically ill patients may have altered albumin binding of valproate IV loading doses have also been used in ICU settings	Contraindicated in active liver disease Monitor for thrombocytopenia (more common in critically ill patients)	Some case reports of its use where antipsychotics and/or benzodiazepines are ineffective; otherwise not recommended

bd, *bis die* (twice a day); ECG, electrocardiogram; EPS, extrapyramidal symptoms; ICU, intensive care unit; IM, intramuscular; IV, intravenous; NMS, neuroleptic malignant syndrome; nocte, at night; od, *omne in die* (once a day).

Pharmacological prophylaxis[53–56]

Data around the use of medication to prevent delirium are sparse and conflicting. Most studies use low-dose haloperidol in patients deemed at high risk of developing delirium (elderly, post-surgical or intensive care patients). Prophylactic low-dose haloperidol (around 3 mg/day) was thought to reduce the severity and duration of delirium episodes and shorten the length of hospital stay in patients at high risk of developing the condition, but a recent study in older subjects found no effect.[18] Cochrane[53] suggests that prophylactic olanzapine may be effective. Rivastigmine may be effective[49] but Cochrane is dismissive.[53] Some evidence exists to support non-drug measures to minimise the risk of delirium.[57] Even low-dose antipsychotic medications have serious adverse effects in elderly patients.

References

1. van Zyl LT et al. Delirium concisely: condition is associated with increased morbidity, mortality, and length of hospitalization. Geriatrics 2006; 61:18–21.
2. American Psychiatric Association. *Diagnostic and Statistical Manual of Mental Disorders*, Fifth Edition (DSM-5). Arlington, VA: American Psychiatric Association; 2013.

3. Inouye SK et al. Clarifying confusion: the confusion assessment method. A new method for detection of delirium. Ann Intern Med 1990; **113**:941–948.

4. Nayeem K et al. Delirium. Clin Med 2003; **3**:412–415.

5. Potter J et al. The prevention, diagnosis and management of delirium in older people: concise guidelines. Clin Med 2006; **6**:303–308.

6. Fong TG et al. Delirium in elderly adults: diagnosis, prevention and treatment. Nat Rev Neurol 2009; **5**:210–220.

7. Inouye SK. Delirium in older persons. N Engl J Med 2006; **354**:1157–1165.

8. Saxena S et al. Delirium in the elderly: a clinical review. Postgrad Med J 2009; **85**:405–413.

9. Naja M et al. Delirium in geriatric medicine is related to anticholinergic burden. Eur Geriatr Med 2013; **4 Suppl 1**:S208.

10. Burns A et al. Delirium. J Neurol Neurosurg Psychiatry 2004; **75**:362–367.

11. Schwartz TL et al. The role of atypical antipsychotics in the treatment of delirium. Psychosomatics 2002; **43**:171–174.

12. Seitz DP et al. Antipsychotics in the treatment of delirium: a systematic review. J Clin Psychiatry 2007; **68**:11–21.

13. National Institute for Health and Care Excellence. Delirium: prevention, diagnosis and management. Clinical Guideline 103, 2010. https://www.nice.org.uk/guidance/cg103.

14. Donders E et al. Effect of haloperidol dosing frequencies on the duration and severity of delirium in elderly hip fracture patients. A prospective randomized trial. Eur Geriatr Med 2012; **3 Suppl 1**:S118–S119.

15. Neufeld KJ et al. Antipsychotic medication for prevention and treatment of delirium in hospitalized adults: a systematic review and meta-analysis. J Am Geriatr Soc 2016; **64**:705–714.

16. Kishi T et al. Antipsychotic medications for the treatment of delirium: a systematic review and meta-analysis of randomised controlled trials. J Neurol Neurosurg Psychiatry 2016; **87**:767–774.

17. Agar MR et al. Efficacy of oral risperidone, haloperidol, or placebo for symptoms of delirium among patients in palliative care: a randomized clinical trial. JAMA Intern Med 2017; **177**:34–42.

18. Schrijver E et al. Haloperidol versus placebo for delirium prevention in acutely hospitalised older at risk patients: a multi-centre double-blind randomised controlled clinical trial. Age Ageing 2018; **47**:48–55.

19. Fricchione GL et al. Postoperative delirium. Am J Psychiatry 2008; **165**:803–812.

20. Lonergan E et al. Antipsychotics for delirium (review). Cochrane Database Syst Rev 2007:CD005594.

21. Page VJ et al. Effect of intravenous haloperidol on the duration of delirium and coma in critically ill patients (Hope-ICU): a randomised, double-blind, placebo-controlled trial. Lancet Respir Med 2013; **1**:515–523.

22. Boettger S et al. Atypical antipsychotics in the management of delirium: a review of the empirical literature. Palliat Support Care 2005; **3**:227–237.

23. Leentjens AF et al. Delirium in elderly people: an update. Curr Opin Psychiatry 2005; **18**:325–330.

24. Boettger S et al. Aripiprazole and haloperidol in the treatment of delirium. Aust NZ J Psychiatry 2011; **45**:477–482.

25. Skrobik YK et al. Olanzapine vs haloperidol: treating delirium in a critical care setting. Intensive Care Med 2004; **30**:444–449.

26. Sipahimalani A et al. Olanzapine in the treatment of delirium. Psychosomatics 1998; **39**:422–430.

27. Duff G. Atypical antipsychotic drugs and stroke – Committee on Safety of Medicines. 2004. http://webarchive.nationalarchives.gov.uk/20141206131857/http://www.mhra.gov.uk/home/groups/pl-p/documents/websiteresources/con019488.pdf.

28. Kim SW et al. Risperidone versus olanzapine for the treatment of delirium. Hum Psychopharmacol 2010; **25**:298–302.

29. Grover S et al. Comparative efficacy study of haloperidol, olanzapine and risperidone in delirium. J Psychosom Res 2011; **71**:277–281.

30. Yoon HJ et al. Efficacy and safety of haloperidol versus atypical antipsychotic medications in the treatment of delirium. BMC Psychiatry 2013; **13**:240.

31. Bourgeois JA et al. Prolonged delirium managed with risperidone. Psychosomatics 2005; **46**:90–91.

32. Gupta N et al. Effectiveness of risperidone in delirium. Can J Psychiatry 2005; **50**:75.

33. Liu CY et al. Efficacy of risperidone in treating the hyperactive symptoms of delirium. Int Clin Psychopharmacol 2004; **19**:165–168.

34. Horikawa N et al. Treatment for delirium with risperidone: results of a prospective open trial with 10 patients. Gen Hosp Psychiatry 2003; **25**:289–292.

35. Han CS et al. A double-blind trial of risperidone and haloperidol for the treatment of delirium. Psychosomatics 2004; **45**:297–301.

36. Hakim SM et al. Early treatment with risperidone for subsyndromal delirium after on-pump cardiac surgery in the elderly: a randomized trial. Anesthesiology 2012; **116**:987–997.

37. Torres R et al. Use of quetiapine in delirium: case reports. Psychosomatics 2001; **42**:347–349.

38. Sasaki Y et al. A prospective, open-label, flexible-dose study of quetiapine in the treatment of delirium. J Clin Psychiatry 2003; **64**:1316–1321.

39. Devlin JW et al. Efficacy and safety of quetiapine in critically ill patients with delirium: a prospective, multicenter, randomized, double-blind, placebo-controlled pilot study. Crit Care Med 2010; **38**:419–427.

40. Hawkins SB et al. Quetiapine for the treatment of delirium. J Hosp Med 2013; **8**:215–220.

41. Tahir TA et al. A randomized controlled trial of quetiapine versus placebo in the treatment of delirium. J Psychosom Res 2010; **69**:485–490.

42. Grover S et al. Comparative effectiveness of quetiapine and haloperidol in delirium: a single blind randomized controlled study. World J Psychiatry 2016; **6**:365–371.

43. Young CC et al. Intravenous ziprasidone for treatment of delirium in the intensive care unit. Anesthesiology 2004; **101**:794–795.

44. Chan D et al. Delirium: making the diagnosis, improving the prognosis. Geriatrics 1999; **54**:28–42.

45. Overshott R et al. Cholinesterase inhibitors for delirium. Cochrane Database Syst Rev 2008:CD005317.

CHAPTER 9

46. Sampson EL et al. A randomized, double-blind, placebo-controlled trial of donepezil hydrochloride (Aricept) for reducing the incidence of postoperative delirium after elective total hip replacement. Int J Geriatr Psychiatry 2007; 22:343–349.

47. Dautzenberg PL et al. Adding rivastigmine to antipsychotics in the treatment of a chronic delirium. Age Ageing 2004; 33:516–517.

48. van Eijk MM et al. Effect of rivastigmine as an adjunct to usual care with haloperidol on duration of delirium and mortality in critically ill patients: a multicentre, double-blind, placebo-controlled randomised trial. Lancet 2010; 376:1829–1837.

49. Youn YC et al. Rivastigmine patch reduces the incidence of postoperative delirium in older patients with cognitive impairment. Int J Geriatr Psychiatry 2017; 32:1079–1084.

50. Chen S et al. Exogenous melatonin for delirium prevention: a meta-analysis of randomized controlled trials. Mol Neurobiol 2016; 53:4046–4053.

51. Sher Y et al. Adjunctive valproic acid in management-refractory hyperactive delirium: a case series and rationale. J Neuropsychiatry Clin Neurosci 2015; 27:365–370.

52. Gagnon DJ et al. Valproate for agitation in critically ill patients: a retrospective study. J Crit Care 2017; 37:119–125.

53. Siddiqi N et al. Interventions for preventing delirium in hospitalised non-ICU patients. Cochrane Database Syst Rev 2016; 3:CD005563.

54. Santos E et al. Effectiveness of haloperidol prophylaxis in critically ill patients with a high risk of delirium: a systematic review. JBI Database System Rev Implement Rep 2017; 15:1440–1472.

55. Fok MC et al. Do antipsychotics prevent postoperative delirium? A systematic review and meta-analysis. Int J Geriatr Psychiatry 2015; 30:333–344.

56. Schrijver EJ et al. Efficacy and safety of haloperidol for in-hospital delirium prevention and treatment: a systematic review of current evidence. Eur J Intern Med 2016; 27:14–23.

57. Clegg A et al. Interventions for preventing delirium in older people in institutional long-term care. Cochrane Database Syst Rev 2014; 1:CD009537.

Chapter 10

Drug treatment of psychiatric symptoms occurring in the context of other disorders

General principles of prescribing in human immunodeficiency virus (HIV)

People living with HIV (PLWH) may experience symptoms of mental illness due to a variety of factors (see Box 10.1). In practice, several of these factors may coexist within an individual.

When prescribing psychotropics, the following principles should be adhered to:

- Start with a low dose and titrate according to tolerability and response.
- Select the simplest dosing regimen possible. (Remember that the patient's drug regimen is likely to be complex already.)
- Select an agent with the fewest adverse effects/interactions. Medical co-morbidity and potential drug interactions must be considered.
- Ensure that management is conducted in close cooperation with the HIV specialists and the rest of the multidisciplinary team.

Box 10.1 Factors contributing to the development of psychiatric symptoms in people living with HIV[1]

- Primary (or pre-existing) psychiatric disorders.
- Neurobiological changes caused by HIV in the central nervous system (CNS).
- Other infections or CNS tumours.
- Antiretroviral drugs and other medical treatments (see section on 'Prescribing psychotropics in HIV' in this chapter).
- Alcohol or substance misuse.
- Adverse psychosocial factors (e.g. stigma).

The Maudsley Prescribing Guidelines in Psychiatry, Thirteenth Edition. David M. Taylor, Thomas R. E. Barnes and Allan H. Young.
© 2018 David M. Taylor. Published 2018 by John Wiley & Sons Ltd.

Although most psychotropic agents are thought to be safe in PLWH, definitive data are lacking in many cases, and it has been suggested that this group may be more sensitive to higher doses, adverse effects and interactions.[2,3] Patients with advanced HIV disease are more likely to have exaggerated adverse reactions to psychotropic medications.

Schizophrenia

In general, there is no difference between the pharmacological treatment of schizophrenia in PLWH and the treatment of an uninfected person,[4] but some specific considerations should be kept in mind (see section on 'Prescribing psychotropics in HIV' in this chapter). PLWH are more susceptible to extrapyramidal symptoms (EPS),[3] particularly during advanced illness, so second-generation antipsychotics (SGAs) are usually used as first-line therapy.[5,6] Quetiapine, risperidone and aripiprazole have been suggested as first-line choices for the treatment of psychosis unrelated to dementia or delirium,[5] though all have interactions with antiretroviral agents that may necessitate dose adjustments.[3] PLWH should be closely monitored for metabolic complications: the combined use of atypical antipsychotics with antiretrovirals increases the risk of metabolic disturbances.[7]

There are only few published reports of the successful use of clozapine for treatment-resistant schizophrenia in PLWH.[8,9] Clozapine may also be helpful in the treatment of individuals with HIV-associated psychosis with drug-induced parkinsonism.[10] Clozapine, certain HIV medications, and the virus itself may all have overlapping suppressive effects on bone marrow[8] and so extremely close monitoring of the white cell count (WCC) is recommended. Treatment with clozapine should only be initiated in patients who are medically well and stable on antiretroviral treatment to avoid any confusion about the aetiology of blood dyscrasias (should they occur).[8]

Delirium

Organic causes should be identified and treated. Short-term symptomatic treatment may include low-dose SGAs (e.g. risperidone[5]). There have been few randomised controlled trials (RCTs) in delirious patients with acquired immune deficiency syndrome (AIDS); earlier studies document the efficacy of typical antipsychotics,[11] and low-dose haloperidol was the agent of choice in one consensus study.[5] However, first-generation antipsychotics (FGAs) should be used cautiously given the increased susceptibility to EPS in this patient group.[11] Benzodiazepines should be used cautiously as they may worsen delirium (except when alcohol or benzodiazepine withdrawal is the precipitating factor).[11]

Depression

Depression is common in PLWH, with an estimated prevalence of 20–40%.[12] Of note, depression is one of the strongest predictors of poor adherence to antiretroviral therapy and poor HIV treatment outcomes.[13] Antidepressants effectively treat depression in PLWH,[14] and may also improve adherence to antiretrovirals,[15] but they remain underutilised.[16]

First-line agents include selective serotonin reuptake inhibitors (SSRIs), especially escitalopram/citalopram[5,17] (because it does not inhibit CYP2D6 or CYP3A4), with further treatment as per standard protocols. Oddly, a study of escitalopram found no difference from placebo,[18] but this seems to be due to a large placebo response, probably because study conditions were markedly different from treatment as usual. Electrocardiogram (ECG) monitoring is recommended when citalopram/escitalopram is co-administered with atazanavir- or lopinavir-based regimens.[12] Mirtazapine is effective,[19,20] with a relatively low risk of drug interactions,[21] and may have a niche in the treatment of coexisting HIV wasting and depression.[22] The use of tricyclic antidepressants (TCAs) may be appropriate in some cases, although adverse effects may limit efficacy and compliance.[3,23] Monoamine oxidase inhibitors (MAOIs) are not recommended in this population. Other agents (bupropion,[24] reboxetine[25] and trazodone[26]) have been investigated, and although these agents were shown to reduce depressive symptoms, adverse effects and drug interactions limit their utility. Their routine use is therefore not recommended. Serotonin–noradrenaline reuptake inhibitors (SNRIs) have not been systematically studied in PLWH but 'dual-action' antidepressants (including duloxetine and venlafaxine) appear equally effective as SSRIs.[27] Testosterone and stimulants have also been successfully used.[3]

Interferon-α-induced depression in HIV/HCV co-infected patients

Citalopram has been shown to be an effective and well-tolerated treatment for emergent depression;[28] however, prophylactic use of citalopram (i.e. before depression emerges) cannot be recommended.[29]

Bipolar affective disorder

Mania in PLWH can be primary (pre-existing bipolar affective disorder) or secondary ('HIV mania'). PLWH may be more sensitive to the adverse effects of mood stabilisers such as neurotoxicity with lithium,[30] especially if they have neurocognitive dysfunction.[31,32] Lithium is also renally excreted, an advantage for drug interactions with antiretrovirals[33] but problematic in patients with renal insufficiencies, which are highly prevalent in this patient population.[5] Lithium may be used cautiously in PLWH for primary bipolar affective disorder with close monitoring, but is best avoided in patients with advanced HIV disease.[33] Carbamazepine should be avoided because of important interactions with antiretrovirals, as well as the risk of blood dyscrasias.[33] Valproate has come into relative favour as a preferred choice for PLWH,[6] mainly because of problems associated with lithium and carbamazepine.[6] PLWH prescribed valproate should be closely monitored for drug interactions, hepatotoxicity, blood dyscrasias and pancreatitis,[6] and use of valproate should be avoided in patients prescribed hepatotoxic drugs (e.g. nevirapine, rifampicin).[33] The use of mood-stabilising antipsychotics such as risperidone, quetiapine and olanzapine is also an option.[5]

Secondary mania ('HIV mania')

Reports of secondary mania, typically occurring in advanced illness in the context of HIV-associated neurocognitive disorders or CNS opportunistic infections,[34] have declined with the widespread use of effective antiretrovirals. The first aim is to identify and treat the potential underlying cause (infections, substance misuse, alcohol withdrawal, metabolic abnormalities). The choice of psychotropic to treat secondary mania is based on case reports and open-label studies, as well as the desire to avoid adverse drug interactions, and the avoidance of HIV-specific adverse effects.[34] Quetiapine, valproate, risperidone, olanzapine and aripiprazole have all been suggested for the treatment of secondary mania.[5]

Anxiety disorders

SSRIs are generally recommended as first-line treatment of anxiety and panic disorders in medically ill patients, including PLWH[35] (see 'Depression' in this section for preferred options). Benzodiazepines may have some utility in the acute treatment of anxiety in PLWH, but caution should be exercised because of the potential for both misuse and, in rare cases, potentially serious interactions. Lorazepam, oxazepam and temazepam have less interaction potential because they are metabolised by non-CYP450 pathways, and so may be preferred options for PLWH.[13] Buspirone may also be useful.[6]

HIV-associated neurocognitive disorders

With the widespread use of effective antiretrovirals, the incidence of severe HIV-associated cerebral disease has declined dramatically; however, more subtle forms of brain disease, known as HIV-associated neurocognitive disorders (HAND), remain prevalent[36] and may occur in individuals who are virally supressed.[37] The diagnosis encompasses three related disorders that range from mild and more common (asymptomatic neurocognitive impairment, mild neurocognitive disorder) to severe and less common (HIV-associated dementia) disorders. HAND is a diagnosis of exclusion; for example, all patients with cognitive impairments should be evaluated for depression and possible treatment[12] as it is a potentially confounding condition. Common behavioural symptoms associated with HAND include apathy, irritability, inertia, lack of spontaneity, social withdrawal, psychomotor slowing, complaints of diminished attention and concentration, emotional lability, and occasionally, 'HIV mania'.[34]

The mainstay of treatment is antiretroviral therapy,[38] which should be commenced immediately in symptomatic individuals.[36] Antiretrovirals penetrate the CNS to varying extents and the inclusion of potentially CNS-active antiretrovirals has been recommended in some circumstances.[12,13] However, this is a controversial area without definitive evidence.[34,36] Treatment of these individuals is carried out primarily by HIV specialists with input from other clinical specialties such as psychiatry, neurology and neuropsychology.[36] A variety of adjunctive treatments for HAND have been studied (minocycline, memantine, selegiline, lithium, valproate, lexipafant, nimodipine, psychostimulants, rivastigmine, and others) but have not demonstrated a significant beneficial effect.[39] Research is ongoing; the most recent study of rivastigmine was also negative[40] but in another recent study paroxetine was associated with neurocognitive improvements (after adjusting for depression).[41] Larger studies are needed to confirm the beneficial effects of adjunctive treatments for HAND.

References

1. Nanni MG et al. Depression in HIV infected patients: a review. Curr Psychiatry Rep 2015; 17:530.

2. Ayuso JL. Use of psychotropic drugs in patients with HIV infection. Drugs 1994; 47:599–610.

3. Hill L et al. Pharmacotherapy considerations in patients with HIV and psychiatric disorders: focus on antidepressants and antipsychotics. Ann Pharmacother 2013; 47:75–89.

4. Cohen M et al. *Comprehensive Textbook of AIDS Psychiatry: A Paradigm for Integrated Care.* Oxford, England: Oxford University Press; 2017.

5. Freudenreich O et al. Psychiatric treatment of persons with HIV/AIDS: an HIV-Psychiatry Consensus Survey of Current Practices. Psychosomatics 2010; 51:480–488.

6. Brogan K et al. Management of common psychiatric conditions in the HIV-positive population. Curr HIV/AIDS Rep 2009; 6:108–115.

7. Ferrara M et al. The concomitant use of second-generation antipsychotics and long-term antiretroviral therapy may be associated with increased cardiovascular risk. Psychiatry Res 2014; 218:201–208.

8. Nejad SH et al. Clozapine use in HIV-infected schizophrenia patients: a case-based discussion and review. Psychosomatics 2009; 50:626–632.

9. Fabrikant A et al. College of Psychiatric and Neurologic Pharmacists 2015 Poster Abstracts. J Pharm Pract 2015; 28:315–375.

10. Lera G et al. Pilot study with clozapine in patients with HIV-associated psychosis and drug-induced parkinsonism. Mov Disord 1999; 14:128–131.

11. Watkins CC et al. Cognitive impairment in patients with AIDS - prevalence and severity. HIV/AIDS (Auckland, NZ) 2015; 7:35–47.

12. European AIDS Clinical Society. Guidelines Version 9.0 October 2017. http://www.eacsociety.org/files/guidelines_9.0-english.pdf.

13. Panel on Antiretroviral Guidelines for Adults and Adolescents. Guidelines for the Use of Antiretroviral Agents in Adults and Adolescents Living with HIV. Department of Health and Human Services. 2017. https://aidsinfo.nih.gov/contentfiles/lvguidelines/AdultandAdolescentGL.pdf.

14. Himelhoch S et al. Efficacy of antidepressant medication among HIV-positive individuals with depression: a systematic review and meta-analysis. AIDS Patient Care STDS 2005; 19:813–822.

15. Sin NL et al. Depression treatment enhances adherence to antiretroviral therapy: a meta-analysis. Ann Behav Med 2014; 47:259–269.

16. Cholera R et al. Mind the gap: gaps in antidepressant treatment, treatment adjustments, and outcomes among patients in routine HIV care in a multisite U.S. clinical cohort. PLoS One 2017; 12:e0166435.

17. Currier MB et al. Citalopram treatment of major depressive disorder in Hispanic HIV and AIDS patients: a prospective study. Psychosomatics 2004; 45:210–216.

18. Hoare J et al. Escitalopram treatment of depression in human immunodeficiency virus/acquired immunodeficiency syndrome: a randomized, double-blind, placebo-controlled study. J Nerv Ment Dis 2014; 202:133–137.

19. Patel S et al. Escitalopram and mirtazapine for the treatment of depression in HIV patients: a randomized controlled open label trial. ASEAN Journal of Psychiatry 2012; 14.

20. Elliott AJ et al. Mirtazapine for depression in patients with human immunodeficiency virus. J Clin Psychopharmacol 2000; 20:265–267.

21. Adams JL et al. Treating depression within the HIV "medical home": a guided algorithm for antidepressant management by HIV clinicians. AIDS Patient Care STDS 2012; 26:647–654.

22. Badowski M et al. Pharmacologic management of human immunodeficiency virus wasting syndrome. Pharmacotherapy 2014; 34:868–881.

23. Elliott AJ et al. Randomized, placebo-controlled trial of paroxetine versus imipramine in depressed HIV-positive outpatients. Am J Psychiatry 1998; 155:367–372.

24. Currier MB et al. A prospective trial of sustained-release bupropion for depression in HIV-seropositive and AIDS patients. Psychosomatics 2003; 44:120–125.

25. Carvalhal AS et al. An open trial of reboxetine in HIV-seropositive outpatients with major depressive disorder. J Clin Psychiatry 2003; 64:421–424.

26. De Wit S et al. Efficacy and safety of trazodone versus clorazepate in the treatment of HIV-positive subjects with adjustment disorders: a pilot study. J Int Med Res 1999; 27:223–232.

27. Mills JC et al. Comparative effectiveness of dual-action versus single-action antidepressants for the treatment of depression in people living with HIV/AIDS. J Affect Disord 2017; 215:179–186.

28. Laguno M et al. Depressive symptoms after initiation of interferon therapy in human immunodeficiency virus-infected patients with chronic hepatitis C. Antivir Ther 2004; 9:905–909.

29. Klein MB et al. Citalopram for the prevention of depression and its consequences in HIV-hepatitis C coinfected individuals initiating pegylated interferon/ribavirin therapy: a multicenter randomized double-blind placebo-controlled trial. HIV Clin Trials 2014; 15:161–175.

30. Tanquary J. Lithium neurotoxicity at therapeutic levels in an AIDS patient. J Nerv Ment Dis 1993; 181:518–519.

31. El-Mallakh RS. Mania in AIDS: clinical significance and theoretical considerations. Int J Psychiatry Med 1991; 21:383–391.

32. Ferrando SJ. Psychopharmacologic treatment of patients with HIV/AIDS. Curr Psychiatry Rep 2009; 11:235–242.

33. Gallego L et al. Psychopharmacological treatments in HIV patients under antiretroviral therapy. AIDS Reviews 2012; 14:101–111.

34. Singer EJ et al. Neurobehavioral Manifestations of Human Immunodeficiency Virus/AIDS: Diagnosis and Treatment. Neurol Clin 2016; 34:33–53.

35. Arseniou S et al. HIV infection and depression. Psychiatry Clin Neurosci 2014; 68:96–109.

36. Waters L et al. British HIV Association guidelines for the treatment of HIV-1-positive adults with antiretroviral therapy 2015 (2016 interim update). http://www.bhiva.org/documents/Guidelines/Treatment/2016/treatment-guidelines-2016-interim-update.pdf.

37. Manji H et al. HIV, dementia and antiretroviral drugs: 30 years of an epidemic. J Neurol Neurosurg Psychiatry 2013; 84:1126–1137.

38. Portegies P et al. Guidelines for the diagnosis and management of neurological complications of HIV infection. Eur J Neurol 2004; **11**:297–304.

39. Eggers C et al. HIV-1-associated neurocognitive disorder: epidemiology, pathogenesis, diagnosis, and treatment. J Neurol 2017; **264**:1715–1727.

40. Munoz-Moreno JA et al. Transdermal rivastigmine for HIV-associated cognitive impairment: a randomized pilot study. PLoS One 2017; **12**:e0182547.

41. Sacktor N et al. Paroxetine and fluconazole therapy for HIV-associated neurocognitive impairment: results from a double-blind, placebo-controlled trial. J Neurovirol 2017:1–12.

Prescribing psychotropics in HIV

Interactions

Pharmacokinetic interactions between antiretroviral and psychotropic drugs occur frequently and are potentially clinically significant. Potential interactions should be checked for all patients receiving antiretrovirals and psychotropics concomitantly. These checks should include alternative non-prescribed treatments (St John's Wort, for example, can lead to subtherapeutic antiretroviral levels). Readers are directed to regularly updated online resources for information about individual pharmacokinetic interactions:

- www.hiv-druginteractions.org
- http://hivinsite.ucsf.edu/

Pharmacodynamic interactions may also occur, usually through overlapping adverse effects. Potential pharmacodynamic interactions are shown in Table 10.1.

Table 10.1 Potential pharmacodynamic interactions with antiretrovirals

Potential adverse effect	Implicated antiretroviral drug(s)[1–3]	Implications for psychotropic prescribing
Bone marrow suppression	Zidovudine	Concurrent use with certain psychotropics (e.g. clozapine) may increase the risk of myelosuppression/neutropenia
Bone mineral density reduction	Tenofovir disoproxil fumarate	May compound the reductions in bone mineral density possible with prolactin-elevating antipsychotics
Creatine kinase (CK) elevations	Dolutegravir, emtricitabine, raltegravir	May be important to acknowledge associated link if diagnosis of NMS is being considered
ECG changes	Atazanavir, darunavir, efavirenz, lopinavir, rilpivirine, ritonavir, saquinavir	May increase risk of arrhythmias associated with certain psychotropic drugs
Gastrointestinal disturbances	Atazanavir, darunavir, dolutegravir, didanosine, elvitegravir/cobicistat, fosamprenavir, indinavir, lopinavir, nelfinavir, raltegravir, saquinavir, tipranavir, zidovudine	May compound gastrointestinal disturbances associated with certain psychotropics (e.g. SSRIs)
Seizure(s)	Darunavir, efavirenz, maraviroc, ritonavir, saquinavir, zidovudine	May increase seizure risk associated with certain psychotropic drugs
Metabolic abnormalities such as hypertriglyceridaemia, hypercholesterolaemia, insulin resistance, hyperglycaemia and hyperlactataemia	All combination antiretroviral therapy	May compound risk of metabolic adverse effects associated with certain psychotropic drugs

ECG, electrocardiogram; NMS, neuroleptic malignant syndrome; SSRI, selective serotonin reuptake inhibitor.

Adverse psychiatric effects of antiretroviral drugs

Psychiatric adverse events have been reported with many antiretroviral drugs, but a causal relationship remains uncertain. Efavirenz has been most commonly implicated, and HIV guidelines suggest avoiding its use in patients with psychiatric illness.[1,2,4] Table 10.2 summarises the most important psychiatric adverse effects of antiretroviral drugs. Note that this is not an exhaustive list; readers are directed to the summaries of product characteristics (SPCs)/product labelling for other possible adverse effects. The differential diagnosis of psychiatric adverse effects is covered elsewhere in the *Guidelines*.

Table 10.2 Summary of psychiatric adverse drug reactions (ADRs) with antiretroviral drugs[1–3,5]

Drug	Adverse psychiatric effects/comment
Nucleoside reverse transcriptase inhibitors	
Abacavir	Depression, anxiety, nightmares, labile mood, mania, psychosis. Very few cases reported; in all reported cases, the patient rapidly returned to baseline after discontinuing drug
Didanosine	Lethargy, nervousness, anxiety, confusion, sleep disturbance, mood disorders, psychosis, mania. Very rare
Emtricitabine	Confusion, irritability, insomnia
Zidovudine	Sleep disturbance, vivid dreams, agitation, mania, depression, psychosis, delirium. Psychiatric ADRs are usually dose-related. The onset varies widely, from <24 hours to 7 months
Non-nucleoside reverse transcriptase inhibitors	
Efavirenz	Somnolence, insomnia, abnormal dreams, impaired concentration, depression, psychosis, and suicidal ideation. Symptoms usually subside or diminish after 2–4 weeks. However, subtler, long-term neuropsychiatric effects may occur. Can exacerbate psychiatric symptoms; avoid in patients with a history of psychiatric illness
Etravirine	Sleep disturbance
Nevirapine	Visual hallucinations, persecutory delusions, mood changes, nightmares and vivid dreams, depression. A small handful of cases have been reported. Onset of symptoms was within the first couple of weeks. Symptoms all resolved on discontinuation of nevirapine
Rilpivirine	Depression, suicidality, sleep disturbances. A similar adverse effect profile to efavirenz but a lower incidence of each event. May exacerbate psychiatric symptoms; consider avoiding in patients with a history of psychiatric illness[2]
Integrase inhibitors	
Dolutegravir, elvitegravir and raltegravir	Depression and suicidal ideation (rare, usually in patients with pre-existing psychiatric conditions)

References

1. European AIDS Clinical Society. Guidelines Version 9.0 October 2017. http://www.eacsociety.org/files/guidelines_9.0-english.pdf.
2. Panel on Antiretroviral Guidelines for Adults and Adolescents. Guidelines for the Use of Antiretroviral Agents in Adults and Adolescents Living with HIV. Department of Health and Human Services. 2017. https://aidsinfo.nih.gov/contentfiles/lvguidelines/AdultandAdolescentGL.pdf.
3. World Health Organization. Consolidated guidelines on the use of antiretroviral drugs for treating and preventing HIV infection. Recommendations for a public health approach Second edition. 2016. http://www.who.int/hiv/pub/arv/arv-2016/en/.
4. Waters L et al. British HIV Association guidelines for the treatment of HIV-1-positive adults with antiretroviral therapy 2015 (2016 interim update). http://www.bhiva.org/documents/Guidelines/Treatment/2016/treatment-guidelines-2016-interim-update.pdf.
5. Parker C. Psychiatric effects of drugs for other disorders. Medicine 2016; **44**:768774.

Epilepsy

Psychiatric co-morbidities in epilepsy

People with epilepsy (PWE) have an elevated prevalence of several psychiatric disorders including depression (22.9%), anxiety (20.2%) and psychosis (5.2%).[1,2] Suicide is five-fold higher in PWE compared to the general population[3] and is an important cause of premature mortality.[4] The link between epilepsy and mental illness is bidirectional as patients with depression, anxiety and psychosis have an increased risk of developing new-onset epilepsy.[5,6] Suicide attempts are also associated with the development of epilepsy.[3] This bidirectional relationship might be explained by a common underlying pathology between mental illness and epilepsy. Disturbances in neurotransmission, neuro-inflammation, and the hypothalamic-pituitary-adrenal (HPA) axis have all been suggested[7] to be the shared pathology.

Interictal psychiatric disorders (with symptoms occurring independently of seizures) are likely to require treatment with psychotropics.[8–10] When prescribing psychotropics to people with epilepsy, the following general principles[11,12] should be adhered to.

- First, rule out other possible causes of psychiatric symptoms (both peri-ictal and iatrogenic, see Table 10.3).
- Optimise the treatment of epilepsy (ideally before prescribing psychotropics).
- Consider using psychotropics with known anticonvulsant properties (e.g. anticonvulsants in bipolar disorder).
- Check for interactions with anticonvulsants.
- Start with a low dose and titrate according to tolerability and response (proconvulsive effects are dose-related).
- If seizures do occur, consider changing the psychotropic drug or optimising the anticonvulsant.

Psychiatric side-effects of anticonvulsants

Virtually all anticonvulsants are known to have psychotropic effects. These effects can be helpful or unhelpful. The adverse and beneficial psychiatric side-effects of anticonvulsants are summarised in Table 10.4. Readers are directed to the "Summary of psychiatric adverse effects of non-psychotropic medications" elsewhere in the *Guidelines* for a more detailed summary of psychiatric symptoms associated with anticonvulsants and for further information about determining causality in any given patient.

Interactions[21]

Pharmacokinetic interactions

Important pharmacokinetic interactions exist in both directions between anticonvulsants and psychotropics, primarily mediated through cytochrome P450 enzymes.[8,22] Psychotropics with enzyme-inhibiting effects (e.g. fluoxetine, fluvoxamine, paroxetine and, at higher doses, sertraline) may increase anticonvulsant plasma levels. This is especially relevant to anticonvulsants with a narrow therapeutic index (e.g. carbamazepine

Table 10.3 Possible causes of psychiatric symptoms in people with epilepsy (PWE) and their management[5]

Cause of symptoms	Description	Management
Interictal psychiatric disorders	■ Symptoms occurring independently of seizures ■ Although common in PWE, other causes and relatedness to seizures should be ruled out first	■ Likely to require treatment with psychotropics ■ See Table 10.5 for more information about the use of specific psychotropics in PWE
Peri-ictal symptoms	■ PWE may experience psychiatric symptoms that are temporally related to seizures	■ All peri-ictal psychiatric symptoms (pre-ictal, postictal and ictal) are initially treated by optimising anticonvulsants[11] ■ Peri-ictal depressive symptoms do not appear to respond to treatment with antidepressants[13,14]
Pre-ictal symptoms	■ Typically presents as a dysphoric mood preceding a seizure by a period of several hours to 3 days	
Postictal symptoms	■ Typically presents between several hours and 7 days following a seizure (depression, anxiety, suicidal ideation and psychosis reported) ■ PWE and interictal psychiatric disorders may experience worsening of symptoms previously in remission (breakthrough symptoms)	■ Postictal psychosis can remit spontaneously or respond to treatment with low doses of antipsychotics.[15] Short-term symptomatic treatment with a benzodiazepine or antipsychotic is recommended for up to 3 months.[16] Taper off carefully after symptom resolution[14]
Ictal symptoms	■ May present as ictal fear/panic (most commonly), depressive symptoms or, rarely, psychosis	■ There is no evidence that psychotropics can prevent ictal symptoms[17]
Para-ictal episodes 'forced normalisation' (psychiatric symptoms emerging as a result of a reduction in seizure frequency)	■ Psychotic or, less commonly, severe affective symptoms following seizure remission in PWE ■ Rapid medication titration schedules, medication-resistant epilepsy, and temporal lobe epilepsy may be risk factors[15]	■ A decision should be made on how to proceed with anticonvulsants and psychotropics through a process of shared decision-making with carers.[14] Symptomatic treatment with antipsychotics or antidepressants may be indicated
Iatrogenic psychiatric symptoms	Recent changes in treatments for seizures could result in psychiatric symptoms after: ■ starting anticonvulsants with known negative psychotropic properties (particularly in those with a psychiatric history) ■ stopping anticonvulsants with beneficial psychotropic properties (e.g. mood stabilisation) ■ starting anticonvulsants with enzyme-inducing properties in people stable on psychotropics ■ surgery for epilepsy: de novo post-surgical episodes of depression, anxiety and, rarely, psychosis have been reported. Exacerbation of pre-existing conditions more common	■ Symptoms are managed by resolving the underlying cause in the first instance ■ Consider switching anticonvulsants with known negative psychotropic properties to better tolerated anticonvulsants (see Table 10.4) ■ Anticonvulsants can lower folate levels which may affect mood. Folate levels should be checked and remedied if necessary ■ If changing anticonvulsants is not suitable, antidepressants can be considered for iatrogenic depressive symptoms[18] ■ Post-surgical neuropsychiatric symptoms may be treated successfully with psychotropics[17]

Table 10.4 Adverse and beneficial psychiatric side-effects of anticonvulsants[5,19,20]

Anticonvulsant drug	Adverse psychiatric symptoms	Psychiatric benefits
Barbiturates, primidone Benzodiazepines	▪ Behavioural disturbance/ADHD symptoms ▪ Depression, cognitive impairment	▪ Anxiolytic
Carbamazepine, oxcarbazepine	▪ Not reported	▪ Mood stabilising, anti-manic
Ethosuximide	▪ Behavioural disturbance, depression, psychosis	▪ None reported
Felbamate	▪ Anxiety, depression	▪ None reported
Gabapentin, pregabalin	▪ None reported	▪ Anxiolytic
Lacosamide	▪ None reported	▪ None reported
Lamotrigine	▪ Anxiogenic in some ▪ Behavioural disturbance in cognitive impairment	▪ Antidepressant ▪ Mood stabilising
Levetiracetam	▪ Anxiety, behavioural disturbance, depression	▪ None confirmed
Perampanel	▪ Behavioural disturbance, depression, psychosis	▪ None reported
Phenytoin	▪ Behavioural disturbance, depression	▪ Anti-manic
Tiagabine	▪ Behavioural disturbance, depression	▪ Anxiolytic
Topiramate	▪ Anxiety, behavioural disturbance, depression	▪ Unclear. Possible anti-manic/ antipsychotic
Valproate	▪ Behavioural disturbance (at high doses in children)	▪ Mood stabilising, anti-manic ▪ Anti-panic
Vigabatrin	▪ Behavioural disturbance/ADHD symptoms ▪ Depression, psychosis	▪ None reported
Zonisamide	▪ Behavioural disturbance, depression	▪ None confirmed

ADHD, attention deficit hyperactivity disorder.

and phenytoin). Plasma levels should be monitored, and dosage adjustment may be required. Citalopram and escitalopram are weak inhibitors of CYPs 1A2 and 2D6.

Some anticonvulsants are potent enzyme inducers (e.g. phenytoin, carbamazepine, phenobarbital, primidone) and others are weak inducers (e.g. oxcarbazepine at doses ≥900 mg/day, topiramate at doses ≥400 mg/day). These drugs can lower plasma levels of multiple psychotropics, possibly leading to treatment failure.

Pharmacodynamic interactions[13]

Adverse effects with anticonvulsants that may overlap with psychotropic adverse effects include:

▪ weight gain: caused by some anticonvulsants (e.g. carbamazepine, gabapentin, pregabalin, valproate)

- sexual adverse effects: with phenobarbital and primidone but possible with all enzyme-inducing anticonvulsants
- hyponatraemia: with carbamazepine, oxcarbazepine (note, if severe can provoke seizures)
- osteoporosis and osteopenia: reported with long-term use of enzyme-inducing anticonvulsants
- blood dyscrasias: reported with valproate and carbamazepine.[10]

Psychotropics and the risk of seizures in people with epilepsy

In the general population, the annual incidence of unprovoked seizures is about 50 per 100,000 persons.[23] It is notable that the incidence of unprovoked seizures in the placebo arms of RCTs of antidepressants and antipsychotics is approximately 15-fold higher, suggesting that both depression and psychosis are risk factors for seizures.[24] More recently, a bidirectional relationship between epilepsy and several psychiatric illnesses has been demonstrated, whereby not only do PWE have a higher risk of developing a psychiatric illness, but people with psychiatric illness have a higher risk of developing epilepsy.[5,6] This bidirectional relationship exists for depression, anxiety, psychosis and suicidality.[3,5,6] Thus, the occurrence of seizures may, in some cases, be the expression of the natural progression of a psychiatric illness, unrelated to the use of psychotropics.

Reports of seizures associated with psychotropics must factor in the existence of a bidirectional relationship between psychiatric illness and epilepsy. For example, although observational studies have reported an association between antidepressant treatment and seizures,[25] a similar association is also found with non-drug treatments for depression (counselling, for example).[26] These findings are consistent with depression itself being the main risk factor for seizures. In fact, one analysis of controlled studies with psychotropics showed that the incidence of seizures was substantially lower among patients receiving most antidepressants (SSRIs, for example) in comparison with those randomised to placebo.[24] Nonetheless, definitive data are lacking in PWE[27,28] and certain psychotropics have a dose-related risk of seizures within usual dose ranges. Most can cause seizures in overdose. Note also that almost all antidepressants and antipsychotics have been associated with hyponatraemia (see sections on hyponatraemia) and seizures may occur if this is severe.[17,29] General guidance on the safety of psychotropics in PWE is summarised in Table 10.5.

Electroconvulsive therapy (ECT) has anticonvulsive properties and is worth considering in the treatment of depression in patients with unstable epilepsy.[8,17,22] ECT does not appear to cause or worsen epilepsy.[17,53]

Epilepsy and driving

In the UK, people with epilepsy may not drive a car if they have had a seizure while awake in the previous year or, if seizures occur only during sleep, this has been an established nocturnal pattern for at least 3 years. The consequences of inducing seizure with antidepressants or antipsychotics can therefore be significant. For further information see www.gov.uk/epilepsy-and-driving.

Table 10.5 Psychotropic drugs in epilepsy

Safety in epilepsy	Drug	Comments
Antidepressants		
Low risk – good choices	SSRIs	Recommended in PWE.[14,18] SSRIs may be anticonvulsant at therapeutic doses[13] and pro-convulsant in overdose.[30] SSRIs with the lowest risk of interactions with anticonvulsants are generally preferred (citalopram/escitalopram, followed by sertraline).[14,18,31,32]. Escitalopram is preferred over citalopram in PWE (lower risk of seizures in overdose).[33] Others have low risk of seizures (e.g. fluoxetine[33]) but drug interactions with anticonvulsants should be considered[14,18]
	Mirtazapine	Recommended in PWE.[18,31] Not known to be pro-convulsive.[24]
Probably low risk – use with caution (limited evidence)	Agomelatine	Not known to be pro-convulsive.[34] Anticonvulsant in animal models[33]
	Duloxetine	Limited data. Has been recommended for PWE[11,18] and risk of seizures is probably negligible[33]
	MAOIs	Not known to be pro-convulsive at therapeutic doses.[33] Low risk of seizures in overdose[17]
	Moclobemide	Not known to be pro-convulsive.[33] Anticonvulsant in animal models[33]
	Reboxetine	Small open-label study suggests no problems in PWE[35]
	Vortioxetine	Not known to be pro-convulsive[33,36] but no experience in PWE[33]
Moderate risk – care required	Lithium	Low risk of seizures.[33] Anticonvulsant in animal models.[33] However, limited data showing increases or decreases in seizure frequency in PWE.[33] For bipolar, consider anticonvulsant mood stabilisers[37]
	Trazodone	Limited data suggest some risk of seizures[33,38]
	Venlafaxine	Effective in PWE[11] and has been recommended[18] but mixed evidence on seizure risk[33]
	Vilazodone	Limited data. Seizure exacerbation in a patient with epilepsy has been reported[33]
Higher risk – avoid (pro-convulsive at therapeutic doses[13])	Amoxapine	Several reports of seizures at therapeutic doses[38]
	Bupropion	Dose-related risk of seizures (particularly with instant-release formulations).[33] Risk is less with slow-release formulations at doses under 300 mg/day[33]
	Maprotiline	Several reports of seizures at therapeutic doses[38]
	TCAs	Most TCAs are epileptogenic at higher doses (particularly clomipramine and amitriptyline[10,24,38]). Doxepin possibly lower risk (one small study in PWE).[33] SNRIs are preferred over TCAs in PWE[17]
Antipsychotics		
Low risk – good choices	Amisulpride/sulpiride	Considered to be safe in PWE.[39] Renally excreted, so low risk of pharmacokinetic interactions with anticonvulsants. Seizures uncommon in overdose[40]
	Aripiprazole Ziprasidone	Rarely lowers seizure threshold.[5] Incidence of seizures similar to placebo in RCTs[24]
	High potency FGAs	e.g. fluphenazine, haloperidol, trifluoperazine, flupentixol. Low risk of lowering the seizure threshold[5]
	Risperidone	Rare to low risk of lowering the seizure threshold.[5] Incidence of seizures similar to placebo in RCTs.[24] Has been recommended for PWE.[31] Evidence of safety in a case series of adolescents with epilepsy[41]

Table 10.5 *(Continued)*

Safety in epilepsy	Drug	Comments
Probably low risk – use with caution (limited evidence)	Asenapine Brexpiprazole Cariprazine Lurasidone	Seizure rate similar to placebo in RCTs.[42] Data and clinical experience of use in PWE are extremely limited
Moderate risk – care required	Olanzapine Quetiapine	Olanzapine and quetiapine both associated with seizures in RCTs.[24] However, olanzapine causes more EEG abnormalities.[40] Overall risk of lowering the seizure threshold is considered to be low[5] and olanzapine has been recommended by some for PWE[31]
Higher risk – care required	Clozapine	Most epileptogenic antipsychotic.[31] However, has been used successfully in PWE stable on anticonvulsants without worsening seizures[43] and even in treatment-resistant epilepsy.[44] Note, should not be used with carbamazepine (risk of blood dyscrasias and reduced clozapine levels). Valproate or lamotrigine are the anticonvulsants of choice
Higher risk – avoid	Low potency FGAs (e.g. chlorpromazine)	Best avoided in PWE.[30] Doses of chlorpromazine above 1 g/day have a 9% incidence of seizures
	Loxapine	Highest rate of seizures amongst the FGAs[45]
	Depot antipsychotics	None of the depot preparations currently available is thought to be epileptogenic, however: ■ The kinetics of depots are complex (seizures may be delayed) ■ If seizures do occur, the offending drug may not be easily withdrawn. Depots should be used with extreme care
	Zotepine	Has established dose-related pro-convulsive effect[40]
Drugs for ADHD		
Low risk	Methylphenidate	Three RCTs support safety and efficacy in children with epilepsy at therapeutic doses (0.3–1 mg/kg/day).[10] A single-dose RCT and open-label extension study demonstrated no effect on seizures in adults[46]
Probably low risk[47,48] – use with caution (limited data)	Amfetamines	Data limited to one small retrospective study in PWE.[10] No patient who had well-controlled epilepsy experienced an increase in seizure frequency.[49] Of note, dexamfetamine was historically used as an adjunctive anticonvulsant agent[50]
	Atomoxetine	Data limited to one small retrospective study in PWE.[10] Discontinuation rates were high (though none due to seizure exacerbation[51]). Seizure rate similar to placebo for patients without epilepsy[52]

This table contains information about the pro-convulsive effects of antidepressants and antipsychotics when used in therapeutic doses. See section on 'Psychotropics in overdose' in Chapter 13 for information about supra-therapeutic doses.

ADHD, attention deficit hyperactivity disorder; ECT, electroconvulsive therapy; EEG, electroencephalogram; FGA, first-generation antipsychotic; MAOI, monoamine oxidase inhibitor; PWE, people with epilepsy; RCT, randomised controlled trial; SNRI, serotonin–noradrenaline reuptake inhibitor; SSRI, selective serotonin reuptake inhibitor; TCA, tricyclic antidepressant.

References

1. Scott AJ et al. Anxiety and depressive disorders in people with epilepsy: a meta-analysis. Epilepsia 2017; **58**:973–982.
2. Clancy MJ et al. The prevalence of psychosis in epilepsy; a systematic review and meta-analysis. BMC Psychiatry 2014; **14**:75.
3. Hesdorffer DC et al. Occurrence and recurrence of attempted suicide among people with epilepsy. JAMA Psychiatry 2016; **73**:80–86.
4. Thurman DJ et al. The burden of premature mortality of epilepsy in high-income countries: a systematic review from the Mortality Task Force of the International League Against Epilepsy. Epilepsia 2017; **58**:17–26.
5. Kanner AM. Management of psychiatric and neurological comorbidities in epilepsy. Nat Rev Neurol 2016; **12**:106–116.
6. Hesdorffer DC. Comorbidity between neurological illness and psychiatric disorders. CNS Spectr 2016; **21**:230–238.
7. Kanner AM. Can neurochemical changes of mood disorders explain the increase risk of epilepsy or its worse seizure control? Neurochem Res 2017; **42**:2071–2076.
8. Curran S et al. Selecting an antidepressant for use in a patient with epilepsy. Safety considerations. Drug Saf 1998; **18**:125–133.
9. Blumer D et al. Treatment of the interictal psychoses. J Clin Psychiatry 2000; **61**:110–122.
10. Mula M. The pharmacological management of psychiatric comorbidities in patients with epilepsy. Pharmacol Res 2016; **107**:147–153.
11. Elger CE et al. Diagnosing and treating depression in epilepsy. Seizure 2017; **44**:184–193.
12. Anbarasan D. Psychoactive medications and seizures—challenges and pitfalls. The Neurology Report 2016; **9**:24–27.
13. Kanner AM. Most antidepressant drugs are safe for patients with epilepsy at therapeutic doses: a review of the evidence. Epilepsy Behav 2016; **61**:282–286.
14. Kerr MP et al. International consensus clinical practice statements for the treatment of neuropsychiatric conditions associated with epilepsy. Epilepsia 2011; **52**:2133–2138.
15. Josephson CB et al. Psychiatric comorbidities in epilepsy. Int Rev Psychiatry 2017; **29**:409–424.
16. Maguire M et al. Epilepsy and psychosis: a practical approach. Pract Neurol 2017; [epub ahead of print]
17. Mula M. *Neuropsychiatric Symptoms of Epilepsy*. Basel, Switzerland: Springer International Publishing; 2016.
18. Barry JJ et al. Consensus statement: the evaluation and treatment of people with epilepsy and affective disorders. Epilepsy Behav 2008; **13 Suppl 1**:S1–29.
19. Schmidt D et al. Drug treatment of epilepsy in adults. BMJ 2014; **348**:g254.
20. Piedad J et al. Beneficial and adverse psychotropic effects of antiepileptic drugs in patients with epilepsy: a summary of prevalence, underlying mechanisms and data limitations. CNS Drugs 2012; **26**:319–335.
21. Spina E et al. Clinically significant pharmacokinetic drug interactions of antiepileptic drugs with new antidepressants and new antipsychotics. Pharmacol Res 2016; **106**:72–86.
22. Harden CL et al. Mood disorders in patients with epilepsy: epidemiology and management. CNS Drugs 2002; **16**:291–302.
23. Ngugi AK et al. Incidence of epilepsy: a systematic review and meta-analysis. Neurology 2011; **77**:1005–1012.
24. Alper K et al. Seizure incidence in psychopharmacological clinical trials: an analysis of Food and Drug Administration (FDA) summary basis of approval reports. Biol Psychiatry 2007; **62**:345–354.
25. Wu CS et al. Seizure risk associated with antidepressant treatment among patients with depressive disorders: a population-based case-crossover study. J Clin Psychiatry 2017; **78**:e1226–e1232.
26. Josephson CB et al. Association of depression and treated depression with epilepsy and seizure outcomes: a multicohort analysis. JAMA Neurol 2017; **74**:533–539.
27. Farooq S et al. Interventions for psychotic symptoms concomitant with epilepsy. Cochrane Database Syst Rev 2015:CD006118.
28. Maguire MJ et al. Antidepressants for people with epilepsy and depression. Cochrane Database Syst Rev 2014:CD010682.
29. Maramattom BV. Duloxetine-induced syndrome of inappropriate antidiuretic hormone secretion and seizures. Neurology 2006; **66**:773–774.
30. Steinert T et al. [Epileptic seizures during treatment with antidepressants and neuroleptics]. Fortschr Neurol Psychiatr 2011; **79**:138–143.
31. Mula M. Epilepsy and psychiatric comorbidities: drug selection. Curr Treat Options Neurol 2017; **19**:44.
32. National Institute for Health and Care Excellence. Depression in adults with a chronic physical health problem: treatment and management. Clinical Guideline 91, 2009. http://www.nice.org.uk/guidance/CG91.
33. Steinert T et al. Epileptic seizures under antidepressive drug treatment: systematic review. Pharmacopsychiatry 2017; [Epub ahead of print]
34. Limited SL. Summary of Product Characteristics. Valdoxan. 2017. https://www.medicines.org.uk/emc/medicine/21830.
35. Kuhn KU et al. Antidepressive treatment in patients with temporal lobe epilepsy and major depression: a prospective study with three different antidepressants. Epilepsy Behav 2003; **4**:674–679.
36. Lundbeck Limited. Summary of Product Characteristics. Brintellix (vortioxetine) tablets 5, 10 and 20 mg. 2017. https://www.medicines.org.uk/emc/medicine/30904.
37. Knott S et al. Epilepsy and bipolar disorder. Epilepsy Behav 2015; **52**:267–274.
38. Johannessen Landmark C et al. Proconvulsant effects of antidepressants - what is the current evidence? Epilepsy Behav 2016; **61**:287–291.
39. Elnazer H et al. Managing aggression in epilepsy. BJPsych Advances 2017; **23**:253.
40. Steinert T, Fröscher W. Chapter 9 – Seizures. In: Manu P, Flanagan RJ, Ronaldson KJ, eds. *Life-threatening Effects of Antipsychotic Drugs*. San Diego: Academic Press; 2016.
41. Gonzalez-Heydrich J et al. No seizure exacerbation from risperidone in youth with comorbid epilepsy and psychiatric disorders: a case series. J Child Adolesc Psychopharmacol 2004; **14**:295–310.
42. Truven Health Analytics. Micromedex. 2018. http://truvenhealth.com/products/micromedex.

43. Langosch JM et al. Epilepsy, psychosis and clozapine. Hum Psychopharmacol 2002; **17**:115–119.
44. Jette Pomerleau V et al. Clozapine safety and efficacy for interictal psychotic disorder in pharmacoresistant epilepsy. Cogn Behav Neurol 2017; **30**:73–76.
45. Habibi M et al. The impact of psychoactive drugs on seizures and antiepileptic drugs. Curr Neurol Neurosci Rep 2016; **16**:71.
46. Adams J et al. Methylphenidate, cognition, and epilepsy: a 1-month open-label trial. Epilepsia 2017; **58**:2124–2132.
47. Besag F et al. Psychiatric and Behavioural Disorders in Children with Epilepsy (ILAE Task Force Report): Epilepsy and ADHD. Epileptic Disord 2016; [Epub ahead of print]
48. Besag F et al. Psychiatric and Behavioural Disorders in Children with Epilepsy (ILAE Task Force Report): When should pharmacotherapy for psychiatric/behavioural disorders in children with epilepsy be prescribed? Epileptic Disord 2016; [Epub ahead of print]
49. Gonzalez-Heydrich J et al. Comparing stimulant effects in youth with ADHD symptoms and epilepsy. Epilepsy Behav 2014; **36**:102–107.
50. Schubert R. Attention deficit disorder and epilepsy. Pediatr Neurol 2005; **32**:1–10.
51. Torres A et al. Tolerability of atomoxetine for treatment of pediatric attention-deficit/hyperactivity disorder in the context of epilepsy. Epilepsy Behav 2011; **20**:95–102.
52. Williams AE et al. Epilepsy and attention-deficit hyperactivity disorder: links, risks, and challenges. Neuropsychiatr Dis Treat 2016; **12**:287–296.
53. Ray AK. Does electroconvulsive therapy cause epilepsy? JECT 2013; **29**:201–205.

Further reading

Kanner AM. Management of psychiatric and neurological comorbidities in epilepsy. Nat Rev Neurol 2016; **12**:106–116.
Mula M. Epilepsy and psychiatric comorbidities: drug selection. Curr Treat Options Neurol 2017; **19**:44.

22q11.2 Deletion syndrome

Clinical features

The commonest autosomal deletion, 22q11.2 deletion syndrome (22q11.2DS), is a multisystem disorder with a heterogeneous presentation which varies greatly in severity between affected individuals.[1,2] Prevalence is estimated to range from 1 per 3000 to 5000 births.[2] The syndrome has been known by many names (including velocardiofacial, DiGeorge or Shprintzen syndrome), in part due to its broad phenotypic range of clinical features (see Box 10.2).

Psychiatric disorders in people with 22q11.2DS

Around 60% of people with 22q11.2DS are estimated to meet the diagnostic criteria for some type of psychiatric disorder at some point during their lives.[3] Children with 22q11.2DS have an elevated prevalence of anxiety, ADHD and autism spectrum disorders.[2] Anxiety disorders are profoundly increased in adults.[2] Schizophrenia is diagnosed in approximately 25% of individuals with 22q11.2DS.[2]

Few studies have evaluated the safety and efficacy of psychotropics in people with 22q11.2DS.[4] However, standard pharmacological (and non-pharmacological) treatments for ADHD, anxiety, mood disorders and schizophrenia appear to be effective and treatment protocols used in the general population should be followed.[2,5] Although most psychotropics are thought to be safe in people with 22q11.2DS, consideration should be given to medical co-morbidities (e.g. cardiovascular disorders), a potentially increased risk of seizures[6] and movement disorders.[2] Endocrine abnormalities (e.g. hypoparathyroidism and hypothyroidism) should be corrected before starting psychotropics because they can mimic psychiatric symptoms and complicate treatment with psychotropics.[5,7] Current evidence and opinion on the treatment of psychiatric disorders in people with 22q11.2DS is summarised in Table 10.6.

Box 10.2   Clinical features of 22q11.2DS[2]

- Cardiovascular abnormalities including tetralogy of Fallot
- Endocrine abnormalities including hypoparathyroidism
- Genitourinary abnormalities including renal agenesis
- Developmental delays and learning disabilities
- Gastrointestinal abnormalities including constipation

- Immunodeficiency and autoimmune disease
- Palatal abnormalities
- Behavioural phenotypes
- Psychiatric disorders
- Skeletal abnormalities

Table 10.6 Management of psychiatric disorders in people with 22q11.2DS[8]

Psychiatric disorder	Treatments
ADHD	■ Although concerns have been raised about the theoretical risk of psychosis with psychostimulants in people with 22q11.2DS, standard treatment protocols are advised[4] ■ Two studies support the efficacy of methylphenidate in children with 22q11.2DS.[4] Treatment was generally well tolerated. A comprehensive cardiovascular assessment prior to and during treatment has been recommended[4]
Depression and anxiety	■ SSRIs: both depression and anxiety appear to respond favourably to SSRIs.[9] Low doses may be sufficient.[10] Further treatment is per standard protocols ■ S-adenosyl-L-methionine was studied in one small RCT and no significant benefit in depressive (or ADHD) symptoms was detected[11]
Obsessive compulsive disorder	■ One study of four people with OCD and 22q11.2DS found a mean rate of improvement of 35% after treatment with fluoxetine (30–60 mg/day). Treatment was well tolerated[8]
Schizophrenia	Standard treatment protocols are generally recommended.[5,12] People with 22q11.2DS may be more susceptible to seizures and EPS with antipsychotics.[8] There is a significantly elevated risk of obesity in 22q11.2DS[13] so metabolic adverse effects should be closely monitored. Patients with cardiac abnormalities have an increased risk of QTc prolongation.[8] Close ECG monitoring is recommended[8] Antipsychotics with a low effect on the QT interval are preferred.[8] Low starting doses and slow dose titrations are widely recommended.[8] Case reports have described the successful use of aripiprazole, olanzapine, risperidone and quetiapine[9] but treatment resistance has been demonstrated in many cases[7,9] ■ **Clozapine:** found to be effective in one retrospective study of 20 patients with 22q11.2DS.[14] Compared to matched controls, lower doses were needed (250 mg/day for those with 22q11.2DS; 450 mg/day for matched controls). However, half of the 22q11.2DS group experienced at least one rare serious adverse effect from clozapine, primarily seizures but also myocarditis and neutropenia. Several case reports further support the efficacy of clozapine at low doses (median of 200 mg/day) for people with 22q11.2DS, but also highlight the risk of seizures[15] (generalised or myoclonic) and agranulocytosis.[14] Overall, clozapine appears to have demonstrable efficacy at lower than usual doses, but the risk of rare, serious adverse events appears to be high.[14] Adjunctive anticonvulsants should be considered[12] ■ **Seizures with antipsychotics:** investigate low calcium and magnesium levels in all cases and ensure adequate treatment.[12] Consider adjunctive anticonvulsants[12] ■ **Other agents:** drugs that act directly against catecholamine excess may also be effective. Metyrosine, used as a monotherapy or as an adjunctive agent, was found to be effective in 22 of 29 patients recruited to one study.[16] Additional positive case reports have been published.[17] There is a single case study where methyldopa was used successfully[18]

ADHD, attention deficit hyperactivity disorder; ECG, electrocardiogram; EPS, extrapyramidal symptoms; OCD, obsessive compulsive disorder; RCT, randomised controlled trial; SSRI, selective serotonin reuptake inhibitor.

References

1. Habel A et al. Towards a safety net for management of 22q11.2 deletion syndrome: guidelines for our times. Eur J Pediatr 2014; 173:757–765.
2. McDonald-McGinn DM et al. 22q11.2 deletion syndrome. Nat Rev Dis Primers 2015; 1:15071.
3. Bertran M et al. Psychiatric manifestations of 22q11.2 deletion syndrome: a literature review. Neurologia 2015; pii: S0213-4853(15)00182-6.

4. Tang KL et al. Behavioral and psychiatric phenotypes in 22q11.2 deletion syndrome. J Dev Behav Pediatr 2015; 36:639–650.

5. Fung WL et al. Practical guidelines for managing adults with 22q11.2 deletion syndrome. Genet Med 2015; 17:599–609.

6. Wither RG et al. 22q11.2 deletion syndrome lowers seizure threshold in adult patients without epilepsy. Epilepsia 2017; 58:1095–1101.

7. Verhoeven WM et al. Atypical antipsychotics and relapsing psychoses in 22q11.2 deletion syndrome: a long-term evaluation of 28 patients. Pharmacopsychiatry 2015; 48:104–110.

8. Baker K et al. Psychiatric illness. Consensus Document on 22q11 Deletion Syndrome (22q11DS) MaxAppeal. 2017. http://www.maxappeal.org.uk/downloads/Consensus_Document_on_22q11_Deletion_Syndrome_Master_2017_(final_draft)_9-end_(1)2018.pdf.

9. Dori N et al. The effectiveness and safety of antipsychotic and antidepressant medications in individuals with 22q11.2 deletion syndrome. J Child Adolesc Psychopharmacol 2017; 27:83–90.

10. Stachon AC et al. Anxiety disorders and perceptual disturbances in adolescents with 22q11.2 deletion syndrome treated with SSRI: a case series. J Can Acad Child Adolesc Psychiatry 2011; 20:305–310.

11. Tang SX et al. Psychiatric disorders in 22q11.2 deletion syndrome are prevalent but undertreated. Psychol Med 2014; 44:1267–1277.

12. Bassett AS et al. Practical guidelines for managing patients with 22q11.2 deletion syndrome. J Pediatr 2011; 159:332–339.

13. Voll SL et al. Obesity in adults with 22q11.2 deletion syndrome. Genet Med 2017; 19:204–208.

14. Butcher NJ et al. Response to clozapine in a clinically identifiable subtype of schizophrenia. Br J Psychiatry 2015; 206:484–491.

15. Aksu H et al. Treatment of schizophrenia by clozapine in an adolescent girl with DiGeorge syndrome. J Child Adolesc Psychopharmacol 2016; 26:652.

16. Faedda GL et al. 4.19 Treatment of velo-cardio-facial syndrome-related psychosis with metyrosine. J Am Acad Child Adolesc Psychiatry 2016; 55:S169.

17. Engebretsen MH et al. Metyrosine treatment in a woman with chromosome 22q11.2 deletion syndrome and psychosis: a case study. Int J Dev Disabil 2017:1–6.

18. O'Hanlon JF et al. Replacement of antipsychotic and antiepileptic medication by L-alpha-methyldopa in a woman with velocardiofacial syndrome. Int Clin Psychopharmacol 2003; 18:117–119.

Further reading

Fung WL et al. Practical guidelines for managing adults with 22q11.2 deletion syndrome. Genet Med 2015; 17:599–609.

Learning disabilities

General considerations[1]

Prescribing psychotropic medications for people with learning disability (LD) is a challenging and controversial area of psychiatric practice.[2,3] There are concerns that psychotropic drugs of all kinds (antipsychotics, antidepressants benzodiazepines (both regular and as required) and anti-epileptics as mood stabilisers) are overprescribed with poor review and assessment of their benefit. The learning disabilities field is notable in having only a small therapeutics research base of its own, with particular ethical and practical considerations regarding how emotional and behavioural disturbances are classified and treated. Although prescribing for individuals with mild or borderline intellectual impairment may be undertaken by mainstream mental health services, the assessment and treatment of behavioural and emotional disorders in people with more marked (or, as in the case of autism, atypical) patterns of significant cognitive impairment should be undertaken in the first instance by, or at least in consultation with, specialist clinicians.

The term 'dual diagnosis' in this context refers to the co-occurrence of an identifiable psychiatric disorder (mental illness, personality disorder) and LD. 'Diagnostic overshadowing' is the misattribution of emotional or behavioural problems to LD itself rather than to a co-morbid condition. LD is an important risk factor for all psychiatric disorders (including dementia, particularly for individuals with Down syndrome).[4] Where it is possible to diagnose a mental illness using conventional or modified criteria then drug treatment in the first instance should, in general, be similar to that in the population at large. Most treatment guidelines are increasingly stating their intended applicability to people with LD in this regard.

Mental illness may present in unusual ways in LD (e.g. depression as self-injurious behaviour, persecutory ideation as complaints of being 'picked on'). Conversely, behaviours such as self-talk may be normal in some individuals but mistakenly identified as a disorder such as psychosis. In general, diagnosis becomes increasingly complex with increasing severity of disability and associated communication impairment.

Co-morbid autistic spectrum disorder has special assessment considerations and in its own right is an important risk factor for psychiatric disorder, in particular anxiety and depression, bipolar spectrum disorder, severe obsessional behaviour, anger disorders and psychosis-like episodes that may not meet criteria for schizophrenia but nonetheless require treatment. Autistic traits are common amongst patients using LD services. Guidance on the treatment of mental health problems in autism can be found in Chapter 5.

Key practice areas

Capacity and consent. It is uncommon for patients in LD services (who often represent a sub-population of those identified with special educational needs in childhood) to have sufficient understanding of their treatment in order to be able to take truly informed decisions. There is inevitably an increased onus on the clinician to bear the weight of decision-making. Decision-making capacity, depending on the severity of intellectual impairment, may be improved through appropriate verbal and written communication. The involvement of carers in this process is generally essential.

Physical co-morbidity, especially epilepsy. Epilepsy is over-represented in LD populations, becoming more prevalent as severity increases: approximately one-third of affected individuals develop a seizure disorder by early adulthood. Special consideration is needed when considering the use of medications that may lower seizure threshold or interact with drugs used for epilepsy.

Assessment of care environments. Behavioural and emotional disturbance may sometimes be a reflection of problems or failings in the care environment. Different staff in a care home may have different thresholds of tolerance (or make different attributions) for these difficulties which can lead to varied reports of their significance and impact. Allowing for a period of prospective assessment and using simple assessment tools (e.g. simple ABC or sleep charts) can be very helpful to the clinician in making judgements about recommending medication. If medication is used in a care home, staff may need special education in its use and anticipated adverse effects and, for 'as required' medications, clear guidelines for their use. This may make it difficult to initiate certain treatments in the community.

Adverse effect sensitivity. It is widely thought that people with LD are especially sensitive to adverse effects of psychotropics and more at risk of long-term effects such as the metabolic syndrome; however this is not supported by study evidence. It is good practice to start at lower doses and increase more slowly than might be usual in general psychiatric practice. Notable adverse effects include worsening of seizures, sedation, extrapyramidal reactions (including with risperidone at normal doses, especially in individuals who already have mobility problems), problems with swallowing (with clozapine and other antipsychotics) and worsening of cognitive function with anticholinergic medications (see section on 'Safer prescribing for physical conditions in dementia' in Chapter 6).

Psychological interventions. In the absence of an identifiable mental illness (including atypical presentations) with clear treatment implications, psychological interventions such as functional behavioural analysis should be considered as first-line intervention for all but the most serious or intractable presentations of behavioural disturbance. In studies where it has been possible to infer severity of challenging behaviour, treatment response is generally associated with more severe problems at baseline.

Some notes on currently and historically used medications for behaviour disorder

Medications used for behaviour disorder in LD are summarised in Table 10.7.

Table 10.7 Currently and historically used medications for behaviour disorder

Drug class	Clinical applications	Notes
Antipsychotics[5]	Use in psychosis with LD is justified Used across a broad range of behavioural disturbances[6] May be useful for aggression and irritability	The most widely used[7,8] yet most controversial medication for behavioural problems.[9,10] Although an RCT[11] cast doubt on their efficacy the study was not without its problems and there is a significant body of other evidence supporting their use including a number of small RCTs in children with LD
		Discontinuation studies in long-term treatment commonly (but not always) show re-emergence of problem behaviours
		NICE suggests considering slow withdrawal of antipsychotics in all those who do not have psychotic symptoms[12]
		Before the advent of SGAs the best evidence was for **haloperidol**[13] in the context of autism and for zuclopenthixol for behavioural disturbance.[14] Zuclopenthixol may reduce aggression and challenging behaviour[15]
		Amongst SGAs the best evidence is for **risperidone**[16,17] at low dose (0.5–2 mg) for aggression and mood instability **(licensed in the UK for short-term use)**, particularly with associated autism though also in non-autistic cases. **Aripiprazole** has an FDA licence for behavioural disturbance in young people with autism[18,19]
		Some evidence to support **olanzapine**[20] and case reports of **clozapine**[21] for very severe cases of aggression though not widely used and unlikely to be used outside highly specialist (in-patient) settings. In 2015, Cochrane uncovered 38 case reports and chart reviews but found no RCT evidence for the use of clozapine in psychosis in LD[22]
		Results for **quetiapine** are modest at best[23]
SSRIs	Helpful for severe anxiety and obsessionality in autistic spectrum disorder. Use here is off-licence unless an additional diagnosis of anxiety disorder or OCD is made	Commonly used in combination with antipsychotics though limited evidence base for combination treatment. Effectiveness in absence of mood or anxiety spectrum disorder is unclear, however, and a 2013 Cochrane review was pessimistic[24] about the evidence for their effectiveness for behaviour disorder in autistic children (who may be at heightened risk of adverse effects) though a little more encouraging in adults
	Also used as a first-line alternative to antipsychotics for aggression and impulsivity	Generally, quality of trials is poor and effects may be exaggerated by use in less severe cases.[25] Caution needed because of the risk of precipitation of hypomania in this population.[26] Also major concerns about overprescribing
		Venlafaxine is probably not effective[27]
Anticonvulsants[28]	Aggression and self-injury	Some uncontrolled studies supporting **sodium valproate**[29] in LD populations though evidence is not strong and research findings contradictory in this population. However, remains best supported of the anticonvulsants for mood lability and aggression partly because of positive studies in non-LD groups[30]
		Limited studies of **lamotrigine**, mostly in children, suggest no effect, at least in autism and in the absence of affective instability[23]
		Data for **carbamazepine** also unconvincing, but it is still widely used[31]

(Continued)

Table 10.7 *(Continued)*

Drug class	Clinical applications	Notes
Lithium[32]	Licensed for the treatment of self-injurious behaviour and aggression	Some RCT evidence[33] for LD though no studies in this population for many years although there has been one more recent positive RCT for aggression in adolescents without developmental impairment.[34] Experience suggests can be very helpful in individual cases where other treatments have failed and is possibly underused though adverse effects can be problematic
		Perhaps best considered where there is a sub-syndromal or nonspecific 'affective component'. Some authorities suggest that, on close examination, challenging behaviour may occur in the context of very rapid cycling bipolar disorder in some individuals with severe and profound LD and that the diagnosis is easily missed
Methylphenidate	Effective in ADHD associated with LD	NICE[12] conducted a meta-analysis and found clear benefit for methylphenidate (and risperidone and clonidine) in ADHD in the context of LD. Insomnia is common
Naltrexone[35]	Has been used for severe self-injurious behaviour[36]	Evidence not strong and results are inconsistent. Use may still be an option in severe and intractable cases

ADHD, attention deficit hyperactivity disorder; FDA, US Food and Drug Administration; LD, learning disability; NICE, National Institute for Health and Care Excellence; OCD, obsessive compulsive disorder; RCT, randomised controlled trial; SGA, second-generation antipsychotic; SSRI, selective serotonin reuptake inhibitor.

References

1. Deb S. The Use of Medications for the Management of Problem Behaviours in Adults who have Intellectual [Learning] Disabilities. 2012. http://www.intellectualdisability.info/mental-health/the-use-of-drugs-for-the-treatment-of-behaviour-disorders-in-adults-who-have-learning-intellectual-disabilities.
2. Sheehan R et al. Psychotropic prescribing in people with intellectual disability and challenging behaviour. BMJ 2017; 358:j3896.
3. Ji NY et al. Pharmacotherapy for mental health problems in people with intellectual disability. Curr Opin Psychiatry 2016; 29:103–125.
4. Cooper SA et al. Mental ill-health in adults with intellectual disabilities: prevalence and associated factors. Br J Psychiatry 2007; 190:27–35.
5. Antochi R et al. Psychopharmacological treatments in persons with dual diagnosis of psychiatric disorders and developmental disabilities. Postgrad Med J 2003; 79:139–146.
6. Lunsky Y et al. Antipsychotic use with and without comorbid psychiatric diagnosis among adults with intellectual and developmental disabilities. Can J Psychiatry 2017:706743717727240.
7. Deb S et al. Characteristics and the trajectory of psychotropic medication use in general and antipsychotics in particular among adults with an intellectual disability who exhibit aggressive behaviour. J Intellect Disabil Res 2015; 59:11–25.
8. Sheehan R et al. Mental illness, challenging behaviour, and psychotropic drug prescribing in people with intellectual disability: UK population based cohort study. BMJ 2015; 351:h4326.
9. Deb S et al. The effectiveness of antipsychotic medication in the management of behaviour problems in adults with intellectual disabilities. J Intellect Disabil Res 2007; 51:766–777.
10. Roy D et al. Pharmacologic management of aggression in adults with intellectual disability. J Intellect Disabil Res 2013; 1:28–43.
11. Tyrer P et al. Risperidone, haloperidol, and placebo in the treatment of aggressive challenging behaviour in patients with intellectual disability: a randomised controlled trial. Lancet 2008; 371:57–63.
12. National Institute for Health and Care Excellence. Mental health problems in people with learning disabilities: prevention, assessment and management. NICE Guideline NG54, 2016. https://www.nice.org.uk/Guidance/NG54.
13. Malone RP et al. The role of antipsychotics in the management of behavioural symptoms in children and adolescents with autism. Drugs 2009; 69:535–548.
14. Malt UF et al. Effectiveness of zuclopenthixol compared with haloperidol in the treatment of behavioural disturbances in learning disabled patients. Br J Psychiatry 1995; 166:374–377.
15. Hassler F et al. Treatment of aggressive behavior problems in boys with intellectual disabilities using zuclopenthixol. J Child Adolesc Psychopharmacol 2014; 24:579–581.

16. Nagaraj R et al. Risperidone in children with autism: randomized, placebo-controlled, double-blind study. J Child Neurol 2006; 21:450–455.
17. Pandina GJ et al. Risperidone improves behavioral symptoms in children with autism in a randomized, double-blind, placebo-controlled trial. J Autism Dev Disord 2007; 37:367–373.
18. Owen R et al. Aripiprazole in the treatment of irritability in children and adolescents with autistic disorder. Pediatrics 2009; 124:1533–1540.
19. Marcus RN et al. A placebo-controlled, fixed-dose study of aripiprazole in children and adolescents with irritability associated with autistic disorder. J Am Acad Child Adolesc Psychiatry 2009; 48:1110–1119.
20. Fido A et al. Olanzapine in the treatment of behavioral problems associated with autism: an open-label trial in Kuwait. Med Princ Pract 2008; 17:415–418.
21. Zuddas A et al. Clinical effects of clozapine on autistic disorder. Am J Psychiatry 1996; 153:738.
22. Ayub M et al. Clozapine for psychotic disorders in adults with intellectual disabilities. Cochrane Database Syst Rev 2015:CD010625.
23. Stigler KA et al. Pharmacotherapy of irritability in pervasive developmental disorders. Child Adolesc Psychiatr Clin N Am 2008; 17:739–752.
24. Williams K et al. Selective serotonin reuptake inhibitors (SSRIs) for autism spectrum disorders (ASD). Cochrane Database Syst Rev 2013; 8:CD004677.
25. Myers SM. Citalopram not effective for repetitive behaviour in autistic spectrum disorders. Evid Based Ment Health 2010; 13:22.
26. Cook EH, Jr. et al. Fluoxetine treatment of children and adults with autistic disorder and mental retardation. J Am Acad Child Adolesc Psychiatry 1992; 31:739–745.
27. Carminati GG et al. Using venlafaxine to treat behavioral disorders in patients with autism spectrum disorder. Prog Neuropsychopharmacol Biol Psychiatry 2016; 65:85–95.
28. Deb S et al. The effectiveness of mood stabilizers and antiepileptic medication for the management of behaviour problems in adults with intellectual disability: a systematic review. J Intellect Disabil Res 2008; 52:107–113.
29. Ruedrich S et al. Effect of divalproex sodium on aggression and self-injurious behaviour in adults with intellectual disability: a retrospective review. J Intellect Disabil Res 1999; 43 (Pt 2):105–111.
30. Donovan SJ et al. Divalproex treatment for youth with explosive temper and mood lability: a double-blind, placebo-controlled crossover design. Am J Psychiatry 2000; 157:818–820.
31. Unwin GL et al. Use of medication for the management of behavior problems among adults with intellectual disabilities: a clinicians' consensus survey. Am J Ment Retard 2008; 113:19–31.
32. Pary RJ Towards defining adequate lithium trials for individuals with mental retardation and mental illness. Am J Ment Retard 1991; 95:681–691.
33. Craft M et al. Lithium in the treatment of aggression in mentally handicapped patients. A double-blind trial. Br J Psychiatry 1987; 150: 685–689.
34. Malone RP et al. A double-blind placebo-controlled study of lithium in hospitalized aggressive children and adolescents with conduct disorder. Arch Gen Psychiatry 2000; 57:649–654.
35. Campbell M et al. Naltrexone in autistic children: an acute open dose range tolerance trial. J Am Acad Child Adolesc Psychiatry 1989; 28:200–206.
36. Barrett RP et al. Effects of naloxone and naltrexone on self-injury: a double-blind, placebo-controlled analysis. Am J Ment Retard 1989; 93:644–651.

Huntington's disease

Huntington's disease (HD) is a genetic disease involving slow progressive degeneration of neurones in the striatum with the involvement of the cerebral cortex as the disease progresses.[1] In Western populations HD has a prevalence of 10.6–13.7 individuals per 100,000.[1] The mutant Huntington protein causes neuronal dysfunction and death through several mechanisms, resulting in a triad of motor, cognitive and neuropsychiatric symptoms. There are currently no disease-modifying treatments[1,2] and so only symptomatic treatment is used, in an attempt to improve quality of life (Box 10.3).

There are few controlled studies to guide practice in this area,[2] though some direction can be drawn from published expert opinion and clinical experience. A summary of the available literature can be found in this section. Readers are directed to the reports cited for details of dosage regimens and further information about tolerability. Clinicians who treat patients with HD are encouraged to publish reports of both positive and negative outcomes to increase the primary literature base.

Box 10.3 General principles of pharmacological symptom management in Huntington's disease[3,4]

- Tailor management to the needs of the individual patient (treatment is typically initiated when symptoms become bothersome, interfering or socially stigmatising).
- Check whether existing medications are causing or exacerbating symptoms before commencing new treatments.
- Prioritise treatment to target the most troublesome symptoms first, with consideration of co-morbid features.
- Balance therapeutic benefit with the potential for adverse effects.
- Start with a low dose and titrate according to tolerability and response (patients are relatively more sensitive to cognitive and motor adverse effects which may also be difficult to distinguish from disease progression).
- Regularly follow up with patients to address changes in treatment (because symptomology evolves with disease progression).

Motor symptoms

Motor disturbances follow a biphasic course: an initial hyperkinetic phase with prominent chorea which tends to plateau over time, and a later hypokinetic phase characterised by bradykinesia, dystonia and balance and gait disturbance.[1] With regards to chorea, the goal of treatment is not to obliterate movements but to reduce their severity to achieve better tolerability.[3] Treatment pathways are available to guide management.[5,6] First-line treatments include tetrabenazine (licensed) or antipsychotics (unlicensed)[3,5–7] (Table 10.8).

Mental and behavioural symptoms

A wide variety of mental and behavioural symptoms occur in HD, including anxiety, depression, suicidality, preservation, disinhibition, irritability, apathy and, rarely, psychosis[14] (Table 10.9). Mental and behavioural symptoms can emerge before motor disturbances and reduce quality of life substantially.[14] In comparison with other HD

Table 10.8 Evidence and experience regarding the pharmacological treatment of motor symptoms in Huntington's disease

Symptom	Treatments
Chorea	■ **Tetrabenazine:** unlike antipsychotics, tetrabenazine's effectiveness is well established;[2,8] however, adverse effects including sedation, depression and parkinsonism may limit its clinical benefit.[8] In clinical practice, many prefer to use tetrabenazine first line in patients without depressive symptoms and suicidal behaviour.[8] Compliance with a multiple daily dosing regimen (e.g. tds) is needed. Deutetrabenazine, recently licensed in the US for chorea in HD, has not been directly compared with tetrabenazine but it may offer an improved pharmacokinetic and adverse-effect profile.[9] ■ **Antipsychotics:** low-dose antipsychotics are considered first-line treatment in the presence of depression, aggression, psychosis, or when poor drug compliance is suspected[3,5–7] despite a lack of data from RCTs.[10] Of note, antipsychotics were associated with a worse prognosis in one recent retrospective analysis;[11] however, further research is needed to assess causality. SGAs such as risperidone or olanzapine are used most commonly.[3,8] Potentially limiting adverse effects include dyskinesia, parkinsonism and metabolic syndrome.[3] Lower starting and maximum doses are recommended.[5,6] Clozapine may be helpful, but it is used infrequently because of the risk of agranulocytosis and the arduous blood monitoring requirements.[3] Typical antipsychotics have been used successfully but are currently less popular in clinical practice because of the risk of EPS.[8] For severe chorea, antipsychotics and tetrabenazine have been used in combination;[3] note that tetrabenazine (and deutetrabenazine[9] have the potential for QT prolongation[3] ■ **Other agents:** amantadine, riluzole and nabilone have been recommended as alternatives to tetrabenazine;[10] the evidence base for beneficial effects with these agents is controversial,[3] and some recent guidelines recommend against using amantadine and riluzole.[7] Nabilone is only used in refractory cases.[4] Clinical trials with other cannabinoids (nabiximols and cannabidiol) showed no difference from placebo.[12] Clonazepam is sometimes used as an adjunctive therapy in the presence of co-morbid features; a small case series reported benefit with high doses.[3] Levetiracetam has been used successfully in two small open-label studies; somnolence led to a 33% dropout in one study and parkinsonism was also reported.[8] Pridopidine has not reached primary endpoints in RCTs so far; further evaluation is required.[8] Recently completed negative studies also include those examining the use of latrepirdine, ethyl-eicosapentaenoic acid and mavoglurant[8]
Hypokinetic rigidity	■ Treatment with levodopa and dopamine agonists has shown variable benefit in case reports[13] but in practice response is often suboptimal.[4] Note the potential for such drugs to exacerbate behavioural disturbances.[13] Dopamine depleters or dopamine blockers should be discontinued in the first instance[3]
Myoclonus	■ Valproate, levetiracetam or clonazepam have been suggested[3]
Dystonia	■ Botulinum toxin injections have been suggested for focal dystonia; clonazepam or baclofen has been suggested for non-focal dystonia[3]

EPS, extrapyramidal symptoms; HD, Huntington's disease; RCT, randomised controlled trial; SGA, second-generation antipsychotic; tds, *ter die sumendum* (three times a day).

features, psychiatric symptoms are perhaps the most amenable to pharmacotherapy.[15] In general, psychiatric treatment choices are selected as they would be in other conditions,[3] though patients are relatively more sensitive to adverse effects.[3] The most commonly prescribed psychotropics are summarised in Table 10.10 (mostly based on low-quality evidence).[14]

Table 10.9 Evidence and experience regarding the pharmacological treatment of mental and behavioural symptoms in Huntington's disease

Symptom	Treatments
Anxiety	■ Reported 16.7–24% lifetime prevalence in HD.[14] There are no RCTs to guide choice, however olanzapine 5 mg/day substantially improved anxiety symptoms in one small open-label pilot study.[14] SSRIs have been suggested as first-line treatment.[3] Some guidelines have recommended considering SGAs (risperidone or olanzapine) for anxiety associated with perseveration, personality or behavioural disturbances.[7] Anxiolytics such as benzodiazepines or buspirone may also be useful[7]
Depression	Reported 20–56% lifetime prevalence in HD.[14] Treatment is typically required: depression is linked to a lower quality of life in HD and increases the risk of suicide.[14] There are no RCTs to guide choice.[16] However, most experts agree that depression in HD responds well to antidepressants;[15] SSRIs are the preferred first-line treatment.[3] ■ **SSRIs:** two controlled trials examined the effects of fluoxetine and citalopram in non-depressed patients with HD; despite excluding depressed patients, both showed near significant improvements in depressive symptoms.[16] Note that tetrabenazine is metabolised by CYP2D6; inhibitors of this enzyme (e.g. fluoxetine) may increase levels ■ **SNRIs:** venlafaxine was effective in an uncontrolled study;[16] however, one in five developed adverse effects such as nausea and irritability[14] ■ **TCAs:** beneficial effects reported in some cases[17] but generally their use should be avoided or limited; the anticholinergic properties of TCAs may worsen hyperkinesias and cognition.[18] Toxicity in overdose may also make them less suitable choices (suicidality is increased in HD[14]) ■ **Others:** mirtazapine was used successfully in a case report of severe depression.[3] In a case registry study it was one of the most frequently prescribed treatments for depression in HD.[14] Lithium produced improvements in suicidality in a small case series[16] but experience is very limited and tolerability may be poor. MAOIs have been used in earlier case studies;[4] a lack of recent experience and important interactions with tetrabenazine make these less suitable.[18] ECT was well tolerated and produced improvement in nine cases of severe depression in HD[14]
Obsessive compulsive behaviours or perseveration	■ There are no RCTs. International consensus supports the use of SSRIs first line; use of clomipramine is also supported[14] but tolerability may be poor. Case studies document the successful use of fluoxetine, paroxetine and sertraline.[3] One study of two patients with perseveration and aggression reported beneficial effects with buspirone[14]
Irritability	■ Initial management is non-pharmacological.[14] There have been no RCTs, but expert consensus supports the use of SSRIs (e.g. citalopram and sertraline) when irritability is accompanied by depression, anxiety or perseveration; antipsychotics are favoured when irritability is accompanied by aggression, hypersexuality or impulsivity[14] ■ **Aggressive behaviours:** a wide variety of psychotropics have been used with reported beneficial effects (e.g. antipsychotics, lithium, valproate, propranolol, medroxyprogesterone, SSRIs, buspirone).[19] Antipsychotics have been used most commonly. The evidence base is too limited to make specific treatment recommendations[19] but low-dose antipsychotics can be considered.[3] ECT was helpful in one case of agitation refractory to pharmacotherapy[20]
Apathy	■ Common in HD and appears to worsen with disease progression.[14] Bupropion was recently studied in one multicentre RCT and found to be ineffective.[21] Other agents, including methylphenidate, atomoxetine, modafinil, amantadine and bromocriptine have been trialled with little success[14]
Psychosis	One of the least prevalent psychiatric manifestations of HD, perhaps due to the use of antidopaminergics for motor symptoms.[14] There are no RCTs to guide choice; treatment is empirical. Note that antipsychotic drugs may exacerbate any underlying movement disorder ■ **SGAs:** olanzapine and risperidone are used most frequently;[14] low starting doses are recommended.[3] Case reports support the efficacy of risperidone,[22–24] quetiapine,[25] aripiprazole and amisulpride[14,26] ■ **FGAs:** used less frequently due to the risk of dystonia and parkinsonism;[3] however, haloperidol has been used when chorea is also problematic to the patient[14]

ECT, electroconvulsive therapy; EPS, extrapyramidal symptoms; FGA, first-generation antipsychotic; HD, Huntington's disease; MAOI, monoamine oxidase inhibitor; RCT, randomised controlled trial; SGA, second-generation antipsychotic; SNRI, serotonin–noradrenaline reuptake inhibitor; SSRI, selective serotonin reuptake inhibitor; TCA, tricyclic antidepressant.

Table 10.10 Summary of available treatments for mental state and behavioural changes in Huntington's disease[14]

Symptom	Most commonly prescribed pharmacological treatments	Alternatives
Anxiety	SSRIs*, mirtazapine, pregabalin, venlafaxine	Olanzapine, benzodiazepines, propranolol, buspirone
Depression or suicidality	SSRIs*, mirtazapine, venlafaxine	TCAs; ECT in refractory cases
Obsessive compulsive behaviours	SSRIs*	Clomipramine
Irritability	SSRIs*, SGAs (olanzapine, risperidone, sulpiride), tiapride	Anticonvulsants (lamotrigine, carbamazepine, valproate), TCAs, buspirone, propranolol
Apathy	None	None
Psychosis	Olanzapine, risperidone, haloperidol, sulpiride, tiapride, injectable antipsychotic medication	Clozapine, quetiapine

*Citalopram typically used first line[4]
ECT, electroconvulsive therapy; SGA, second-generation antipsychotic; SSRI, selective serotonin reuptake inhibitor; TCA, tricyclic antidepressant.

Cognitive symptoms

Cognitive disturbances may emerge many years before motor disturbances;[1] the progression of cognitive decline is gradual[27] and dementia is inevitable in late stages. Although a wide variety of agents have been studied, none has become an established treatment and the benefit of most remains unclear.[28] There is insufficient evidence to support the use of acetylcholinesterase inhibitors[29] and no evidence to support any other medications to treat dementia in HD.[30]

References

1. McColgan P et al. Huntington's disease: a clinical review. Eur J Neurol 2018; 25:24–34.
2. Mestre T et al. Therapeutic interventions for symptomatic treatment in Huntington's disease. Cochrane Database Syst Rev 2009:CD006456.
3. Killoran A et al. Current therapeutic options for Huntington's disease: good clinical practice versus evidence-based approaches? Mov Disord 2014; 29:1404–1413.
4. Mason SL et al. Advancing pharmacotherapy for treating Huntington's disease: a review of the existing literature. Expert Opin Pharmacother 2016; 17:41–52.
5. Reilmann R. Pharmacological treatment of chorea in Huntington's disease – good clinical practice versus evidence-based guideline. Mov Disord 2013; 28:1030–1033.
6. Burgunder JM et al. An international survey-based algorithm for the pharmacologic treatment of chorea in Huntington's disease. PLoS Curr 2011; 3:RRN1260.
7. Desamericq G et al. Guidelines for clinical pharmacological practices in Huntington's disease. Rev Neurol (Paris) 2016; 172:423–432.
8. Coppen EM et al. Current Pharmacological Approaches to Reduce Chorea in Huntington's Disease. Drugs 2017; 77:29–46.
9. Heo YA et al. Deutetrabenazine: A review in chorea associated with Huntington's disease. Drugs 2017; 77:1857–1864.
10. Armstrong MJ et al. Evidence-based guideline: pharmacologic treatment of chorea in Huntington disease: report of the guideline development subcommittee of the American Academy of Neurology. Neurology 2012; 79:597–603.
11. Tedroff J et al. Antidopaminergic medication is associated with more rapidly progressive Huntington's disease. J Huntingtons Dis 2015; 4:131–140.
12. Lim K et al. A systematic review of the effectiveness of medical cannabis for psychiatric, movement and neurodegenerative disorders. Clin Psychopharmacol Neurosci 2017; 15:301–312.
13. Wyant KJ et al. Huntington's disease – update on treatments. Curr Neurol Neurosci Rep 2017; 17:33.

14. Eddy CM et al. Changes in mental state and behaviour in Huntington's disease. Lancet Psychiatry 2016; 3:1079–1086.

15. Dayalu P et al. Huntington disease: pathogenesis and treatment. Neurol Clin 2015; 33:101–114.

16. Moulton CD et al. Systematic review of pharmacological treatments for depressive symptoms in Huntington's disease. Mov Disord 2014; 29:1556–1561.

17. Ossig C et al. *Neuropsychiatric Symptoms of Movement Disorders - Depression in Huntington's Disease.* Basel, Switzerland: Springer International Publishing; 2015, pp. 201–209.

18. Schiefer J et al. Clinical diagnosis and management in early Huntington's disease: a review. Degen Neurol Neuromusc Dis 2015; 5:37–50.

19. Fisher CA et al. Aggression in Huntington's disease: a systematic review of rates of aggression and treatment methods. J Huntingtons Dis 2014; 3:319–332.

20. Shah RP et al. Treatment of agitation in Huntington's disease with electroconvulsive therapy. J Neuropsychiatry Clin Neurosci 2017; 29:293–294.

21. Gelderblom H et al. Bupropion for the treatment of apathy in Huntington's disease: a multicenter, randomised, double-blind, placebo-controlled, prospective crossover trial. PLoS One 2017; 12:e0173872.

22. Dallocchio C et al. Effectiveness of risperidone in Huntington chorea patients. J Clin Psychopharmacol 1999; 19:101–103.

23. Duff K et al. Risperidone and the treatment of psychiatric, motor, and cognitive symptoms in Huntington's disease. Ann Clin Psychiatry 2008; 20:1–3.

24. Madhusoodanan S et al. Use of risperidone in psychosis associated with Huntington's disease. Am J Geriatr Psychiatry 1998; 6:347–349.

25. Seitz DP et al. Quetiapine in the management of psychosis secondary to Huntington's disease: a case report. Can J Psychiatry 2004; 49:413.

26. Bonelli RM et al. A systematic review of the treatment studies in Huntington's disease since 1990. Expert Opin Pharmacother 2007; 8:141–153.

27. Ross CA et al. Huntington disease: natural history, biomarkers and prospects for therapeutics. Nat Rev Neurol 2014; 10:204–216.

28. van der Vaart T et al. Treatment of cognitive deficits in genetic disorders: a systematic review of clinical trials of diet and drug treatments. JAMA Neurol 2015; 72:1052–1060.

29. Li Y et al. Cholinesterase inhibitors for rarer dementias associated with neurological conditions. Cochrane Database Syst Rev 2015:CD009444.

30. O'Brien JT et al. Clinical practice with anti-dementia drugs: a revised (third) consensus statement from the British Association for Psychopharmacology. J Psychopharmacol 2017; 31:147–168.

Multiple sclerosis

Multiple sclerosis (MS) is a common cause of neurological disability, affecting approximately 85,000 people in the UK. Onset is usually between 20 and 50 years of age. Individuals with MS experience a variety of psychiatric/neurological disorders such as depression, anxiety, pathological laughter and crying (pseudobulbar affect, PBA), mania and euphoria, psychosis/bipolar disorder, fatigue and cognitive impairment. Psychiatric disorders result from the psychological impact of MS diagnosis and prognosis, perceived lack of social support or unhelpful coping styles,[1] increased stress,[2] iatrogenic effects of treatments commonly used with MS,[3] or damage to neuronal pathways.[3] According to some studies, shorter duration of illness confers a greater risk of depression.

Depression

In people with MS, depression is common with a point prevalence of 14–31%[4–6] and lifetime prevalence of up to 50%.[5,7] Suicide rates are 2–7.5 times higher than the general population.[8] Depression is often associated with fatigue and pain, though the relationship direction is unclear. Overlapping symptoms of depression, PBA and MS can complicate diagnosis and so cooperation between neurologists and psychiatrists is essential to ensure optimal treatment for individuals with MS.

The role of interferon-β in the aetiology of MS depression is unclear, but it is now thought that depression occurs no more frequently in people treated with interferon-β.[9–11] Standard care for initiation of interferon-β should include assessment for depression and, for those with a past history of depressive illness, prophylactic treatment with an antidepressant.[3]

Recommendations for treatment

Depression in MS

Treatment of depression in MS is summarised in Table 10.11.

Anxiety

Anxiety affects many people with MS, with a point prevalence of up to 50%[34] and lifetime incidence of 35–37%.[35] Elevated rates in comparison with the general population are seen for generalised anxiety disorder, panic disorder, obsessive compulsive disorder[35] and social anxiety. Anxiety appears to be linked to perceived lack of support, increased pain, fatigue, sleep disturbance, depression, alcohol misuse and suicidal ideas. There are no published trials for the treatment of anxiety in MS, but SSRIs can be used, and in nonresponsive cases venlafaxine might be an option (based on practice in non-MS patients).

Benzodiazepines may be used for acute and severe anxiety of less than 4 weeks duration but should not be prescribed in the long term. Buspirone and beta blockers could also be considered although there is unproven efficacy in MS. Pregabalin is also licensed for anxiety and may be useful in this population group, especially where pain relief is required.[36,37] People with MS may also respond to CBT. Generally treatment is as for non-MS anxiety disorders (see Anxiety section, Chapter 3).

Table 10.11 Treatment of depression in multiple sclerosis

Step	Intervention
1	Screen for depression with PHQ-9 HADS/BDI[12]/CES-D.[13] Exclude and treat any organic causes. Consider iatrogenic effects of medications as potential cause of depression. Ensure there is no past history of mania or bipolar disorder. People with mild depression could be considered for CBT[14] or self-help[15]
2	SSRIs should be first-line treatment[3,13,16] because of their relatively benign adverse-effect profile
	Sertraline was as effective as CBT in one trial,[17] but paroxetine was found to be no more effective than placebo in another study.[18] Fluoxetine was effective in MS-related depression in a small case series.[19] Because of reduced tolerability of adverse effects in this patient group, medications should be titrated from an initial half dose. Many MS patients are prescribed low-dose TCAs for pain/bladder disturbance and so SSRIs should be used with caution and patients should be observed for serotonin syndrome. For those with co-morbid pain, consideration should be given to treating with an SNRI such as duloxetine[20] or venlafaxine.[21] One RCT of desipramine showed it was more effective than placebo but TCAs are often poorly tolerated.[22] Cochrane is not convinced by the studies cited here,[23] but there is no reason to suppose that antidepressants are any less effective in depression associated with physical illness.[24] CBT is the most appropriate psychological intervention with best efficacy in comparison to supportive therapy or usual care, and should be used in conjunction with medication for those who are moderately to severely depressed.[16,17,25] Mindfulness training may also help.[26] Omega-3 fatty acids are ineffective[27]
3	If SSRIs are not tolerated or there is no response there are limited data that moclobemide is effective and well tolerated.[28,29] There are no published trials on venlafaxine, duloxetine and mirtazapine but these are used widely. Mirtazapine may worsen fatigue, at least initially
4	ECT could be considered for people who are actively suicidal or severely depressed and at high risk, but it may trigger an exacerbation of MS symptoms, although some studies suggest that no neurological disturbance occurs[30]
5	Other treatments that have shown some effect in depression in MS are zinc,[31] vitamin A[32] and co-enzyme Q10[33]

BDI, Beck Depression Inventory; CBT, cognitive behavioural therapy; CES-D, Centre for Epidemiological Studies Depression Scale; ECT, electroconvulsive therapy; HADS, Hospital Anxiety and Depression Scale; MS, multiple sclerosis; PHQ-9, Patient Health Questionnaire-9; RCT, randomised controlled trial; SNRI, serotonin–noradrenaline reuptake inhibitor; SSRI, selective serotonin reuptake inhibitor; TCA, tricyclic antidepressant.

Pseudobulbar affect (PBA)

Up to 10% of individuals with MS experience pathological laughing or crying (PLC) or other incongruence of affect. It is more common in the advanced stages of the disease and is associated with cognitive impairment.[35] There have been a few open-label trials recommending the use of small doses of TCAs (e.g. amitriptyline) or SSRIs (e.g. fluoxetine[38,39]) in MS. Citalopram[40] and sertraline[41] have been investigated in people with post-stroke PLC and shown reasonable efficacy and rapid response. Valproic acid may be effective.[42] The combination of dextromethorphan and low-dose quinidine (DMq) is effective.[43] Dextromethorphan plus fluoxetine may show similar effects.[44]

Bipolar disorder

The incidence of bipolar disorder can be as high as 13% in MS patients[2] compared with 1–6% in the general population. Mania can be induced by drugs such as steroids or baclofen.[45]

Anecdotal evidence suggests that patients presenting with mania/bipolar disorder should be treated with mood stabilisers such as sodium valproate as these are better tolerated than lithium.[46]

Lithium can cause diuresis and thus lead to increased difficulties with tolerance in people with bladder disorder. Mania accompanied by psychosis could be treated with low-dose atypical antipsychotics such as risperidone, olanzapine,[2] and ziprasidone.[47] Patients requiring psychiatric treatment for steroid-induced mania with psychosis have been known to respond well to olanzapine;[48] further case reports suggest risperidone is also useful. There have been no trials in this area.

Psychosis

Psychosis occurs in 1.1% of the MS population and is relatively uncommon compared with other psychiatric disorders.[47] There have been few published trials, but risperidone or clozapine have been recommended because of their low risk of EPS.[45] On this basis, olanzapine, aripiprazole and quetiapine might also, in theory at least, be possible options.

Psychosis may rarely be the presentation of an MS relapse, in which case steroids may be beneficial but would need to be given under close supervision. Note also the small risk of psychotic reactions in patients receiving cannabinoids for MS.[49]

Cognitive impairment

Cognitive impairment occurs in at least 40–65% of people with MS. Some of the effects of commonly prescribed medications can worsen cognition (e.g. tizanidine, diazepam, gabapentin[50]). Although there are no published trials, evidence from clinical case studies suggests that the treatment of sleep difficulties, depression and fatigue can enhance cognitive function.[50] There have been two small, underpowered trials with donepezil for people with mild to moderate cognitive impairment showing moderate efficacy.[51,52] A larger study found no effect.[53] Similarly, data supporting the use of memantine are weak.[54] Overall, no symptomatic treatment has proven efficacy and disease-modifying agents offer greater promise.[55]

Fatigue

Fatigue is a common symptom in MS: up to 80% of people with MS are affected.[56] The aetiology of fatigue is unclear but there have been suggestions that disruption of neuronal networks,[57] depression or psychological reactions,[45] sleep disturbances or medication may play a role in its development. Pharmacological and non-pharmacological strategies[56] should be used in a treatment strategy.

Non-pharmacological strategies include reviewing the patient's history for any possible contributing factors, assessment and treatment of underlying depression if present, medication, pacing activities and appropriate exercise. One trial suggests that CBT reduces fatigue scores.[58]

Pharmacological strategies include the use of amantadine[59] or modafinil. NICE guidelines suggest no medicine should be used routinely but that amantadine could have a small benefit and should be offered.[60] A Cochrane review of amantadine in people with MS suggests that the quality and outcomes of the amantadine trials are inconsistent and therefore efficacy remains unclear.[59] In the only study published since then,[61] amantadine outperformed placebo on some measures of fatigue. Modafinil has mixed results in clinical trials. Early studies[62,63] showed statistically significant improvements in fatigue, but these studies were subject to some bias. A later randomised placebo-controlled double-blind study[64] found no improvement in fatigue compared with placebo. Another study[65] showed distinct advantages for modafinil over placebo. Most recently, a small study showed no benefit for modafinil on fatigue or cognition.[66] Despite doubts over its efficacy, modafinil is widely used in MS.[67]

Other pharmacological agents recommended for use in MS fatigue include pemoline, aspirin and ginseng. A double-blind crossover study of aspirin compared with placebo favoured aspirin but further studies are required.[68] An RCT of pemoline showed double the rate of symptom relief compared with placebo.[69] Data relating to ginseng are mixed.[70,71]

References

1. Ron MA. Do neurologists provide adequate care for depression in patients with multiple sclerosis? Nat Clin Pract Neurol 2006; 2:534–535.
2. Patten SB et al. Biopsychosocial correlates of lifetime major depression in a multiple sclerosis population. Mult Scler 2000; 6:115–120.
3. Servis ME. Psychiatric comorbidity in parkinson's disease, multiple sclerosis, and seizure disorder. Continuum 2006; 12:72–86.
4. Gottberg K et al. A population-based study of depressive symptoms in multiple sclerosis in Stockholm county: association with functioning and sense of coherence. J Neurol Neurosurg Psychiatry 2007; 78:60–65.
5. Patten SB et al. Major depression in multiple sclerosis: a population-based perspective. Neurology 2003; 61:1524–1527.
6. Boeschoten RE et al. Prevalence of depression and anxiety in multiple sclerosis: a systematic review and meta-analysis. J Neurol Sci 2017; 372:331–341.
7. Patten SB et al. Depression in multiple sclerosis. Int Rev Psychiatry 2017; 29:463–472.
8. Sadovnick AD et al. Cause of death in patients attending multiple sclerosis clinics. Neurology 1991; 41:1193–1196.
9. Zephir H et al. Multiple sclerosis and depression: influence of interferon beta therapy. Mult Scler 2003; 9:284–288.
10. Patten SB et al. Anti-depressant use in association with interferon and glatiramer acetate treatment in multiple sclerosis. Mult Scler 2008; 14:406–411.
11. Schippling S et al. Incidence and course of depression in multiple sclerosis in the multinational BEYOND trial. J Neurol 2016; 263: 1418–1426.
12. Moran PJ, Mohr DC. The validity of Beck Depression Inventory and Hamilton Rating Scale for Depression items in the assessment of depression among patients with multiple sclerosis. J Behav Med 2005; 28:35–41.
13. Pandya R et al. Predictive value of the CES-D in detecting depression among candidates for disease-modifying multiple sclerosis treatment. Psychosomatics 2005; 46:131–134.
14. Minden SL et al. Evidence-based guideline: assessment and management of psychiatric disorders in individuals with MS: report of the Guideline Development Subcommittee of the American Academy of Neurology. Neurology 2014; 82:174–181.
15. Rickards H. Depression in neurological disorders: Parkinson's disease, multiple sclerosis, and stroke. J Neurol Neurosurg Psychiatry 2005; 76 Suppl 1:i48–i52.
16. Siegert RJ et al. Depression in multiple sclerosis: a review. J Neurol Neurosurg Psychiatry 2005; 76:469–475.
17. Mohr DC et al. Comparative outcomes for individual cognitive-behavior therapy, supportive-expressive group psychotherapy, and sertraline for the treatment of depression in multiple sclerosis. J Consult Clin Psychol 2001; 69:942–949.
18. Ehde DM et al. Efficacy of paroxetine in treating major depressive disorder in persons with multiple sclerosis. Gen Hosp Psychiatry 2008; 30:40–48.
19. Flax JW et al. Effect of fluoxetine on patients with multiple sclerosis. Am J Psychiatry 1991; 148:1603.
20. Vollmer TL et al. A randomized, double-blind, placebo-controlled trial of duloxetine for the treatment of pain in patients with multiple sclerosis. Pain Pract 2014; 14:732–744.
21. Hilty DM et al. Psychopharmacology for neurologists: principles, algorithms, and other resources. Continuum 2006; 12:33–46.
22. Barak Y et al. Treatment of depression in patients with multiple sclerosis. Neurologist 1998; 4:99–104.
23. Koch MW et al. Pharmacologic treatment of depression in multiple sclerosis. Cochrane Database Syst Rev 2011; 2:CD007295.
24. Taylor D et al. Pharmacological interventions for people with depression and chronic physical health problems: systematic review and meta-analyses of safety and efficacy. Br J Psychiatry 2011; 198:179–188.

25. Larcombe NA et al. An evaluation of cognitive-behaviour therapy for depression in patients with multiple sclerosis. Br J Psychiatry 1984; 145:366–371.

26. Grossman P et al. MS quality of life, depression, and fatigue improve after mindfulness training: a randomized trial. Neurology 2010; 75:1141–1149.

27. Shinto L et al. Omega-3 fatty acids for depression in multiple sclerosis: a randomized pilot study. PLoS One 2016; 11:e0147195.

28. Schiffer RB et al. Antidepressant pharmacotherapy of depression associated with multiple sclerosis. Am J Psychiatry 1990; 147:1493–1497.

29. Barak Y et al. Moclobemide treatment in multiple sclerosis patients with comorbid depression: an open-label safety trial. J Neuropsychiatry Clin Neurosci 1999; 11:271–273.

30. Rasmussen KG et al. Electroconvulsive therapy in patients with multiple sclerosis. JECT 2007; 23:179–180.

31. Salari S et al. Zinc sulphate: a reasonable choice for depression management in patients with multiple sclerosis: a randomized, double-blind, placebo-controlled clinical trial. Pharmacol Rep 2015; 67:606–609.

32. Bitarafan S et al. Effect of Vitamin A supplementation on fatigue and depression in multiple sclerosis patients: a double-blind placebo-controlled clinical trial. Iran J Allergy Asthma Immunol 2016; 15:13–19.

33. Sanoobar M et al. Coenzyme Q10 as a treatment for fatigue and depression in multiple sclerosis patients: a double blind randomized clinical trial. Nutr Neurosci 2016; 19:138–143.

34. Jones KH et al. A large-scale study of anxiety and depression in people with multiple sclerosis: a survey via the web portal of the UK MS Register. PLoSOne 2012; 7:e41910.

35. Korostil M et al. Anxiety disorders and their clinical correlates in multiple sclerosis patients. Mult Scler 2007; 13:67–72.

36. Solaro C et al. Pregabalin for treating paroxysmal painful symptoms in multiple sclerosis: a pilot study. J Neurol 2009; 256:1773–1774.

37. Bittner S et al. [Pregabalin and gabapentin in multiple sclerosis: clinical experiences and therapeutic implications]. Nervenarzt 2011; 82:1273–1280.

38. Feinstein A et al. The effects of anxiety on psychiatric morbidity in patients with multiple sclerosis. Mult Scler 1999; 5:323–326.

39. Feinstein A et al. Prevalence and neurobehavioral correlates of pathological laughing and crying in multiple sclerosis. Arch Neurol 1997; 54:1116–1121.

40. Andersen G et al. Citalopram for post-stroke pathological crying. Lancet 1993; 342:837–839.

41. Burns A et al. Sertraline in stroke-associated lability of mood. Int J Geriatr Psychiatry 1999; 14:681–685.

42. Johnson B et al. Crying and suicidal, but not depressed. Pseudobulbar affect in multiple sclerosis successfully treated with valproic acid: case report and literature review. Palliat Support Care 2015; 13:1797–1801.

43. Pioro EP et al. Dextromethorphan plus ultra low-dose quinidine reduces pseudobulbar affect. Ann Neurol 2010; 68:693–702.

44. McGrane I et al. Treatment of pseudobulbar affect with fluoxetine and dextromethorphan in a woman with multiple sclerosis. Ann Pharmacother 2017:1060028017720746.

45. Jefferies K. The neuropsychiatry of multiple sclerosis. Adv Psychiatr Treat 2006; 12:214–220.

46. Stip E et al. Valproate in the treatment of mood disorder due to multiple sclerosis. Can J Psychiatry 1995; 40:219–220.

47. Davids E et al. Antipsychotic treatment of psychosis associated with multiple sclerosis. Prog Neuropsychopharmacol Biol Psychiatry 2004; 28:743–744.

48. Budur K et al. Olanzapine for corticosteroid-induced mood disorders. Psychosomatics 2003; 44:353.

49. Aragona M et al. Psychopathological and cognitive effects of therapeutic cannabinoids in multiple sclerosis: a double-blind, placebo controlled, crossover study. Clin Neuropharmacol 2009; 32:41–47.

50. Pierson SH et al. Treatment of cognitive impairment in multiple sclerosis. Behav Neurol 2006; 17:53–67.

51. Krupp LB et al. Donepezil improved memory in multiple sclerosis in a randomized clinical trial. Neurology 2004; 63:1579–1585.

52. Greene YM et al. A 12-week, open trial of donepezil hydrochloride in patients with multiple sclerosis and associated cognitive impairments. J Clin Psychopharmacol 2000; 20:350–356.

53. Krupp LB et al. Multicenter randomized clinical trial of donepezil for memory impairment in multiple sclerosis. Neurology 2011; 76:1500–1507.

54. Lovera JF et al. Memantine for cognitive impairment in multiple sclerosis: a randomized placebo-controlled trial. Mult Scler 2010; 16:715–723.

55. Patti F. Treatment of cognitive impairment in patients with multiple sclerosis. Expert Opin Investig Drugs 2012; 21:1679–1699.

56. Bakshi R. Fatigue associated with multiple sclerosis: diagnosis, impact and management. Mult Scler 2003; 9:219–227.

57. Sepulcre J et al. Fatigue in multiple sclerosis is associated with the disruption of frontal and parietal pathways. Mult Scler 2009; 15: 337–344.

58. van KK et al. A randomized controlled trial of cognitive behavior therapy for multiple sclerosis fatigue. Psychosom Med 2008; 70: 205–213.

59. Pucci E et al. Amantadine for fatigue in multiple sclerosis. Cochrane Database Syst Rev 2007:CD002818.

60. National Institute for Health and Care Excellence. Multiple sclerosis in adults: management. Clinical Guideline 186, 2014. https://www.nice.org.uk/guidance/cg186.

61. Ashtari F et al. Does amantadine have favourable effects on fatigue in Persian patients suffering from multiple sclerosis? Neurol Neurochir Pol 2009; 43:428–432.

62. Rammohan KW et al. Efficacy and safety of modafinil (Provigil) for the treatment of fatigue in multiple sclerosis: a two centre phase 2 study. J Neurol Neurosurg Psychiatry 2002; 72:179–183.

63. Zifko UA et al. Modafinil in treatment of fatigue in multiple sclerosis. Results of an open-label study. J Neurol 2002; 249:983–987.

64. Stankoff B et al. Modafinil for fatigue in MS: a randomized placebo-controlled double-blind study. Neurology 2005; **64**:1139–1143.

65. Lange R et al. Modafinil effects in multiple sclerosis patients with fatigue. J Neurol 2009; **256**:645–650.

66. Ford-Johnson L et al. Cognitive effects of modafinil in patients with multiple sclerosis: a clinical trial. Rehabil Psychol 2016; **61**:82–91.

67. Davies M et al. Safety profile of modafinil across a range of prescribing indications, including off-label use, in a primary care setting in England: results of a modified prescription-event monitoring study. Drug Saf 2013; **36**:237–246.

68. Wingerchuk DM et al. A randomized controlled crossover trial of aspirin for fatigue in multiple sclerosis. Neurology 2005; **64**:1267–1269.

69. Weinshenker BG et al. A double-blind, randomized, crossover trial of pemoline in fatigue associated with multiple sclerosis. Neurology 1992; **42**:1468–1471.

70. Kim E et al. American ginseng does not improve fatigue in multiple sclerosis: a single center randomized double-blind placebo-controlled crossover pilot study. Mult Scler 2011; **17**:1523—1526.

71. Etemadifar M et al. Ginseng in the treatment of fatigue in multiple sclerosis: a randomized, placebo-controlled, double-blind pilot study. Int J Neurosci 2013; **123**:480–486.

Parkinson's disease

Parkinson's disease (PD) is a progressive, degenerative neurological disorder character-ised by resting tremor, cogwheel rigidity, bradykinesia and postural instability. The prevalence of co-morbid psychiatric disorders is high. Approximately 25% will suffer from major depression at some point during the course of their illness, a further 25% from milder forms of depression, 25% from anxiety spectrum disorders and 25% from psychosis; up to 80% will develop dementia.[1-3] While depression and anxiety can occur at any time, psychosis, dementia and delirium are more prevalent in the later stages of the illness. Close cooperation between the psychiatrist and neurologist is required to optimise treatment for this group of patients.

Depression in Parkinson's disease

Depression in PD predicts greater cognitive decline, deterioration in functioning and progression of motor symptoms,[4] possibly reflecting more advanced and widespread neurodegeneration involving multiple neurotransmitter pathways.[5] Depression may also occur after the withdrawal of dopamine agonists.[6] Pre-existing dementia is an established risk factor for the development of depression.

Treatment recommendations for depression in PD are summarised in Table 10.12.

Table 10.12 Depression in Parkinson's disease – recommendations for treatment

Step	Intervention
1	Exclude/treat organic causes such as hypothyroidism (the prevalence of which is relatively high in Parkinson's disease[4])
2	**SSRIs** are considered to be first-line treatment although the effect size is modest.[7-9] Some patients may experience a worsening of motor symptoms although the absolute risk is low.[10,11] Care must be taken when combining SSRIs with selegiline, as the risk of serotonin syndrome is increased.[4] The SNRIs venlafaxine[12] and duloxetine[13] also appear to have some effect although venlafaxine may modestly worsen motor symptoms[12]
	TCAs are generally poorly tolerated because of their anticholinergic (can worsen cognitive problems; constipation) and alpha-blocking effects (can worsen symptoms of autonomic dysfunction). Note though that several meta-analyses[8,9] have reported low-dose TCAs to be more effective than SSRIs,[14-16] although low-dose amitriptyline and sertraline seem to be equally effective.[17,18] Limited evidence supports the safe use of agomelatine.[19,20] Atomoxetine is not effective.[21] CBT should always be considered[22]
3	Consider augmentation with dopamine agonists/releasers such as pramiprexole.[23] Note though that these drugs increase the risk of impulse control disorders.[24,25] They have also rarely been associated with the development of psychosis[26]
4	Consider **ECT**. Depression and motor symptoms generally respond well[4] but the risk of inducing delirium is high,[27] particularly in patients with pre-existing cognitive impairment
5	Follow the algorithm for treatment-resistant depression (see Chapter 3) from this point. Be aware of the increased propensity for adverse effects and drug interactions in this patient group

CBT, cognitive behavioural therapy; ECT, electroconvulsive therapy; SNRI, serotonin–noradrenaline reuptake inhibitor; SSRI, selective serotonin reuptake inhibitor; TCA, tricyclic antidepressant.

Psychosis in Parkinson's disease

Psychosis in PD is often characterised by visual hallucinations.[28] Auditory hallucinations and delusions occur far less frequently,[29] and usually in younger patients.[30] Psychosis and dementia frequently co-exist. Having one predicts the development of the other.[31] Sleep disorders are also an established risk factor for the development of psychosis.[32]

Abnormalities in dopamine, serotonin and acetylcholine neurotransmission have all been implicated, but the exact aetiology of psychosis in PD is poorly understood. In the majority of patients, psychotic symptoms are thought to be secondary to dopaminergic medication rather than part of PD itself; psychosis secondary to medication may be determined at least in part through polymorphisms of the ACE gene.[33] From the limited data available, anticholinergics and dopamine agonists seem to be associated with a higher risk of inducing psychosis than levodopa or catechol-O-methyltransferase (COMT) inhibitors.[29,34] Psychosis is a major contributor to caregiver distress and a risk factor for institutionalisation and early death.[31]

Treatment recommendations for psychosis in PD are summarised in Table 10.13.

Table 10.13 Psychosis in Parkinson's disease – recommendations for treatment

Step	Intervention
1	Exclude organic causes (delirium)
2	Optimise the environment to maximise orientation and minimise problems due to poor caregiver–patient interactions
3	If the patient has insight and hallucinations are infrequent and not troubling, do not treat
4	Consider reducing or stopping anticholinergics and dopamine agonists. Monitor for signs of motor deterioration. Be prepared to restart/increase the dose of these drugs again to achieve the best balance between psychosis and mobility
5	Try an atypical antipsychotic. The efficacy of clozapine (see below, 7) is supported by placebo-controlled RCTs.[28] In contrast, there are several negative placebo-controlled trials each for quetiapine and olanzapine.[28] Low-dose quetiapine is the best tolerated, although EPS and stereotypical movements can occur. It is probably reasonable to try quetiapine[35] before clozapine but the success rate may be low. Olanzapine, ziprasidone and aripiprazole are all likely to have greater adverse effects on motor function than quetiapine, although one small trial[36] supports the safe use of ziprasidone. Risperidone and typical antipsychotics should be avoided completely. Severe rebound psychosis has been described when antipsychotic drugs (quetiapine or clozapine) are discontinued
	Note that all antipsychotics may be even less effective in managing psychotic symptoms in patients with dementia, and such patients may be more prone to developing motor and cognitive adverse effects.[37] Antipsychotics have been associated with an increased risk of vascular events in the elderly. In PD all antipsychotics are linked to increased mortality[38] although the effect of clozapine is not known
6	Consider a **cholinesterase inhibitor**, particularly if the patient has co-morbid dementia.[28,39] Cholinesterase inhibitors may also reduce the risk of falls[40]
7	Try **clozapine**. Start at 6.25 mg – usual dose 25–35 mg/day.[28,36] Usually safe but NMS has been reported[41]
	Monitor as for clozapine in schizophrenia. The elderly are more prone to develop serious blood dyscrasia. A case of aplastic anaemia has been reported[42]
8	Consider **ECT**.[43] Psychotic and motor symptoms usually respond well[44] but the risk of inducing delirium is high,[27] particularly in patients with pre-existing cognitive impairment

ECT, electroconvulsive therapy; EPS, extrapyramidal symptoms; NMS, neuroleptic malignant syndrome; PD, Parkinson's disease; RCT, randomised controlled trial.

Pimavanserin

Pimavanserin is a 5-HT2A receptor inverse agonist available in the USA and some other countries. It is effective in PD psychosis but has no dopamine receptor activity and does not worsen PD movement disorder or seem to increase mortality.[45]

Pimavanserin and clozapine are the only drugs recommended for PD psychosis.[46]

Cholinesterase inhibitors in Parkinson's disease

Cholinesterase inhibitors have been shown to improve cognition, delusions and hallucinations in patients with Lewy body dementia (which has many similarities to PD). Motor function may deteriorate.[47,48] Improvements in cognitive functioning are modest.[49–51] A Cochrane review and some large RCTs[50,52,53] concluded that there is evidence that cholinesterase inhibitors lead to improvements in global functioning, cognition, behavioural disturbance and activities of daily living in PD. Again, motor function may deteriorate[53,54] with particular increase in tremor.[51] Evidence for memantine is mixed.[55,56] Discontinuation of anticholinergic drugs should improve cognition and psychosis – PD patients often have a very high anticholinergic burden, often unrelated to treatment of PD itself.[57]

Many patients with PD use complementary therapies, some of which may be modestly beneficial (see Zesiewicz et al.[58]). Caffeine may offer a protective effect against the development of PD and also modestly improves motor function in established disease.[59]

References

1. Hely MA et al. The Sydney multicenter study of Parkinson's disease: the inevitability of dementia at 20 years. Mov Disord 2008; 23:837–844.
2. Riedel O et al. Frequency of dementia, depression, and other neuropsychiatric symptoms in 1,449 outpatients with Parkinson's disease. J Neurol 2010; 257:1073–1082.
3. Reijnders JS et al. A systematic review of prevalence studies of depression in Parkinson's disease. Mov Disord 2008; 23:183–189.
4. McDonald WM et al. Prevalence, etiology, and treatment of depression in Parkinson's disease. Biol Psychiatry 2003; 54:363–375.
5. Palhagen SE et al. Depressive illness in Parkinson's disease indication of a more advanced and widespread neurodegenerative process? Acta Neurol Scand 2008; 117:295–304.
6. Rabinak CA et al. Dopamine agonist withdrawal syndrome in Parkinson disease. Arch Neurol 2010; 67:58–63.
7. Rocha FL et al. Antidepressants for depression in Parkinson's disease: systematic review and meta-analysis. J Psychopharmacol 2013; 27:417–423.
8. Liu J et al. Comparative efficacy and acceptability of antidepressants in Parkinson's disease: a network meta-analysis. PLoS One 2013; 8:e76651.
9. Troeung L et al. A meta-analysis of randomised placebo-controlled treatment trials for depression and anxiety in Parkinson's disease. PLoS One 2013; 8:e79510.
10. Gony M et al. Risk of serious extrapyramidal symptoms in patients with Parkinson's disease receiving antidepressant drugs: a pharmacoepidemiologic study comparing serotonin reuptake inhibitors and other antidepressant drugs. Clin Neuropharmacol 2003; 26:142–145.
11. Kulisevsky J et al. Motor changes during sertraline treatment in depressed patients with Parkinson's disease. Eur J Neurol 2008; 15:953–959.
12. Richard IH et al. A randomized, double-blind, placebo-controlled trial of antidepressants in Parkinson disease. Neurology 2012; 78:1229–1236.
13. Bonuccelli U et al. A non-comparative assessment of tolerability and efficacy of duloxetine in the treatment of depressed patients with Parkinson's disease. Expert Opin Pharmacother 2012; 13:2269–2280.
14. Serrano-Duenas M. A comparison between low doses of amitriptyline and low doses of fluoxetine used in the control of depression in patients suffering from Parkinson's disease (Spanish). Rev Neurol 2002; 35:1010–1014.
15. Menza M et al. A controlled trial of antidepressants in patients with Parkinson disease and depression. Neurology 2009; 72:886–892.
16. Devos D et al. Comparison of desipramine and citalopram treatments for depression in Parkinson's disease: a double-blind, randomized, placebo-controlled study. Mov Disord 2008; 23:850–857.
17. Antonini A et al. Randomized study of sertraline and low-dose amitriptyline in patients with Parkinson's disease and depression: effect on quality of life. Mov Disord 2006; 21:1119–1122.
18. Goodarzi Z et al. Guidelines for dementia or Parkinson's disease with depression or anxiety: a systematic review. BMC Neurol 2016; 16:244.
19. Avila A et al. Agomelatine for depression in Parkinson disease: additional effect on sleep and motor dysfunction. J Clin Psychopharmacol 2015; 35:719–723.

20. De Berardis D et al. Agomelatine treatment of major depressive disorder in Parkinson's disease: a case series. J Neuropsychiatry Clin Neurosci 2013; 25:343–345.

21. Weintraub D et al. Atomoxetine for depression and other neuropsychiatric symptoms in Parkinson disease. Neurology 2010; 75:448–455.

22. Dobkin RD et al. Cognitive-behavioral therapy for depression in Parkinson's disease: a randomized, controlled trial. Am J Psychiatry 2011; 168:1066–1074.

23. Barone P et al. Pramipexole versus sertraline in the treatment of depression in Parkinson's disease: a national multicenter parallel-group randomized study. J Neurol 2006; 253:601–607.

24. Antonini A et al. A reassessment of risks and benefits of dopamine agonists in Parkinson's disease. Lancet Neurol 2009; 8:929–937.

25. Weintraub D et al. Impulse control disorders in Parkinson disease: a cross-sectional study of 3090 patients. Arch Neurol 2010; 67:589–595.

26. Li CT et al. Pramipexole-induced psychosis in Parkinson's disease. Psychiatry Clin Neurosci 2008; 62:245.

27. Figiel GS et al. ECT-induced delirium in depressed patients with Parkinson's disease. J Neuropsychiatry Clin Neurosci 1991; 3:405–411.

28. Friedman JH. Parkinson's disease psychosis 2010: a review article. Parkinsonism Relat Disord 2010; 16:553–560.

29. Ismail MS et al. A reality test: how well do we understand psychosis in Parkinson's disease? J Neuropsychiatry Clin Neurosci 2004; 16:8–18.

30. Kiziltan G et al. Relationship between age and subtypes of psychotic symptoms in Parkinson's disease. J Neurol 2007; 254:448–452.

31. Factor SA et al. Longitudinal outcome of Parkinson's disease patients with psychosis. Neurology 2003; 60:1756–1761.

32. Reich SG et al. Ten most commonly asked questions about the psychiatric aspects of Parkinson's disease. Neurologist 2003; 9:50–56.

33. Lin JJ et al. Genetic polymorphism of the angiotensin converting enzyme and L-dopa-induced adverse effects in Parkinson's disease. J Neurol Sci 2007; 252:130–134.

34. Stowe RL et al. Dopamine agonist therapy in early Parkinson's disease. Cochrane Database Syst Rev 2008:Cd006564.

35. Divac N et al. The efficacy and safety of antipsychotic medications in the treatment of psychosis in patients with Parkinson's disease. Behav Neurol 2016; 2016:4938154.

36. Pintor L et al. Ziprasidone versus clozapine in the treatment of psychotic symptoms in Parkinson disease: a randomized open clinical trial. Clin Neuropharmacol 2012; 35:61–66.

37. Prohorov T et al. The effect of quetiapine in psychotic Parkinsonian patients with and without dementia. An open-labeled study utilizing a structured interview. J Neurol 2006; 253:171–175.

38. Weintraub D et al. Association of antipsychotic use with mortality risk in patients with Parkinson disease. JAMA Neurol 2016; 73:535–541.

39. Marti M et al. Dementia in Parkinson's disease. J Neurol 2007; 254 Suppl 1:41–48.

40. Chung KA et al. Effects of a central cholinesterase inhibitor on reducing falls in Parkinson disease. Neurology 2010; 75:1263–1269.

41. Mesquita J et al. Fatal neuroleptic malignant syndrome induced by clozapine in Parkinson's psychosis. J Neuropsychiatry Clin Neurosci 2014; 26:E34.

42. Ziegenbein M et al. Clozapine-induced aplastic anemia in a patient with Parkinson's disease. Can J Psychiatry 2003; 48:352.

43. Factor SA et al. Combined clozapine and electroconvulsive therapy for the treatment of drug-induced psychosis in Parkinson's disease. J Neuropsychiatry Clin Neurosci 1995; 7:304–307.

44. Martin BA. ECT for Parkinson's? CMAJ 2003; 168:1391–1392.

45. Sarva H et al. Evidence for the use of pimavanserin in the treatment of Parkinson's disease psychosis. Ther Adv Neurol Disord 2016; 9:462–473.

46. Wilby KJ et al. Evidence-based review of pharmacotherapy used for Parkinson's disease psychosis. Ann Pharmacother 2017; 51:682–695.

47. Richard IH et al. Rivastigmine-induced worsening of motor function and mood in a patient with Parkinson's disease. Mov Disord 2001; 16 Suppl 1:33–34.

48. McKeith I et al. Efficacy of rivastigmine in dementia with Lewy bodies: a randomised, double-blind, placebo-controlled international study. Lancet 2000; 356:2031–2036.

49. Emre M et al. Rivastigmine for dementia associated with Parkinson's disease. N Engl J Med 2004; 351:2509–2518.

50. Aarsland D et al. Donepezil for cognitive impairment in Parkinson's disease: a randomised controlled study. J Neurol Neurosurg Psychiatry 2002; 72:708–712.

51. Pagano G et al. Cholinesterase inhibitors for Parkinson's disease: a systematic review and meta-analysis. J Neurol Neurosurg Psychiatry 2015; 86:767–773.

52. Rolinski M et al. Cholinesterase inhibitors for dementia with Lewy bodies, Parkinson's disease dementia and cognitive impairment in Parkinson's disease. Cochrane Database Syst Rev 2012; 3:CD006504.

53. Dubois B et al. Donepezil in Parkinson's disease dementia: a randomized, double-blind efficacy and safety study. Mov Disord 2012; 27:1230–1238.

54. Connolly BS et al. Pharmacological treatment of Parkinson disease: a review. JAMA 2014; 311:1670–1683.

55. Emre M et al. Memantine for patients with Parkinson's disease dementia or dementia with Lewy bodies: a randomised, double-blind, placebo-controlled trial. Lancet Neurol 2010; 9:969–977.

56. Seppi K et al. The Movement Disorder Society Evidence-Based Medicine Review Update: Treatments for the non-motor symptoms of Parkinson's disease. Mov Disord 2011; 26 Suppl 3:S42–S80.

57. Lertxundi U et al. Anticholinergic burden in Parkinson's disease inpatients. Eur J Clin Pharmacol 2015; 71:1271–1277.

58. Zesiewicz TA et al. Potential influences of complementary therapy on motor and non-motor complications in Parkinson's disease. CNS Drugs 2009; 23:817–835.

59. Postuma RB et al. Caffeine for treatment of Parkinson disease: a randomized controlled trial. Neurology 2012; 79:651–658.

Atrial fibrillation

Atrial fibrillation (AF) is the most common cardiac arrhythmia. It particularly affects older people but may occur in an important proportion of people under 40. Risk factors include anxiety, obesity, diabetes, hypertension, long-standing aerobic exercise and high alcohol consumption.[1-3] AF itself is not usually life-threatening but stasis of blood in the atria during fibrillation predisposes to clot formation and substantially increases the risk of stroke.[4] The use of warfarin or novel oral anticoagulants is therefore essential.[3]

AF can be defined as 'lone' or **paroxysmal** (occurring infrequently and spontaneously reverting to sinus rhythm), **persistent** (repeated and prolonged [>1 week] episodes usually, if temporarily, responsive to treatment) or **permanent** (unresponsive). Risk of stroke is increased in all three conditions.[3]

Treatment may involve DC conversion, rhythm control (usually flecainide, propafenone or amiodarone) or rate control (with diltiazem, verapamil or sotalol). With rhythm control the aim is to maintain sinus rhythm, although this is not always achieved. With rate control, AF is allowed to continue but ventricular response is controlled and the ventricles are filled passively. Many people with paroxysmal or persistent AF can now be effectively cured of the condition by catheter- or cryo-ablation of aberrant electrical pathways,[5,6] an increasingly routine procedure.

AF is commonly encountered in psychiatry, not least because of the high rates of obesity, diabetes and alcohol misuse seen in mental health patients. When considering the use of psychotropics, several factors need to be taken into account:

- interactions between psychotropics and anticoagulant therapy (see section on SSRIs and bleeding in Chapter 3)
- arrhythmogenicity of psychotropics prescribed (AF usually results from cardiovascular disease; drugs affecting cardiac ion channels may increase mortality in these patients, especially those with ischaemic disease[7,8])
- effect on ventricular rate (some drugs induce reflex tachycardia via postural hypotension, others [clozapine, quetiapine] directly increase heart rate)
- reported association between individual psychotropics and AF
- risk of interaction with co-prescribed anti-arrhythmics or rate-controlling drugs
- whether AF is paroxysmal (aim to avoid precipitating AF), persistent (aim to avoid prolonging AF) or permanent (aim to avoid increasing ventricular rate).

Recommendations on the use of psychotropics in AF are summarised in Table 10.14.

Table 10.14 Recommendations on the use of psychotropics in atrial fibrillation

Condition	Suggested drugs	Drugs to avoid
Schizophrenia/schizoaffective disorder The condition itself may be associated with an increased risk of AF[9] One case-control study suggested antipsychotics increase risk of AF by 17%[10]	In paroxysmal or persistent AF, **aripiprazole** or **lurasidone** may be appropriate choices In permanent AF with rate control, drug choice is less crucial but probably best to avoid drugs with potent effects on the ECG (ziprasidone, pimozide, sertindole, etc.) and those which increase heart rate	AF reported with clozapine,[11,12] olanzapine[13,14] and paliperidone.[15] Causation not established but avoid use in paroxysmal or persistent AF Avoid QT-prolonging drugs in ischaemic heart disease (see section on 'Antipsychotic-related QT prolongation' in Chapter 1) Association with AF may be linked to metabolic disturbance[16]
Bipolar disorder	**Valproate** **Lithium** **Carbamazepine**	Mood stabilisers appear not to affect risk of AF One case of AF following lithium overdose[17]
Depression Note – untreated depression predicts recurrence of AF[18] Presence of AF increases risk of depression and anxiety[19]	**SSRIs** but beware interaction with warfarin and other anticoagulants[20] Animal studies suggest an anti-arrhythmic effect for SSRIs[21,22] **Paroxetine** improved paroxysmal AF in a series of non-depressed patients[23] **Venlafaxine** does not directly affect atrial conduction[24] and may cardiovert paroxysmal AF[25] No evidence that **agomelatine** affects cardiac conduction or clotting	Avoid tricyclics in coronary disease[26] Tricyclics may provoke AF[27,28] but do not increase risk of haemorrhage when combined with warfarin[20] A database study suggests antidepressants in general do not increase risk of AF[29]
Anxiety disorders (anxiety symptoms increase risk of AF)[30]	**Benzodiazepines** **SSRIs** (see above)	Tricyclics (see above) One case of pregabalin-associated AF[31]
Alzheimer's disease	**Acetylcholinesterase inhibitors** (but beware bradycardic effects in patients with paroxysmal 'vagal' AF [paroxysmal AF provoked by low heart rate]) **Rivastigmine** has least interaction potential **Memantine**	Avoid cholinesterase inhibitors in paroxysmal 'vagal' AF

AF, atrial fibrillation; ECG, electrocardiogram; SSRI, selective serotonin reuptake inhibitor.

References

1. Chen LY et al. Epidemiology of atrial fibrillation: a current perspective. Heart Rhythm 2007; 4:S1–S6.
2. Tully PJ et al. Anxiety, depression, and stress as risk factors for atrial fibrillation after cardiac surgery. Heart Lung 2011; 40:4–11.
3. National Institute for Health and Care Excellence. Atrial fibrillation: management. Clinical Guideline 180, 2014. http://www.nice.org.uk/guidance/cg180.
4. Lakshminarayan K et al. Clinical epidemiology of atrial fibrillation and related cerebrovascular events in the United States. Neurologist 2008; 14:143–150.

5. Rodgers M et al. Curative catheter ablation in atrial fibrillation and typical atrial flutter: systematic review and economic evaluation. Health Technol Assess 2008; 12:iii–xiii, 1.

6. Latchamsetty R et al. Catheter ablation of atrial fibrillation. Cardiol Clin 2014; 32:551–561.

7. Cardiac Arrhythmia Suppression Trial II Investigators. Effect of the antiarrhythmic agent moricizine on survival after myocardial infarction. N Engl J Med 1992; 327:227–233.

8. Epstein AE et al. Mortality following ventricular arrhythmia suppression by encainide, flecainide, and moricizine after myocardial infarction. The original design concept of the Cardiac Arrhythmia Suppression Trial (CAST). JAMA 1993; 270:2451–2455.

9. Emul M et al. P wave and QT changes among inpatients with schizophrenia after parenteral ziprasidone administration. Pharmacol Res 2009; 60:369–372.

10. Chou RH et al. Antipsychotic treatment is associated with risk of atrial fibrillation: a nationwide nested case-control study. Int J Cardiol 2017; 227:134–140.

11. Cam B et al. [Clozapine and olanzapine associated atrial fibrillation: a case report]. Turk Psikiyatri Derg 2015; 26:221–226.

12. Low RA, Jr. et al. Clozapine induced atrial fibrillation. J Clin Psychopharmacol 1998; 18:170.

13. Waters BM et al. Olanzapine-associated new-onset atrial fibrillation. J Clin Psychopharmacol 2008; 28:354–355.

14. Yaylaci S et al. Atrial fibrillation due to olanzapine overdose. Clin Toxicol (Phila) 2011; 49:440.

15. Schneider RA et al. Apparent seizure and atrial fibrillation associated with paliperidone. Am J Health Syst Pharm 2008; 65:2122–2125.

16. Zeng J et al. Metabolic disorder caused by antipsychotic treatment may facilitate the development of atrial fibrillation. Int J Cardiol 2017; 239:14.

17. Kalcik MDM et al. Acute atrial fibrillation as an unusual form of cardiotoxicity in chronic lithium overdose. J Atr Fibrillation 2014; 6:1009.

18. Lange HW et al. Depressive symptoms predict recurrence of atrial fibrillation after cardioversion. J Psychosom Res 2007; 63:509–513.

19. Patel D et al. A systematic review of depression and anxiety in patients with atrial fibrillation: the mind-heart link. Cardiovasc Psychiatry Neurol 2013; 2013:159850.

20. Quinn GR et al. Effect of selective serotonin reuptake inhibitors on bleeding risk in patients with atrial fibrillation taking warfarin. Am J Cardiol 2014; 114:583–586.

21. Pousti A et al. Effect of sertraline on ouabain-induced arrhythmia in isolated guinea-pig atria. Depress Anxiety 2009; 26:E106–E110.

22. Pousti A et al. Effect of citalopram on ouabain-induced arrhythmia in isolated guinea-pig atria. Hum Psychopharmacol 2003; 18:121–124.

23. Shirayama T et al. Usefulness of paroxetine in depressed men with paroxysmal atrial fibrillation. Am J Cardiol 2006; 97:1749–1751.

24. Emul M et al. The influences of depression and venlafaxine use at therapeutic doses on atrial conduction. J Psychopharmacol 2009; 23:163–167.

25. Finch SJ et al. Cardioversion of persistent atrial arrhythmia after treatment with venlafaxine in successful management of major depression and posttraumatic stress disorder. Psychosomatics 2006; 47:533–536.

26. Taylor D. Antidepressant drugs and cardiovascular pathology: a clinical overview of effectiveness and safety. Acta Psychiatr Scand 2008; 118:434–442.

27. Moorehead CN et al. Imipramine-induced auricular fibrillation. Am J Psychiatry 1965; 122:216–217.

28. Rosen BH. Case report of auricular fibrillation following the use of imipramine (Tofranil). J Mt Sinai Hosp NY 1960; 27:609–611.

29. Lapi F et al. The use of antidepressants and the risk of chronic atrial fibrillation. J Clin Pharmacol 2015; 55:423–430.

30. Eaker ED et al. Tension and anxiety and the prediction of the 10-year incidence of coronary heart disease, atrial fibrillation, and total mortality: the Framingham Offspring Study. Psychosom Med 2005; 67:692–696.

31. Chilkoti G et al. Could pregabalin premedication predispose to perioperative atrial fibrillation in patients with sepsis? Saudi J Anaesth 2014; 8:S115–116.

Bariatric surgery

Psychiatric illness and the use of psychotropics is relatively common in patients who have undergone bariatric surgery.[1,2] Almost half of those seeking bariatric surgery are prescribed psychotropics, a prevalence that is six times higher than the general population.[3] Bariatric surgery can be associated with clinically important changes in drug pharmacokinetics, although it is difficult to predict how psychotropics will be affected because of interindividual differences and limited data. Current research supports the need for close treatment monitoring and the ongoing monitoring of symptoms after bariatric surgery.[4]

Surgical procedures can be classified as:

- **predominantly restrictive:** sleeve gastrectomy and gastric banding
- **predominantly malabsorptive:** biliopancreatic diversion and jejunoileal bypass
- **mixed restrictive/malabsorptive:** Roux-en-Y gastric bypass (RYGB).

Malabsorptive procedures (including RYGB) have a relatively greater potential to alter drug absorption. Most data are derived from studies of patients undergoing RYGB. It is not clear how these data relate to the consequences of other procedures.

Pharmacokinetic changes following bariatric surgery

All procedures may alter:

- tablet disintegration and dissolution times via changes in gastric pH and mixing
- rate of absorption via changes in the gastric emptying rate
- drug distribution via loss of adipose tissue (especially lipid soluble drugs) and altered protein binding
- drug metabolism owing to improvements in hepatic function after weight loss
- drug excretion via changes in renal function after weight loss.

Malabsorptive surgical procedures may further lead to:

- decreased area for drug absorption (reduced functional intestinal length)
- altered lipophilic drug solubilisation (bypassing proximal small intestine bile salts)
- reduced intestinal wall drug metabolism via decreased intestinal length.

Drug formulations

Any drug formulation that prolongs drug disintegration and dissolution can potentially impair drug absorption following bariatric surgery.[5] Switching to immediate-release formulations before surgery is generally recommended[5,6] (based more on expert consensus rather than any objective data[7]). Orodispersible and liquid preparations do not go through a disintegration phase and may be preferred if reduced absorption from solid tablets is suspected.[8] Very large tablets (e.g. those over 10 mm in diameter) should be avoided as passage may be impeded by restrictive procedures.

Drugs

Antidepressants

Recommendations on the use of psychotropic drugs after bariatric surgery are summarised in Table 10.15.

Antipsychotics

Recommendations on the use of antipsychotics in bariatric surgery are summarised in Table 10.16.

Table 10.15 Antidepressants in bariatric surgery

Drug	Specific evidence and considerations
SSRIs[9–14]	■ Evidence demonstrates that plasma levels may be significantly reduced following RYGB ■ Malabsorption has been implicated in cases of discontinuation symptoms and loss of efficacy
SNRIs[11,15]	■ Duloxetine levels 42% lower after RYGB compared with matched controls ■ The absorption of venlafaxine MR capsules seems not to be altered by RYGB[16]
Mirtazapine[17,18]	■ Increased appetite and weight gain are possible ■ Has been used successfully for non-mechanical vomiting after RYGB
TCAs[19,20]	■ Single case report suggests therapeutic plasma levels can be achieved within usual dose range after RYGB ■ Plasma levels may be increased after significant weight loss; consider monitoring levels and reducing dose

General summary

- Antidepressants are the best studied psychotropics in the bariatric population. Current evidence suggests that antidepressant absorption is reduced after surgery (though studies are mostly limited to SSRIs after RYGB)
- Signs of reduced absorption may include the rapid development of discontinuation symptoms and later loss of efficacy
- Patients require close monitoring as those at risk of reduced absorption cannot be reliably predicted
- The risk of gastric bleeds with bariatric surgery will probably be increased by serotonergic antidepressants

RYGB, Roux-en-Y gastric bypass; SNRI, serotonin–noradrenaline reuptake inhibitor; SSRI, selective serotonin reuptake inhibitor; TCA, tricyclic antidepressant.

Table 10.16 Antipsychotics in bariatric surgery

Drug	Specific evidence and considerations
Asenapine[21]	■ Primarily absorbed via oral mucosa; problems after bariatric surgery are not expected ■ One case report of successful use after RYGB
Clozapine[22–24]	■ One case report of relapse after RYGB ■ Take drug plasma levels before surgery and regularly monitor afterwards ■ Constipation is common after surgery; the manufacturer recommends close monitoring and active treatment ■ Check smoking status (quitting before surgery is encouraged); adjust dose accordingly
Haloperidol[25]	■ Single case report suggests levels after RYGB are similar to those generally reported in the literature
Lurasidone	■ Must be taken with food for absorption (350 kcal); risk of reduced absorption with reduced/inconsistent calorific intake peri-operatively. Consider switching to alternatives before surgery
Olanzapine[26,27]	■ Conflicting information on site of absorption; follow general recommendations
Quetiapine[8,26]	■ May be absorbed via the stomach and duodenum; monitor mental state ■ Switching to immediate-release preparation and dividing doses ≥300 mg has been recommended
Risperidone[28]	■ Consider switching stable patients to an equivalent dose of paliperidone LAI ■ Risperidone LAI has been used successfully when oral treatment was not tolerated after bariatric surgery
Ziprasidone[29]	■ Must be taken with food for absorption (500 kcal); risk of reduced absorption with reduced/inconsistent calorific intake peri-operatively. Consider switching to alternatives before surgery

General summary

■ Antipsychotics are not well studied in bariatric surgery; data are limited to case reports or theoretical concerns
■ Depot antipsychotics avoid the risk of reduced absorption after surgery. Given the limited data on pharmacokinetic changes after surgery and interindividual variability, routinely switching to depot antipsychotics before surgery may not be justified.[8] However, depot preparations remain an option for those stabilised on treatment available as a depot or in patients demonstrating signs of reduced bioavailability after surgery
■ Bariatric surgery may contribute additional cardiac stressors to patients with QT prolongation;[30] ECG monitoring before surgery is recommended

ECG, electrocardiogram; LAI, long-acting injection; RYGB, Roux-en-Y gastric bypass.

Mood stabilisers

Recommendations on the use of mood stabilisers in bariatric surgery are summarised in Table 10.17.

Other drugs

Recommendations on the use of other drugs in bariatric surgery are summarised in Table 10.18.

Table 10.17 Mood stabilisers in bariatric surgery

Drug	Summary of evidence and considerations
Carbamazepine[31]	■ Single case report of agranulocytosis possibly related to increased plasma levels after sleeve gastrectomy
Lamotrigine[26]	■ Possibly absorbed from the stomach and proximal small intestine; monitor for loss of efficacy
Lithium[32–37] (see Box 10.4)	■ Cases of lithium toxicity following RYGB and sleeve gastrectomy have been reported ■ Switch to an equivalent dose of lithium citrate solution ■ In the pre-operative period, plasma levels may be affected by prescribed dietary changes ■ In the post-operative period, plasma levels may be affected by malabsorption (mainly absorbed via small intestine), fluid shifts and weight loss (lithium clearance increased in obesity)
Valproate[8,38]	■ Single case report suggests that absorption may be significantly reduced after malabsorptive procedures; no data on restrictive procedures ■ Dose reductions may be necessary after weight loss (plasma levels related to body weight) ■ Switch to liquid preparation before surgery or if malabsorption suspected on controlled-release/enteric-coated tablets ■ Baseline plasma valproate levels, FBC and LFTs with ongoing monitoring recommended ■ Monitor for clinical signs of poor tolerability, possibly occurring at normal plasma levels

General summary

- The literature on mood stabilisers after bariatric surgery is limited to a few case reports; the use of lithium requires particular care owing to its narrow therapeutic index
- The absorption of oral contraceptives may be reduced after bariatric surgery.[39] In patients prescribed teratogenic mood stabilisers, non-oral methods of contraception are recommended

FBC, full blood count; LFT, liver function test; RYGB, Roux-en-Y gastric bypass.

Box 10.4 Lithium around the time of bariatric surgery

The continued use of lithium throughout the peri-operative phases of bariatric surgery requires particularly close monitoring. The following guidance is based on available case reports and expert opinion.[37]

- Monitor lithium plasma levels weekly during pre-operative phase and for 6 weeks post surgery (as fluid intake gradually increases), 2-weekly for 6 months and monthly thereafter. Resume usual lithium monitoring 1 year post bariatric surgery.
- If plasma levels increase by >25% or approach 1.2 mmol/L, consider decreasing lithium dose.
- Withhold lithium if signs of toxicity are present and review dose.
- Monitor mental state periodically, using formal rating scales if possible.
- Encourage patient to drink 2.5–3 litres of fluid per day in the pre-operative phase (including liquid meal replacement).

General recommendations

General recommendations on prescribing after bariatric surgery are summarised in Table 10.19.

Table 10.18 Miscellaneous agents in bariatric surgery

Drug	Summary of evidence and considerations
Benzodiazepines[40–43]	▪ Bioavailability probably unaffected, shorter time to peak concentration
Methadone[44]	▪ Substantial increase in bioavailability after sleeve gastrectomy in one case report, possibly related to increased rate of gastric emptying; consider plasma level and QT monitoring
Methylphenidate[45,46]	▪ Conflicting limited data: one case report of reduced treatment efficacy after RYGB that resolved after switching to transdermal patch suggesting reduced oral bioavailability; another reports signs of toxicity

RYGB, Roux-en-Y gastric bypass.

Table 10.19 General recommendations for prescribing in bariatric surgery[8]

Before surgery	After surgery (0–6 weeks)	After surgery (>6 weeks after)
▪ Do not routinely increase doses; clinically relevant malabsorption cannot be reliably predicted ▪ Assess mental state before surgery and consider measuring baseline drug plasma levels ▪ Switch modified-release/enteric-coated preparations to immediate-release tablets or liquid preparations	▪ Closely monitor for signs of adverse effects and drug malabsorption (symptom re-emergence, discontinuation symptoms) ▪ Regularly monitor drug plasma levels if clinically indicated ▪ If malabsorption suspected, consider the recommended strategies ▪ If medication toxicity suspected, withhold and reassess dose	▪ Continue regular monitoring for the first year post-operatively, although frequency can be reduced if stable ▪ Monitor for an increase in adverse effects, especially if doses were increased in the acute post-operative period ▪ Consider returning to pre-surgical treatment regimen after 1 year (depending on clinical history)

General management strategies for patients demonstrating signs of reduced bioavailability

▪ Consider non-oral routes of administration where available (e.g. depots for patients stable on antipsychotics)
▪ Dividing doses may improve malabsorption related to a reduced stomach capacity after surgery
▪ Switching modified/prolonged/delayed-release to immediate-release formulations
▪ Switching solid tablets to liquid or orodispersible preparations to bypass disintegration phase
▪ Switching large tablets to smaller ones
▪ In cases where doses have been increased to account for reduced bioavailability, monitor for emergent adverse effects as bioavailability may normalise over time

Psychotropics with a risk of weight gain after bariatric surgery

It is estimated that 10–20% of patients regain a significant amount of weight after bariatric surgery.[47] There is no information on how psychotropics associated with weight gain affect outcomes after surgery, but high-risk drugs should probably be avoided. Patients' individual clinical circumstances should be considered (especially if stable on treatment and at a high risk of relapse) as there is evidence that uncontrolled mental illness is a risk factor for weight regain.[47]

Alcohol[48]

Gastric bypass surgery is associated with accelerated alcohol absorption, higher maximum alcohol concentrations and a longer time to elimination. There is also an increased risk of alcohol misuse disorders after gastric bypass. Data are less clear for sleeve gastrectomy and there is no evidence that gastric banding leads to any changes.

Wider considerations[49]

In practice, many patients may not require significant changes to drug treatment after surgery. Relapse of symptoms after surgery may not be related to altered drug pharmacokinetics. Although improvements in mental health are to be anticipated, deterioration can also occur due to a range of factors, including unmet weight-loss expectations, poor tolerability and dissatisfaction after surgical treatment.

References

1. Dawes AJ et al. Mental health conditions among patients seeking and undergoing bariatric surgery: a meta-analysis. JAMA 2016; 315: 150–163.
2. Cunningham JL et al. Investigation of antidepressant medication usage after bariatric surgery. Obes Surg 2012; 22:530–535.
3. Pawlow LA et al. Findings and outcomes of psychological evaluations of gastric bypass applicants. Surg Obes Relat Dis2005; 1:523–527; discussion 528–529.
4. Gondek W. Psychiatric suitability assessment for bariatric surgery. In: Sockalingam S, Hawa R, eds. *Psychiatric Care in Severe Obesity: An Interdisciplinary Guide to Integrated Care*. Cham: Springer International Publishing; 2017, pp. 173–186.
5. Padwal R et al. A systematic review of drug absorption following bariatric surgery and its theoretical implications. Obes Rev 2010; 11:41–50.
6. Macgregor AM et al. Drug distribution in obesity and following bariatric surgery: a literature review. Obes Surg 1996; 6:17–27.
7. Roerig JL et al. Psychopharmacology and bariatric surgery. Eur Eat Disord Rev 2015; 23:463–469.
8. Bingham KS et al. Psychopharmacology in bariatric surgery patients. In: Sockalingam S, Hawa R, eds. *Psychiatric Care in Severe Obesity: An Interdisciplinary Guide to Integrated Care*. Cham: Springer International Publishing; 2017, pp. 313–333.
9. Faye E et al. Antidepressant agents in short bowel syndrome. Clin Ther 2014; 36:2029–2033.e2023.
10. Marzinke MA et al. Decreased escitalopram concentrations post-Roux-en-Y gastric bypass surgery. Ther Drug Monit 2015; 37:408–412.
11. Hamad GG et al. The effect of gastric bypass on the pharmacokinetics of serotonin reuptake inhibitors. Am J Psychiatry 2012; 169:256–263.
12. Seaman JS et al. Dissolution of common psychiatric medications in a Roux-en-Y gastric bypass model. Psychosomatics 2005; 46:250–253.
13. Bingham K et al. SSRI discontinuation syndrome following bariatric surgery: a case report and focused literature review. Psychosomatics 2014; 55:692–697.
14. Roerig JL et al. Preliminary comparison of sertraline levels in postbariatric surgery patients versus matched nonsurgical cohort. Surg Obes Relat Dis 2012; 8:62–66.
15. Roerig JL et al. A comparison of duloxetine plasma levels in postbariatric surgery patients versus matched nonsurgical control subjects. J Clin Psychopharmacol 2013; 33:479–484.
16. Krieger CA et al. Comparison of bioavailability of single-dose extended-release venlafaxine capsules in obese patients before and after gastric bypass surgery. Pharmacotherapy 2017; 37:1374–1382.
17. Teixeira FV et al. Mirtazapine (Remeron) as treatment for non-mechanical vomiting after gastric bypass. Obes Surg 2005; 15:707–709.
18. Huerta S et al. Intractable nausea and vomiting following Roux-en-Y gastric bypass: role of mirtazapine. Obes Surg 2006; 16:1399.
19. Broyles JE et al. Nortriptyline absorption in short bowel syndrome. JPEN J Parenter Enteral Nutr 1990; 14:326–327.
20. Jobson K et al. Weight loss and a concomitant change in plasma tricyclic levels. Am J Psychiatry 1978; 135:237–238.
21. Tabaac BJ et al. Pica patient, status post gastric bypass, improves with change in medication regimen. Ther Adv Psychopharmacol 2015; 5:38–42.
22. Kaltsounis J et al. Intravenous valproate treatment of severe manic symptoms after gastric bypass surgery: a case report. Psychosomatics 2000; 41:454–456.
23. Afshar S et al. The effects of bariatric procedures on bowel habit. Obes Surg 2016; 26:2348–2354.
24. Mylan Products Limited. Summary of Product Characteristics. Clozaril. 2016. https://www.medicines.org.uk/emc/medicine/32564.
25. Fuller AK et al. Haloperidol pharmacokinetics following gastric bypass surgery. J Clin Psychopharmacol 1986; 6:376–378
26. Miller AD et al. Medication and nutrient administration considerations after bariatric surgery. Am J Health Syst Pharm 2006; 63:1852–1857.
27. Tran PV et al. *Olanzapine (Zyprexa): A Novel Antipsychotic*. Philadelphia: Lippincott Williams & Wilkins; 2001.

28. Brietzke E et al. Long-acting injectable risperidone in a bipolar patient submitted to bariatric surgery and intolerant to conventional mood stabilizers. Psychiatry Clin Neurosci 2011; **65**:205.

29. Gandelman K et al. The impact of calories and fat content of meals on oral ziprasidone absorption: a randomized, open-label, crossover trial. J Clin Psychiatry 2009; **70**:58–62.

30. Woodard G et al. Cardiac arrest during laparoscopic Roux-en-Y gastric bypass in a bariatric patient with drug-associated long QT syndrome. Obes Surg 2011; **21**:134–137.

31. Koutsavlis I et al. Dose-dependent carbamazepine-induced agranulocytosis following bariatric surgery (sleeve gastrectomy): a possible mechanism. Bariatr Surg Pract Patient Care 2015; **10**:130–134.

32. Reiss RA et al. Lithium pharmacokinetics in the obese. Clin Pharmacol Ther 1994; **55**:392–398.

33. Tripp AC. Lithium toxicity after Roux-en-Y gastric bypass surgery. J Clin Psychopharmacol 2011; **31**:261–262.

34. Musfeldt D et al. Lithium toxicity after Roux-en-Y bariatric surgery. BMJ Case Rep 2016; **2016**.

35. Walsh K et al. Lithium toxicity following Roux-en-Y gastric bypass. Bariatr Surg Pract Patient Care 2014; **9**:77–80.

36. Alam A et al. Lithium toxicity following vertical sleeve gastrectomy: a case report. Clin Psychopharmacol Neurosci 2016; **14**:318–320.

37. Bingham KS et al. Perioperative lithium use in bariatric surgery: a case series and literature review. Psychosomatics 2016; **57**:638–644.

38. Wolter S et al. P098 Valproic Acid Dosage in the Post Bariatric Surgery Patient in Abstracts from the XVII World Congress of International Federation for the Surgery of Obesity and Metabolic Disorders (IFSO), New Delhi 11 -15 September, 2012. Obes Surg 2012; **22**:1315–1419.

39. Merhi ZO. Challenging oral contraception after weight loss by bariatric surgery. Gynecol Obstet Invest 2007; **64**:100–102.

40. Tandra S et al. Pharmacokinetic and pharmacodynamic alterations in the Roux-en-Y gastric bypass recipients. Ann Surg 2013; **258**:262–269.

41. Chan LN et al. Proximal Roux-en-Y gastric bypass alters drug absorption pattern but not systemic exposure of CYP3A4 and P-glycoprotein substrates. Pharmacotherapy 2015; **35**:361–369.

42. Brill MJ et al. The pharmacokinetics of the CYP3A substrate midazolam in morbidly obese patients before and one year after bariatric surgery. Pharm Res 2015; **32**:3927–3936.

43. Ochs HR et al. Diazepam absorption: effects of age, sex, and Billroth gastrectomy. Dig Dis Sci 1982; **27**:225–230.

44. Strømmen M et al. Bioavailability of methadone after sleeve gastrectomy: a planned case observation. Clin Ther 2016; **38**:1532–1536.

45. Azran C et al. Impaired oral absorption of methylphenidate after Roux-en-Y gastric bypass. Surg Obes Relat Dis 2017; **13**:1245–1247.

46. Ludvigsson M et al. Methylphenidate toxicity after Roux-en-Y gastric bypass. Surg Obes Relat Dis 2016; **12**:e55–e57.

47. Karmali S et al. Weight recidivism post-bariatric surgery: a systematic review. Obes Surg 2013; **23**:1922–1933.

48. Parikh M et al. ASMBS position statement on alcohol use before and after bariatric surgery. Surg Obes Relat Dis 2016; **12**:225–230.

49. Stevens T et al. Your patient and weight-loss surgery. Adv Psychiatr Treat 2012; **18**:418–425.

Part 4

Other aspects of psychotropic drug use

Pharmacokinetics

Plasma level monitoring of psychotropic drugs

Plasma drug concentration or plasma 'level' monitoring is a process often subject to some confusion and misunderstanding. Drug level monitoring, when appropriately used, is of considerable help in optimising treatment and assuring adherence. However, in psychiatry, as in other areas of medicine, plasma level determinations are frequently undertaken without good cause and results acted upon inappropriately.[1] In other instances, therapeutic drug monitoring is underused.

Before taking a blood sample for plasma concentration assay, make sure that the following criteria are satisfied:

- **Is there a clinically useful assay method available?**
  Only a minority of drugs have available assays. The assay must be clinically validated and results available within a clinically useful timescale. Check with your local laboratory.
- **Is the drug at 'steady state'?**
  Plasma levels are usually meaningful only when samples are taken after steady-state levels have been achieved. This takes 4–5 drug half-lives. A clear exception to this advice is suspected overdose; in such situations attainment of steady state is of no relevance.
- **Is the timing of the sample correct?**
  Sampling time is vitally important for many but not all drugs. If the recommended sampling time is, say, 12 hours post dose, then the sample should be taken 11–13 hours post dose if possible; 10–14 hours post dose, if absolutely necessary. For trough or 'pre-dose' samples, take the blood sample immediately before the next dose is due. Do not, under any circumstances, withhold the next dose for more than 1 or (possibly) 2 hours until the sample is taken. Withholding for longer than this will inevitably give a misleading result (it will give a lower result than that ever seen in the usual, regular dosing), and this may lead to an inappropriate dose increase. Sampling time

The Maudsley Prescribing Guidelines in Psychiatry, Thirteenth Edition. David M. Taylor, Thomas R. E. Barnes and Allan H. Young.
© 2018 David M. Taylor. Published 2018 by John Wiley & Sons Ltd.

is less critical with drugs with a long half-life (e.g. olanzapine) but, as an absolute minimum, prescribers should always record the time of sampling and time of last dose. This cannot be emphasised enough.

- If a sample is not taken within 1–2 hours of the required time, it has the potential to mislead rather than inform. The only exception to this is if toxicity is suspected – sampling at the time of suspected toxicity is obviously appropriate.
- **Will the level have any inherent meaning?**
  Is there a target range of plasma levels? If so, then plasma levels (from samples taken at the right time) will usefully guide dosing. If there is not an accepted target range, plasma levels can only indicate adherence or potential toxicity. However, if the sample is being used to check compliance, then bear in mind that a plasma level of zero indicates only that the drug has not been taken in the past several days. Plasma levels above zero may indicate erratic compliance, full compliance or even long-standing non-compliance disguised by recent taking of prescribed doses. Note also that target ranges have their limitations: patients may respond to lower levels than the quoted range and tolerate levels above the range; also, ranges quoted by different laboratories vary sometimes widely, often without explanation.
- **Is there a clear reason for plasma level determination?**
  Only the following reasons are valid:
  - to confirm compliance (see previous passage)
  - if toxicity is suspected
  - if a pharmacokinetic drug interaction is suspected
  - if clinical response is difficult to assess directly (and where a target range of plasma levels has been established)
  - if the drug has a narrow therapeutic index and toxicity concerns are considerable.

Interpreting sample results

The basic rule for sample level interpretation is to act upon assay results only in conjunction with reliable clinical observation (*'treat the patient, not the level'*). For example, if a patient is responding adequately to a drug but has a plasma level below the accepted target range, then the dose should not normally be increased. If a patient has intolerable adverse effects but a plasma level within the target range, then a dose decrease may be appropriate.

Where a plasma level result is substantially different from previous results, a repeat sample is usually advised. Check dose, timing of dose and recent compliance but ensure, in particular, the correct timing of the sample. Many anomalous results are the consequence of changes in sample timing.

Table 11.1 shows the target ranges for some commonly prescribed psychotropic drugs.

Amisulpride

Amisulpride plasma levels are closely related to dose with insufficient variation to make routine plasma level monitoring prudent. Higher levels observed in women[22–24] seem to have little significant clinical implication for either therapeutic response or adverse effects.

Table 11.1 Interpreting sample results

Drug	Target range	Sample timing	Time to steady state	Comments
Amisulpride	200–320 µg/L 20–60 µg/L (elderly)	Trough	3 days	See text
Aripiprazole	150–210 µg/L	Trough	15–16 days	See text
Carbamazepine[2–4]	>7 mg/L bipolar disorder	Trough	2 weeks	Carbamazepine induces its own metabolism. Time to steady state dependent on auto-induction
Clozapine	350–500 µg/L Upper limit of target range is ill-defined	Trough	2–3 days	See text
Lamotrigine[5–7]	Not established but suggest 2.5–15 mg/L	Trough	5 days Auto-induction is thought to occur, so time to steady state may be longer	Some debate over utility of lamotrigine levels, especially in bipolar disorder. In treatment-resistant unipolar depression, plasma levels of above 12.7 µmol/L (3.3 mg/L) are associated with response.[8,9] Toxicity may be increased above 15 mg/L but normally well tolerated
Lithium[10–14]	0.6–1.0 mmol/L (0.4 mmol may be sufficient for some patients/indications; >1.0 mmol/L required for mania)	12 hours	5 days post dose	Well-established target range, albeit derived from ancient data sources. A study published in 2013[15] suggested 0.6 mmol/L was the minimum level for a prophylactic effect
Olanzapine	20–40 µg/L	12 hours	1 week	See text
Paliperidone[16]	20–60 µg/L (9-OH risperidone)	Trough	2–3 days oral 2 months depot	No obvious reason to suspect range should be any different from risperidone. Some practical confirmation. As with risperidone, plasma level monitoring is not recommended
Phenytoin[3]	10–20 mg/L	Trough	Variable	Follows zero-order kinetics Free levels may be useful in some circumstances
Quetiapine	Around 50–100 µg/L?	Trough?	2–3 days oral	Target range not defined. Plasma level monitoring not recommended. See text
Risperidone	20–60 µg/L (active moiety – risperidone + 9-OH risperidone)	Trough	2–3 days oral 6–8 weeks injection	Plasma level monitoring is not recommended See text

CHAPTER 11

(Continued)

Table 11.1 (*Continued*)

Drug	Target range	Sample timing	Time to steady state	Comments
Tricyclics[17]	Nortriptyline 50–150 µg/L Amitriptyline 100–200 µg/L	Trough	2–3 days	Rarely used and of dubious benefit Use electrocardiogram to assess toxicity
Valproate[2,3,18–20]	50–100 mg/L Epilepsy and bipolar	Trough	2–3 days	Some doubt over value of levels in epilepsy and in bipolar disorder. Some evidence that, in mania, levels up to 125 mg/L are tolerated and more effective than lower concentrations. Valproate plasma levels are linearly related to plasma ammonia[21]

A (trough) threshold for clinical response has been suggested to be approximately 100 µg/L[25] and mean levels of 367 µg/L[24] have been noted in responders in individual studies. Adverse effects (notably extrapyramidal symptoms; EPS) have been observed at mean levels of 336 µg/L,[22] 377 µg/L[25] and 395 µg/L.[23] A plasma level threshold of below 320 µg/L has been found to predict avoidance of EPS.[25] A review[26] has suggested an approximate range of **200–320 µg/L** for optimal clinical response and avoidance of adverse effects. In older patients with psychosis, recent studies suggest plasma concentrations of **20–60 µg/L** may give optimal D_2 occupancy and clinical response.[27,28]

In practice, only a minority of treated patients have 'therapeutic' plasma levels (probably because of poor adherence[29]) so plasma monitoring may be of some benefit. However, amisulpride plasma level monitoring is rarely undertaken and few laboratories offer amisulpride assays. The dose–response relationship is sufficiently robust (in trials, at least) to obviate the need for plasma sampling within the licensed dose range (although note that in older patients doses of 50–100 mg/day may be sufficient) and adverse effects are usually well managed by dose adjustment alone. Plasma level monitoring is best reserved for those in whom clinical response is poor, adherence is questioned or drug interactions or physical illness may make adverse effects more likely.

Aripiprazole

Plasma level monitoring of aripiprazole is rarely undertaken in practice. The dose–response relationship for aripiprazole is well established with a plateau in clinical response and D_2 dopamine occupancy seen in doses above approximately 10 mg/day.[30] Plasma levels of aripiprazole, its metabolite, and the total moiety (parent plus metabolite) strongly relate linearly to dose, making it possible to predict, with some certainty, an approximate plasma level for a given dose.[31] Target plasma level ranges for optimal clinical response have been suggested as 146–254 µg/L[32] and 150–300 µg/L,[33] with adverse effects observed above 210 µg/L.[33] Inter-individual variation in aripiprazole plasma levels has been observed but not fully investigated, although gender appears to have little influence.[34,35] Age, metabolic enzyme genotype and interacting medications seem likely causes of variation,[33–36] however there are too few reports regarding their clinical implication to recommend specific monitoring in respect to these factors. A putative range of between **150 µg/L and 210 µg/L**[31] has been suggested as a target for patients taking aripiprazole and these are broadly the concentrations seen in patients receiving depot aripiprazole at 300 mg and 400 mg monthly.[37] However, for reasons described here, plasma level monitoring is not advised in routine practice.

Clozapine

Clozapine plasma levels are broadly related to daily dose,[38] but there is sufficient variation to make impossible any precise prediction of plasma level. Plasma levels are generally lower in younger patients, males,[39] and smokers[40] and higher in Asians.[41] A series of algorithms has been developed for the approximate prediction of clozapine levels according to patient factors and these are strongly recommended.[42] Algorithms cannot, however, account for other influences on clozapine plasma levels such as changes in adherence, inflammation[43] and infection.[44,45]

The plasma level threshold for acute response to clozapine has been suggested to be 200 µg/L,[46] 350 µg/L,[47–49] 370 µg/L,[50] 420 µg/L,[51] 504 µg/L[52] and 550 µg/L.[53] Limited data suggest a level of at least 200 µg/L is required to prevent relapse.[54] Substantial variation in clozapine plasma level may also predict relapse.[55] Changes in an individual's plasma clozapine are common with a tendency for concentrations to decrease slightly over time.[56]

Despite these somewhat varied estimates of response threshold, plasma levels can be useful in optimising treatment. In those not responding to clozapine, dose should be adjusted to give plasma levels in the range **350–500 µg/L** (a range reflecting a consensus of the above findings). Those not tolerating clozapine may benefit from a reduction to a dose giving plasma levels in this range. An upper limit to the clozapine target range has not been defined. Any upper limit must take into account two components: the level above which no therapeutic advantage is gained and the level at which toxicity/tolerability is unacceptable. Plasma levels do seem to predict electroencephalogram (EEG) changes[57,58] and seizures occur more frequently in patients with levels above 1000 µg/L,[59] so levels should probably be kept well below this. Other non-neurological clozapine-related adverse effects also seem to be plasma-level related[60] as might be expected. An upper limit of concentrations around 600–800 µg/L has been proposed.[61]

A further consideration is that placing an upper limit on the target range for clozapine levels may discourage potentially worthwhile dose increases within the licensed dose range. Before plasma levels were widely used, clozapine was fairly often given in doses up to 900 mg/day, with valproate being added when the dose reached 600 mg/day. It remains unclear whether using these high doses can benefit patients with plasma levels already above the accepted threshold. Nonetheless, it is prudent to use an anticonvulsant as prophylaxis against seizures and myoclonus when plasma levels are above 600 µg/L (a level based more on repeated recommendation than on a clear evidence-based threshold[61]) and certainly when levels approach 1000 µg/L.

Norclozapine is the major metabolite of clozapine. The ratio of clozapine to norclozapine averages 1.25 in populations[62] but may differ for individuals. In chronic dosing, the ratio should remain the same for a given patient. A decrease in ratio may suggest enzyme induction; an increase suggests enzyme inhibition, a non-trough sample or recent missed doses. Note also that clozapine metabolism may become saturated at higher doses: the ratio of clozapine to norclozapine increases with increasing plasma levels, suggesting saturation.[63–65] The effect of fluvoxamine also suggests that metabolism via CYP1A2 to norclozapine can be overwhelmed.[66] Norclozapine has muscarinic M_1 agonist activity and relatively higher concentrations are associated with better working memory performance.[67]

Olanzapine

Plasma levels of olanzapine are linearly related to daily dose,[68] but there is substantial variation,[69] with higher levels seen in women,[52] non-smokers[70] and those on enzyme-inhibiting drugs.[70,71] With once-daily dosing, the threshold level for response in schizophrenia has been suggested to be 9.3 µg/L (trough sample),[72] 23.2 µg/L (12-hour post-dose sample)[52] and 23 µg/L at a mean of 13.5 hours post dose.[73] There is evidence to suggest that levels greater than around 40 µg/L (12-hour sampling) produce no further therapeutic benefit than lower levels.[74] Severe toxicity is uncommon but may be associated with levels above 100 µg/L, and death is occasionally seen at levels above 160 µg/L[75] (albeit when other drugs or physical factors are relevant). A target range for therapeutic use of **20–40 µg/L** (12-hour post-dose sample) has been proposed[76] for schizophrenia; the range for mania is probably similar.[77]

Notably, significant weight gain seems most likely to occur in those with plasma levels above 20 µg/L.[78] Constipation, dry mouth and tachycardia also seem to be plasma level-related.[79]

In practice, the dose of olanzapine should be largely governed by response and tolerability. However, a survey of UK sample assay results suggested that around 20% of patients on 20 mg/day will have sub-therapeutic plasma levels and more than 40% have levels above 40 µg/L.[80] Plasma level determinations might then be useful for those suspected of non-adherence, those showing poor tolerability or those not responding to the maximum licensed dose. Where there is poor response and plasma levels are below 20 µg/L, dose may then be adjusted to give 12-hour plasma levels of 20–40 µg/L; where there is good response and poor tolerability, the dose should be tentatively reduced to give plasma levels below 40 µg/L. Changes in dose give proportionate changes in plasma levels.[81]

Quetiapine (IR)

Dose of quetiapine is weakly related to trough plasma samples.[82] Mean levels reported within the dose range 150–800 mg/day range from 27 µg/L to 387 µg/L,[83–88] although the highest and lowest levels are not necessarily found at the lowest and highest doses. Age, gender and co-medication may contribute to the significant inter-individual variance observed in therapeutic drug monitoring studies, with female gender,[88,89] older age[87,88] and CYP3A4-inhibiting drugs[83,87,88] likely to increase quetiapine concentration. Reports of these effects are conflicting[89] and not sufficient to support the routine use of plasma level monitoring based on these factors alone. Despite the substantial variation in plasma levels at each dose, there is insufficient evidence to suggest a target therapeutic range to aim for (although a target range of 100–500 µg/L has been proposed[90]), thus plasma level monitoring is likely to have little value. Moreover, the metabolites of quetiapine have major therapeutic effects and their concentrations are only loosely associated with parent drug levels.[91]

Most current reports of quetiapine concentration associations are derived from analysis of trough samples. Because of the short half-life of quetiapine, trough levels tend to drop to within a relatively small range regardless of dose and previous peak level. Thus peak plasma levels may be more closely related to dose and clinical response,[82] although monitoring of such is not currently justified in the absence of an established peak plasma target range. Interestingly, a study of quetiapine in patients with borderline personality disorder or drug-induced psychosis showed a linear relationship between response and 12-hour plasma level.[89]

Quetiapine has an established dose–response relationship and appears to be well tolerated at doses well beyond the licensed dose range.[92] In practice, dose adjustment should be based on patient response and tolerability.

Risperidone

Risperidone plasma levels are rarely measured in the UK and very few laboratories have developed assay methods for its determination. In any case, plasma level monitoring is probably unproductive (dose–response is well described) except where compliance is in doubt and in such cases measurement of prolactin will give some idea of compliance.

The therapeutic range for risperidone is generally agreed to be **20–60 µg/L** of the active moiety (risperidone + 9-OH-risperidone)[93,94] although other ranges (25–150 µg/L and 25–80 µg/L) have been proposed.[95] Plasma levels of 20–60 µg/L are usually afforded by oral doses of between 3 mg and 6 mg a day.[93,96–98] Occupancy of striatal dopamine D_2 receptors has been shown to be around 65% (the minimum required for acute therapeutic effect) at plasma levels of approximately 20 µg/L.[94,99]

Risperidone long-acting injection (RLAI) (25 mg/2 weeks) appears to afford plasma levels averaging between 4.4 and 22.7 µg/L.[97] Dopamine D_2 occupancies at this dose have been variously estimated at between 25% and 71%.[94,100,101] There is considerable inter-individual variation around these mean values with a substantial minority of patients with plasma levels above those shown. Nonetheless, these data do cast doubt on the efficacy of a dose of 25 mg/2 weeks,[97] although it is noteworthy that there is some evidence that long-acting antipsychotic preparations are effective despite apparently sub-therapeutic plasma levels and dopamine occupancies.[102] Indeed, evidence continues to grow that sustained high dopamine occupancy is not necessary to prevent recurrence in longer-term treatment[103–105] (as opposed to providing acute effects).

Disturbingly, however, a report of assay results for patients receiving RLAI[106] found that 50% of patients had levels below 20 µg/L, and for 10% no risperidone/9-OH-risperidone was detected. Thus therapeutic drug monitoring might be clinically helpful for those on RLAI but this rather defeats the object of a long-acting injection.

Limited data for paliperidone palmitate 1-monthly long-acting injection suggest that standard loading doses give plasma levels of 25–45 µg/L; at steady state, plasma levels ranged from 10 to 25 µg/L for 100 mg/month and 15 to 35 µg/L for 150 mg/month.[107] For the 3-monthly injection, steady state plasma concentrations range from 30 to 55 µg/L for 525 mg every 3 months, 25 to 55 µg/L for 350 mg every 3 months and 20 to 35 µg/L for 263 mg every 3 months.[108]

References

1. Mann K et al. Appropriateness of therapeutic drug monitoring for antidepressants in routine psychiatric inpatient care. Ther Drug Monit 2006; 28:83–88.
2. Taylor D et al. Doses of carbamazepine and valproate in bipolar affective disorder. Psychiatr Bull 1997; 21:221–223.
3. Eadie MJ. Anticonvulsant drugs. Drugs 1984; 27:328–363.
4. Chbili C et al. Relationships between pharmacokinetic parameters of carbamazepine and therapeutic response in patients with bipolar disease. Ann Biol Clin (Paris) 2014; 72:453–459.
5. Cohen AF et al. Lamotrigine, a new anticonvulsant: pharmacokinetics in normal humans. Clin Pharmacol Ther 1987; 42:535–541.
6. Kilpatrick ES et al. Concentration-effect and concentration-toxicity relations with lamotrigine: a prospective study. Epilepsia 1996; 37:534–538.
7. Johannessen SI et al. Therapeutic drug monitoring of the newer antiepileptic drugs. Ther Drug Monit 2003; 25:347–63.
8. Kagawa S et al. Relationship between plasma concentrations of lamotrigine and its early therapeutic effect of lamotrigine augmentation therapy in treatment-resistant depressive disorder. Ther Drug Monit 2014; 36:730–733.
9. Nakamura A et al. Prediction of an optimal dose of lamotrigine for augmentation therapy in treatment-resistant depressive disorder from plasma lamotrigine concentration at week 2. Ther Drug Monit 2016; 38:379–382.
10. Schou M. Forty years of lithium treatment. Arch Gen Psychiatry 1997; 54:9–13.
11. Anon. Using lithium safely. Drug Ther Bull 1999; 37:22–24.
12. Nicholson J, Fitzmaurice B. Monitoring patients on lithium – a good practice guideline. Psychiatr Bull 2002; 26:348–351.
13. National Institute for Health and Care Excellence. Bipolar disorder: assessment and management: Clinical Guidance 185, 2014. Last updated February 2016. https://www.nice.org.uk/guidance/cg185.
14. Severus WE et al. What is the optimal serum lithium level in the long-term treatment of bipolar disorder – a review? Bipolar Disord 2008; 10:231–237.
15. Nolen WA et al. The association of the effect of lithium in the maintenance treatment of bipolar disorder with lithium plasma levels: a post hoc analysis of a double-blind study comparing switching to lithium or placebo in patients who responded to quetiapine (Trial 144). Bipolar Disord 2013; 15:100–109.
16. Nazirizadeh Y et al. Serum concentrations of paliperidone versus risperidone and clinical effects. Eur J Clin Pharmacol 2010; 66:797–803.
17. Taylor D et al. Plasma levels of tricyclics and related antidepressants: are they necessary or useful? Psychiatr Bull 1995; 19:548–550.
18. Perucca E. Pharmacological and therapeutic properties of valproate. CNS Drugs 2002; 16:695–714.
19. Allen MH et al. Linear relationship of valproate serum concentration to response and optimal serum levels for acute mania. Am J Psychiatry 2006; 163:272–275.
20. Bowden CL et al. Relation of serum valproate concentration to response in mania. Am J Psychiatry 1996; 153:765–770.
21. Vazquez M et al. Hyperammonemia associated with valproic acid concentrations. BioMed Res Int 2014; 2014:217269.
22. Muller MJ et al. Amisulpride doses and plasma levels in different age groups of patients with schizophrenia or schizoaffective disorder. J Psychopharmacol 2008; 23:278–286.
23. Muller MJ et al. Gender aspects in the clinical treatment of schizophrenic inpatients with amisulpride: a therapeutic drug monitoring study. Pharmacopsychiatry 2006; 39:41–46.
24. Bergemann N et al. Plasma amisulpride levels in schizophrenia or schizoaffective disorder. Eur Neuropsychopharmacol 2004; 14:245–250.
25. Muller MJ et al. Therapeutic drug monitoring for optimizing amisulpride therapy in patients with schizophrenia. J Psychiatr Res 2007; 41:673–679.
26. Sparshatt A et al. Amisulpride – dose, plasma concentration, occupancy and response: implications for therapeutic drug monitoring. Acta Psychiatr Scand 2009; 120:416–428.
27. Reeves S et al. Therapeutic window of dopamine D2/3 receptor occupancy to treat psychosis in Alzheimer's disease. Brain 2017; 140:1117–1127.
28. Reeves S et al. Therapeutic D2/3 receptor occupancies and response with low amisulpride blood concentrations in very late-onset schizophrenia-like psychosis (VLOSLP). Int J Geriatr Psychiatry 2017 [Epub ahead of print].
29. Bowskill SV et al. Plasma amisulpride in relation to prescribed dose, clozapine augmentation, and other factors: data from a therapeutic drug monitoring service, 2002-2010. Hum Psychopharmacol 2012; 27:507–513.
30. Mace S et al. Aripiprazole: dose-response relationship in schizophrenia and schizoaffective disorder. CNS Drugs 2008; 23:773–780.
31. Sparshatt A et al. A systematic review of aripiprazole – dose, plasma concentration, receptor occupancy and response: implications for therapeutic drug monitoring. J Clin Psychiatry 2010; 71:1447–1456.

32. Kirschbaum KM et al. Therapeutic monitoring of aripiprazole by HPLC with column-switching and spectrophotometric detection. Clin Chem 2005; 51:1718–1721.

33. Kirschbaum KM et al. Serum levels of aripiprazole and dehydroaripiprazole, clinical response and side effects. World J Biol Psychiatry 2008; 9:212–218.

34. Molden E et al. Pharmacokinetic variability of aripiprazole and the active metabolite dehydroaripiprazole in psychiatric patients. Ther Drug Monit 2006; 28:744–749.

35. Bachmann CJ et al. Large variability of aripiprazole and dehydroaripiprazole serum concentrations in adolescent patients with schizophrenia. Ther Drug Monit 2008; 30:462–466.

36. Hendset M et al. Impact of the CYP2D6 genotype on steady-state serum concentrations of aripiprazole and dehydroaripiprazole. Eur J Clin Pharmacol 2007; 63:1147–1151.

37. Mallikaarjun S et al. Pharmacokinetics, tolerability and safety of aripiprazole once-monthly in adult schizophrenia: an open-label, parallel-arm, multiple-dose study. Schizophr Res 2013; 150:281–288.

38. Haring C et al. Influence of patient-related variables on clozapine plasma levels. Am J Psychiatry 1990; 147:1471–1475.

39. Haring C et al. Dose-related plasma levels of clozapine: influence of smoking behaviour, sex and age. Psychopharmacology (Berl) 1989; 99 Suppl:S38–S40.

40. Taylor D. Pharmacokinetic interactions involving clozapine. Br J Psychiatry 1997; 171:109–112.

41. Ng CH et al. An inter-ethnic comparison study of clozapine dosage, clinical response and plasma levels. Int Clin Psychopharmacol 2005; 20:163–168.

42. Rostami-Hodjegan A et al. Influence of dose, cigarette smoking, age, sex, and metabolic activity on plasma clozapine concentrations: a predictive model and nomograms to aid clozapine dose adjustment and to assess compliance in individual patients. J Clin Psychopharmacol 2004; 24:70–78.

43. Haack MJ et al. Toxic rise of clozapine plasma concentrations in relation to inflammation. Eur Neuropsychopharmacol 2003; 13:381–385.

44. de Leon J et al. Serious respiratory infections can increase clozapine levels and contribute to side effects: a case report. Prog Neuropsychopharmacol Biol Psychiatry 2003; 27:1059–1063.

45. Espnes KA et al. A puzzling case of increased serum clozapine levels in a patient with inflammation and infection. Ther Drug Monit 2012; 34:489–492.

46. VanderZwaag C et al. Response of patients with treatment-refractory schizophrenia to clozapine within three serum level ranges. Am J Psychiatry 1996; 153:1579–1584.

47. Perry PJ et al. Clozapine and norclozapine plasma concentrations and clinical response of treatment refractory schizophrenic patients. Am J Psychiatry 1991; 148:231–235.

48. Miller DD. Effect of phenytoin on plasma clozapine concentrations in two patients. J Clin Psychiatry 1991; 52:23–25.

49. Spina E et al. Relationship between plasma concentrations of clozapine and norclozapine and therapeutic response in patients with schizophrenia resistant to conventional neuroleptics. Psychopharmacology (Berl) 2000; 148:83–89.

50. Hasegawa M et al. Relationship between clinical efficacy and clozapine concentrations in plasma in schizophrenia: effect of smoking. J Clin Psychopharmacol 1993; 13:383–390.

51. Potkin SG et al. Plasma clozapine concentrations predict clinical response in treatment-resistant schizophrenia. J Clin Psychiatry 1994; 55 Suppl B:133–136.

52. Perry PJ. Therapeutic drug monitoring of antipsychotics. Psychopharmacol Bull 2001; 35:19–29.

53. Llorca PM et al. Effectiveness of clozapine in neuroleptic-resistant schizophrenia: clinical response and plasma concentrations. J Psychiatry Neurosci 2002; 27:30–37.

54. Xiang YQ et al. Serum concentrations of clozapine and norclozapine in the prediction of relapse of patients with schizophrenia. Schizophr Res 2006; 83:201–210.

55. Stieffenhofer V et al. Clozapine plasma level monitoring for prediction of rehospitalization schizophrenic outpatients. Pharmacopsychiatry 2011; 44:55–59.

56. Lee J et al. Quantifying intraindividual variations in plasma clozapine levels: a population pharmacokinetic approach. J Clin Psychiatry 2016; 77:681–687.

57. Khan AY et al. Examining concentration-dependent toxicity of clozapine: role of therapeutic drug monitoring. J Psychiatr Pract 2005; 11:289–301.

58. Varma S et al. Clozapine-related EEG changes and seizures: dose and plasma-level relationships. Ther Adv Psychopharmacol 2011; 1:47–66.

59. Greenwood-Smith C et al. Serum clozapine levels: a review of their clinical utility. J Psychopharm 2003; 17:234–238.

60. Yusufi B et al. Prevalence and nature of side effects during clozapine maintenance treatment and the relationship with clozapine dose and plasma concentration. Int Clin Psychopharmacol 2007; 22:238–243.

61. Remington G et al. Clozapine and therapeutic drug monitoring: is there sufficient evidence for an upper threshold? Psychopharmacology (Berl) 2013; 225:505–518.

62. Couchman L et al. Plasma clozapine, norclozapine, and the clozapine:norclozapine ratio in relation to prescribed dose and other factors: data from a therapeutic drug monitoring service, 1993-2007. Ther Drug Monit 2010; 32:438–447.

63. Volpicelli SA et al. Determination of clozapine, norclozapine, and clozapine-N-oxide in serum by liquid chromatography. Clin Chem 1993; 39:1656–1659.

64. Guitton C et al. Clozapine and metabolite concentrations during treatment of patients with chronic schizophrenia. J Clin Pharmacol 1999; 39:721–728.

CHAPTER 11

65. Palego L et al. Clozapine, norclozapine plasma levels, their sum and ratio in 50 psychotic patients: influence of patient-related variables. Prog Neuropsychopharmacol Biol Psychiatry 2002; **26**:473–480.

66. Wang CY et al. The differential effects of steady-state fluvoxamine on the pharmacokinetics of olanzapine and clozapine in healthy volunteers. J Clin Pharmacol 2004; **44**:785–792.

67. Rajji TK et al. Prediction of working memory performance in schizophrenia by plasma ratio of clozapine to N-desmethylclozapine. Am J Psychiatry 2015; **172**:579–585.

68. Bishara D et al. Olanzapine: a systematic review and meta-regression of the relationships between dose, plasma concentration, receptor occupancy, and response. J Clin Psychopharmacol 2013; **33**:329–335.

69. Aravagiri M et al. Plasma level monitoring of olanzapine in patients with schizophrenia: determination by high-performance liquid chromatography with electrochemical detection. Ther Drug Monit 1997; **19**:307–313.

70. Gex-Fabry M et al. Therapeutic drug monitoring of olanzapine: the combined effect of age, gender, smoking, and comedication. Ther Drug Monit 2003; **25**:46–53.

71. Bergemann N et al. Olanzapine plasma concentration, average daily dose, and interaction with co-medication in schizophrenic patients. Pharmacopsychiatry 2004; **37**:63–68.

72. Perry PJ et al. Olanzapine plasma concentrations and clinical response in acutely ill schizophrenic patients. J Clin Psychopharmacol 1997; **17**:472–477.

73. Fellows L et al. Investigation of target plasma concentration–effect relationships for olanzapine in schizophrenia. Ther Drug Monit 2003; **25**:682–689.

74. Mauri MC et al. Clinical outcome and olanzapine plasma levels in acute schizophrenia. Eur Psychiatry 2005; **20**:55–60.

75. Rao ML et al. Olanzapine: pharmacology, pharmacokinetics and therapeutic drug monitoring. Fortschr Neurol Psychiatr 2001; **69**:510–517.

76. Robertson MD et al. Olanzapine concentrations in clinical serum and postmortem blood specimens – when does therapeutic become toxic? J Forensic Sci 2000; **45**:418–421.

77. Bech P et al. Olanzapine plasma level in relation to antimanic effect in the acute therapy of manic states. Nord J Psychiatry 2006; **60**:181–182.

78. Perry PJ et al. The association of weight gain and olanzapine plasma concentrations. J Clin Psychopharmacol 2005; **25**:250–254.

79. Kelly DL et al. Plasma concentrations of high-dose olanzapine in a double-blind crossover study. Hum Psychopharmacol 2006; **21**:393–398.

80. Patel MX et al. Plasma olanzapine in relation to prescribed dose and other factors: data from a therapeutic drug monitoring service, 1999-2009. J Clin Psychopharmacol 2011; **31**:411–417.

81. Tsuboi T et al. Predicting plasma olanzapine concentration following a change in dosage: a population pharmacokinetic study. Pharmacopsychiatry 2015; **48**:286–291.

82. Sparshatt A et al. Relationship between daily dose, plasma concentrations, dopamine receptor occupancy, and clinical response to quetiapine: a review. J Clin Psychiatry 2011; **72**:1108–1123.

83. Hasselstrom J et al. Quetiapine serum concentrations in psychiatric patients: the influence of comedication. Ther Drug Monit 2004; **26**:486–491.

84. Winter HR et al. Steady-state pharmacokinetic, safety, and tolerability profiles of quetiapine, norquetiapine, and other quetiapine metabolites in pediatric and adult patients with psychotic disorders. J Child Adolesc Psychopharmacol 2008; **18**:81–98.

85. Li KY et al. Multiple dose pharmacokinetics of quetiapine and some of its metabolites in Chinese suffering from schizophrenia. Acta Pharmacol Sin 2004; **25**:390–394.

86. McConville BJ et al. Pharmacokinetics, tolerability, and clinical effectiveness of quetiapine fumarate: an open-label trial in adolescents with psychotic disorders. J Clin Psychiatry 2000; **61**:252–260.

87. Castberg I et al. Quetiapine and drug interactions: evidence from a routine therapeutic drug monitoring service. J Clin Psychiatry 2007; **68**:1540–1545.

88. Aichhorn W et al. Influence of age, gender, body weight and valproate comedication on quetiapine plasma concentrations. Int Clin Psychopharmacol 2006; **21**:81–85.

89. Mauri MC et al. Two weeks' quetiapine treatment for schizophrenia, drug-induced psychosis and borderline personality disorder: a naturalistic study with drug plasma levels. Expert Opin Pharmacother 2007; **8**:2207–2213.

90. Patteet L et al. Therapeutic drug monitoring of common antipsychotics. Ther Drug Monit 2012; **34**:629–651.

91. Fisher DS et al. Plasma concentrations of quetiapine, N-desalkylquetiapine, o-desalkylquetiapine, 7-hydroxyquetiapine, and quetiapine sulfoxide in relation to quetiapine dose, formulation, and other factors. Ther Drug Monit 2012; **34**:415–421.

92. Sparshatt A et al. Quetiapine: dose-response relationship in schizophrenia. CNS Drugs 2008; **22**:49–68.

93. Olesen OV et al. Serum concentrations and side effects in psychiatric patients during risperidone therapy. Ther Drug Monit 1998; **20**:380–384.

94. Remington G et al. A PET study evaluating dopamine D2 receptor occupancy for long-acting injectable risperidone. Am J Psychiatry 2006; **163**:396–401.

95. Seto K et al. Risperidone in schizophrenia: is there a role for therapeutic drug monitoring? Ther Drug Monit 2011; **33**:275–283.

96. Lane HY et al. Risperidone in acutely exacerbated schizophrenia: dosing strategies and plasma levels. J Clin Psychiatry 2000; **61**:209–214.

97. Taylor D. Risperidone long-acting injection in practice – more questions than answers? Acta Psychiatr Scand 2006; **114**:1–2.

98. Nyberg S et al. Suggested minimal effective dose of risperidone based on PET-measured D2 and 5-HT2A receptor occupancy in schizophrenic patients. Am J Psychiatry 1999; **156**:869–875.

CHAPTER 11

99. Uchida H et al. Predicting dopamine D receptor occupancy from plasma levels of antipsychotic drugs: a systematic review and pooled analysis. J Clin Psychopharmacol 2011; 31:318–325.

100. Medori R et al. Plasma antipsychotic concentration and receptor occupancy, with special focus on risperidone long-acting injectable. Eur Neuropsychopharmacol 2006; 16:233–240.

101. Gefvert O et al. Pharmacokinetics and D2 receptor occupancy of long-acting injectable risperidone (Risperdal Consta™) in patients with schizophrenia. Int J Neuropsychopharmacol 2005; 8:27–36.

102. Nyberg S et al. D2 dopamine receptor occupancy during low-dose treatment with haloperidol decanoate. Am J Psychiatry 1995; 152:173–178.

103. Moriguchi S et al. Estimated dopamine D(2) receptor occupancy and remission in schizophrenia: analysis of the CATIE data. J Clin Psychopharmacol 2013; 33:682–685.

104. Tsuboi T et al. Challenging the need for sustained blockade of dopamine D(2) receptor estimated from antipsychotic plasma levels in the maintenance treatment of schizophrenia: a single-blind, randomized, controlled study. Schizophr Res 2015; 164:149–154.

105. Takeuchi H et al. Dose reduction of risperidone and olanzapine and estimated dopamine D(2) receptor occupancy in stable patients with schizophrenia: findings from an open-label, randomized, controlled study. J Clin Psychiatry 2014; 75:1209–1214.

106. Bowskill SV et al. Risperidone and total 9-hydroxyrisperidone in relation to prescribed dose and other factors: data from a therapeutic drug monitoring service, 2002-2010. Ther Drug Monit 2012; 34:349–355.

107. Pandina GJ et al. A randomized, placebo-controlled study to assess the efficacy and safety of 3 doses of paliperidone palmitate in adults with acutely exacerbated schizophrenia. J Clin Psychopharmacol 2010; 30:235–244.

108. Berwaerts J et al. Efficacy and safety of the 3-month formulation of paliperidone palmitate vs placebo for relapse prevention of schizophrenia: a randomized clinical trial. JAMA Psychiatry 2015; 72:830–839.

CHAPTER 11

Interpreting post-mortem blood concentrations

Much is known about the distribution of drugs in the body during life but relatively little about these same parameters after death. A great many drugs are subject to post-mortem distribution changes but, for obvious practical reasons, research into the mechanisms and extent of these effects is very limited. The best that can be said is that a drug *plasma* concentration measured during life may be very different from the (usually *whole blood*) concentration measured some time after death.

A number of processes are responsible for these changes in concentrations. In life, active mechanisms serve to concentrate some drugs in certain organs or tissues. After death, passive diffusion occurs as cell membranes break down and this will mean that post-mortem blood samples will, for some drugs, show higher concentrations than were seen during life. (This is known as post-mortem redistribution (PMR) and has been described as a 'toxicological nightmare'[1] because of the number of different processes involved.) In addition, central blood vessels surrounding major organs often demonstrate much higher drug concentrations than relatively distant peripheral samples.[2] PMR and other processes are temperature- and time-dependent and so time since death and conditions of storage are important determinants of blood concentration changes.[3] Post-mortem redistribution tends to be greater with drugs with a large volume of distribution (i.e. those for which tissue concentrations in life vastly exceed blood concentrations), especially when given over a long period during life.

Other processes of importance[4] include the post-mortem synthesis of certain compounds. For example, the body is able to generate γ-hydroxybutyrate, and trauma may allow the introduction of yeasts that metabolise glucose to alcohol. Another phenomenon is the degradation of drugs by bacteria (e.g. clonazepam and nitrazepam) or fungi. Also, the metabolism of some drugs (cocaine, for example) appears to continue after death (although this may be simple chemical instability of the parent compound).

Table 11.2 lists some of the factors relevant to drug concentration changes after death and the possible consequences of these processes. Generally speaking, an isolated post-mortem blood concentration cannot be sensibly interpreted. Even where in-life levels are available, experts agree that, for most drugs in most circumstances, interpretation of blood levels after death is near impossible: high concentrations should certainly not be taken, in the absence of other evidence, to indicate death by overdose, for example. Expert advice should always be sought when considering the role of medication in a death.[20]

Table 11.2 Factors affecting post-mortem blood concentrations

Factor	Examples	Consequences
Redistribution of drug from tissues to blood compartment	Most drugs with large volume of distribution, e.g. clozapine,[5,6] olanzapine,[7] methadone,[8] SSRIs,[9] TCAs, mirtazapine,[10] lithium[11] May not occur to any significant extent with risperidone,[12] aripiprazole[13] or quetiapine[13]	Post-mortem levels up to 10 × higher than in-life levels, sometimes higher still
Uneven distribution of drugs in the blood compartment and in organs (i.e. site of blood collection affects concentration)	Most drugs,[14,15] e.g. clozapine, TCAs, SSRIs, duloxetine,[16] benzodiazepines	Concentrations may vary several-fold according to site of collection at post mortem, e.g. femoral blood versus heart blood
Decay of drugs in post-mortem tissue (usually by bacterial degradation)	Not widely studied but known to occur with olanzapine, risperidone[17] and some benzodiazepines. Fungi can metabolise amitriptyline, mirtazapine and zolpidem[18,19]	Post-mortem levels may be lower than in-life levels
Post-mortem metabolism/ degradation	Cocaine metabolised/degraded post mortem. Many other drugs are unstable in post-mortem samples Yeasts may produce ethanol following trauma[4]	Post-mortem levels may be lower (cocaine) or higher (alcohol) than in-life levels

SSRI, selective serotonin reuptake inhibitor; TCA, tricyclic antidepressant.

References

1. Pounder DJ et al. Post-mortem drug redistribution – a toxicological nightmare. Forensic Sci Int 1990; 45:253–263.
2. Ferner RE. Post-mortem clinical pharmacology. Br J Clin Pharmacol 2008; 66:430–443.
3. Flanagan RJ et al. Analytical toxicology: guidelines for sample collection postmortem. Toxicol Rev 2005; 24:63–71.
4. Kennedy MC. Post-mortem drug concentrations. Intern Med J 2010; 40:183–187.
5. Flanagan RJ et al. Effect of post-mortem changes on peripheral and central whole blood and tissue clozapine and norclozapine concentrations in the domestic pig (Sus scrofa). Forensic Sci Int 2003; 132:9–17.
6. Flanagan RJ et al. Suspected clozapine poisoning in the UK/Eire, 1992-2003. Forensic Sci Int 2005; 155:91–99.
7. Saar E et al. The time-dependant post-mortem redistribution of antipsychotic drugs. Forensic Sci Int 2012; 222:223–227.
8. Caplehorn JR et al. Methadone dose and post-mortem blood concentration. Drug Alcohol Rev 2002; 21:329–333.
9. Lewis RJ et al. Paroxetine in postmortem fluids and tissues from nine aviation accident victims. J Anal Toxicol 2015; 39:637–641.
10. Launiainen T et al. Drug concentrations in post-mortem femoral blood compared with therapeutic concentrations in plasma. Drug Test Anal 2014; 6:308–316.
11. Soderberg C et al. Reference values of lithium in postmortem femoral blood. Forensic Sci Int 2017; 277:207–214.
12. Linnet K et al. Postmortem femoral blood concentrations of risperidone. J Anal Toxicol 2014; 38:57–60.
13. Skov L et al. Postmortem femoral blood reference concentrations of aripiprazole, chlorprothixene, and quetiapine. J Anal Toxicol 2015; 39:41–44.
14. Rodda KE et al. The redistribution of selected psychiatric drugs in post-mortem cases. Forensic Sci Int 2006; 164:235–239.
15. Han E et al. Evaluation of postmortem redistribution phenomena for commonly encountered drugs. Forensic Sci Int 2012; 219:265–271.
16. Scanlon KA et al. Comprehensive duloxetine analysis in a fatal overdose. J Anal Toxicol 2016; 40:167–170.
17. Butzbach DM et al. Bacterial degradation of risperidone and paliperidone in decomposing blood. J Forensic Sci 2013; 58:90–100.
18. Martinez-Ramirez JA et al. Search for fungi-specific metabolites of four model drugs in postmortem blood as potential indicators of postmortem fungal metabolism. Forensic Sci Int 2016; 262:173–178.
19. Martinez-Ramirez JA et al. Studies on drug metabolism by fungi colonizing decomposing human cadavers. Part II: biotransformation of five model drugs by fungi isolated from post mortem material. Drug Test Anal 2015; 7:265–279.
20. Flanagan RJ. Poisoning: fact or fiction? Med Leg J 2012; 80:127–148.

CHAPTER 11

Acting on clozapine plasma concentration results

In most developed countries, clozapine plasma concentration monitoring is widely employed. Table 11.1 gives some general advice about actions that should be taken when clozapine levels fall within a certain range. The ranges shown are somewhat arbitrary and convenient – the concentration at which a particular patient might respond cannot be known without a trial of clozapine. Most adverse effects are linearly related to dose or plasma level. That is, there is no step change in risk of seizures, for example, at a particular dose or plasma concentration.[1] As a consequence, Table 11.3 should be considered more an aid to decision-making rather than a rigorous, unbending evidence-based instruction. Note also the effect of tolerance to adverse effects – many patients have a significant adverse-effect burden before therapeutic levels are reached.[2]

Table 11.3 Acting on clozapine plasma concentration results*

Plasma concentration	Response status	Tolerability status	Suggest action
<350 µg/L	Poor	Poor	Increase dose very slowly to give level of 350 µg/L
	Poor	Good	Increase dose to give level of 350 µg/L
	Good	Poor	Maintain dose. Consider dose reduction if tolerability does not improve
	Good	Good	Continue to monitor. No action required
350–500 µg/L	Poor	Poor	Increase dose slowly, according to tolerability, to give level of >500 µg/L. Consider prophylactic anticonvulsant.** If no improvement, consider augmentation
	Poor	Good	Increase dose slowly, according to tolerability, to give level of >500 µg/L. Consider prophylactic anticonvulsant.** If no improvement, consider augmentation
	Good	Poor	Maintain dose to see if tolerability improves. Consider dose reduction to give plasma level of around 350 µg/L
	Good	Good	Continue to monitor. No action required
500–1000 µg/L	Poor	Poor	Consider use of prophylactic anticonvulsant.** Consider augmentation Attempt dose reduction if augmentation successful
	Poor	Good	Consider use of prophylactic anticonvulsant.** Consider augmentation
	Good	Poor	Attempt slow dose reduction to give plasma level of 350–500 µg/L unless there is known non-response at lower level. If this is the case, maintain dose and consider adding anticonvulsant.** Optimise treatment of adverse effects
	Good	Good	Consider use of prophylactic anticonvulsant.** Maintain dose if good tolerability continues

Table 11.3 (*Continued*)

Plasma concentration	Response status	Tolerability status	Suggest action
>1000 μg/L	Poor	Poor	Add anticonvulsant. Attempt augmentation. Reduce dose to give level of <1000 μg/L Consider abandoning clozapine treatment
	Poor	Good	Add anticonvulsant. Attempt augmentation If augmentation successful, reduce dose to give level <1000 μg/L. If unsuccessful, consider abandoning clozapine treatment
	Good	Poor	Add anticonvulsant. Attempt slow dose reduction to give plasma level <1000 μg/L
	Good	Good	Add anticonvulsant. Monitor closely; attempt dose reduction only if tolerability declines

Notes

Poor response	No response or unsatisfactory response to clozapine. Not sufficiently well to be discharged
Good response	Obvious positive changes related to use of clozapine. Patient likely to be suitable for discharge to supported or unsupported care in the community
Poor tolerability	Dose constrained by adverse effects such as tachycardia, sedation, hypersalivation, hypotension (see Chapter 1 for suggestions of treatment for adverse effects)
Good tolerability	Patient tolerates treatment well and there are no signs of serious toxicity
Augmentation	Adding another antipsychotic or mood stabiliser (see Chapter 1)

- In all situations, ensure adequate treatment for clozapine-induced constipation. Constipation is dose-related. Ensure regular bowel movements and record bowel function. Stimulant laxatives such as senna often required (see Chapter 1).
- Seizures are dose- and plasma level-dependent. Suitable anticonvulsants are valproate, lamotrigine and, rarely, topiramate. Use lamotrigine if response poor; valproate if affective symptoms present (see Chapter 1). Note that use of valproate increases risk of neutropenia with clozapine.[3]

* This table applies to results for patients on a stable clozapine dose with confirmed good adherence.
** Anticonvulsants should be used in patients whose plasma level exceeds 600 μg/L, unless electroencephalogram (EEG) is normal.

References

1. Varma S et al. Clozapine-related EEG changes and seizures: dose and plasma-level relationships. Ther Adv Psychopharmacol 2011; 1:47–66.
2. Yusufi B et al. Prevalence and nature of side effects during clozapine maintenance treatment and the relationship with clozapine dose and plasma concentration. Int Clin Psychopharmacol 2007; 22:238–243.
3. Malik S et al. Sodium valproate and clozapine induced neutropenia: a case control study using register data. Schizophr Res 2017:Epub ahead of print.

Psychotropic drugs and cytochrome (CYP) function

Information on the effect of drugs on cytochrome function helps predict or confirm suspected interactions which may not have been uncovered in regulatory trials or in clinical use (sometimes called prediction from 'first principles'). Using 'first principles' essentially means understanding and interpreting pharmacokinetic information and anticipating the net effect of combining two or more drugs *in vivo*.

In addition to the effect of co-administered drugs on CYP function, genetic polymorphism associated with some enzyme pathways (e.g. 2D6, 2C9, 2C19 enzymes) may also account for inter-individual variations in metabolism of certain drugs.

The effects of polymorphism and pharmacokinetic interaction are difficult to predict because some drugs are metabolised by more than one enzyme and an alternative pathway(s) may compensate if other enzyme pathways are inhibited.

Also note that the function of CYPs is not the only consideration. P-glycoprotein (P-gp) is a drug transporter protein found in the gut wall. P-gp can eject (active process) drugs that diffuse (passive process) across the gut wall. P-gp is also found in testes and in the blood–brain barrier. Drugs that inhibit P-gp are anticipated to increase the uptake of other drugs (that are substrates for P-gp) and drugs that induce P-gp are anticipated to reduce the uptake of drugs (that are substrates for P-gp). Many drugs that are substrates for CYP3A4 have also been found to be substrates for P-gp.

UDP-glucuronosyl transferase (UGT) has been identified as an enzyme that is responsible for phase II (conjugation) reactions. Valproate is a potent inhibitor of UGT, hence its interaction with lamotrigine.

Table 11.4 summarises the interactions of psychotropic drugs with cytochromes. It does not include details of the effects of non-psychotropic drugs on CYP function.

Table 11.4 Interactions of psychotropic drugs with cytochromes

Substrates	Inhibitors	Inducers
CYP1A2		
Agomelatine	**Fluvoxamine**	**'Barbiturates'**
Amitriptyline*	Moclobemide	Carbamazepine
Asenapine	Perphenazine	Modafinil*
Bupropion*		**Phenobarbital**
Chlorpromazine		Phenytoin
Clomipramine*		
Clozapine		
Duloxetine		
Fluphenazine		
Fluvoxamine		
Imipramine*		
Melatonin		
Mirtazapine*		
Olanzapine		
Perphenazine		
?Pimozide*		
Zolpidem*		

Table 11.4 (*Continued*)

Substrates	Inhibitors	Inducers
CYP2A6		
Bupropion*	Tranylcypromine	Phenobarbital
Nicotine		
CYP2B6		
Bupropion	Fluoxetine*	Carbamazepine*
Methadone*	Fluvoxamine	Modafinil*
Nicotine	Memantine	Phenobarbital
Sertraline*	Paroxetine*	Phenytoin
	Sertraline*	
CYP2B7		
Buprenorphine*	Not known	Not known
CYP2C8		
Zopiclone*	Not known	Not known
CYP2C9		
Agomelatine*	Fluoxetine*	Carbamazepine
Amitriptyline	Fluvoxamine	St John's wort
Bupropion*	Modafinil	
Fluoxetine*	Valproate	
Lamotrigine		
Phenobarbital		
Phenytoin		
Sertraline*		
Valproic acid		
CYP2C19		
Agomelatine*	Escitalopram*	Carbamazepine
Amitriptyline	Fluvoxamine	St John's wort
Carbamazepine*	Moclobemide	
Citalopram	Modafinil	
Clomipramine*	Topiramate	
Diazepam		
Escitalopram		
Fluoxetine*		
Imipramine*		
?Melatonin		
?Methadone		
Moclobemide		
Phenytoin		
Sertraline*		
Trimipramine*		

(Continued)

Table 11.4 (*Continued*)

Substrates	Inhibitors	Inducers
CYP2D6		
Amitriptyline	**Amitriptyline**	Not known
'Amfetamines'	**Asenapine**	
Atomoxetine	**Bupropion**	
Aripiprazole	Chlorpromazine	
Brexipiprazole	Citalopram*	
Cariprazine	Clomipramine	
Chlorpromazine	Clozapine	
Citalopram	**Duloxetine**	
Clomipramine	Escitalopram	
Clozapine*	**Fluoxetine**	
Donepezil*	Fluphenazine	
Duloxetine	Fluvoxamine*	
Escitalopram	Haloperidol	
Fluoxetine	Levomepromazine	
Fluvoxamine	Methadone*	
Fluphenazine	Moclobemide	
Galantamine	**Paroxetine**	
Haloperidol	Perphenazine	
Iloperidone	Reboxetine*	
Imipramine	Risperidone	
Methadone*	Sertraline	
Mianserin	Venlafaxine*	
Mirtazapine*		
Moclobemide		
Nortriptyline		
Olanzapine		
Paroxetine		
Perphenazine		
Pimozide*		
Quetiapine*		
Risperidone		
Sertraline		
Trazodone*		
Trimipramine		
Venlafaxine		
Vortioxetine		
Zuclopenthixol		
CYP2E1		
Bupropion	**Disulfiram**	Ethanol
Ethanol	Paracetamol	

Table 11.4 (*Continued*)

Substrates	Inhibitors	Inducers
CYP3A4		
Alfentanyl	**Fluoxetine**	**Asenapine?**
Alprazolam	Fluvoxamine	**Carbamazepine**
Amitriptyline	**Paroxetine**	**Modafinil**
Aripiprazole	Perphenazine	**Phenobarbital** 'and probably other
Brexipiprazole	Reboxetine*	barbiturates'
Buprenorphine		**Phenytoin**
Bupropion*		St John's wort
Buspirone		Topiramate
Carbamazepine		
Cariprazine		
Chlorpromazine		
Citalopram		
Clomipramine*		
Clonazepam		
Clozapine*		
Diazepam		
Donepezil		
Dosulepin		
Escitalopram*		
Fentanyl		
Fluoxetine*		
?**Flurazepam**		
Galantamine		
Haloperidol		
Imipramine		
Lurasidone		
Methadone		
Midazolam		
Mirtazapine		
Modafinil		
Nitrazepam		
Perphenazine		
Pimozide		
Quetiapine		
Reboxetine		
Risperidone*		
Sertindole		
Sertraline*		
Trazodone		
Trimipramine*		
Venlafaxine		
Zaleplon		
Ziprasidone		
Zolpidem		
Zopiclone		

Drugs highlighted in **bold** indicate:
- predominant metabolic enzyme pathway or
- predominant enzyme activity (inhibition or induction).

Drugs annotated with * indicate:
- known to be a minor metabolic enzyme pathway or activity (i.e. not demonstrated to be clinically significant).

Drugs in normal font (not bold and without *) indicate:
- metabolic enzyme pathway(s) or activity where significance is unclear or unknown.

Note: Information on CYP function is derived from individual Summaries of Product Characteristics and US labelling (accessed November 2017).

Smoking and psychotropic drugs

Tobacco smoke contains polycyclic aromatic hydrocarbons that induce (increase the activity of) certain hepatic enzymes (CYP1A2 in particular).[1] The extent of enzyme induction is determined by the number and type of cigarettes smoked and the degree of smoke inhalation.[2] For some drugs used in psychiatry, smoking significantly reduces drug plasma levels and higher doses are required than in non-smokers. Smoking may also affect alcohol metabolism by inducing CYP2E1.[2]

When people stop smoking, enzyme activity reduces over a week or so. (Nicotine replacement or vaping has no effect on this process.) Plasma levels of affected drugs will then rise, sometimes substantially. Dose reduction will usually be necessary. If smoking is re-started, enzyme activity increases, plasma levels fall and dose increases are then required. The process is complicated and effects are difficult to predict. Of course, few people manage to give up smoking completely, so additional complexity is introduced by intermittent smoking and repeated attempts at stopping completely. Close monitoring of plasma levels (where useful), clinical progress and adverse effect severity is essential.

Table 11.5 gives details of psychotropic drugs known to be affected by smoking status.

Table 11.5 Psychotropic drugs affected by smoking status

Drug	Effect of smoking	Action to be taken on stopping smoking	Action to be taken on re-starting
Agomelatine[3]	Plasma levels reduced	Monitor closely Dose may need to be reduced	Consider re-introducing previous smoking dose
Benzodiazapines[2,4]	Plasma levels reduced by 0–50% (depends on drug and smoking status)	Monitor closely. Consider reducing dose by up to 25% over 1 week	Monitor closely. Consider re-starting 'normal' smoking dose
Carbamazepine[2]	Unclear, but smoking may reduce carbamazepine plasma levels to a small extent	Monitor for changes in severity of adverse effects	Monitor plasma levels
Chlorpromazine[2,4,5]	Plasma levels reduced. Varied estimates of exact effect	Monitor closely, consider dose reduction	Monitor closely, consider re-starting previous smoking dose
Clozapine[6–11]	Reduces plasma levels by up to 50% Plasma level reduction may be greater in those receiving valproate	Take plasma level before stopping. On stopping, reduce dose gradually (over 1 week) until around 75% of original dose reached (i.e. reduce by 25%). Repeat plasma level 1 week after stopping. Anticipate further dose reductions	Take plasma level before re-starting. Increase dose to previous smoking dose over 1 week. Repeat plasma level

Table 11.5 (*Continued*)

Drug	Effect of smoking	Action to be taken on stopping smoking	Action to be taken on re-starting
Duloxetine[12]	Plasma levels may be reduced by up to 50%	Monitor closely Dose may need to be reduced	Consider re-introducing previous smoking dose
Fluphenazine[13]	Reduces plasma levels by up to 50%	On stopping, reduce dose by 25%. Monitor carefully over following 4–8 weeks. Consider further dose reductions	On re-starting, increase dose to previous smoking dose
Fluvoxamine[14]	Plasma levels decreased by around a third	Monitor closely Dose may need to be reduced	Dose may need to be increased to previous level
Haloperidol[15,16]	Reduces plasma levels by around 25–50%	Reduce dose by around 25%. Monitor carefully. Consider further dose reductions	On re-starting, increase dose to previous smoking dose
Loxapine[17] (inhaled)	Half-life reduced from 15.7 h to 13.6 h	Monitor	Monitor
Mirtazapine[18]	Unclear, but effect probably minimal	Monitor	Monitor
Olanzapine[11,19–22]	Reduces plasma levels by up to 50%	Take plasma level before stopping. On stopping, reduce dose by 25%. After 1 week, repeat plasma level. Consider further dose reductions	Take plasma level before restarting. Increase dose to previous smoking dose over 1 week. Repeat plasma level
Trazodone[23]	Around 25% reduction	Monitor for increased sedation. Consider dose reduction	Monitor closely. Consider increasing dose
Tricyclic antidepressants[2,4]	Plasma levels reduced by 25–50%	Monitor closely. Consider reducing dose by 10–25% over 1 week. Consider further dose reductions	Monitor closely. Consider re-starting previous smoking dose
Zuclopentixol[24,25]	Unclear, but effect probably minimal	Monitor	Monitor

Note: Only cigarette smoking induces hepatic enzymes in the manner described above; nicotine replacement, vaping devices and electronic cigarettes (which do not contain polycyclic aromatic compounds) have no effect on enzyme activity.

References

1. Kroon LA. Drug interactions with smoking. Am J Health Syst Pharm 2007; **64**:1917–1921.
2. Desai HD et al. Smoking in patients receiving psychotropic medications: a pharmacokinetic perspective. CNS Drugs 2001; **15**:469–494.
3. Servier Laboratories Limited. Summary of Product Characteristics. Valdoxan (Agomelatine). 2016. https://www.medicines.org.uk/emc/medicine/21830.
4. Miller LG. Recent developments in the study of the effects of cigarette smoking on clinical pharmacokinetics and clinical pharmacodynamics. Clin Pharmacokinet 1989; **17**:90–108.
5. Goff DC et al. Cigarette smoking in schizophrenia: relationship to psychopathology and medication side effects. Am J Psychiatry 1992; **149**:1189–1194.
6. Haring C et al. Influence of patient-related variables on clozapine plasma levels. Am J Psychiatry 1990; **147**:1471–1475.
7. Haring C et al. Dose-related plasma levels of clozapine: influence of smoking behaviour, sex and age. Psychopharmacology (Berl) 1989; **99** Suppl:S38–S40.
8. Diaz FJ et al. Estimating the size of the effects of co-medications on plasma clozapine concentrations using a model that controls for clozapine doses and confounding variables. Pharmacopsychiatry 2008; **41**:81–91.
9. Murayama-Sung L et al. The impact of hospital smoking ban on clozapine and norclozapine levels. J Clin Psychopharmacol 2011; **31**:124–126.
10. Cormac I et al. A retrospective evaluation of the impact of total smoking cessation on psychiatric inpatients taking clozapine. Acta Psychiatr Scand 2010; **121**:393–397.
11. Tsuda Y et al. Meta-analysis: the effects of smoking on the disposition of two commonly used antipsychotic agents, olanzapine and clozapine. BMJ Open 2014; **4**:e004216.
12. Fric M et al. The influence of smoking on the serum level of duloxetine. Pharmacopsychiatry 2008; **41**:151–155.
13. Ereshefsky L et al. Effects of smoking on fluphenazine clearance in psychiatric inpatients. Biol Psychiatry 1985; **20**:329–332.
14. Spigset O et al. Effect of cigarette smoking on fluvoxamine pharmacokinetics in humans. Clin Pharmacol Ther 1995; **58**:399–403.
15. Jann MW et al. Effects of smoking on haloperidol and reduced haloperidol plasma concentrations and haloperidol clearance. Psychopharmacology (Berl) 1986; **90**:468–470.
16. Shimoda K et al. Lower plasma levels of haloperidol in smoking than in nonsmoking schizophrenic patients. Ther Drug Monit 1999; **21**:293–296.
17. Takahashi LH et al. Effect of smoking on the pharmacokinetics of inhaled loxapine. Ther Drug Monit 2014; **36**:618–623.
18. Grasmader K et al. Population pharmacokinetic analysis of mirtazapine. Eur J Clin Pharmacol 2004; **60**:473–480.
19. Carrillo JA et al. Role of the smoking-induced cytochrome P450 (CYP)1A2 and polymorphic CYP2D6 in steady-state concentration of olanzapine. J Clin Psychopharmacol 2003; **23**:119–127.
20. Gex-Fabry M et al. Therapeutic drug monitoring of olanzapine: the combined effect of age, gender, smoking, and comedication. Ther Drug Monit 2003; **25**:46–53.
21. Bigos KL et al. Sex, race, and smoking impact olanzapine exposure. J Clin Pharmacol 2008; **48**:157–165.
22. Lowe EJ et al. Impact of tobacco smoking cessation on stable clozapine or olanzapine treatment. Ann Pharmacother 2010; **44**:727–732.
23. Ishida M et al. Effects of various factors on steady state plasma concentrations of trazodone and its active metabolite m-chlorophenylpiperazine. Int Clin Psychopharmacol 1995; **10**:143–146.
24. Jann MW et al. Clinical pharmacokinetics of the depot antipsychotics. Clin Pharmacokinet 1985; **10**:315–333.
25. Jorgensen A et al. Zuclopenthixol decanoate in schizophrenia: serum levels and clinical state. Psychopharmacology (Berl) 1985; **87**:364–367.

Drug interactions with alcohol

Drug interactions with alcohol are complex. Many patient-related and drug-related factors need to be considered. It can be difficult to predict outcomes accurately because a number of processes may occur simultaneously or consecutively.

Pharmacokinetic interactions[1-4]

Alcohol (ethanol) is absorbed from the gastrointestinal tract and distributed in body water. The volume of distribution is smaller in women and the elderly where plasma levels of alcohol will be higher for a given 'dose' of alcohol than in young males. Approximately 10% of ingested alcohol is subjected to first pass metabolism by alcohol dehydrogenase (ADH). A small proportion of alcohol is metabolised by ADH in the stomach. The remainder is metabolised in the liver by ADH and CYP2E1. Women have less capacity to metabolise via ADH than men. CYP2E1 plays a minor role in occasional drinkers but is an important and inducible metabolic route in chronic, heavy drinkers. CYP1A2, CYP3A4 and many other CYP enzymes also play a minor role.[5,6]

CYP2E1 and ADH convert alcohol to acetaldehyde which is both the toxic substance responsible for the unpleasant symptoms of the 'Antabuse reaction' (e.g. flushing, headache, nausea, malaise), and the compound implicated in hepatic damage. It may also have psychotropic effects – ethanol is metabolised to acetaldehyde by CYP2E1 in the brain.[7] The enzyme catalase is also known to metabolise alcohol to acetaldehyde in the brain and elsewhere.[8] Acetaldehyde is further metabolised by aldehyde dehydrogenase to acetic acid and then to carbon dioxide and water.

All of the enzymes involved in the metabolism of alcohol exhibit genetic polymorphism. For example, the majority of people of north Asian origin are poor metabolisers via aldehyde dehydrogenase.[9] Chronic consumption of alcohol induces CYP2E1 and CYP3A4. The effects of alcohol on other hepatic metabolising enzymes have been poorly studied.

Metabolism of alcohol

The metabolism of alcohol is summarised in Figure 11.1.

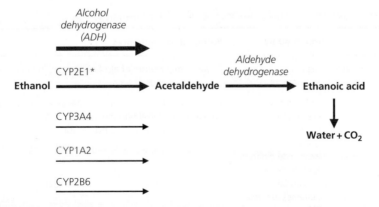

Figure 11.1 Metabolism of alcohol. *Minor route in occasional drinkers, major route in misusers and at higher blood alcohol concentration. The ubiquitous enzyme catalase is also able to metabolise ethanol but its overall contribution is not known.

Interactions are difficult to predict in alcohol misusers because two opposing processes may be at work: competition for enzymatic sites during periods of intoxication (increasing drug plasma levels) and enzyme induction prevailing during periods of sobriety (reducing drug plasma levels[8]). See Tables 11.6 and 11.7. In chronic drinkers, particularly those who binge drink, serum levels of prescribed drugs may reach toxic

Table 11.6 Co-administration of alcohol and substrates for CYP2E1 and CYP3A4

	Substrates for enzyme (note: this is not an exhaustive list)	Effects in an intoxicated patient	Effects in a chronic, sober drinker
CYP2E1	Paracetamol Isoniazid Phenobarbitone Warfarin Zopiclone	Competition between alcohol and drug leading to reduced rates of metabolism of both compounds. Increased plasma levels may lead to toxicity	Activity of CYP2E1 is increased up to 10-fold Increased metabolism of drugs potentially leading to therapeutic failure
CYP3A4	Aripiprazole Benzodiazepines Carbamazepine Clozapine Donepezil Galantamine Haloperidol Methadone Mirtazapine Quetiapine Risperidone Sildenafil Tricyclics Valproate Venlafaxine Z-hypnotics	Competition between alcohol and drug leading to reduced rates of metabolism of both compounds. Increased plasma levels may lead to toxicity	Increased rate of drug metabolism potentially leading to therapeutic failure Enzyme induction can last for several weeks after alcohol consumption ceases

Table 11.7 Drugs that inhibit alcohol dehydrogenase and aldehyde dehydrogenase

Enzyme	Inhibited by	Potential consequences
Alcohol dehydrogenase	Aspirin H$_2$ antagonists	Reduced metabolism of alcohol resulting in higher plasma levels for longer periods of time
Aldehyde dehydrogenase	Chlorpropamide Disulfiram Griseofulvin Isoniazid Isosorbide dinitrate Metronidazole Nitrofurantoin Sulfamethoxazole Tolbutamide	Reduced ability to metabolise acetaldehyde leading to 'Antabuse' type reaction: facial flushing, headache, tachycardia, nausea and vomiting, arrhythmias and hypotension

levels during periods of intoxication with alcohol and then be sub-therapeutic when the patient is sober. This makes it very difficult to optimise treatment of physical or mental illness.

Interactions of uncertain aetiology include increased blood alcohol concentrations in people who take verapamil and decreased metabolism of methylphenidate in people who consume alcohol.

Pharmacodynamic interactions[2–4]

Alcohol enhances inhibitory neurotransmission at γ-aminobutyric acid (GABA$_A$) receptors and reduces excitatory neurotransmission at glutamate N-methyl-D-aspartate (NMDA) receptors. It also increases dopamine release in the mesolimbic pathway and may have some effects on serotonin and opiate pathways. Given these actions, alcohol would be expected to cause sedation, amnesia and ataxia and give rise to feelings of pleasure (and/or worsen psychotic symptoms in vulnerable individuals) (Table 11.8).

Alcohol can cause or worsen psychotic symptoms by increasing dopamine release in mesolimbic pathways. The effect of antipsychotic drugs may be competitively antagonised, rendering them less effective.

Table 11.8 Pharmacodynamic interactions with alcohol

Effect of alcohol	Effect exacerbated by	Potential consequences
Sedation	Other sedative drugs, e.g.: Antihistamines Antipsychotics Baclofen Benzodiazepines Lofexidine Opiates Tizanidine Tricyclics Z-hypnotics	Increased CNS depression ranging from increased propensity to be involved in accidents through to respiratory depression and death
Amnesia	Other amnesic drugs, e.g.: Barbiturates Benzodiazepines Z-hypnotics	Increased amnesic effects ranging from mild memory loss to total amnesia
Ataxia	ACE inhibitors Beta blockers Calcium channel blockers Nitrates Adrenergic alpha receptor antagonists, e.g. Clozapine Risperidone Tricyclics	Increased unsteadiness and falls

ACE, angiotensin-converting enzyme; CNS, central nervous system.

Electrolyte disturbances secondary to alcohol-related dehydration can be exacerbated by other drugs that cause electrolyte disturbances such as diuretics.

Note that heavy alcohol consumption can lead to hypoglycaemia in people with diabetes who take insulin or oral hypoglycaemics. Theoretically there is an increased risk of lactic acidosis in patients who take metformin with alcohol. Alcohol can also increase blood pressure.

Chronic drinkers are particularly susceptible to the gastrointestinal irritant effects of aspirin and non-steroidal anti-inflammatory drugs (NSAIDs).

Note: In the presence of pharmacokinetic interactions, pharmacodynamic interactions will be more marked. For example, in a chronic heavy drinker who is sober, enzyme induction will increase the metabolism of diazepam which may lead to increased levels of anxiety (treatment failure). If the same patient becomes intoxicated with alcohol, the metabolism of diazepam will be greatly reduced as it will have to compete with alcohol for the metabolic capacity of CYP3A4. Plasma levels of alcohol and diazepam will rise (toxicity). As both alcohol and diazepam are sedative (via $GABA_A$ affinity), loss of consciousness and respiratory depression may occur.

Note: Be aware of the possibility of hepatic failure or reduced hepatic function in chronic alcohol misusers. See section on 'Hepatic impairment' in Chapter 8. Also note the risk of hepatic toxicity with some recommended drugs (e.g. valproate). Table 11.9 lists psychotropic drugs that can be used in patients who continue to drink.

Table 11.9 Psychotropic drugs: choice in patients who continue to drink

	Safest choice	Best avoided
Antipsychotics	**Sulpiride** and **amisulpride** **Paliperidone,** if depot required (non-sedative and renally excreted)	**Very sedative antipsychotics** such as chlorpromazine and clozapine
Antidepressants	**SSRI – citalopram, sertraline** Potent inhibitors of CYP3A4 (fluoxetine, paroxetine) may decrease alcohol metabolism in chronic drinkers	**TCAs,** because impairment of metabolism by alcohol (while intoxicated) can lead to increased plasma levels and consequent signs and symptoms of overdose (profound hypotension, seizures, arrhythmias and coma) Cardiac effects can be exacerbated by electrolyte disturbances Combinations of TCAs and alcohol profoundly impair psychomotor skills **MAOIs** can cause profound hypotension. Also potential interaction with tyramine-containing drinks which can lead to hypertensive crisis
Mood stabilisers	**Valproate** **Carbamazepine** Note: higher plasma levels achieved during periods of alcohol intoxication may be poorly tolerated	**Lithium,** because it has a narrow therapeutic index and alcohol-related dehydration and electrolyte disturbance can precipitate lithium toxicity

MAOI, monoamine oxidase inhibitor; SSRI, selective serotonin reuptake inhibitor; TCA, tricyclic antidepressant.

References

1. Zakhari S. Overview: how is alcohol metabolized by the body? Alcohol Res Health 2006; **29**:245–254.
2. Tanaka E. Toxicological interactions involving psychiatric drugs and alcohol: an update. J Clin Pharm Ther 2003; **28**:81–95.
3. Wan Chih T. Alcohol-related drug interactions. Pharmacist's Letter/Prescriber's Letter 2008; **24**:240106.
4. Smith RG. An appraisal of potential drug interactions in cigarette smokers and alcohol drinkers. J Am Podiatr Med Assoc 2009; **99**:81–88.
5. Salmela KS et al. Respective roles of human cytochrome P-4502E1, 1A2, and 3A4 in the hepatic microsomal ethanol oxidizing system. Alcohol Clin Exp Res 1998; **22**:2125–2132.
6. Hamitouche S et al. Ethanol oxidation into acetaldehyde by 16 recombinant human cytochrome P450 isoforms: role of CYP2C isoforms in human liver microsomes. Toxicol Lett 2006; **167**:221–230.
7. Koster M et al. Seizures during antidepressant treatment in psychiatric inpatients – results from the transnational pharmacovigilance project "Arzneimittelsicherheit in der Psychiatrie" (AMSP) 1993-2008. Psychopharmacology (Berl) 2013; **230**:191–201.
8. Cederbaum AI. Alcohol metabolism. Clin Liver Dis 2012; **16**:667–685.
9. Wall TL et al. Biology, genetics, and environment: underlying factors influencing alcohol metabolism. Alcohol Res 2016; **38**:59–68.

References

Chapter 12

Other substances

Caffeine

Caffeine is probably the most popular psychoactive substance in the world. Mean daily consumption in the UK is 350–620 mg.[1] A quarter of the general population and half of those with psychiatric illness regularly consume over 500 mg caffeine/day.[2] Consumption of caffeine should be routinely discussed with an individual to assess its effect on their symptoms and presentation.[3] In particular, caffeine withdrawal can have a marked effect on mental and physical health. See Table 12.1 for the caffeine content of various drinks.

Chocolate also contains caffeine. Martindale lists over 600 medicines that contain caffeine.[4] Most are available without prescription and are marketed as analgesics or appetite suppressants.

Table 12.1 Caffeine content of drinks

Drink	Caffeine content
Brewed coffee	100 mg/cup
Red Bull	80 mg/can (other energy drinks may contain substantially more)
Instant coffee	60 mg/cup
Black tea	45 mg/cup
Green tea	20–30 mg/cup
Soft drinks	25–50 mg/can

The Maudsley Prescribing Guidelines in Psychiatry, Thirteenth Edition. David M. Taylor, Thomas R. E. Barnes and Allan H. Young.
© 2018 David M. Taylor. Published 2018 by John Wiley & Sons Ltd.

Table 12.2 Psychotropic effects of caffeine

Dose	Psychotropic effect
Generally	Central nervous system stimulation Increased catecholamine release, particularly dopamine[7]
Low to moderate dose[2,8]	Elation Impulsivity Peacefulness
Large doses >600 mg/day[9] (Sensitive (non-tolerant) individuals may experience effects at lower doses; tolerance develops in long-term users)	Anxiety Insomnia Psychomotor agitation Excitement Rambling speech Delirium Psychosis

General effects of caffeine

- Acute use can increase systolic and diastolic blood pressure (BP) by up to 10 mmHg for up to 4 hours.[3] Chronic moderate use probably has little effect on BP.[5]
- May enhance reinforcing effects of nicotine and possibly other drugs of misuse.[4,6]
- Caffeine has *de novo* psychotropic effects (Table 12.2), may worsen existing psychiatric illness, and may interact with psychotropic drugs.
- Caffeine is an antagonist at adenosine A_1 and A_{2A} receptors, thus stimulating dopamine pathways.

An established withdrawal syndrome exists. Symptoms include: headache, depressed mood, anxiety, fatigue, irritability, nausea, dysphoria and craving.[10]

Pharmacokinetics

- **Absorption**
  - Rapid after oral administration, especially in liquid form.
  - Half-life of 2.5–4.5 hours.
- **Metabolism**
  - Metabolised by CYP1A2, a hepatic cytochrome enzyme that exhibits genetic polymorphism, which may partially account for the large inter-individual differences that are seen in the ability to tolerate caffeine.[11] Note that CYP1A2 is induced by smoking and inhibited by a number of drugs such as fluvoxamine.
  - Metabolic pathways also become saturated at higher doses.[12]
- **Interactions** (Table 12.3)
  - The potential effects of caffeine on the metabolism of other drugs, as well as the potential to induce a caffeine withdrawal syndrome, should always be considered before substituting caffeine-free drinks.
  - Caffeine competitively inhibits CYP1A2. Plasma levels of some drugs may be reduced if caffeine is withdrawn.

Table 12.3 Interactions of caffeine

Interacting substance	Effect	Comment

CYP1A2 inhibitors:
  Oestrogens
  Cimetidine
  Fluvoxamine (may decrease caffeine clearance by 80%)[13]
  Disulfiram
	Reduce caffeine clearance	Effects of caffeine may be prolonged or increased
		Adverse effects may be increased
		May precipitate caffeine toxicity

Cigarette smoke	CYP1A2 inducer – increasing caffeine metabolism[7]	Smokers may require higher doses of caffeine to gain desired effects[7]
Lithium	High doses of caffeine may reduce lithium levels	Caffeine withdrawal may cause a lithium level rise[14]
MAOIs	May enhance stimulant CNS effects	
Clozapine	Caffeine may increase clozapine plasma concentrations by up to 60%[15]	Thought to be via competitive inhibition of CYP1A2. Other drugs affected by caffeine-induced inhibition of the enzyme include olanzapine, imipramine and clomipramine
SSRIs	Large doses of caffeine may increase risk of serotonin syndrome[16]	
Benzodiazepines	Caffeine may act as an antagonist	Reduces the efficacy of benzodiazepines[9]

CNS, central nervous system; MAOI, monoamine oxidase inhibitor; SSRI, selective serotonin reuptake inhibitor.

Caffeine intoxication

The *Diagnostic and Statistical Manual of Mental Disorders* DSM-V[17] defines caffeine intoxication as the recent consumption of caffeine, usually in excess of 250 mg, accompanied by five or more of the symptoms listed in Box 12.1.

In caffeine intoxication, these symptoms cause significant distress or impairment in social, occupational or other important areas of functioning and are not due to a general medical condition or better accounted for by another mental disorder (e.g. an anxiety disorder).

Caffeine abuse or dependence as a clinical syndrome has been reported[3] and caffeine use disorder and caffeine withdrawal are both DSM-V diagnoses.

Box 12.1 Symptoms of caffeine intoxication

- Restlessness
- Nervousness
- Excitement
- Insomnia
- Flushed face
- Diuresis

- Gastrointestinal disturbance
- Muscle twitching
- Rambling flow of thought and speech
- Tachycardia or cardiac arrhythmia
- Periods of inexhaustibility
- Psychomotor agitation

Energy drinks

So-called 'energy drinks' contain large amounts of caffeine along with sugar, vitamins and a number of other ingredients such as guarana and taurine. There is some evidence that these drinks can improve attention and short-term memory.[18] Marketing is targeted at adolescents and young adults, some of whom consume large volumes of these drinks and seem to be particularly vulnerable to developing signs and symptoms of caffeine intoxication. Symptoms of anxiety and depression, frank suicidal behaviour and seizures have been associated with use of these products by young people.[19–21] When combined with alcohol, aggressive behaviour may result.[22]

Schizophrenia

- Patients with schizophrenia often consume large amounts of caffeine-containing drinks[1] and they are twice as likely as controls to consume >200 mg caffeine/day.[7]
- Caffeine-containing drinks may be used to relieve dry mouth (as an adverse effect of antipsychotic drugs), for the stimulant effects of caffeine (to relieve dysphoria/sedation/negative symptoms)[7] or simply because coffee/tea drinking structures the day or relieves boredom.
- Schizophrenia may increase sensitivity to drug-related cues.[7]
- Large doses of caffeine can worsen psychotic symptoms[7,23] (in particular elation and conceptual disorganisation) and result in the prescription of larger doses of antipsychotic drugs.
- The removal of caffeine from the diets of chronically disturbed (challenging behaviour) patients may ultimately lead to decreased levels of hostility, irritability and suspiciousness[24] and may be of benefit in clozapine-resistant schizophrenia,[25] although this may not hold true in less disturbed populations.[26]

Mood disorders

- Caffeine may elevate mood through increasing noradrenaline release[27] and modest caffeine consumption may protect against depression in those who do not have a pre-existing mood disorder.[28,29]
- People with mood disorders are more likely to consume caffeine, particularly when depressed.[14,30]
- Depressed patients may be more sensitive to the anxiogenic effects of caffeine.[31,32]
- Excessive consumption of caffeine may precipitate mania.[32–34]
- Caffeine can increase cortisol secretion (gives a false positive in the dexamethasone-suppression test),[35] increase seizure length during electroconvulsive therapy[36] and increase the clearance of lithium by promoting diuresis.[37]

Anxiety disorders

- Caffeine increases vigilance, decreases reaction times, increases sleep latency and worsens subjective estimates of sleep quality – effects that may be more marked in poor metabolisers.

- Caffeine may precipitate or worsen generalised anxiety and panic attacks;[38] vulnerability to these effects may be genetically determined.[6]
- Effects are so marked that caffeine intoxication should always be considered when patients complain of anxiety symptoms or insomnia.
- Symptoms may diminish considerably or even abate completely if caffeine is avoided.[39]

Other disorders

Weak evidence supports the benefit of caffeine in ADHD[40] and that high caffeine consumption may protect against late-life cognitive decline.[41]

Summary

Caffeine:

- Is present in high quantities in coffee and some soft drinks, particularly energy drinks.
- May worsen psychosis and anxiety. Young people may be particularly vulnerable.
- Can increase plasma clozapine levels.
- May induce intoxication which is characterised by psychomotor agitation and rambling speech.
- May be associated with toxicity when co-administered with CYP1A2 inhibitors such as fluvoxamine.
- Can enhance the reinforcing effects of nicotine and possibly other drugs of abuse.

References

1. Rihs M et al. Caffeine consumption in hospitalized psychiatric patients. Eur Arch Psychiatry Clin Neurosci 1996; **246**:83–92.
2. Clementz GL et al. Psychotropic effects of caffeine. Am Fam Physician 1988; **37**:167–172.
3. Ogawa N et al. Clinical importance of caffeine dependence and abuse. Psychiatry Clin Neurosci 2007; **61**:263–268.
4. Pharmaceutical Press. Martindale: The Complete Drug Reference (online). 2017. https://www.medicinescomplete.com/.
5. O'Keefe JH et al. Effects of habitual coffee consumption on cardiometabolic disease, cardiovascular health, and all-cause mortality. J Am Coll Cardiol 2013; **62**:1043–1051.
6. Bergin JE et al. Common psychiatric disorders and caffeine use, tolerance, and withdrawal: an examination of shared genetic and environmental effects. Twin Res Hum Genet 2012; **15**:473–482.
7. Adolfo AB et al. Effects of smoking cues on caffeine urges in heavy smokers and caffeine consumers with and without schizophrenia. Schizophr Res 2009; **107**:192–197.
8. Grant JE et al. Caffeine's influence on gambling behavior and other types of impulsivity. Addict Behav 2018; **76**:156–160.
9. Sawynok J. Pharmacological rationale for the clinical use of caffeine. Drugs 1995; **49**:37–50.
10. Silverman K et al. Withdrawal syndrome after the double-blind cessation of caffeine consumption. N Engl J Med 1992; **327**:1109–1114.
11. Butler MA et al. Determination of CYP1A2 and NAT2 phenotypes in human populations by analysis of caffeine urinary metabolites. Pharmacogenetics 1992; **2**:116–127.
12. Kaplan GB et al. Dose-dependent pharmacokinetics and psychomotor effects of caffeine in humans. J Clin Pharmacol 1997; **37**:693–703.
13. Medicines Complete. Stockley's Drug Interactions. 2017. https://www.medicinescomplete.com/.
14. Baethge C et al. Coffee and cigarette use: association with suicidal acts in 352 Sardinian bipolar disorder patients. Bipolar Disord 2009; **11**:494–503.
15. Carrillo JA et al. Effects of caffeine withdrawal from the diet on the metabolism of clozapine in schizophrenic patients. J Clin Psychopharmacol 1998; **18**:311–316.
16. Shioda K et al. Possible serotonin syndrome arising from an interaction between caffeine and serotonergic antidepressants. Hum Psychopharmacol 2004; **19**:353–354.
17. American Psychiatric Association. *Diagnostic and Statistical Manual of Mental Disorders*, 5th edn (DSM-5). Arlington, VA: American Psychiatric Association; 2013.
18. Wesnes KA et al. An evaluation of the cognitive and mood effects of an energy shot over a 6h period in volunteers: a randomized, double-blind, placebo controlled, cross-over study. Appetite 2013; **67**:105–113.

19. Szpak A et al. A case of acute suicidality following excessive caffeine intake. J Psychopharmacol 2012; **26**:1502–1510.

20. Trapp GS et al. Energy drink consumption among young Australian adults: associations with alcohol and illicit drug use. Drug Alcohol Depend 2014; **134**:30–37.

21. Pennington N et al. Energy drinks: a new health hazard for adolescents. J Sch Nurs 2010; **26**:352–359.

22. Sheehan BE et al. Caffeinated and non-caffeinated alcohol use and indirect aggression: the impact of self-regulation. Addict Behav 2016; **58**:53–59.

23. Wang HR et al. Caffeine-induced psychiatric manifestations: a review. Int Clin Psychopharmacol 2015; **30**:179–182.

24. De Freitas B et al. Effects of caffeine in chronic psychiatric patients. Am J Psychiatry 1979; **136**:1337–1338.

25. Dratcu L et al. Clozapine-resistant psychosis, smoking, and caffeine: managing the neglected effects of substances that our patients consume every day. Am J Ther 2007; **14**:314–318.

26. Koczapski A et al. Effects of caffeine on behavior of schizophrenic inpatients. Schizophr Bull 1989; **15**:339–344.

27. Achor MB et al. Diet aids, mania, and affective illness. Am J Psychiatry 1981; **138**:392.

28. Lucas M et al. Coffee, caffeine, and risk of depression among women. Arch Intern Med 2011; **171**:1571–1578.

29. Wang L et al. Coffee and caffeine consumption and depression: a meta-analysis of observational studies. Aust N Z J Psychiatry 2016; **50**:228–242.

30. Maremmani I et al. Are "social drugs" (tobacco, coffee and chocolate) related to the bipolar spectrum? J Affect Disord 2011; **133**:227–233.

31. Lee MA et al. Anxiogenic effects of caffeine on panic and depressed patients. Am J Psychiatry 1988; **145**:632–635.

32. Rizkallah E et al. Could the use of energy drinks induce manic or depressive relapse among abstinent substance use disorder patients with comorbid bipolar spectrum disorder? Bipolar Disord 2011; **13**:578–580.

33. Machado-Vieira R et al. Mania associated with an energy drink: the possible role of caffeine, taurine, and inositol. Can J Psychiatry 2001; **46**:454–455.

34. Ogawa N et al. Secondary mania caused by caffeine. Gen Hosp Psychiatry 2003; **25**:138–139.

35. Uhde TW et al. Caffeine-induced escape from dexamethasone suppression. Arch Gen Psychiatry 1985; **42**:737–738.

36. Cantu TG et al. Caffeine in electroconvulsive therapy. Ann Pharmacother 1991; **25**:1079–1080.

37. Mester R et al. Caffeine withdrawal increases lithium blood levels. Biol Psychiatry 1995; **37**:348–350.

38. Bruce MS. The anxiogenic effects of caffeine. Postgrad Med J 1990; **66** Suppl 2:S18–S24.

39. Bruce MS et al. Caffeine abstention in the management of anxiety disorders. Psychol Med 1989; **19**:211–214.

40. Ioannidis K et al. Ostracising caffeine from the pharmacological arsenal for attention-deficit hyperactivity disorder – was this a correct decision? A literature review. J Psychopharmacol 2014; **28**:830–836.

41. Panza F et al. Coffee, tea, and caffeine consumption and prevention of late-life cognitive decline and dementia: a systematic review. J Nutr Health Aging 2015; **19**:313–328.

Nicotine

The most common method of consuming nicotine is by smoking cigarettes. One-quarter of the general population, 40–50% of those with depression[1] and 70–80% of those with schizophrenia smoke.[2] Nicotine causes peripheral vasoconstriction, tachycardia and increased blood pressure.[3] Smokers are at increased risk of developing cardiovascular disease. People with schizophrenia who smoke are more likely to develop metabolic syndrome, compared with those who do not smoke.[4] As well as nicotine, cigarettes also contain tar (a complex mixture of organic molecules, many carcinogenic), a cause of cancers of the respiratory tract, chronic bronchitis and emphysema.[5] Electronic cigarettes, it is claimed, contain only nicotine (alongside some necessary excipients), which has very limited toxicity and is not thought to be carcinogenic. Vaping is thus preferred for all smokers, albeit with some reservations in regard to quality control of content and the so-called 're-normalisation' of smoking.

Nicotine is highly addictive; an effect which may be at least partially genetically determined.[6] People with mental illness are 2–3 times more likely than the general population to develop and maintain a nicotine addiction.[1] Chronic smoking contributes to the increased morbidity and mortality from respiratory and cardiovascular disease that is seen in this patient group. Nicotine also has psychotropic effects. Smoking can affect the metabolism (and therefore the efficacy and toxicity) of drugs prescribed to treat psychiatric illness,[7] see section on 'Smoking and psychotropic drugs' in Chapter 11. Nicotine use may be a gateway drug to experimenting with other psychoactive substances.

Psychotropic effects

Nicotine is highly lipid-soluble and rapidly enters the brain after inhalation. Nicotine receptors are found on dopaminergic cell bodies and stimulation of these receptors leads to dopamine release.[1] Dopamine release in the limbic system is associated with pleasure: dopamine is the brain's 'reward' neurotransmitter. Nicotine may be used by people with mental health problems as a form of 'self-medication' (e.g. to alleviate the negative symptoms of schizophrenia or antipsychotic-induced dysphoria or for its anxiolytic effect[8]). Drugs that increase the release of dopamine reduce the craving for nicotine. They may also worsen psychotic illness (see Chapter 4).

Nicotine improves concentration and vigilance.[1] It also enhances the effects of glutamate, acetylcholine and serotonin.[8]

Schizophrenia

Seventy to eighty per cent of people with schizophrenia regularly smoke cigarettes[2] (with increasing numbers switching to vaping[9]) and this increased tendency to smoke predates the onset of psychiatric symptoms.[10] Possible explanations are as follows: smoking causes dopamine release, leading to feelings of well-being and a reduction in negative symptoms;[8] to alleviate some of the adverse effects of antipsychotics such as drowsiness and extrapyramidal symptoms (EPS)[1] and cognitive slowing;[11,12] as a means of structuring the day (a behavioural filler); a familial vulnerability;[13] or as a means of alleviating the deficit in auditory gating that is found in schizophrenia.[14] Nicotine may also improve working memory and attentional deficits.[15-17] Nicotinic receptor agonists may have beneficial effects on neurocognition,[18,19] although none is yet licensed for this purpose. Note, though, that cholinergic drugs may exacerbate nicotine dependence.[20] A single-photon emission computed tomography (SPECT) study has shown that the greater the occupancy of striatal D_2 receptors by antipsychotic drugs, the more likely the patient is to smoke.[21] This may partly explain the clinical observation that smoking cessation may be more achievable when clozapine (a weak dopamine antagonist) is prescribed in place of a conventional antipsychotic. It has been suggested that people with schizophrenia find it particularly difficult to tolerate nicotine withdrawal symptoms.[7] Switching to nicotine replacement therapy or vaping may thus be a preferred option.[22]

Depression and anxiety

In 'normal' individuals a moderate consumption of nicotine is associated with pleasure and a decrease in anxiety and feelings of anger.[23] The mechanism of this anxiolytic effect is not understood. People who suffer from anxiety and/or depression are more likely to smoke[24,25] and find it more difficult to stop.[23,26] This is compounded by the observation that nicotine withdrawal can precipitate or exacerbate depression in those with a history of the illness,[23] and cigarette smoking may directly increase the risk of symptoms of depression.[27] In marked contrast, recent studies suggest that stopping smoking actually improves depression and anxiety.[28,29] These contradictory findings might be explained by the fact that early withdrawal worsens depression whereas successful cessation improves depression in the longer term. A Cochrane review[30] suggested that smoking cessation is achievable in depressed smokers.

Patients with depression are at increased risk of cardiovascular disease. By directly causing tachycardia and hypertension,[3] nicotine may, in theory, exacerbate this problem. More importantly, smoking is a well-known independent risk factor for cardiovascular disease, probably because it hastens atherosclerosis. Vaping, while not carcinogenic, probably does increase risk of cardiovascular disease.[31]

Movement disorders and Parkinson's disease

By increasing dopaminergic neurotransmission, nicotine provides a protective effect against both drug-induced EPS and idiopathic Parkinson's disease. Smokers are less likely to suffer from antipsychotic-induced movement disorders than non-smokers[1] and use anticholinergics less often.[7] Parkinson's disease occurs less frequently in smokers than in non-smokers and the onset of clinical symptoms is delayed.[1,32] This may reflect the inverse association between Parkinson's disease and sensation-seeking behavioural traits, rather than a direct effect of nicotine.[33]

Drug interactions

Polycyclic hydrocarbons in cigarette smoke are known to stimulate the hepatic microsomal enzyme system, particularly P4501A2,[8] the enzyme responsible for the metabolism of many psychotropic drugs. Smoking can lower the blood levels of some drugs by up to 50%.[8] This can affect both efficacy and adverse effects and needs to be taken into account when making clinical decisions. The drugs most likely to be affected are: clozapine,[34] fluphenazine, haloperidol, chlorpromazine, olanzapine, many tricyclic antidepressants, mirtazapine, fluvoxamine and propranolol. Vaping has no effect on hepatic enzyme function. See section on 'Smoking and psychotropic drugs' in Chapter 11.

Withdrawal symptoms

Withdrawal symptoms[7] occur within 6–12 hours of stopping smoking and include intense craving, depressed mood, insomnia, anxiety, restlessness, irritability, difficulty in concentrating and increased appetite. Nicotine withdrawal can be confused with depression, anxiety, sleep disorders and mania. Withdrawal can also exacerbate the symptoms of schizophrenia.

Smoking cessation

See section on 'Nicotine and smoking cessation' in Chapter 4.

References

1. Goff DC et al. Cigarette smoking in schizophrenia: relationship to psychopathology and medication side effects. Am J Psychiatry 1992; **149**:1189–1194.
2. Winterer G. Why do patients with schizophrenia smoke? Curr Opin Psychiatry 2010; **23**:112–119.
3. Benowitz NL et al. Cardiovascular effects of nasal and transdermal nicotine and cigarette smoking. Hypertension 2002; **39**:1107–1112.
4. Yevtushenko OO et al. Influence of 5-HT2C receptor and leptin gene polymorphisms, smoking and drug treatment on metabolic disturbances in patients with schizophrenia. Br J Psychiatry 2008; **192**:424–428.
5. Anderson JE et al. Treating tobacco use and dependence: an evidence-based clinical practice guideline for tobacco cessation. Chest 2002; **121**:932–941.
6. Berrettini W. Nicotine addiction. Am J Psychiatry 2008; **165**:1089–1092.
7. Ziedonis DM et al. Schizophrenia and nicotine use: report of a pilot smoking cessation program and review of neurobiological and clinical issues. Schizophr Bull 1997; **23**:247–254.
8. Lyon ER. A review of the effects of nicotine on schizophrenia and antipsychotic medications. Psychiatr Serv 1999; **50**:1346–1350.
9. Sharma R et al. Motivations and limitations associated with vaping among people with mental illness: a qualitative analysis of Reddit discussions. Int J Environ Res Public Health 2017; **14**:7.
10. Weiser M et al. Higher rates of cigarette smoking in male adolescents before the onset of schizophrenia: a historical-prospective cohort study. Am J Psychiatry 2004; **161**:1219–1223.
11. Harris JG et al. Effects of nicotine on cognitive deficits in schizophrenia. Neuropsychopharmacology 2004; **29**:1378–1385.
12. Gupta T et al. Nicotine usage is associated with elevated processing speed, spatial working memory, and visual learning performance in youth at ultrahigh-risk for psychosis. Psychiatry Res 2014; **220**:687–690.
13. Ferchiou A et al. Exploring the relationships between tobacco smoking and schizophrenia in first-degree relatives. Psychiatry Res 2012; **200**:674–678.
14. McEvoy JP et al. Smoking and therapeutic response to clozapine in patients with schizophrenia. Biol Psychiatry 1999; **46**:125–129.
15. Jacobsen LK et al. Nicotine effects on brain function and functional connectivity in schizophrenia. Biol Psychiatry 2004; **55**:850–858.
16. Sacco KA et al. Effects of cigarette smoking on spatial working memory and attentional deficits in schizophrenia: involvement of nicotinic receptor mechanisms. Arch Gen Psychiatry 2005; **62**:649–659.
17. Smith RC et al. Effects of nicotine nasal spray on cognitive function in schizophrenia. Neuropsychopharmacology 2006; **31**:637–643.
18. Olincy A et al. Proof-of-concept trial of an alpha7 nicotinic agonist in schizophrenia. Arch Gen Psychiatry 2006; **63**:630–638.
19. Lieberman JA et al. Cholinergic agonists as novel treatments for schizophrenia: the promise of rational drug development for psychiatry. Am J Psychiatry 2008; **165**:931–936.
20. Kelly DL et al. Lack of beneficial galantamine effect for smoking behavior: a double-blind randomized trial in people with schizophrenia. Schizophr Res 2008; **103**:161–168.
21. de Haan L et al. Occupancy of dopamine D2 receptors by antipsychotic drugs is related to nicotine addiction in young patients with schizophrenia. Psychopharmacology (Berl) 2006; **183**:500–505.
22. Caponnetto P et al. Impact of an electronic cigarette on smoking reduction and cessation in schizophrenic smokers: a prospective 12-month pilot study. Int J Environ Res Public Health 2013; **10**:446–461.

CHAPTER 12

23. Glassman AH. Cigarette smoking: implications for psychiatric illness. Am J Psychiatry 1993; 150:546–553.

24. Nunes SO et al. The shared role of oxidative stress and inflammation in major depressive disorder and nicotine dependence. Neurosci Biobehav Rev 2013; 37:1336–1345.

25. Tsuang MT et al. Genetics of smoking and depression. Hum Genet 2012; 131:905–915.

26. Wilhelm K et al. Clinical aspects of nicotine dependence and depression. Med Today 2004; 5:40–47.

27. Boden JM et al. Cigarette smoking and depression: tests of causal linkages using a longitudinal birth cohort. Br J Psychiatry 2010; 196:440–446.

28. Taylor G et al. Change in mental health after smoking cessation: systematic review and meta-analysis. BMJ 2014; 348:g1151.

29. Almadana Pacheco V et al. Anxiety, depression and tobacco abstinence. Adicciones 2017; 29:233–244.

30. van der Meer RM et al. Smoking cessation interventions for smokers with current or past depression. Cochrane Database Syst Rev 2013; 8:CD006102.

31. Schweitzer RJ et al. E-cigarette use and indicators of cardiovascular disease risk. Current Epidemiology Reports 2017; 4:248–257.

32. Scott WK et al. Family-based case-control study of cigarette smoking and Parkinson disease. Neurology 2005; 64:442–447.

33. Evans AH et al. Relationship between impulsive sensation seeking traits, smoking, alcohol and caffeine intake, and Parkinson's disease. J Neurol Neurosurg Psychiatry 2006; 77:317–321.

34. Derenne JL et al. Clozapine toxicity associated with smoking cessation: case report. Am J Ther 2005; 12:469–471.

Chapter 13

Psychotropic drugs in special conditions

Psychotropic drugs in overdose

Suicide attempts and suicidal gestures are frequently encountered in psychiatric and general practice, and psychotropic drugs are often taken in overdose. Table 13.1 gives brief details of the toxicity in overdose of commonly used psychotropic drugs. It is intended to help guide drug choice in those thought to be at risk of suicide and to help identify symptoms of overdose. This section gives no information on the treatment of psychotropic overdose and readers are directed to specialist poisons units. In all cases of suspected overdose, urgent referral to acute medical facilities is, of course, strongly advised.

Table 13.1 Psychotropic drugs in overdose

Drug or drug group	Toxicity in overdose	Smallest dose likely to cause death	Signs and symptoms of overdose
Antidepressants			
Agomelatine[1,2]	Low	No deaths reported	Sedation, agitation, stomach pains
		In early trials, 800 mg was maximum tolerated dose. EU SPC reports no serious effects from 2.45 g overdose	
Bupropion[3–6]	Moderate	Around 4.5 g, although largest overdose of 13.5 g was not fatal[7]	Tachycardia, seizures, QRS prolongation, QT prolongation, arrhythmia

(Continued)

The Maudsley Prescribing Guidelines in Psychiatry, Thirteenth Edition. David M. Taylor, Thomas R. E. Barnes and Allan H. Young.
© 2018 David M. Taylor. Published 2018 by John Wiley & Sons Ltd.

Table 13.1 (*Continued*)

Drug or drug group	Toxicity in overdose	Smallest dose likely to cause death	Signs and symptoms of overdose
Duloxetine[8–11]	Low	Unclear – no deaths from single overdose reported but involved in numerous mixed overdose deaths	Drowsiness, bradycardia, hypotension. May be asymptomatic
Lofepramine[12–14]	Low	Unclear. Fatality unlikely if lofepramine taken alone	Sedation, coma, tachycardia, hypotension
MAOIs (not moclobemide)[12,15–17]	High	Phenelzine: 400 mg Tranylcypromine: 200 mg	Tremor, weakness, confusion, sweating, tachycardia, hypertension
Mianserin[18–20]	Low	Unclear but probably more than 1000 mg Fatality unlikely if mianserin taken alone	Sedation, coma, hypotension, hypertension, tachycardia, possible QT prolongation
Mirtazapine[3,21–23]	Low	Fatality unlikely in overdose of mirtazapine alone. One death reported (following overdose with 990 mg[24])	Sedation; even large overdose may be asymptomatic. Tachycardia/hypertension sometimes seen. Agitation
Moclobemide[25,26]	Low	Unclear, but probably more than 8 g Fatality unlikely if moclobemide taken alone	Vomiting, sedation, disorientation
Reboxetine[3,27]	Low	Not known Fatality unlikely in overdose of reboxetine alone	Sweating, tachycardia, changes in blood pressure
SSRIs[13,14,28–30]	Low	Unclear. Probably above 1–2 g Fatality unlikely if SSRI taken alone	Vomiting, tremor, drowsiness, tachycardia, ST depression. Seizures and QT prolongation possible. Citalopram most toxic of SSRIs in overdose[31] (coma, seizures, arrhythmia); escitalopram is less toxic[32,33]
Trazodone[9,34–37]	Low	Unclear but probably more than 10 g Fatality unlikely in overdose of trazodone alone	Drowsiness, nausea, hypotension, dizziness. Rarely QT prolongation, arrhythmia
Tricyclics[12,15,16,38,39] (not lofepramine)	High	Around 500 mg Doses over 50 mg/kg usually fatal	Sedation, coma, tachycardia, arrhythmia (QRS, QT prolongation), hypotension, seizures
Venlafaxine[3,40–42] (desvenlafaxine* causes similar effects but may be less toxic[43])	Moderate	Probably above 5 g, but seizures may occur after ingestion of 1 g	Vomiting, sedation, tachycardia, hypertension, seizures, acidosis. Rarely QT prolongation, arrhythmia, rhabdomyolysis. Very rarely cardiac arrest/MI, heart failure
Vilazodone*[44,45]	Probably low	Doses below 300 mg are not fatal	Drowsiness, agitation, vomiting, seizures

Table 13.1 (Continued)

Drug or drug group	Toxicity in overdose	Smallest dose likely to cause death	Signs and symptoms of overdose
Vortioxetine[46]	Low	Unclear	Nausea, somnolence, diarrhoea, pruritus
Antipsychotics			
Amisulpride[47–49]	Moderate	Around 16 g	QT prolongation, arrhythmia, cardiac arrest
Aripiprazole[50–52]	Low	Unclear Fatality unlikely when taken alone	Sedation, lethargy, GI disturbance, drooling
Asenapine[53]	Probably low	Unclear. No deaths from overdose reported	Sedation, confusion, facial dystonia, benign ECG changes
Butyrophenones,[54–56] e.g. haloperidol	Moderate	Haloperidol – probably above 500 mg Arrhythmia may occur at 300 mg	Sedation, coma, dystonia, NMS, QT prolongation, arrhythmia
Clozapine[57,58]	Moderate	Around 2 g; much lower in those not tolerant[59]	Lethargy, coma, tachycardia, hypotension, hypersalivation, pneumonia, seizures
Iloperidone[60–62]	Probably moderate	Unclear but probably more than 500 mg	Potent effect on QT interval. Sedation, tachycardia, respiratory depression, hypotension likely
Lurasidone[63]	Probably low	Unclear. An overdose of 1360 mg was not fatal[64]	Very limited information. Minimal effect on QT interval
Olanzapine[57,65–67]	Moderate	Unclear. Probably substantially more than 200 mg	Lethargy, confusion, myoclonus, myopathy, hypotension, tachycardia, delirium. Possibly QT prolongation
Phenothiazines,[54,68–70] e.g. chlorpromazine, fluphenazine	Moderate	Chlorpromazine 5–10 g	Sedation, coma, tachycardia, arrhythmia, pulmonary oedema, hypotension, QT prolongation, seizures, dystonia, NMS
Quetiapine[57,71–76]	Moderate	Unclear. Probably more than 5 g. Fatalities rare in single substance overdose	Lethargy, delirium, tachycardia, QT prolongation, respiratory depression, hypotension, rhabdomyolysis, NMS
Risperidone[57,77,78] (assume same for paliperidone)	Low	Unclear Fatality rare in those taking risperidone alone	Lethargy, dystonia, tachycardia, changes in blood pressure, QT prolongation. Renal failure with paliperidone
Ziprasidone[79–84]	Low	Around 10 g. Fatality unlikely when taken alone	Drowsiness, lethargy. QT prolongation, torsades de pointes
Mood stabilisers			
Carbamazepine[85,86]	Moderate	Around 20 g, but seizures may occur at around 5 g	Somnolence, coma, respiratory depression, ataxia, seizures, tachycardia, arrhythmia, electrolyte disturbance

(Continued)

CHAPTER 13

Table 13.1 (*Continued*)

Drug or drug group	Toxicity in overdose	Smallest dose likely to cause death	Signs and symptoms of overdose
Lamotrigine[87]	Low	At least 4 g Two deaths reported – one after 4 g, the other after 7.5 g, but overdoses of >40 g have not proved fatal	Drowsiness, vomiting, ataxia, seizures, tachycardia, dyskinesia, QT prolongation
Lithium[88–91]	Low (acute overdose)	Acute overdose does not normally result in fatality. Insidious, chronic toxicity is more dangerous	Nausea, diarrhoea, tremor, confusion, weakness, lethargy, seizures, coma, cardiovascular collapse, bradycardia, arrhythmia, heart block
Valproate[92–96]	Moderate	Unclear but probably more than 20 g. Doses over 400 mg/kg cause severe toxicity	Somnolence, coma, cerebral oedema, respiratory depression, blood dyscrasia, hypotension, hypothermia, seizures, electrolyte disturbance (hyperammonaemia)
Others			
Benzodiazepines[97,98]	Low	Probably more than 100 mg diazepam equivalents Fatality unusual if taken alone Alprazolam is most toxic	Drowsiness, ataxia, nystagmus, respiratory dysarthria, depression, coma
Methadone[99,100]	High	20–50 mg may be fatal in non-users. Co-ingestion of benzodiazepines increases toxicity	Drowsiness, nausea, hypotension, respiratory depression, coma, rhabdomyolysis
Modafinil[101,102]	Low	Unclear Overdoses of >6 g have not caused death	Tachycardia, insomnia, agitation, anxiety, nausea, hypertension, dystonia
Pregabalin[103,104]	Low	No deaths reported One overdose of 8.4 g caused unconsciousness and coma	May be asymptomatic. Sedation and coma may occur
Zolpidem[105,106]	Low	Unclear. Probably >200 mg Fatality rare in those taking zolpidem alone	Drowsiness, agitation, respiratory depression, tachycardia, coma
Zopiclone[97,107,108]	Low	Unclear. Probably >100 mg Fatality rare in those taking zopiclone alone	Ataxia, nausea, diplopia, drowsiness, coma

*Not licensed in UK or EU.

ECG, electrocardiogram; GI, gastrointestinal; MAOI, monoamine oxidase inhibitor; MI, myocardial infarction; NMS, neuroleptic malignant syndrome; SPC, summary of product characteristics; SSRI, selective serotonin reuptake inhibitor.

High = less than 1 week's supply likely to cause serious toxicity or death.
Moderate = 1–4 weeks' supply likely to cause serious toxicity or death.
Low = death or serious toxicity unlikely even if more than 1 month's supply taken.

References

1. Howland RH. Critical appraisal and update on the clinical utility of agomelatine, a melatonergic agonist, for the treatment of major depressive disease in adults. Neuropsychiatr Dis Treat 2009; 5:563–576.
2. Servier Laboratories Limited. Summary of Product Characteristics. Valdoxan (Agomelatine). 2016. https://www.medicines.org.uk/emc/medicine/21830.
3. Buckley NA et al. 'Atypical' antidepressants in overdose: clinical considerations with respect to safety. Drug Saf 2003; 26:539–551.
4. Paris PA et al. ECG conduction delays associated with massive bupropion overdose. J Toxicol Clin Toxicol 1998; 36:595–598.
5. Curry SC et al. Intraventricular conduction delay after bupropion overdose. J Emerg Med 2005; 29:299–305.
6. Mercerolle M et al. A fatal case of bupropion (Zyban) overdose. J Anal Toxicol 2008; 32:192–196.
7. Zhu Y et al. Atypical findings in massive bupropion overdose: a case report and discussion of psychopharmacologic issues. J Psychiatr Pract 2016; 22:405–409.
8. Menchetti M et al. Non-fatal overdose of duloxetine in combination with other antidepressants and benzodiazepines. World J Biol Psychiatry 2009; 10(4 Pt 2):385–389.
9. White N et al. Suicidal antidepressant overdoses: a comparative analysis by antidepressant type. J Med Toxicol 2008; 4:238–250.
10. Darracq MA et al. A retrospective review of isolated duloxetine-exposure cases. Clin Toxicol (Phila) 2013; 51:106–110.
11. Scanlon KA et al. Comprehensive duloxetine analysis in a fatal overdose. J Anal Toxicol 2016; 40:167–170.
12. Cassidy S et al. Fatal toxicity of antidepressant drugs in overdose. Br Med J 1987; 295:1021–1024.
13. Henry JA et al. Relative mortality from overdose of antidepressants. BMJ 1995; 310:221–224.
14. Cheeta S et al. Antidepressant-related deaths and antidepressant prescriptions in England and Wales, 1998-2000. Br J Psychiatry 2004; 184:41–47.
15. Crome P. Antidepressant overdosage. Drugs 1982; 23:431–461.
16. Henry JA. Epidemiology and relative toxicity of antidepressant drugs in overdose. Drug Saf 1997; 16:374–390.
17. Waring WS et al. Acute myocarditis after massive phenelzine overdose. Eur J Clin Pharmacol 2007; 63:1007–1009.
18. Chand S et al. One hundred cases of acute intoxication with mianserin hydrochloride. Pharmacopsychiatry 1981; 14:15–17.
19. Scherer D et al. Inhibition of cardiac hERG potassium channels by tetracyclic antidepressant mianserin. Naunyn Schmiedebergs Arch Pharmacol 2008; 378:73–83.
20. Koseoglu Z et al. Bradycardia and hypotension in mianserin intoxication. Hum Exp Toxicol 2010; 29:887–888.
21. Bremner JD et al. Safety of mirtazapine in overdose. J Clin Psychiatry 1998; 59:233–235.
22. LoVecchio F et al. Outcomes after isolated mirtazapine (Remeron) supratherapeutic ingestions. J Emerg Med 2008; 34:77–78.
23. Berling I et al. Mirtazapine overdose is unlikely to cause major toxicity. Clin Toxicol (Phila) 2014; 52:20–24.
24. Vignali C et al. Mirtazapine fatal poisoning. Forensic Sci Int 2017; 276:e8–e12.
25. Hetzel W. Safety of moclobemide taken in overdose for attempted suicide. Psychopharmacology (Berl) 1992; 106 Suppl:S127–S129.
26. Myrenfors PG et al. Moclobemide overdose. J Intern Med 1993; 233:113–115.
27. Baldwin DS et al. Tolerability and safety of reboxetine. Rev Contemp Pharmacother 2000; 11:321–330.
28. Barbey JT et al. SSRI safety in overdose. J Clin Psychiatry 1998; 59 Suppl 15:42–48.
29. Jimmink A et al. Clinical toxicology of citalopram after acute intoxication with the sole drug or in combination with other drugs: overview of 26 cases. Ther Drug Monit 2008; 30:365–371.
30. Tarabar AF et al. Citalopram overdose: late presentation of torsades de pointes (TdP) with cardiac arrest. J Med Toxicol 2008; 4:101–105.
31. Kraai EP et al. Citalopram overdose: a fatal case. J Med Toxicol 2015; 11:232–236.
32. Yilmaz Z et al. Escitalopram causes fewer seizures in human overdose than citalopram. Clin Toxicol (Phila) 2010; 48:207–212.
33. van GF et al. Clinical and ECG effects of escitalopram overdose. Ann Emerg Med 2009; 54:404–408.
34. Gamble DE et al. Trazodone overdose: four years of experience from voluntary reports. J Clin Psychiatry 1986; 47:544–546.
35. Martinez MA et al. Investigation of a fatality due to trazodone poisoning: case report and literature review. J Anal Toxicol 2005; 29:262–268.
36. Dattilo PB et al. Prolonged QT associated with an overdose of trazodone. J Clin Psychiatry 2007; 68:1309–1310.
37. Service JA et al. QT Prolongation and delayed atrioventricular conduction caused by acute ingestion of trazodone. Clin Toxicol (Phila) 2008; 46:71–73.
38. Power BM et al. Antidepressant toxicity and the need for identification and concentration monitoring in overdose. Clin Pharmacokinet 1995; 29:154–171.
39. Caksen H et al. Acute amitriptyline intoxication: an analysis of 44 children. Hum Exp Toxicol 2006; 25:107–110.
40. Howell C et al. Cardiovascular toxicity due to venlafaxine poisoning in adults: a review of 235 consecutive cases. Br J Clin Pharmacol 2007; 64:192–197.
41. Hojer J et al. Fatal cardiotoxicity induced by venlafaxine overdosage. Clin Toxicol (Phila) 2008; 46:336–337.
42. Taylor D. Venlafaxine and cardiovascular toxicity. BMJ 2010; 340:327.
43. Cooper JM et al. Desvenlafaxine overdose and the occurrence of serotonin toxicity, seizures and cardiovascular effects. Clin Toxicol (Phila) 2017; 55:18–24.
44. Russell JL et al. Pediatric ingestion of vilazodone compared to other selective serotonin reuptake inhibitor medications. Clin Toxicol (Phila) 2017; 55:352–356.
45. Allergan USA I. Highlights of Prescribing Information: VIIBRYD (vilazodone hydrochloride) tablets. 2017. https://www.allergan.com/assets/pdf/viibryd_pi.

CHAPTER 13

46. Lundbeck Limited. Summary of Product Characteristics. Brintellix (vortioxetine) tablets 5, 10 and 20mg. 2017. https://www.medicines.org.uk/emc/medicine/30904.

47. Isbister GK et al. Amisulpride deliberate self-poisoning causing severe cardiac toxicity including QT prolongation and torsades de pointes. Med J Aust 2006; 184:354–356.

48. Ward DI. Two cases of amisulpride overdose: a cause for prolonged QT syndrome. Emerg Med Australas 2005; 17:274–276.

49. Isbister GK et al. Amisulpride overdose is frequently associated with QT prolongation and torsades de pointes. J Clin Psychopharmacol 2010; 30:391–395.

50. Lofton AL et al. Atypical experience: a case series of pediatric aripiprazole exposures. Clin Toxicol (Phila) 2005; 43:151–153.

51. Carstairs SD et al. Overdose of aripiprazole, a new type of antipsychotic. J Emerg Med 2005; 28:311–313.

52. Forrester MB. Aripiprazole exposures reported to Texas poison control centers during 2002-2004. J Toxicol Environ Health A 2006; 69:1719–1726.

53. Taylor JE et al. A case of intentional asenapine overdose. Prim Care Companion CNS Disord 2013; 15.

54. Haddad PM et al. Antipsychotic-related QTc prolongation, torsade de pointes and sudden death. Drugs 2002; 62:1649–1671.

55. Levine BS et al. Two fatalities involving haloperidol. J Anal Toxicol 1991; 15:282–284.

56. Henderson RA et al. Life-threatening ventricular arrhythmia (torsades de pointes) after haloperidol overdose. Hum Exp Toxicol 1991; 10:59–62.

57. Trenton A et al. Fatalities associated with therapeutic use and overdose of atypical antipsychotics. CNS Drugs 2003; 17:307–324.

58. Flanagan RJ et al. Suspected clozapine poisoning in the UK/Eire, 1992-2003. Forensic Sci Int 2005; 155:91–99.

59. Shigeev SV et al. [Clozapine intoxication: theoretical aspects and forensic-medical examination]. Sud Med Ekspert 2013; 56:41–46.

60. Vigneault P et al. Iloperidone (Fanapt®), a novel atypical antipsychotic, is a potent HERG blocker and delays cardiac ventricular repolarization at clinically relevant concentration. Pharmacol Res 2012; 66:60–65.

61. Vanda Pharmaceuticals Inc. Highlights of Prescribing Information: FANAPT® (iloperidone) tablets. 2016. https://www.fanapt.com/product/pi/pdf/fanapt.pdf.

62. Amon J et al. A case of iloperidone overdose in a 27-year-old man with cocaine abuse. SAGE Open Med Case Rep 2016; 4:2050313x16660485.

63. Sunovion Pharmaceuticals Europe Ltd. Latuda 18.5mg, 37mg and 74mg film-coated tablets. 2016. https://www.medicines.org.uk/emc/medicine/29125.

64. Molnar GP et al. Acute lurasidone overdose. J Clin Psychopharmacol 2014; 34:768–770.

65. Chue P et al. A review of olanzapine-associated toxicity and fatality in overdose. J Psychiatry Neurosci 2003; 28:253–261.

66. Waring WS et al. Olanzapine overdose is associated with acute muscle toxicity. Hum Exp Toxicol 2006; 25:735–740.

67. Morissette P et al. Olanzapine prolongs cardiac repolarization by blocking the rapid component of the delayed rectifier potassium current. J Psychopharmacol 2007; 21:735–741.

68. Buckley NA et al. Cardiotoxicity more common in thioridazine overdose than with other neuroleptics. J Toxicol Clin Toxicol 1995; 33:199–204.

69. Li C et al. Acute pulmonary edema induced by overdosage of phenothiazines. Chest 1992; 101:102–104.

70. Flanagan RJ. Fatal toxicity of drugs used in psychiatry. Hum Psychopharmacol 2008; 23 Suppl 1:43–51.

71. Langman LJ et al. Fatal overdoses associated with quetiapine. J Anal Toxicol 2004; 28:520–525.

72. Hunfeld NG et al. Quetiapine in overdosage: a clinical and pharmacokinetic analysis of 14 cases. Ther Drug Monit 2006; 28:185–189.

73. Strachan PM et al. Mental status change, myoclonus, electrocardiographic changes, and acute respiratory distress syndrome induced by quetiapine overdose. Pharmacotherapy 2006; 26:578–582.

74. Ngo A et al. Acute quetiapine overdose in adults: a 5-year retrospective case series. Ann Emerg Med 2008; 52:541–547.

75. Khan KH et al. Neuroleptic malignant syndrome induced by quetiapine overdose. Br J Hosp Med 2008; 69:171.

76. Alexander J. Delirium as a symptom of quetiapine poisoning. Aust N Z J Psychiatry 2009; 43:781.

77. Liang CS et al. Acute renal failure after paliperidone overdose: a case report. J Clin Psychopharmacol 2012; 32:128.

78. Lapid MI et al. Acute dystonia associated with paliperidone overdose. Psychosomatics 2011; 52:291–294.

79. Gomez-Criado MS et al. Ziprasidone overdose: cases recorded in the database of Pfizer-Spain and literature review. Pharmacotherapy 2005; 25:1660–1665.

80. Arbuck DM. 12,800-mg ziprasidone overdose without significant ECG changes. Gen Hosp Psychiatry 2005; 27:222–223.

81. Insa Gomez FJ et al. Ziprasidone overdose: cardiac safety. Actas Esp Psiquiatr 2005; 33:398–400.

82. Klein-Schwartz W et al. Prospective observational multi-poison center study of ziprasidone exposures. Clin Toxicol (Phila) 2007; 45:782–786.

83. Tan HH et al. A systematic review of cardiovascular effects after atypical antipsychotic medication overdose. Am J Emerg Med 2009; 27:607–616.

84. Alipour A et al. Torsade de pointes after ziprasidone overdose with coingestants. J Clin Psychopharmacol 2010; 30:76–77.

85. Spiller HA. Management of carbamazepine overdose. Pediatr Emerg Care 2001; 17:452–456.

86. Schmidt S et al. Signs and symptoms of carbamazepine overdose. J Neurol 1995; 242:169–173.

87. Alabi A et al. Safety profile of lamotrigine in overdose. Ther Adv Psychopharmacol 2016; 6:369–381.

88. Tuohy K et al. Acute lithium intoxication. Dial Transplant 2003; 32:478–481.

89. Chen KP et al. Implication of serum concentration monitoring in patients with lithium intoxication. Psychiatry Clin Neurosci 2004; 58:25–29.

90. Serinken M et al. Rarely seen cardiotoxicity of lithium overdose: complete heart block. Int J Cardiol 2009; 132:276–278.

91. Offerman SR et al. Hospitalized lithium overdose cases reported to the California Poison Control System. Clin Toxicol (Phila) 2010; 48:443–448.

92. Isbister GK et al. Valproate overdose: a comparative cohort study of self poisonings. Br J Clin Pharmacol 2003; 55:398–404.

93. Spiller HA et al. Multicenter case series of valproic acid ingestion: serum concentrations and toxicity. J Toxicol Clin Toxicol 2000; 38:755–760.

94. Sztajnkrycer MD. Valproic acid toxicity: overview and management. J Toxicol Clin Toxicol 2002; 40:789–801.

95. Eyer F et al. Acute valproate poisoning: pharmacokinetics, alteration in fatty acid metabolism, and changes during therapy. J Clin Psychopharmacol 2005; 25:376–380.

96. Robinson P et al. Severe hypothermia in association with sodium valproate overdose. N Z Med J 2005; 118:U1681.

97. Reith DM et al. Comparison of the fatal toxicity index of zopiclone with benzodiazepines. J Toxicol Clin Toxicol 2003; 41:975–980.

98. Isbister GK et al. Alprazolam is relatively more toxic than other benzodiazepines in overdose. Br J Clin Pharmacol 2004; 58:88–95.

99. Gable RS. Comparison of acute lethal toxicity of commonly abused psychoactive substances. Addiction 2004; 99:686–696.

100. Caplehorn JR et al. Fatal methadone toxicity: signs and circumstances, and the role of benzodiazepines. Aust N Z J Public Health 2002; 26:358–362.

101. Spiller HA et al. Toxicity from modafinil ingestion. Clin Toxicol (Phila) 2009; 47:153–156.

102. Carstairs SD et al. A retrospective review of supratherapeutic modafinil exposures. J Med Toxicol 2010; 6:307–310.

103. Miljevic C et al. A case of pregabalin intoxication. Psychiatriki 2012; 23:162–165.

104. Wood DM et al. Significant pregabalin toxicity managed with supportive care alone. J Med Toxicol 2010; 6:435–437.

105. Gock SB et al. Acute zolpidem overdose – report of two cases. J Anal Toxicol 1999; 23:559–562.

106. Garnier R et al. Acute zolpidem poisoning – analysis of 344 cases. J Toxicol Clin Toxicol 1994; 32:391–404.

107. Pounder D et al. Zopiclone poisoning. J Anal Toxicol 1996; 20:273–274.

108. Bramness JG et al. Fatal overdose of zopiclone in an elderly woman with bronchogenic carcinoma. J Forensic Sci 2001; 46:1247–1249.

CHAPTER 13

Driving and psychotropic drugs

Everyone has a duty to drive reasonably and all drivers are legally responsible for accidents they cause.[1] In the UK, the driver is responsible for ensuring that they are not unfit to drive through drink or drugs.

Many factors have been shown to affect driving performance. These include age, gender, personality, physical and mental state and being under the influence of alcohol, prescribed medicines, street drugs or over-the-counter medicines.[2,3] Studying the effects of any of these factors in isolation is extremely difficult. Some studies have attempted to categorise medicinal drugs according to how they affect driving performance.[4] Some studies have assessed the effect of medication on tests such as response time and attention,[5] but these tests do not directly measure ability or inability to drive.

It has been estimated that up to 10% of people killed or injured in road traffic accidents (RTAs) are taking psychotropic medication.[5] See Table 13.2. Patients with personality disorders and alcoholism have the highest rates of motoring offences and are more likely to be involved in accidents.[5] People whose driving ability may be impaired through their illness or prescribed medication should inform their insurance company. Failure to do so is considered to be 'withholding a material fact' and may render the insurance policy void.

Effects of mental illness

In the UK, severe mental disorder is a prescribed disability for the purposes of the Road Traffic Act 1988.[24] Regulations define mental disorder as including mental illness, arrested or incomplete development of the mind, psychopathic disorder or severe impairment of intelligence or social functioning. The licence restrictions that apply to each disorder can be found at https://www.gov.uk/government/publications/assessing-fitness-to-drive-a-guide-for-medical-professionals. Note also that licence restrictions may also apply to people with diabetes, particularly if treated with insulin or if there are established micro- or macro-vascular complications.

Many people with early dementia are capable of driving safely.[25,26] In the UK, all drivers with new diagnoses of Alzheimer's disease and other dementias must notify the Driver and Vehicle Licensing Agency (DVLA).[25] The doctor may need to make an immediate decision on safety to drive and ensure that the licensing agency is notified.[27] There are no data to support ongoing driving assessments as a way of maintaining driving ability or improving road safety of drivers with dementia.[28]

Psychiatric medicines, driving and UK law

Drug-driving law gives the threshold blood concentration for eight drugs associated with illicit use (zero tolerance approach – threshold set to reveal any recent use) and eight medicinal drugs.[29] For the latter group, Table 13.3 gives the legal limit and expected plasma concentrations in clinical use.

In regards to methadone, doses of up to 80 mg a day generally give plasma levels below the legal limit.[39]

Table 13.2 Psychotropic drugs and driving

Drug	Effect
Alcohol	Alcohol causes sedation and impaired coordination, vision, attention and information processing. Alcohol-dependent drivers are twice as likely to be involved in traffic accidents and offences than licensed drivers as a whole,[5] and a third of all fatal RTAs involve alcohol-dependent drivers.[5] Young drivers who use alcohol in combination with illicit drugs are particularly high risk[6,7]
Anticonvulsants	Initial, dose-related adverse effects may affect driving ability (e.g. blurred vision, ataxia and sedation). There are strict rules regarding epilepsy and driving. Lamotrigine may have limited effects on driving ability[8]
Antidepressants	People who are prescribed an antidepressant have an increased risk of being involved in a RTA, particularly at treatment initiation. SSRIs may have some advantages over TCAs but driving ability is still diminished compared with healthy individuals,[9] suggesting that depression itself may make a major contribution.[10,11] Initiation effects caused by mirtazapine diminish to an extent when it is given as a single dose at night but many people experience substantial hangover which can impair driving.[12] Trazodone appears to impair driving ability.[13] Agomelatine and venlafaxine may actually improve driving performance[14]
Antipsychotics	Sedation and EPS can impair coordination and response time.[2] A high proportion of patients treated with antipsychotics may have an impaired ability to drive.[15,16] One study found that patients with schizophrenia taking atypical antipsychotics or clozapine performed better in tests of skills related to car-driving ability than patients with schizophrenia taking first-generation antipsychotics[17]
Hypnotics and anxiolytics	Benzodiazepines cause sedation and impaired attention, information processing, memory and motor coordination, and along with opiates are the medicines most frequently implicated in RTAs.[18,19] When used as anxiolytics and hypnotics, benzodiazepines, zopiclone and zolpidem are associated with an increased risk of RTAs.[18] There is some gender variation in the pharmacokinetics of zolpidem with females having higher drug plasma concentrations than males for any given dose; the driving ability of females may therefore be particularly impaired.[3] Zaleplon and the newer hypnotics acting at melatonin or serotonin receptors have not been found to have any negative residual effects on driving ability[20]
Lithium	Lithium may impair visual adaptation to the dark[2] but the implications for driving safety are unknown. Many patients treated with lithium can be shown to be unfit to drive,[8] although the exact contribution of lithium is difficult to determine. Elderly people who take lithium may be at increased risk of being involved in an injurious motor vehicle crash[21]
Methylphenidate	Some studies have demonstrated that reaction time is longer in patients with ADHD, which may in turn be associated with increased driving risks.[22] Other studies have found that methylphenidate improved driving performance in adults with ADHD,[23] again suggesting that illness may make a bigger contribution to fitness to drive than the specific pharmacology of the treatment[23]

ADHD, attention deficit hyperactivity disorder; EPS, extrapyramidal symptoms; RTA, road traffic accident; SSRI, selective serotonin reuptake inhibitor; TCA, tricyclic antidepressant.

Other medicines

Many psychotropic drugs can impair alertness, concentration and driving performance. Medicines that block H_1, α_1-adrenergic or cholinergic receptors may be particularly problematic. Effects are particularly marked at the start of treatment and after

CHAPTER 13

Table 13.3 Benzodiazepines concentration in normal dosing and the legal limit

Drug/daily dose	Range of concentrations reported (legal limit)
Clonazepam 0.5–6.0 mg[30,31]	5–80 µg/L (50)
Diazepam 5–30 mg[32]	50–1000 µg/L (550)
Flunitrazepam 0.5–2.0 mg[33,34]	10–20 µg/L (300)
Lorazepam 1–4 mg[35,36]	10–70 µg/L (100)
Oxazepam 15–30 mg[37]	250–600 µg/L (300)
Temazepam 10–20 mg[38]	200–900 µg/L (1000)

increasing the dose. Drivers must be made aware of any potential for impairment and are advised to evaluate their driving performance at these times. They must stop driving if adversely affected.[40] The use of alcohol will further increase any impairment.

Many antipsychotics and antidepressants lower the seizure threshold. In the UK, the DVLA advises that this be taken into consideration when prescribing for a driver. Further information about the effects of psychotropic drugs on driving can be found in Table 13.2.

Medication-induced sedation

Many psychotropic drugs are sedating. The more sedating a medicine is, the more likely it is to impair driving ability. Other medicines, either prescribed or bought over the counter, may also be sedative and/or affect driving ability (e.g. antihistamines[5]). One study found that 89% of patients taking other psychotropic drugs in addition to antidepressants failed a battery of 'fitness to drive' tests.[41] Since the degree of sedation any individual will experience is very difficult to predict, patients prescribed sedating medicines should be advised not to drive if they feel sedated.

DVLA – duty of the driver

It is the legal responsibility of the licence holder or applicant to notify the DVLA of any medical condition which may affect safe driving. A list of relevant medical conditions can be found in the DVLA guidance 'Assessing fitness to drive: a guide for medical professionals'.[25] Drivers must recognise signs of impaired driving performance due to medication or illness.

DVLA – duty of the prescriber

Make sure the patient understands that their condition may impair their ability to drive. If the patient is incapable of understanding, notify the DVLA immediately. Explain to the patient that they have a legal duty to inform the DVLA.

Note: The DVLA guidance specifies that patients under S17 of the Mental Health Act must be able to satisfy the standards of fitness for their respective conditions and be free from any effects of medication which would affect driving adversely, before resuming driving. Very few patients will fulfil these criteria.

General Medical Council guidelines for prescribers[42]

- Patients who disagree with the diagnosis or the effect of the condition on their ability to drive should seek a second opinion and refrain from driving until this has been obtained.
- If the patient continues to drive while unfit, you should make every reasonable effort to persuade them to stop. This may include telling their next of kin if they agree you may do so.
- If they continue to drive, inform the DVLA. Tell the patient you are going to do this and write to the patient to confirm you have done so. Clearly document the advice given in the patient's notes.

References

1. Annas GJ. Doctors, drugs, and driving – tort liability for patient-caused accidents. N Engl J Med 2008; 359:521–525.
2. Metzner JL et al. Impairment in driving and psychiatric illness. J Neuropsychiatry Clin Neurosci 1993; 5:211–220.
3. Farkas RH et al. Zolpidem and driving impairment – identifying persons at risk. N Engl J Med 2013; 369:689–691.
4. Alvarez J et al. ICADTS Working Group: Categorization system for medicinal drugs affecting driving performance. 2007. http://www.icadts.nl/medicinal.html.
5. Noyes R, Jr. Motor vehicle accidents related to psychiatric impairment. Psychosomatics 1985; 26:569–580.
6. Biecheler MB et al. SAM survey on "drugs and fatal accidents": search of substances consumed and comparison between drivers involved under the influence of alcohol or cannabis. Traffic Inj Prev 2008; 9:11–21.
7. Oyefeso A et al. Fatal injuries while under the influence of psychoactive drugs: a cross-sectional exploratory study in England. BMC Public Health 2006; 6:148.
8. Segmiller FM et al. Driving ability according to German guidelines in stabilized bipolar I and II outpatients receiving lithium or lamotrigine. J Clin Pharmacol 2013; 53:459–462.
9. Brunnauer A et al. The effects of most commonly prescribed second generation antidepressants on driving ability: a systematic review: 70th Birthday Prof. Riederer. J Neural Transm 2013; 120:225–232.
10. Bramness JG et al. Minor increase in risk of road traffic accidents after prescriptions of antidepressants: a study of population registry data in Norway. J Clin Psychiatry 2008; 69:1099–1103.
11. Verster JC et al. Psychoactive medication and traffic safety. Int J Environ Res Public Health 2009; 6:1041–1054.
12. Verster JC et al. Mirtazapine as positive control drug in studies examining the effects of antidepressants on driving ability. Eur J Pharmacol 2015; 753:252–256.
13. Ip EJ et al. The effect of trazodone on standardized field sobriety tests. Pharmacotherapy 2013; 33:369–374.
14. Brunnauer A et al. Driving performance and psychomotor function in depressed patients treated with agomelatine or venlafaxine. Pharmacopsychiatry 2015; 48:65–71.
15. Grabe HJ et al. The influence of clozapine and typical neuroleptics on information processing of the central nervous system under clinical conditions in schizophrenic disorders: implications for fitness to drive. Neuropsychobiology 1999; 40:196–201.
16. Wylie KR et al. Effects of depot neuroleptics on driving performance in chronic schizophrenic patients. J Neurol Neurosurg Psychiatry 1993; 56:910–913.
17. Brunnauer A et al. The impact of antipsychotics on psychomotor performance with regards to car driving skills. J Clin Psychopharmacol 2004; 24:155–160.
18. Dassanayake T et al. Effects of benzodiazepines, antidepressants and opioids on driving: a systematic review and meta-analysis of epidemiological and experimental evidence. Drug Saf 2011; 34:125–156.
19. Rudisill TM et al. Medication use and the risk of motor vehicle collisions among licensed drivers: a systematic review. Accid Anal Prev 2016; 96:255–270.
20. Verster JC et al. Hypnotics and driving safety: meta-analyses of randomized controlled trials applying the on-the-road driving test. Curr Drug Saf 2006; 1:63–71.
21. Etminan M et al. Use of lithium and the risk of injurious motor vehicle crash in elderly adults: case-control study nested within a cohort. BMJ 2004; 328:558–559.
22. Hashemian F et al. A comparison of the effects of reboxetine and placebo on reaction time in adults with Attention Deficit-Hyperactivity Disorder (ADHD). Daru 2011; 19:231–235.

23. Classen S et al. Evidence-based review on interventions and determinants of driving performance in teens with attention deficit hyperactivity disorder or autism spectrum disorder. Traffic Inj Prev 2013; **14**:188–193.

24. The National Archives. Road Traffic Act 1991. 1991. http://www.legislation.gov.uk/ukpga/1991/40/contents.

25. Driver and Vehicle Licensing Agency. Assessing fitness to drive: a guide for medical professionals. https://www.gov.uk/government/publications/assessing-fitness-to-drive-a-guide-for-medical-professionals.

26. Piersma D et al. Prediction of fitness to drive in patients with alzheimer's dementia. PLoS One 2016; **11**:e0149566.

27. Breen DA et al. Driving and dementia. BMJ 2007; **334**:1365–1369.

28. Martin AJ et al. Driving assessment for maintaining mobility and safety in drivers with dementia. Cochrane Database Syst Rev 2013; 8:CD006222.

29. Department for Transport. Changes to drug driving law. 2013. Last updated August 2017. https://www.gov.uk/government/collections/drug-driving.

30. Sjo O et al. Pharmacokinetics and side-effects of clonazepam and its 7-amino-metabolite in man. Eur J Clin Pharmacol 1975; **8**:249–254.

31. Berlin A et al. Pharmacokinetics of the anticonvulsant drug clonazepam evaluated from single oral and intravenous doses and by repeated oral administration. Eur J Clin Pharmacol 1975; **9**:155–159.

32. Rutherford DM et al. Plasma concentrations of diazepam and desmethyldiazepam during chronic diazepam therapy. Br J Clin Pharmacol 1978; **6**:69–73.

33. Wickstrom E et al. Pharmacokinetic and clinical observations on prolonged administration of flunitrazepam. Eur J Clin Pharmacol 1980; **17**:189–196.

34. Mattila MA et al. Flunitrazepam: a review of its pharmacological properties and therapeutic use. Drugs 1980; **20**:353–374.

35. Greenblatt DJ et al. Single- and multiple-dose kinetics of oral lorazepam in humans: the predictability of accumulation. J Pharmacokinet Biopharm 1979; **7**:159–179.

36. Greenblatt DJ et al. Pharmacokinetic comparison of sublingual lorazepam with intravenous, intramuscular, and oral lorazepam. J Pharm Sci 1982; **71**:248–252.

37. Smink BE et al. The concentration of oxazepam and oxazepam glucuronide in oral fluid, blood and serum after controlled administration of 15 and 30 mg oxazepam. Br J Clin Pharmacol 2008; **66**:556–560.

38. Greenblatt DJ et al. Clinical pharmacokinetics of the newer benzodiazepines. Clin Pharmacokinet 1983; **8**:233–252.

39. Ferrari A et al. Methadone – metabolism, pharmacokinetics and interactions. Pharmacol Res 2004; **50**:551–559.

40. Department for Transport. Medication and Road Safety: A Scoping Study. Road Safety Research Report No. 116. 2010. http://webarchive.nationalarchives.gov.uk/20101007211118/http://www.dft.gov.uk/pgr/roadsafety/research/rsrr/theme3/report16findings.pdf.

41. Grabe HJ et al. The influence of polypharmacological antidepressive treatment on central nervous information processing of depressed patients: implications for fitness to drive. Neuropsychobiology 1998; **37**:200–204.

42. General Medical Council. Good practice in prescribing and managing medicines and devices. 2013. https://www.gmc-uk.org/guidance/ethical_guidance/14316.asp.

Psychotropic drugs and surgery

There are few worthwhile studies of the effects of non-anaesthetic drugs on surgery and the anaesthetic process.[1,2] Practice is therefore largely based on theoretical considerations, case reports, clinical experience and personal opinion. Any guidance given in this area is therefore somewhat speculative.

The decision as to whether or not to continue a drug during surgery and the peri-operative period should take into account a number of interacting factors. Some general considerations include:

- Patients are at risk of aspirating their stomach contents during general anaesthesia. For this reason they are usually prevented from eating for at least 6 hours before surgery. However, clear fluids leave the stomach within 2 hours of ingestion and so fluids that enable a patient to take routine medication may be allowed up to 2 hours before surgery. A clear fluid is defined as one through which newspaper print can be read.[3]
- There are some drug interactions between drugs used during surgery and routine medication that require the drugs not to be administered concurrently. This is usually managed by the anaesthetist through their choice of anaesthetic technique. Significant drug interactions between medicines used during surgery and psychotropic drugs include:
  - Enflurane may precipitate seizures in patients taking tricyclic antidepressants.[4-6]
  - Pethidine and other serotonergic opioids may precipitate fatal 'excitatory' reactions in patients taking MAOIs and may cause serotonin syndrome in patients taking SSRIs.[4-7]
- Major procedures induce profound physiological changes, which include electrolyte disturbances and the release of cortisol and catecholamines.
- Postoperatively, surgical stress and some agents used in anaesthesia often lead to gastric or gastrointestinal stasis. Oral absorption is therefore likely to be compromised.

For the most part, psychotropic drugs should be continued during the peri-operative period, assuming agreement of the anaesthetist concerned. Table 13.4 provides some discussion of the merits or otherwise of continuing individual psychotropic drugs during surgery. Note, however, that psychotropic and other drugs are frequently (accidentally and/or unthinkingly) withheld from pre-operative patients simply because they are 'nil by mouth'.[1] Patients may be labelled 'nil by mouth' for several reasons, including pre-operative preparation, unconsciousness, to rest the gut postoperatively or as a result of the surgery itself. Patients may also develop an intolerance to oral medicines at any time during a stay in hospital, often because of nausea and vomiting. When it is decided to continue a psychotropic drug, this decision needs to be explicitly outlined to appropriate medical and nursing staff.

For many patients undergoing surgery and recovery in a hospital there will be little or no opportunity to smoke. Abrupt cessation is likely to affect mental state and may also result in drug toxicity if psychotropic drugs are continued (see section on 'Smoking and psychotropic drugs').

Alternative routes and formulations may be sought. When changing the route or formulation, care should be taken to ensure the appropriate dose and frequency is

Table 13.4 Psychotropic drugs and surgery

Drug or drug group	Considerations	Safe in surgery?	Alternative formulations
Anticonvulsants[4,8-10]	■ CNS depressant activity may reduce anaesthetic requirements ■ Drug level monitoring may be required ■ Reduced dose of propofol may be required ■ Lamotrigine has been used pre-operatively and has analgesic properties	Probably, usually continued for people with epilepsy	Carbamazepine liquid or suppositories are available: 100 mg tablet = 125 mg suppository. Maximum by rectum 1 g daily in four divided doses Phenytoin is available IV or liquid: IV dose = oral dose Sodium valproate is available IV or liquid: IV dose = oral dose Before crushing tablets and mixing with water, confirm stability with either local guidelines or the drug company Lamotrigine liquid and dispersible tablets fairly widely available
Antidepressants – MAOIs[3,4,11-15]	■ Dangerous, potentially fatal interaction with pethidine and dextromethorphan (serotonin syndrome or coma/respiratory depression may occur) ■ Action of inhaled anaesthetics and neuromuscular blockers is reduced ■ Sympathomimetic agents may result in hypertensive crisis ■ Phenylephrine only agent safe for hypotension ■ MAO inhibition lasts for up to 2 weeks: early withdrawal is required ■ Switching to moclobemide 2 weeks before surgery allows continued treatment up until day of surgery (do not give moclobemide on the day of surgery)	Probably not, but careful selection of anaesthetic agents may reduce risks if continuation is essential	None
Antidepressants – SSRIs[4-7,14,16-18]	■ Danger of serotonin syndrome if administered with pethidine, fentanyl, pentazocine or tramadol ■ Occasional seizures reported ■ Cessation may result in withdrawal syndrome ■ Rule out hyponatraemia in all surgical patients[19] ■ Various interactions with drugs used in surgery ■ Venlafaxine may provoke opioid-induced rigidity ■ Increases risk of peri-operative bleeding	Probably, but avoid other serotonergic agents	Liquid escitalopram, fluoxetine and paroxetine are available Oral disintegrating tablets of mirtazapine have been used peri-operatively (for nausea)[20]

Drug			
Antidepressants – TCAs[4-6,16,18,21]	• α$_1$ blockade may lead to hypotension and interfere with effects of epinephrine/norepinephrine • Danger of serotonin syndrome (clomipramine, amitriptyline) if administered with pethidine, pentazocine or tramadol • Many drugs prolong QT interval so arrhythmia more likely • Most drugs lower seizure threshold • May decrease core hypothermia • Sympathomimetic agents may give exaggerated response • Effects persist for several days after cessation so will need to be stopped some time before surgery • Clomipramine, amitriptyline may increase bleeding risk	Unclear, but anaesthetic agents need to be carefully chosen Some authorities recommend slow discontinuation before surgery	Liquid amitriptyline is available. It is acidic and may interact with enteral feeds Dosulepin (dothiepin) capsules can be opened and mixed with water before flushing well. This is preferred over crushing tablets Most TCAs have potent local anaesthetic effects – oral delivery in liquid form is likely to cause local anaesthesia
Antipsychotics[4,14,22-26]	• Some antipsychotics widely used in anaesthetic practice • Increased risk of arrhythmia with most drugs • α$_1$ blockade may lead to hypotension and interfere with effects of epinephrine/norepinephrine • Most drugs lower seizure threshold • May enhance intra-operative core hypothermia • Some evidence of safe use in surgery[27] • Clozapine may delay recovery from anaesthesia • Gaseous anaesthetics may affect dopamine metabolism • Pre-operative olanzapine reduces risk of delirium[28]	Probably, usually continued to avoid relapse	Liquid preparations of some antipsychotics are available Some 'specials' liquids can be made for nasogastric delivery Before crushing tablets and mixing with water, confirm stability with either local guidelines or the drug company
Benzodiazepines[4,8]	• Reduced requirements for induction and maintenance anaesthetics • Many have prolonged action (days or weeks), so early withdrawal is necessary • Withdrawal symptoms possible	Probably; usually continued	Liquid, IM, IV and rectal diazepam are available (do not use IM route) Buccal liquid available for midazolam Sublingual (use normal tablets), IM, IV and lorazepam are available

(Continued)

Table 13.4 (*Continued*)

Drug or drug group	Considerations	Safe in surgery?	Alternative formulations
Lithium[3,4,11,14]	■ Prolongs the action of both depolarising and non-depolarising muscle relaxants ■ Surgery-related electrolyte disturbance and reduced renal function may precipitate lithium toxicity. Avoid dehydration and NSAIDs ■ Possible increased risk of arrhythmia	Probably safe in minor surgery but usually discontinued before major procedures and re-started once electrolytes normalise Slow discontinuation is essential – anaesthetists may not appreciate this[29]	The bioavailability of lithium varies between brands. Care is needed with equivalent doses of salts: lithium carbonate 200 mg = lithium citrate 509 mg Liquid lithium citrate is available and is usually administered twice daily
Methadone[3,8]	■ May reduce opiate requirements ■ Naloxone may induce withdrawal ■ Methadone prolongs QT interval ■ When using opiates, use only full agonists (avoid buprenorphine)	Probably, usually continued	IM dose = oral dose
Modafinil[30,31]	■ Limited data suggest no interference with anaesthesia ■ Improves recovery after anaesthesia	Probably, data limited	None
Pregabalin[32]	■ Pre-operative pregabalin reduces post-operative nausea	Yes	None

CNS, central nervous system; IM, intramuscular; IV, intravenous; MAOI, monoamine oxidase inhibitor; NSAID, non-steroidal anti-inflammatory drug; SSRI, selective serotonin reuptake inhibitor; TCA, tricyclic antidepressant.

prescribed as these may not be the same as for the oral route or previous formulation. Oral preparations may sometimes be administered via a nasogastric (NG), percutaneous endoscopic gastrostomy (PEG) or jejunostomy tube.

Risks associated with discontinuing psychotropic drugs

- Relapse (especially if treatment ceased for more than a few days).[33]
- Worsening of condition. For example, abrupt cessation of lithium worsens outcome in bipolar affective disorder,[34] as does abrupt stopping of antidepressants.[35]
- Suicide. Cessation of antidepressants may increase risk of suicide.[36]
- Discontinuation symptoms. These may complicate diagnosis in the peri-operative period.
- Delirium. May be more common in those discontinuing antipsychotics[37] or antidepressants.[6]

Risks associated with continuing psychotropic drugs

- Potential for interactions with anaesthetic and peri-operative drugs, both pharmacokinetic and pharmacodynamic.
- Increased likelihood of bleeding (e.g. with SSRIs).[38]
- Hypo/hypertension (depending on psychotropic).[21,22]
- Effects on core body temperature (e.g. with phenothiazines).

References

1. Noble DW et al. Interrupting drug therapy in the perioperative period. Drug Saf 2002; 25:489–495.
2. Noble DW et al. Risks of interrupting drug treatment before surgery. BMJ 2000; 321:719–720.
3. Anon. Drugs in the peri-operative period: 1 – Stopping or continuing drugs around surgery. Drug Ther Bull 1999; 37:62–64.
4. Smith MS et al. Perioperative management of drug therapy, clinical considerations. Drugs 1996; 51:238–259.
5. Chui PT et al. Medications to withhold or continue in the preoperative consultation. Curr Anaesth Crit Care 1998; 9:302–306.
6. Kudoh A et al. Antidepressant treatment for chronic depressed patients should not be discontinued prior to anesthesia. Can J Anaesth 2002; 49:132–136.
7. Spivey KM et al. Perioperative seizures and fluvoxamine. Br J Anaesth 1993; 71:321.
8. Morrow JI et al. Essential drugs in the perioperative period. Curr Pract Surg 1990; 90:106–109.
9. Bloor M et al. Antiepileptic drugs and anesthesia. Paediatr Anaesth 2017; 27:248–250.
10. Bhosale UA et al. Comparative pre-emptive analgesic efficacy study of novel antiepileptic agents gabapentin, lamotrigine and topiramate in patients undergoing major surgeries at a tertiary care hospital: a randomized double blind clinical trial. J Basic Clin Physiol Pharmacol 2017; 28:59–66.
11. Rahman MH et al. Medication in the peri-operative period. Pharm J 2004; 272:287–289.
12. Blom-Peters L et al. Monoamine oxidase inhibitors and anesthesia: an updated literature review. Acta Anaesthesiol Belg 1993; 44:57–60.
13. Hill S et al. MAOIs to RIMAs in anaesthesia – a literature review. Psychopharmacology (Berl) 1992; 106 Suppl:S43–S45.
14. Huyse FJ et al. Psychotropic drugs and the perioperative period: a proposal for a guideline in elective surgery. Psychosomatics 2006; 47:8–22.
15. Bajwa SJ et al. Psychiatric diseases: need for an increased awareness among the anesthesiologists. J Anaesthesiol Clin Pharmacol 2011; 27:440–446.
16. Takakura K et al. Refractory hypotension during combined general and epidural anaesthesia in a patient on tricyclic antidepressants. Anaesth Intensive Care 2008; 34:111–114.
17. Roy S et al. Fentanyl-induced rigidity during emergence from general anesthesia potentiated by venlafaxine. Can J Anaesth 2003; 50:32–35.
18. Mahdanian AA et al. Serotonergic antidepressants and perioperative bleeding risk: a systematic review. Expert Opin Drug Saf 2014; 13:695–704.
19. Levine SM et al. Selective serotonin reuptake inhibitor-induced hyponatremia and the plastic surgery patient. Plast Reconstr Surg 2017; 139:1481–1488.
20. Chang FL et al. Efficacy of mirtazapine in preventing intrathecal morphine-induced nausea and vomiting after orthopaedic surgery*. Anaesthesia 2010; 65:1206–1211.
21. Kudoh A et al. Chronic treatment with antidepressants decreases intraoperative core hypothermia. Anesth Analg 2003; 97:275–279.
22. Kudoh A et al. Chronic treatment with antipsychotics enhances intraoperative core hypothermia. Anesth Analg 2004; 98.111–115.

23. Doherty J et al. Implications for anaesthesia in a patient established on clozapine treatment. Int J Obstet Anesth 2006; 15:59–62.

24. Geeraerts T et al. Delayed recovery after short-duration, general anesthesia in a patient chronically treated with clozapine. Anesth Analg 2006; 103:1618.

25. Adachi YU et al. Isoflurane anesthesia inhibits clozapine- and risperidone-induced dopamine release and anesthesia-induced changes in dopamine metabolism was modified by fluoxetine in the rat striatum: an in vivo microdialysis study. Neurochem Int 2008; 52:384–391.

26. Parlow JL et al. Single-dose haloperidol for the prophylaxis of postoperative nausea and vomiting after intrathecal morphine. Anesth Analg 2004; 98:1072–1076, table.

27. Kim DH et al. Adverse events associated with antipsychotic use in hospitalized older adults after cardiac surgery. J Am Geriatr Soc 2017; 65:1229–1237.

28. Larsen KA et al. Administration of olanzapine to prevent postoperative delirium in elderly joint-replacement patients: a randomized, controlled trial. Psychosomatics 2010; 51:409–418.

29. Attri JP et al. Psychiatric patient and anaesthesia. Indian J Anaesth 2012; 56:8–13.

30. Larijani GE et al. Modafinil improves recovery after general anesthesia. Anesth Analg 2004; 98:976–981, table.

31. Doyle A et al. Day case general anaesthesia in a patient with narcolepsy. Anaesthesia 2008; 63:880–882.

32. Grant MC et al. The effect of preoperative pregabalin on postoperative nausea and vomiting: a meta-analysis. Anesth Analg 2016; 123:1100–1107.

33. De Baerdemaeker L et al. Anaesthesia for patients with mood disorders. Curr Opin Anaesthesiol 2005; 18:333–338.

34. Faedda GL et al. Outcome after rapid vs gradual discontinuation of lithium treatment in bipolar disorders. Arch Gen Psychiatry 1993; 50:448–455.

35. Baldessarini RJ et al. Illness risk following rapid versus gradual discontinuation of antidepressants. Am J Psychiatry 2010; 167:934–941.

36. Yerevanian BI et al. Antidepressants and suicidal behaviour in unipolar depression. Acta Psychiatr Scand 2004; 110:452–458.

37. Copeland LA et al. Postoperative complications in the seriously mentally ill: a systematic review of the literature. Ann Surg 2008; 248:31–38.

38. Paton C et al. SSRIs and gastrointestinal bleeding. BMJ 2005; 331:529–530.

Miscellany

Enhancing medication adherence

Recommendations made in clinical guidelines regarding the use of medicines are based on evidence from clinical trials supplemented by clinicians' opinions of the balance between the potential benefits and potential risks of treatment. In clinical practice, however, a range of patient-related factors such as insight, health beliefs and the perceived efficacy and tolerability of treatment influence whether or not medication is taken and, if so, for how long.

Generally speaking, the patient and prescriber should agree jointly on the goals of treatment and how these can be reached. Sticking to this mutually agreed plan is termed concordance or adherence; non-adherence indicates that the treatment plan should be renegotiated, and not that the patient is at fault.

How common is non-adherence?

Reviews of adherence generally conclude that approximately 50% of people do not take their medication as prescribed, and that this proportion is similar across chronic physical and mental disorders.[1] This however may be an over-simplification in that it is probable that only a very small proportion of patients are fully adherent, the majority are partially adherent to varying degrees, and a few never take any medication at all of their own volition.[2]

There is some **variation in adherence** rates both **over time** and **across settings**. For example, 10 days after discharge from hospital, up to 25% of patients with schizophrenia are partially or completely non-adherent and this figure rises to 50% at 1 year and 75% by 2 years.[3] In some mental health-care settings the rate of non-adherence may be up to 90%.[4] A great deal of poor adherence occurs without the knowledge of the prescriber. In one study,[5] prescribers identified only half of those who were non-adherent.

In another, 35% of patients referred for treatment of refractory schizophrenia had a sub-therapeutic plasma concentration.[6]

Poor adherence to medication is a major risk factor for poor outcomes, including relapse, in people with schizophrenia,[7–9] bipolar disorder[10] and depression.[11,12] Wider health benefits are also lost. For example, compared with depressed patients who take an antidepressant, those who do not have a 20% increased risk of an incident myocardial infarction.[12] As a rule of thumb, the lower the amount of prescribed medication that is taken, the poorer the outcome. There is no evidence that newer (presumed better tolerated) medicines are consistently associated with increased adherence.[2]

According to the World Health Organization, 'increasing the effectiveness of adherence interventions may have far greater impact on the health of the population than any improvements in specific medical treatments'; it has therefore been suggested that non-adherence should be a diagnosable condition for which active interventions are provided.[13] Indeed, analyses of data collected as part of the national confidential inquiry into suicide and homicide by people with mental illness revealed that health-care providers that had a policy in place regarding how to manage patients who are not taking their medication as prescribed had 20% fewer suicides than providers that did not have such a policy.[14]

Not surprisingly, non-adherence is known to be more common when the patient disagrees with the need for treatment, the medication regime is complex, or the patient perceives the adverse effects of treatment to be unacceptable (see Box 14.1).[11]

Box 14.1 Why don't people take medication?

Non-adherence can be intentional (sometimes termed 'intelligent' non-adherence) or unintentional or a mixture of both. Most non-adherence is intentional. Individual influences (which can change in any given patient over time) include:[15]

- **Illness-related factors** such as denial of illness stigma, specific symptoms such as grandiose or persecutory thoughts or delusions, or the impact of illness on lifestyle (e.g. cognitive deficits, disorganisation).
- **Treatment-related factors** such as the drug being perceived not to be effective or the adverse effects intolerable; akathisia, weight gain and sexual dysfunction feature prominently here.
- **Clinician-related factors** such as not feeling listened to or consulted, perceiving the clinician as authoritative or dismissive, being given a poor explanation of treatment or having infrequent contact.
- **Patient-related factors** such as personal beliefs about illness, denial of illness/or lack of insight, perception of illness severity, being young and male, having co-morbid personality disorder(s) and/or substance misuse, personal beliefs about treatment such as concerns about dependency, concerns about long-term adverse effects, a lack of knowledge about treatment, misunderstanding instructions or simply forgetting. Also, up to 25% of people with schizophrenia report missing their psychotic experiences,[16] when effectively treated.
- **Environmental and cultural factors** such as the family's beliefs about illness and treatment, religious beliefs and peer pressure.
- Cognitive function is strongly linked to adherence in bipolar disorder.[17]

NICE (2009)[18] recommended that, as long as the patient has capacity to consent, their right not to take medication should be respected. If the prescriber considers that this decision may have an adverse effect, the reasons for the patient's decision and the prescriber's concerns should be recorded.

Adherence may also therefore be **medication specific,** where some medicines are taken regularly, others intermittently and others not at all. Notably, half of those who stop treatment do not tell their doctor. Psychiatrists generally prefer to use direct questioning over the use of more intrusive/objective methods of assessing adherence,[19] and so partial or non-adherence may go undetected, as discussed earlier in this section.

Assessing attitudes to medication

A number of rating scales and checklists are available that help to guide and structure discussion around attitudes to medication. The most widely used is the Drug Attitude Inventory (DAI),[20] which consists of a mix of positive and negative statements about medication – 30 statements in its full form and 10 in its abbreviated form. It is designed to be completed by the patient, who simply agrees or disagrees with each statement. The total score is an indicator of the patient's overall perception of the balance between the benefits and harms associated with taking medication, and therefore likely adherence. Attitudes to medication as measured using the DAI have been shown to be a useful predictor of compliance over time.[21] Other available checklists include the Rating of Medication Influences Scale (ROMI),[22] the Beliefs about Medicines Questionnaire[23] and the Medication Adherence rating Scale (MARS).[9]

How can you assess adherence?

It is very difficult to be certain about whether or not a patient is taking prescribed medicines; partial and non-adherence are almost always covert until the patient relapses. Clinicians are known to overestimate adherence rates and patients may not openly acknowledge that they are not taking all or any of their medication. NICE recommend that the patient should be asked in a non-judgemental way if they have missed any doses over a specific time period such as the previous week.[18]

It is also important to ask the patient about perceived effectiveness and adverse effects. More intrusive methods include checks that prescriptions have been collected, asking to see the patient's medication (pill counts) and asking family or carers. For some antipsychotic drugs such as clozapine, olanzapine and risperidone, blood tests can be useful to directly assess plasma levels. It is important to note that plasma levels of these drugs achieved with a fixed dose vary somewhat and it is not possible to accurately determine partial non-adherence (i.e. total non-adherence will be readily revealed but partial and full adherence may be difficult to tell apart).

Strategies for improving adherence

Note that few studies specifically recruit non-adherent patients (the refusal rate in such patients is likely to be high) and the specific barriers to adherence are rarely identified. The small effect size seen in many studies may simply be a consequence of this unfocused approach. Where barriers to adherence are identified and targeted interventions delivered, adherence is more likely to improve.[24]

NICE has reviewed the evidence for adherence over a range of health conditions.[18] They conclude that no specific intervention can be recommended for all patients but, in general, **adherence is maximised if:**

- The patient is **offered information about medicines** before the decision is taken to prescribe.
- This information is actively **discussed**, taking into account the patient's understanding and beliefs about diagnosis and treatment.
- The information includes the **name** of the medicine, how it works, the likely benefits and adverse effects, and how long it should be continued.
- The patient is given the opportunity to be **involved in making decisions** about prescribed medicines[25] (interestingly, one study found no effect on adherence for shared decision-making in depression[26]).
- At each contact, the patient is asked if they have any concerns about their medicines, and any identified **concerns are addressed.**
- Specific to schizophrenia, **good social and family support** has been shown to have a positive impact on adherence,[25] as has participation in dedicated early intervention services.[27]

NICE further recommend that any intervention that is used to increase adherence should be tailored to overcome the specific difficulties experienced or reported by a patient.

It is essential that the **patient's perspective is understood and respected and a treatment plan agreed jointly.** The following strategies may help to achieve this.

- Explore aspirations for the future and **how medication could help**, e.g. staying out of hospital or not getting into trouble with the police.
- Help the patient and carer **understand** their experiences in a culturally sensitive way that recognises the place of medication in recovery.
- Work with the patient to elicit and explore the **positive and negative** things about taking/not taking medication.
- Talk through past experiences of medication and explore which medicines were helpful and less helpful **from the patient's perspective.**
- **Listen** to and **acknowledge** the **concerns** of patients and their carers about the use of medication and address any false beliefs.
- **Work collaboratively** with the patient to find a medication that the patient perceives to be helpful.
- **Systematically monitor the effectiveness and adverse effects** of medication so that the patient feels listened to and respected.
- **Manage adverse effects when they occur.** Consider dosage reduction, change of medication, alteration of the timing of doses, or additional medication for adverse effects.

Overcoming **practical difficulties** can also help. Potentially useful strategies include:

- ensuring the patient knows how to **obtain medication** and is able to do this[28]
- keeping **medication regimes** as **simple** as possible
- using **reminders and prompts**, including electronic pill dispensers,[29] telephone follow-up or mobile phone text messaging[30,31]

- **maximising engagement** with services by introducing patients to their community team before discharge from hospital
- providing support, encouragement and **regular planned follow-up.**

The need to consider multiple strategies tailored to the needs of individual patients is also the conclusion of a Cochrane review that examined medication adherence over a wide range of medical conditions.[1] Almost all of the interventions that were effective in improving adherence in long-term care were complex, and even the most effective interventions did not lead to large improvements in adherence and treatment outcomes. Nieuwlaat et al[1] emphasised that there is no evidence that low adherence can be 'cured'; efforts to improve adherence must be maintained for as long as treatment is needed.

'Compliance therapy' for schizophrenia

After early promise of compliance therapy in improving insight, adherence, attitudes towards medication and re-hospitalisation rates in an in-patient sample,[32] further studies have failed to replicate this finding. Compliance therapy has been shown to have no advantage over non-specific counselling in either in-patients[21] or out-patients,[33] or those who have been clinically unstable in the last year.[34] More recently a programme based on the theory of 'reasoned action' showed a five-fold improvement in rates of adherence compared with treatment as usual.[35]

Compliance aids

Compliance aids that contain compartments that accommodate up to four doses of multiple medicines each day may be helpful in patients who are clearly motivated to take medication but find this difficult because of disorganisation or cognitive deficits. It should be noted that only 10% of non-compliant patients say that they forgot to take medication[36] and that compliance aids are not a substitute for lack of insight or lack of motivation to take medication. Some medicines are unstable when removed from blister packaging and placed in a compliance aid. These include oro-dispersible formulations which are often prescribed for non-adherent patients. In addition, compliance aids are labour intensive (expensive) to fill, it can be difficult to change prescriptions at short notice and the filling of these devices is particularly error-prone.[37]

Depot antipsychotics

Meta-analyses of clinical trials have shown that the relative and absolute risks of relapse with depot maintenance treatment were 30% and 10% lower, respectively, than with oral treatment.[38,39] In clinical practice, covert non-adherence is avoided; if the patient defaults from treatment, it will be immediately apparent. Risk of treatment change or discontinuation is lower with depots than with oral treatment.[40] NICE recommends that depots are an option in patients who are known to be non-adherent to oral treatment and/or those who prefer this method of administration.[41] Depots are likely to be underused, for example a US study found that depot preparations were prescribed for fewer than one in five patients with a recent episode of non-adherence.[42]

CHAPTER 14

Financial incentives

There is evidence from controlled trials across a number of disease areas supporting the potential of financial incentives to enhance medication adherence. Paying people to take their medication is extremely controversial, though some clinicians have found this strategy to be successful in high-risk patients with psychotic illness.[43] A randomised controlled trial (RCT) has demonstrated that modest payments improve adherence in patients with psychotic illness.[44]

References

1. Nieuwlaat R et al. Interventions for enhancing medication adherence. Cochrane Database Syst Rev 2014:CD000011.
2. Masand PS et al. Partial adherence to antipsychotic medication impacts the course of illness in patients with schizophrenia: a review. Prim Care Companion J Clin Psychiatry 2009; 11:147–154.
3. Leucht S et al. Epidemiology, clinical consequences, and psychosocial treatment of nonadherence in schizophrenia. J Clin Psychiatry 2006; 67 Suppl 5:3–8.
4. Cramer JA et al. Compliance with medication regimens for mental and physical disorders. Psychiatr Serv 1998; 49:196–201.
5. Remington G et al. The use of electronic monitoring (MEMS) to evaluate antipsychotic compliance in outpatients with schizophrenia. Schizophr Res 2007; 90:229–237.
6. McCutcheon R et al. Antipsychotic plasma levels in the assessment of poor treatment response in schizophrenia. Acta Psychiatr Scand 2018; 137:39–46.
7. Morken G et al. Non-adherence to antipsychotic medication, relapse and rehospitalisation in recent-onset schizophrenia. BMC Psychiatry 2008; 8:32.
8. Knapp M et al. Non-adherence to antipsychotic medication regimens: associations with resource use and costs. Br J Psychiatry 2004; 184:509–516.
9. Jaeger S et al. Adherence styles of schizophrenia patients identified by a latent class analysis of the Medication Adherence Rating Scale (MARS): a six-month follow-up study. Psychiatry Res 2012; 200:83–88.
10. Lang K et al. Predictors of medication nonadherence and hospitalization in Medicaid patients with bipolar I disorder given long-acting or oral antipsychotics. J Med Econ 2011; 14:217–226.
11. Mitchell AJ et al. Why don't patients take their medicine? Reasons and solutions in psychiatry. Adv Psychiatr Treat 2007; 13:336–346.
12. Scherrer JF et al. Antidepressant drug compliance: reduced risk of MI and mortality in depressed patients. Am J Med 2011; 124:318–324.
13. Marcum ZA et al. Medication nonadherence: a diagnosable and treatable medical condition. JAMA 2013; 309:2105–2106.
14. Appleby L et al. National Confidential Inquiry into Suicide and Homicide by People with Mental Illness. 2013. http://research.bmh.manchester.ac.uk/cmhs/research/centreforsuicideprevention/nci.
15. Wade M et al. A systematic review of service-user reasons for adherence and nonadherence to neuroleptic medication in psychosis. Clin Psychol Rev 2017; 51:75–95.
16. Moritz S et al. Beyond the usual suspects: positive attitudes towards positive symptoms is associated with medication noncompliance in psychosis. Schizophr Bull 2013; 39:917–922.
17. Correard N et al. Neuropsychological functioning, age, and medication adherence in bipolar disorder. PLoS One 2017; 12:e0184313.
18. National Institute for Health and Care Excellence. Medicines adherence: involving patients in decisions about prescribed medicines and supporting adherence. Clinical Guideline CG76, 2009. https://www.nice.org.uk/guidance/cg76.
19. Vieta E et al. Psychiatrists' perceptions of potential reasons for non- and partial adherence to medication: results of a survey in bipolar disorder from eight European countries. J Affect Disord 2012; 143:125–130.
20. Hogan TP et al. A self-report scale predictive of drug compliance in schizophrenics: reliability and discriminative validity. Psychol Med 1983; 13:177–183.
21. O'Donnell C et al. Compliance therapy: a randomised controlled trial in schizophrenia. BMJ 2003; 327:834.
22. Weiden P et al. Rating of medication influences (ROMI) scale in schizophrenia. Schizophr Bull 1994; 20:297–310.
23. Horne R et al. The beliefs about medicines questionnaire: The development and evaluation of a new method for assessing the cognitive representation of medication. Psychology & Health 1999; 14:1–24.
24. Staring AB et al. Treatment adherence therapy in people with psychotic disorders: randomised controlled trial. Br J Psychiatry 2010; 197:448–455.
25. Wilder CM et al. Medication preferences and adherence among individuals with severe mental illness and psychiatric advance directives. Psychiatr Serv 2010; 61:380–385.
26. LeBlanc A et al. Shared decision making for antidepressants in primary care: a cluster randomized trial. JAMA Int Med 2015; 175:1761–1770.
27. Randall J et al. Increasing medication adherence and income assistance access for first-episode psychosis patients. PLoS One 2017; 12:e0179089.

28. Valenstein M et al. Using a pharmacy-based intervention to improve antipsychotic adherence among patients with serious mental illness. Schizophr Bull 2011; 37:727–736.

29. Velligan D et al. A randomized trial comparing in person and electronic interventions for improving adherence to oral medications in schizophrenia. Schizophr Bull 2013; 39:999–1007.

30. Granholm E et al. Mobile Assessment and Treatment for Schizophrenia (MATS): a pilot trial of an interactive text-messaging intervention for medication adherence, socialization, and auditory hallucinations. Schizophr Bull 2012; 38:414–425.

31. Montes JM et al. A short message service (SMS)-based strategy for enhancing adherence to antipsychotic medication in schizophrenia. Psychiatry Res 2012; 200:89–95.

32. Kemp R et al. Randomised controlled trial of compliance therapy. 18-month follow-up. Br J Psychiatry 1998; 172:413–419.

33. Byerly MJ et al. A trial of compliance therapy in outpatients with schizophrenia or schizoaffective disorder. J Clin Psychiatry 2005; 66:997–1001.

34. Gray R et al. Adherence therapy for people with schizophrenia. European multicentre randomised controlled trial. Br J Psychiatry 2006; 189:508–514.

35. Sirey JA et al. Adherence to depression treatment in primary care: a randomized clinical trial. JAMA Psychiatry 2017; 74:1129–1135.

36. Perkins DO. Predictors of noncompliance in patients with schizophrenia. J Clin Psychiatry 2002; 63:1121–1128.

37. Barber ND et al. Care homes' use of medicines study: prevalence, causes and potential harm of medication errors in care homes for older people. Qual Saf Health Care 2009; 18:341–346.

38. Leucht C et al. Oral versus depot antipsychotic drugs for schizophrenia – a critical systematic review and meta-analysis of randomised long-term trials. Schizophr Res 2011; 127:83–92.

39. Leucht S et al. Antipsychotic drugs versus placebo for relapse prevention in schizophrenia: a systematic review and meta-analysis. Lancet 2012; 379:2063–2071.

40. Verdoux H et al. Risk of discontinuation of antipsychotic long-acting injections vs. oral antipsychotics in real-life prescribing practice: a community-based study. Acta Psychiatr Scand 2017; 135:429–438.

41. National Institute for Health and Care Excellence. Psychosis and schizophrenia in adults: treatment and management. Clinical Guideline 178, 2014; last updated March 2014. https://www.nice.org.uk/guidance/cg178.

42. West JC et al. Use of depot antipsychotic medications for medication nonadherence in schizophrenia. Schizophr Bull 2008; 34:995–1001.

43. Claassen D et al. Money for medication: financial incentives to improve medication adherence in assertive outreach. Psychiatr Bull 2007; 31:4–7.

44. Priebe S et al. Effectiveness of financial incentives to improve adherence to maintenance treatment with antipsychotics: cluster randomised controlled trial. BMJ 2013; 347:f5847.

CHAPTER 14

Re-starting psychotropic medications after a period of non-compliance

A common scenario when a patient is admitted to hospital is that they have been non-compliant with their medications for some time before admission. The clinical question of whether to re-start the medication, and at which dose, is a complex one. The risk of withdrawal symptoms and relapse when there is reticence to re-prescribe must be balanced against the risk of adverse drug reactions when medications are re-introduced too quickly. There is little published evidence on this area, with most guidance (of undeclared provenance) coming from manufacturers, so the guidance provided here should be followed with caution.

Summary of Product Characteristics (SPC) documents tend not to deal with this clinical scenario, but official Patient Information Leaflets often do. These leaflets are unanimous in advising that on no account should a double dose be given to make up for a missed dose. The vast majority advise only on what to do if a single dose has been missed. In this case, some leaflets advise taking the missed dose later (provided it is not too close to the next dose), whereas others recommend skipping the missed dose altogether and waiting for the next dose.

In the event that more than one dose has been missed, the first question is whether this is the appropriate drug for a patient to be taking. If it is a drug with a short half-life or one that requires lengthy re-titration, it may not be appropriate for a patient who is frequently non-compliant. Similarly, if a patient is intoxicated with alcohol or drugs, it may not be appropriate to re-start a medication at that time. Find out if there are any particular reasons for non-compliance. Consider the appropriateness of an antipsychotic long-acting injection in the future.

Regarding the question as to whether to re-start the drug at the same dose or to re-titrate from a lower dose, clearly the time since the last dose is important – if more than a week or two has passed, then all drugs will probably need to be re-started as if new treatment (although for many drugs this will mean starting back on the same dose as before).

Table 14.1 summarises our recommendations. The drugs in column A have specific safety issues that mean they require re-titration after the specified length of time. The drugs in column B are thought to be safe because the maximum dose is usually no higher than the highest recommended starting dose. Drugs in column C are thought to be safe to re-start at the prior dose because a similar drug appears in column B and clinical experience suggests they are safe or the risks associated with giving untitrated high doses are thought to be low.

Lamotrigine

Lamotrigine has been associated with life-threatening cutaneous reactions, especially with high initial doses. The manufacturer's product information therefore advises that if five half-lives have elapsed since the last lamotrigine dose was given, lamotrigine should be titrated as if for the first time. The half-life in healthy subjects on no other medication is 33 hours. This is affected by other medications and is approximately 14 hours when given with glucuronidation-inducing drugs such as carbamazepine or phenytoin. The half-life is increased to approximately 70 hours

Table 14.1 Recommendations for re-starting psychotropic medications after a period of non-compliance

A. Drugs that require re-titration			B. Drugs that are usually safe for restarting at the previous dose	C. Drugs that are probably safe for restarting at the previous dose
Drug	**Time after which re-titration must be performed**	**Further guidance**		
Clozapine	48 h	See 'Restarting clozapine' section in Chapter 1	Acamprosate[1]	Antipsychotics (except restarting clozapine)[12–27]
			Asenapine[2]	Carbamazepine[28,29]
			Fluoxetine[3]	Cholinesterase inhibitors[30–35]
			Haloperidol[4]	CNS stimulants[36–41]
Lamotrigine	3–7 days	See text.	Isocarboxazid[5]	Disulfiram[42,43]
Methadone	3 days	See section	Lofepramine[6]	Lithium[44,45]
Buprenorphine	3 days	on 'Opioid dependence' in Chapter 4	Methylphenidate[7]	MAOIs[46,47]
			Phenelzine[8]	Memantine[48,49]
			Sulpiride[9]	Naltrexone[50,51]
			Tranylcypromine[10]	Other antidepressants[52–63]
			Valproate[11]	Pregabalin[64,65]
				SSRIs[66–77]
				TCAs[78–91]

CNS, central nervous system; MAOI, monoamine oxidase inhibitor; SSRI, selective serotonin reuptake inhibitor; TCA, tricyclic antidepressant.

when given with valproate. This means that the time before complete re-titration is necessary therefore varies between 3 and 7 days, depending on the other drugs prescribed.[92]

References

1. BNF Online. Acamprosate. 2017. https://www.medicinescomplete.com/mc/bnf/current/PHP3181-acamprosate-calcium.htm.
2. BNF Online. Asenapine. 2017. https://www.medicinescomplete.com/mc/bnf/current/PHP2327-asenapine.htm.
3. BNF Online. Fluoxetine. 2017. https://www.medicinescomplete.com/mc/bnf/current/PHP2426-fluoxetine.htm.
4. BNF Online. Haloperidol. 2017. https://www.medicinescomplete.com/mc/bnf/current/PHP2226-haloperidol.htm.
5. BNF Online. Isocarboxazid. 2017. https://www.medicinescomplete.com/mc/bnf/current/PHP2404-isocarboxazid.htm.
6. BNF Online. Lofepramine. 2017. https://www.medicinescomplete.com/mc/bnf/current/PHP2381-lofepramine.htm.
7. BNF Online. Methylphenidate. 2017. https://www.medicinescomplete.com/mc/bnf/current/PHP2479-methylphenidate-hydrochloride.htm.
8. BNF Online. Phenelzine. 2017. https://www.medicinescomplete.com/mc/bnf/current/PHP2399-phenelzine.htm.
9. BNF Online. Sulpiride. 2017. https://www.medicinescomplete.com/mc/bnf/current/PHP2253-sulpiride.htm.
10. BNF Online. Tranylcypromine. 2017. https://www.medicinescomplete.com/mc/bnf/current/PHP2406-tranylcypromine.htm.
11. BNF Online. Sodium valproate. 2017. https://www.medicinescomplete.com/mc/bnf/current/PHP2978-sodium-valproate.htm.
12. BNF Online. Amisulpride. 2017. https://www.medicinescomplete.com/mc/bnf/current/PHP2268-amisulpride.htm.
13. Generics UK T/A Mylan. Patient Information Leaflet. Amisulpride 50 mg, 100 mg, 200 mg, 400 mg tablets. 2017. https://www.medicines.org.uk/emc/medicine/33548.
14. BNF Online. Aripiprazole. 2017. https://www.medicinescomplete.com/mc/bnf/current/PHP2271-aripiprazole.htm.
15. Actavis UK Ltd. Patient Information Leaflet. Aripiprazole 5 mg,10 mg, 15 mg, 30 mg Tablets. 2017. https://www.medicines.org.uk/emc/medicine/29797.
16. BNF Online. Chlorpromazine hydrochloride. 2017. https://www.medicinescomplete.com/mc/bnf/current/PHP2213-chlorpromazine-hydrochloride.htm.
17. Dr. Reddy's Laboratories (UK) Ltd. Patient Information Leaflet. Chlorpromazine 25 mg, 50 mg, 100 mg Tablets. 2017. https://www.medicines.org.uk/emc/medicine/29573.
18. BNF Online. Lurasidone hydrochloride. 2017. https://www.medicinescomplete.com/mc/bnf/current/PHP93592-lurasidone-hydrochloride.htm.

19. Sunovion Pharmaceuticals Europe Ltd. Patient Information Leaflet. Latuda 18.5 mg, 37 mg and 74 mg film-coated tablets (lurasidone). 2016. https://www.medicines.org.uk/emc/medicine/29131.
20. BNF Online. Olanzapine. 2017. https://www.medicinescomplete.com/mc/bnf/current/PHP2277-olanzapine.htm.
21. Dr. Reddy's Laboratories (UK) Ltd. Patient Information Leaflet. Olanzapine 2.5, 5, 7.5, 10, 15 and 20 mg film-coated Tablets. 2016. https://www.medicines.org.uk/emc/medicine/29655.
22. BNF Online. Quetiapine. 2017. https://www.medicinescomplete.com/mc/bnf/current/PHP2284-quetiapine.htm.
23. Actavis UK Ltd. Patient Information Leaflet. Quetiapine 25 mg, 100 mg, 150 mg, 200 mg, 300 mg Film-coated Tablets. 2016. https://www.medicines.org.uk/emc/PIL.26238.latest.pdf.
24. BNF Online. Risperidone. 2017. https://www.medicinescomplete.com/mc/bnf/current/PHP2288-risperidone.htm.
25. Accord Healthcare Limited. Risperidone 0.5/1/2/3/4/6 mg film coated tablets. 2016. https://www.medicines.org.uk/emc/PIL.25958.latest.pdf.
26. BNF Online. Trifluoperazine. 2017. https://www.medicinescomplete.com/mc/bnf/current/PHP2258-trifluoperazine.htm.
27. Concordia International. Patient Information Leaflet. Trifluoperazine 1 mg and 5 mg tablets. 2016. https://www.medicines.org.uk/emc/medicine/31520.
28. BNF Online. Carbamazepine. 2017. https://www.medicinescomplete.com/mc/bnf/current/PHP2909-carbamazepine.htm.
29. Novartis Pharmaceuticals UK Ltd. Patient Information Leaflet. Tegretol Tablets 100 mg, 200 mg, 400 mg (carbamazepine). 2015. https://www.medicines.org.uk/emc/medicine/4095.
30. BNF Online. Donepezil hydrochloride. 2017. https://www.medicinescomplete.com/mc/bnf/current/PHP3239-donepezil-hydrochloride.htm.
31. Accord Healthcare Limited. Patient Information Leaflet. Donepezil Hydrochloride 5 mg and 10 mg Film-coated tablets. 2017. https://www.medicines.org.uk/emc/medicine/25794.
32. BNF Online. Galantamine. 2017. https://www.medicinescomplete.com/mc/bnf/current/PHP3242-galantamine.htm.
33. Shire Pharmaceuticals Limited. Patient Information Leaflet. Reminyl Tablets (galantamine). 2017. https://www.medicines.org.uk/emc/medicine/10338.
34. BNF Online. Rivastigmine. 2017. https://www.medicinescomplete.com/mc/bnf/current/PHP3250-rivastigmine.htm.
35. Actavis UK Ltd. Patient Information Leaflet. Rivastigmine Actavis 1.5 mg, 3 mg, 4.5 mg, 6 mg hard capsules. 2016. https://www.medicines.org.uk/emc/medicine/25885.
36. BNF Online. Atomoxetine. 2017. https://www.medicinescomplete.com/mc/bnf/current/PHP2473-atomoxetine.htm.
37. Eli Lilly and Company Limited. Patient Information Leaflet. Strattera 10 mg, 18 mg, 25 mg, 40 mg, 60 mgm, 80 mg or 100 mg hard capsules (atomoxetine). 2015. https://www.medicines.org.uk/emc/medicine/14549.
38. BNF Online. Dexamfetamine sulfate (Dexamphetamine sulfate). 2017. https://www.medicinescomplete.com/mc/bnf/current/PHP2475-dexamfetamine-sulfate.htm.
39. Flynn Pharma Ltd. Summary of Product Characteristic. Amfexa 5mg Tablets (dexamfetamine sulphate). 2016. https://www.medicines.org.uk/emc/product/5004.
40. BNF Online. Lisdexamfetamine mesilate. 2017. https://www.medicinescomplete.com/mc/bnf/current/PHP2478-lisdexamfetamine-mesilate.htm.
41. Shire Pharmaceuticals Limited. Patient Information Leaflet. Elvanse 20 mg, 30 mg, 40 mg, 50 mg, 60 mg & 70 mg Capsules, hard (lisdexamfetamine). 2016. https://www.medicines.org.uk/emc/medicine/27443.
42. BNF Online. Disulfiram. 2017. https://www.medicinescomplete.com/mc/bnf/current/PHP3185-disulfiram.htm.
43. Actavis UK Ltd. Patient Information Leaflet. Disulfiram Tablets 200 mg. 2015. https://www.medicines.org.uk/emc/medicine/3048.
44. BNF Online. Lithium carbonate. 2017. https://www.medicinescomplete.com/mc/bnf/current/PHP2337-lithium-carbonate.htm.
45. Sanofi. Patient Information Leaflet. Priadel 200 mg & 400 mg prolonged release tablets (lithium). 2017. https://www.medicines.org.uk/emc/medicine/11006.
46. BNF Online. Moclobemide. 2017. https://www.medicinescomplete.com/mc/bnf/current/PHP2410-moclobemide.htm.
47. Meda Pharmaceuticals. Patient Information Leaflet. Manerix 150 mg and 300 mg (moclobemide). 2014. https://www.medicines.org.uk/emc/medicine/22283.
48. BNF Online. Memantine hydrochloride. 2017. https://www.medicinescomplete.com/mc/bnf/current/PHP3248-memantine-hydrochloride.htm.
49. Accord Healthcare Limited. Patient Information Leaflet. Memantine Accord 5, 10, 15 & 20 mg film-coated tablets. 2016. https://www.medicines.org.uk/emc/medicine/28653.
50. BNF Online. Naltrexone hydrochloride. 2017. https://www.medicinescomplete.com/mc/bnf/current/PHP3233-naltrexone-hydrochloride.htm.
51. Accord Healthcare Limited. Patient Information Leaflet. Naltrexone Hydrochloride 50 mg Film-coated Tablets. 2014. https://www.medicines.org.uk/emc/medicine/25828.
52. BNF Online. Agomelatine. 2017. https://www.medicinescomplete.com/mc/bnf/current/PHP2440-agomelatine.htm.
53. Servier Laboratories Limited. Patient Information Leaflet. Valdoxan (agomelatine). 2016. https://www.medicines.org.uk/emc/medicine/21841.
54. BNF Online. Duloxetine. 2017. https://www.medicinescomplete.com/mc/bnf/current/PHP2442-duloxetine.htm7.
55. Consilient Health Ltd. Patient Information Leaflet. Duloxetine 20 mg & 40 mg gastro-resistant capsules. 2015. https://www.medicines.org.uk/emc/medicine/30379.
56. BNF Online. Mianserin hydrochloride. 2017. https://www.medicinescomplete.com/mc/bnf/current/PHP2390-mianserin-hydrochloride.htm.
57. Generics UK T/A Mylan. Patient Information Leaflet. Mianserin 30 mg film-coated tablets. 2017. https://www.medicines.org.uk/emc/medicine/33541.
58. BNF Online. Reboxetine. 2017. https://www.medicinescomplete.com/mc/bnf/current/PHP2454-reboxetine.htm.
59. Pfizer Limited. Patient Information Leaflet. Edronax 4 mg Tablets (reboxetine). 2017. https://www.medicines.org.uk/emc/medicine/8082.
60. BNF Online. Trazodone hydrochloride. 2017. https://www.medicinescomplete.com/mc/bnf/current/PHP2392-trazodone-hydrochloride.htm.
61. Concordia International. Patient Information Leaflet. Trazodone 50 mg & 100 mg Capsules. 2017. https://www.medicines.org.uk/emc/medicine/31059.

CHAPTER 14

62. BNF Online. Venlafaxine. 2017. https://www.medicinescomplete.com/mc/bnf/current/PHP2459-venlafaxine.htm.

63. Dexcel Pharma Ltd. Patient Information Leaflet. Venlafaxine 37.5 mg, 75 mg Tablets. 2017. https://www.medicines.org.uk/emc/medicine/26862.

64. BNF Online. Pregabalin. 2017. https://www.medicinescomplete.com/mc/bnf/current/PHP2933-pregabalin.htm.

65. Aurobindo Pharma - Milpharm Ltd. Patient Information Leaflet. Pregabalin 25 mg, 50 mg, 75 mg, 100 mg, 150 mg, 200 mg, 225 mg, & 300 mg capsules. 2015. https://www.medicines.org.uk/emc/medicine/30646.

66. BNF Online. Citalopram. 2017. https://www.medicinescomplete.com/mc/bnf/current/PHP2421-citalopram.htm.

67. Aurobindo Pharma - Milpharm Ltd. Patient Information Leaflet. Citalopram 10 mg/20 mg/40 mg Tablets. 2017. https://www.medicines.org.uk/emc/PIL.23219.latest.pdf.

68. BNF Online. Escitalopram. 2017. https://www.medicinescomplete.com/mc/bnf/current/PHP2424-escitalopram.htm.

69. Consilient Health Ltd. Escitalopram 5 mg, 10 mg and 20 mg film-coated tablets. 2016. https://www.medicines.org.uk/emc/PIL.31930.latest.pdf.

70. BNF Online. Fluvoxamine maleate. 2017. https://www.medicinescomplete.com/mc/bnf/current/PHP2429-fluvoxamine-maleate.htm.

71. Wockhardt UK Ltd. Patient Information Leaflet. Fluvoxamine 50 mg & 100 mg Film-Coated Tablets. 2017. https://www.medicines.org.uk/emc/PIL.18758.latest.pdf.

72. BNF Online. Paroxetine. 2017. https://www.medicinescomplete.com/mc/bnf/current/PHP2432-paroxetine.htm.

73. GlaxoSmithKline UK. Patient Information Leaflet. Seroxat 10 mg, 20 mg and 30 mg film-coated tablets (paroxetine). 2015. http://www.medicines.org.uk/emc/PIL.3185.latest.pdf.

74. BNF Online. Sertraline. 2017. https://www.medicinescomplete.com/mc/bnf/current/PHP2435-sertraline.htm.

75. Ranbaxy (UK) Limited. Patient Information Leaflet. Sertraline 50 mg & 100 mg Film-coated Tablets. 2016. https://www.medicines.org.uk/emc/PIL.32459.latest.pdf.

76. BNF Online. Vortioxetine. 2017. https://www.medicinescomplete.com/mc/bnf/current/PHP200772-vortioxetine.htm.

77. Lundbeck Limited. Summary of Product Characteristics. Brintellix (vortioxetine) tablets 5, 10 and 20 mg. 2017. https://www.medicines.org.uk/emc/medicine/30904.

78. BNF Online. Amitriptyline hydrochloride. 2017. https://www.medicinescomplete.com/mc/bnf/current/PHP2362-amitriptyline-hydrochloride.htm.

79. Actavis UK Ltd. Patient Information Leaflet. Amitriptyline 10 mg, 25 mg and 50 mg tablets. 2017. https://www.medicines.org.uk/emc/medicine/18030.

80. BNF Online. Clomipramine hydrochloride. 2017. https://www.medicinescomplete.com/mc/bnf/current/PHP2369-clomipramine-hydrochloride.htm.

81. Generics UK T/A Mylan. Patient Information Leaflet. Clomipramine 10 mg, 25 mg and 50 mg Capsules, Hard. 2017. https://www.medicines.org.uk/emc/medicine/33269.

82. BNF Online. Dosulepin hydrochloride (Dothiepin hydrochloride). 2017. https://www.medicinescomplete.com/mc/bnf/current/PHP2374-dosulepin-hydrochloride.htm.

83. Medicines and Healthcare Products Regulatory Agency. Dosulepin 75 mg tablets and Dosulepin 25 mg Capsules Dosulepin hydrochloride. 2010. http://www.mhra.gov.uk/home/groups/spcpil/documents/spcpil/con1473654797484.pdf.

84. BNF Online. Doxepin. 2017. https://www.medicinescomplete.com/mc/bnf/current/PHP2377-doxepin.htm.

85. Marlborough Pharmaceuticals Ltd. Patient Information Leaflet. Doxepin 25 mg and 50 mg Capsules. 2014. https://www.medicines.org.uk/emc/medicine/28800.

86. BNF Online. Imipramine hydrochloride. 2017. https://www.medicinescomplete.com/mc/bnf/current/PHP2379-imipramine-hydrochloride.htm.

87. Actavis UK Ltd. Patient Information Leaflet. Imipramine Tablets 10 mg, 25 mg. 2017. https://www.medicines.org.uk/emc/medicine/18094.

88. BNF Online. Nortriptyline. 2017. https://www.medicinescomplete.com/mc/bnf/current/PHP2383-nortriptyline.htm.

89. Auden Mckenzie (Pharma Division) Ltd. Patient Information Leaflet. Nortriptyline 10 mg and 25 mg Tablets (Lime Pharma). 2016. https://www.medicines.org.uk/emc/medicine/31448.

90. BNF Online. Trimipramine. 2017. https://www.medicinescomplete.com/mc/bnf/current/PHP2386-trimipramine.htm.

91. Concordia International. Patient Information Leaflet. Trimipramine 10 mg and 25 mg tablets. 2017. https://www.medicines.org.uk/emc/medicine/31037.

92. Actavis UK Ltd. Summary of Product Characteristics. Lamotrigine 25 mg Tablets. 2015. https://www.medicines.org.uk/emc/medicine/23986.

Biochemical and haematological effects of psychotropic medications

Almost all psychotropic medications have haematology- or biochemistry-related adverse effects that may be detected using routine blood tests. While many of these changes are idiosyncratic and not clinically significant, others, such as the agranulocytosis associated with agents such as clozapine, will require regular monitoring of the full blood count. In general, where an agent has a high incidence of biochemical/haematological adverse effects or a rare but potentially fatal effect, regular monitoring is required as discussed in other sections.

For other agents, laboratory-detectable adverse effects are comparatively rare (prevalence usually less than 1%), often reversible upon cessation of the putative offending agent and not always clinically significant. It should further be noted that medical comorbidity, polypharmacy and the effects of non-prescribed agents including substances of abuse and alcohol may also influence biochemical and haematological parameters. In some cases, where a clear temporal association between starting the agent and the onset of laboratory changes is unclear, then withdrawal and re-challenge with the agent in question may be considered. Where there is doubt as to the aetiology and significance of the effect, the appropriate source of expert advice should always be consulted.

Tables 14.2 and 14.3 summarise those agents with identified biochemical and haematological effects, with information compiled from various sources.[1–8] In many cases the evidence for these various effects is limited, with information obtained mostly from case reports, case series and information supplied by manufacturers. For further details about each individual agent, the reader is encouraged to consult the appropriate section of the *Guidelines* as well as other specialist sources, particularly product literature relating to individual drugs.

References

1. BMJ Group and Pharmaceutical Press. British National Formulary. 2017. https://www.medicinescomplete.com/.
2. Aronson J. *Meyler's Side Effects of Drugs: The International Encyclopedia of Adverse Drug Reactions and Interactions*. Oxford: Elsevier Science; 2015.
3. Foster R. *Clinical Laboratory Investigation and Psychiatry. A Practical Handbook*. New York: Informa; 2008.
4. Oyesanmi O et al. Hematologic side effects of psychotropics. Psychosomatics 1999; 40:414–421.
5. Stubner S et al. Blood dyscrasias induced by psychotropic drugs. Pharmacopsychiatry 2004; 37 Suppl 1:S70–S78.
6. Pharmaceutical Press. Martindale: The Complete Drug Reference (online). 2017. https://www.medicinescomplete.com/.
7. National Institutes of Health. Clinical and Research Information on Drug-Induced Liver Injury. 2017. https://livertox.nih.gov.
8. Medicines Complete (Online). AHFS Drug Information. 2017. https://www.medicinescomplete.com/mc/ahfs/current/.
9. Association for Clinical Biochemistry and Laboratory Medicine. Analyte Monographs Alongside the National Library of Medicine Catalogue. 2017. http://www.acb.org.uk/whatwedo/science/amalc.aspx.

Table 14.2 Summary of biochemical changes associated with psychotropic agents

Parameter	Reference range[9]	Agents reported to raise levels	Agents reported to lower levels
Alanine aminotransferase (ALT)	Females: ≤34 U/L Males: ≤45 U/L (may be higher in obese subjects)	**Antipsychotics:** asenapine, benperidol, cariprazine, clozapine, haloperidol, loxapine, olanzapine, phenothiazines, quetiapine, risperidone/ paliperidone **Antidepressants:** agomelatine, bupropion, MAOIs, mianserin, mirtazapine, SNRIs, SSRIs (especially paroxetine and sertraline), TCAs, trazodone, vortioxetine **Anxiolytics/hypnotics:** barbiturates, benzodiazepines, buspirone, clomethiazole, promethazine, suvorexant, tasimelteon, zolpidem **Mood stabilisers:** carbamazepine, lamotrigine, valproate **Other:** alcohol, atomoxetine, beta blockers, caffeine, cocaine, disulfiram, naltrexone, opioids, stimulants (abused)	Vigabatrin
Albumin	35–50 g/L (gradually decreases after age 40)	Microalbuminuria may be a feature of metabolic syndrome secondary to psychotropic use (especially phenothiazines, clozapine, olanzapine and possibly quetiapine)	Chronic use of amphetamine or cocaine
Alkaline phosphatase	50–120 U/L	Baclofen, beta blockers, benzodiazepines, caffeine (excess/chronic use), carbamazepine, citalopram, clozapine, disulfiram, duloxetine, galantamine, haloperidol, loxapine, memantine, modafinil, nortriptyline, olanzapine, phenytoin, sertraline, topiramate, trazodone, valproate; also associated with agents causing NMS	Buprenorphine, fluoxetine (in children), zolpidem (rarely)
Ammonia	11–32 µmol/L (increased following meals and exercise)	Barbiturates, carbamazepine, tobacco smoking, topiramate, valproate (may present with signs of encephalopathy)	None known

(Continued)

CHAPTER 14

Table 14.2 (*Continued*)

Parameter	Reference range[9]	Agents reported to raise levels	Agents reported to lower levels
Amylase	28–100 U/L	Alcohol (acute), donepezil, opioids, pregabalin, rivastigmine, SSRIs (rarely) **Agents associated with pancreatitis:** alcohol, carbamazepine, clozapine, olanzapine, valproate	None known
Aspartate aminotransferase (AST)	Females: ≤34 U/L Males: ≤45 U/L	As for alanine transferase; baclofen. Note: ALT is preferred as an indicator of liver damage	Trifluoperazine, vigabatrin
Bicarbonate	22–29 mmol/L	Laxative abuse	Agents associated with SIADH: all antidepressants, antipsychotics (clozapine, haloperidol, olanzapine, phenothiazines, pimozide, risperidone/paliperidone, quetiapine); carbamazepine; also associated with agents causing metabolic acidosis (alcohol, cocaine, topiramate, zonisamide)
Bilirubin	≤21 µmol/L (total)	Amitriptyline, atomoxetine, benzodiazepines, carbamazepine, chlordiazepoxide, chlorpromazine, citalopram, clomethiazole, clozapine, disulfiram, imipramine, fluphenazine, lamotrigine, meprobamate, milnacipran, olanzapine, phenothiazines, phenytoin, promethazine, sertraline, valproate; also associated with agents causing cholestasis/hepatic damage	Barbiturates
C-reactive protein	<10 mg/L	Buprenorphine (rare); also associated with agents causing myocarditis (clozapine)	None known
Calcium	2.20–2.60 mmol/L (total, adjusted) 1.15–1.34 mmol/L (ionised)	Lithium (rare)	Barbiturates, carbamazepine, haloperidol, valproate
Carbohydrate-deficient transferrin (CDT)	≤1.5%	Alcohol (CDT levels of 1.6–1.9% suggest high intake; levels ≥2% suggest excessive intake)	None known

Table 14.2 (*Continued*)

Parameter	Reference range[9]	Agents reported to raise levels	Agents reported to lower levels
Chloride	95–108 mmol/L	Agents causing hyperchloraemic metabolic acidosis: topiramate, zonisamide	Medications associated with SIADH: all antidepressants, antipsychotics (clozapine, haloperidol, olanzapine, phenothiazines, pimozide, risperidone/paliperidone, quetiapine); carbamazepine, laxative abuse
Cholesterol (total)	≤5.2 mmol/L (usually compared to recommended action limits rather than reference ranges)	Antipsychotics, especially those implicated in the metabolic syndrome (phenothiazines, clozapine, olanzapine and quetiapine). Rarely: aripiprazole, beta blockers (additive effects with clozapine), carbamazepine, disulfiram, duloxetine, memantine, mirtazapine, modafinil, phenytoin, rivastigmine, sertraline, venlafaxine	Prazosin, thyroid agents
Creatine kinase	Females: 25–200 U/L Males: 40–320 U/L (range for Caucasians; may be higher in other ethnic groups)	Brexpiprazole, cariprazine, clonidine, clozapine (when associated with seizures), cocaine, dexamfetamine, donepezil, olanzapine, pregabalin; also associated with agents causing NMS and SIADH; agents administered intramuscularly	None known
Creatinine	Females: 55–100 µmol/L Males: 60–120 µmol/L	Clozapine, lithium, lurasidone, thioridazine, valproate, medications associated with rhabdomyolysis (benzodiazepines, dexamfetamine, pregabalin, thioridazine); also associated with agents causing renal impairment, NMS and SIADH	None known
Ferritin	Females: 15–150 µg/L Males: 30–400 µg/L (increases with age)	Alcohol (acutely and in alcoholic liver disease)	None known

(*Continued*)

CHAPTER 14

Table 14.2 (*Continued*)

Parameter	Reference range[9]	Agents reported to raise levels	Agents reported to lower levels
γ-Glutamyl transferase (GGT)	Females: ≤38 U/L Males: ≤55 U/L (limits two-fold higher in persons of African ancestry)	**Antidepressants:** mirtazapine, SSRIs (paroxetine and sertraline implicated), TCAs, trazodone, venlafaxine **Anticonvulsants/mood stabilisers:** carbamazepine, lamotrigine, phenytoin, phenobarbitone, valproate **Antipsychotics:** benperidol, chlorpromazine, clozapine, fluphenazine, haloperidol, olanzapine, quetiapine **Other:** alcohol, barbiturates, clomethiazole, dexamphetamine, modafinil, tobacco smoking	None known
Glucose	Fasting: 2.8–6.1 mmol/L Random: <11.1 mmol/L	**Antidepressants:** MAOIs*, SSRIs/SNRIs*, TCAs* **Antipsychotics:** chlorpromazine, clozapine, haloperidol*, olanzapine*, quetiapine and others **Substances of abuse:** amfetamine, methadone, opioids **Other:** baclofen, beta blockers*, bupropion*, caffeine* (in diabetics), clonidine, donepezil, gabapentin, galantamine, lithium*, nicotine, sympathomimetics, thyroid agents	Alcohol; rarely with duloxetine, haloperidol, pregabalin, TCAs Medications associated with metabolic syndrome may result in raised or decreased glucose levels
HbA$_{1c}$	20–39 mmol/mol		Lithium, MAOIs, SSRIs
Lactate dehydrogenase	90–200 U/L (levels rise gradually with age)	Benzodiazepines, clozapine, methadone, TCAs (especially imipramine), valproate, also associated with agents causing NMS	None known
Lipoproteins: HDL	>1.2 mmol/L	Carbamazepine, nicotine, phenobarbital, phenytoin	Beta blockers, olanzapine, phenothiazines, valproate
Lipoproteins: LDL	<3.5 mmol/L	Beta blockers, caffeine (controversial), carbamazepine, chlorpromazine, clozapine, iloperidone, memantine, mirtazapine, modafinil, olanzapine, phenothiazines, quetiapine, risperidone/ paliperidone, rivastigmine, venlafaxine	Prazosin

Table 14.2 (*Continued*)

Parameter	Reference range[9]	Agents reported to raise levels	Agents reported to lower levels
Phosphate	0.8–1.5 mmol/L	Dexamfetamine; also associated with agents causing NMS	Carbamazepine, lithium, mianserin, topiramate
Potassium	3.5–5.3 mmol/L	Beta blockers, lithium	Alcohol, disulfiram, caffeine, cocaine, haloperidol, lithium, mianserin, pregabalin, reboxetine, rivastigmine, sodium oxybate, sympathomimetics, topiramate, zonisamide; may also be a feature of delirium tremens
Prolactin	Normal: <350 mU/L Abnormal: >600 mU/L;	**Antidepressants:** especially amoxapine, MAOIs and TCAs; SSRIs and venlafaxine also implicated **Antipsychotics:** amisulpride, haloperidol, pimozide, risperidone/paliperidone, sulpiride and others (aripiprazole[†], asenapine, brexpiprazole, cariprazine, clozapine, lurasidone, olanzapine, quetiapine and ziprasidone have minimal effects on prolactin levels) **Other:** benzodiazepines, buspirone, opioids, ramelteon, tetrabenazine	Aripiprazole, dopamine agonists, pirenzepine
Protein (total)	60–80 g/L	None known	Olanzapine (rarely)
Sodium	133–146 mmol/L	Lithium (in overdose)	**Antidepressants:** especially SSRIs/SNRIs; others also implicated **Antipsychotics:** all (via SIADH) **Mood stabilisers:** carbamazepine, lithium, valproate **Other:** benzodiazepines, clonidine, donepezil, memantine, rivastigmine Hyponatraemia should be considered in any patient on an antidepressant who develops confusion, convulsions or drowsiness
Testosterone	Males: 9.9–27.8 nmol/L Females: 0.22–2.9 nmol/L	Diazepam	Opioids, ramelteon
Thyroid-stimulating hormone	0.3–4.0 mU/L	Aripiprazole, carbamazepine, lithium, quetiapine, rivastigmine, sertraline, valproate (slightly)	Moclobemide, thyroid agents

(*Continued*)

Table 14.2 (*Continued*)

Parameter	Reference range[9]	Agents reported to raise levels	Agents reported to lower levels
Thyroxine	Free: 9–26 pmol/L Total: 60–150 nmol/L	Rarely; amfetamine (heavy abuse), moclobemide, propranolol	Barbiturates, carbamazepine, liothyronine, lithium (causes decreased T4 secretion), opioids, phenytoin, valproate. Rarely implicated: aripiprazole, clozapine, quetiapine, rivastigmine, sertraline
Triglycerides			None known
Tri-iodothyronine	Free 3.0–6.8 pmol/L; total 1.2–2.9 nmol/L	Heroin, methadone	Free T3: valproate; total T3: carbamazepine, lithium, propranolol
Urate (uric acid)	Females: 0.16–0.36 mmol/L Males: 0.21–0.43 mmol/L (increases with age)	Alcohol (acute), caffeine (false positive), clozapine, levodopa, olanzapine, pindolol, prazosin, topiramate, zonisamide	Sertraline (slightly)
Urea	2.5–7.8 mmol/L (increases with age)	Carbamazepine, levodopa; rarely with agents associated with anticonvulsant hypersensitivity syndrome and rhabdomyolysis	None known

* May also be associated with hypoglycaemia.
† May also be associated with subnormal prolactin levels.
HDL, high-density lipoprotein; LDL, low-density lipoprotein; MAOI, monoamine oxidase inhibitor; NMS, neuroleptic malignant syndrome; SIADH, syndrome of inappropriate antidiuretic hormone; SNRI, serotonin–noradrenaline reuptake inhibitor; SSRI, selective serotonin reuptake inhibitor; TCA, tricyclic antidepressant.

Table 14.3 Summary of haematological changes associated with psychotropic agents

Parameter	Reference range	Agents reported to raise levels	Agents reported to lower levels
Activated partial thromboplastin time	23–33 seconds	Phenothiazines (especially chlorpromazine)	Modafinil (rare)
Basophils	$0.0–0.1 \times 10^9$/L	Clozapine, TCAs (especially desipramine)	None known
Eosinophils	$0.04–0.40 \times 10^9$/L	Amoxapine, beta blockers, bupropion, buspirone, carbamazepine, chloral hydrate, chlorpromazine, clonazepam, clozapine, donepezil, fluphenazine, haloperidol, loxapine, meprobamate, maprotiline, methylphenidate (IV abuse only), modafinil, naltrexone (parenterally administered), olanzapine, promethazine, quetiapine, risperidone/paliperidone, SSRIs, TCAs, tetrazepam, tryptophan*, valproate, venlafaxine; may also be a feature of agents causing a hypersensitivity syndrome	None known
Erythrocyte sedimentation rate	Females: 1–12 mm/h Males: 1–10 mm/h (increases with age)	Clozapine, dexamfetamine, levomepromazine, maprotiline, SSRIs	Buprenorphine
Haemoglobin	Females: 115–165 g/L Males: 130–180 g/L	Clozapine, testosterone, tobacco smoking	Aripiprazole, barbiturates, buprenorphine, bupropion, carbamazepine, chlordiazepoxide, chlorpromazine, donepezil, duloxetine, galantamine, MAOIs, memantine, meprobamate, mianserin, phenytoin, promethazine, rivastigmine, tramadol, trifluoperazine, vigabatrin
Lymphocytes	$1.5–4.5 \times 10^9$/L	Naltrexone, opioids, tobacco smoking, valproate; may also be a feature of drugs causing hypersensitivity syndrome	Alcohol (chronic), chloral hydrate, clozapine, lithium, mirtazapine (rarely)

(*Continued*)

Table 14.3 (*Continued*)

Parameter	Reference range	Agents reported to raise levels	Agents reported to lower levels
Mean cell haemoglobin	27–32 pg	Medications associated with megaloblastic anaemia, e.g. all anticonvulsants, nitrous oxide	None known
Mean cell haemoglobin concentration	320–360 g/L		
Mean cell volume	80–100 fL	Alcohol	
Monocytes	0.2–0.8 × 10⁹/L	Haloperidol	None known
Neutrophils	2.0–7.5 × 10⁹/L (may be lower in people of African descent due to benign ethnic neutropenia)	Bupropion, carbamazepine†, chlorpromazine, citalopram, clozapine†, duloxetine, fluoxetine, fluphenazine, haloperidol, lamotrigine, lithium, maprotiline, olanzapine, quetiapine, risperidone/ paliperidone, rivastigmine, tiotixene, trazodone, venlafaxine	**Agents associated with agranulocytosis:** amoxapine, aripiprazole, barbiturates, carbamazepine, chlordiazepoxide, chlorpromazine, clozapine‡, cocaine (adulterated), diazepam, fluphenazine, haloperidol, meprobamate, mianserin, mirtazapine, olanzapine, pirenzepine, promethazine, risperidone/paliperidone, TCAs (especially imipramine), tranylcypromine, valproate **Agents associated with leucopenia:** amitriptyline, amoxapine, asenapine, bupropion, carbamazepine, cariprazine, chlorpromazine, citalopram, clomipramine, clonazepam, clozapine, duloxetine, fluoxetine, fluphenazine, galantamine, haloperidol, lamotrigine, lorazepam, lurasidone, memantine, meprobamate, mianserin, mirtazapine, modafinil, nitrous oxide, olanzapine, oxazepam, phenelzine, pregabalin, promethazine, quetiapine, tranylcypromine, valproate, venlafaxine, ziprasidone **Agents associated with neutropenia:** sertraline, trazodone, valproate
Packed cell volume	Females: 0.37–0.47 L/L Males: 0.40–0.52 L/L	Clozapine (rare), testosterone	Benzodiazepines (rare), buprenorphine, naltrexone, vigabatrin

Table 14.3 (*Continued*)

Parameter	Reference range	Agents reported to raise levels	Agents reported to lower levels
Platelets	$150–450 \times 10^9$/L	Lamotrigine, lithium[†]	Alcohol, barbiturates, beta blockers, benzodiazepines, bupropion, buspirone, carbamazepine, chlordiazepoxide, chlorpromazine, clonazepam, clonidine, clozapine[†], cocaine, diazepam, donepezil, duloxetine, fluoxetine, fluphenazine, lamotrigine, meprobamate, methadone, methylphenidate, mirtazapine, naltrexone, nitrous oxide, olanzapine, pirenzepine, promethazine, quetiapine, risperidone/paliperidone, rivastigmine, sertraline, TCAs, tranylcypromine, trazodone, trifluoperazine, valproate, venlafaxine, ziprasidone; may also be a feature of drugs causing hypersensitivity syndrome **Agents associated with impaired platelet aggregation:** chlordiazepoxide, citalopram, diazepam, fluoxetine, fluvoxamine, paroxetine, piracetam, sertraline, valproate
Prothrombin time (PT)/international normalised ratio (INR)	PT: 10–13 seconds INR: 0.8–1.2	Chloral hydrate, disulfiram, fluoxetine, fluvoxamine, mirtazapine, valproate; also agents interacting with warfarin	Barbiturates, carbamazepine, phenytoin, tiotixene
Red blood count	Males: $4.5–6.5 \times 10^{12}$/L Females: $3.8–5.8 \times 10^{12}$/L	Lithium, testosterone	Buprenorphine, carbamazepine, chlordiazepoxide, chlorpromazine, donepezil, haloperidol, meprobamate, phenytoin, quetiapine, trifluoperazine
Red cell distribution width	11.5–14.5%	Agents associated with anaemia, e.g. carbamazepine, chlordiazepoxide, citalopram, clonazepam, diazepam, lamotrigine, memantine, mirtazapine, sertraline, tranylcypromine, trazodone, valproate, venlafaxine	None known
Reticulocyte count	0.5–2.5% (or $50–100 \times 10^9$/L)	None known	Carbamazepine, chlordiazepoxide, chlorpromazine, meprobamate, phenytoin, trifluoperazine **Agents associated with pure red cell aplasia:** carbamazepine, clozapine, valproate

* Previous reports of eosinophilia–myalgia syndrome may have been due to a contaminant from a single manufacturer.
† May raise or lower levels.
‡ Note that in rare cases clozapine has been associated with a 'morning pseudo-neutropenia' with lower levels of circulating neutrophil levels. As neutrophil counts may show circadian rhythms, repeating the full blood count at a later time of day may be instructive.
IV, intravenous; MAOI, monoamine oxidase inhibitor; SSRI, selective serotonin reuptake inhibitor; TCA, tricyclic antidepressant.

Summary of psychiatric adverse effects of non-psychotropic medications

It is increasingly recognised that non-psychotropic medications can induce a wide range of psychiatric symptoms.[1] Up to two-thirds of all drugs have potential psychiatric adverse effects listed in their product labelling,[2] although in most cases the evidence supporting a causal link is limited. Psychiatric adverse effects are poorly characterised in drug clinical trials, often only becoming apparent during post-marketing surveillance.[3] Given this level of uncertainty, suspected psychiatric adverse effects should be diagnosed and managed on a case-by-case basis. As a general guide, the psychiatric adverse effects of non-psychotropic medications are shown in Table 14.4. For individual drugs and agents not listed below, additional sources of information and the product literature should be consulted. Note that psychiatric adverse effects of drugs used in psychiatry and drugs for human immunodeficiency virus (HIV) are summarised elsewhere in the *Guidelines*.

Table 14.4 Summary of psychiatric adverse drug reactions (ADRs) with non-psychotropic medications[4-7]

Drug	Psychiatric adverse effect	Comment
ACE inhibitors		
e.g. captopril, lisinopril	Fatigue, hallucinations, delirium, mood disturbances	Captopril most closely associated with mood effects. Overall, limited psychiatric ADRs
Analgesics		
Opioids	Sedation, dysphoria, confusion, mood changes including euphoria, sleep disturbances, hallucinations, psychosis, delirium, dependence	Psychiatric ADRs are relatively common with opioids. Psychosis during opioid withdrawal has also been reported rarely[8]
5-HT$_1$ agonists (e.g. sumatriptan)	Fatigue, anxiety, panic attacks	
Antibiotics		
Cephalosporins, penicillins, quinolones (including fluoroquinolones), tetracyclines	Sleep disturbances (insomnia and somnolence, abnormal dreams, nightmares), anxiety, delirium and confusional states, depression and agitation, psychotic symptoms (e.g. hallucinations, suicidal ideation)	All antibiotics can cause delirium. Patients with underlying medical conditions can be at higher risk of developing psychiatric ADRs. Of the quinolones, ciprofloxacin causes the most psychiatric ADRs, including mood disturbances, agitation and confusion. Onset of psychiatric ADRs can be very fast, e.g. after one dose
Metronidazole	Psychosis	Rare but established association
Anticonvulsants		
Carbamazepine	Depression, agitation, sedation, psychosis, cognitive impairment, delirium	Psychosis also reported with oxcarbazepine
Ethosuximide	Mood changes, irritability, sleep disturbances, psychosis, delirium	

Table 14.4 (*Continued*)

Drug	Psychiatric adverse effect	Comment
Levetiracetam	Irritability, depression, mood disturbances, sedation, insomnia, sleep disturbances, aggression, psychosis	
Perampanel	Aggression, anger, anxiety and confusional states. Suicidal ideation and attempts	In up to 20% of patients. Effects may be dose-related and tend to occur nearer the onset of treatment
Phenytoin	Agitation, insomnia, delirium, psychosis	Psychosis also reported with fosphenytoin
Tiagabine	Depression and labile mood, anxiety, insomnia, confusion, nervousness, concentration difficulties, aggression, psychosis	
Topiramate	Psychosis, depression and emotional lability, sleep disturbances, cognitive dysfunction, paraesthesia, behavioural changes	Psychosis is much more common with topiramate (6%) than with other anticonvulsants. Cognitive complaints are the most common psychiatric adverse effect
Vigabatrin	Agitation, lethargy, irritability, depression, sleep disturbances, mood disturbances including mania, psychosis, cognitive impairment	Psychosis is more common with vigabatrin (2–4%) than with other anti-epileptic drugs although it can be transient
Zonisamide	Agitation, irritability, confusion, depression, labile affect (mood), anxiety, insomnia, sleep disturbances, psychosis, anger and aggression, suicidal ideation and attempt	
Antimalarial agents		
Chloroquine, mefloquine	Psychosis including hallucinations, panic attacks, suicidal ideation and attempts, anxiety, depression, restlessness, confusion. Abnormal dreams/nightmares are very common with mefloquine	Symptoms begin very early in treatment. Patients should be advised to stop treatment if these develop, and seek medical advice. Psychiatric ADRs are more common with mefloquine than chloroquine. Reactions can even occur after discontinuation of the drug. Mefloquine should not be prescribed for patients with an active or a history of a psychiatric diagnosis
Antiparkinsonian treatments		
Levodopa	Visual hallucinations, depression, hypomania, sleep disturbances, abnormal dreams, cognitive impairment, agitation, psychosis, delirium	

CHAPTER 14

(*Continued*)

Table 14.4 (*Continued*)

Drug	Psychiatric adverse effect	Comment
Dopamine agonists	Sedation, psychomotor agitation, anxiety, akathisia, sleep disturbances, psychosis, cognitive impairment, delirium, visual hallucinations	These are associated with more psychiatric adverse effects than levodopa
Amantadine	Decreased concentration, sleep disturbances, visual hallucinations, irritability, anxiety, depression, euphoria, fatigue, psychosis, delirium	
Selegiline (MAO-B inhibitor)	Sleep disturbances, agitation, psychosis	Primary metabolites include levoamfetamines
Entacapone (COMT inhibitor)	Sleep disturbances, hallucinations, delirium	
Cardiovascular agents		
Beta blockers	Fatigue, sedation, sleep disturbances and nightmares, cognitive impairment, depression, hallucinations, psychosis, delirium	Disturbances more common with lipophilic beta blockers (e.g. propranolol, metoprolol) than with hydrophilic beta blockers (e.g. atenolol, sotalol, nadolol). Propranolol most commonly associated with depressive symptoms, but even with this drug, causality has not clearly been established. Reports of psychiatric ADRs from numerous clinical trials are equivocal
Calcium channel blockers (e.g. diltiazem, amlodipine)	Mood changes, lethargy, dysphoria, mania, psychosis, delirium, akathisia	Causal association not clearly demonstrated
Statins[9-11] (e.g. simvastatin, atorvastatin)	Cognitive impairment, memory impairment, depression, emotional lability, irritability, sleep disturbance	Causal associations between statins and changes in mood, sleep and cognition have not been established in systematic reviews of RCTs. Statins penetrate the blood–brain barrier; simvastatin has the highest permeability. Switching to hydrophilic statins (e.g. pravastatin, rosuvastatin) has been suggested in suspected cases of moderate–severe psychiatric ADRs
Corticosteroids		
Glucocorticoids (e.g. betamethasone, prednisolone, prednisone)	Mood disorders, suicidal ideation, euphoria, agitation, sleep disturbances, psychosis and delirium, dementia, cognitive impairment	Clear causal association. Onset of psychiatric ADRs is often very sudden, and within the first 1–2 weeks of starting treatment. Symptoms generally respond to dose decreases, and have been reported in association with several routes of administration (including oral, parenteral and inhaled), although are probably less common with inhalation. Symptoms usually resolve on gradual discontinuation, although duration of symptoms varies considerably

Table 14.4 (Continued)

Drug	Psychiatric adverse effect	Comment
Other agents		
Chemotherapeutic agents (e.g. 5-fluorouracil, asparaginase, bortezomib, ifosfamide, vincristine)	More commonly: cognitive impairment, delirium, psychosis Less commonly: depression, anxiety, suicidal ideation	Almost all chemotherapeutic agents are associated with significant psychiatric ADRs which may be multifactorial in origin (i.e. secondary to the disease process, ADRs and psychological distress). Cancer therapy-associated cognitive changes include difficulty in executive functions, multitasking, short-term memory recall and attention. Cognitive changes seem to be dose dependent, and certain drugs (methotrexate, fludarabine, cytarabine, 5-fluorouracil, cisplatin) are associated with worse cognitive effects
Cimetidine	Cognitive impairment, delirium	
Interferons α and β	Depression, loss of efficacy of previously effective antidepressants, suicidal ideation, delirium, non-specific psychiatric symptoms. Rare case reports of psychosis and mania with interferon-α	Psychiatric ADRs are relatively unlikely with interferon-β but much more widely reported with interferon-α. Interferon-α-associated depression responds to antidepressants, use of which can be preventive. Novel diagnostic biomarkers have been investigated to predict which patients are likely to develop interferon-α-associated psychiatric ADRs
Isotretinoin[12]	Depression, suicide, psychosis	Sporadic reports of psychiatric ADRs but a causal link between isotretinoin therapy and depression, anxiety, mood changes, or suicidal ideation/suicide has not been established. Rare, idiosyncratic reactions cannot be ruled out; if they occur the drug should be discontinued. Risk is no higher in those with prior suicide attempts and is not dose or treatment duration related

COMT, catechol-O-methyltransferase; MAO, monoamine oxidase; RCT, randomised controlled trial.

Differential diagnosis of psychiatric adverse effects

A wide range of confounding factors complicate the diagnosis (and perhaps also the recognition) of psychiatric adverse effects. For example, physical illness, co-prescribed medication, non-prescribed agents and pre-existing mental illness may all influence the clinical presentation and outcome. Factors determining the probability of a causal relationship between drugs and psychiatric adverse effects are shown in Box 14.2. To further support clinical decision-making, the Naranjo scale can be used to assess the likelihood of any adverse reaction being drug-related (Table 14.5). Although cessation of the implicated non-psychotropic drug might be indicated in some cases, such decisions require individual considerations beyond the scope of this book.

CHAPTER 14

> **Box 14.2** Factors determining the probability of a causal relationship between drugs and psychiatric adverse effects[4,13]
>
> - Temporal relationship between the drug exposure and the psychiatric adverse effect.
> - Evidence of the specific psychiatric adverse effects occurring with the suspected drug.
> - Plausible pharmacological mechanism for the psychiatric adverse effect (e.g. dopamine agonists and psychosis).
> - Presence of alternative explanations for symptoms (e.g. pre-existing mental illness, *de novo* psychiatric illness, other drugs).
> - Response of symptoms to the withdrawal of the drug.
> - Effect of re-challenge with the same drug.

Table 14.5 Adapted Naranjo adverse drug reactions (ADR) probability scale criteria[14]

Questions	Yes	No	NA/unknown
1. Are there previous *conclusive* reports on this reaction?	+1	0	0
2. Did the ADR appear after the suspected drug was administered?	+2	−1	0
3. Did the ADR improve when the drug was discontinued?	+1	0	0
4. Did the ADR appear with re-challenge?	+2	−1	0
5. Are there alternative causes for the ADR?	−1	+2	0
6. Did the reaction appear when placebo was given?	−1	+1	0
7. Was the drug detected in the blood at toxic levels?	+1	0	0
8. Was the ADR more severe when the dose was increased, or less severe when the dose was decreased?	+1	0	0
9. Did the patient have a similar reaction to the same or similar drugs in *any* previous exposure?	+1	0	0
10. Was the ADR confirmed by any objective evidence?	+1	0	0

Probability score: ≥9 = definite; 5–8 = probable; 1–4 = possible; ≤0 = doubtful.
NA, not applicable.

References

1. Rudorfer MV et al. Assessing psychiatric adverse effects during clinical drug development. Pharmaceut Med 2012; 26:363–394.
2. Smith DA. Psychiatric side effects of non-psychiatric drugs. S D J Med 1991; 44:291–292.
3. Holvey C et al. Psychiatric side effects of non-psychiatric drugs. Br J Hosp Med (Lond) 2010; 71:432–436.
4. Gupta A et al. Adverse psychiatric effects of non-psychotropic medications. B J Psych Advances 2016; 22:325–334.
5. Huffman JC et al. Neuropsychiatric consequences of cardiovascular medications. Dialogues Clin Neurosci 2007; 9:29–45.
6. Munjampalli SK et al. Medicinal-induced behavior disorders. Neurol Clin 2016; 34:133–169.
7. Parker C. Psychiatric effects of drugs for other disorders. Medicine 2016; 44:768–774.
8. Maremmani AG et al. Substance abuse and psychosis. The strange case of opioids. Eur Rev Med Pharmacol Sci 2014; 18:287–302.
9. Ott BR et al. Do statins impair cognition? A systematic review and meta-analysis of randomized controlled trials. J Gen Intern Med 2015; 30:348–358.
10. Swiger KJ et al. Statins, mood, sleep, and physical function: a systematic review. Eur J Clin Pharmacol 2014; 70:1413–1422.
11. Tuccori M et al. Neuropsychiatric adverse events associated with statins: epidemiology, pathophysiology, prevention and management. CNS Drugs 2014; 28:249–272.
12. Liu M et al. Neurological and neuropsychiatric adverse effects of dermatologic medications. CNS Drugs 2016; 30:1149–1168.
13. World Health Organization and Uppsala Monitoring Centre. The use of the WHO-UMC system for standardised case causality assessment. 2004. http://www.who.int/medicines/areas/quality_safety/safety_efficacy/WHOcausality_assessment.pdf.
14. Naranjo CA et al. A method for estimating the probability of adverse drug reactions. Clin Pharmacol Ther 1981; 30:239–245.

Prescribing drugs outside their licensed indications ('off-label' prescribing)

A Product Licence (PL) is granted when regulatory authorities are satisfied that the drug in question has proven efficacy in the treatment of a specified disorder, along with an acceptable adverse-effect profile, relative to the severity of the disorder being treated and other available treatments. Licensed indications are preparation specific, outlined in the SPC, and may be different for branded and generic formulations of the same drug.[1] In the USA, product 'labelling' has a similar legal status to EU licensing.

The decision of a manufacturer to seek a PL for a given indication is essentially a commercial one; potential sales are balanced against the cost of conducting the necessary clinical trials. It therefore follows that drugs may be effective outside their licensed indications for different disease states, age ranges, doses and durations. The absence of a formal PL or labelling may simply reflect the absence of controlled trials supporting the drug's efficacy in these areas. In other cases (e.g. sertraline or quetiapine in generalised anxiety disorder) there is sufficient evidence but a licence has not been sought by the manufacturer. Importantly, however, it is possible that trials have been conducted but have given negative results. Clinicians often assume that drugs with a similar mode of action will be similarly effective for a given indication, and in many cases this may be true. For example, the efficacy of aripiprazole, olanzapine, quetiapine and risperidone in reducing behavioural and psychological symptoms in dementia (BPSD) is similar,[2] yet only risperidone is licensed for this indication.

Prescribing a drug within its licence or labelling does not guarantee that the patient will come to no harm. Likewise, prescribing outside a licence does not mean that the risk–benefit ratio is automatically adverse. In the BPSD example given above, risperidone is not clearly better tolerated than other antipsychotic drugs.[2] Prescribing outside a licence, usually called 'off-label', does confer extra responsibilities on prescribers, who will be expected to be able to show that they acted in accordance with a respected body of medical opinion (the Bolam test)[3] and that their action was capable of withstanding logical analysis (the Bolitho test).[4] Both need to be considered alongside the Montgomery versus Lanarkshire Health Board appeal case decision,[5] which stated:

> An adult person of sound mind is entitled to decide which, if any, of the available forms of treatment to undergo, and her consent must be obtained before treatment interfering with her bodily integrity is undertaken. The doctor is therefore under a duty to take reasonable care to ensure that the patient is aware of any material risks involved in any recommended treatment, and of any reasonable alternative or variant treatments. The test of materiality is whether, in the circumstances of the particular case, a reasonable person in the patient's position would be likely to attach significance to the risk, or the doctor is or should reasonably be aware that the particular patient would be likely to attach significance to it.

Thus, in the UK, the prescriber has a duty to make a patient aware of any material risks associated with the prescribing of any medicines and to outline alternatives.

It has been suggested that off-label prescribing in psychiatry is less likely to be supported by a strong evidence base than off-label prescribing in other areas of medicine.[6]

CHAPTER 14

In psychiatry, small (underpowered) studies (with wide confidence intervals) often influence practice, particularly with respect to treatment-resistant illness. When these small studies are combined in the form of a meta-analysis, considerable heterogeneity is often found suggesting publication bias (that is, that some negative studies are not published). Treatments may therefore become incorporated into 'routine custom and practice' in the absence of any evidence supporting efficacy and/or tolerability, and these treatments may sometimes continue to be used despite the findings of later, larger, and more definitive negative studies and meta-analyses. The use of omega-3 fatty acids in schizophrenia is a good example of this.

The psychopharmacology special interest group at the Royal College of Psychiatrists has published a consensus statement on the use of licensed medicines for unlicensed uses[7] which was updated in late 2017.[8] They note that unlicensed use is common in general adult psychiatry, with cross-sectional studies showing that up to 50% of patients are prescribed at least one drug outside the terms of its licence. They also note that the prevalence of this type of prescribing is likely to be higher in patients under the age of 18 or over 65, in those with a learning disability, in women who are pregnant or lactating and in those patients who are cared for in forensic psychiatry settings. The main recommendations in the consensus statement are summarised in Box 14.3.

Box 14.3 Recommendations of the Royal College of Psychiatrists' consensus statement

Before prescribing 'off-label':

- Exclude licensed alternatives (e.g. they have proved ineffective or poorly tolerated).
- Ensure familiarity with the evidence base for the intended unlicensed use. If unsure, seek advice from another clinician (and possibly a specialist pharmacist).
- Consider and document the potential risks and benefits of the proposed treatment. Share this risk assessment with the patient, and carers if applicable. Document the discussion and the patient's consent or lack of capacity to consent.
- If prescribing responsibility is to be shared with primary care, ensure that the risk assessment and consent issues are shared with the GP.
- Monitor for efficacy and adverse effects; start a low dose and increase slowly.
- Withdraw any treatment that is ineffective or where emergent risks outweigh the benefits.

Examples of acceptable use of drugs outside their Product Licences/labels

Table 14.6 gives examples of common unlicensed uses of drugs in psychiatric practice. These examples would all fulfil the Bolam and Bolitho criteria in principle. An exhaustive list of unlicensed uses is impossible to prepare because:

- The evidence base is constantly changing.
- The expertise and experience of prescribers vary. A particular strategy may be justified in the hands of a specialist in psychopharmacology based in a tertiary referral centre but much more difficult to justify if initiated by someone with a special interest in psychotherapy who rarely prescribes.

Table 14.6 Examples of common unlicensed uses of drugs in psychiatric practice

Drug/drug group	Unlicensed use(s)	Further information
Second-generation antipsychotics	Psychotic illness other than schizophrenia	Licensed indications vary markedly, and in most cases are unlikely to reflect real differences in efficacy between drugs
Clozapine	Rapid-cycling bipolar disorder	Some evidence to support efficacy when standard treatments have failed to control symptoms
Cyproheptadine	Akathisia	Some evidence to support efficacy in this distressing and difficult to treat adverse effect of antipsychotics
Fluoxetine/sertraline	Generalised anxiety disorder	Substantial supporting evidence
Melatonin (Circadin)	Insomnia in children	Licence covers adults >55 years only. Probably preferable to unlicensed formulations of melatonin
Methylphenidate	ADHD in children under 6	Established clinical practice
Naltrexone	Self-injurious behaviour in people with learning disabilities	Limited evidence base. Acceptable in specialist hands
Sodium valproate	Treatment and prophylaxis of bipolar disorder	Established clinical practice

ADHD, attention deficit hyperactivity disorder.

Note that some drugs do not have a UK licence for any indication. Two commonly prescribed examples in psychiatric practice are immediate-release formulations of melatonin (used to treat insomnia in children and adolescents) and pirenzepine (used to treat clozapine-induced hypersalivation). Awareness of the evidence base and documentation of potential benefits, adverse effects and patient consent are especially important here.

References

1. Datapharm Communications Ltd. Summary of Product Characteristics. Electronic Medicines Compendium. 2014. http://www.medicines.org.uk/emc/.
2. Maher AR et al. Efficacy and comparative effectiveness of atypical antipsychotic medications for off-label uses in adults: a systematic review and meta-analysis. JAMA 2011; 306:1359–1369.
3. Bolam v Friern Barnet Hospital Management Committee. The Weekly Law Reports 1957; 1:582.
4. Bolitho v City and Hackney Health Authority. The Weekly Law Reports 1997; 3:1151.
5. British and Irish Legal Information Institute. Montgomery (Appellant) v Lanarkshire Health Board (Respondent) (Scotland). 2015. http://www.bailii.org/uk/cases/UKSC/2015/11.html.
6. Epstein RS et al. The many sides of off-label prescribing. Clin Pharmacol Ther 2012; 91:755–758.
7. Royal College of Psychiatrists. College Report 210. Use of licensed medicines for unlicensed applications in psychiatric practice (2nd edition). 2007. http://www.rcpsych.ac.uk/files/pdfversion/CR210.pdf.
8. Royal College of Psychiatrists Psychopharmacology Committee. Use of licensed medicines for unlicensed applications in psychiatric practice, 2nd edn. College Report CR210. 2017. http://www.rcpsych.ac.uk/files/pdfversion/CR210.pdf.

Further reading

Frank B et al. Psychotropic medications and informed consent: a review. Ann Clin Psychiatry 2008; 20:87–95.
General Medical Council. Good practice in prescribing and managing medicines and devices. 2013. http://www.gmc-uk.org/guidance/ethical_guidance/14316.asp.

CHAPTER 14

The Mental Health Act in England and Wales

The 1983 Mental Health Act (MHA), as amended by the 2007 MHA, is the legislation within England and Wales that provides the framework for detaining and treating people with mental disorder in hospital. It also allows for the supervision of people in the community.

The guidance here provides a quick summary of the sections that prescribers are likely to come across in their day-to-day work. It is not an exhaustive list. The Act has a statutory Code of Practice for practitioners, and Chapter 25 of the Code provides detailed guidance on the treatment rules of the Act.[1] The MHA may be accessed at www.legislation.gov.uk.

Civil and forensic detention sections

Section 2   Admission for assessment which lasts for up to 28 days.
Section 3   Admission for treatment which may last up to 6 months and is renewable.
Section 36   Remand to hospital for treatment.
Section 37   Hospital Order made by the courts (runs like an S3).
Notional 37   Treat as if subject to S37. This term is used informally under a number of different circumstances. One example is where a patient was previously detained under S47/49 and their restriction order expires.
Section 38   Interim Hospital Order.
Section 41   Restriction Order – an order made by the Crown Court restricting discharge. Accompanies S37 and is written as S37/41.
Section 47   Transfer to hospital of prisoners.
Section 49   A restriction order which usually accompanies S47. (Written as S47/49.)
Section 48   Applies to unsentenced prisoners in need of urgent treatment and is accompanied by S49. (Written as S48/49.)
Section 58   **Treatment requiring consent or a second opinion.** Please note **in law it is the Responsible Clinician (RC) who is accountable for the operation of S58.**

It is important to note that the power to treat under Section 58 is only for treatment of mental disorder. Physical treatment (generally) is governed by the normal rules of consent or, if the person lacks capacity, the authority of the Mental Capacity Act.

The RC is usually the patient's consultant. For the first 3 months of detention the RC may give medication (with or without consent) to a person under one of the detention sections named above for the treatment of their mental disorder. Thereafter the patient's consent or a second opinion must be sought. The 3 months countdown starts when medication for mental disorder is first administered while the patient is detained. Be aware that this includes a patient detained under S2 who is then, without a break, changed to and detained under S3. For practical purposes the 3-month rule is usually calculated from the date of first detention.

If a patient consents to treatment, the RC completes a form **T2**.

If a patient has not given consent or has not got the capacity to consent, a second opinion appointed doctor (SOAD) is called. The SOAD then completes a form **T3**.

A copy of the forms T2 and T3 should be kept with the patient's medication chart as recommended in paragraph 25.75 of the Code of Practice.[1]

Completion of forms T2 and T3

The following should be stated on the forms:

- the name of the drug **or** the class of drug
- if the class of drug is stated, the number of drugs allowed at any one time
- the route of administration
- the maximum dosage with reference to BNF guidance.

e.g. Antipsychotic, second generation × 1 (oral) within BNF maximum dose limits.

For a patient who has capacity and is consenting to treatment and is only willing to take a particular drug, it is appropriate for the RC to write the name of the drug instead of the name of the class of drug on the T2.

e.g. Olanzapine tablets only (oral) within BNF maximum dose limits.

A psychotropic drug not found in the BNF may be written on a T2 or T3 with its indication.

e.g. Melperone tablets (oral) up to a maximum of 25 mg daily for the treatment of schizophrenia.

Non-psychotropic drugs used for the treatment of mental disorder should be included on the T2 and T3, for example omega-3 fatty acids (fish oils) in schizophrenia. Antimuscarinic drugs used to treat hypersalivation and the extrapyramidal adverse effects of antipsychotic drugs should be included too.

Arranging and preparing for SOAD visits

The Code at paragraph 25.51 states:

> Clinicians should consider seeking a review by a specialist mental health pharmacist before seeking a SOAD certificate, particularly if the patient's medication regime is complex or unusual.

Statutory consultees

SOADs should consult with two people before issuing a T3. One must be a nurse. The other must not be a nurse or a doctor. Both must have been involved with the patient's treatment. These two people are known as statutory consultees. Mental health pharmacists can perform this role where they have been involved in any recent review of a patient's medication.

CHAPTER 14

The Code of Practice 24.52 states:

Statutory consultees may expect to have a private discussion with the SOAD and to be listened to with consideration. Issues that the consultees may be asked about include, but are not limited to:

- the proposed treatment and the patient's ability to consent to it;
- their understanding of the past and present views and wishes of the patient;
- other treatment options and the way in which the decision on the treatment proposal was arrived at;
- the patient's progress and the views of the patient's carers; and
- where relevant, the implications of imposing treatment on a patient who does not want it and the reasons why the patient is refusing treatment.

What is consent?

The Code of 24.34 defines consent as:

...the voluntary and continuing permission of a patient to be given a particular treatment, based on a sufficient knowledge of the purpose, nature, likely effects and risks of that treatment, including the likelihood of its success and any alternatives to it. Permission given under any unfair or undue pressure is not consent.

For a patient to consent formally they must have the 'capacity' to make a decision.

What is capacity?

The Mental Capacity Act 2005 states that:

- People must be assumed to have capacity unless it is established that they lack capacity.
- People are not to be treated as unable to make a decision unless all practicable steps to help them do so have been taken without success.
- People are not to be treated as unable to make a decision merely because they make an unwise decision.

A patient is deemed to lack capacity if they cannot:

- understand relevant information about the decision to be made,
  or
- retain that information in their mind,
  or
- use or weigh that information as part of the decision-making process,
  or
- communicate their decision (by talking, using sign language or any other means).

The patient needs to fail on only one of the four points above to be deemed not to have capacity. Capacity may change over time so reassessment is important. A person may lack capacity about one decision but not about another.

Section 62 urgent treatment

If, after 3 months, medication is needed urgently to treat a patient's mental disorder and it is not covered by a T2 or T3, S62 may be applied.

The Code of Practice 25.38 states:

This applies only if the treatment in question is immediately necessary to:

- save the patient's life;
- prevent a serious deterioration of the patient's condition, and the treatment does not have unfavourable physical or psychological consequences which cannot be reversed;
- alleviate serious suffering by the patient, and the treatment does not have unfavourable physical or psychological consequences which cannot be reversed and does not entail significant physical hazard; or
- prevent patients behaving violently or being a danger to themselves or others, and the treatment represents the minimum interference necessary for that purpose, does not have unfavourable physical or psychological consequences which cannot be reversed and does not entail significant physical hazard.

Each Trust should design a form for the clinician in charge of treatment (usually the consultant) to state what the treatment is, why it is immediately necessary and the length of treatment.

Section 132 duty of managers of hospitals to give information to detained patients

With regards to S132 and consent to treatment the Code of Practice 4.20 states:

Patients must be told what the Act says about treatment for their mental disorder. In particular they must be told:

- the circumstances (if any) in which they can be treated without their consent – and the circumstances in which they have the right to refuse treatment;
- the role of second opinion appointed doctors (SOADs) and the circumstances in which they may be involved; and
- (where relevant) the rules on electro-convulsive therapy (ECT) and medication administered as part of ECT.

Electroconvulsive therapy (ECT)

Section 58a deals with ECT. Treatment for ECT is authorised on forms:

T4   For consenting adults 18 and over, may be written by the RC or SOAD
T5   For consenting patients under 18, to be written by a SOAD only
T6   For patients who lack capacity. To be written by a SOAD only.

All patients under the age of 18 who are to receive ECT, whether or not they are detained under the MHA, must have treatment authorised on a T5 or T6.

CHAPTER 14

Patients who have the capacity to consent must not receive ECT unless they do consent (in emergencies this can, however, be overridden under Section 62 of the Act). There is no 3-month rule with regards to ECT and this also applies to medication given as part of ECT. Hence a form for ECT must always be in place regardless of the first date of detention. The forms should indicate the maximum number of treatments the patient is to receive (Code of Practice paragraph 25.23).

Community patients

Patients on a Community Treatment Order (CTO) should have treatment authorised on one of the following forms:

CTO11   Written by a SOAD, after one month on a CTO, when the patient lacks capacity

CTO12   Written by the RC when the patient has capacity and is consenting to treatment, after one month on a CTO.

There is no legal authority to give patients medication in the community if they refuse it.

Reference

1. Department of Health. Code of practice: Mental Health Act 1983. Last updated 31 October 2017. https://www.gov.uk/government/publications/code-of-practice-mental-health-act-1983#history.

Site of administration of intramuscular injections

Table 14.7 gives the sites of administration formally indicated in the individual product's EU licence. Other routes and sites may be possible but pharmacokinetic analysis of administration via these sites is generally not available.

Table 14.7 Site of administration of intramuscular injections[1-7]

Antipsychotic generic name and formulation	Site(s) of administration
Typical antipsychotic (FGA) depots	
Flupentixol decanoate (in thin vegetable oil derived from coconuts)	Deep intramuscular injection into the **upper outer buttock** (dorsogluteal) or **lateral thigh** (vastus lateralis)
Fluphenazine decanoate (in sesame oil)	Deep intramuscular injection into the **gluteal region.** Can also be administered into the **lateral surface of the thigh muscle** but this is **unlicensed use.** Administration into the deltoid is not recommended by manufacturer
Haloperidol decanoate (in sesame oil)	Deep intramuscular injection into the **gluteal region** using an appropriate needle, preferably 2–2.5 inches long, of at least 21 gauge. Can also be administered into the **deltoid muscle according to the manufacturer.** Although this is an **unlicensed use** one trial suggests it is safe and effective[8]
Zuclopentixol decanoate (in thin vegetable oil derived from coconuts)	Deep intramuscular injection into the **upper outer buttock** (dorsogluteal) or **lateral thigh** (vastus lateralis)
Atypical antipsychotic (SGA) depots	
Aripiprazole (Abilify Maintena) Powder and vehicle for prolonged-release suspension for deep intramuscular injection	***Gluteal muscle*** administration. The recommended needle for gluteal administration is a 38 mm (1.5 inch), 22 gauge hypodermic safety needle; for obese patients (body mass index >28 kg/m²), a 50 mm (2 inch), 21 gauge hypodermic safety needle should be used. Gluteal injections should be alternated between the two gluteal muscles. ***Deltoid muscle*** administration. The recommended needle for deltoid administration is a 25 mm (1 inch), 23 gauge hypodermic safety needle; for obese patients, a 38 mm (1.5 inch), 22 gauge hypodermic safety needle should be used. Deltoid injections should be alternated between the two deltoid muscles. The powder and vehicle vials and the pre-filled syringe are for single use only
Olanzapine pamoate monohydrate (ZypAdhera) Powder and vehicle for prolonged-release suspension for deep intramuscular injection	Olanzapine pamoate monohydrate should only be administered by deep intramuscular **gluteal** injection by a health-care professional trained in the appropriate injection technique and in locations where post-injection observation and access to appropriate medical care in the case of overdose can be assured
Paliperidone palmitate (Xeplion) Prolonged-release suspension for injection	Injected slowly, deep into the **deltoid or gluteal muscle** (the two initial loading doses should be administered in the deltoid muscle so as to attain therapeutic concentrations rapidly). Administration should be in a single injection. The dose should not be given in divided injections

(Continued)

CHAPTER 14

Table 14.7 (*Continued*)

Antipsychotic generic name and formulation	Site(s) of administration
Paliperidone palmitate (Trevicta) Prolonged-release suspension for injection every 3 months	*Deltoid muscle administration* The specified needle for administration of Trevicta into the deltoid muscle is determined by the patient's weight. • For those ≥90 kg, the thin wall 1½ inch, 22 gauge (0.72 mm × 38.1 mm) needle should be used. • For those <90 kg, the thin wall 1 inch, 22 gauge (0.72 mm × 25.4 mm) needle should be used. The injection should be administered into the centre of the deltoid muscle. Deltoid injections should be alternated between the two deltoid muscles *Gluteal muscle administration* The needle to be used for administration of Trevicta into the gluteal muscle is the thin wall 1½ inch, 22 gauge (0.72 mm × 38.1 mm) needle regardless of body weight. It should be administered into the upper-outer quadrant of the gluteal muscle. Gluteal injections should be alternated between the two gluteal muscles
Risperidone (Risperdal Consta) Powder and vehicle for prolonged-release suspension for intramuscular injection	Deep intramuscular **deltoid or gluteal** injection using the appropriate safety needle. For deltoid administration, use the 1 inch needle alternating injections between the two arms. For gluteal administration, use the 2 inch needle alternating injections between the two buttocks
Intramuscular injections for rapid tranquillisation	
Aripiprazole (Abilify) Solution for injection	To enhance absorption and minimise variability, injection into the **deltoid** or **deep within the gluteus maximus muscle**, avoiding adipose regions, is recommended
Haloperidol Solution for injection	Intramuscular administration Preferably, **gluteal muscle** is selected when the dosage volume is high. **Deltoid muscle** is preferred for low doses of the injection. However, there is no information on the dosage limit for these specific muscle groups. Choice of site is at the discretion of the prescriber, according to the manufacturer
Lorazepam Solution for injection	Intramuscular administration Can be administered into the **gluteal, deltoid** or **frontal thigh area** according to the manufacturer A 1:1 dilution of Ativan Injection with normal saline or Sterile Water for Injection BP is recommended in order to facilitate intramuscular administration and absorption
Olanzapine (Zyprexa) Powder for solution for injection	Inject slowly, deep into the muscle mass. The exact site of administration is not specified and choice of muscle site should be a clinical decision, according to the manufacturer Dissolve the contents of the vial using 2.1 mL of Sterile Water for Injection to provide a solution containing approximately 5 mg/mL of olanzapine The resulting solution should appear clear and yellow. Use immediately (within 1 hour) after reconstitution. *Discard any unused portion*
Promethazine hydrochloride Solution for injection	By deep intramuscular injection Can be administered into the **thigh, upper arm** or **gluteal region**. Ensure muscle mass is sufficient for the volume being injected

References

1. Datapharm Ltd. Electronic Medicines Compendium. 2017. https://www.medicines.org.uk/emc/.
2. Janssen UK. Guidance on the Administration to Adults of Oil-based Depot and other Long-Acting Intramuscular Antipsychotic Injections. 2016. https://hydra.hull.ac.uk/assets/hull:13659/content.
3. Sanofi. Medical Information department – verbal and written communication, 2017.
4. Janssen. Medical Information department – verbal and written communication, 2017.
5. Concordia International. Medical Information department – verbal and written communication, 2017.
6. Pfizer. Medical Information department – verbal and written communication, 2017.
7. Lilly UK. Medical Information department – verbal and written communication, 2017.
8. McEvoy JP et al. Effectiveness of paliperidone palmitate vs haloperidol decanoate for maintenance treatment of schizophrenia: a randomized clinical trial. JAMA 2014; **311**:1978–1987.

Treatment of tardive dyskinesia (TD)

Tardive dyskinesia is probably a somewhat less commonly encountered problem than in previous decades[1,2], probably because of the introduction and widespread use of second generation antipsychotics[3–6]. Nonetheless, SGAs do present an important risk of TD[7]. Treatment of established TD is often unsuccessful, so prevention, early detection and early treatment are essential. TD is associated with greater cognitive impairment[8], more severe psychopathology[9] and higher mortality[10].

There is fairly good evidence that SGAs are less likely to cause TD[7,11–15] although, as noted above, TD certainly does occur with these drugs and at quite different rates with individual SGAs[16–20]. The observation that SGAs produce less TD than typical drugs is consistent with the long-held belief that early acute movement disorders and akathisia predict later TD[21–23]. TD can occur after minuscule doses of conventional drugs (and in the absence of prior acute movement disorder[24]) and following the use of other dopamine antagonists such as metoclopramide[25]. It can also occur in never-medicated patients with both first-episode[26] and established[27] schizophrenia. FGA depot treatments may be particularly likely to bring about TD[20]. Risk of TD may be related to the extent of D_2 receptor occupancy (higher occupancy, higher risk)[28]. It follows that the lower doses of FGAs that are now routine in clinical practice may be associated with a lower risk of TD, perhaps approaching that seen with SGAs, but this has not yet been systematically explored. Interestingly, a relatively low prevalence of TD was reported before the advent of SGAs in areas where low dose FGA treatment was common[29].

Treatment – first steps

Most authorities recommend the withdrawal of any anticholinergic drugs and a reduction in the dose of antipsychotic as initial steps in those with early signs of TD[30,31] (dose reduction may initially worsen TD). Cochrane, however found little support for dose reduction[32] or anticholinergic withdrawal[33] and the American Academy of Neurology does not recommend dose reduction[34]. It is however common practice to withdraw the antipsychotic prescribed when TD was first observed and to substitute another drug; one thought less likely to cause TD. The use of clozapine[30] is probably best supported in this regard, but quetiapine, another weak striatal dopamine antagonist, is also effective[35–41]. Olanzapine[39–42,42,43] and aripiprazole[44] are also options. There are a few supporting data for risperidone[45] but this might not be considered a logical choice in a patient with established TD, given that risperidone is more likely than clozapine, olanzapine and quetiapine to be associated with acute movement disorder. Again, the evidence for benefit in switching to particular SGAs is considered rather inconclusive[34].

Treatment – additional agents

Switching or withdrawing antipsychotics is not always effective or advisable and so additional agents are often used. The table below describes the most frequently prescribed add-on drugs for TD, in order of preference.

Table 14.8 First line treatments for tardive dyskinesia (in order of preference)

Drug	Comments
Valbenazine[46–48]	Licensed in USA and some other countries. A dose of 80 mg once daily is effective with a benign cardiovasular profile. Low incidence of depression and akathisia.
Deutetrabenazine[49,50]	Licensed for Huntingtons in some countries but effective in TD. Better supporting evidence than for tetrabenazine. Longer half-life than tertrabenazine but still needs to be taken twice a day. Low incidence of psychiatric and neurological effects. Dose is 12-48 mg/day.
Tetrabenazine[51,52]	Only licensed treatment for TD in UK. Depression, drowsiness, parkinsonism and akathisia may occur[53,54]. Dose is 25-200 mg/day. Reserpine (similar mode of action) also effective but rarely, if ever, used.
Benzodiazepines[30,31]	Widely used and considered effective but Cochrane review suggests benzodiazepines are 'experimental'[55]. Intermittant use may be necessary to avoid tolerance to effects. Most used are clonazepam 1-4 mg/day and diazepam 6-25 mg/day. Better supporting evidence for clonazepam[34,54]
Vitamin E[56,57]	Numerous studies but efficacy remains to be conclusively established. Cochrane suggest that there is evidence only for slowing deterioration of TD[58]. Dose is in the range 400-1600 IU/day.
Ginkgo biloba[59]	Well tolerated. There are three Chinese RCTs showing good effect for 240 mg/day[60].
Propranolol[61,62]	Open label studies only but formerly a widely used treatment. Dose is 40-120 mg/day. Beware contra-indications (asthma, bradycardia, hypotension)

Treatment – other possible options

The large number of proposed treatments for TD undoubtedly reflects the somewhat limited effectiveness of standard remedies, at least before the introduction of valbenazine and deutetrabenazine. The following table lists some of these putative treatments in alphabetical order.

Table 14.9 Other treatments for tardive dyskinesia (in alphabetical order)

Drug	Comments
Amantadine[63,64]	Rarely used but apparently effective at 100-300 mg a day
Amino acids[65]	Use is supported by a small randomised, placebo-controlled trial. Low risk of toxicity
Botulinum toxin[66–69]	Case reports of success for localised dyskinesia. Probably now treatment of choice for disabling or distressing focal symptoms
Calcium antagonists[70]	A few published studies but not widely used. Cochrane is dismissive[71]
Donepezil[72–74]	Supported by a single open study and case series. One negative RCT (n = 12). Dose is 10 mg/day. No clear evidence of efficacy for rivastigmine or galantamine[75].
Fish oils[76,77]	Very limited support for use of EPA at dose of 2G/day
Fluvoxamine[78]	Three case reports. Dose is 100 mg/day. Beware interactions.
Gabapentin[79]	Adds weight to theory that GABAergic mechansims improve TD. Dose is 900-1200 mg/day. Inconclusive data on other GABA agonists[80].
Levetiracetam[81–84]	Three published case studies. One RCT. Dose up to 3000 mg/day

(Continued)

CHAPTER 14

Table 14.9 (*Continued*)

Drug	Comments
Melatonin[85]	Use is supported by a meta-analysis of four trials[86]. Usually well tolerated. Dose is 10 mg/day. Some evidence that melatonin receptor genotype determines risk of TD[87]
Naltrexone[88]	May be effective when added to benzodiazepines. Well tolerated. Dose is 200 mg/day
Ondansetron[89,90]	Limited evidence but low toxicity. Dose – up to 12 mg/day
Pyridoxine[91]	Supported by a well conducted trial. Dose – up to 400 mg/day
Quercetin[92]	Plant compound which is thought to be an antioxidant. Some promising case reports[92–94].
Sodium oxybate[95]	One case report. Dose was 8G/day
Transcranial magnetic stimulation[96] (rTMS)	Single case report
Zolpidem[97]	Three case reports. Dose 10-30 mg a day

References

1. Merrill RM, Lyon JL, Matiaco PM. Tardive and spontaneous dyskinesia incidence in the general population. BMC Psychiatry 2013; 13:152.
2. Kane JM, Woerner M, Lieberman J. Tardive dyskinesia: prevalence, incidence, and risk factors. J Clin Psychopharmacol 1988; 8:52 s–56 s.
3. de Leon J. The effect of atypical versus typical antipsychotics on tardive dyskinesia : A naturalistic study. Eur Arch Psychiatry Clin Neurosci 2007; 257:169–172.
4. Halliday J, Farrington S, Macdonald S, et al. Nithsdale Schizophrenia Surveys 23: movement disorders. 20-year review. Br J Psychiatry 2002; 181:422–427.
5. Kane JM. Tardive dyskinesia circa 2006. Am J Psychiatry 2006; 163:1316–1318.
6. Eberhard J, Lindstrom E, Levander S. Tardive dyskinesia and antipsychotics: a 5-year longitudinal study of frequency, correlates and course. Int Clin Psychopharmacol 2006; 21:35–42.
7. Carbon M, Hsieh CH, Kane JM, et al. Tardive Dyskinesia Prevalence in the Period of Second-Generation Antipsychotic Use: A Meta-Analysis. J Clin Psychiatry 2017; 78:e264–e278.
8. Wu JQ, Chen da C, Xiu MH, et al. Tardive dyskinesia is associated with greater cognitive impairment in schizophrenia. Prog Neuropsychopharmacol Biol Psychiatry 2013; 46:71–77.
9. Ascher-Svanum H, Zhu B, Faries D, et al. Tardive dyskinesia and the 3-year course of schizophrenia: results from a large, prospective, naturalistic study. J Clin Psychiatry 2008; 69:1580–1588.
10. Chong SA, Tay JA, Subramaniam M, et al. Mortality rates among patients with schizophrenia and tardive dyskinesia. J Clin Psychopharmacol 2009; 29:5–8.
11. Beasley C, Dellva M, Tamura R. Randomised double-blind comparison of the incidence of tardive dyskinesia in patients with schizophrenia during long-term treatment with olanzapine or haloperidol. Br J Psychiatry 1999; 174:23–30.
12. Glazer WM. Expected incidence of tardive dyskinesia associated with atypical antipsychotics. J Clin Psychiatry 2000; 61 Suppl 4:21–26.
13. Correll CU, Leucht S, Kane JM. Lower risk for tardive dyskinesia associated with second-generation antipsychotics: a systematic review of 1-year studies. Am J Psychiatry 2004; 161:414–425.
14. Dolder CR, Jeste DV. Incidence of tardive dyskinesia with typical versus atypical antipsychotics in very high risk patients. Biol Psychiatry 2003; 53:1142–1145.
15. Correll CU, Schenk EM. Tardive dyskinesia and new antipsychotics. Current opinion in psychiatry 2008; 21:151–156.
16. Gafoor R, Brophy J. Three case reports of emergent dyskinesia with clozapine. Eur Psychiatry 2003; 18:260–261.
17. Keck ME, Muller MB, Binder EB, et al. Ziprasidone-related tardive dyskinesia (Letter). Am J Psychiatry 2004; 161:175–176.
18. Maytal G, Ostacher M, Stern TA. Aripiprazole-related tardive dyskinesia. CNS Spectr 2006; 11:435–439.
19. Fountoulakis KN, Panagiotidis P, Siamouli M, et al. Amisulpride-induced tardive dyskinesia. Schizophr Res 2006; 88:232–234.
20. Novick D, Haro JM, Bertsch J, et al. Incidence of extrapyramidal symptoms and tardive dyskinesia in schizophrenia: thirty-six-month results from the European schizophrenia outpatient health outcomes study. J Clin Psychopharmacol 2010; 30:531–540.
21. Sachdev P. Early extrapyramidal side-effects as risk factors for later tardive dyskinesia: a prospective study. Aust N Z J Psychiatry 2004; 38:445–449.
22. Miller DD, McEvoy JP, Davis SM, et al. Clinical correlates of tardive dyskinesia in schizophrenia: baseline data from the CATIE schizophrenia trial. Schizophr Res 2005; 80:33–43.

23. Tenback DE, van Harten PN, Slooff CJ, et al. Evidence that early extrapyramidal symptoms predict later tardive dyskinesia: a prospective analysis of 10,000 patients in the European Schizophrenia Outpatient Health Outcomes (SOHO) Study. Am J Psychiatry 2006; 163:1438–1440.

24. Oosthuizen PP, Emsley RA, Maritz JS, et al. Incidence of tardive dyskinesia in first-episode psychosis patients treated with low-dose haloperidol. J Clin Psychiatry 2003; 64:1075–1080.

25. Kenney C, Hunter C, Davidson A, et al. Metoclopramide, an increasingly recognized cause of tardive dyskinesia. J Clin Pharmacol 2008; 48:379–384.

26. Puri BK, Barnes TR, Chapman MJ, et al. Spontaneous dyskinesia in first episode schizophrenia. J Neurol Neurosurg Psychiatry 1999; 66:76–78.

27. McCreadie RG, Padmavati R, Thara R, et al. Spontaneous dyskinesia and parkinsonism in never-medicated, chronically ill patients with schizophrenia: 18-month follow-up. Br J Psychiatry 2002; 181:135–137.

28. Yoshida K, Bies RR, Suzuki T, et al. Tardive dyskinesia in relation to estimated dopamine D2 receptor occupancy in patients with schizophrenia: analysis of the CATIE data. Schizophr Res 2014; 153:184–188.

29. Ko GN, Zhang LD, Yan WW, et al. The Shanghai 800: prevalence of tardive dyskinesia in a Chinese psychiatric hospital. Am J Psychiatry 1989; 146:387–389.

30. Duncan D, H M. Tardive dyskinesia: how is it prevented and treated? Psychiatric Bulletin 1997; 21:422–425.

31. Simpson GM. The treatment of tardive dyskinesia and tardive dystonia. J Clin Psychiatry 2000; 61 Suppl 4:39–44.

32. Bergman H, Rathbone J, Agarwal V, et al. Antipsychotic reduction and/or cessation and antipsychotics as specific treatments for tardive dyskinesia. The Cochrane database of systematic reviews 2018; 2:Cd000459.

33. Bergman H, Soares-Weiser K. Anticholinergic medication for antipsychotic-induced tardive dyskinesia. The Cochrane database of systematic reviews 2018; 1:Cd000204.

34. Bhidayasiri R, Fahn S, Weiner WJ, et al. Evidence-based guideline: treatment of tardive syndromes: report of the Guideline Development Subcommittee of the American Academy of Neurology. Neurology 2013; 81:463–469.

35. Vesely C, Kufferle B, Brucke T, et al. Remission of severe tardive dyskinesia in a schizophrenic patient treated with the atypical antipsychotic substance quetiapine. Int Clin Psychopharmacol 2000; 15:57–60.

36. Alptekin K, Kivircik AK. Quetiapine-induced improvement of tardive dyskinesia in three patients with schizophrenia. Int Clin Psychopharmacol 2002; 17:263–264.

37. Nelson MW, Reynolds RR, Kelly DL, et al. Adjunctive quetiapine decreases symptoms of tardive dyskinesia in a patient taking risperidone. Clin Neuropharmacol 2003; 26:297–298.

38. Emsley R, Turner HJ, Schronen J, et al. A single-blind, randomized trial comparing quetiapine and haloperidol in the treatment of tardive dyskinesia. J Clin Psychiatry 2004; 65:696–701.

39. Bressan RA, Jones HM, Pilowsky LS. Atypical antipsychotic drugs and tardive dyskinesia: relevance of D2 receptor affinity. Journal of psychopharmacology (Oxford, England) 2004; 18:124–127.

40. Sacchetti E, Valsecchi P. Quetiapine, clozapine, and olanzapine in the treatment of tardive dyskinesia induced by first-generation antipsychotics: a 124-week case report. Int Clin Psychopharmacol 2003; 18:357–359.

41. Gourzis P, Polychronopoulos P, Papapetropoulos S, et al. Quetiapine in the treatment of focal tardive dystonia induced by other atypical antipsychotics: a report of 2 cases. Clin Neuropharmacol 2005; 28:195–196.

42. Soutullo CA, Keck PE, Jr., McElroy SL. Olanzapine in the treatment of tardive dyskinesia: a report of two cases. J Clin Psychopharmacol 1999; 19:100–101.

43. Kinon BJ, Jeste DV, Kollack-Walker S, et al. Olanzapine treatment for tardive dyskinesia in schizophrenia patients: a prospective clinical trial with patients randomized to blinded dose reduction periods. Prog Neuropsychopharmacol Biol Psychiatry 2004; 28:985–996.

44. Chan CH, Chan HY, Chen YC. Switching antipsychotic treatment to aripiprazole in psychotic patients with neuroleptic-induced tardive dyskinesia: a 24-week follow-up study. Int Clin Psychopharmacol 2018; 33:155–162.

45. Bai YM, Yu SC, Lin CC. Risperidone for severe tardive dyskinesia: a 12-week randomized, double-blind, placebo-controlled study. J Clin Psychiatry 2003; 64:1342–1348.

46. Hauser RA, Factor SA, Marder SR, et al. KINECT 3: A Phase 3 Randomized, Double-Blind, Placebo-Controlled Trial of Valbenazine for Tardive Dyskinesia. Am J Psychiatry 2017; 174:476–484.

47. Kane JM, Correll CU, Liang GS, et al. Efficacy of Valbenazine (NBI-98854) in Treating Subjects with Tardive Dyskinesia and Schizophrenia or Schizoaffective Disorder. Psychopharmacol Bull 2017; 47:69–76.

48. Josiassen RC, Kane JM, Liang GS, et al. Long-Term Safety and Tolerability of Valbenazine (NBI-98854) in Subjects with Tardive Dyskinesia and a Diagnosis of Schizophrenia or Mood Disorder. Psychopharmacol Bull 2017; 47:61–68.

49. Cummings MA, Proctor GJ, Stahl SM. Deuterium Tetrabenazine for Tardive Dyskinesia. Clin Schizophr Relat Psychoses 2018; 11:214–220.

50. Solmi M, Pigato G, Kane JM, et al. Treatment of tardive dyskinesia with VMAT-2 inhibitors: a systematic review and meta-analysis of randomized controlled trials. Drug Des Devel Ther 2018; 12:1215–1238.

51. Jankovic J, Beach J. Long-term effects of tetrabenazine in hyperkinetic movement disorders. Neurology 1997; 48:358–362.

52. Leung JG, Breden EL. Tetrabenazine for the treatment of tardive dyskinesia. Ann Pharmacother 2011; 45:525–531.

53. Kenney C, Hunter C, Jankovic J. Long-term tolerability of tetrabenazine in the treatment of hyperkinetic movement disorders. Mov Disord 2007; 22:193–197.

54. Rana AQ, Chaudry ZM, Blanchet PJ. New and emerging treatments for symptomatic tardive dyskinesia. Drug Des Devel Ther 2013; 7:1329–1340.

55. Bergman H, Bhoopathi PS, Soares-Weiser K. Benzodiazepines for antipsychotic-induced tardive dyskinesia. The Cochrane database of systematic reviews 2018; 1:Cd000205.

CHAPTER 14

56. Adler LA, Rotrosen J, Edson R, et al. Vitamin E treatment for tardive dyskinesia. Arch Gen Psychiatry 1999; 56:836–841.

57. Zhang XY, Zhou DF, Cao LY, et al. The effect of vitamin E treatment on tardive dyskinesia and blood superoxide dismutase: a double-blind placebo-controlled trial. J Clin Psychopharmacol 2004; 24:83–86.

58. Soares-Weiser K, Maayan N, Bergman H. Vitamin E for antipsychotic-induced tardive dyskinesia. The Cochrane database of systematic reviews 2018; 1:Cd000209.

59. Zhang WF, Tan YL, Zhang XY, et al. Extract of Ginkgo biloba treatment for tardive dyskinesia in schizophrenia: a randomized, double-blind, placebo-controlled trial. J Clin Psychiatry 2011; 72:615–621.

60. Zheng W, Xiang YQ, Ng CH, et al. Extract of Ginkgo biloba for Tardive Dyskinesia: Meta-analysis of Randomized Controlled Trials. Pharmacopsychiatry 2016; 49:107–111.

61. Perenyi A, Farkas A. Propranolol in the treatment of tardive dyskinesia. Biol Psychiatry 1983; 18:391–394.

62. Pitts FN, Jr. Treatment of tardive dyskinesia with propranolol. J Clin Psychiatry 1982; 43:304.

63. Angus S, Sugars J, Boltezar R, et al. A controlled trial of amantadine hydrochloride and neuroleptics in the treatment of tardive dyskinesia. J Clin Psychopharmacol 1997; 17:88–91.

64. Pappa S, Tsouli S, Apostolou G, et al. Effects of amantadine on tardive dyskinesia: a randomized, double-blind, placebo-controlled study. Clin Neuropharmacol 2010; 33:271–275.

65. Richardson MA, Bevans ML, Read LL, et al. Efficacy of the branched-chain amino acids in the treatment of tardive dyskinesia in men. Am J Psychiatry 2003; 160:1117–1124.

66. Tarsy D, Kaufman D, Sethi KD, et al. An open-label study of botulinum toxin A for treatment of tardive dystonia. Clin Neuropharmacol 1997; 20:90–93.

67. Brashear A, Ambrosius WT, Eckert GJ, et al. Comparison of treatment of tardive dystonia and idiopathic cervical dystonia with botulinum toxin type A. Mov Disord 1998; 13:158–161.

68. Hennings JM, Krause E, Botzel K, et al. Successful treatment of tardive lingual dystonia with botulinum toxin: case report and review of the literature. Prog Neuropsychopharmacol Biol Psychiatry 2008; 32:1167–1171.

69. Beckmann YY, Secil Y, Saka S, et al. Treatment of intractable tardive lingual dyskinesia with botulinum toxin. J Clin Psychopharmacol 2011; 31:250–251.

70. Essali A, Deirawan H, Soares-Weiser K, et al. Calcium channel blockers for neuroleptic-induced tardive dyskinesia. The Cochrane database of systematic reviews 2011:Cd000206.

71. Essali A, Soares-Weiser K, Bergman H, et al. Calcium channel blockers for antipsychotic-induced tardive dyskinesia. The Cochrane database of systematic reviews 2018; 3:Cd000206.

72. Caroff SN, Campbell EC, Havey JC, et al. Treatment of tardive dyskinesia with donepezil. J Clin Psychiatry 2001; 62:128–129.

73. Bergman J, Dwolatzky T, Brettholz I, et al. Beneficial effect of donepezil in the treatment of elderly patients with tardive movement disorders. J Clin Psychiatry 2005; 66:107–110.

74. Ogunmefun A, Hasnain M, Alam A, et al. Effect of donepezil on tardive dyskinesia. J Clin Psychopharmacol 2009; 29:102–104.

75. Tammenmaa-Aho I, Asher R, Soares-Weiser K, et al. Cholinergic medication for antipsychotic-induced tardive dyskinesia. The Cochrane database of systematic reviews 2018; 3:Cd000207.

76. Emsley R, Niehaus DJ, Koen L, et al. The effects of eicosapentaenoic acid in tardive dyskinesia: a randomized, placebo-controlled trial. Schizophr Res 2006; 84:112–120.

77. Vaddadi K, Hakansson K, Clifford J, et al. Tardive dyskinesia and essential fatty acids. International review of psychiatry (Abingdon, England) 2006; 18:133–143.

78. Albayrak Y, Hashimoto K. Benefical effects of sigma-1 agonist fluvoxamine for tardive dyskinesia and tardive akathisia in patients with schizophrenia: report of three cases. Psychiatry Investig 2013; 10:417–420.

79. Hardoy MC, Carta MG, Carpiniello B, et al. Gabapentin in antipsychotic-induced tardive dyskinesia: results of 1-year follow-up. J Affect Disord 2003; 75:125–130.

80. Alabed S, Latifeh Y, Mohammad HA, et al. Gamma-aminobutyric acid agonists for antipsychotic-induced tardive dyskinesia. The Cochrane database of systematic reviews 2018; 4:Cd000203.

81. McGavin CL, John V, Musser WS. Levetiracetam as a treatment for tardive dyskinesia: a case report. Neurology 2003; 61:419.

82. Meco G, Fabrizio E, Epifanio A, et al. Levetiracetam in tardive dyskinesia. Clin Neuropharmacol 2006; 29:265–268.

83. Woods SW, Saksa JR, Baker CB, et al. Effects of levetiracetam on tardive dyskinesia: a randomized, double-blind, placebo-controlled study. J Clin Psychiatry 2008; 69:546–554.

84. Chen PH, Liu HC. Rapid improvement of neuroleptic-induced tardive dyskinesia with levetiracetam in an interictal psychotic patient. J Clin Psychopharmacol 2010; 30:205–207.

85. Shamir E, Barak Y, Shalman I, et al. Melatonin treatment for tardive dyskinesia: a double-blind, placebo-controlled, crossover study. Arch Gen Psychiatry 2001; 58:1049–1052.

86. Sun CH, Zheng W, Yang XH, et al. Adjunctive Melatonin for Tardive Dyskinesia in Patients with Schizophrenia: A Meta-Analysis. Shanghai archives of psychiatry 2017; 29:129–136.

87. Lai IC, Chen ML, Wang YC, et al. Analysis of genetic variations in the human melatonin receptor (MTNR1A, MTNR1B) genes and antipsychotics-induced tardive dyskinesia in schizophrenia. World J Biol Psychiatry 2011; 12:143–148.

88. Wonodi I, Adami H, Sherr J, et al. Naltrexone treatment of tardive dyskinesia in patients with schizophrenia. J Clin Psychopharmacol 2004; 24:441–445.

89. Sirota P, Mosheva T, Shabtay H, et al. Use of the selective serotonin 3 receptor antagonist ondansetron in the treatment of neuroleptic-induced tardive dyskinesia. Am J Psychiatry 2000; 157:287–289.

CHAPTER 14

90. Naidu PS, Kulkarni SK. Reversal of neuroleptic-induced orofacial dyskinesia by 5-HT3 receptor antagonists. Eur J Pharmacol 2001; **420**:113–117.

91. Lerner V, Miodownik C, Kaptsan A, et al. Vitamin B(6) in the treatment of tardive dyskinesia: a double-blind, placebo-controlled, crossover study. Am J Psychiatry 2001; **158**:1511–1514.

92. Naidu PS, Singh A, Kulkarni SK. Reversal of haloperidol-induced orofacial dyskinesia by quercetin, a bioflavonoid. Psychopharmacology (Berl) 2003; **167**:418–423.

93. Naidu PS, Singh A, Kulkarni SK. Quercetin, a bioflavonoid, attenuates haloperidol-induced orofacial dyskinesia. Neuropharmacology 2003; **44**:1100–1106.

94. Naidu PS, Singh A, Kulkarni SK. Reversal of reserpine-induced orofacial dyskinesia and cognitive dysfunction by quercetin. Pharmacology 2004; **70**:59–67.

95. Berner JE. A case of sodium oxybate treatment of tardive dyskinesia and bipolar disorder. J Clin Psychiatry 2008; **69**:862.

96. Brambilla P, Perez J, Monchieri S, et al. Transient improvement of tardive dyskinesia induced with rTMS. Neurology 2003; **61**:1155.

97. Waln O, Jankovic J. Zolpidem improves tardive dyskinesia and akathisia. Mov Disord 2013; **28**:1748–1749.

CHAPTER 14

Index

Note: page numbers in *italics* refer to figures; those in **bold** to tables or boxes.

The Maudsley Prescribing Guidelines in Psychiatry, Thirteenth Edition. David M. Taylor,
Thomas R. E. Barnes and Allan H. Young.
© 2018 David M. Taylor. Published 2018 by John Wiley & Sons Ltd.

opioid antagonists
  borderline personality disorder 665
  see also naloxone; naltrexone
opioid dependence 405–430
  acute in-patient settings 419–421, 420
  alcohol dependence with 401
  assessment 407, 407
  detoxification and reduction regimes
    422–425
  NICE guidelines 408, 422
  pain management 426
  pregnancy and 409, 427–428
  prescribing for 405
  psychotropic prescribing 421–422
  relapse prevention 424–425, 425
  substitute prescribing *see* opioid
    substitution treatment
opioid overdose/toxicity 405
  clinical features 405
  starting methadone therapy
    and 410–411
  treatment 405, 406
opioid substitution treatment (OST) 405,
  406–419
  acute in-patient settings 419–421, 420
  alternative oral preparations 418
  buprenorphine 414–418
  buprenorphine with naloxone 418
  discharge home 421
  goals 406
  induction and stabilisation 408
  injectable diamorphine 419
  methadone 408–413
  methadone vs buprenorphine 408, 409
  pain control for patients on 426
  pregnancy 409, 427
  principles 407–408
opioid withdrawal 407–408
  acute ward settings 419–421
  community setting 423
  lofexidine-mediated 424
  naltrexone-treated patients 425
  precipitated by buprenorphine 414,
    416, 416
  regimes 422–424
  scales 407, 408
  specialist addiction in-patient
    setting 423–424
  symptomatic treatment 420, 424
oral glucose tolerance test (OGTT)
  125, 126
orgasm 141
  disorders 144
  effects of antidepressants 344
orlistat 101, 195
orthopaedic surgery, SSRI-treated
  patients 351, 351
orthostatic hypotension *see* postural
  hypotension
osteopenia 323
osteoporosis 668, 691

overactivity, autism spectrum
  disorders 505–506
overdose, psychotropic drug 769–772,
  769–775
oxazepam
  alcohol withdrawal 393
  breastfeeding 629
  diazepam equivalent dose 378
  driving and 778
  hepatic impairment 641
  HIV infection 682
  renal impairment 655
oxcarbazepine
  adverse effects 691
  bipolar disorder 222, 237
  child and adolescent bipolar illness 473
  dementia 579
  drug interactions 690
  mechanism of action 221
  psychiatric side-effects 690
oxybutynin
  clozapine-induced hypersalivation 190
  cognitive effects in dementia 557, 562
oxycodone, older people 565
oxytocin, autism spectrum disorders 505

Pabrinex 395–396, 396
packed cell volume 806
Paediatric Acute-onset Neuropsychiatric
  Syndrome (PANS) 514–515
Paediatric Autoimmune Neuropsychiatric
  Disorder Associated with
  Streptococcus (PANDAS) 514–515
paediatric patients *see* children and
  adolescents
pain management
  dementia 571
  opioid-dependent patients 409, 426
  see also analgesic agents
paliperidone
  adverse effects 39
  alcohol misusers 756
  atrial fibrillation 720
  bipolar disorder 229
  breastfeeding 626
  children and adolescents 478
  equivalent doses 80
  hepatic impairment 638, 641
  hyponatraemia 134
  maximum licensed dose 12
  monitoring physical health 38
  neuroleptic malignant syndrome 105
  overdose 771
  palmitate long-acting injection (LAI) 67,
    79–81
    1-monthly 68, 79, 79
    3-monthly 68, 81, 81
    dose equivalents 80, 82
    dose reduction 73
    equivalent dose 15
    intramuscular injection site 821, 822

    maximum licensed dose 12
    older people 590, 591
    pharmacokinetics 71
    switching to 80
    vs haloperidol decanoate 45, 79
  plasma level monitoring 733, 738
  renal impairment 650
  sexual adverse effects 143
  weight gain risk 97
palliative care, substance misusers 426
pancreatitis 120, 179, 800
PANDAS 514–515
panic disorder 362, 365, 367
  NICE guidance 368
  non-psychotropics causing 808, 809
PANS (Paediatric Acute-onset
  Neuropsychiatric
  Syndrome) 514–515
paracetamol, in dementia 564, 571
parkinsonism
  antipsychotic-induced 39, 91–92
  never-medicated schizophrenia 90
  switching antipsychotics 150
  valproate-induced 216
  see also extrapyramidal symptoms
Parkinson's disease 715–718
  beta-agonist bronchodilators 563
  cognitive enhancers 550, 551, 717
  dementia 550, 715, 716
  depression 715
  psychiatric adverse effects of
    medications 809–810
  psychosis 716, 716–717
  smoking 766
parotid gland swelling, clozapine-
  induced 179
paroxetine
  adverse effects 258, 358
  alcohol dependence 403
  anxiety disorders 367
  atrial fibrillation 720
  breastfeeding 623
  cardiac effects 327
  children and adolescents
    anxiety disorders 481, 482
    depression 464
    obsessive compulsive disorder 485
  discontinuation symptoms 311, 312
  drug interactions 259, 321
  hepatic impairment 639, 641
  HIV-associated neurocognitive
    disorders 682
  Huntington's disease 706
  hyperprolactinaemia and 337
  minimum effective dose 262
  multiple sclerosis 710
  obsessive compulsive disorder 367
  older people 294
  post-stroke depression 291
  pregnancy 606–607
  renal impairment 653